A	Strong scientific evidence for this use
B	Good scientific evidence for this use
C	Unclear scientific evidence for this use
D	Fair scientific evidence against this use (it may not work)
F	Strong scientific evidence against this use (it likely does not work)

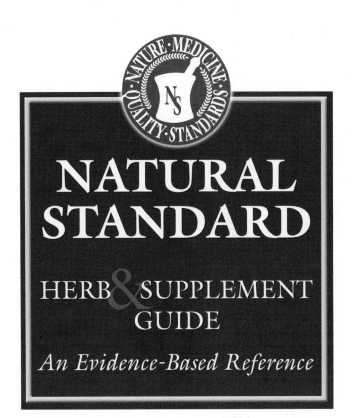

NATURE · MEDICINE · QUALITY · STANDARDS

NATURAL STANDARD

HERB & SUPPLEMENT GUIDE

An Evidence-Based Reference

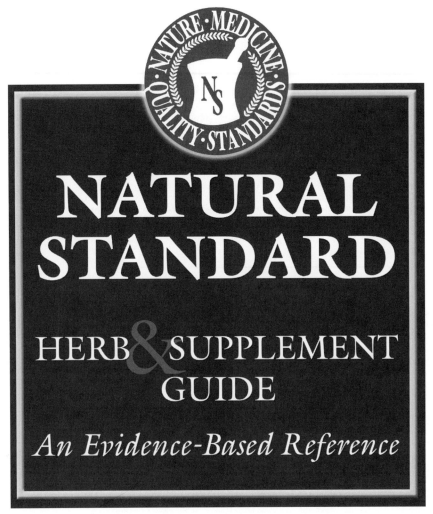

NATURAL STANDARD

HERB & SUPPLEMENT GUIDE

An Evidence-Based Reference

Catherine Ulbricht, PharmD

Senior Attending Pharmacist, Massachusetts General Hospital
Founder, Natural Standard Research Collaboration

www.naturalstandard.com

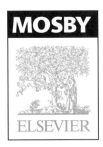

MOSBY

ELSEVIER

3251 Riverport Lane
Maryland Heights, Missouri 63043

NATURAL STANDARD HERB & SUPPLEMENT GUIDE: ISBN: 978-0-323-07295-3
AN EVIDENCE-BASED REFERENCE

Notices

Knowledge and best practice in this field are constantly changing. As new research and experience broaden our understanding, changes in research methods, professional practices, or medical treatment may become necessary. Practitioners and researchers must always rely on their own experience and knowledge in evaluating and using any information, methods, compounds, or experiments described herein. In using such information or methods they should be mindful of their own safety and the safety of others, including parties for whom they have a professional responsibility. With respect to any drug or pharmaceutical products identified, readers are advised to check the most current information provided (i) on procedures featured or (ii) by the manufacturer of each product to be administered, to verify the recommended dose or formula, the method and duration of administration, and contraindications. It is the responsibility of practitioners, relying on their own experience and knowledge of their patients, to make diagnoses, to determine dosages and the best treatment for each individual patient, and to take all appropriate safety precautions. To the fullest extent of the law, neither the Publisher nor the authors, contributors, or editors, assume any liability for any injury and/or damage to persons or property as a matter of products liability, negligence or otherwise, or from any use or operation of any methods, products, instructions, or ideas contained in the material herein.

Library of Congress Cataloging-in-Publication Data
Natural Standard herb & supplement guide : an evidence-based reference/Catherine E. Ulbricht, chief editor. – 1st ed.
   p. ; cm.
   Includes bibliographical references.
   ISBN 978-0-323-07295-3 (hardback : alk. paper)
  1. Herbs–Therapeutic use–Handbooks, manuals, etc. 2. Materia medica, Vegetable–Handbooks, manuals, etc. 3. Dietary supplements–Handbooks, manuals, etc. I. Ulbricht, Catherine E. II. Natural Standard (Firm) III. Title: National Standard herb and supplement guide. IV. Title: Herb & supplement guide.
   [DNLM: 1. Plants, Medicinal–Handbooks. 2. Dietary Supplements–Handbooks. 3. Evidence-Based Medicine–Handbooks. 4. Phytotherapy–Handbooks. 5. Plant Preparations–Handbooks. QV 735 N2848 2010]
   RM666.H33N385 2010
   615′.321–dc22   2009047860

Vice President and Publisher: Linda Duncan
Senior Editor: Kellie White
Associate Developmental Editor: Kelly Milford
Publishing Services Managers: Hemamalini Rajendrababu, Pat Joiner-Myers
Project Manager: Sukanthi Sukumar
Design Direction: Kim Denando

Printed in United States of America

Last digit is the print number: 9 8 7 6 5 4 3 2 1

Disclaimer

The content in this book is for general informational purposes only and is not intended as a substitute for medical advice, treatment, or diagnosis. Consumers should consult a physician or other competent medical provider for specific advice applicable to you. Seek immediate medical care in case of illness. Any use of this book or reliance on its content or information is solely at the user's risk.

Although some complementary and alternative techniques have been studied scientifically, high-quality data regarding safety, effectiveness, dosage, and mechanism of action are limited or controversial for most therapies. Whenever possible, a practitioner of complementary and alternative techniques should be licensed by a recognized professional organization that adheres to clearly published and generally accepted standards. Before starting any new technique or engaging such a practitioner, an individual should consult with his or her own primary health care provider(s). Among other factors, you and your health care provider should evaluate the potential risks, benefits, costs, scientific and evidence-based support, and alternatives for the proposed complementary and alternative technique.

As of the date of this publication, the U.S. Food and Drug Administration does not strictly regulate herbs and supplements. There is no guarantee of strength, purity, or safety of unregulated products, and the effects of any such products may vary. Always read product labels fully. Consumers with medical conditions or taking prescription drugs or over-the-counter drugs, herbs, or supplements should speak with a qualified health care provider about contraindications, interactions, side effects, and other adverse reactions before starting any new therapy. Immediately consult with a health care provider if any unintended side effects or adverse reactions are experienced.

In reading and using this book, users agree that the book and its content are provided "as is, where is" and with all faults and that Natural Standard, its shareholders, officers, directors, staff, editors, authors, contributors, and consultants (the "affiliated parties") make no representations or warranties of any kind with respect to the book and its content, including without limitation, as to matters of safety, effectiveness, accuracy, reliability, completeness, timeliness, or results. To the fullest extent allowed by law, Natural Standard and the affiliated parties hereby expressly disclaim any and all representations, guarantees, conditions, and warranties of any and every kind, express or implied or statutory, including without limitation, warranties of title or infringement, and implied warranties of merchantability or fitness for a particular purpose. Readers and users of this book assume full responsibility for the appropriate use of the information it contains and agree to hold Natural Standard and the affiliated parties harmless from and against any and all liabilities, claims, and actions arising from the reader's or user's use of the work or its content. Some jurisdictions do not allow exclusions or limitations of implied warranties, so certain of the above exclusions might not apply.

Natural Standard Editorial Board and Contributors

FOUNDERS

Catherine (Kate) Ulbricht, PharmD, MBA[c]
Ethan Basch, MD, MSc, MPhil.

SENIOR EDITORIAL BOARD

Glen F. Aukerman, MD
Jason Barker, ND
Ernie-Paul Barrette, MD, FACP
Brent A. Bauer, MD
William Benda, MD, FACEP, FAAEM
Deena Beneda-Khosh, ND
Samuel D. Benjamin, MD, MD (H)
Stephen Bent, MD
Lee S. Berk, DrPH, MPH, FACSM, CHES, CLS
Timothy C. Birdsall, N.D.
Reid B. Blackwelder, MD
Heather Boon, BScPhm, PhD
Thomas Brendler
Stefan Bughi, MD
Mark S. Chambers, DMD, MS
Theresa Charrois, BScPharm, MSc
Richard Philip Cohan, DDS, MS, MBA
William Collinge, MPH, PhD
Julie Conquer, BSc, MSc, PhD
B.H. Cook, MD, PhD
Cathi Dennehy, PharmD
J. Donald Dishman, DC, MSc
John Douillard, PhD
Sarah Elsabagh, BSc, PhD
Joan Engebretson, DrPH, RN
Edzard Ernst, MD, PhD, FRCP
Mitchell A. Fleisher, MD, DHt, FAAFP, DcABCT
Daniel Gagnon, RH (AHG)
Harley Goldberg, DO
Joerg Gruenwald, PhD
Ruoling Guo, BSc MSc PhD
William R. Hamilton, PharmD
Paul Hammerness, MD
Donna Hebbeler, MPH, DrPH
Evelyn Hermes-DeSantis, PharmD, BCPS
Kevin Hoehn, BS, PharmD, MBA, CGP
Charles Holmes, MD, MPH
Stephen Holt, MD
Karen Hopenwasser, MD
Ionela O. Hubbard, LAc, MAOM, QME
Paul Ingraham, RMT
Courtney Jarvis, PharmD
Joseph K. Jordan, PharmD, BCPS
Karta Purkh Singh Khalsa, CDN, RH (AHG)
Catherine DeFranco Kirkwood, MPH, CCCJS-MAC
Benjamin Kligler, MD, MPH
David J. Kroll, PhD
Vasant Lad, MASc
Dana J. Lawrence, DC
Shulamit Lazarus, RN, CCH, CHt, EFT-adv
Zhongxing Liao, MD
Richard Liebowitz, MD

Yanze Liu, PhD
Ann M. Lynch, RPh, AE-C
John S. Markowitz, Pharm.D.
Danik M. Martirosyan, PhD
Sonia Elisa Masocco
Jörg Melzer, MD
Jennifer Minigh, PhD
Shri Kant Mishra, ABMS (BHU), MD, MS, FAAN, FIAA
Wadie Najm, MD, MSEd
Susan A. Nyanzi, DrPH, MPH, CHES, ACSM
Carolyn Williams Orlando, MA, PhD candidate
Steven G. Ottariano, BS Pharm, RPh
Drew Peterson, DC
Todd D. Porter, PhD
Pamela Hemrajani Ramer, DC, PhD[c]
John Redwanski, PharmD
Adrianne Rogers, MD
Aviva Romm, BSc, RH (AHG), CPM
Anthony L. Rosner, PhD, LLD [Hon.]
Michael Rotblatt, MD, PharmD
Andrew L. Rubman, ND
Nancy C. Russell, DrPH (retired)
Kenneth Sancier, PhD
Elad Schiff, MD
Robb Scholten, MSLIS
David Shannahoff-Khalsa
Hari Sharma, MD, FRCPC
Amy Heck Sheehan, PharmD
Charles A. Simpson, DC, DABCO
Judith Smith, PharmD, FCCP, BCOP
Michael Smith, MRPharmS, ND
Ivan Solà, Bs C
David Sollars, MAc, HMC
Philippe Szapary, MD
Candy Tsourounis, PharmD
René Vega, MD
Andrew Weil, MD
Wynn Werner
James Whedon, DC
Roger Wood, LMT, Dipl. ABT (NCCAOM)
Jen Woods
Jay Woosaree, MAg, P Ag
Steven H. Yale, MD, FACP
Youko Yeracaris, MD
Mario M. Zeolla, PharmD, BCPS.
Robert Zori, MD

AUTHORS/CONTRIBUTORS

Clement Abedamowo, MD: Harvard School of Public Health
Lena Abraham, PharmD: Massachusetts College of Pharmacy
Winnie Abrahamson, ND: Private Practice
Tracee Abrams, PharmD: University of Rhode Island
James David Adams, Jr., PhD: University of Southern California School of Pharmacy
Imtiaz Ahmad, MD: Harvard School of Public Health
Qlaitan Akinade, PharmD: Massachusetts College of Pharmacy
Aceele Al-Saleh, PharmD: MCPHS - Worcester

BRIEF BACKGROUND

Complementary and alternative medicine (CAM) encompasses a broad group of healing philosophies, diagnostic approaches, and therapeutic interventions outside of the politically dominant (conventional) health system of a particular society.[1,2] In the United States and other Western countries, CAM therapies are often defined functionally as interventions that are neither taught in medical schools nor available in hospital-based practices.[3] Some authors separately define "alternative" therapies as those used in place of conventional practices, whereas "complementary" or "integrative" medicine can be combined with mainstream approaches.[2,4] Other terms used to refer to CAM include *folkloric, holistic, irregular, non-conventional, non-Western, traditional, unconventional, unorthodox,* and *unproven medicine.*

Major types of CAM therapies include herb, supplement, vitamin supplementation, therapeutic modalities (such as manipulative therapies, mind-body medicine, and energy/bioelectromagnetic-based approaches), spiritual healing, special diets, exercise, and beauty regimens. Boundaries between CAM and conventional therapies are not always clear and often change over time. Published scientific evidence has led to broader acceptance of some CAM therapies and their integration into mainstream medicine, whereas others have been refuted.

RESEARCH

For many CAM approaches, safety and efficacy are not well established; however, the body of research is growing. In 1991, the U.S. Congress allocated funds to establish the Office of Alternative Medicine (OAM) within the National Institutes of Health (NIH), with a budget of $2 million to "investigate and evaluate promising unconventional medical practices." In 1998, Congress elevated the OAM to an NIH Center, thus creating the National Center for Complementary and Alternative Medicine (NCCAM).

The budget of NCCAM has progressively increased, from $50 million in fiscal year 1999 to about $125 million in 2009, toward its mission to "support rigorous research on CAM, to train researchers in CAM, and to disseminate information to the public and professionals on which CAM modalities work, which do not, and why."[5]

PREVALENCE

In 2007, NCCAM (in conjunction with the National Center for Health Statistics, a part of the Centers for Disease Control and Prevention) conducted the National Health Interview Survey (NHIS); according to NCCAM director Dr. Josephine Briggs, this survey contains "the most current, comprehensive and reliable source of information" on CAM use in the United States.[6] According to the 2007 NHIS,[7] the prevalence of CAM use in the United States was approximately 38% for adults and 12% for children. The most popular CAM therapies were nonvitamin, nonmineral natural products for adults as well as for children (Figure 1).

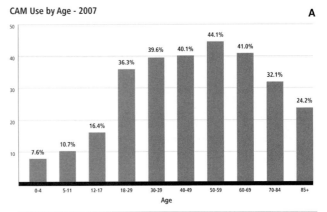

CAM Use by Age - 2007   **A**

Source: Barnes PM, Bloom B, Nahin R. CDC *National Health Statistics Report #12: Complementary and Alternative Medicine Use Among Adults and Children: United States, 2007.* December 2008.

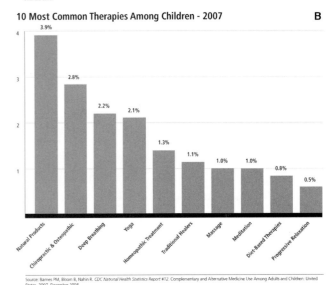

10 Most Common Therapies Among Children - 2007   **B**

Source: Barnes PM, Bloom B, Nahin R. CDC *National Health Statistics Report #12: Complementary and Alternative Medicine Use Among Adults and Children: United States, 2007.* December 2008.

FIGURE 1 *Ten Most Common CAM Therapies Among Adults and Children—2007.* **A,** Percentage of adults in 2007 who used the 10 most common complementary and alternative medicine (CAM) therapies. **B,** Percentage of children in 2007 who used the 10 most common CAM therapies. (From National Center for Complementary and Alternative Medicine, NIH, DHHS.)

Among adults who used nonvitamin, nonmineral natural products in the last year, the most popular natural products were fish oils/omega-3 fatty acids, glucosamine, Echinacea, and flaxseed (Figure 2, *A*). Among children, the most common were Echinacea, fish oil/omega-3 fatty acids, combination herb pills, and flaxseed oil (Figure 2, *B*).

Of the 20 most popular nonvitamin, nonmineral natural products used by adults, 15 had herbal components (Table 1). For children under age 18, 11 of the top 15 nonvitamin, nonmineral natural products had herbal components (Table 2).

According to the 2007 NHIS,[7] the most common medical problems treated with CAM were musculoskeletal conditions. Back problems were the most common indications (17.1%), followed distantly by neck problems (5.9%). In children, the

10 Most Common Natural Products Among Adults* - 2007   **A**

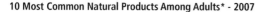

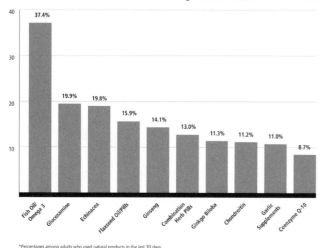

*Percentages among adults who used natural products in the last 30 days.

Source: Barnes PM, Bloom B, Nahin R. CDC *National Health Statistics Report #12: Complementary and Alternative Medicine Use Among Adults and Children: United States, 2007.* December 2008.

Most Common Natural Products Among Children* - 2007   **B**

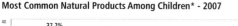

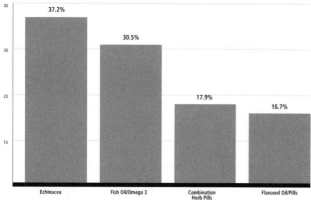

*Percentages among children who used natural products in the last 30 days.

Source: Barnes PM, Bloom B, Nahin R. CDC *National Health Statistics Report #12: Complementary and Alternative Medicine Use Among Adults and Children: United States, 2007.* December 2008

FIGURE 2 *Ten Most Common Natural Products Among Adults and Children—2007.* **A,** The most popular natural products among adults who used nonvitamin, nonmineral natural products in the last year. **B,** The top 10 natural products used in last 30 days among children who used nonvitamin, nonmineral natural products in the past 12 months. (From National Center for Complementary and Alternative Medicine, NIH, DHHS.)

top medical conditions treated with CAM were back or neck problems (6.7%) and head or chest colds (6.6%). The cost of conventional medical care was a significant factor in CAM usage. CAM usage among children was more likely if the parents also used CAM; likelihood of use in children also increased with the education level of the parents.

Herbs and dietary supplements, which are often categorized as CAM but are commonly used in mainstream health care, currently constitute a multibillion dollar industry. According to the American Botanical Council, total estimated herb sales in the United States rose from $4 billion in 1998 to $4.8 billion in 2008.[8] Herbs and other natural products have also served as principal sources of pharmacologically active compounds for over 5,000 years[9,10] In fact, many conventional drugs used today are derived from plant sources. Aspirin, which has been called "the most popular painkiller in the world" and is the world's first-ever synthetic drug, is derived from salicylic acid, a constituent found in the bark of the

TABLE 1. Frequencies and Age-Adjusted Percentages of Adults 18 Years and Over Who Used Selected Types of Nonvitamin, Nonmineral, Natural Products for Health Reasons in the Past 30 Days, by Type of Product Used: United States—2007

Nonvitamin, Nonmineral, Natural Products	Used Selected Nonvitamin, Nonmineral, Natural Products[a]	
	Number in Thousands	Percent[b] (Standard Error)
Fish oil or omega-3 or DHA	10,923	37.4 (1.13)
Glucosamine	6,132	19.9 (0.91)
Echinacea	4,848	19.8 (1.01)
Flaxseed oil or pills	4,416	15.9 (0.87)
Ginseng	3,345	14.1 (0.87)
Combination herb pill	3,446	13.0 (0.83)
Ginkgo biloba	2,977	11.3 (0.88)
Chondroitin	3,390	11.2 (0.82)
Garlic supplements	3,278	11.0 (0.66)
Coenzyme Q-10	2,691	8.7 (0.60)
Fiber or psyllium	1,791	6.6 (0.61)
Green tea pills	1,528	6.3 (0.65)
Cranberry (pills, gelcaps)	1,560	6.0 (0.63)
Saw palmetto	1,682	5.1 (0.46)
Soy supplements or isoflavones	1,363	5.0 (0.53)
Melatonin	1,296	4.6 (0.48)
Grapeseed extract	1,214	4.3 (0.43)
MSM (methylsulfonylmethane)	1,312	4.1 (0.37)
Milk thistle	1,001	3.7 (0.49)
Lutein	1,047	3.4 (0.38)

NOTE: Estimates were age adjusted using the projected 2000 U.S. population as the standard population and using four age groups: 18-24 years, 25-44 years, 45-64 years, and 65 years and over.
[a]Respondents may have used more than one nonvitamin, nonmineral, natural product.
[b]The denominator used in the calculation of percentages was the number of adults who used nonvitamin, nonmineral, natural products within the past 30 days, excluding persons with unknown information for usage of the specified nonvitamin, nonmineral, natural product.
From National Center for Complementary and Alternative Medicine, NIH, DHHS. Data from CDC/NCHS, National Health Interview Survey, 2007. Estimates are based on household interviews of a sample of the civilian, noninstitutionalized population.

willow tree (*Salix* spp.) and some other plant species.[11] The narcotic alkaloids found in the latex sap of the opium poppy (*Papaver somniferum*) are used to make drugs in the class known as opiates, such as morphine, codeine, and heroin.[12] Metformin, the most popular antidiabetic drug and the eleventh most commonly prescribed generic drug in the country,[13] is a biguanide derivative of the guanidines found in galega

TABLE 2. Frequencies and Age-Adjusted Percentages of Children Under 18 Years of Age Who Used Selected Types of Nonvitamin, Nonmineral, Natural Products, for Health Reasons in the Past 30 Days, by Type of Product Used: United States, 2007

Nonvitamin, Nonmineral, Natural Products	Used Selected Nonvitamin, Nonmineral, Natural Products[a]	
	Number in Thousands	Percent[b] (Standard Error)
Echinacea	524	37.2 (4.94)
Fish oil or omega-3 or DHA	441	30.5 (4.88)
Combination herb pill	296	17.9 (3.94)
Flaxseed oil or pills	233	16.7 (4.85)
Prebiotics or probiotics	199	*13.6 (4.49)
Goldenseal	143	*8.6 (3.83)
Garlic supplements	84	*5.9 (1.85)
Melatonin	92	*5.8 (2.02)
Fiber or psyllium	33	†
Cranberry (pills, gelcaps)	33	*1.8 (0.83)
Ginkgo biloba	24	†
Creatine	24	†
Ginseng	19	†
Soy supplements or isoflavones	15	†
DHEA	15	†

DHEA, Dehydroepiandrosterine.
*Estimates preceded by an asterisk have a relative standard error of greater than 30% and less than or equal to 50% and do not meet the standard of reliability or precision.
†Estimates with a relative standard error greater than 50% are indicated with a dagger but are not shown.
aRespondents may have used more than one nonvitamin, nonmineral, natural product.
bThe denominator used in the calculation of percentages was the number of children who used nonvitamin, nonmineral, natural products within the past 30 days, excluding persons with unknown information for usage of the specified nonvitamin, nonmineral, natural product.
NOTE: Estimates were age adjusted using the projected 2000 U.S. population as the standard population using three age groups: 0-4 years, 5-11 years, and 12-17 years. From National Center for Complementary and Alternative Medicine, NIH, DHHS. Data from CDC/NCHS, National Health Interview Survey, 2007. Estimates are based on household interviews of a sample of the civilian, noninstitutionalized population.

(Galega officinalis) and considered to be an "essential medicine" by the World Health Organization.[14] Other notable herb-derived drugs include digoxin, extracted from foxglove *(Digitalis purpurea);* paclitaxel (Taxol), isolated from the bark of the Pacific yew tree *(Taxus brevifolia);* and oseltamivir (Tamiflu), synthesized using shikimic acid found in Chinese star anise *(Illicium verum).*[15]

SAFETY CONCERNS

Although many herbs and supplements have known pharmacological effects, their "natural" origin has led to a widespread notion that all natural products are safe. Rather, adverse and toxic effects have been documented for many herbal products—sometimes caused by contaminants but often caused by the constituents of the herbs themselves. The potential interactions between herbs and conventional drugs are also often overlooked when many herbs not only possess known pharmacological effects, but also serve as sources for conventional drugs. Significant potential morbidity and cost have been associated with herb- and supplement-drug interactions, including increased numbers of emergency room visits, outpatient clinic visits, and perioperative complications.[16-18] However, the true direct and indirect costs, morbidity, and mortality associated with CAM-related interactions and adverse effects are not yet well studied.

There is limited systematic research or published data regarding potential interactions between specific herbs and vitamins and prescription drugs.[19-27] However, Natural Standard has compiled both theoretical and clinical evidence for numerous interactions between drugs, herbs, and dietary supplements to aid in safe decision-making.[28]

STANDARDIZATION

Preparation of herbs and supplements may vary from manufacturer to manufacturer and from batch to batch within one manufacturer. Because it is often not clear what active components are contained in a product, standardization may not be possible, and the clinical effects of different brands may not be comparable.

PATIENT-CLINICIAN COMMUNICATION

Some studies have revealed that neither adult[23,29] nor pediatric[30] patients receive sufficient information or discuss CAM therapies with a physician, pharmacist, nurse, or CAM practitioner; other studies have found that over 60% of patients discuss CAM with their physicians.[31] These discrepancies likely reflect an overall heterogeneity in clinicians' styles of managing patients who use CAM.

Most physicians do not receive formal training regarding the safety and effectiveness of CAM and have limited knowledge in this area.[32] There appears to be significant concern among practitioners about potential safety risks and patient out-of-pocket expenses associated with CAM use.[33,34] Surveys suggest a desire by clinicians for access to quality CAM information, both to improve quality of care and to enhance communication with patients.[35,36] Because of potential adverse effects and interactions associated with CAM use, clinicians are often encouraged to ask patients about CAM use.

Recommended approaches for clinicians to patients who use CAM have been published[37,38] and generally include suggestions to encourage patients to discuss their reasons for seeking CAM, to provide patients with evidence-based information about specific CAM therapies (or explain when available evidence is insufficient), to explain known safety concerns and note that "natural" does not always equate with safety, to support patients emotionally and psychologically even if they choose a CAM therapy with which the clinician does not agree, and to provide close clinical follow-up of patients using CAM therapies.

NATURAL STANDARD BACKGROUND

As the volume of CAM information increases, clinicians and patients are faced with progressively complex therapeutic decisions. These issues, coupled with a growing consciousness among practitioners that many patients use CAM therapies, has created a need for high-quality information services and decision support utilities.

However, rigorous, peer-reviewed, evidence-based resources in this area before the founding of Natural Standard were scarce. Sources of CAM information are often not updated with appropriate frequency; moreover, unlike Natural Standard, these sources may rely on anecdotal evidence rather than scientific evidence that is rigorous, is rooted in academic health centers, and provides multidisciplinary consensus.

In response to this need, the Natural Standard Research Collaboration was formed as a multidisciplinary, multicenter initiative in 1999. Natural Standard's rigorous research methodologies (and the health care content that results) address issues of safety and efficacy that directly pertain to the questions raised by clinicians, patients, and health care institutions.

Natural Standard Research Collaboration now serves as a clearinghouse for evidence-based integrative medicine information. This international effort involves hundreds of prestigious health care providers and scientists who contribute as authors, editors, and peer reviewers toward making trustworthy content for clinicians and consumers. Natural Standard provides high quality time- and life-saving health care information to hospitals, clinics, universities, health maintenance organizations, research organizations, manufacturers, journals, magazines, and textbooks worldwide. Millions of professionals and consumers rely on Natural Standard's help to make informed healthcare decisions.

Natural Standard maintains the online decision support tool www.naturalstandard.com——The Authority on Integrative Medicine. This epic resource aggregates thousands of evidence-based systematic reviews, housing them in searchable, user-friendly databases. Topics include the following:

- Herbs, supplements, and functional foods
- Diets, exercise, and beauty therapies
- Therapeutic modalities (such as chiropractic or acupuncture)
- Environmental and global health topics
- Medical conditions (an integrative approach)
- Genomics and proteomics

Additional resources include daily news stories, events, practitioner listings, continuing education courses plus interactive tools such as the following:

- Interactions and nutrient depletion checkers
- Comparative effectiveness charts
- Brand names database

CAM is one part of a larger health care context that is becoming progressively integrated. Natural Standard aspires to raise the standards for CAM information, thus improving the overall quality of health care delivery overall.

This book collates over a decade of cumulative research found on www.naturalstandard.com and summarizes it into over 360 concise monographs on popular herbs and supplements. Therapies have been selected based on utilization data, sales trends, safety concerns, and requests by institutional or individual users of Natural Standard. Each Natural Standard monograph is painstakingly created, involving numerous contributors and an extensive research methodology (described next). Natural Standard regularly adds new topics and updates, thus constantly expanding this rich portal. Now, print readers can easily access the clinical bottom line on popular therapies in this consolidated reference guide.

RESEARCH METHODOLOGY: SYSTEMATIC AGGREGATION, ANALYSIS, AND REVIEW OF THE LITERATURE

Search Strategy

Natural Standard provides high-quality, reliable information about CAM therapies to clinicians, patients, and health care institutions. Through systematic aggregation and analysis of scientific data, incorporation of historic and folkloric perspectives, consultation with multidisciplinary editorial experts, use of validated grading scales (Table 3), and blinded peer-review processes, Natural Standard builds evidence-based and consensus-based content. This content is designed to support safe and educated therapeutic decisions.

Systematic Aggregation of Research

To prepare each Natural Standard monograph, electronic searches are conducted in multiple databases, including AMED, CANCERLIT, CINAHL, CISCOM, the Cochrane Library, EMBASE, HerbMed, International Pharmaceutical Abstracts, Medline, and NAPRALERT. Search terms include the common names, scientific names, and known synonyms for all topics. Hand searches are conducted in more than 20 additional journals that are not indexed in common databases, as well as in bibliographies from over 50 selected secondary references. No restrictions are placed on language or quality of publications. Researchers in the CAM field are consulted for access to additional references or ongoing research.

Selection Criteria

All literature is collected pertaining to efficacy in humans (regardless of study design, quality, or language), dosing, precautions, adverse effects, use in pregnancy or lactation, interactions, effects on clinical testing, and mechanism of action (in vitro, animal research, human data). Standardized inclusion/exclusion criteria are used in the selection.

Data Analysis

Health care experts perform data extraction and analysis using standardized instruments that pertain to each monograph section (defining inclusion and exclusion criteria and analytic techniques, including validated measures of study quality). Data verification is performed by independent reviewers.

Review Process

Blinded review of each monograph is conducted by multidisciplinary research-clinical faculty at major academic centers with expertise in epidemiology and biostatistics, pharmacology, toxicology, CAM research, and clinical practice. In cases of editorial disagreement, a three-member panel of the editorial board addresses conflicts and consults experts when applicable. Authors of studies are contacted when clarification is required.

Natural Standard Evidence-based Validated Grading Rationale

Multiple grading scales have been developed over the past decade to evaluate the level of available scientific evidence supporting the efficacy of medical interventions. Based on existing grading scales (e.g., U.S. Preventive Services Task Force [USPTF]), as well as the unique challenges involved in the evaluation of CAM therapies, the Natural Standard grading scale was developed through a multidisciplinary consensus group, widely reviewed, piloted, and validated. This scale has been found to produce consistent grades among different raters; it has been used in numerous publications, and has been

TABLE 3. Natural Standard Evidence-Based Validated Grading Rationale™

Level of Evidence Grade	Criteria
A (strong scientific evidence)	Statistically significant evidence of benefit from more than two properly randomized trials (RCTs), OR evidence from one properly conducted RCT AND one properly conducted meta-analysis, OR evidence from multiple RCTs with a clear majority of the properly conducted trials showing statistically significant evidence of benefit AND with supporting evidence in basic science, animal studies, or theory.
B (good scientific evidence)	Statistically significant evidence of benefit from one or two properly randomized trials, OR evidence of benefit from more than one properly conducted meta-analysis OR evidence of benefit from more than one cohort/case-control/nonrandomized trial AND with supporting evidence in basic science, animal studies, or theory. This grade applies to situations in which a well-designed randomized, controlled trial reports negative results but stands in contrast to the positive efficacy results of multiple other less well-designed trials or a well-designed meta-analysis, while awaiting confirmatory evidence from an additional well designed randomized controlled trial.
C (unclear or conflicting scientific evidence)	Evidence of benefit from more than one small RCT without adequate size, power, statistical significance, or quality of design by objective criteria,* OR conflicting evidence from multiple RCTs without a clear majority of the properly conducted trials showing evidence of benefit or ineffectiveness, OR evidence of benefit from more than one cohort/case-control/nonrandomized trial AND without supporting evidence in basic science, animal studies, or theory, OR evidence of efficacy only from basic science, animal studies, or theory.
D (fair negative scientific evidence)	Statistically significant negative evidence (i.e., lack of evidence of benefit) from cohort/case-control/nonrandomized trials, AND evidence in basic science, animal studies, or theory suggesting a lack of benefit. This grade also applies to situations in which more than one well-designed randomized, controlled trial reports negative results, notwithstanding the existence of positive efficacy results reported from other less well designed trials or a meta-analysis. (Note: if there is more than one negative randomized controlled trial that is well-designed and highly compelling, this will result in a grade of "F" notwithstanding positive results from other less well designed studies.)
F (strong negative scientific evidence)	Statistically significant negative evidence (i.e., lack of evidence of benefit) from more than one properly randomized adequately powered trial(s) of high-quality design by objective criteria.*
Lack of evidence†	Unable to evaluate efficacy due to lack of adequate available human data.

*Objective criteria are derived from validated instruments for evaluating study quality, including the 5-point scale developed by Jadad et al., in which a score below 4 is considered to indicate lesser quality methodologically (Jadad AR, Moore RA, Carroll D, Jenkinson C, Reynolds DJ, Gavaghan DJ, McQuay HJ. Assessing the quality of reports of randomized clinical trials: is blinding necessary? *Controlled Clinical Trials* 1996; 17[1]:1–12).
†Listed separately in monographs in the "Historical or Theoretical Uses which Lack Sufficient Evidence" section.

presented for discussion at the Agency for Healthcare Research and Quality (AHRQ).

These grades are used in all Natural Standard reviews (monographs). Specific grades reflect the level of available scientific evidence supporting the efficacy of a specific therapy for a given indication. Expert opinion and folkloric precedent are not included in this assessment but are discussed in a separate section of each monograph. Evidence of harm is considered separately, and the grades apply only to evidence of benefit (Table 3).

HOW TO USE THIS BOOK

Over 360 monographs constitute this book. Each is formatted in the same way. Monograph sections are summarized below. Because of space constraints, the disclaimers have been removed from each monograph but are reproduced here.

Title

Natural Standard Monograph, Copyright © 2009 (www. naturalstandard.com). Commercial distribution prohibited. This monograph is intended for informational purposes only, and should not be interpreted as specific medical advice. Consumers should consult with a qualified health care professional before making decisions about therapies and/or health conditions.

Related Terms

- *Related Terms* contains a comprehensive alphabetical list of constituents, related substances, synonyms, branded and/ or combination products, and common, scientific, and foreign language names pertaining to the herb or supplement.

Background

- *Background* provides an overview of the herb or supplement, including the origin, history, and popular and science-based uses. Available scientific evidence is thoroughly summarized, and promising future uses or pertinent safety information may be indicated.

Evidence

- *Evidence* provides a summary of the scientific evidence on the use of an herb or supplement to prevent or treat a disease or medical condition. Using a comprehensive methodology and the **Natural Standard evidence-based validated grading rationale™** to evaluate the quality of available research, a simple letter grade from A to F is assigned to each use for an herb or supplement. Grade A reflects strong scientific evidence; Grade B, good scientific evidence; Grade C, unclear or conflicting scientific evidence; Grade D, fair negative scientific evidence; and Grade F, strong scientific evidence against this use (it likely does not work).

Uses Based on Scientific Evidence

These uses have been tested in humans or animals. Safety and effectiveness have not always been proven. Some of these conditions are potentially serious, and should be evaluated by a qualified healthcare professional.

Uses Based on Tradition or Theory

Below uses are based on tradition or scientific theories. They often have not been thoroughly tested in humans, and safety and effectiveness have not always been proven. Some of these conditions are potentially serious and should be evaluated by a qualified health care professional.

- Contains a comprehensive alphabetical list of traditional or theoretical uses of the herb or supplement. These indications may reflect use by natural medicine practitioners, have not been sufficiently evaluated in scientific studies, and do not meet criteria for the **Natural Standard evidence-based validated grading rationale™.**

Dosing

Below are based on scientific research, secondary or manufacturer publications, traditional use, or expert opinion. Many herbs and supplements have not been thoroughly tested, and safety and effectiveness may not be proven. Brands may be made differently, with variable ingredients, even within the same brand. The below doses may not apply to all products. Consumers should read product labels, and discuss doses with a qualified health care professional before starting therapy.

- Contains dosing of the herb or supplement for adults and children, categorized by route of administration and specific use.

  Adults (18 Years and Older)
  Children (Younger than 18 Years)

Safety

The U.S. Food and Drug Administration does not strictly regulate herbs and supplements. There is no guarantee of strength, purity, or safety of products, and effects may vary. Consumers should always read product labels. People with medical conditions or taking other drugs, herbs, or supplements should speak with a qualified health care professional before starting a new therapy. Consult a healthcare professional immediately side effects are experienced.

Allergies
Side Effects and Warnings
Pregnancy and Breastfeeding

Interactions

Most herbs and supplements have not been thoroughly tested for interactions with other herbs, supplements, drugs, or foods. The interactions listed below are based on reports in scientific publications, laboratory experiments, or traditional use. Consumers should always read product labels. People with medical conditions or taking other drugs, herbs, or supplements should speak with a qualified health care professional before starting a new therapy.

Interactions with Drugs

- Provides a summary of potential interactions between the therapy and drugs and other agents. Examples include interactions with agents that may increase the risk of bleeding, alter blood sugar levels or blood pressure, or interfere with metabolism.

Interactions with Herbs and Dietary Supplements

- Provides a summary of potential interactions between the therapy and other herbs or supplements. Examples include interactions with agents that may increase the risk of bleeding, alter blood sugar levels or blood pressure, or interfere with metabolism.

Selected References

Natural Standard developed the above evidence-based information based on a thorough systematic review of the available scientific articles. For comprehensive information about alternative and complementary therapies on the professional level, go to www.naturalstandard.com and enter the monograph title into the search box. When results appear, click on the Limit Search link located on the right-hand side at the top of the page. Click the References box to limit the search to only references, and then click Go. A document titled Selected References will appear. Click the title link and you'll be taken to the selected references for that particular monograph.

- Includes a list of selected references that can be used to obtain further research on the herb or supplement.

Acknowledgments

We are sincerely grateful for the ongoing contributions of Natural Standard's authors, peer reviewers, and editors since the founding of our international research collaboration. The hard work and dedication of internal content team members Dawn Costa and Wendy Weissner deserve special recognition for helping make this particular book available. Additionally, we thank our operational, outreach, member services, and technical teams, along with our Board of Directors for their support of evidence-based integrative medicine research. Please visit www.naturalstandard.com to learn more about our work. We welcome additional members, including students, to participate in our academic research programs.

Contents

5-HTP
(5-Hydroxytryptophan, L-5 Hydroxytryptophan)

RELATED TERMS

- 5-Hydroxytryptophan, *Griffonia simplicifolia*, L-5-HTP, L-5 hydroxytryptophan, oxitriptan, Tript-OH, tryptophan.
- **Note:** 5-Hydroxytryptophan should not be confused with L-tryptophan.

BACKGROUND

- 5-HTP is the precursor of the neurotransmitter serotonin. It is obtained commercially from the seeds of the plant *Griffonia simplicifolia*.
- 5-HTP has been suggested as a treatment for many conditions. There is some research to support the use of 5-HTP in treating cerebellar ataxia, headache, depression, psychiatric disorders, fibromyalgia, and as an appetite suppressant or weight loss agent. There is not enough scientific evidence to support the use of 5-HTP for any other medical condition.
- 5-HTP may cause gastrointestinal disturbances, including nausea, vomiting, diarrhea, and loss of appetite. There is also concern that 5-HTP may cause eosinophilia myalgia syndrome (EMS). 5-HTP should not be used with serotonergic drugs (e.g., SSRIs) due to increased risk of serotonin syndrome.

EVIDENCE

Uses Based on Scientific Evidence	Grade
Cerebellar Ataxia Cerebellar ataxia results from the failure of part of the brain to regulate body posture and limb movements. 5-HTP has been observed to have benefits in some people who have difficulty standing or walking because of cerebellar ataxia. However, current evidence is mixed.	B
Depression The results of numerous studies in humans suggest that 5-HTP may aid in the treatment of depression. However, it is not known whether 5-HTP is as effective as commonly prescribed antidepressant drugs.	B
Fibromyalgia There is a small amount of research evaluating the use of 5-HTP for fibromyalgia, and early evidence suggests that 5-HTP may reduce the number of tender points, anxiety, and intensity of pain, and may improve sleep, fatigue, and morning stiffness.	B
Headaches There is evidence from several studies in children and adults that 5-HTP may be effective in reducing the severity and frequency of headaches, including tension headaches and migraines. Further research is needed.	B
Obesity Studies suggest that 5-HTP may reduce eating behaviors, lessen caloric intake, and promote weight loss in obese individuals.	B

Alcoholism (Withdrawal Symptoms) Early studies suggest that 5-HTP may lessen alcohol withdrawal symptoms. Further research is needed to confirm these results.	B
Anxiety Although 5-HTP has been proposed as a possible treatment for anxiety disorders, there is not enough human evidence to make a firm recommendation.	C
Down's Syndrome Preliminary studies of 5-HTP in children with Down's syndrome have yielded insignificant results. Further research is necessary.	C
Neurological Disorders (Lesch-Nyhan Syndrome) Lesch-Nyhan syndrome (LNS) is a rare genetic disorder affecting mostly males that often causes mental retardation and self-mutilation. Small studies of 5-HTP in Lesch-Nyhan syndrome show conflicting results. Additional studies are needed.	C
Psychiatric Disorders It has been suggested that 5-HTP may reduce psychotic symptoms and mania or aid in panic disorder, but studies in people with schizophrenia have shown differing results.	C
Sleep Disorders There is insufficient evidence regarding the use of 5-HTP for sleep disorders. Additional studies are needed before a conclusion can be drawn.	C
Seizures/Epilepsy (Myoclonic Disorders) Although 5-HTP has been studied as a treatment for various myoclonic syndromes and epilepsy, available research does not support the use of 5-HTP for these conditions.	D

Uses Based on Tradition or Theory

Aggression, agoraphobia (fear of open/public spaces), Alzheimer's disease, amyotrophic lateral sclerosis (fatal progressive neurological disease), anorexia, attention-deficit/hyperactivity disorder (ADHD), autism, bipolar disorder, bulimia nervosa, cough, deficiency (aromatic-L-amino acid decarboxylase deficiency; serotonin deficiency), delirium tremens (DTs), diabetes, digestion, dizziness, dystonia (muscle spasms), eating disorders (binge eating), endocrine disorders (Cushing syndrome), eye disorders (ophthalmoplegia), hepatitis, herpesvirus infection (Ramsey-Hunt syndrome), hormonal disorders, inflammation, insomnia, menopausal symptoms, mood disorder, myoclonic disorders (Lance-Adams syndrome), obsessive-compulsive disorder, pain, panic disorder, Parkinson's disease, phenylketonuria, premenstrual syndrome, psychosis (LSD-induced), restless legs syndrome, seasonal affective disorder, sexual dysfunction, temperature regulation.

DOSING
Adults (18 Years and Older)

- In general, most studies have administered 5-HTP at low doses and for a short duration. A common dose used is 300 mg/day, which has been taken for depression or headache. Doses of 1600 mg/day or 16 mg/kg/day over 12 months have been studied. Starting with low doses (50 mg three times daily) and increasing the dosage gradually may minimize side effects such as nausea.

Children (Younger than 18 Years)

- There is not enough scientific data to recommend 5-HTP for use in children, and 5-HTP is not usually recommended because of potential side effects. However, for headache, 100 mg daily for 12 weeks has been used.

SAFETY
Allergies

- 5-HTP should be avoided in individuals with a known allergy or hypersensitivity to 5-HTP. Signs of allergy may include rash, itching, or shortness of breath. Urticaria (hives) has been reported.

Side Effects and Warnings

- Although 5-HTP seems to be generally well tolerated, because of potential serious adverse effects, a physician should supervise the use of 5-HTP. Cases of eosinophilia myalgia syndrome (EMS) have been reported, and although the precise role of 5-HTP in these cases is unclear, it has been suggested that contaminants in certain batches were responsible for these adverse effects. Several thousand cases of EMS and deaths were linked to the ingestion of contaminated L-tryptophan in 1989. 5-HTP should be avoided in patients with eosinophilia syndromes.
- Palpitations, lowered blood pressure, myalgia (muscle pain), weakness, rhabdomyolysis (breakdown of skeletal muscle), eosinophilia (increased number of white blood cells), nausea, vomiting, abdominal pain, heartburn, diarrhea, gas, and taste alteration have been reported. Slow initiation of treatment and enteric-coated tablets have decreased gastrointestinal side effects.
- Drowsiness, dizziness, vertigo, somnolence (sleepiness), insomnia, and headache are occasionally reported. Mania and euphoria have also been noted. Seizure syndrome has occurred in patients with Down's syndrome. Despite possible efficacy of 5-HTP for Down's syndrome, 5-HTP is not recommended in Down's syndrome patients.
- Other potential side effects of taking 5-HTP by mouth include transient disinhibition, euphoria, irritability, depressed mood, restlessness, rapid speech, anxiety, aggressiveness, and agitation. Weight gain has been reported in a few cases. In contrast, loss of appetite has also been reported. Amenorrhea (absence of menstruation) was noted in one case.
- Patients receiving carbidopa (a drug for Parkinson's disease) and 5-HTP long-term had reductions in total cholesterol, bradycardia (slowed heart rate), hypomania (mild mania), pseudobullous morphea (chronic, degenerative disease that affects the joints, skin, and internal organs), and scleroderma-like illness.
- An intravenous derivative of 5-HTP called gamma-L-glutamyl 5-HTP administered over 1 hour resulted in sodium retention. It is unknown if this effect was the result of the formulation, the route of administration, or the rate of infusion.
- 5-HTP should be used cautiously in patients with kidney insufficiency because 5-HTP is eliminated through the kidneys.
- 5-HTP should be used cautiously in patients with human immunodeficiency virus (HIV-1) infection, in patients with existing gastrointestinal disorders, or in patients with a history of mental disorders.

Pregnancy and Breastfeeding

- 5-HTP is not recommended in pregnant or breastfeeding women because of a lack of available scientific evidence. The risk of contaminants found in 5-HTP products further precludes use during pregnancy. 5-HTP may increase prolactin, a necessary hormone for milk production; 5-HTP should be avoided while breastfeeding.

INTERACTIONS
Interactions with Drugs

- Concomitant use of 5-HTP and sertonergic drugs (e.g., selective serotonin reuptake inhibitors [SSRIs], tricyclic antidepressants [TCAs], and monoamine oxidase inhibitors [MAOIs]) may increase the risk of serotonergic effects, including serotonin syndrome.
- When 5-HTP is used with CNS depressants, there may be an increased risk of adverse effects.
- Drugs such as methysergide and cyproheptadine may reduce the effects of 5-HTP.
- Losartan, an angiotensin receptor blocker, may cause a decrease in pineal serotonin levels.
- Administration of 5-HTP with decarboxylase inhibitors can increase the plasma concentration and half-life of 5-HTP.
- 5-HTP, when taken with fenfluramine, may cause suppression in food intake.
- Lithium carbonate may enhance serotonin receptor sensitivity, whereas tricyclic antidepressants (TCA) and second-generation antidepressants may diminish serotonin receptor sensitivity.
- Anecdotally, concomitant use of reserpine and 5-HTP may result in hypertensive (high blood pressure) reactions.
- The 5-HTP-induced increase in plasma cortisol can be blocked by the administration of ritanserin, a $5-HT_2$/$5-HT_{1C}$ antagonist.
- Although human evidence is lacking, 5-HTP may interact with angiotensin II receptor antagonists (A2R blockers) and thyroid-stimulating hormones. 5-HTP has also been shown to increase luteinizing hormone, although the effects on hormones in humans are unclear.
- In theory, 5-HTP may have additive effects with sedatives or medications taken for epilepsy or seizures.
- 5-HTP has produced weight loss in the obese. In theory, 5-HTP may interact additively or synergistically with other weight loss agents.
- It has been suggested that 5-HTP may reduce psychotic symptoms and mania or aid in panic disorder, but studies in people with schizophrenia have shown differing results. Caution is advised.
- 5-HTP may alter the effects of cytochrome P450 substrates.

Interactions with Herbs and Dietary Supplements

- In theory, L-tyrosine, adenosyl-L-methionine, tryptophan, vitamin B_6, chromium, melatonin, niacin, S-adenosyl-L

methionine (SAMe), and magnesium may increase the effects or side effects associated with 5-HTP.
- Concomitant use of 5-HTP and serotonergic herbs and supplements (e.g., St. John's wort) may increase the risk of serotonergic effects, including serotonin syndrome.
- When 5-HTP is used with sedative herbs and supplements, there may be an increased risk of adverse effects.

- It has been suggested that 5-HTP may reduce psychotic symptoms and mania or aid in panic disorder, but studies in people with schizophrenia have shown different results. Caution is advised.
- 5-HTP may alter the effects of cytochrome P450 substrates.

For a complete list of references, please visit www.naturalstandard.com.

Abuta

RELATED TERMS

- *Abuta fluminum, Abuta grandifolia, Abuta grisebachii, Abuta panurensis,* abutua, aristoloche lobee, barbasco, bejuco de cerca, bejuco de raton, butua, false pareira, feuille coeur, gasing-gasing, ice vine, imchich masha, liane patte cheval, Menispermaceae, pareira, pareira brava, patacon, velvetleaf.

BACKGROUND

- Abuta grows in the Amazon basin and other humid, tropical areas of the world. It is known as a "midwife's herb" in South America and is used to treat various women's complaints. In some parts of the world, abuta is used to reduce fever, inflammation, and pain. In the United States, abuta is used mainly for minor reproductive tract conditions such as menstrual cramping.
- Abuta may function as an emmenagogue (menstrual flow stimulant). However, there are no human trials that have determined the safety and effectiveness of the abuta plant on the menstrual cycle. Further research is needed before a recommendation can be made.
- Documented uses in traditional medicine show that abuta is used as a diuretic (increases urine flow), expectorant (expels phlegm), emmenagogue, and antipyretic (reduces fever). It is also used to prevent abortion, relieve heavy menstrual bleeding, and stop uterine hemorrhages (bleeding). Powdered abuta bark has also been used for menstrual complaints.

EVIDENCE

Uses Based on Scientific Evidence

No available studies qualify for inclusion in the evidence table.

Uses Based on Tradition or Theory

Acne, anemia, antiplasmoidal, aphrodisiac, asthma, boils, bronchitis, burns, cerebral tonic, chills, cholera, colds, colic, constipation, convulsions, cough, cystitis (inflammation of the bladder), delirium, dental analgesia (dental pain), diabetes, diarrhea, digestion, diuretic, dog bites, dropsy (edema), dysentery (severe diarrhea), dyspepsia (upset stomach), erysipelas (bacterial skin infection), expectorant (expels phlegm), eye infections, fertility (in women), fever, hematuria (blood in the urine), hemorrhage (bleeding), hypercholesterolemia (high cholesterol), hypertension (high blood pressure), insecticide, itching, jaundice, kidney stones, leukorrhea (vaginal discharge), malaria, menstrual discomfort, nephritis, palpitations, parturition (childbirth), purgative, prenatal and postnatal pain, rabies, rheumatism, snake bites, sores, stimulant, stimulating menstrual flow, stomach ache, tonic, toothache, typhoid, venereal diseases, wounds.

DOSING

Adults (18 Years and Older)

- Safety and effectiveness have not been proven for any dose. For menstrual complaints, 1-2 g of powdered abuta bark in tablets or capsules has been used twice daily. Abuta has also been taken as a 4:1 tincture in a dose of 2-4 mL twice daily.

Children (Younger than 18 Years)

- There is insufficient evidence to recommend a dose for abuta in children.

SAFETY

Allergies

- Individuals with a known allergy or hypersensitivity to abuta or any component of the formulation should not take abuta.

Side Effects and Warnings

- Currently, there is not enough available evidence about the safety of abuta. Use in pregnant women is not advised because of possible abortion-inducing effects, although there is controversy in this area.
- Many plants related to abuta look alike. Some abuta products may be contaminated with these similar plants.

Pregnancy and Breastfeeding

- Abuta is not recommended in pregnant or breastfeeding women. Abuta may cause abortion, although there is controversy in this area.

INTERACTIONS

Interactions with Drugs

- Currently, available scientific evidence describing drug interactions with abuta is lacking.

Interactions with Herbs and Dietary Supplements

- Currently, available scientific evidence describing herb and supplement interactions with abuta is lacking.

For a complete list of references, please visit www.naturalstandard.com.

RELATED TERMS

- *Acacia arabica*, *Acacia arabica gum*, *Acacia aulacocarpa*, *Acacia auriculiformis*, *Acacia baileyana*, acacia bark, *Acacia catechu*, *Acacia caven*, *Acacia concinna*, *Acacia confusa* (ACTI), *Acacia coriacea*, *Acacia dealbata*, *Acacia farnesiana*, *Acacia floribunda*, *Acacia glaucoptera*, *Acacia greggii*, acacia gum, *Acacia lenticularis*, *Acacia longifolia*, *Acacia melanoxylon*, *Acacia mellifera*, *Acacia nilotica*, *Acacia pilispina*, *Acacia pycnantha*, *Acacia senegal*, *Acacia senegal* (L.) Willd., *Acacia seyal*, *Acacia tenuifolia*, *Acacia tortilis* sp. raddiana, *Acacia tortuoso*, *Acacia victoriae* (Bentham), black wattle, blackwood, catclaw acacia, espinillo negro, Fabaceae (family), gastrilis, gomme arabique, gomme de Senegal, gum arabic, gum senegal, huizache, ker, khadira, kikar, Leguminosae (family), mimosa, miswaki, *Robinia pseudoacacia*, silver wattle, Sydney golden wattle, wattles, white acacia seeds.

BACKGROUND

- The name *acacia* is derived from the Greek word *akis* meaning "sharp point," and relates to the sharp thorny shrubs and trees of tropical Africa and Western Asia that were the only known acacias at the time the name was published. The Australian acacias are commonly called "wattles" because of their pliable branches that were woven into the structure of early wattle houses and fences.
- Acacia is commonly present in chewing sticks, mainly as an antimicrobial with activity against *Streptococcus faecalis*. Acacia has also shown some cholesterol-lowering and antidiabetic properties, although there is insufficient evidence in support of these uses.
- Acacia is generally considered to be safe. Adverse reactions seem to be mild, with occasional gastrointestinal symptoms.
- Acacia has been used to treat high cholesterol, diabetes, cancer, gingivitis, stomatitis (mouth sores), pharyngitis, and indigestion in children. Acacia gum is used as a food additive. *Acacia concinna* is often used in cosmetics.

EVIDENCE

Uses Based on Scientific Evidence	Grade
Plaque The available data shows promising results; however, further studies are warranted.	C
Hypercholesterolemia (High Cholesterol) There is preliminary evidence that acacia may not be helpful for hypercholesterolemia.	D

Uses Based on Tradition or Theory
Astringent, blood clots, cancer, contraception, cosmetic, dandruff, diabetes, flavoring agent, food additive, gingivitis, hepatitis, human immunodeficiency virus (HIV), indigestion, infection, inflammation, leprosy, lice, parasites (visceral leishmaniasis), pharyngitis, renal failure, sexually transmitted diseases (*Acacia nilotica*), stomatitis (mouth sores).

DOSING

Adults (18 Years and Older)

- There is no proven safe or effective dose for acacia. Traditionally, 5 g twice daily for 4 weeks has been used.
- Daily use of a chewing stick of *Acacia arabica* may be effective for plaque; studies have shown positive results in 7 days.

Children (Younger than 18 Years)

- There is insufficient evidence to recommend a dose for acacia in children.

SAFETY

Allergies

- Avoid in individuals with a known allergy or hypersensitivity to acacia or the Fabaceae or Leguminosae family. There is cross-sensitivity between acacia and rye grass, pollen allergens, and date palm.
- Avoid in individuals with a known allergy or hypersensitivity to pollen, particularly mimosa, other pollens, bee pollen, other inhalants, and foods containing related substances.

Side Effects and Warnings

- Acacia gum is regarded as safe when used orally and in amounts commonly found in foods. Acacia has generally recognized as safe (GRAS) status for use in foods in the United States.
- When sucked or chewed, acacia may cause gastrointestinal disturbances and neurological side effects.
- Allergic reactions, including asthma, rhinitis, conjunctivitis, and rash, may occur.
- *Acacia senegal* can cause minor gastrointestinal disturbances, such as bloating, loose stools, and flatulence. Side effects may diminish with continued use.
- Iridocyclitis, a type of anterior uveitis, can be caused by acacia thorns.
- Use cautiously in patients taking amoxicillin or iron.
- Use cautiously in patients with respiratory disorders.
- Be aware that the fiber of acacia may impair the absorption of oral drugs.
- Be aware that tannins from *Acacia catechu* L. plant may contribute to oral and esophageal cancer when combined with other substances that also contain high amounts of tannins.

Pregnancy and Breastfeeding

- Acacia is not recommended in pregnant or breastfeeding women due to a lack of available scientific evidence.

INTERACTIONS

Interactions with Drugs

- Acacia may affect the absorption of amoxicillin when taken concurrently; doses should be separated by at least 4 hours.
- Use of acacia as a surfactant may increase the intestinal absorption of some anticancer drugs through P-glycoprotein (P-gp) inhibition and thus improve drug bioavailability for P-gp substrate.
- Mixing acacia with a substance containing more than 50% concentration of ethyl alcohol may cause acacia to become insoluble.

- Acacia can be gelatinized by solutions of iron salts.
- Theoretically, the fiber in acacia may impair the absorption of oral drugs.

Interactions with Herbs and Dietary Supplements

- Theoretically, the fiber in acacia may impair the absorption of oral herbs and supplements.

- Theoretically, tannins from *Acacia catechu* L. plant may contribute to oral and esophageal cancer when combined with other substances that also contain high amounts of tannins.

For a complete list of references, please visit www. naturalstandard.com.

Acai
(Euterpe oleracea)

RELATED TERMS

- Acai flour, acai palm, Amazonian palm, *Euterpe oleracea*, *Euterpe oleracea* Mart., heart of palm, OptiAcai, palm heart.

BACKGROUND

- The acai palm tree (*Euterpe oleracea*) is native to tropical Central and South America, and grows mainly in flood-plains and swamps. Although the soft interior stem can be used as a source for heart of palm, acai is better known for its inch-long reddish purple fruit. Acai has been a traditional food of the native people of the Amazon for hundreds of years. Acai beverages are prepared by extracting juice from the fruit pulp and skin.
- Currently, research on acai fruit has been centered on its potential antioxidant properties. Acai fruit has also shown antiproliferative and anti-inflammatory activity. Acai may also show promise as an agent for use in magnetic resonance imaging (MRI), which is a non-invasive procedure that produces a two-dimensional view of internal organs or structures, especially the brain and spinal cord. Currently, insufficient evidence is available in humans to support the use of acai for any indication.

EVIDENCE

Uses Based on Scientific Evidence

No available studies qualify for inclusion in the evidence table.

Uses Based on Tradition or Theory

Alternative oral contrast agent in MRI, anti-inflammatory, antioxidant, cancer, food uses.

DOSING

Adults (18 Years and Older)

- There is insufficient evidence to recommend a dose for acai in adults.

Children (Younger than 18 Years)

- There is insufficient evidence to recommend a dose for acai in children.

SAFETY

Allergies

- Acai should be avoided in individuals with a known allergy or hypersensitivity to acai (*Euterpe oleracea*) or its constituents.

Side Effects and Warnings

- Acai is likely safe when used in food amounts.
- Acai should be avoided in patients undergoing MRI or using oral contrast agents for MRI because acai has been used as an experimental clinical oral contrast agent for MRI of the gastrointestinal tract.
- Acai may aggravate or initiate hypertension (high blood pressure) or edema (swelling). It may also aggravate or initiate gastrointestinal disorders (ulcers or intestinal bleeding).
- Acai should be used cautiously in patients taking antineoplastics (anticancer agents).

Pregnancy and Breastfeeding

- Acai is not recommended in pregnant or breastfeeding women due to a lack of available scientific evidence.

INTERACTIONS

Interactions with Drugs

- Acai may have cyclooxygenase COX-1 and COX-2 inhibition properties. Theoretically, concurrent use may have additive effects.
- Acai may have antiproliferative effects. Theoretically, concurrent use may have additive effects.

Interactions with Herbs and Dietary Supplements

- Acai may have cyclooxygenase COX-1 and COX-2 inhibition properties. Theoretically, concurrent use may have additive effects.
- Acai may have antiproliferative effects. Theoretically, concurrent use may have additive effects.
- Freeze-dried acai fruit pulp/skin powder may have antioxidant capacity. Theoretically, concurrent use may have additive effects.

For a complete list of references, please visit www.naturalstandard.com.

RELATED TERMS

- Acerola fruits, Antilles cherry, Barbados cherry, cerea-do-para, cereja-das-antillhas, cereso, *Malpighia emarginata* DC, *Malpighia glabra* L., *Malpighia punicifolia*, *Malpighia punicifolia* L., Puerto Rican cherry, West Indian cherry wild crapemyrtle.

BACKGROUND

- Acerola (*Malphighia glabra*), also known as Barbados cherry, is the fruit of a small tree known as *Malphighia glabra* L. in the Antilles and north of South America. In 1945, the School of Medicine at the University of Puerto Rico found that the Barbados cherry was a very rich source of vitamin C.
- Folk healers have used acerola to treat liver ailments, diarrhea, dysentery, coughs, colds, and sore throat. As one of the richest sources of vitamin C, acerola may be used as an immune stimulator and modulator.
- Acerola has been used as a supplement for adults and infants. The Barbados cherry extract, the fruit of *Malpighia emarginata* DC, has been reported to prevent age-related diseases. The Barbados cherry has been shown to exhibit cytotoxic effects and may be useful in the treatment of cancer. It has high antibacterial activity and shows multi-drug resistance reversal activity.
- Currently, available scientific evidence is lacking, and additional study is needed to evaluate the safety, effectiveness, and dosing of acerola.

EVIDENCE

Uses Based on Scientific Evidence

No available studies qualify for inclusion in the evidence table.

Uses Based on Tradition or Theory

Aging, antibacterial, antioxidant, atherosclerosis (hardening of the arteries), blood clot prevention, cancer, colds, coughs, depression, diabetes, diarrhea, dysentery (severe diarrhea), exercise performance, fungal infections, gum disease, hay fever, heart disease, hemorrhage (retinal), hypercholesterolemia (high cholesterol), immunostimulation, liver disorders, pressure ulcers, scurvy, skin conditions, sore throat, tooth disease, vitamin C deficiency.

DOSING

Adults (18 Years and Older)

- Safety, efficacy, and dosing have not been systematically studied in adults.

Children (Younger than 18 Years)

- Safety, efficacy, and dosing have not been systematically studied in children.

SAFETY

Allergies

- Individuals with a known allergy or hypersensitivity to acerola or species in the Malpighiaceae family should not use acerola.

Side Effects and Warnings

- Acerola seems to be generally well tolerated in recommended amounts in otherwise healthy individuals. High doses may cause diarrhea, nausea, abdominal cramps, insomnia, fatigue, or sleeplessness owing to the vitamin C content.
- Patients with gout should not take acerola because the vitamin C in acerola might increase uric acid levels.
- Patients with a history of kidney stones (nephrolithiasis) should not take acerola because large doses of vitamin C in acerola may cause the production of urate, cystine, or oxalate stones.

Pregnancy and Breastfeeding

- Acerola is not recommended in pregnant or breastfeeding women due to a lack of available scientific evidence.

INTERACTIONS

Interactions with Drugs

- The vitamin C in acerola may interact with acidic or basic drugs, acidify urine, and affect excretion. Patients taking medications should consult with a qualified health care professional, including a pharmacist.
- Vitamin C seems to interfere with the "blood thinning" effects of warfarin by lowering prothrombin time. In theory, acerola may reduce the effectiveness of anticoagulant or antiplatelet agents. Examples include heparin (Hepalean), lepirudin (Refludan), warfarin (Coumadin), abciximab (ReoPro), and clopidogrel (Plavix).
- Use of acerola with medications containing estrogen or birth control pills may increase the absorption and therapeutic effects owing to the vitamin C content. Caution is advised.
- Use of fluphenazine (Prolixin) with acerola may decrease blood levels owing to vitamin C content. Patients taking fluphenazine should consult with a qualified health care professional, including a pharmacist.

Interactions with Herbs and Dietary Supplements

- Acerola cherry extract may increase the antioxidant effects of alfalfa or soy. Caution is advised.
- Vitamin C seems to interfere with the "blood thinning" effects of warfarin (Coumadin) by lowering prothrombin time. In theory, acerola may reduce the effectiveness of herbs and supplements that are used for their "blood thinning" effects, such as willow bark.
- When taken together, the vitamin C in acerola may increase the absorption of iron in the gastrointestinal tract. Caution is advised.
- Due to acerola's high vitamin C content, taking vitamin C supplements in addition to acerola may increase the total amount of vitamin C in the body and lead to adverse effects. Caution is advised.

For a complete list of references, please visit www.naturalstandard.com.

Acetyl-L-Carnitine
(L-Carnitine)

RELATED TERMS

- AcCn, acetyl-L-carnitine, B (t) Factor, beta-hydroxy-gamma-N-trimethylamino butyrate, carnitene, carnitine, carnitor, canitor, D-carnitine, D,L-carnitine, LAC, L-acetyl-carnitine, LCLT, L-carnitina, L-carnitine L-tartrate, L-CARNIPURE, levacecarnine, levocarnitine, levocarnitine chloride, LK-80, L-propionylcarnitine, propionil-L-carnitine, propionyl-L-carnitine, VitaCarn, vitamin B(t), vitamin B_t.

BACKGROUND

- The main function of L-carnitine is to transfer long-chain fatty acids in the form of their acyl-carnitine esters across the inner mitochondrial membrane before beta-oxidation. In humans, it is synthesized in the liver, kidney, and brain, and actively transported to other areas of the body. For example, 98% of the total body L-carnitine is confined to the skeletal and cardiac muscle at concentrations approximately 70 times higher than in the blood serum.
- Supplementation may be necessary in rare cases of primary carnitine deficiency, which may be caused by a defect in carnitine biosynthesis, a defect in carnitine active transport into tissue, or a defect in renal (kidney) conservation of carnitine. Known conditions of secondary deficiency of carnitine (insufficiency) in which L-carnitine is effective include chronic stable angina and intermittent claudication characterized by distinct tissue hypoxia (low oxygen levels). Another condition that may benefit from carnitine supplementation is decreased sperm motility.
- Although use in preterm infants suggests carnitine supplementation may aid in maintaining or increasing plasma carnitine levels and possibly weight gain, carnitine is not routinely added to preterm total parenteral nutrition (TPN). However, soy-based infant formulas are fortified with carnitine to levels found in breast milk.
- In 1986, the U.S. Food and Drug Administration (FDA) approved L-carnitine for use in primary carnitine deficiency. D-carnitine or D,L-carnitine may cause secondary L-carnitine deficiency and should not be used.

EVIDENCE

Uses Based on Scientific Evidence	Grade
Nutritional Deficiencies (Primary and Secondary Carnitine Deficiency in Adults) Intravenous (injection) and oral (by mouth) carnitine supplementation is indicated for cases of primary and secondary carnitine deficiency. Use of L-carnitine in primary carnitine deficiency restores plasma carnitine levels to nearly normal levels. Muscle carnitine levels may increase only slightly; however, muscle function can be normalized.	A
Angina (Chronic Stable) Evidence from clinical trials suggests that L-carnitine and L-propionyl-carnitine (propionyl-L-carnitine) are effective in reducing symptoms of angina. Carnitine may not offer further benefit when patients continue conventional therapies. Additional study is needed to confirm these findings.	B
Attention-Deficit/Hyperactivity Disorder (ADHD) Only one study has examined the effects of L-carnitine in boys with ADHD. Although results were promising, additional study is needed before a strong recommendation can be made.	C
AIDS Carnitine may be beneficial in AIDS treatment by increasing proliferation of mononuclear cells and increasing CD4 counts. Additional study is needed to make a firm recommendation.	C
Alcoholism L-Carnitine or acetyl-L-carnitine may be beneficial to alcoholics. Additional study is needed to make a firm recommendation.	C
Alzheimer's Disease Early evidence suggests the effectiveness of L-carnitine or acetyl-L-carnitine for Alzheimer's disease. However, the evidence is mixed.	C
Arrhythmia (Abnormal Heart Rhythms) Although preliminary results are promising, available evidence is insufficient to recommend for or against this use.	C
Cerebral Ischemia (Lack of Adequate Blood Flow to the Brain) A few studies show a positive effect of acetyl-L-carnitine on cerebral blood flow and metabolism of the brain in patients who have had a stroke. Additional study is required before a firm recommendation can be made.	C
Congestive Heart Failure Although preliminary results are promising, available evidence is insufficient to recommend for or against the use of carnitine for congestive heart failure.	C
Dementia (Elderly) Most studies related to dementia have various weaknesses. Although preliminary evidence is promising, available evidence is insufficient to recommend for or against this use.	C
Depression Although preliminary evidence is promising, available evidence is insufficient to recommend for or against the use of carnitine in the treatment of depression.	C

(Continued)

Uses Based on Scientific Evidence	Grade
Diabetes Mellitus It has been suggested that L-carnitine under constant infusion is able to increase insulin sensitivity in patients with type 2 diabetes mellitus and enhance glucose oxidation. Carnitine may also decrease fasting blood glucose and Lp(a). Additional study is needed before a firm recommendation can be made.	C
Diabetic Neuropathy Early evidence suggests that acetyl-L-carnitine may be beneficial for individuals with diabetic neuropathy. Additional study is needed before a firm recommendation can be made.	C
Dialysis (CAPD) L-Carnitine taken by mouth has been used in patients receiving continuous ambulatory peritoneal dialysis (CAPD), but does not seem to lead to the resolution of hypertriglyceridemia. Additional study is needed before a firm recommendation can be made.	C
Dialysis (Hemodialysis) Although preliminary evidence is promising, available evidence is insufficient to recommend for or against the use of carnitine for hemodialysis patients.	C
Diphtheria (Throat Disease) Early studies suggest that carnitine may be beneficial for patients with diphtheria, mainly in terms of myocardial (heart) damage. However, additional study is needed to confirm these findings.	C
Erectile Dysfunction Preliminary studies suggest that propionyl-L-carnitine with acetyl-L-carnitine or sildenafil may be beneficial for patients with erectile dysfunction. However, more rigorous trials should be performed, in order to recommend carnitine for routine use in erectile dysfunction.	C
Exercise Performance Overall, data are mixed in terms of the benefits of L-carnitine for exercise performance. Until confirmed, a strong recommendation for L-carnitine cannot be made for increased exercise endurance.	C
Fatigue There are several promising reports on the use of L-carnitine for fatigue. However, additional study is warranted in this area.	C
Fragile X Syndrome Evidence is insufficient to support the use of carnitine in the treatment of hyperactive behavior of children with fragile X syndrome.	C
Hepatic Encephalopathy (Brain Disease) Preliminary evidence suggests L-carnitine may be beneficial to individuals with hepatic encephalopathy,	C

Uses Based on Scientific Evidence	Grade
in terms of ammonia levels and psychometric functioning. Additional study is needed to make a firm recommendation.	
Huntington's Chorea/Disease One preliminary study showed that L-acetyl-carnitine possesses neither efficacy nor toxicity in patients with Huntington's disease. Further trials are required before a firm recommendation can be made.	C
Hyperlipoproteinemia (High Levels of Lipoprotein and Cholesterol in the Blood) Although preliminary evidence is promising, available evidence is insufficient to recommend for or against the use of carnitine for hyperlipoproteinemia.	C
Hyperthyroidism Although preliminary evidence is promising, available evidence is insufficient to recommend for or against the use of carnitine for hyperthyroidism.	C
Infertility (Asthenospermia) Early evidence shows a positive effect for carnitine or acetyl-L-carnitine or both in terms of increased sperm motility. However, additional study is needed before a firm conclusion can be made.	C
Lactic Acidosis Although early evidence seems promising, currently evidence is insufficient to recommend carnitine in the treatment of lactic acidosis.	C
Liver Disease (Cirrhosis) Although early evidence seems promising, currently evidence is insufficient to recommend carnitine in the treatment of liver cirrhosis.	C
Memory Studies relevant to the use of carnitine for memory are limited. Carnitine does not seem to have any effect on memory. Additional study is needed before a firm recommendation can be made.	C
Myocardial Infarction (Heart Attack) Currently evidence is insufficient to support the use of carnitine for myocardial infarction. Additional study is needed in this area.	C
Nutritional Deficiencies (Adults) Currently evidence is insufficient to support the use of carnitine in TPN for adults. Additional study is needed in this area.	C
Nutritional Deficiencies (Full-Term Infants) Despite a large number of studies, it is not clear what effect, if any, the addition of carnitine has on weight gain in full-term infants. Additional study is needed.	C

Uses Based on Scientific Evidence	Grade
Nutritional Deficiencies (Premature Infants) Despite a large number of studies, it is not clear what effect, if any, the addition of carnitine has on weight gain in premature infants. Additional study is needed.	C
Obesity Early evidence shows that L-carnitine may have no effect on weight loss in obese patients. Further studies are needed before a firm recommendation can be made.	C
Peripheral Neuropathy (Nerve Damage) Currently evidence is insufficient to support the use of carnitine for peripheral neuropathy.	C
Peripheral Vascular Disease Propionyl-L-carnitine and L-carnitine may treat peripheral vascular disease, especially in patients with severe limitations in peripheral circulation. The comparative effectiveness of propionyl-L-carnitine and other recognized treatments is unclear. More study is needed to make a firm recommendation.	C
Peyronie's Disease Although early evidence is promising, more study is needed before a firm recommendation can be made.	C
Pregnancy (Miscarriage) Currently evidence is insufficient to support the use of carnitine for miscarriage.	C
Respiratory Distress (Adults) Currently evidence is insufficient to support the use of carnitine for respiratory distress in adults.	C
Respiratory Distress (Infants) Currently evidence is insufficient to support the use of carnitine for respiratory distress in infants.	C
Rett's Syndrome There are promising results on the use of carnitine for this condition. Before a strong recommendation can be made, however, additional well-designed trials are needed.	C
Sickle Cell Disease Preliminary evidence suggests the absence of any therapeutic effect of propionyl-L-carnitine for sickle cell disease. Additional studies are required before a firm recommendation can be made.	C
Surgical Uses (Bypass) The results of studies on the use of carnitine in improving the functioning of myocardium (heart muscle) during open-heart surgery are controversial. Currently, available evidence is insufficient to recommend for or against the use of carnitine.	C

	Grade
Tuberculosis A preliminary study suggests antibacterial activity may be increased in patients with tuberculosis given acetyl-L-carnitine. Additional study is needed to confirm these findings.	C

Uses Based on Tradition or Theory

Acidosis (acidemia), acne, anorexia, blood circulation, cocaine withdrawal, gonarthrosis (chronic wear of the cartilage in the knee joint), hypertension (high blood pressure), immunomodulator, macular degeneration, metabolic abnormalities (propionate), metabolic disorders (acquired total lipodystrophy), myocarditis/endocarditis (heart infections), neurological disorders (children), retinal protection.

DOSING
Adults (18 Years and Older)

- Various oral doses have been used, with 3 g/day in divided doses for 2-4 months being the most common; however, doses range from 1-9 g/day. Conditions treated with L-carnitine include acquired immunodeficiency syndrome (AIDS), memory in alcoholics, Alzheimer's disease, angina (chest pain), congestive heart failure, depression, diabetes, diabetic neuropathy, dialysis, exercise performance, hepatic encephalopathy (brain disease), hyperlipidemia (high cholesterol), hyperthyroidism, myocardial infarction (heart attack), peripheral neuropathy (nerve damage), and peripheral vascular disease.
- The FDA recommends 1 g of L-carnitine three times per day, intravenously (injected), for primary and secondary carnitine deficiency; this dose should not exceed 3 g/day. Other intravenous (needle into a vein) injections have also been used, with doses typically ranging from 15-50 mg/kg twice daily. Injections have been given for 7 days up to 1 year. Higher doses (9 g/day) have been studied. Injections should be given only under the supervision of a qualified health care professional.

Children (Younger than 18 Years)

- The FDA does not recommend exceeding 3 g carnitine daily for primary and secondary carnitine deficiency. A typical dose for these deficiencies and for Rett's syndrome is 100-200 mg/kg taken daily divided into two or three doses. For hyperlipidemia (high cholesterol), 3 g of L-carnitine for 6 weeks has been used. For TPN in infants, 50 μmol/kg for 2 weeks has been used. Injections should be given only under the supervision of a qualified health care professional.

SAFETY
Allergies

- L-Carnitine should be avoided in individuals with a known allergy or hypersensitivity to carnitine.

Side Effects and Warnings

- In general, L-carnitine is safe, and no significant complications have been reported in available human clinical studies. Minor adverse effects have been reported with the use of L-carnitine or acetyl-L-carnitine, such as skin rash, body odor, "fishy smell," diarrhea, gastric pyrosis (heartburn), nausea, gastralgia (stomachache), loose bowel movement, nonspecific abdominal discomfort, and vomiting. Euphoria, insomnia, nervousness, mania, depression, and aggression have also been reported, but primarily in patients with pre-existing psychiatric conditions.

- Transient hair loss was reported in 1% of cases. Less birth weight was regained in low-birth-weight infants treated with L-carnitine.
- Carnitine supplements should be used cautiously in patients with peripheral vascular disease, patients with hypertension (high blood pressure), patients with alcohol-induced liver cirrhosis, low-birth-weight infants, diabetics, and patients on hemodialysis.

Pregnancy and Breastfeeding

- L-Carnitine is not recommended in pregnant or breastfeeding women due to a lack of available scientific evidence.

INTERACTIONS
Interactions with Drugs

- Several drugs may affect the levels of carnitine in the body. For example, adefovir dipivoxil (Hepsera), which is given for hepatitis B, may reduce free carnitine levels. Cephalosporin antibiotics may reduce plasma carnitine levels. Anticonvulsants (e.g., phenobarbital, phenytoin, carbamazepine) may decrease serum carnitine in children. Cisplatin may increase urinary excretion of carnitine. Ifosfamide (Mitoxana), a chemotherapy drug, may increase urinary loss of carnitine; however, use of carnitine plus ifosfamide may help reduce fatigue (side effect of ifosfamide treatment). Patients with neuropathy (nerve damage) induced by nucleosides may have reduced levels of acetyl-L-carnitine. Penicillin derivatives (e.g., pivaloyloxymethyl esterified, pivampicillin, and pivmecillinam) may increase L-carnitine loss from the body and reduces carnitine in muscle.
- L-Carnitine may decrease the need for certain drugs, such as glycosides, digoxin, diuretics, beta blockers, channel blockers, hypolipidemic (cholesterol-altering) drugs, and nitro derivatives.
- L-Carnitine supplementation may reduce side effects associated with interleukin-2 (IL-2) or nortriptyline (Pamelor, Aventyl). It may also improve liver and muscular side effects associated with isotretinoin (Accutane) in patients with acne. Carnitine may reduce nerve damage symptoms associated with paclitaxel (Taxol) use.
- Carnitine may prevent doxorubicin (Adriamycin)-induced cardiotoxicity.
- L-Carnitine may decrease the need for antiarrhythmics (medications used to treat abnormal rhythms in the heart).

Carnitine plus propafenone may improve arrhythmia (heart rhythm) better than propafenone alone.

- L-Carnitine may decrease the need for anticoagulants ("blood thinners") such as warfarin (Coumadin) or heparin.
- Several combinations have shown positive interactions. For example, Sildenafil and propionyl-L-carnitine may be more effective than sildenafil alone. Although not well studied in humans, L-carnitine used concurrently with antiviral agents such as zidovudin (Retrovir) or carnitine used with nortriptyline may also have a positive interaction that reduces side effects. The combination L-carnitine plus acetyl-L-carnitine plus cinnoxicam has been found more effective in improving sperm parameters compared with L-carnitine plus acetyl-L-carnitine alone.
- Patients with diabetes should use caution because L-carnitine may decrease blood glucose. However, carnitine levels did not change in diabetics using insulin or sulfonylurea therapy. It is unclear whether L-carnitine would have similar effects when combined with other medications that reduce blood glucose. A qualified health care professional, including a pharmacist, should be consulted before combining therapies.
- Although not well studied in humans, carnitine may increase valproic acid concentrations in the brain, which might increase the effects of valproic acid. Caution is advised.

Interactions with Herbs and Dietary Supplements

- L-Carnitine may decrease the need for herbs or supplements with anticoagulant effects ("blood thinners"). L-carnitine may also decrease the need for herbs or supplements with diuretic effects. Dosing adjustments may be necessary.
- Patients with diabetes should use caution because L-carnitine may decrease blood glucose. However, carnitine levels did not change in diabetics using insulin or sulfonylurea therapy. It is unclear whether L-carnitine would have similar effects when combined with other herbs and supplements that reduce blood glucose. A qualified health care professional, including a pharmacist, should be consulted before combining therapies.
- Choline supplementation may reduce excretion, renal (kidney) clearance, and fractional clearance of nonesterified carnitine.
- L-Carnitine chloride and potassium chloride may minimize rhabdomyolysis, a side effect of taking licorice by mouth.

For a complete list of references, please visit www.naturalstandard.com.

Acidophilus
(Lactobacillus acidophilus)

RELATED TERMS

- Acidophilus, Acidophilus Extra Strength, acidophilus milk, Actimel, Bacid, Cultura, DDS-Acidophilus, Endolac, Enpac, Fermalac (Canadian), Florajen, fresh poi, Gynoflor, Infloran, Kala, Kyo-Dophilus, L-92, *Lactobacillus acidophilus, Lactobacillus acidophilus* OLL2769, *Lactobacillus acidophilus* milk, *Lactobacillus acidophilus* yogurt, Lacteol Fort, lactic acid–producing bacteria (LAB), Lactinex, Lactobacillaceae (family), lactobacilli, lactobacillus, *Lactobacillus acidophilus* 145, *Lactobacillus acidophilus* DDS-1, *Lactobacillus acidophilus* LA 02, *Lactobacillus acidophilus* La5, *Lactobacillus acidophilus* L-92, *Lactobacillus acidophilus* NCFM, *Lactobacillus acidophilus* NCK56, *Lactobacillus acidophilus* strain 27L, *Lactobacillus acidophilus* strain LB (LaLB), Lacto Bacillus, MoreDophilus, Narine, poi, Probiata, Pro-Bionate, probiotic, sour poi, Superdophilus, yogurt.

BACKGROUND

- Lactobacilli are bacteria that normally live in the human small intestine and vagina. *Lactobacillus acidophilus* is generally considered to be beneficial because it produces vitamin K; lactase; and antimicrobial substances such as acidolin, acidolphilin, lactocidin, and bacteriocin. Multiple human trials report benefits of *Lactobacillus acidophilus* for bacterial vaginosis. Other medicinal uses of *Lactobacillus acidophilus* are not sufficiently studied to form clear conclusions.
- The term *probiotic* is used to describe organisms that are used medicinally, including bacteria such as *Lactobacillus acidophilus* and yeast such as *Saccharomyces boulardii*.
- Although generally believed to be safe with few side effects, oral *Lactobacillus acidophilus* should be avoided in people with intestinal damage, a weakened immune system, or with overgrowth of intestinal bacteria.

EVIDENCE

Uses Based on Scientific Evidence	Grade
Bacterial Vaginosis Multiple human studies report that *Lactobacillus acidophilus* vaginal suppositories are effective in the treatment of bacterial vaginosis. A few studies suggest that eating yogurt enriched with *Lactobacillus acidophilus* may be similarly beneficial. Additional research is necessary before a firm conclusion can be reached. Patients with persistent vaginal discomfort are advised to seek medical attention.	B
Allergy Treatment (Japanese Cedar Pollen) A small study was conducted to evaluate the effects of *Lactobacillus acidophilus* strain L-92 on the symptoms of Japanese cedarpollen allergy with positive results. Further research is needed before a decision can be made.	C
Asthma There is limited research in this area, with unclear results.	C
Diarrhea Prevention A small amount of human research suggests that *Lactobacillus acidophilus* may not be effective when used to prevent diarrhea in travelers or in people taking antibiotics. Several studies report that the related species *Lactobacillus* GG may be helpful for the prevention of diarrhea in children and travelers. Additional study is needed in these areas before a firm conclusion can be drawn.	C
Diarrhea Treatment (Children) A small amount of research in children, using different forms of acidophilus, reports no improvement in diarrhea. Future studies should use a viable *Lactobacillus acidophilus* culture to assess effects on diarrhea. *Lactobacillus* GG, a different species, is suggested by multiple human studies to be a safe and effective treatment for diarrhea in otherwise healthy infants and children. *Lactobacillus acidophilus* may aid in the management of chronic or persistent diarrhea and bacterial overgrowth–related diarrhea. Further research is needed to determine what dose may be safe and effective.	C
Hepatic Encephalopathy (Confused Thinking Due to Liver Disorders) There is limited study in this area, with mixed results.	C
High Cholesterol There is conflicting information from several human studies regarding the effects of *Lactobacillus acidophilus*–enriched dairy products on lowering blood levels of total cholesterol or low-density lipoprotein ("bad cholesterol").	C
Irritable Bowel Syndrome Human studies report mixed results in the improvement of bowel symptoms after taking *Lactobacillus acidophilus* by mouth.	C
Lactose Intolerance There is conflicting information from several human studies as to whether using *Lactobacillus acidophilus* by mouth improves digestion of lactose. More research is needed in this area before a conclusion can be drawn.	C
Necrotizing Enterocolitis Prevention in Infants One human study using *Lactobacillus acidophilus* in combination with another bacterium (*Bifidobacterium infantis*) in infants reported fewer cases of necrotizing enterocolitis (severe inflammation of the gut) and no complications related to treatment. Additional research is necessary in this area before a conclusion can be drawn.	C

(Continued)

Uses Based on Scientific Evidence	Grade
Vaginal Candidiasis (Yeast Infection) *Lactobacillus acidophilus* taken by mouth or as a vaginal suppository has not been adequately assessed for the prevention or treatment of vaginal yeast infections. More research is needed in this area before a conclusion can be drawn.	C

Uses Based on Tradition or Theory

Acne, acquired immunodeficiency syndrome (AIDS), cancer, canker sores, colitis, colon cancer prevention, constipation, diaper rash, Crohn's disease, diverticulitis, *Escherichia coli* infection in cancer patients, fever blisters, heart disease, heartburn, hives, immune enhancer, indigestion, infection, overgrowth of bacteria in the small bowel, preoperative prevention of infections or gut bacteria loss, stomach ulcer, thrush, ulcerative colitis, urinary tract infection.

DOSING
Adults (18 Years and Older)

- **Tablets/capsules/liquid/yogurt:** Expert opinion suggests that a dose between 1 and 10 billion viable (live) *Lactobacillus acidophilus* bacteria taken daily in divided doses is sufficient for most people. Higher doses may cause mild abdominal discomfort, and smaller doses may not be able to establish a stable population in the gut. For vaginal bacterial infections, a dose that has been used is 8 oz of yogurt containing *Lactobacillus acidophilus* in a concentration of 100 million colony-forming units (10^8 CFU) in each milliliter. Capsules containing 1.5 g of *Lactobacillus acidophilus* were used in one study.
- **Vaginal suppository:** One to two tablets of 10^7-10^9 CFU per tablet (Gynoflor or Vivag), inserted intravaginally once or twice daily up to three months.
- **Rectal suppository:** Capsules containing 1.5 g of *Lactobacillus acidophilus* have been used to treat diarrhea.

Children (Younger than 18 Years)

- **Tablets/capsules/liquid:** Some natural medicine textbooks and experts suggest that one quarter teaspoon or one quarter capsule of commercially available *Lactobacillus acidophilus* may be safe for use in children for the replacement of gut bacteria destroyed by antibiotics. Up to 12 billion lyophilized heat-killed *Lactobacillus acidophilus* has been given every 12 hours for 5 days. It is often recommended that *Lactobacillus acidophilus* supplements be taken 2 hours after antibiotic doses because antibiotics may kill *Lactobacillus acidophilus* if taken at the same time. A qualified health care practitioner should be consulted before using *Lactobacillus acidophilus* in children, and it should be used cautiously in children younger than 3 years.
- **Applied to the skin:** Liquid preparations have been used on the diaper area to treat yeast infections, although safety and effectiveness are not well studied. A qualified health care practitioner should be consulted before using *Lactobacillus acidophilus* in children, and it should be used cautiously in children younger than 3 years.

SAFETY
Allergies

- Lactose-sensitive people may develop abdominal discomfort from dairy products containing *Lactobacillus acidophilus*.

Side Effects and Warnings

- Studies report few side effects from *Lactobacillus acidophilus* when used at recommended doses. The most common complaint is abdominal discomfort or gas, which usually resolves with continued use. Some experts recommend limiting the daily dose of living *Lactobacillus acidophilus* organisms to reduce the risk of abdominal discomfort. Some women have reported burning of the vagina after using *Lactobacillus acidophilus* vaginal tablets.
- There are rare reports of infections of heart valves with *Lactobacillus acidophilus*, and the risk may be greater in people with artificial heart valves. People with severely weakened immune systems (as a result of disease or drugs such as cancer chemotherapy and organ transplant immunosuppressants) may develop serious infections or bacteria in the blood from taking *Lactobacillus acidophilus*. Therefore, *Lactobacillus acidophilus* should be avoided in such individuals. People with intestinal damage or recent bowel surgery should avoid taking lactobacilli.

Pregnancy and Breastfeeding

- There is not enough scientific study available to establish safety during pregnancy. Therefore, pregnant women should use *Lactobacillus acidophilus* cautiously and under medical supervision, if at all. A small number of pregnant women have taken part in studies investigating *Lactobacillus acidophilus* vaginal tablets and a culture of *Lactobacillus acidophilus* with no negative effects reported. Further research is necessary.

INTERACTIONS
Interactions with Drugs

- Some experts believe that *Lactobacillus acidophilus* taken by mouth should be used 2-3 hours after antibiotic doses, to prevent killing the *Lactobacillus acidophilus*. It has also been suggested that lactobacilli are damaged by alcohol and should not be taken at the same time. Scientific research is limited in these areas.
- In theory, *Lactobacillus acidophilus* taken by mouth might not survive the acidic environment of the stomach. Some experts have suggested that antacids should be taken 30-60 minutes before taking lactobacilli. However, this has not been well studied in humans.
- In theory, *Lactobacillus acidophilus* may prolong the effects on some drugs, including birth control pills or benzodiazepines such as diazepam (Valium). Based on laboratory experiments, *Lactobacillus acidophilus* may reduce the effectiveness of sulfasalazine (Azulfidine), a drug used for inflammatory bowel disease.

Interactions with Herbs and Dietary Supplements

- Fructo-oligosaccharides (FOS, also called "prebiotics") are nondigestible sugar chains that are nutrients for lactobacilli. Some experts believe that FOS, taken by mouth, may help the growth of lactobacilli. Natural food sources of FOS include banana, Jerusalem artichoke, onion, asparagus, and garlic.
- *Lactobacillus casei, Saccharomyces boulardii,* or other probiotics may add to the effects of *Lactobacillus acidophilus*.

For a complete list of references, please visit www.naturalstandard.com.

RELATED TERMS

- Achee, ackee apple, akee, akee apple, ankye, arilli, *Blighia sapida*, *Cupania sapida*, *Blighia sapida*, hypoglycin A, hypoglycin B, ishin, Sapindaceae (soapberry family), vegetable brain, vegetable brains.

BACKGROUND

- Ackee (*Blighia sapida*) is the national fruit of Jamaica and grows in clusters on evergreen trees. Hypoglycin A (the causative toxic substance in ackee) is contained in the aril, seeds, and husks of ackee fruit, at various stages of ripeness.
- The ingestion of unripe ackee for the purpose of medicinal or nutritional purposes can give rise to acute poisoning called "Jamaican vomiting sickness" or toxic hypoglycemic syndrome. Adverse effects include loss of muscle tone, vomiting, convulsions, coma, and death. Deaths have occurred after unintentional poisoning with ackee; most of these deaths have occurred in small children 2-6 years old. The fruit may be eaten only when it ripens and opens naturally on the tree; however, the membrane at the base should be removed.
- Various parts of the ackee tree have been used medicinally to expel parasites and to treat dysentery (severe diarrhea), ophthalmic conjunctivitis (eye inflammation), and headache. More research is needed to make a recommendation of the therapeutic benefits of ackee.
- Because of its toxicity, the importation of this fruit into the United States is forbidden by the U.S. Food and Drug Administration (FDA).

EVIDENCE

Uses Based on Scientific Evidence

No available studies qualify for inclusion in the evidence table.

Uses Based on Tradition or Theory

Conjunctivitis (eye inflammation), digestive disorders, dysentery (severe diarrhea), epilepsy, food flavoring, food uses, headache, pain relief, stimulant, ulcers, yellow fever.

DOSING

Adults (18 Years and Older)

- Safety, efficacy, and dosing have not been systematically studied in adults.

Children (Younger than 18 Years)

- Safety, efficacy, and dosing have not been systematically studied in children.

SAFETY

Allergies

- Individuals with a known allergy or hypersensitivity to ackee (*Blighia sapida*), its constituents, or other members of the Sapindaceae family should not take ackee.
- There have been reports of anaphylaxis reactions to ackee fruit.

Side Effects and Warnings

- Ackee is likely safe when tree-ripened fruit is consumed as a food. Individuals should be cautious, however, when consuming imported canned products. There have been numerous cases of toxic levels of hypoglycin detected in cans containing ackee fruit that were imported to the United States. Eating unripe or overripe fruit is not recommended because of potential toxicity.
- Ingestion of unripe ackee fruit may cause abdominal pain, intermittent diarrhea, hypotonia (decreased muscle tone), weakness, nausea, vomiting, stupor, hemorrhages (bleeding), confusion, headache, convulsions, tachypnea (rapid breathing), tachycardia (fast heartbeat), and intense itching.
- Multiple cases of "Jamaican vomiting sickness," also known as toxic hypoglycemic syndrome (lowered blood glucose levels in the body), have been reported after the ingestion of unripe ackee fruit. Unripe ackee fruit may also be toxic to the brain, kidneys, and liver. Coma and death have occurred.
- Unripe ackee arillus (oil) may decrease the number of neutrophils in the blood and increase platelets.
- Cholestatic jaundice, steatosis (fatty liver), vomiting, and abdominal pain have been noted with chronic ackee fruit ingestion.
- Use cautiously in patients with diabetes, liver disease, or compromised kidney function.

Pregnancy and Breastfeeding

- Ackee is not recommended in pregnant or breastfeeding women due to a lack of available scientific evidence.

INTERACTIONS

Interactions with Drugs

- Ackee may lower blood glucose levels. Caution is advised when using medications that may also lower blood glucose. Patients taking drugs for diabetes by mouth or insulin should be monitored closely by a qualified health care professional, including a pharmacist. Medication adjustments may be necessary.

Interactions with Herbs and Dietary Supplements

- Ackee may lower blood glucose levels. Caution is advised when using herbs or supplements that may also lower blood glucose.

For a complete list of references, please visit www.naturalstandard.com.

Aconite
(Aconitum napellus)

RELATED TERMS

- Acetylbenzoylaconin, aconite root, aconiti frus, Aconiti Herba, aconiti lateralis preparata, aconiti tuber, aconitine, aconitknollen, aconito, *Aconitum angustius, Aconitum anthoroideum, Aconitumartemisiifolium, Aconitum austroyunnanense, Aconitum balfourii, Aconitum barbatum, Aconitumbrachypodum, Aconitum brunneum, Aconitum carmichaelii, Aconitum chasmanthum, Aconitumchilienshanicum, Aconitum columbianum, Aconitum coreanum, Aconitum episcopale, Aconitumferox, Aconitum flavum, Aconitum gymnandrum, Aconitum hemsleyanum, Aconitum japonicum, Aconitum karakolicum, Aconitum kongboense, Aconitum kusnezoffii, Aconitum longilobum, Aconitum moldavicum, Aconitum nagarum, Aconitum napellus, Aconitum naviculare, Aconitum ouvrardianum, Aconitum paniculigerum, Aconitum pendulum, Aconitum polyschistum, Aconitum pomeense, Aconitum pterocaule, Aconitum racemulosum, Aconitum richardsonianum, Aconitum rotundifolium, Aconitum scaposum, Aconitum sczukinii, Aconitum sessiliflorum, Aconitum sinomantanum* Nakai, *Aconitum soongaricum, Aconitum spicatum, Aconitum stylosum, Aconitum sungpanense, Aconitum taipeicum, Aconitum tanguticum, Aconitum transectum, Aconitum uncinatum, Aconitum vilmorinianum, Aconitum vulparia*, autumn monkshood, bachnag, bear's foot, bikh, bikhroot, bish, bishma, blauer eisenhut, blue monkshood, blue monkshood herb, blue monkshood root, blue rocket, brute killer, bushi, cao wu (Chinese), chan-wu (Chinese), ch'uan wu (Chinese), cuanwu (Chinese), dudhia bish (Indian), eisenhutknollen (German), friar's cap, friar's cowl, fuchswurz (German), futzu (Chinese), fu zi (Chinese), garden monkshood, garden wolfsbane (German), giftwurzel (German), helmet flower, higenamine, house bane, hsüeh shang i chih hao (Chinese), Indian aconite, kako-bushi (Japanese), kuan pai fu (Chinese), lang tu (Chinese), leopard killer, mithazahar (Indian), moenchswurz (German), monkshood, monkshood herb, monkshood root, monkshood tuber, monnikskap, monsebane, mouse-bane, mousebane, old wife's hood, pao-fuzi (Japanese), racine d'aconit (French), soldier's cap, storkjelm (German), sturmhutknollen (German), teufelswurz (German), Turk's cap, ts'ao wu (Chinese), venusvogn (Danish), visha, wolfbane, wolf's bane, wolfsbane, wolfshbone, wolfswurzel (German), wu hui (Chinese), wu t'ou (Chinese).

BACKGROUND

- The word *Aconitum* comes from "akone," meaning "rocky," which is the type of area where the aconite plant grows. Cured aconite preparations have a long history of use in Chinese medicine. Processed aconite was used to treat heart failure and other heart diseases. However, aconite has been repeatedly associated with cardiovascular (heart) adverse events. For this reason, the German Commission E does not recommend its use.
- Aconite is well known for its extreme toxicity. The tuberous root is used in traditional medicine, although all parts of the plant are considered to be toxic. Aconite also has an almost worldwide historical usage as an arrow poison and as a poison in executions, homicides, and suicides. Aconite is also said to be an ingredient of "flying ointments" used by witches to imitate the sensation of flying.
- Aconite has been used in very low doses to treat neuralgia (nerve pain), sciatica, and rheumatism. Aconite is also an ingredient in homeopathic preparations used for cold and flu symptoms, heart palpitations with anxiety, acute inflammatory illness, and peripheral nerve pain. Overall, the efficacy has not been established.

EVIDENCE

Uses Based on Scientific Evidence	Grade
Arrhythmia (Abnormal Heart Rhythms) Toxic effects associated with aconitine (a poisonous alkaloid and the active principle of aconite) limit its ability to be used to treat bradycardia (slow heartbeat). Additional study is needed in this area to make a strong recommendation.	C
Heart Failure Toxic effects associated with aconite limit its ability to be used to treat heart failure, including renocardiovascular disease and left ventricular function. Further study is needed to confirm these results.	C
Postoperative Pain (in Infants) Data on the use of aconite or any of its derivatives in treating pain are limited. Homeopathic aconite may help relieve postoperative agitation, but further information is needed to confirm these results.	C

Uses Based on Tradition or Theory

Abortifacient (induces abortion), agitated behavior, analgesia (pain reliever), antibacterial, antifungal, anxiety, arthritis, ascites (fluid in the abdomen), asthma, blindness (amaurosis, transient monocular blindness), bronchitis, bruises, cancer, catalepsy (trancelike state), central nervous system depressant (large doses), central nervous system stimulant, chickenpox, cholera, chronic low back pain, common cold, convulsions, cough, croup, cystitis (bladder infection), dandruff, dengue ("break bone fever"), depression, diabetes mellitus, diarrhea, dysentery (severe diarrhea), eclampsia (pregnancy-induced high blood pressure), enlarged glands, esophagitis (inflamed esophagus), fever, fractures, glossitis (inflamed tongue), gonorrhea (sexually transmitted disease), gout (inflamed foot), hair loss, headache, heart disorders, hemorrhage (purpura), hemorrhoids, hepatitis, Hodgkin's disease, hypertension (high blood pressure), hypocalcemic tetany, immunodeficiency, inflammation (pleurodynia), inflammatory conditions (of the mouth and pharyngeal area), influenza, insomnia, intermittent claudication (pain or fatigue in arms and legs owing to poor supply of oxygen to the muscles), joint pain, laryngitis, lice, malaise, mania, measles, meningitis, menstrual disorders, migraine, miscarriages, mumps, musculoskeletal disorders, myalgia (muscle pain), neck stiffness, nephritis (inflamed kidneys), neuralgia (nerve pain),

Uses Based on Tradition or Theory—Cont'd

neurological disorders, ophthalmological (eye) disorders, otitis media (middle ear infection), pain, paralysis, peripheral neuropathy pain, peritonitis (infection of abdominal cavity), pertussis (whooping cough), phlegmasia alba dolens (milk leg syndrome), pleurisy (inflamed lungs), pneumonia, polydipsia (excessive thirst), prolapsed uterus, rash (heat), respiratory disease, rheumatoid arthritis, roseola (viral illness), scarlet fever, sciatica, scirrhus (hard tumor), seizure disorder (epilepsy), septicemia (blood poisoning), skin pigmentation disorders (chronic exanthemas), sleep disorders, smell disorders, spine problems (myelitis), stroke, sweating, teething, testicular damage, tetanus, tonsillitis, toothache, trigeminal neuralgia (nerve pain), tuberculosis, urinary retention, vertigo, yellow fever.

DOSING
Adults (18 Years and Older)
- There is no proven safe or effective dose for aconite. Topical (application on the skin) use is not recommended. Aconite is sometimes used in liniments (rubifacients) with belladonna. Historically, a 1.3% aconitine topical liniment has been used.
- Taking 1-5 drops of a tincture of the fresh leaf by mouth four times a day to relieve pain has been used. Also, homeopathic preparations of 6-30 c have been used. A 6 c potency strength is made by diluting 1 part of aconite tincture to 99 parts of alcohol or water, then the solution is taken and diluted again with 99 parts of alcohol or water. This process is repeated six additional times, resulting in a 6 c potency.

Children (Younger than 18 Years)
- There is no proven safe or effective dose for aconite, and use in children is not recommended. Homeopathic aconite has been studied in infants to help relieve postoperative agitation, but further information is needed to confirm these results.

SAFETY
Allergies
- Aconite is highly toxic and is not safe for human consumption.

Side Effects and Warnings
- Based on widespread use, many experts believe aconite to be unsafe even in recommended amounts in otherwise healthy individuals. Aconite is not recommended for children because of known toxic effects; however, a homeopathic preparation containing aconite has been studied in infants with no toxicity reported.
- Severe poisoning has been reported after ingestion of aconitine (found in aconite) or processed and cured aconite. Aconite is not approved by the German Commission E for use in any patients. The American Herbal Product Association rated aconite a class 3 (to be used only under the supervision of an expert qualified in the appropriate use of this substance).
- Aconite may cause hypotension (low blood pressure), irregular pulse, various arrhythmias (altered heartbeats), or first-degree heart block. Aconite poisoning can cause prolonged repolarization of the myocardium, which leads to triggered automaticity and ventricular tachyarrhythmias including ventricular ectopy, ventricular tachycardia (fast

heartbeat), and ventricular fibrillation. Aconite has also been reported to cause nausea; vomiting; epigastric pain; diarrhea; muscle cramps; retrosternal discomfort; dizziness; vertigo; variations in motor and sensory skills of limbs; ataxia (loss of coordination); paresthesia (altered sensation); "stiffness" in face, trunk, and limbs; clonic convulsions; coma; leukocytosis (elevated white blood cell count); dimness of vision; blackouts; blurred or double vision; agitation; hyperventilation; difficulty breathing; and respiratory depression.
- In theory, aconite may cause liver or kidney damage, hypersalivation, throat constriction, hypokalemia (low potassium in the blood), and hypothermia (low body temperature).
- Tingling and numbness have occurred when aconite is applied to the skin (topically).
- Aconite may lower blood glucose levels. Caution is advised in patients with diabetes or hypoglycemia, and in those taking drugs, herbs, or supplements that affect blood glucose. Serum glucose levels may need to be monitored by a health care provider, and medication adjustments may be necessary.
- Aconite is contraindicated in patients with coronary disease, cardiac dysfunction, and arrhythmias or hemodynamic instability. Use cautiously in patients with suicidal tendencies due to the abuse potential associated with aconite. Avoid aconite in patients younger than 18 years due to a lack of research in this patient population. Avoid aconite use in patients with gastrointestinal disorders, stomach ulcers, duodenal ulcers, reflux esophagitis, ulcerative colitis, spastic colitis, and diverticulosis.

Pregnancy and Breastfeeding
- The use of aconite during pregnancy or breastfeeding should be avoided because it is known to be toxic even at therapeutic doses. Studies suggest it is unsafe when used orally (taken by mouth) or topically (applied to the skin) in pregnant women.

INTERACTIONS
Interactions with Drugs
- Aconite activates sodium channels in the cardiac muscle. Theoretically, aconite may alter or interfere with the effects of antiarrhythmic drugs.
- Aconitine, a constituent of aconite, may lower blood glucose levels. Caution is warranted, as concurrent use with antidiabetic agents can increase the risk of hypoglycemic effects. Patients taking drugs for diabetes by mouth or insulin should be monitored closely by a qualified health care provider. Medication adjustments may be necessary.
- Aconitine, a constituent of aconite, may lower blood pressure. Caution is warranted, as concurrent use with antihypertensive agents can increase the risk of hypotension. Caution is also advised with diuretic agents (medications that increase urine flow) due to increased risk of additive effects and electrolyte imbalances.
- Theoretically, digoxin may interfere with aconitine effects on the heart. Combined use of these medications could be extremely dangerous and result in additive effects of both agents. A qualified health care professional, including a pharmacist, should be consulted.

Interactions with Herbs and Dietary Supplements
- Aconitine, a constituent of aconite, may lower blood pressure. Caution is warranted, as concurrent use with

antihypertensive herbs/supplements can increase the risk of hypotension. Caution is also advised with diuretic herbs/supplements (medications that increase urine flow) due to increased risk of additive effects and electrolyte imbalances.

- Aconitine, a constituent of aconite, may lower blood glucose levels. Caution is warranted, as concurrent use with hypoglycemic herbs/supplements can increase the risk of hypoglycemic effects. Patients taking herbs/supplements for diabetes by mouth or insulin should be monitored closely by a qualified health care provider. Medication adjustments may be necessary.

- Theoretically, digoxin-like herbs or supplements (foxglove, Siberian ginseng) may interfere with aconite effects on the heart, producing an unknown and potentially dangerous effect. A qualified health care professional, including a pharmacist, should be consulted before combining therapies.

For a complete list of references, please visit www.naturalstandard.com.

S-Adenosyl methionine (SAMe)
($C_{15}H_{22}N_6O_5S^+$)

RELATED TERMS

- Ademetionin, ademetionine, adenosylmethionine, Ade-SD4, AdoMet, Geptral (Russian), Gumbaral (German), Heptral (Russian), S-adenosylmethionine, SAM-e, Sammy, Samyr (Italian), sulfoadenosilmethionina (Italian), sulfo-adenosil-L-metionina (Spanish), sulfo-adenosyl-L-methionine sulfate-p-toluenesulfonate (stable salt form), sulfo-adenosyl-methionine.

BACKGROUND

- SAMe was first discovered in 1953 by a researcher named Cantoni. It is formed in the body from methionine and adenosine triphosphate in a reaction catalyzed by methionine adenosyltransferase. SAMe functions as a primary methyl group donor in a variety of reactions in the body. After donating a methyl group, SAMe is converted to S-adenosyl-homocysteine.
- SAMe is used for psychiatric illnesses, infertility, liver concerns, premenstrual disorders, and musculoskeletal disorders, among others.
- SAMe has been studied extensively in the treatment of osteoarthritis and depression. Many trials provide evidence that SAMe reduces the pain associated with osteoarthritis and is well tolerated in this patient population. Some evidence is available for the use of SAMe for intrahepatic cholestasis of pregnancy, although additional study is needed in this area. Antiinflammatory and analgesic (pain-relieving) activity has also been attributed to SAMe.
- Future well-designed clinical trials are required in the areas of depression, fibromyalgia, and liver cholestasis before a strong recommendation can be made in these areas.

EVIDENCE

Uses Based on Scientific Evidence	Grade
Osteoarthritis SAMe has been studied extensively in the treatment of osteoarthritis. SAMe reduces the pain associated with osteoarthritis and is well-tolerated in this patient population. Although an optimal dose has yet to be determined, SAMe appears as effective as the nonsteroidal antiinflammatory drugs (NSAIDs).	B
Attention Deficit Hyperactivity Disorder (ADHD) Preliminary evidence from an open trial suggests that SAMe may be of benefit for adults with ADHD. However, the evidence thus far is insufficient to recommend this use.	C
Cholestasis (Pregnancy) Currently, there is insufficient available evidence to recommend for or against the use of SAMe for cholestasis (build up of bile in the liver) in pregnant women. It is important to note that there is no information on the use of SAMe before the third trimester.	C
Cholestasis (Nonpregnant) SAMe may be beneficial for pruritus (severe itching) and serum bilirubin levels associated with nonpregnancy cholestasis. However, the evidence thus far has not been conclusive.	C
Depression SAMe has been studied for use in depression for many decades; however, currently available trials are inconclusive.	C
Fibromyalgia Because fibromyalgia is characterized by chronic pain and depressive symptoms, there is an increased interest in studying SAMe for this indication. Current available evidence, however, does not appear to show any benefit of SAMe over placebo in reducing the number of tender points and in alleviating depression.	C
Liver Disease (General) Preliminary evidence suggests that SAMe may normalize levels of liver enzymes in individuals with liver disease.	C

Uses Based on Tradition or Theory

Acetaminophen metabolism (hepatic cirrhosis), adjustment disorder, aging, alcoholism, Alzheimer's disease, anxiety, bilirubin and porphyrin metabolism disorders, bursitis, cirrhosis (primary biliary), dementia, bipolar disorder, drug/toxin-induced hepatotoxicity (liver damage), gastritis (hemorrhagic), Gilbert's syndrome, heart disease, hepatitis, high cholesterol levels, infertility, intrahepatic cholestasis (oral contraceptive–induced), intrahepatic cholestasis (total parenteral nutrition–induced), ischemic stroke, lead toxicity, male sterility, migraine, multiple sclerosis, pancreatitis, myelopathy (spinal cord injury), Parkinson's disease, postconcussive syndrome, postpartum depression, premenstrual syndrome, premenstrual dysphoric disorder, psychiatric illness, rheumatoid arthritis, seizures, Sjögren's syndrome, systemic sclerosis, tendonitis.

DOSING
Adults (18 Years and Older)

- Both oral (taken by mouth) and intravenous (injection) preparations of SAMe have been studied in clinical trials with some evidence of benefit for certain conditions. SAMe appears effective for osteoarthritis, and 600-1200 mg has been taken daily in one to three divided doses for 10-84 days. Up to 1600 mg has been taken for up to 2 weeks for the treatment of cholestasis. For depression, 800-1600 mg daily was the most commonly used dosage range in clinical studies, for up to 6 weeks. For fibromyalgia, 400 mg twice daily has been used. For intrahepatic cholestasis of pregnancy, 500 mg given twice daily has been used. For general liver disease, 600-1200 mg daily has also been used.

- As an injection into the muscle, the most common dose of SAMe is 200-400 mg for 2-4 weeks. Both S-adenosyl-L-methionine 1,4-butanedisulfonate stable salt and disulfate-p-toluenesulfonate stable salt have been studied as injections. In addition, 500 mg SAMe twice daily has been delivered in a slow-running infusion for 12 days followed by oral administration of 500 mg twice daily. Injections should be given only under the supervision of a qualified health care professional, including a pharmacist.

Children (Younger than 18 Years)

- There is insufficient evidence to recommend a dose for SAMe in children.

SAFETY

Allergies

- Avoid in individuals with a known allergy or hypersensitivity to S-adenosyl-L-methionine. Flushing, erythema (reddening of the skin), palpitations, dizziness, and nausea (symptoms of an anaphylactic reaction) have been reported.

Side Effects and Warnings

- SAMe has been well-tolerated in the majority of clinical trials conducted. The most common adverse effects reported are gastrointestinal in nature with nausea being the most frequently reported. Skin rashes have also been reported. Anxiety and hypomania have been reported mainly in trials that have included patients with bipolar disorder. The use of SAMe has not been adequately studied in the pediatric and elderly population, in pregnancy other than the third trimester, or during breastfeeding.
- When given as an injection, diluted SAMe has caused superficial phlebitis (inflammation of a vein) and tachycardia (increased heart rate), increased perspiration, transient pain at the injection site, arm soreness, flushing, erythema (reddening of the skin), palpitations, dizziness, nausea, pruritus (itching), urticaria ("hives"), and epigastric pain.
- SAMe may lower blood sugar levels. Caution is advised in patients with diabetes or hypoglycemia and in those taking drugs, herbs, or supplements that affect blood sugar. Serum glucose levels may need to be monitored by a qualified health care professional, including a pharmacist, and medication adjustments may be necessary.

- When taken by mouth or by injection, SAMe may cause a hot sensation, itchiness of the ear, nausea, vomiting, dry mouth, heartburn, blood in the stool, anorexia, mild diarrhea, stomachaches, slight constipation, increased thirst, increased salivation, urinary frequency, intolerable bowel symptoms, gas, and decreased appetite. Anxiety, insomnia, hypomania, hostility, insomnia, elevated mood, psychoactivation, headache, suicidal ideation, hyperactivity, a reduced need for sleep, and bursts of energy have also been reported.

Pregnancy and Breastfeeding

- SAMe crosses the placenta. SAMe is not recommended in the first trimester or during breastfeeding because of a lack of available scientific evidence. However, SAMe has been used in the third trimester for the treatment of intrahepatic cholestasis with no reported adverse effects in the pregnant women or their newborn babies. A single study of SAMe included women in their second trimester with no adverse effects noted. Use cautiously in women in their third trimester of pregnancy; SAMe should be used in pregnancy only if the benefits clearly outweigh the risks.

INTERACTIONS

Interactions with Drugs

- SAMe may lower blood sugar levels. Caution is advised when medications that may also lower blood sugar are used. Patients taking drugs for diabetes by mouth or using insulin should be monitored closely by a qualified health care professional, including a pharmacist. Medication adjustments may be necessary.
- Use cautiously in patients using tricyclic antidepressant drugs, such as clomipramine. Combination of SAMe and tricyclic antidepressant drugs may increase the likelihood of adverse effects.

Interactions with Herbs and Dietary Supplements

- SAMe may lower blood sugar levels. Caution is advised when herbs or supplements that may also lower blood sugar are used. Blood glucose levels may require monitoring, and doses may need adjustment.

For a complete list of references, please visit www.naturalstandard.com.

Adrenal Extract

RELATED TERMS

- ACE, Adrena Support, adrenal, adrenal complex, adrenal concentrate, adrenal cortex extract, adrenal factors, adrenal substance, glandular, protomorphogen (adrenal), suprarenal extract, whole adrenal extract.

BACKGROUND

- Adrenal extracts are derived from the adrenal glands of cows, pigs, or sheep gathered from slaughterhouses. The adrenal glands, which are above the kidneys, secrete adrenal hormones. The adrenal medulla secretes epinephrine (adrenaline) and norepinephrine (noradrenaline); the adrenal cortex secretes a group of hormones called corticosteroids.
- Adrenal extracts have been used medicinally since 1931, primarily in the injectable form. Today, adrenal extract is available only in the form of capsules or tablets. Commercially available adrenal extracts are made from the whole gland (whole or total adrenal extracts) or just from the outer part of the gland (adrenal cortex extracts). Although adrenal extract has been used to treat fatigue and low adrenal function, currently no human trials of adrenal extract have been performed to support these claims.

EVIDENCE

Uses Based on Scientific Evidence

No available studies qualify for inclusion in the evidence table.

Uses Based on Tradition or Theory

Adrenal insufficiency, alcohol withdrawal, allergies, asthma, autoimmune disorders, blood disorders, bone healing, burns, cholesterol, colds, coughs, depression, drug withdrawal, dyspepsia, eczema, enlarged glands (status thymicolymphaticus), exhaustion, fatigue, fibromyalgia, high blood potassium level, hypoglycemia (low blood glucose), hypotension (low blood pressure), immune enhancement, infections, inflammation, long-term debility, miscarriage (prevention), psoriasis, purification procedure for chromogranin A, rheumatoid arthritis, spermatogenesis, stress (physical or emotional), ulcerative colitis.

DOSING

Adults (18 Years and Older)

- There is insufficient evidence to recommend a dose for adrenal extract in adults. Commercially available adrenal extracts are made from the whole gland (whole or total adrenal extracts) or just from the outer part of the gland (adrenal cortex extracts).

Children (Younger than 18 Years)

- There is insufficient evidence to recommend a dose for adrenal extract in children.

SAFETY

Allergies

- Use of adrenal extract should be avoided in individuals with a known allergy or hypersensitivity to adrenal extract.

Side Effects and Warnings

- When adrenal extract is taken by mouth, no adverse reactions have been reported. However, adrenal extracts are derived from raw cow, pig, or sheep adrenal glands, so there is concern about contamination with diseased animal parts. To date, no reports of disease transmission to humans due to use of contaminated adrenal extracts have been documented. Bovine spongiform encephalitis (BSE) has been reported in some countries, and adrenal extract products should be avoided in these areas.
- Adrenal extract is likely unsafe when used parenterally. Use of injectable adrenal extract has been associated with serious bacterial infections and abscesses at injection sites, when contaminated with diseased animal parts. In 1996, the U.S. Food and Drug Administration (FDA) issued a nationwide alert regarding an injectable adrenal cortex extract after more than 50 cases of serious bacterial infections were reported.
- Adrenal extract should be avoided in immunocompromised patients. Theoretically, adrenal extracts may increase the risk of infection because the extracts might harbor pathogens. Injectable adrenal extract reportedly caused serious infections.

Pregnancy and Breastfeeding

- Adrenal extract is not recommended in pregnant or breastfeeding women due to a lack of available scientific evidence.

INTERACTIONS

Interactions with Drugs

- Insufficient available evidence.

Interactions with Herbs and Dietary Supplements

- In theory, taking hypophysis extract with adrenal extract (cortine) may augment the preputial glands.
- Adrenal extract might affect mineral metabolism.

For a complete list of references, please visit www.naturalstandard.com.

African Wild Potato

RELATED TERMS

- African potato, Afrika patat, agglutinins, aglucones, bantu tulip, beta-sitosterin, beta-sitosterol, diglucuronide, disulfate, glucuronide-sulfate conjugates, glycosides, Hypoxis, *Hypoxis colchicifolia, Hypoxis hemerocallidea, Hypoxis hemerocallidea corm, Hypoxis latifolia, Hypoxis rooperi, Hypoxis roperi*, hypoxoside, lectin-like proteins, norlignans picea, phytosterols, pinus, rooperol analogues, sitoserin, South African star grass, star grass, sterretjie.

BACKGROUND

- The African wild potato is native to South Africa. It is a bitter plant used for a wide variety of conditions including diabetes mellitus, hemorrhage, and prostate problems.
- Traditional healers have used the African wild potato tea for its medicinal properties. In southern Mozambique, the tea was widely used during the Civil War (1976-1992) by soldiers and civilians who lost blood through injuries. It is said to quickly replace the loss of blood. The tea is also used in conjunction with other plants to combat "bad blood" in patients with diabetes mellitus.
- The Shangaan used African wild potato in a mixture with other plants for endometriosis and premenstrual syndrome (PMS). The rootstock was one of the ingredients of an infusion taken as an "internal parasiticide" and purgative. The Manyika used the rootstock for medicinal and ceremonial purposes. The Karanga used the rootstock as a remedy for vomiting, loss of appetite, abdominal pains, and fevers. It was also used to treat delirium.
- African wild potato may boost immune function, based on indirect evidence that sterols and sterolins in *Hypoxis* root have the potential to enhance immunity. Some believe its nutrient values are 50,000 times greater than modern vegetables. Today, sterols and sterolins are still sought after and are preferred immune system boosters.

EVIDENCE

Uses Based on Scientific Evidence	Grade
Benign Prostatic Hyperplasia African wild potato may be a potentially effective treatment option for benign prostatic hyperplasia. Additional study is needed to make a firm recom-mendation.	C

Uses Based on Tradition or Theory
Abdominal pain, arthritis, bladder disorders, cancer, chronic fatigue syndrome, convulsions, coronary disease, cystitis (inflammation of the bladder), delirium, diabetes, endometriosis, epilepsy, fevers, hemorrhage, high cholesterol, HIV/AIDS, immune enhancement, inflammation, insecticide, loss of appetite, lung cancer, lung disease, lupus erythematosus, multiple sclerosis, premenstrual syndrome (PMS), pesticide, prostate cancer, psoriasis (skin disease), rheumatoid arthritis, tuberculosis, urinary disorders, viral infections, vomiting, wound healing.

DOSING

Adults (18 Years and Older)

- For benign prostatic hyperplasia, 60-130 mg of beta-sitosterol divided into two to three doses daily has been taken by mouth. For lung cancer, 1200-3200 mg of standardized *Hypoxis* plant extract (200-mg capsules) per day divided into three doses has been taken by mouth. African wild potato has also been taken as a tumoricidal agent in a dose of 2400 mg daily (12 × 200-mg capsules), although safety and effectiveness have not been proven.

Children (Younger than 18 Years)

- There is insufficient evidence to recommend a dose for adrenal extract in children.

SAFETY

Allergies

- African wild potato should be avoided in individuals with a known allergy or hypersensitivity to African wild potato. Allergy to the plant may manifest as a skin rash.

Side Effects and Warnings

- African wild potato is likely safe when consumed as a source of vitamins and nutrients such as phytosterols, as well as a tea. However, African wild potato is possibly unsafe when used by patients with diabetes, liver disorders, and autoimmune diseases, and during concurrent use with cytochrome P450 substrates.
- Adverse effects may cause gastrointestinal adverse effects including mild abdominal cramps, nausea, vomiting, and diarrhea. It may also lower blood glucose levels. Caution is advised in patients with diabetes or those taking drugs, herbs, or supplements that affect blood glucose. Blood glucose levels should be monitored and medication adjustments may be necessary.
- When taken by mouth, beta-sitosterol, a constituent of African wild potato, has been associated with erectile dysfunction and loss of libido. In theory, African wild potato aqueous extract may impair kidney function, reduce urine output, and reduce potassium and sodium excretion. It should be used cautiously in patients with impaired kidney function.

Pregnancy and Breastfeeding

- African wild potato is not recommended in pregnant and breastfeeding women due to a lack of available scientific evidence.

INTERACTIONS

Interactions with Drugs

- African wild potato may lower blood glucose levels. Caution is advised in patients who have diabetes or who are using medications that may lower blood glucose. Patients should be monitored closely by a qualified health care provider. Medication adjustments may be necessary.

- African wild potato may inhibit the P-glycoprotein. Patients taking antiretroviral agents should consult with a qualified health care professional, including a pharmacist. Combined use may put patients at risk of treatment failure, viral resistance, or drug toxicity.
- African wild potato extracts may alter the effects of CYP450 and P-glycoprotein substrates. Caution is warranted, as drug levels may be altered.
- Aqueous extracts of African wild potato may impair kidney function. African wild potato should be used cautiously in patients taking nephrotoxic (kidney-damaging) drugs.
- Aqueous extracts of African wild potato may reduce urination and excretion of potassium and sodium. African wild potato should be used cautiously in patients taking drugs that increase urine flow (diuretics).
- Aqueous extracts of African wild potato may reduce urination and excretion of potassium and sodium. Caution is advised when combining with other herbs and supplements that increase urine flow (diuretics).

Interactions with Herbs and Dietary Supplements

- African wild potato extracts may alter the effects of CYP450 and P-glycoprotein substrates. Caution is warranted, as herb/supplement levels may be altered.
- African wild potato may lower blood glucose levels. Caution is advised in patients who have diabetes or who are using herbs/supplements that may lower blood glucose. Patients should be monitored closely by a qualified health care provider. Medication adjustments may be necessary.
- Patients taking antiretroviral agents should consult with a qualified health care professional, including a pharmacist. Combined use may put patients at risk of treatment failure, viral resistance, or drug toxicity.
- Aqueous extracts of African wild potato may reduce urination and excretion of potassium and sodium. Caution is advised when combining with other herbs and supplements that increase urine flow (diuretics).

For a complete list of references, please visit www.naturalstandard.com.

Agaric

RELATED TERMS

- AA, Agaricaceae, Agaricales, agaric acid, agaric fungus, Agaric aux mouches (French), agaricinic acid, *Agaric basidiomycete*, Amanitaceae, *Amanita flavivolvata, Amanita formosa*, Amanita matamoscas (Spanish), *Amanita muscaria, Amanita pantherina, Amanita regalis, Amanita virosa*, Amanitaceae, Amanite tue-mouche (French), basidiomycete agaric, bitter fungus, brown fly agaric, *Clitocybula dusenii, Coprinus cinereus, Cortinarius orellanus* Fr., *Crepidotus fulvotomentosus*, ectomycorrhizal fungi, falsa oronja (Spanish), fausse oronge (French), Fliegenpilz (German), fly agaric, *Hebeloma cylindrosporum, Hypholomafasciculare* Fries, ibotenic acid, laricic, magic mushrooms, muchomor czerwony (Polish), muscarine, muscazone, muscimol, ovulo malefico (Italian), pantherina poisoning, Roter fliegenpilz (German), selenium, Soma, toadstool, tufted agaric, uovolaccio (Italian), white agaric (*Fomes officinalis* Neum.).

BACKGROUND

- Fly agaric, or Amanita muscaria, is a basidiomycete mushroom that produces hallucinogenic effects (although not a true hallucinogen). Fly agaric contains isoxazole compounds (e.g., ibotenic acid, muscimol, muscazone, muscarine) that are responsible for the psychotropic effects. Toxic effects occur about 30-90 minutes after consumption of the fungi and primarily cause euphoria, special distortion, increased sensitivity to visual and auditory stimuli, mydriasis, anxiety, drowsiness, confusion, mania, and illusions. Death, although rare, can result.
- Fully grown, the cap is usually around 12 cm in diameter (up to 30 cm) with a distinctive blood-red color (crimson, fading to yellow with age), scattered with white-to-yellow, removable flecks (warts). It is often referred to as fly agaric because of use in Europe as an insecticide and its ability to stun or kill flies.
- Agaric has traditionally been used in rituals as a hallucinogen. Religious and ceremonial usage of agaric has been documented in Buddhist, Native American, Japanese, Siberian, ancient Greek, and proto-Hindi texts. Gathering and consuming mushrooms and other plants containing psychoactive substances have become increasingly popular among some people experimenting with drugs.
- Agaric is considered poisonous, although rarely fatal. Several studies document the toxicity and neurological effects of taking agaric by mouth. No formal trials regarding agaric toxicity or therapeutic benefit are currently available.
- Note: Not to be confused with *Agaricus* mushroom.

EVIDENCE

Uses Based on Scientific Evidence

No available studies qualify for inclusion in the evidence table.

Uses Based on Tradition or Theory

Antipyretic (fever reducer), hallucinogenic, insecticide, sweating, tuberculosis (intestinal).

DOSING

Adults (18 Years and Older)

- Safety, efficacy, and dosing have not been systematically studied. However, due to adverse effects, use in adults is not recommended.

Children (Younger than 18 Years)

- Safety, efficacy, and dosing have not been systematically studied. However, due to adverse effects, use in children is not recommended.

SAFETY

Allergies

- Agaric should be avoided in individuals with a known allergy or hypersensitivity to basidiomycetes.

Side Effects and Warnings

- Fly agaric should not be ingested due to risk of toxicity. Taking agaric may cause visual and auditory hallucinations that appear after 30-90 minutes and peak within 3 hours, with certain effects lasting for up to 10 hours. The effect per volume consumed is highly variable, and individuals can react quite differently to the same dose.
- In a moderate dose, agaric acid may have no effect on the central nervous system (CNS) except to paralyze the nerves of the sweat glands. In higher doses, CNS dysfunction has occurred. Agaric may cause alternating CNS depression and stimulation. Symptoms usually begin with drowsiness followed by a state of confusion, with ataxia (loss of coordination), dizziness, and euphoria resembling alcohol intoxication, and may proceed to increased activity, illusions, or manic excitement. These periods of excitement may alternate with periods of somnolence, deep sleep, or stupor.
- Given in large doses, fly agaric first increases and then decreases blood pressure. An increase in respiratory rate, followed by a decrease, has also been noted. Skin may be warm and flushed. Fly agaric toxicity is characterized by nausea, heavy vomiting, and severe diarrhea. In near-fatal doses, *Amanita muscarina* causes swollen features, rage, and madness, characterized by bouts of mania, followed by periods of hallucination.
- Theoretically, airborne agaric may cause chronic sinusitis (inflammation of the sinuses) or other respiratory conditions.
- Liver damage, liver failure, and death have occurred in people taking related mushroom species, such as *Amanita phalloides* (death cap) or *Amanita virosa* (deadly agaric). There are no available reports of liver damage from *Amanita muscarina*.

Pregnancy and Breastfeeding

- Agaric is not recommended for pregnant or lactating women because of potential adverse effects.

INTERACTIONS

Interactions with Drugs

- Based on reported adverse effects of agaric, significant interactions may occur. Patients taking any medications should consult with a qualified health care professional, including a pharmacist.

- Agaric may cause changes in blood pressure. Patients using blood pressure–lowering medications should consult with a qualified health care professional, including a pharmacist.

Interactions with Herbs and Dietary Supplements

- Based on reported adverse effects of agaric, significant interactions may occur. Patients taking herbs and supplements should consult with a qualified health care professional, including a pharmacist.
- Agaric is abundant in selenium and may have additive effects when taken with other herbs and supplements that contain selenium. Caution is advised.

For a complete list of references, please visit www.naturalstandard.com.

Agave
(Agave americana)

RELATED TERMS

- Agavaceae, American aloe, Arizona agave, Arizona century plant, bald agave, blue agave, cantala, century plant, Chisos agave, Chisos mountain century plant, coastal agave, corita, cow's horn agave, desert agave, desert century plant, dragon tree agave, drunkard agave, dwarf century plant, dwarf octopus agave, eggers' century plant, false sisal, foxtail agave, golden flowered agave, golden flower century plant, hardy century plant, Havard's century plant, henequen, hohokam agave, ixtle de jaumave, leather agave, lecheguilla, little princess agave, maguey, Maguey bandeado, Maguey chato, Maguey del Bravo, Maguey de Desierto, Maguey de Havard, Maguey de la India, Maguey de montana, Maguey de pastizal, Maguey de Sisal, Maguey de tlalcoyote, Maguey diente de tiburn, Maguey Henequen, Maguey lechuguilla, Maguey liso, Maguey mezortillo, Maguey pajarito, Maguey primavera, Maguey spero, Maguey sbari, McKelvey agave, McKelvey's century plant, mescal ceniza, mescalito, Mexican sisal, Mezcal azul tequilero, Mezcal yapavai, Murphey agave, Murphey's century plant, Octopus Agave, palmer agave, palmer century plant, palmer's century plant, Parry agave, Parry's agave, Puerto Rico century plant, pulque, Queen Victoria's Agave, Rough century plant, smallflower agave, smallflower century plant, Schott agave, Schott's century plant, sisal, sisal hemp, shindagger, smooth agave, squid agave, St. Croix agave, slimfoot century plant, swan's neck agave, tequila, tequila agave, thorncrest century plant, thread-leaf agave, Toumey agave, Toumey's century plant, Utah agave, Weber agave, Weber blue agave, Weber's century plant, wild century plant.

BACKGROUND

- Agaves are succulent plants from the family Agavaceae, which includes *Beschorneria, Furcraea, Hesperaloe, Manfreda, Polianthes, Prochnyanthes,* and *Yucca.* Agave plants are common in the American southwest, Mexico, central and tropical South America, the Mediterranean, and some parts of India. There are more than 200 known species of agave; many produce musky odors that attract bats, which serve to pollinate them, whereas others produce sweet odors to attract insects.
- *Agave americana* is also known as the American aloe, although it is not related to the true aloes. The leaves of the agave plant yield fibers suitable for textile production. The native people in Mexico used the agave spikes to make pens, nails, and needles. *Agave sisalana,* the source of sisal fiber, is cultivated in plantations in Africa and Asia. The flowering stem can be dried or roasted and eaten; the seeds can be ground into flour to make bread or used as a thickener for soups. A sweet liquid (sap) called agua miel (honey water) gathers in the plant if the stem is cut before flowering. This sap is collected over a period of about 2 months and can then be fermented to produce the alcoholic beverage pulque (octili), which Native Americans use in religious ceremonies. Further distillation creates Mescal (mezcal). A form of tequila is made when Mescal is produced from the blue agave (*Agave tequilana*) plant within the Tequila region of Mexico. This is the most important economic use of agave, worth millions of dollars to the Mexican economy. Mescal is often sold with the caterpillar of the agave moth in the bottle.
- Agave is also useful as a sugar alternative because with 90% fructose, it has a low glycemic index. Steroid hormone precursors are obtained from the leaves. Pulque prepared from *Agave* species was a food item studied intensively for nutrition potential among traditional and indigenous peoples and is an example of how local food-based strategies can be used to ensure micronutrient nutrition. Traditional food strategies could be used not only for alleviating malnutrition, but also for developing locally relevant programs for stemming the nutrition transition and preventing chronic disease, particularly among indigenous and traditional peoples who retain knowledge of using food species in their local ecosystems.

EVIDENCE

Uses Based on Scientific Evidence

No available studies qualify for inclusion in the evidence table.

Uses Based on Tradition or Theory

Antibacterial, bruises, constipation, diabetes, diuretic, dysentery, flatulence (gas), hair-restorer, hemolytic activities, indigestion, insulin resistance, jaundice, laxative, nutritional supplement, parasites, steroid source, swelling, syndrome X.

DOSING
Adults (18 Years and Older)

- There is no proven safe or effective dose for agave in adults.

Children (Younger than 18 Years)

- There is no proven safe or effective dose for agave in children.

SAFETY
Allergies

- Avoid use in patients who have allergies to plants in the Agavaceae family. In rare cases, contact dermatitis after exposure to the sap of *Agave americana* has been reported.
- Significant increases in homocysteine levels and a tendency to increase blood glucose concentration and to decrease insulin sensitivity were found in healthy, nonobese young men who consumed tequila agave daily.

Side Effects and Warnings

- The stiff, erect leaves of some agave plants are tipped with sharp needles, which can cause injury on contact. Multiple reports of skin rash from *Agave americana* exist.

- Vascular damage from crystals in agave has been reported. There are reports of irritant contact dermatitis from *Agave americana* when used incorrectly as a hair-restorer.
- Pulque consumption may be associated with liver disease (cirrhosis) and increased death rate.
- Some constituents of *Agave sisalana* have high hemolytic activity and may be potentially toxic.
- Calcium oxalate crystals, found in prickly pear and agave, may have caused microwear of human teeth.
- Significant increases in homocysteine levels and a tendency to increase blood glucose concentration and to decrease insulin sensitivity were found in healthy, nonobese young men who consumed tequila daily.

Pregnancy and Breastfeeding

- Women from rural areas of the central plateau of Mexico drink a mild alcoholic beverage called pulque to stimulate breast milk flow (as a galactogogue). The relatively small amount of ethanol taken in by infants through milk is unlikely to have harmful effects. However, pulque intake during breastfeeding may have adverse influences on postnatal growth in some Mexican populations.
- Anordin and dinordin, prepared with steroids derived from the sisal plants *Agave sisalana* and *Agave americana*, have been used for their antifertility effects. These agents, whose antifertility properties have been confirmed by scientists in Sweden and the United States, constitute a potential new family of contraceptives promising the advantage of having to be taken only once or twice a month instead of the 20 times per month necessary with the ordinary oral contraceptive pill.

INTERACTIONS
Interactions with Drugs

- Steroid hormone precursors are obtained from agave leaves. Caution is advised when taking agave with other steroidal agents.
- Contraceptive and antifertility effects have been reported with the use of agave. In theory, caution is advised when taking agave with other contraceptive agents, such as birth control pills.
- Agave may alter blood glucose levels. Caution is advised in patients with diabetes and in those taking drugs that affect blood glucose. Serum glucose levels may need to be monitored by a qualified health care professional, including a pharmacist, and medication adjustments may be necessary.

Interactions with Herbs and Dietary Supplements

- Steroid hormone precursors are obtained from agave leaves. Caution is advised when taking agave with other herbs with steroidal properties.
- Agave may alter blood glucose levels. Caution is advised in patients with diabetes and in those taking herbs or supplements that affect blood glucose. Patients taking drugs for diabetes by mouth or insulin should be monitored closely by a qualified health care professional, including a pharmacist. Medication adjustments may be necessary.

For a complete list of references, please visit www. naturalstandard.com.

Agrimony
(*Agrimonia eupatoria, Agrimonia procera*)

RELATED TERMS

- Agrimonia, *Agrimonia asiatica, Agrimonia eupatoria* L., *Agrimonia parviflora, Agrimonia pilosa* Ledeb, *Agrimonia striata, Agrimonia procera,* Ackerkraut, Agrimoniae herba, agrimony, Agrimony eupatoria, Church Steeples, cockeburr, cocklebur, common agrimony, fragrant agrimony, Funffing, Funffingerkraut, Herba eupatoriae, herbe d'aigremoine, herbe de saint-guillaume, liverwort, longyacao, odermenning, philanthropos, Potentilla, roadside rosaceae, sticklewort, stickwort, woodland groovebur.
- **Note:** Other plants that are not related botanically to agrimony are given a similar name by older herbalists because of similarities in properties. These include the common hemp agrimony (common Dutch agrimony, *Eupatorium aquaticum mas, Eupatorium cannabinum*) and the water agrimony (bastard agrimony, bastard hemp, *Bidens tripartita,* trifid bur-marigold).

BACKGROUND

- The name *agrimonia* may have its origin in the Greek word *agremone,* which refers to plants that supposedly healed cataracts of the eye. The species name *eupatoria* relates to Mithradates Eupator, King of Pontus, who is credited with introducing many herbal remedies. *The Doctrine of Signatures,* developed in Europe in the 16th and 17th centuries, has listed agrimony as 1 of the 23 substances with medicinal uses, bearing witness to the extent of its influence at the time.
- Germany's Commission E has approved the use of agrimony (when prepared as a tea) for controlling diarrhea and as a throat gargle to reduce inflammation and relieve sore throat pain (cooled tea).
- Agrimony was one of the most famous vulnerary (healing) herbs with anti-inflammatory and diuretic properties. The tannin content is responsible for many of its medicinal uses. The dried leaves can be used to make tea for drinking or as a throat gargle. Preliminary studies suggest that agrimony may be useful against certain bacterial and viral infections, for inhibition of tumor growth, for diabetes, and for hypertension (high blood pressure). Available clinical trials looked at its use in treating certain skin and gastrointestinal disorders. More human studies are needed to confirm these and other reported uses for agrimony.

EVIDENCE

Uses Based on Scientific Evidence	Grade
Cutaneous Disorders Many skin conditions, wounds, and bruises have been treated with agrimony. Additional study is needed in this area to make a strong recommendation.	C
Gastrointestinal Disorders Agrimony has been used for many gastrointestinal conditions, such as appendicitis, mild diarrhea, stimulation of appetite, and ulcers. Additional human study is needed to make a firm recommendation.	C

Uses Based on Tradition or Theory

Anemia (red blood cell deficiency), antihistamine, antitumor agent, antiviral, appendicitis, appetite stimulant, astringent, bleeding, corns, cardiotonic (restores heart strength), diabetes (high blood glucose), diarrhea (mild and acute), diuretic, enlargement of the heart, exudative atopic dermatitis, fevers, gallbladder disorders, gargle, gout (foot inflammation), indigestion, jaundice and other liver complaints, kidney and bladder disorders, pimples, rheumatism, skin conditions such as blotches and scrofulous sores, sedative, sore throat, taeniasis (parasitic disease), tonic, ulcers, upper respiratory tract astringent, tuberculosis, upset stomach, warts.

DOSING
Adults (18 Years and Older)

- There is no proven safe or effective dose for agrimony. Agrimony has traditionally been given as a tea, tincture, infusion, or extract. Examples of traditional doses that have been used include 1-3 mL of liquid extract (1:1 in 25% alcohol) per day, 2-4 g of dried herb infusion three times per day, and 1-4 mL of tincture (1:5 in 45% alcohol) three times daily.
- When applied on the skin, a poultice has been applied several times daily using approximately 10% water extract, which is prepared by boiling agrimony at low heat for 10-20 minutes.

Children (Younger than 18 Years)

- There is insufficient evidence to recommend a dose for agrimony in children.

SAFETY
Allergies

- Use of agrimony should be avoided in individuals with a known allergy or hypersensitivity to agrimony.

Side Effects and Warnings

- Agrimony is likely safe because its leaves are used as a substitute for tea. It is also likely safe when applied on the skin. No significant adverse effects for agrimony have been documented. When used as recommended for a short time, agrimony is considered to be safe.
- Agrimony is listed by the Council of Europe as a natural source of food flavoring. This use is possibly safe because agrimony can be added to foodstuffs in small quantities with a possible limitation of an active principle (not yet specified) in the final product.
- Agrimony is possibly unsafe when used orally (by mouth) or topically (applied on the skin) in excessive amounts because of its high tannin content. In theory, agrimony may cause photodermatitis, low blood pressure, and nausea.
- The high amount of tannins (up to 21%) in agrimony may lead to gastrointestinal upset, hepatic necrosis (death of liver cells), nephrotoxicity (damage to the kidneys), or increased risk of developing esophageal (of the esophagus) cancer with long-term use. Use of agrimony should be

avoided in patients with diarrhea caused by an underlying disease. Agrimony should be used only for mild and acute diarrhea. Patients who tend to develop constipation easily should also avoid agrimony.

- Isocoumarins have been found in the roots of agrimony; there may be an increased risk for bleeding. Caution is advised in patients with bleeding disorders or taking agents that may increase the risk of bleeding. Dosing adjustments may be necessary.

Pregnancy and Breastfeeding

- Oral use of agrimony should be avoided during pregnancy due to its effects on the menstrual cycle. The effects in breastfeeding are not well understood.

INTERACTIONS

Interactions with Drugs

- Because of isocoumarins found in the roots of agrimony, agrimony may increase the risk of bleeding when taken with drugs that increase the risk of bleeding. Examples include aspirin, anticoagulants ("blood thinners") such as warfarin (Coumadin) or heparin, antiplatelet drugs such as clopidogrel (Plavix), and nonsteroidal anti-inflammatory drugs such as ibuprofen (Motrin, Advil) or naproxen (Naprosyn, Aleve).
- Agrimony may lower blood glucose levels. Caution is advised in patients who have diabetes or who are using medications that may lower blood glucose. Patients should be monitored closely by a qualified health care provider. Medication adjustments may be necessary.
- Agrimony may lower blood pressure. The hypotensive (blood pressure–lowering) effect possibly may be additive with drugs used to treat hypertension (high blood pressure). Excessive doses of agrimony might cause hypotension, interfering with therapy for hypertension or hypotension.

- Agrimony may contain estrogenic constituents. Caution is warranted in patients using estrogens, hormone replacement therapy, or birth control pills.
- Because agrimony contains up to 21% tannins, chronic ingestion may result in nephrotoxicity (damage to the kidneys). Agrimony should not be used with other nephrotoxic agents.

Interactions with Herbs and Dietary Supplements

- Because of isocoumarins found in the roots of agrimony, agrimony possibly may increase the risk of bleeding when taken with herbs and supplements that are believed to increase the risk of bleeding. Multiple cases of bleeding have been reported with the use of *Ginkgo biloba,* and fewer cases have been reported with garlic and saw palmetto. Numerous other agents may theoretically increase the risk of bleeding, although this has not been proven in most cases.
- Agrimony may lower blood glucose levels. Caution is advised in patients who have diabetes or who are using medications that may also lower blood glucose. Patients should be monitored closely by a qualified health care provider. Medication adjustments may be necessary.
- Agrimony may lower blood pressure. The hypotensive (blood pressure–lowering) effect possibly may be additive with drugs used to treat hypertension (high blood pressure). Excessive doses of agrimony might cause hypotension, interfering with therapy for hypertension or hypotension.
- Agrimony may contain estrogenic constituents. Caution is warranted in patients using phytoestrogens.
- Because agrimony contains up to 21% tannins, chronic ingestion may result in nephrotoxicity (damage to the kidneys). Agrimony should not be used with other nephrotoxic agents.

For a complete list of references, please visit www. naturalstandard.com.

Alfalfa
(Medicago sativa)

RELATED TERMS

- Al-fac-facah, alfalfa weevil, arc, buffalo herb, California clover, Chilean clover, Fabaceae (family), feuille de luzerne (French), isoflavone, jatt, kaba yonca, Leguminosae (family), lucerne, medicago, mielga, mu su, phytoestrogen, purple medic, purple medick, purple medicle, sai pi li ka, saranac, Spanish clover, team, weevelchek, yonja.

BACKGROUND

- Alfalfa is a legume that has a long history of dietary and medicinal uses. A few animal and preliminary human studies report that alfalfa supplements may lower cholesterol and glucose. However, most research has not been well-designed. Therefore, there is not enough reliable evidence available to form clear conclusions in these areas.
- Alfalfa supplements taken by mouth seem to be generally well tolerated. However, ingestion of alfalfa tablets has been associated with reports of a lupus-like syndrome or lupus flares. These reactions may be due to the amino acid L-canavanine, which appears to be present in alfalfa seeds and sprouts, but not in the leaves. There are also rare cases of pancytopenia (low blood counts), dermatitis (skin inflammation), and gastrointestinal upset.

EVIDENCE

Uses Based on Scientific Evidence	Grade
Atherosclerosis (Cholesterol Plaques in Heart Arteries) Several studies in animals report reductions in cholesterol plaques of the arteries after use of alfalfa. Well-designed research in humans is necessary before a firm conclusion can be drawn.	C
Diabetes A few animal studies report reductions in blood glucose levels after ingestion of alfalfa. Human data are limited, and it remains unclear if alfalfa can aid in the control of glucose levels in patients with diabetes or hyperglycemia.	C
High Cholesterol Reductions in blood levels of total cholesterol and low-density lipoprotein ("bad cholesterol") have been reported in animal studies and in a few human cases. High-density lipoprotein ("good cholesterol") has not been altered in these cases. Although this evidence is promising, better research is needed before a firm conclusion can be reached.	C

Uses Based on Tradition or Theory
Allergies, antifungal, antimicrobial, antioxidant, appetite stimulant, asthma, bladder disorders, blood-clotting disorders, boils, breast cancer, cervical cancer, cough, diuresis (increased urination), estrogen replacement, gastrointestinal tract disorders, gum healing after dental procedures, increasing breast milk, indigestion, inflammation, insect bites, jaundice, kidney disorders, menopausal symptoms, nutritional support, peptic ulcer disease, prostate disorders, radiotherapy-induced skin damage, rheumatoid arthritis, scurvy, skin damage from radiation, stomach ulcers, thrombocytopenic purpura, uterine stimulant, vitamin supplementation (vitamins A, C, E, K), wound healing.

DOSING

Adults (18 Years and Older)

- A dose of 5-10 g of dried herb three times daily has been taken by mouth.
- Two tablets (1 g each) of Cholestaid (esterin processed alfalfa) three times daily, then 1 tablet three times daily, by mouth, has been recommended by the manufacturer.
- A dose of 5-10 mL (1-2 teaspoonfuls) of a 1:1 solution in 25% alcohol three times daily by mouth has been taken.
- For treating high cholesterol, 40 g of heated seeds prepared three times daily by mouth with food has been taken.

Children (Younger than 18 Years)

- There is insufficient evidence to recommend a dose for alfalfa in children.

SAFETY

Allergies

- Alfalfa should be avoided in people with allergies to members of the Fabaceae or Leguminosae plant families. Caution is warranted in individuals with grass allergies.

Side Effects and Warnings

- Alfalfa seems to be well tolerated by most individuals, although rare serious adverse effects have been reported.
- Mild gastrointestinal symptoms may occur, such as stomach discomfort, diarrhea, gas, or larger or more frequent stools. Dermatitis (skin inflammation or redness) has been reported and may be due to alfalfa allergy.
- Alfalfa may reduce blood glucose levels. Caution is warranted in patients who have diabetes or who are using drugs, herbs, or supplements that may alter glucose levels. Blood glucose levels should be monitored and medication adjustments may be necessary.
- Lupus-like effects have been associated with alfalfa use, including antinuclear antibodies in the blood, muscle pains, fatigue, abnormal immune system function, and kidney abnormalities. Therefore, people with a history of systemic lupus erythematosus or a family history of lupus should avoid alfalfa supplements.
- Rarely, alfalfa may cause abnormal blood cell counts (pancytopenia) and lowered potassium levels (hypokalemia), increased thyroid hormone levels, gout flares, and estrogen-like effects.
- Contamination of alfalfa products with potentially dangerous bacteria (including *Escherichia coli*, 0157:H7 *Salmonella*, and *Listeria monocytogenes*) has been reported. In one case report, vomiting occurring after the consumption of seaweed

and organic alfalfa was attributed to contamination of the capsules with high amounts of entospore-forming and *Streptomyces*-like bacteria. Copper, arsenic, and antimony have been found in alfalfa plants.

- Many tinctures and liquid extracts contain high levels of alcohol and should be avoided when driving or operating heavy machinery.

Pregnancy and Breastfeeding

- Alfalfa supplements are not recommended during pregnancy due to possible estrogenic effects. Anecdotally, alfalfa may increase the risk of birth defects and spontaneous abortion. Amounts found in food are generally believed to be safe. Traditionally, alfalfa is believed to stimulate breast milk production, although this has not been well studied.
- Tinctures and liquid extracts may contain high levels of alcohol and should be avoided during pregnancy.

INTERACTIONS

Interactions with Drugs

- Blood glucose levels may be reduced. Caution is advised in patients with diabetes or hypoglycemia and in those taking drugs that affect blood glucose. Serum glucose levels may need to be monitored by a health care provider, and medication adjustments may be necessary.
- Alfalfa contains vitamin K and therefore may reduce the "blood-thinning" effects of the drug warfarin (Coumadin). Alfalfa may add to the effects of cholesterol-lowering medications such as atorvastatin (Lipitor) or simvastatin (Zocor).
- Alfalfa may increase the risk of sun sensitivity. Concurrent use of alfalfa with other photosensitizing agents (e.g., chlorpromazine) may increase the risk of sun-damaging effects.
- Alfalfa contains estrogen-like components. Alfafla may cause additive effects when used with other estrogens, hormone replacement therapy, or contraceptives.
- Alfalfa may increase thyroid hormone levels. Alfalfa may alter the effects of thyroid hormones.
- Alfalfa is used as a source of various minerals, including calcium, potassium, phosphorus, and iron. Concurrent use with these agents may affect levels of calcium, potassium, phosphorus, and iron in the body.

- Many tinctures and liquid extracts contain high levels of alcohol and may cause nausea or vomiting when taken with metronidazole (Flagyl) or disulfiram (Antabuse).
- Alfalfa may have immune-stimulating effects. Theoretically, alfalfa may alter or interfere with the effects of immunosuppressants.
- Alfalfa may lower cholesterol levels. The use of alfalfa with cholesterol-lowering agents may have additive effects

Interactions with Herbs and Dietary Supplements

- Blood glucose levels may be reduced. Caution is advised in patients with diabetes or hypoglycemia, and in those taking herbs or supplements that affect blood glucose. Serum glucose levels may need to be monitored by a health care provider, and medication adjustments may be necessary.
- Alfalfa may lower cholesterol levels. The use of alfalfa with cholesterol-lowering agents may have additive effects.
- Alfalfa has been reported to contain vitamin K and may reduce the effects of herbs and supplements that have blood-thinning effects that rely on depletion of vitamin K.
- Alfalfa contains estrogen-like components. Alfalfa may cause additive effects when used with other phytoestrogens (e.g., black cohosh).
- Alfalfa may increase thyroid hormone levels. Alfalfa may alter the effects of thyroid herbs/supplements (e.g. bladderwrack).
- Alfalfa is used as a source of various minerals, including calcium, potassium, phosphorus, and iron. Concurrent use with these agents may affect levels of calcium, potassium, phosphorus, and iron in the body. Alfalfa may also contain significant levels of zinc, copper, manganese, and selenium. Concurrent use with these supplements may cause additive effects and increase levels.
- Alfalfa may have immune-stimulating effects. Theoretically, alfalfa may alter or interfere with the effects of immunosuppressants.
- Alfalfa may increase the risk of sun sensitivity. Concurrent use of alfalfa with other photosensitizing agents may increase the risk of sun-damaging effects.

For a complete list of references, please visit www. naturalstandard.com.

Algin

RELATED TERMS

- Alginates, alginic acid, *Ascophyllum nodosum*, Fermion gas, *Laminaria digitata*, Lessoniaceae (family), *Macrocystis pyrifera*, sodium alginate.

BACKGROUND

- Algin is a polysaccharide (a type of carbohydrate) derived from brown seaweed (from the genera *Ascophyllum, Macrocystis,* and *Laminaria*) currently found in the North Atlantic basin. Seaweed has been used as food for humans and animals for thousands of years. Its derivatives have wide application in the food industry, the cosmetic industry, and medicine and dentistry. In Asia, seaweed is relied on as a vegetable and fiber source, whereas the Western world has developed a tablet form to obtain the nutrients.
- In folk medicine, algin is taken by mouth to prevent and treat high blood pressure. It is also used in foods such as candy, gelatins, puddings, condiments, relish, processed vegetables, fish products, and imitation products. In manufacturing, algin is used as a binding and disintegrating agent in tablets, as a binding and demulcent in lozenges, and as a film in peel-off facial masks.
- Algin is often used to normalize bowel function. It has also been studied in combination with dietary fibers. Additional study is needed before any firm recommendations can be made about the safety or effectiveness of algin.

EVIDENCE

Uses Based on Scientific Evidence

No available studies qualify for inclusion in the evidence table.

Uses Based on Tradition or Theory

Abortion, bowel function improvement, cervical dilation, diabetes, gastric ulcers, healing of colonic anastomoses, hyperlipidemia (high cholesterol), hypertension (high blood pressure), ocular fillings, reducing absorption of strontium/barium/tin/cadmium/manganese/zinc/mercury, tissue replacement, wound healing, wound infection.

DOSING

Adults (18 Years and Older)

- There is insufficient evidence to recommend a dose for algin in adults.

Children (Younger than 18 Years)

- There is insufficient evidence to recommend a dose for algin in children.

SAFETY

Allergies

- Use of algin should be avoided in individuals with a known allergy or hypersensitivity to algin or its derivatives.

Side Effects and Warnings

- Currently, available scientific evidence is lacking regarding algin's safety and potential side effects. Algin is likely safe when taken by mouth in amounts typically found in foods. However, It is possibly unsafe when used in pregnant women. *Laminaria digitata*, a species from which algin can be derived, has been used as an aid in cervical dilation.

Pregnancy and Breastfeeding

- Algin is not recommended in pregnant or breastfeeding women due to lack of available scientific evidence. Algin may cause abortion or dilate the cervix.

INTERACTIONS

Interactions with Drugs

- The fiber in algin may impair the body's ability to absorb oral drugs. Patients taking any medications should consult with a qualified health care professional, including a pharmacist, before taking algin.

Interactions with Herbs and Dietary Supplements

- The fiber in algin may impair the body's ability to absorb oral herbs and supplements. Patients taking any herbs or supplements should consult with a qualified health care professional, including a pharmacist, before taking algin.

For a complete list of references, please visit www.naturalstandard.com.

Alizarin

RELATED TERMS

- Alizarin fluorine blue, alizarin red, alizarin red S (ARS), alizarin S, alizarin sulfonic acid, alizarin yellow GG, alizarine, anthraquine, dyer's madder, faberrote, garance, Krapp, madder, madder plant, robbia, rubia, *Rubia tintorum*, *Rubia tinctorum* L., *Rubia tinctorum* radix.

BACKGROUND

- Alizarin has been used as a staining agent for centuries. Originally, alizarin vegetable dye was prepared from the madder plant *Rubia tinctorum*, but now a synthetic preparation is used that is chemically identical. Madder or alizarin has been regarded as a mild diuretic.
- The Ministry of Health of Russian Federation has approved alizarin as an antiviral preparation for acute and recurring forms of herpes simplex infection of extragenital and genital areas, herpetiform Kaposi's eczema, viral diseases of the oral cavity, herpes zoster, and chickenpox in children and adults.
- Currently, there are no well-established therapeutic uses of alizarin. It is potentially carcinogenic and mutagenic if consumed orally. Precautions should be taken while handling this dye because of the lack of safety data.

EVIDENCE

Uses Based on Scientific Evidence	Grade
Viral Infections Limited available evidence suggests that alizarin may improve various herpes infections. Additional study is needed before a firm recommendation can be made.	C

Uses Based on Tradition or Theory
Anemia, aphrodisiac, blood disorders, bone healing (ectopic), bruises, chickenpox, coloration of articular fluids, diuretic, eczema, edema (swelling), expectorant, flavoring agent, food additive, human immunodeficiency virus (HIV), jaundice, kidney or bladder stones, leukemia, liver and gallbladder tonic, liver disease, menstrual disorders, paralysis, sciatica (leg pain), skin conditions, spleen disorders, tonic, urinary disorders, urinary tract inflammation, weight gain, wound healing.

DOSING

Adults (18 Years and Older)

- No dose is proven safe or effective in adults. Madder bark has been prepared by using 1 teaspoon boiled in a covered container with 3 cups of water for 30 minutes. The liquid is cooled slowly in the closed container and taken cold, 1-2 cups per day. For herpes simplex lesions, a 0.2%-0.5% ointment has been applied on the skin.

Children (Younger than 18 Years)

- No dose is proven safe or effective in children. Nonetheless, 0.1-g tablets of alizarin three times a day has been taken by mouth within 5 days of exposure to chickenpox. A 0.2% ointment applied on the skin has also been used.

SAFETY

Allergies

- Patients with a known allergy or hypersensitivity to alizarin, *Rubia tinctorum*, or other plants from the Rubiaceae family should not take alizarin preparations.
- Contact dermatitis from handling stems and roots of *Rubia tinctorum* has been reported.

Side Effects and Warnings

- There are few reports of adverse effects in humans associated with alizarin. However, alizarin may be toxic and should not be handled for long periods, rubbed in the eyes, or eaten. Alizarin is potentially carcinogenic (cancer-causing) and mutagenic (capable of causing genetic changes). When taken by mouth, madder can cause red-colored urine, saliva, perspiration, and breast milk. There is some concern that madder can stain contact lenses.
- Contact dermatitis has been reported in two women, handling wild madder (*Rubia peregrina*) and madder (*Rubia tinctorum*).
- Other side effects noted include nausea, vomiting, transient weakness, loss of muscle control, subacute toxicity, progressive listlessness, hyperirritability, insomnia, and abnormal breathing.

Pregnancy and Breastfeeding

- Alizarin is not recommended in pregnant or breastfeeding women. Alizarin dye may cross the placenta. Extracts from madder plant (*Rubia tinctorum*) are likely unsafe when taken by mouth in pregnant women because of potential menstrual stimulation and genotoxic (damaging to the DNA) effects. The extract can also cause red-colored breast milk.

INTERACTIONS

Interactions with Drugs

- Parts of the chemical structure of alizarin are similar to those in the tetracycline molecule. Therefore, there is a possibility of an additive interaction between alizarin and tetracyclines such as demeclocycline.

Interactions with Herbs and Dietary Supplements

- Currently, available scientific evidence describing herb and supplement interactions with alizarin is lacking.

For a complete list of references, please visit www. naturalstandard.com.

RELATED TERMS

- *Alcanna d'Oriente, Alcanna vera,* alkanet, alkanet root, *Alkanna lehmannii, Alkanna orientalis, Alkanna sempervireus, Alkanna tinctoria, Alkanna tinctoria* Tausch, *Alkanna tuberculata,* Alkannawurzel (German), anchusa, *Anchusae radix, Anchusa tinctoria, Anchusa tuberculata,* ancusa (Spanish), Boraginaceae (family), bugloss, dyer's bugloss, havaciva, *henna, Lithospermum tinctorium,* onoquiles, orcanette (French), orchanet, Schminkwurz (German), Spanish bugloss.

BACKGROUND

- Alkanna is grown in the south of France and on the shores of the Levant (the mountainous region paralleling the eastern shore of the Mediterranean, including parts of Turkey, Syria, Lebanon, and Israel). Its root yields a fine red coloring, which has been used as a cloth dye and a tint for tinctures, oils, wines, and varnishes. It is commonly used today as a food coloring.
- Alkanna has been used traditionally for its wound healing and anti-inflammatory effects. Historically, alkanna has been referred to as henna and used as a fabric dye.
- Currently, no scientific evidence is available to recommend use, safety, or effectiveness of alkanna for any medical condition.
- Some products may contain hepatotoxic pyrrolizidine alkaloid that may also be potentially carcinogenic.

EVIDENCE

Uses Based on Scientific Evidence

No available studies qualify for inclusion in the evidence table.

Uses Based on Tradition or Theory

Antiaging, antibacterial, anti-inflammatory, antimicrobial, antipruritic (prevents/relieves itching), antiviral (*Alkanna orientalis*), astringent, back pain, bed sores, bruises, cancer, jaundice, kidney disorders, measles, poisonous snake bites, rash, smallpox, varicose veins, vulnerary (skin regenerative), wound healing.

DOSING

Adults (18 Years and Older)

- There is insufficient evidence to recommend a dose for alkanna in adults.

Children (Younger than 18 Years)

- There is insufficient evidence to recommend a dose for alkanna in children.

SAFETY

Allergies

- Individuals with a known allergy or hypersensitivity to alkanna, its constituents, or potentially any member of the family Boraginaceae should not take alkanna.

Side Effects and Warnings

- In general, the lack of available scientific evidence makes it difficult to comment on the potential adverse effects of alkanna. Nevertheless, certain constituents (pyrrolizidine alkaloids) found in alkanna may be potentially damaging to the liver and lungs and may be carcinogenic (cancer-causing). Pyrrolizidine alkaloids may also cause pneumonitis (inflammation of the lungs) or pulmonary hypertension (high blood pressure).
- Caution is advised in patients with hepatic or pulmonary insufficiency. Patients with cancer should use alkanna cautiously because the quantity of pyrrolizidine alkaloids in some herbal teas and dietary supplements may worsen the condition.

Pregnancy and Breastfeeding

- Alkanna is not recommended in pregnant or breastfeeding women due to lack of available scientific evidence.

INTERACTIONS

Interactions with Drugs

- Constituents of alkanna include pyrrolizidine alkaloids. These are potentially liver toxic. Concurrent use of alkanna with other liver toxic agents may increase the risk of toxicity. Patients taking any medications should consult with a qualified health care professional, including a pharmacist, before using alkanna.

Interactions with Herbs and Dietary Supplements

- Constituents of alkanna include pyrrolizidine alkaloids. These are potentially liver toxic. Concurrent use of alkanna with other liver toxic herbs/supplements may increase the risk of toxicity. Patients taking any herbs or supplements should consult with a qualified health care professional, including a pharmacist, before using alkanna.

For a complete list of references, please visit www.naturalstandard.com.

Allspice
(Pimenta dioica)

RELATED TERMS

- Allyl alkoxybenzenes, castalagin, casuariin, casuarinin, dietary polyphenols, ellagic acid, estragole, gallic acid, galloylglucosides, grandinin, grandininol, glycosidic tannins, Jamaica pepper, methyl eugenol, methyl-flavogallonate, methyl gallate, Myrtaceae (family), myrtle pepper, nilocitin, pedunculagin, phenolic glycosides, *Pimenta dioica*, pimentol, polyphenols, vascalagin, vascalaginone.

BACKGROUND

- Allspice is produced from the fruit of the *Pimenta dioica* plant and originates primarily from Jamaica, the West Indies, and South America. The fruits are picked when they are green, dried in the sun or in a kiln, and sold either as whole dried fruit or in powdered form. Allspice has a complex, peppery taste similar to a mix of cinnamon, juniper, clove, and nutmeg.
- Historically, allspice was used to treat indigestion and intestinal gas. It was also taken by mouth to treat stomach aches, heavy menstrual bleeding, vomiting, diarrhea, fever, flu, and colds. Allspice has been used commercially to flavor toothpastes.
- Currently, there is limited high-quality evidence supporting any clinical use of allspice.

EVIDENCE

Uses Based on Scientific Evidence

No available studies qualify for inclusion in the evidence table.

Uses Based on Tradition or Theory

Age-related nerve damage, antioxidant, antiseptic (teeth and gums), cancer, colds, diarrhea, dyspepsia, excessive menstrual bleeding, fever, flavoring (to compensate for low-salt foods), flu, gas, heart disease, indigestion, muscle pain, toothache (topical), vomiting.

DOSING

Adults (18 Years and Older)

- There is insufficient evidence to recommend a dose for allspice in adults.

Children (Younger than 18 Years)

- There is insufficient evidence to recommend a dose for allspice in children.

SAFETY

Allergies

- Avoid with known allergy or hypersensitivity to allspice. There have been reports of allergic reactions of the skin to spices and flavorings including allspice in people who work in restaurants or other food-service jobs. People with such allergies may also have cross-reactivity to foods such as tomatoes, lettuce, and carrots. There have been reports of cross-reactivity among people allergic to Balsam of Peru.

Side Effects and Warnings

- Data on reactions to allspice are limited. Most reported side effects were mild and affected the skin. Allspice and many other herbs, spices, and foods contain naturally occurring agents called estragole and methyl eugenol, which may cause cancer.

Pregnancy and Breastfeeding

- Allspice is not recommended in pregnant or breastfeeding women due to a lack of available scientific evidence.

INTERACTIONS

Interactions with Drugs

- Allspice may interfere with the way the body processes certain drugs using the cytochrome P450 enzyme system of the liver. As a result, the levels of these drugs may be increased or decreased in the blood and may cause increased effects of potentially serious adverse reactions. Patients using any medications should check the package insert and speak with a qualified health care professional, including a pharmacist, about possible interactions.
- Allspice may have immune stimulating effects. Theoretically concurrent use of allspice may interfere or alter the effects of immunosuppressants.

Interactions with Herbs and Dietary Supplements

- Allspice may interfere with the way the body processes certain herbs or supplements using the cytochrome P450 enzyme system of the liver. As a result, the levels of these drugs may be increased or decreased in the blood and may cause increased effects of potentially serious adverse reactions. Patients using any medications should check the package insert and speak with a qualified health care professional, including a pharmacist, about possible interactions.
- Allspice may have immune-stimulating effects. Theoretically concurrent use of allspice may interfere or alter the effects of immunosuppressants.

For a complete list of references, please visit www.naturalstandard.com.

Aloe
(Aloe vera)

RELATED TERMS

- Acemannan, *Aloe africana*, *Aloe arborescens* Miller, *Aloe barbadensis*, *Aloe barbadesis*, *Aloe capensis*, aloe-coated gloves, *Aloe ferox*, aloe latex, aloe mucilage, *Aloe perfoliata*, *Aloe perryi* Baker, *Aloe saponaria*, *Aloe spicata*, *Aloe vulgari*, anthraquinones Barbados aloe, bitter aloe, burn plant, Cape aloe, Carrisyn, Curaçao aloe, elephant's gall, first-aid plant, Ghai kunwar, Ghikumar, hirukattali, Hsiang-Dan, hydroxy-anthraquinones jelly leek, kumari, lahoi, laloi, lily of the desert, Lu-Hui, medicine plant, Mediterranean aloe, miracle plant, mocha aloes, musabbar, natal aloes, nohwa, plant of immortality, plant of life, rokai, sabilla, Savila, Socotrine aloe, subr, true aloe, Venezuela aloe, Za'bila, Zanzibar aloe.

BACKGROUND

- Transparent gel from the pulp of the meaty leaves of *Aloe vera* has been used topically for thousands of years to treat wounds, skin infections, burns, and numerous other dermatological conditions. Dried latex from the inner lining of the leaf has traditionally been used as an oral laxative.
- There is strong scientific evidence in support of the laxative properties of aloe latex, based on the well-established cathartic properties of anthroquinone glycosides (found in aloe latex). However, aloe's therapeutic value compared with other approaches to constipation remains unclear.
- There is promising preliminary support from laboratory, animal, and human studies that topical aloe gel has immunomodulatory properties that may improve wound healing and skin inflammation.

EVIDENCE

Uses Based on Scientific Evidence	Grade
Constipation (Laxative) Dried latex from the inner lining of aloe leaves has been used traditionally as a laxative taken by mouth. Although few studies have been conducted to assess this effect of aloe in humans, the laxative properties of aloe components such as aloin are well supported by scientific evidence. A combination herbal remedy containing aloe was found to be an effective laxative, although it is not clear if this effect was due to aloe or to other ingredients in the product. Further study is needed to establish dosing and to compare the effectiveness and safety of aloe with other commonly used laxatives.	B
Genital Herpes Limited evidence from human studies suggests that extract from *Aloe vera* in a hydrophilic cream may be an effective treatment of genital herpes in men (better than aloe gel or placebo). Additional research is needed in this area before a strong recommendation can be made.	B
Psoriasis Vulgaris Early evidence suggests that an extract from aloe in a hydrophilic cream may be an effective treatment of psoriasis vulgaris. Additional research is needed in this area before a strong recommendation can be made.	B
Seborrheic Dermatitis (Seborrhea, Dandruff) Early study of aloe lotion suggests effectiveness for treating seborrheic dermatitis when applied to the skin. Further study is needed in this area before a strong recommendation can be made.	B
Cancer Prevention There is early evidence that oral aloe may reduce the risk of developing lung cancer. Further study is needed in this area to clarify whether it is aloe itself or other factors that may cause this benefit.	C
Canker Sores (Aphthous Stomatitis) There is weak evidence that treatment of recurrent aphthous ulcers of the mouth with aloe gel may reduce pain and increase the amount of time between the appearance of new ulcers. Further study is needed before a firm recommendation can be made.	C
Diabetes (Type 2) Study results are mixed. More research is needed to explore the effectiveness and safety of aloe in diabetics.	C
Dry Skin Traditionally, aloe has been used as a moisturizer. Early low-quality studies suggest aloe may effectively reduce skin dryness. Higher quality studies are needed in this area.	C
HIV Infection Without further human trials, the evidence cannot be considered convincing either in favor or against use of aloe in HIV disease.	C
Lichen Planus Limited study suggests that aloe may be a helpful, safe treatment for lichen planus, which is a chronic inflammatory disease that affects the lining of the mouth. Additional study is needed.	C
Skin Burns Early evidence suggests that aloe may aid healing of mild to moderate skin burns. Further study is needed in this area.	C
Skin Ulcers Early studies suggest aloe may help heal skin ulcers. High-quality studies comparing aloe alone with placebo are needed.	C

Uses Based on Scientific Evidence	Grade
Ulcerative Colitis (including Inflammatory Bowel Disease) There is limited but promising research of the use of oral aloe vera in ulcerative colitis (UC), compared with placebo. It is not clear how aloe vera compares with other treatments used for UC.	C
Wound Healing Study results of aloe on wound healing are mixed, with some studies reporting positive results and others showing no benefit or potential worsening of the condition. Further study is needed because wound healing is a popular use of topical aloe.	C
Mucositis There is early evidence that oral *Aloe vera* does not prevent or improve mucositis (mouth sores) associated with radiation therapy.	D
Pressure Ulcers Early well-designed studies in humans found no benefit of topical acemannan hydrogel (a component of aloe gel) in the treatment of pressure ulcers.	D
Radiation Dermatitis Reports in the 1930s of the beneficial effects of topical aloe on skin after radiation exposure led to widespread use of aloe in skin products. Currently, aloe gel is sometimes recommended for skin irritation caused by prolonged exposure to radiation, although scientific evidence suggests a lack of benefit in this area.	D

Uses Based on Tradition or Theory

Alzheimer's disease, antifungal, antimicrobial, antioxidant, antitumor, antiviral, arthritis (osteoarthritis, rheumatoid arthritis), asthma, bacterial skin infections, birth control, blood vessel disorders, bowel disorders, chronic fatigue syndrome, congestive heart failure, frostbite, gingivitis, hair loss, heart disease prevention, hepatitis, high cholesterol, human papillomavirus (HPV), itchiness (skin), kidney or bladder stones, leukemia, lichen planus (skin condition), parasitic worm infections, Parkinson's disease, periodontal surgical rinse, scratches or superficial wounds of the eye, stomach acid reduction, sunburn, systemic lupus erythematosus (SLE), tic douloureux (trigeminal neuralgia, severe facial pain), untreatable tumors, vaginal contraceptive, yeast infections of the skin.

DOSING
Adults (18 Years and Older)

- Pure *Aloe vera* gel is often used liberally on the skin three to four times per day for the treatment of sunburn and other minor burns. Creams and lotions are also available. There are no reports that using aloe on the skin causes absorption of chemicals into the body that may cause significant side effects. Skin products are available that contain aloe alone or aloe combined with other active ingredients.
- The dose often recommended for constipation is the minimum amount to maintain a soft stool, typically 0.04-0.17 g of dried juice (corresponds to 10-30 mg of hydroxyanthraquinones) by mouth. Alternatively, in combination with celandine (300 mg) and psyllium (50 mg), 150 mg of the dried juice per day of aloe has been found to be effective as a laxative in research.
- Deaths have been associated with *Aloe vera* injections under unclear circumstances. Injected use is not recommended due to a lack of safety data.
- Other uses of aloe from scientific studies include the treatment of genital herpes (0.5% cream applied to lesions for 5 consecutive days per week for 2 weeks) and psoriasis (0.5% cream applied to skin three times per day for 5 consecutive days per week for 4 weeks).

Children (Younger than 18 Years)

- Topical (skin) use of aloe gel in children is common and seems to be well tolerated. However, a dermatologist and pharmacist should be consulted before starting therapy. Aloe taken by mouth has not been studied in children and theoretically may have harmful effects, such as lowering reducing blood glucose levels. Therefore, it is not recommended.

SAFETY
Allergies

- People with known allergy to garlic, onions, tulips, or other plants of the Liliaceae family may have allergic reactions to aloe. Individuals using aloe gel for prolonged times have developed allergic reactions, including hives and eczema-like rash. Aloe injections have caused severe reactions and should be avoided.

Side Effects and Warnings

- The use of aloe on surgical wounds has been reported to slow healing; redness and burning have been reported after aloe juice was applied to the face after a skin-peeling procedure (dermabrasion). Application of aloe before sun exposure may lead to rash in sun-exposed areas.
- The use of aloe or aloe latex by mouth for laxative effects can cause cramping or diarrhea. Use for more than 7 days may cause dependency or worsening of constipation after the aloe is stopped. Ingestion of aloe for more than 1 year has been reported to increase the risk of colorectal cancer. Individuals with severe abdominal pain, appendicitis, ileus (temporary paralysis of the bowel), or a prolonged period without bowel movements should not take aloe. Hepatitis (liver inflammation) has been reported with the use of oral aloe.
- Electrolyte imbalances in the blood, including low potassium levels, may be caused by the laxative effect of aloe. This effect may be greater in people with diabetes or kidney disease. Low potassium levels can lead to abnormal heart rhythms or muscle weakness. People with heart disease, kidney disease, or electrolyte abnormalities should not take aloe by mouth. Health care professionals should monitor for changes in potassium and other electrolytes in individuals who take aloe by mouth for more than a few days.
- Aloe taken by mouth may lower reduce blood glucose levels. Caution is advised in patients with diabetes or hypoglycemia and in those taking drugs, herbs, or supplements that affect blood glucose. Serum glucose levels may need to be monitored by a health care professional, and medication adjustments may be necessary. People with thyroid disorders, kidney disease, heart disease, or electrolyte abnormalities should also use oral aloe only under medical supervision.

- *Aloe vera* injections have been associated with cases of death under unclear circumstances and should be avoided.

Pregnancy and Breastfeeding

- Although topical (skin) use of aloe is unlikely to be harmful during pregnancy or breastfeeding, oral (by mouth) use is not recommended due to theoretical stimulation of uterine contractions. It is not known whether active ingredients of aloe may be present in breast milk. The dried juice of aloe leaves should not be consumed by breastfeeding mothers.

INTERACTIONS
Interactions with Drugs

- Aloe taken by mouth may lower blood glucose levels. Caution is advised in patients who are using medication that may lower blood glucose due to increased risk of hypoglycemia (low blood sugar). Blood glucose should be monitored.
- Aloe latex may cause losses of potassium. Aloe should not be used with drugs such as digoxin and diuretics, as this may increase potassium loss.
- Use of aloe with laxative drugs may increase the risk of dehydration, potassium depletion, electrolyte imbalance, and changes in blood pH. Due to its laxative effect, aloe may also reduce the absorption of some drugs.
- Application of aloe to skin may increase the absorption of steroid creams, such as hydrocortisone. Oral use of aloe and steroids such as prednisone may also increase the risk of potassium depletion.
- There is one report of excess bleeding in a patient undergoing surgery receiving the anesthetic drug sevoflurane, who was also taking aloe by mouth. It is not clear that aloe or this specific interaction was the cause of bleeding.

- Preliminary reports suggest that levels of AZT, a drug prescribed in human immunodeficiency virus (HIV) infection, may be increased by intake of aloe.
- Aloe may alter the effects of cancer drugs. Caution is warranted with concurrent use.
- Aloe may alter the effects with phytoestrogens. Caution is warranted with concurrent use.

Interactions with Herbs and Dietary Supplements

- Based on the laxative properties of oral aloe, prolonged use may result in potassium depletion. Aloe may increase the potassium-lowering effects of other herbs, such as licorice (*Glycyrrhiza glabra*). Theoretically, use of oral aloe and other laxative herbs such as senna may increase the risk of dehydration, potassium depletion, electrolyte imbalance, and changes in blood pH.
- Oral aloe can reduce blood glucose. Caution is advised when using herbs or supplements such as bitter melon that may also lower blood glucose. Blood glucose levels may require monitoring, and doses may need adjustment.
- Aloe should not be used with cardiac glycosides–containing herbs (e.g., oleander) due to increase risk of toxicity and adverse effects such as potassium depletion. Use with diuretic herbs (e.g., horsetail) may also increase the risk of potassium depletion.
- Aloe may alter the effects of cancer drugs. Caution is warranted with concurrent use.
- Aloe may alter the effects of antiviral agents. Caution is warranted with concurrent use.
- Aloe may alter the effects with phytoestrogens. Caution is warranted with concurrent use.
- Aloe may improve the absorption of vitamins C and E.

For a complete list of references, please visit www.naturalstandard.com.

Alpha-Lipoic Acid
(1,2-dithiolane-3-pentanoic acid)

RELATED TERMS

- 1, 2-diathiolane-3 valeric acid, 6, 8 alpha lipoic acid, 5-(1, 2 dithiolan-3-yl) valeric acid, acetate replacing factor, ALA, alpha lipoate, alpha-lipoic acid, Berlition, Biletan, DHLA, dihydrolipoic acid, lipoic acid, lipoicin, liponsäure (German), thioctamide, thioctan, thioctic acid, Thiogamma, Tiobec, tioctic acid.
- **Note:** Alpha-lipoic acid should not be confused with alpha linolenic acid, which is also abbreviated as ALA.

BACKGROUND

- Alpha-lipoic acid (ALA) is made naturally in the body and may protect against cell damage in various conditions. Food sources rich in ALA include spinach, broccoli, and yeast.
- ALA, known as the "universal oxidant," has been used for decades in Europe, especially Germany, to treat nerve conditions, including nerve damage resulting from poorly controlled diabetes (peripheral neuropathy).
- There is strong evidence that ALA may help treat type 2 diabetes and neuropathy. According to a survey of 685 herbalists, ALA was 1 of the 10 most frequently recommended dietary supplements because of its efficacy in reducing high blood glucose levels.
- Data are insufficient to support the use of ALA in *Amanita* poisoning, which has reportedly been a common practice for many years.
- The therapeutic use of ALA is not approved by the U.S. Food and Drug Administration (FDA) or corresponding regulatory agencies in other countries.

EVIDENCE

Uses Based on Scientific Evidence	Grade
Diabetes Many studies have shown that ALA may improve blood glucose levels in patients with type 2 diabetes. Higher quality studies are needed to provide more definitive answers in the future. Diabetes is a serious illness and should be treated under the supervision of a qualified health care provider.	A
Neuropathy (Nerve Pain or Damage) Many studies have shown that ALA is an effective treatment for nerve pain or damage (neuropathy) associated with diabetes or cancer treatment.	A
Alcoholic Liver Disease ALA has been studied as a treatment for alcohol-related liver disease. Benefits have not been observed so far, however. More research is needed in this area.	C
Cognitive Function (HIV) ALA has been studied as a treatment for cognitive impairment caused by nerve damage in HIV patients. At this time, there is not enough scientific evidence to recommend ALA for treating this condition.	C
Glaucoma There are some human studies of ALA as a treatment for glaucoma, but scientific evidence is inadequate to make a recommendation at this time.	C
Kidney Disease ALA may provide some benefit in kidney disease, but there is not enough evidence to recommend this use.	C
Pain (Burning Mouth Syndrome) ALA shows some promise as a treatment for burning mouth syndrome, a condition that causes the mouth to feel hot or tingly. Additional research is needed before any recommendations can be made.	C
Pancreatic Cancer ALA has not been well studied for pancreatic cancer in humans. A case report shows that ALA may help prevent cancer progression. However, high-quality studies are needed before a conclusion can be made.	C
Postoperative Tissue Injury Prevention (Ischemia-Reperfusion Injury after Liver Surgery) When blood supply to an organ is blocked, it is called ischemia. When the blood supply is restored (called reperfusion), the resulting swelling and stress can lead to organ damage. Treatment with ALA before liver surgery may help prevent this type of damage. However, more research is needed.	C
Radiation Injuries Early evidence suggests that ALA may be beneficial to people exposed to high levels of radiation. Well-designed studies are needed before ALA can be recommended for this use.	C
Skin Aging Early research shows that a skin cream containing ALA may help improve signs of skin aging. More research is needed before any recommendations can be made.	C
Wound Healing (in Patients Undergoing Hyperbaric Oxygen Therapy) ALA may reduce tissue damage that is often caused by long-term exposure to high levels of oxygen. While early studies are promising, more research is needed to fully understand how this might work.	C

Uses Based on Tradition or Theory
Age-associated memory impairment, altitude (mountain) sickness, Alzheimer's dementia, *Amanita phalloides* mushroom toxicity, antioxidant, appetite/weight loss in cancer patients, atherosclerosis (clogged arteries), atopic dermatitis, bile flow stimulation, blood

(Continued)

Uses Based on Tradition or Theory—Cont'd

disorders (erythropoietic protoporphyria), blood vessel disease (brain, endothelium), bone loss, brain damage (degenerative, copper-induced oxidative damage), cancer, cardiovascular disorders (cerebrovascular disease), central nervous system disorders, chemotherapy adverse effects, cirrhosis, constipation, contact dermatitis, deficiency (zinc), dementia, depression, Down's syndrome, endocrine disorders (metabolic syndrome), gastrointestinal conditions (gastric mucosa protection), hearing damage (from certain drugs), heart damage from doxorubicin (Adriamycin, Doxil), hepatitis C, high blood pressure, high cholesterol, HIV/AIDS, immune system stimulant, inflammation, inflammatory conditions (inflammatory vascular diseases), kidney protection, lactic acidosis (lipoamide dehydrogenase deficiency), lead toxicity, liver disease, memory, metabolic disorders (Leigh's disease, porphyria, Krabbe disease), mitochondrial diseases, multiple sclerosis, muscular dystrophy (facioscapulohumeral dystrophy), neural tube defects, neuroprotection, nutritional supplement, obesity, Parkinson's disease, postoperative pain, psoriasis, retinal protection (leukostasis, retinal ischemia-reperfusion), retinopathy, scurvy, sepsis (prevention and treatment), sickle cell anemia, smell disorders, stomach problems, stroke, toxic kidney damage (oxaliplatin-induced, cyclophosphamide cytotoxicity, mercury-induced), vitamin E deficiency, Wilson's disease (a hereditary disorder).

DOSING

Adults (18 Years and Older)

- **General:** Experts believe it is safe to use ALA at recommended doses for 2 years.
- **Alcoholic liver disease:** A dose of 300 mg of thioctic acid has been taken daily in three divided doses for 24 weeks.
- **Cognitive function (human immunodeficiency virus [HIV]):** A dose of 600 mg of ALA has been taken twice daily for 10 weeks.
- **Diabetes:** Doses of 600-1800 mg of ALA have been taken by mouth daily. Doses of 500-1000 mg of ALA per 50-500 mL of sodium chloride have been injected.
- **Drug-induced cardiotoxicity:** A dose of 100 mg/kg of ALA reportedly reduced heart damage caused by the anticancer drug doxorubicin in a poorly described study.
- **Glaucoma:** A dose of 150 mg of ALA has been taken for 1 month.
- **Ischemia-reperfusion injury protection:** A dose of 600 mg of ALA in 50 mL of sodium chloride has been injected.
- **Kidney disease:** Patients undergoing hemodialysis took 600 mg of ALA daily for 12 weeks.
- **Neuropathy:** In divided doses, 600-1800 mg of ALA has been taken by mouth daily from 3 weeks to 2 years. A dose of 600 mg of ALA has been injected daily for 5-10 days.
- **Pain (burning mouth syndrome):** A daily dose of 200-600 mg of ALA has been taken by mouth for 2 months.
- **Wound healing (in patients undergoing hyperbaric oxygen therapy):** A dose of 300 mg of ALA has been used 1 hour before exposure to oxygen and immediately after therapy. Patients then took 300 mg twice daily for the next 30 treatments.

Children (Younger than 18 Years)

- The dosing and safety of ALA have not been well studied in children, and ALA cannot be recommended.

SAFETY

Allergies

- People with allergies or hypersensitivities to ALA should avoid use of ALA. Pain and redness have occurred around a needle site when ALA was injected through a vein. Allergic skin reactions (contact dermatitis) have occurred after an ALA antiwrinkle cream was used.

Side Effects and Warnings

- Few side effects have been reported from ALA. The most common complaints include nausea, vomiting, and dizziness, all of which occurred with doses of 1200-1800 mg.
- Caution should be used among patients with type 2 diabetes because of the possibility of changes in insulin sensitivity and trace element deficiency. A case of insulin autoimmune syndrome, a rare disease that causes the immune system to attack insulin mistakenly, leading to low blood glucose levels, was reported after ALA use. Blood glucose levels may need to be monitored by a qualified health care professional, including a pharmacist, and medication adjustments may be necessary.
- Although not well studied in humans, ALA should be used with caution in people with thyroid diseases, as ALA may interfere with the conversion of thyroid hormones.
- Avoid in patients with thiamin deficiency (commonly seen in alcoholics), as fatal cases of thiamin deficiency has been reported in animals.

Pregnancy and Breastfeeding

- There is not enough scientific evidence available to recommend using ALA during pregnancy or breastfeeding.

INTERACTIONS

Interactions with Drugs

- ALA may lower blood glucose levels. Caution is warranted in patients who have diabetes or who are using drugs that lower blood sugar due to increased risk of hypoglycemia (low blood sugar). Blood glucose levels should be monitored. Medication adjustments may be necessary.
- ALA may alter thyroid levels. Caution is advised in people diagnosed with thyroid disease or who are using thyroid hormones. Thyroid levels should be monitored. Dosing adjustments may be necessary.
- ALA, when given with doxorubicin, provides a protective effect against heart damage. This effect may improve the therapeutic index of doxorubicin when given with ALA.
- ALA may block the effects of cisplatin (chemotherapy) and reduce the effectiveness of cisplatin.
- ALA may reduce body weight and food intake. Concurrent use with weight-loss agents may have additive effects.
- ALA may cause vasodilation (widening of blood vessels). Concurrent use with vasodilators may cause additive effects.
- ALA may affect the way in which the liver breaks down certain drugs.

Interactions with Herbs and Dietary Supplements

- ALA may lower blood glucose levels. Caution is warranted in patients who have diabetes or who are using herbs and supplements that lower blood sugar due to increased risk of hypoglycemia (low blood sugar). Blood glucose levels should be monitored. Medication adjustments may be necessary.
- ALA may alter thyroid levels. Caution is advised in people diagnosed with thyroid disease or who are using thyroid hormones. Thyroid levels should be monitored. Dosing adjustments may be necessary.
- ALA may block the effects of cancer treatments. Caution is warranted.

- ALA may reduce body weight and food intake. Concurrent use with weight-loss agents may have additive effects.
- ALA may cause vasodilation (widening of blood vessels). Concurrent use with vasodilators may cause additive effects.
- Vitamin C levels may be increased when taken with ALA.
- ALA may affect the way in which the liver breaks down certain herbs or supplements.

For a complete list of references, please visit www.naturalstandard.com.

RELATED TERMS

- Adkham, Alpinetin, *Alpinia allughas, Alpinia blepharocalyx, Alpinia calcarata* Roscoe, *Alpinia conchigera,* alpinia epoxide, *Alpinia flabellata, Alpinia formosana, Alpinia galanga, Alpinia galanga* Wild, Alpínia galangová, *Alpinia hainanensis, Alpinia henryi, Alpinia japonica, Alpinia javanica, Alpinia jianganfeng, Alpinia katsumadai, Alpinia katsumadai* Hayata, *Alpinia kumatake* Makino, Alpínia liecivá, *Alpinia mutica,* alpinia nigra, *Alpinia nutans,* alpinia officinalis, *Alpinia officinarum, Alpinia officinarum* Hance, *Alpinia oxyphylla* Miquel, *Alpinia pupurata, Alpinia rafflesiana, Alpinia sanderae, Alpinia smithiae, Alpinia speciosa, Alpinia speciosa* Schum, *Alpinia tonkinensis, Alpinia zerumbet,* Alpiniae fructus, Alpinija, Arrata, Arattai, baidukou, blepharcalyxins A and B, calyxin H, calyxin I, caodoukou, Cao khuong huong, Cao luong khuong, cardamonin, catarrh root, chewing john, China root, Chinese ginger, colic root, colonia, colony, Da gao liang jiang, daaih gou lèuhng geung, dehydrokawain, Djus rishe, Dok kha, East India catarrh root, East India root, epicalyxin F, epicalyxin H, fingerroot, galanga, galanga maggiore, Galangagyökér, galangal, galangal root, galangarot, galangin, galango, galanki, galgán, galgán lekársky, galgan obecný, galgán veliký, galgán vetší, galgant, galigaan, gao liang, gao liang jiang, garanga, gargaut, gengibre do laos, gengibre tailandés, gettou, ginza, gou lèuhng geung, greater galangal, großer Galgant, grote galanga, havlican, hong dou kou, hùhng dáu kau, India root, jouz rishe, junça ordinária, kacchuramu, kalgan, kalkán, kallengal, khaa, kha ta deng, khaa-ling, khulanjan, kolinjan, koshtkulinjan, kulanja, kulanjam, kulinjan, langkwas, languas speciosa, laos, lengkuas, lengoewas, lesser galangal, lèuhng geung, liang jiang, little john chew, madeng, mot loai gung, nankyo, nootkatol, orchid ginger, pa de gaw gyi, padagoji, palla, pras sva, puar, punnagchampa, rasmi, rasna, red ginger, Renealmia alpinia, *Rhizoma galangae,* rieng, rieng nep, romdeng, sannadumparashtramu, saan geung, sga-skya, shallflower, shan jiang, shellflower, shell ginger, Siamese ginger, siam-Ingwer, small shell ginger, son nai, souchet long, souchet odorant, suur kalganirohi, Thai alpinia galangal, variegated ginger, wild ginger, yakuchinone A, yakuchinone B, Zingiberaceae (family).
- **Note:** Alpinia should not be confused with ginger (*Zingiber officinale*).

BACKGROUND

- *Alpinia* is a large genus from the ginger family (Zingiberaceae). Alpinia has been known in Europe for several centuries longer than its botanical origin. It was recognized in 1870, when specimens were examined that had been found near Tung-sai, in the extreme south of China, and later, on the island of Hainan.
- Traditional uses have included treatment of flatulence (gas), dyspepsia (stomach upset), vomiting, high blood pressure, gastrointestinal complaints, and sea sickness.
- Alpinia has been studied for its diuretic (increasing urine flow) effects. Although alpinia is generally believed to be well tolerated, safety is not well studied. Currently, there is not enough available scientific evidence for or against the use of alpinia for any indication.

EVIDENCE

Uses Based on Scientific Evidence

No available studies qualify for inclusion in the evidence table.

Uses Based on Tradition or Theory

Allergic disorders, anaphylaxis, antibiotic, antifungal, anthelmintic, antihypertensive (lowering high blood pressure), anti-inflammatory, antimicrobial, antioxidant, antiparasitic, antiplatelet, antispasmodic, arthritis, cancer, cardiovascular disease, chemoprotectant, dementia, diabetes, diuresis, dyspepsia (upset stomach), expectorant (expels phlegm), fever, flatulence (gas), gastrointestinal disorders, *Helicobacter pylori,* hyperlipidemia, hypertension (high blood pressure), immune stimulant, inflammation, insect repellant, insecticide, intestinal disorders, leukemia, nausea and vomiting, neurological disorders, pain, sea sickness, skin disorders, snake bites, stimulant, ulcers, vasorelaxant.

DOSING

Adults (18 Years and Older)

- Based on available scientific evidence, there is no proven safe or effective dosing for alpinia. A typical dose of alpinia is 2-4 g of the herb per day or 1 cup of the tea, 30 minutes before meals. The tea is prepared by steeping 0.5-1 g in 150 mL hot water for 10 minutes and then straining. To increase the flow of urine, 0.8 g of *Alpinia speciosa* in 100 mL of water over 7 days has been used.

Children (Younger than 18 Years)

- There is insufficient evidence to recommend a dose for alpinia in children.

SAFETY

Allergies

- Avoid in patients with known allergy to alpinia or the ginger (Zingiberaceae) family.

Side Effects and Warnings

- Alpinia is generally considered to be well tolerated, with few adverse effects. Alpinia has generally recognized as safe (GRAS) status in the United States, and is likely safe when taken by mouth in amounts commonly found in foods.
- Decreased blood pressure, pruritus (itching), abnormally slow movements or alterations in movement, diuresis, and prolonged sleep time have been reported after use of *Alpinia speciosa.*
- Adverse effects of taking *Alpinia galanga* may include decreased blood glucose levels or mild gastrointestinal complaints.
- Elevated red blood cell levels have been noted.
- Caution is advised in patients with diabetes, in patients taking blood glucose–lowering medications, in patients with electrolyte imbalance, in patients with low blood pressure,

and in patients with known allergy to the ginger (Zingiberaceae) family.

Pregnancy and Breastfeeding

- Alpinia is not recommended in pregnant or breastfeeding women due to lack of available scientific evidence.

INTERACTIONS

Interactions with Drugs

- Alpinia may increase stomach acid and may decrease the effectiveness of antacids, including H_2 blockers. Alpinia may also interact with proton pump inhibitors (PPIs). Caution is advised.
- Small reductions in systolic and diastolic blood pressure have been associated with the use of alpinia. Caution is advised in patients taking medications that alter blood pressure due to the risk of additive effects. A qualified health care professional, including a pharmacist, should be consulted before taking alpinia.
- *Alpinia speciosa* may act as a diuretic and increase urine flow. Patients taking other medications that have a similar effect should use caution because an additive effect may occur.

- Alpinia may decrease blood glucose levels. Caution is advised in patients with diabetes who are taking medications that alter blood glucose or insulin. Blood glucose levels should be monitored.

Interactions with Herbs and Dietary Supplements

- *Alpinia speciosa* may act as a diuretic and increase urine flow. Patients taking other herbs or supplements that have a similar effect should use caution because an additive effect may occur.
- Alpinia may decrease blood glucose levels. Caution is advised in patients taking herbs and supplements that alter blood glucose. Blood glucose levels should be monitored. A qualified health care professional, including a pharmacist, should be consulted before taking alpinia.
- Small reductions in systolic and diastolic blood pressure have been associated with the use of alpinia. Caution is advised in patients taking herbs and supplements that alter blood pressure due to the risk of additive effects. A qualified health care professional, including a pharmacist, should be consulted before taking alpinia.

For a complete list of references, please visit www.naturalstandard.com.

Amaranth Oil
(Amaranthus L.)

RELATED TERMS

- Achis, achita, African amaranth, African spinach, alegra, amarante, amarante, amaranth grain, amaranth hybrid, amaranth seed oil, amaranth tender, Amaranthaceae (family), amaranthoideae, *Amaranthus acanthochiton, Amaranthus acutilobius, Amaranthus albus, Amaranthus arenicola, Amaranthus australis, Amaranthus bigelovii, Amaranthus blitoides, Amaranthus blitum, Amaranthus brownie, Amaranthus californicus, Amaranthus cannabinus, Amaranthus caudatus, Amaranthus chihuahuensis, Amaranthus chlorostachys, Amaranthus crassipes, Amaranthus crispus, Amaranthus cruentus, Amaranthus deflexus, Amaranthus dubius, Amaranthus edulis, Amaranthus fimbriatus, Amaranthus floridanus, Amaranthus gangeticus, Amaranthus graecizans, Amaranthus greggii, Amaranthus hybridus, Amaranthus hypochondriacus, Amaranthus leucocarpus, Amaranthus lineatus, Amaranthus lividus, Amaranthus mantegazzianus, Amaranthus minimus, Amaranthus muricatus, Amaranthus obcordatus, Amaranthus palmeri, Amaranthus paniculus, Amaranthus polygonoides, Amaranthus powelii, Amaranthus pringlei, Amaranthus pumilus, Amaranthus quitensis, Amaranthus retroflexus, Amaranthus rudis, Amaranthus scleropoides, Amaranthus spinosus, Amaranthus standleyanus, Amaranthus thunbergii, Amaranthus torreyi, Amaranthus tricolor, Amaranthus tuberculatus, Amaranthus viridis, Amaranthus watsonii, Amaranthus wrightii,* amaranto, amarantos, arowo jeta, ataco, Australian amaranth, azorubin, bayam, bayam bhaji, bayam hedjo, bigelow's amaranth, biteku teku, bledos, blero spinach, bondue, bone-bract amaranth, brown's amaranth, buautli, bush greens, calaloo, calalu, California amaranth, California pigweed, callaloo, careless weed, chihuahuan amaranth, Chinese spinach, choito, coimicoyo, common amaranth, common waterhemp, crispleaf amaranth, cuime, efo tete, elephant head amaranth, Florida amaranth, foxtail amaranth, fringed amaranth, fringed pigweed, fuchsschwanz, golden grain of the Gods, green amaranth, greenstripe, Gregg's amaranth, guegui, hinn choy, huautli, Indian spinach, Joseph's coat, khada sag, kiwicha, komo, kulitis, lady bleeding, large-fruit amaranth, lenga lenga, linoleic acid, livid amaranth, love-lies-bleeding, lovely bleeding, mat amaranth, mchicha, Mexican grain amaranth, millmi, mystical grains of the Aztecs, oleic acid, pale-seeded amaranth, palmer pigweed, Palmer's amaranth, palmitic acid, pendant amaranth, pigweed amaranth, pilewort, Powell amaranth, Powell pigweed, prickly amaranth, Prince-of-Wales-feather, Prince's feather, princess feather, Pringle's amaranth, prostrate amaranth, prostrate pigweed, purple amaranth, quilete, quinoa de castilla, quintonil, ramdana, red amaranth, red cockscomb, red-root amaranth, redroot pigweed, Reuzen amaranth, rough-fruit amaranth, sandhill amaranth, sangorache, seaside amaranth, sharp-lobe amaranth, slender amaranth, smooth amaranth, smooth pigweed, southern amaranth, spinach grass, spiny amaranth, spleen amaranth, spreading amaranth, squalene, stearic acid, super grain of the Aztecs, surinam spinach, tall amaranth, tall waterhemp, tampala, tassel flower, thorny amaranth, thotakura, Thunberg's amaranth, tidal-marsh amaranth, Torrey's amaranth, Trans-Pecos amaranth, tropical amaranth, tumble pigweed, tumbleweed, vegetable amaranth, velvet flower, vitamin E, Watson's amaranth, white pigweed, wild beet, wild blite, Wright's amaranth, yin choi.

BACKGROUND

- Amaranth is grown in Asia and the Americas, and harvested primarily for its grain, which is used as a food source for bread, pasta, and infant food.
- Amaranth oil has been shown to decrease cholesterol and lipid levels when taken with a low-sodium, heart-healthy diet. However, other studies have shown that amaranth in conjunction with a low-fat diet has no effect on cholesterol levels in patients with high cholesterol. Early research has also shown that amaranth oil may lower reduce blood glucose.
- Scientific evidence of an effect of amaranth for any indication is inadequate. High-quality research is needed before a recommendation can be made.

EVIDENCE

Uses Based on Scientific Evidence	Grade
Antioxidant Limited evidence suggests that amaranth may have antioxidant properties when combined with a heart-healthy diet. Additional studies are needed before conclusions can be drawn.	C
Heart Disease Amaranth plus a low-sodium, heart-healthy diet decreased cholesterol and blood pressure in patients with heart disease. However, additional evidence is needed before a recommendation can be made in this area.	C
Immune System Function Limited evidence suggests that amaranth may stimulate the immune system when combined with a heart-healthy diet in patients with heart disease and high cholesterol. However, additional studies of amaranth alone are needed in this area.	C
Night Vision Early research suggests that consuming amaranth greens may improve night blindness. However, more studies are needed before a recommendation can be made.	C

Uses Based on Tradition or Theory
Abnormal menstrual bleeding, allergies, antibacterial, antifungal, antiviral, arthritis, asthma, astringent, bed sores, burns, cancer, canker sores, cosmetic uses, diabetes, diarrhea, digestion, diuretic, eczema, energy, high blood pressure, high cholesterol, inflammation,

insect bites, leukorrhea (vaginal discharge), lung cancer prevention, nosebleed, nutritional supplement (infant formulas/cereal, pediatric, preschool children), pain, psoriasis, rash, ulcers, wound care.

DOSING
Adults (18 Years and Older)

- A tea may be prepared by adding 1 teaspoon of amaranth leaves to 1 cup of cold water and consuming 1-2 cups per day. As an antioxidant, 200-400 mg of squalene, a constituent of amaranth, has been used daily. To enhance immune function, 600 mg of squalene has been used daily. A daily dose of 18 mg of amaranth oil has been used for 3 weeks for heart disease. For night vision, a daily dose of 850 µg retinol equivalents in the form of amaranth leaves has been used in pregnant women for 6 days per week for 6 weeks.

Children (Younger than 18 Years)

- There is insufficient evidence to recommend a dose for amaranth in children.

SAFETY
Allergies

- Individuals with allergy or sensitivity to amaranth should avoid use of amaranth.

Side Effects and Warnings

- Evidence is limited regarding adverse effects of amaranth. Amaranth may contain high levels of cadmium, nitrates, antitrypsin proteins, and heat-labile factors, which may affect the nervous system. In addition, amaranth grown in nitrogen-rich soil may cause health problems. Amaranth should be used cautiously in those with kidney disorders due to its high oxalate content.
- Amaranth may increase or decrease immune function and should be used with caution in patients with immune disorders and in those taking drugs, herbs, or supplements that affect the immune system.
- Amaranth may lower blood glucose levels. Caution is advised in patients with diabetes or hypoglycemia and in those taking drugs, herbs, or supplements that affect blood glucose. Blood glucose levels may need to be monitored. Medication adjustments may be necessary.

- Amaranth may lower blood pressure. Caution is advised in patients with low blood pressure and in those taking drugs, herbs, or supplements that affect blood pressure. Blood pressure may need to be monitored, and medication adjustments may be necessary.

Pregnancy and Breastfeeding

- Amaranth is not recommended in pregnant or breastfeeding women due to a lack of available scientific evidence.

INTERACTIONS
Interactions with Drugs

- Amaranth may lower blood glucose levels. Caution is advised when using medications that may also lower blood glucose. Blood glucose levels may need to be monitored. Medication adjustments may be necessary.
- Amaranth may lower blood pressure. Caution is advised when using medications that may also lower blood pressure. Blood pressure may need to be monitored, and medication adjustments may be necessary.
- Amaranth may alter the effects of antihistamines.
- Amaranth may increase or decrease the immune system. Caution is advised with immunosuppressants.
- Amaranth may have cholesterol-lowering effects. Use with other cholesterol-lowering agents may have additive effects.

Interactions with Herbs and Dietary Supplements

- Amaranth may lower blood glucose levels. Caution is advised when using herbs or supplements that may also lower blood glucose. Blood glucose levels should be monitored closely, and dosage adjustments may be necessary.
- Amaranth may blood pressure. Caution is advised when using herbs or supplements that may also lower blood pressure. Blood pressure may need to be monitored, and medication adjustments may be necessary.
- Amaranth may alter the effects of antihistamines.
- Amaranth may increase or decrease the immune system. Caution is advised with immunosuppressants.
- Amaranth may have cholesterol-lowering effects. Use with other cholesterol-lowering agents may have additive effects.
- Amaranth may affect the levels of amino acid–containing supplements and some essential fatty acids.

For a complete list of references, please visit www.naturalstandard.com.

RELATED TERMS

- American false hellebore, American white hellebore, cevadine, corn lily, cryptenamine, cyclopamine, false hellebore, germidine, germitrine, green corn lily, green false hellebore, green hellebore, green veratrum, hellebore, Indian poke, itch weed, jervine, jervine alkaloids, Liliaceae (family), Melanthiaceae (subfamily), muldamine, O-acetyljervine, protoveratrine, poison lily, proveratrine, swamp hellebore, verat-v., veratramine, veratridine, *Veratrum viride*, Veratrone, veriloid, Vergitryl, Vertavis, white American hellebore.
- **Note:** Much of the toxicological data in this monograph is based on the European white hellebore (*Veratrum album*) because American hellebore and European white hellebore contain jervine alkaloids, the constituents responsible for the plants' toxic cardiovascular effects.

BACKGROUND

- American hellebore is a perennial plant native to the swampy areas and moist meadows of the eastern and western United States. The root and rhizome of American hellebore has been used historically for fever, pain, and high blood pressure, with a decoction (boiled in water) of the root being used for chronic coughs and constipation. Historically, the whole plant was not routinely used medicinally, only the root and rhizome. Although American hellebore was formerly used as a tea or tincture, potentially toxic and irritating constituents preclude its modern-day use by ingestion.
- The toxic effects associated with American hellebore limit its ability to be used as an agent to treat hypertension (high blood pressure), related kidney/heart diseases, and hypertension associated with preeclampsia in pregnancy.
- Currently, scientific information is lacking regarding the safety or effectiveness of American hellebore as a whole plant, or homeopathically. Most studies have investigated the isolated jervine alkaloids.

EVIDENCE

Uses Based on Scientific Evidence	Grade
Cardiovascular and Renal Dysfunction Isolated jervine alkaloids found in American hellebore have been studied for use in cardiovascular and renal (kidney) dysfunction. Additional study is needed before a firm recommendation can be made.	C
Hypertension (High Blood Pressure) Isolated jervine alkaloids found in American hellebore have been used to treat hypertension; however, other herbs and prescription drugs that can treat this condition have fewer toxic side effects. Additional study is needed in this area.	C
Preeclampsia and Pregnancy-Induced Hypertension Isolated jervine alkaloids found in American hellebore may be beneficial for preeclampsia and pregnancy-induced hypertension, but other herbs and prescription drugs that can treat this condition have fewer toxic side effects. Additional study is needed in this area.	C

Uses Based on Tradition or Theory

Antioxidant, arrhythmia (abnormal heart rhythms), bruises, cardiac conditions, cerebrovascular accident (stroke), diaphoretic (promotes sweating), emetic (induces vomiting), expectorant, fever reducer, fractures, heart rate reduction (homeopathic), lice, mental illness, pain, pesticide, skin care (topical rubefacient), snake bite, sprains.

DOSING

Adults (18 Years and Older)

- Currently, scientific information about safe or effective dosing of American hellebore in adults is unavailable. Most preparations used in studies contain isolated jervine alkaloids from American hellebore (Vertavis, Veratrone); no doses of whole American hellebore have been noted.

Children (Younger than 18 Years)

- There is insufficient evidence to recommend a dose for American hellebore in children.

SAFETY

Allergies

- Use of American hellebore should be avoided in individuals with a known allergy or hypersensitivity to plants in the lily family (Liliaceae) or a known allergy to American hellebore or any related species of *Veratrum*.

Side Effects and Warnings

- American hellebore does not seem to be well tolerated in humans. Even at recommended doses, American hellebore may cause toxicity that may result in death. The isolated chemical constituents (steroidal alkaloids) have been reported to cause arrhythmias (irregular heartbeat), bradycardia (slowed heart rate), hypotension (low blood pressure), headache, nausea, vomiting, diarrhea, gastrointestinal upset, and altered renal (kidney) function. Patients with cardiovascular disorders should use caution when taking American hellebore.
- Homeopathic American hellebore may be safe for use, but currently there is a lack of available information regarding side effects.

Pregnancy and Breastfeeding

- American hellebore should be avoided in pregnant and breastfeeding women because it may be toxic even at therapeutic doses.

INTERACTIONS
Interactions with Drugs

- The use of American hellebore or its alkaloidal constituents could cause arrhythmia (irregular heartbeat), and combination with antiarrhythmic drugs may be unsafe. Caution is advised.
- American hellebore or its alkaloidal constituents may lower blood pressure. Combined use with blood pressure–lowering agents (antihypertensives) may result in dangerously low blood pressure.
- American hellebore or its alkaloidal constituents may cause a decrease in glomerular filtration rate (GFR) and effective renal blood flow. Thus, American hellebore may interact with certain medications that increase urine flow (diuretics), such as chlorothiazide (Diuril). Preparations of American hellebore may also interact with drugs that are excreted through the kidneys or that are potentially toxic to the kidneys.

- Isolated constituents found in American hellebore may have beta-agonist or beta-antagonist activity. Caution is warranted in patients taking beta-agonists and beta-antagonist agents.

Interactions with Herbs and Dietary Supplements

- The use of American hellebore or its alkaloidal constituents could cause arrhythmia (irregular heartbeat), and combination with antiarrhythmic herbs and supplements may be unsafe. Caution is advised.
- American hellebore or its alkaloidal constituents may lower blood pressure. Combined use with blood pressure–lowering herbs and supplements may result in dangerously low blood pressure.
- American hellebore or its alkaloidal constituents may cause a decrease in GFR and effective renal blood flow. Thus, American hellebore may interact with certain herbs and supplements that increase urine flow (diuretics). Preparations may also interact with herbs and supplements that are excreted through the kidneys or that are potentially toxic to the kidneys.

For a complete list of references, please visit www.naturalstandard.com.

RELATED TERMS

- Acetogenin, alkaloids, American paw paw, annomontacin, Annonaceae (family), Annonaceous acetogenins, *Annona cherimola, Annona diversifolia, Annona glabra, Annona muricata, Annona palustris, Annona purpurea, Annona reticulata, Annona squamosa, Annona squamosa* X *Annona cherimola, Annona triloba* L., annonacin, annonacin-A, asimicin, asimilobin, asimin, *Asimina incarna, Asimina longifolia, Asimina obovata, Asimina parviflora, Asimina pygmaea, Asimina reticulata, Asimina tetramera, Asimina triloba* (L.) Dunal, *Asimina* X *nashii,* asiminacin, asiminecin, asiminocin, asimitrin, asitrocin, asitrilobins, atemoya, benzyltetrahydroisoquinolone alkaloids, biriba, Brazilian pawpaw, bullanin, bullatacin, bullatacinone, bullatetrocin, bulletin, *Carica papaya,* cherimoya, coumaroyltyramine, custard apple, *Deeringothamnus rugelii, Deeringothamnus puchellus, Disepalum,* dog banana, dwarf pawpaw, feruloyltyramine, flag pawpaw, flavonoids, gigantetrocinone, *Goniothalanus,* graviola, guanabana, Hoosier banana, ilama, Indiana banana, isoannonacin, murisolinone, nicotiflorine, octanoate, opossum pawpaw, Ozark banana, papaya, paw paw, Paw Paw Cell-Reg, poor man's banana, prairie banana, *Rollinia mucosa,* rutin, soncoya, soursop, squamolone, sugar apple, sweetsop, syringaresinol, trilobacin, trilobalicin, *Uvaria,* West Virginia banana, xylomaticin, *Xylopia.*
- **Note:** American pawpaw (*Asimina triloba*) is not a papaya and should not be confused with *Carica papaya* or *Annona muricata* (graviola), although the species have similar common names and may be called pawpaw.

BACKGROUND

- American pawpaw (*Annona triloba*) is a fruiting tree native to North America. However, plantings of the tree can be found in Asia, Australia, and Europe. Pawpaw extract is made from the twigs of the tree.
- In the 1980s and 1990s, researchers at Purdue University isolated compounds from pawpaw bark extracts. Many of these compounds were found to have cytotoxic effects on cancer cell lines. Currently, there is a lack of available scientific evidence supporting the safety or effectiveness of pawpaw for any condition.

EVIDENCE

Uses Based on Scientific Evidence	Grade
Cancer Treatment Pawpaw extract may have some anticancer activity, but additional study is needed to make a firm recommendation.	C
Lice Pawpaw extract in combination with thymol and tea tree oil in a shampoo formulation may be effective for the eradication of lice. Studies of better quality using pawpaw alone are needed before a firm recommendation can be made.	C

Uses Based on Tradition or Theory

Antibacterial, antifungal, anti-inflammatory (for the mouth and throat), antiprotozoal, antiviral, emetic (induced vomiting), fat substitute, fever reducer, food uses, insecticide (nematodes), pesticide, scarlet fever, skin rashes.

DOSING
Adults (18 Years and Older)

- Dosing from scientific studies has not been proven safe or effective. For cancer, 12.5-50 mg of extract has been taken by mouth four times a day with food for 18 months. For lice, 40 mL of Paw Paw Lice Remover Shampoo (0.5% pawpaw extract, 1% thymol, and 0.5% tea tree oil) applied three times to dry hair, once every 8 days for up to 24 days, has been used.

Children (Younger than 18 Years)

- Dosing from scientific trials has not been proven safe or effective. For lice, 40 mL of Paw Paw Lice Remover Shampoo (0.5% pawpaw extract, 1% thymol, and 0.5% tea tree oil) applied three times to dry hair, once every 8 days for up to 24 days, has been used.

SAFETY
Allergies

- Pawpaw should be avoided in individuals with a known allergy or hypersensitivity to *Annona triloba,* or any other members of the Annonaceae plant family (including other species of *Asimina* and species in the genera *Annona, Deeringothamnus, Disepalum, Goniothalanus, Rollinia, Uvaria,* and *Xylopia*).

Side Effects and Warnings

- Safety information about pawpaw extracts is lacking. The constituents in pawpaw extract are cytotoxic. Taking pawpaw extract by mouth is not recommended without the supervision of a qualified health care professional, including a pharmacist.
- Patients with gastrointestinal problems or a history of skin reactions should use pawpaw cautiously because nausea, vomiting, and adverse skin reaction have been reported after taking pawpaw by mouth.
- Patients with known allergy or hypersensitivity to *Annona triloba* or any other members of the Annonaceae plant family should avoid pawpaw due to the possibility of developing urticaria (hives), reddening of the skin, or itching.

Pregnancy and Breastfeeding

- Use of pawpaw during pregnancy or breastfeeding is not recommended due to the cytotoxic effects of pawpaw extract.

INTERACTIONS
Interactions with Drugs

- Insufficient available evidence.

Interactions with Herbs and Dietary Supplements

- The combined use of 7-keto (a metabolite of the hormone DHEA) and pawpaw extract may lessen the effect of 7-keto, and combined use of these agents may be ineffective. Patients taking herbs and supplements should consult with a qualified health care professional, including a pharmacist, before combining therapies.

- Pawpaw may interact with coenzyme Q10. It may also interact with antioxidant herbs and supplements. Caution is advised.

For a complete list of references, please visit www. naturalstandard.com.

Amylase Inhibitors

RELATED TERMS

- AAI, alphaAI-1, alphaAI-2, arcelin-5, bean amylase inhibitors, Calorex, Fabaceae (family), Phase 2, Phase 2 Starch Neutralizer, phaseolamin, *Phaseolus vulgaris* extract, starch blockers, Starchex, wheat amylase inhibitor, wheat proteinaceous alpha-amylase inhibitors (alpha-AIs), white kidney bean extract.

BACKGROUND

- Amylase is an enzyme that breaks down carbohydrates or starches in the body. Because of their purported ability to prevent starch breakdown and absorption, alpha amylase inhibitors have been used for weight loss. At this time, commercially available amylase inhibitors are extracted from wheat or white kidney bean (*Phaseolus vulgaris*).
- In humans, amylase inhibitors have been shown to decrease intestinal absorption of carbohydrates by reducing intestinal amylase activity. However, there are few high-quality human studies that support the use of amylase inhibitors for any indication.

EVIDENCE

Uses Based on Scientific Evidence	Grade
Diabetes Amylase inhibitors have been shown to decrease levels of blood glucose. Large, well-designed studies are needed before a firm recommendation can be made.	C
Obesity and Weight Loss Preliminary studies have shown that taking an amylase inhibitor with meals may lead to weight loss. However, well-designed clinical studies are needed in this area.	C

Uses Based on Tradition or Theory
Antibacterial, antifungal, insecticide.

DOSING

Adults (18 Years and Older)

- Various doses of amylase inhibitors have been studied, but no dose has been proven effective. Typically, 1500-6000 mg of amylase inhibitors has been used before meals.
- For diabetes, 4-6 g has been used for 7 days. For weight loss, a dose of 3000 amylase inhibitor units from Phase 2 (white kidney bean–derived amylase inhibitor) has been used daily for 30 days. A dose of 1500 mg Phase 2 has been used twice daily for 8 weeks without effect.

Children (Younger than 18 Years)

- There is insufficient evidence to recommend a dose for amylase inhibitors in children.

SAFETY

Allergies

- Amylase inhibitors should be avoided in individuals with known allergy or sensitivity to amylase inhibitors or sources of amylase inhibitors, such as wheat or legumes.

Side Effects and Warnings

- Amylase inhibitors may lower blood glucose levels. Caution is advised in patients with diabetes or hypoglycemia and in those taking drugs, herbs, or supplements that affect blood glucose. Blood glucose levels may need to be monitored, and medication adjustments may be necessary.
- Amylase inhibitors should be used with caution in individuals with gastrointestinal disorders, kidney disorders, or liver problems. When used in combination with other weight loss agents, amylase inhibitors may have additive effects.

Pregnancy and Breastfeeding

- Amylase inhibitors are not recommended in pregnant or breastfeeding women due to a lack of available scientific evidence.

INTERACTIONS

Interactions with Drugs

- Amylase inhibitors may lower blood glucose levels. Caution is advised when using medications that may also lower blood glucose. Patients taking drugs for diabetes by mouth or injection should be monitored closely. Medication adjustments may be necessary.
- When taken with other weight loss agents, amylase inhibitors may have additive effects.

Interactions with Herbs and Dietary Supplements

- Amylase inhibitors may lower blood glucose levels. Caution is advised when using herbs or supplements that may also lower blood glucose. Blood glucose levels may require monitoring, and doses may need to be adjusted.
- When taken with other weight loss agents, including *Garcinia cambogia*, inulin, and rosmarinic acid, amylase inhibitors may have additive effects. Amylase inhibitors may also interact with guar gum.

For a complete list of references, please visit www.naturalstandard.com.

Andrographis paniculata
(Nees, Kan Jang, SHA-10)

RELATED TERMS

- Andrographolide, Chuan Xin Lin, Green chiretta, Kalmegh leaf extract, Kan Jang, King of Bitters, Kold Kare, Remdex.

BACKGROUND

- The leaves of *Andrographis paniculata* have been used in Indian folk medicine and Ayurveda for centuries. The Chinese and Thai herbal medicine systems have also used this herb, mostly for its "bitter" properties, as a treatment for digestive problems and for various fever-causing illnesses. More recently, this herb has become popular in Scandinavia as a remedy for upper respiratory infections (URIs) and the flu.
- The most widely tested product is a product called Kan Jang (Swedish Herbal Institute). This product is available with andrographis alone and in combination with *Eleutherococcus senticosus*. Kan jang has been studied for upper respiratory tract infections and male fertility.
- There is reasonably strong evidence from clinical trials to suggest that andrographis effectively reduces the severity and the duration of URIs. It has also been studied in human clinical trials for the flu and familial Mediterranean fever. Based on animal and laboratory studies, andrographis may have many other potential therapeutic uses, including as an anti-inflammatory agent and as a treatment for chemically induced liver damage.

EVIDENCE

Uses Based on Scientific Evidence	Grade
Upper Respiratory Tract Infection: Treatment Research suggests that andrographis may reduce symptom severity and duration in active URIs if started within 36-48 hours after symptoms develop. Additional studies are needed, especially studies that test the effects of andrographis alone.	A
Familial Mediterranean Fever Familial Mediterranean fever is a genetic disorder that mainly affects ethnic groups around the Mediterranean, causing recurrent episodes of fever and swelling of serous membranes. Although early studies suggest that a combination product containing andrographis may reduce the duration, frequency, and severity of attacks among children, more studies using andrographis alone are needed.	C
Influenza Early studies suggest that andrographis may reduce the duration and severity of flu symptoms and the amount of sick time taken off work by patients with the flu. More research is needed to confirm these results.	C
Upper Respiratory Tract Infection: Prevention Early studies suggest that andrographis extract may help prevent URIs during the winter months if taken daily. Larger studies are required to confirm these results.	C

Uses Based on Tradition or Theory

Allergies, antioxidant, atherosclerosis (clogged arteries), blood purifier, blood vessel dilation, cancer, cholera, diabetes, dysentery, fever, gonorrhea, human immunodeficiency virus (HIV), increasing sperm count, indigestion, inflammation, intestinal worms (*Ascaris lumbricoides*), jaundice, liver protection, malaria, male contraception, multiple sclerosis, postoperative recovery, prevention of blood clots, prevention of heart muscle injury, reperfusion injury (prevention), shock, snake bite, vitiligo.

DOSING

Adults (18 Years and Older)

- Preparations that contain 48-60 mg of andrographolide constituents have been taken in divided doses three or four times daily for respiratory infections. A 300-mg Kan Jang tablet containing 4% andrographolides has been taken four times daily for cold treatment (for a total daily dose of 48 mg of andrographolides). Smaller daily doses (e.g., 200-300 mg) have been tested for prevention of respiratory infections. Use seems to be safe for 2 weeks. Larger doses may be unsafe and cause side effects. Long-term use of andrographis preparations (>2 weeks) has not been well studied.
- Doses of 500-3000 mg of andrographis leaf have been taken by mouth three times daily.
- For digestive problems, a tea made with 1 teaspoon of herb per 1 cup of water, steeped for 5-10 minutes, has been taken with meals.

Children (Younger than 18 Years)

- There is limited research available in children. Children 4-11 years old have taken 2 tablets three times daily (about 30 mg daily of andrographolide and deoxyandrographolide) for 10 days.
- In Indian Ayurvedic formulas, andrographis leaves and juice are mixed with cardamom, clove, and cinnamon to treat colic and other stomach ailments in infants. However, these uses are not well supported by scientific evidence.

SAFETY

Allergies

- There have been cases of severe allergic reactions (anaphylaxis), including one case of shock associated with andrographis.

Side Effects and Warnings

- Andrographis taken at common doses appears to be relatively safe. Reported side effects include nausea, vomiting, and abdominal discomfort. At high doses (5-10 mg/kg body weight), patients have experienced nausea, diarrhea, and metallic taste. Rare side effects include headache, dizziness, drowsiness, fatigue, chest discomfort, increased nasal discharge, "blocked nose," and lymph node pain.

- Andrographis should be used cautiously in patients with low blood pressure, diabetes, or bleeding disorders.

Pregnancy and Breastfeeding

- Andrographis is not recommended during pregnancy due to possible contraceptive effects observed in animal studies. Safety during breastfeeding is unknown. In theory, andrographis may decrease sperm count.

INTERACTIONS

Interactions with Drugs

- Andrographis may increase the risk of bleeding. It should be used cautiously in patients taking anticoagulant agents, such as warfarin (Coumadin) or heparin, or antiplatelet agents, such as ibuprofen (Motrin, Advil) or clopidogrel (Plavix). Andrographis use should be stopped before some surgeries; this should be discussed with a health care professional.
- Andrographis may lower blood pressure and may add to the effects of drugs taken to lower blood pressure. Patients with high or low blood pressure who are considering taking any of these agents should discuss options with health care professionals. Dosing adjustments may be necessary.
- Andrographis may decrease blood glucose levels. Concurrent use of andrographis with drugs that lower blood glucose may cause additive effects and increase the risk of hypoglycemia. Blood glucose should be monitored. Dosing adjustments may be necessary.

- Andrographis may also interact with allergy, anti-inflammatory, anticancer, antiviral, fertility, and immunomodulatory drugs.

Interactions with Herbs and Dietary Supplements

- Andrographis may increase the risk of bleeding, and should be used cautiously in patients taking anticoagulant agents. Multiple cases of bleeding have been reported with the use of *Ginkgo biloba*; fewer cases have been reported with garlic and saw palmetto. Numerous other agents may theoretically increase the risk of bleeding, although this has not been proven in most cases.
- In theory, andrographis may lower blood pressure and may add to the effects of other agents that also lower blood pressure. Patients with high or low blood pressure who are considering taking any of these agents should discuss options with their health care professionals.
- Andrographis may decrease blood glucose levels. Concurrent use of andrographis with herbs and supplements that lower blood glucose, such as bitter melon (*Momordica charantia*), may cause additive effects and increase the risk of hypoglycemia. Blood glucose should be monitored. Dosing adjustments may be necessary.
- Andrographis may also interact with anti-inflammatory, anticancer, antiviral, immunomodulatory, and fertility herbs and supplements.

For a complete list of references, please visit www. naturalstandard.com.

Angostura
(Galipea officinalis, Angostura trifoliata)

RELATED TERMS

- Allocspariene, *Angostura trifoliata, Angostura trifoliate, Bonplandia trifoliata* Willd., candicine, *Cusparia febrifuga* Humb. ex DC., *Cusparia felorifuga, Cusparia trifoliata* (Willd.) Engl., *Galipea, Galipea officinalis,* galipinine, quinolones, Rutaceae (family), tetrahydroquinolines.

BACKGROUND

- Angostura (*Galipea officinalis, Angostura trifoliata*) is a shrublike tree that has been studied for its potential antibiotic and cytotoxic (cell-killing) activity. The bark is thought to be the main source of its medicinal properties.
- Although the angostura tree and Angostura aromatic bitters bear the same name, the bitters were named after the city, Angostura, Venezuela, and the proprietary formula is not said to contain angostura.
- There is not enough human data available to support the use of angostura for any indication.

EVIDENCE

Uses Based on Scientific Evidence

No available studies qualify for inclusion in the evidence table.

Uses Based on Tradition or Theory

Antibacterial, cancer, digestive, malaria, tuberculosis.

DOSING

Adults (18 Years and Older)

- There is no proven safe or effective dose for angostura.

Children (Younger than 18 Years)

- There is no proven safe or effective dose for angostura.

SAFETY

Allergies

- Angostura should be avoided with known allergy or hypersensitivity to angostura, its constituents, or members of the Rutaceae family.

Side Effects and Warnings

- Angostura should be used with caution in patients taking antibiotics or being treated for tuberculosis.
- Angostura should be used with caution in patients taking anticancer or antimalaria drugs.

Pregnancy and Breastfeeding

- Angostura cannot be recommended during pregnancy or breastfeeding because scientific safety data are lacking.

INTERACTIONS

Interactions with Drugs

- Angostura may interact with antimalaria or anticancer drugs.
- Angostura may interact with antibiotics that fight tuberculosis-causing bacteria.

Interactions with Herbs and Dietary Supplements

- Angostura may interact with herbs and supplements that have activity against malaria and the bacteria that cause tuberculosis.
- Angostura may interact with herbs and supplements with anticancer activity.

For a complete list of references, please visit www.naturalstandard.com.

Anhydrous Crystalline Maltose

RELATED TERMS

- ACM, disaccharide.

BACKGROUND

- Anhydrous crystalline maltose (ACM) has been used as a food stabilizer and a desiccant (chemical agent used to absorb moisture) for use in foods, cosmetics, and pharmaceuticals.
- ACM has been studied in patients with Sjögren's syndrome (inflammatory autoimmune disorder) for treatment of dry mouth.
- Limited information is currently available about the effects of ACM for the treatment of any indication in humans.

EVIDENCE

Uses Based on Scientific Evidence	Grade
Dry Mouth (Sjögren's Syndrome) ACM has been studied and may be effective for relieving symptoms of dry mouth associated with Sjögren's syndrome (inflammatory autoimmune disorder characterized by dry mouth and dry eyes). Additional study is needed.	C

Uses Based on Tradition or Theory
Available evidence is insufficient.

DOSING

Adults (18 Years and Older)

- There is no proven effective dose for ACM. However, for relief of dry mouth, 200-mg lozenges by mouth three times daily for up to 24 weeks has been used.

Children (Younger than 18 Years)

- There is no proven safe or effective dose for ACM in children.

SAFETY

Allergies

- Avoid in individuals with a known allergy or hypersensitivity to ACM.

Side Effects and Warnings

- ACM seems to be safe, although there is a lack of available reports on adverse events. Avoid in patients with a known allergy or hypersensitivity to anhydrous crystalline maltose.

Pregnancy and Breastfeeding

- ACM is not recommended in pregnant or breastfeeding women due to a lack of available scientific evidence.

INTERACTIONS

Interactions with Drugs

- Insufficient available evidence.

Interactions with Herbs and Dietary Supplements

- Insufficient available evidence.

For a complete list of references, please visit www.naturalstandard.com.

Anise

RELATED TERMS

- Anace, anason, aneys, anice, anis, anís, aniseed, anise seed, anisi, anisi fructus, anisi vulgaris, anison (Greek), anissame, anisu, anisum (Latin), anisun, anisur, anis vert (French), anny, annyle, anysum (Arabic), Apiaceae (family), fruto de anis (Spanish), fructus anisi, graines d'anis (French), p-anisaldehyde, *Pimpinella anisetum*, *Pimpinella anisum*, saunf, sconio, semi d'Aniso (Italian), simiente de anis (Spanish), sompf, souf, sweet Alice, sweet cumin, Tut-te See-Hau.

BACKGROUND

- Anise is native to the eastern Mediterranean and is one of the oldest known spice plants used for medicinal purposes and for cooking. It is a member of the Apiaceae family, which includes carrot, parsley, dill, fennel, coriander, cumin, and caraway.
- The Greek name *anison* and the Latin name *anisum* were derived from the early Arabic name *anysum*. Evidence has shown that anise was used in Egypt in 1500 B.C. The Romans used anise-spiced cakes after heavy meals to aid digestion. Because of its strong licorice flavor, the oil of anise is mixed with wine to form the liqueur anisette. It is also found in raki, a Turkish alcoholic beverage, and ouzo, a Greek alcoholic beverage.
- Anise is mostly used as a spice in cooking. It is used medicinally to promote digestion and to increase urine flow. Anise oil is also used in flavoring artificial licorice candies, cough lozenges, and syrups.
- Anise is used in Europe to aid in the treatment of cancer. In Mexico, Turkey, and China, it is used as a carminative (promotes digestion) and galactagogue (lactation stimulant). Elsewhere, it is used to induce abortions and to treat respiratory illnesses, such as asthma, bronchitis, and cough. Anise is recognized by the U.S. Food and Drug Administration (FDA) as generally recognized as safe (GRAS).

EVIDENCE

Uses Based on Scientific Evidence

No available studies qualify for inclusion in the evidence table.

Uses Based on Tradition or Theory

Abortifacient (induces abortion), andropause/andrenopause (male climacteric symptoms), anemia, antibacterial, anticonvulsant, antidepressant, antifungal, anti-inflammatory, antioxidant, antiparasitic, antispasmodic, anxiety, asthma, bronchitis, bronchodilator, cancer, carminative (promotes digestion), catarrh (inflammation of mucous membrane), cathartic, childbirth facilitation/induction, chronic diarrhea, common cold, cough, diaphoretic (promotes sweating), diuretic (increases urine flow), dropsy (edema), dyspepsia (stomach upset), emmenagogue (menstrual flow stimulant), estrogenic effects, expectorant (expels phlegm), flatulence (gas), flavoring, fragrance, galactagogue (lactation stimulant), gallbladder disorders, heart disease, *Helicobacter pylori* infection, hernia, hiccups, influenza, insecticide (house dust mites), insecticide (mosquitoes), insomnia, intestinal colic, kidney problems, laxative, libido, lice, menopausal symptoms, mental performance, mosquito repellent, muscle aches, osteoporosis prevention, pain (eye), pain relief, psoriasis (chronic skin disease), respiratory disorders, rheumatic disorders, scabies, sedative, sore throat, vascular problems (decreased vascular wall tension), whooping cough.

DOSING

Adults (18 Years and Older)

- Based on the available scientific evidence, there is no proven safe or effective dose for anise. As a digestive aid, essence of aniseed in hot water at bedtime has been used.

Children (Younger than 18 Years)

- Based on the available scientific evidence, there is no proven safe or effective dose for anise in children. For runny nose, half a pint of boiling water poured on 2 teaspoons of bruised anise seed, sweetened and frequently given cold in doses of 1-3 teaspoons has been used. For colic, 10-30 grains of bruised (lightly ground) or powdered seeds steeped in distilled hot water, taken in "wineglassful" doses, has been used; 4-20 drops of anise essential oil on sugar has also been used.

SAFETY

Allergies

- Individuals with a known allergy or hypersensitivity to anise (*Pimpinella anisum*) or any of its constituents should not take anise. Individuals with a known allergy to any members of the Apiaceae family (formerly known as the Umbelliferae family) also should not take anise because of cross-sensitivity to spices. Urticaria (hives) has been reported.

Side Effects and Warnings

- Anise is possibly safe when used as a flavoring agent and in doses found in foods. A nationwide outbreak of *Salmonella* serotype Agona caused by aniseed-containing herbal tea occurred from October 2002 through July 2003 among infants in Germany. Consumers should adhere strictly to brewing instructions.
- Cardiorespiratory arrest, hypertension (high blood pressure), and muscle weakness have been reported after consumption of an alcohol-free anise-flavored beverage. It is unclear whether these side effects were due to anise flavoring or glycyrrhizinic acid, which is the active ingredient in licorice root. Many anise-flavored beverages contain licorice root, which has been associated with the above adverse effects. Many anise-containing beverages also contain alcohol, which may cause nausea and vomiting when taken with metronidazole (Flagyl) or disulfiram (Antabuse).
- Anise may increase sensitivity to light when applied on the skin because it contains coumarin constituents. Anise may have diuretic (increases urine flow), anticoagulant ("thins" the blood), and alter blood glucose levels. Anise oil should not be ingested because it may cause nausea, pulmonary edema (fluid in lungs), seizures, and vomiting.

- Caution is advised in patients with endometriosis, estrogen-dependent cancers, and diabetes.

Pregnancy and Breastfeeding

- Anise is not recommended in pregnant or breastfeeding women because scientific evidence is lacking. Traditionally, anise has been used to induce abortions and as a galactagogue (stimulates lactation).

INTERACTIONS
Interactions with Drugs

- Anise contains coumarins and may increase the risk of bleeding when taken with drugs that also increase the risk of bleeding. Examples include aspirin, anticoagulants ("blood thinners") such as warfarin (Coumadin) and heparin, antiplatelet drugs such as clopidogrel (Plavix), and non-steroidal anti-inflammatory drugs (NSAIDs) such as ibuprofen (Motrin, Advil) and naproxen (Naprosyn, Aleve).
- Anise may have diuretic (increase flow of urine) effects and may have additive effects and increase the risk of electrolyte imbalances when used with other diuretic medications. Patients taking any diuretic medications should consult with a qualified health care professional, including a pharmacist.
- Aniseed oil has been shown to increase glucose absorption. Caution is advised when using medications that may lower blood glucose. Patients taking drugs for diabetes should be monitored closely by a qualified health care professional. Medication adjustments may be necessary.

- Many anise-containing beverages contain alcohol and may cause nausea or vomiting when taken with metronidazole (Flagyl) or disulfiram (Antabuse).
- Anise may increase sensitivity to light when applied on the skin. Caution is advised when using with other medications that increase light sensitivity.

Interactions with Herbs and Dietary Supplements

- Anise contains coumarins, and may increase the risk of bleeding when taken with herbs or supplements that also increase the risk of bleeding. Multiple cases of bleeding have been reported with the use of *Ginkgo biloba*, and two cases have been reported with saw palmetto. Numerous other agents may theoretically increase the risk of bleeding, although this has not been proven in most cases.
- Anise may have diuretic (increase flow of urine) effects and may have additive effects and increase the risk of electrolyte imbalances when used with other diuretic herbs/supplements. Patients taking any diuretic herbs/supplements should consult with a qualified health care professional, including a pharmacist.
- Aniseed oil has been shown to increase glucose absorption. Caution is advised when using herbs or supplements that may lower blood glucose.
- Anise may increase sensitivity to light when applied on the skin because it contains coumarin constituents. Caution is advised when using anise with other herbs and supplements that increase light sensitivity.

For a complete list of references, please visit www.naturalstandard.com.

Antineoplastons

RELATED TERMS

- A1, A2, A3, A4, A5, A10, A10-1, AS2-1, AS2-5, AS5, antineoplaston A, antineoplaston Ch, antineoplaston F, antineoplaston H, antineoplaston K, antineoplaston L, antineoplaston O, 3-N-phenylacetylaminopiperidine-2,6 dione, phenylacetylglutamine (PAG), phenylacetylisoglutamine (PAIG), phenylacetic acid (PAA), 3-phenylacetylamino-2,6-piperidinedione, sodium phenylacetate.

BACKGROUND

- Antineoplastons are a group of naturally occurring peptide fractions, which were observed by Burzynski in the late 1970s to be absent in the urine of cancer patients. It was hypothesized that these substances may have antitumor properties. In the 1980s, Burzynski identified chemical structures for several of these antineoplastons and developed a process to prepare them synthetically. Antineoplaston A10, identified as 3-phenylacetylamino-2,6-piperidinedione, was the first to be synthesized.

- The use of antineoplastons in the treatment of various cancer types has been studied in the laboratory and in animals, and in limited preliminary human research. In 1991, the Cancer Therapy Evaluation Program of the National Cancer Institute (NCI) examined records of seven patients with brain tumors treated at the Burzynski Clinic in Texas. Based on their findings, the NCI sponsored a brain tumor clinical trial. However, due to difficulty recruiting patients and a disagreement over study design, this research was canceled. The results in nine patients included before cancellation were reported, but were not conclusive. In 1997, Burzynski had legal troubles for permitting antineoplastons to be shipped out of Texas.

- Sufficient evidence from randomized, controlled trials in support of antineoplastons as a cancer treatment is lacking, and antineoplastons are not U.S. Food and Drug Administration (FDA) approved therapies. Antineoplastons are not widely available in the United States, and safety and efficacy are not proven. Multiple studies of antineoplastons in various cancers have been sponsored by the Burzynski Research Institute. In recent years, antineoplastons have also been suggested as treatment for other conditions, such as Parkinson's disease, sickle cell anemia, and thalassemia.

EVIDENCE

Uses Based on Scientific Evidence	Grade
Cancer There is inconclusive scientific evidence regarding the effectiveness of antineoplastons in the treatment of cancer. Several preliminary human studies (case series, phase I/II trials) have examined antineoplaston types A2, A5, A10, AS2-1, and AS2-5 for various cancer types. It remains unclear if antineoplastons are effective, or what doses may be safe. Until better research is available, no clear conclusion can be drawn.	C
HIV A small preliminary study published by Burzynski and colleagues in 1992 reported increased energy and weight in patients with human immunodeficiency virus (HIV), and a decreased number of opportunistic infections and increased CD4$^+$ counts overall. These patients were treated with antineoplaston AS2-1. However, this evidence cannot be considered conclusive. Currently, there are drug therapy regimens available for HIV with clearly demonstrated effects (highly active antiretroviral therapy [HAART]); patients with HIV are recommended to consult with a physician about treatment options.	C
Sickle Cell Anemia and Thalassemia A small preliminary study reported positive findings related to sickle cell anemia and thalassemia, but currently evidence is insufficient to make a clear recommendation in this area.	C

Uses Based on Tradition or Theory

Acute lymphocytic leukemia, adenocarcinoma, aging, astrocytoma, basal cell epithelioma, brain and central nervous system tumors, cholesterol and triglyceride abnormalities, chronic lymphocytic leukemia, encephalitis, glioblastoma, hepatocellular carcinoma, leukocytosis, malignant melanoma, medulloblastoma, metastatic synovial sarcoma, Parkinson's disease, promyelocytic leukemia, recurrent glioma, thrombocytosis.

DOSING

Adults (18 Years and Older)

- Various doses of antineoplastons have been used in preliminary studies. Safety and efficacy are not proven for any specific dose or use. Doses of antineoplaston A10 used by mouth in studies range from 10-40 g daily or 100-288 mg/kg body weight per day. Duration of use has varied. Antineoplaston AS2-1 has been studied at doses ranging from 12-30 g daily or 97-130 mg/kg body weight per day. Antineoplastons have also been studied when applied to the skin, injected through the veins (intravenous), and injected into muscles (intramuscular).

Children (Younger than 18 Years)

- There is insufficient evidence to recommend a dose for antineoplastons in children.

SAFETY

Allergies

- Allergic skin rash has been reported after injection of antineoplaston AS2-1. Individuals who have reacted to antineoplastons in the past should avoid this therapy.

Side Effects and Warnings

- Adverse effects are reported in several preliminary studies. It is not clear how common these reactions are, or if they occur more frequently than with placebo. Because many patients taking antineoplastons have been diagnosed with serious illnesses such as advanced cancers, it is not clear if these effects are from the illnesses themselves or caused by antineoplastons.

- Antineoplaston therapy has been associated with drowsiness, headache, fatigue, mild dizziness and vertigo, and confusion. Antineoplaston A10 is retained in the brain tissue of animals, although the importance of this in humans is not known. Weakness, nausea, vomiting, upset stomach, abdominal pain, and increased flatulence (gas) have been reported.
- Various types of antineoplastons administered for periods ranging from weeks to years have been associated with sore throat, fever, chills, reduced blood albumin levels, liver function test abnormalities, low blood glucose levels (hypoglycemia), low potassium, and a strong body odor similar to urine.
- Palpitations, high blood pressure (hypertension), and water retention (mild peripheral edema) have been noted. Chest pressure and irregular or fast heartbeat have also been observed. Joint swelling, muscle and joint pain, muscle

contractions in the throat, weakness, and finger rigidity have been reported in clinical trials.
- Decreases in blood platelets, red blood cells, and white blood cells have been observed. Other serious reported effects include slow or abnormal breathing, metabolic and electrolyte abnormalities, brain swelling (cerebral edema), dangerously low blood pressure (hypotension), and death.

Pregnancy and Breastfeeding

- The safety of antineoplastons during pregnancy or breastfeeding is not known, and therefore cannot be recommended.

INTERACTIONS

Interactions with Drugs, Herbs, and Dietary Supplements

- Limited information is available about interactions with antineoplastons. Agents with effects similar to antineoplastons and that may have additive effects when used concurrently include agents that lower potassium or glucose levels or that cause liver damage. It is not known if antineoplastons add to the effects of chemotherapeutic drugs.

For a complete list of references, please visit www.naturalstandard.com.

Apple Cider Vinegar

RELATED TERMS

- Acetic acid, ACV, apple cider vinegar plus honey cocktail, apple cider vinegar tablets, cider vinegar, *Malus sylvestris*, Mother Nature's perfect food.

BACKGROUND

- Apple cider vinegar (ACV) is prepared by pulverizing apples into a slurry of juice and pulp and then adding yeast and sugars.
- Reports of the healing properties of apple cider vinegar date to 3300 B.C. In 400 B.C., Hippocrates supposedly used apple cider vinegar as a healing elixir, an antibiotic, and for general health. Samurai warriors purportedly used a vinegar tonic for strength and power. U.S. Civil War soldiers used a vinegar solution to prevent gastric upset and as a treatment for pneumonia and scurvy.
- Apple cider vinegar has been used alone and in combination with other agents for many health conditions. Anecdotally, ancient Egyptians used apple cider vinegar for weight loss. During the diet "craze" of the 1970s, proponents suggested that a combination of apple cider, kelp, vitamin B_6, and lecithin could "trick" the body's metabolism into burning fat faster. Claims of preventing viral and bacterial infections, and allergic reactions to pollen, dander, and dust stem from the proposed ability of apple cider vinegar to prevent alkalinization of the body. However, there is not enough scientific evidence to form a clear conclusion about the efficacy or safety of apple cider vinegar for any health condition.
- There may be long-term risks associated with the acidity of apple cider vinegar, including low blood potassium levels (hypokalemia) or diminished bone mineral density.

EVIDENCE

Uses Based on Scientific Evidence

No available studies qualify for inclusion in the evidence table.

Uses Based on Tradition or Theory

Acne (topical), amino acid source, antiaging (alone or with honey), antiseptic (for gastrointestinal tract), appetite suppression, arthritis, asthma, bladder cleanser, bowel stone prevention in horses, circulation improvement, colitis, dandruff prevention (topical), decongestant, dental conditions, detoxification, diarrhea, digestion aid, dizziness, ear discharge, eczema, fatigue, flavoring agent, food poisoning, hair loss (topical), hair rinse, hay fever, headache, hearing impairment, heartburn, hemorrhage, hiccoughs, high blood pressure, high cholesterol, household sanitizer, immune enhancement, infections, insect bites (topical), insomnia, itchy scalp (topical), kidney cleanser, leg cramps, menstruation regulation, mental alertness, mineral source, nail problems, nervousness, nosebleeds, obesity, osteoporosis, queasy stomach, scurvy prevention, shingles (topical), sinus congestion, skin toner (topical), sore eyes, sore throat, strength enhancement, stuffy nose, sunburn (topical), tired eyes, vaginitis (added to baths), varicose veins, viral hepatitis, vitamin source, weight loss.

DOSING

Adults (18 Years and Older)

- No specific doses are supported by well-designed clinical trials. In general, 2 teaspoons of cider vinegar have been taken in 1 cup water three times daily. Also, 285-mg tablets have been taken with meals. Topical and rectal preparations have also been used, but their safety is unclear.

Children (Younger than 18 Years)

- There is insufficient evidence to recommend a dose for apple cider vinegar in children.

SAFETY

Allergies

- Caution should be exercised in patients with known allergy or hypersensitivity to apple cider vinegar or any of its ingredients, including apples and pectin.

Side Effects and Warnings

- There are few scientific studies of the safety of apple cider vinegar. The acidity of undiluted apple cider vinegar may destroy tooth enamel when sipped orally. Apple cider vinegar should be used cautiously in patients with low potassium levels and patients taking potassium-lowering medications. It should be used cautiously in patients with diabetes because apple cider vinegar may contain chromium, which may affect insulin levels. Apple cider vinegar should be used cautiously in patients with osteoporosis, based on one case report. Sipping or drinking undiluted apple cider vinegar should be avoided.

Pregnancy and Breastfeeding

- Use of apple cider vinegar is not recommended in pregnant and breastfeeding women because of lack of sufficient data. Apple cider vinegar is likely safe when taken orally as food flavoring, but possibly unsafe when used in larger amounts.

INTERACTIONS

Interactions with Drugs

- Theoretical interactions are based on potential pH-altering effects of apple cider vinegar. The degree to which apple cider vinegar affects blood pH is currently not established.
- Theoretically, long-term oral use of apple cider vinegar can decrease potassium levels, increasing the risk of toxicity of cardiac glycoside drugs such as digoxin (Lanoxin). Long-term use may also add to the potassium-lowering effects of insulin, laxatives, and diuretics such as furosemide (Lasix).

Interactions with Herbs and Dietary Supplements

- Theoretical interactions are based on potential pH-altering effects of apple cider vinegar. The degree to which apple cider vinegar affects blood pH is currently not established.
- Theoretically, long-term oral use of apple cider vinegar can decrease potassium levels; this may increase the risk of toxicity of cardiac glycoside herbs, add to the potassium-lowering effects of diuretics, and add to the potassium-lowering effects of laxative herbs.

For a complete list of references, please visit www.naturalstandard.com.

Arabinogalactan

RELATED TERMS

- AG, alpha-arabinofuranose, Ambrotose, amphotericin B-arabinogalactan conjugates, *Andrographis paniculata*, arabinans, arabinogalactan protein, arabinogalactan pectin, arabinose, BCG-CWS, *Biophytum petersianum* Klotzsch, Biophytum sensitivum (L.) DC, *Codium dwarkense, Codium tomentosum*, D-arabino-D-galactan, D-galactopyranose, D-galactose, D-glucose, D-rhamnose, *Euonymus sieboldiana* seeds, fiber, galactan, galactosamine, galactose, galacturonic acid, GalN, glucuronic acid, *Juniperus scopolorum* cones, Kaki fruits, L-arabinofuranose, L-arabinose, larch, larch arabinogalactan, larch gum, larch tree, *Larix, Larix decidua, Larix kaempferi, Larix laricina, Larix occidentalis,* Lch, Mongolian larch, Mongolian larchwood, mountain larch, mugwort pollen, *Mycobacterium avium, Mycobacterium bovis* BCG, *Mycobacterium bovis bacillus* Calmette-Guerin, *Mycobacterium leprae, Mycobacterium tuberculosis, Mycobacterium vaccae*, neutral arabinogalactan, Nocardia, pectic arabinogalactan, Pinaceae (family), polysaccharide, ragweed pollen, rhamno-arabinogalactans, rhamnose, *Silene vulgaris,* soluble fiber, stractan, sulfated arabinogalactan, tamarack, *Trichilia emetica*, ukonan C, Vk2a, Vk100A2a, *Vernonia kotschyana, Viscum album,* western larch, western tamarack, wild indigo *(Baptisia tinctoria)*, wood gum, wood sugar, xylose.
- **Note:** Arabinogalactan is found in many species of plants and is thought to be the primary active compound in the larch tree (*Larix* spp.). This monograph includes studies on arabinogalactan isolated from other species of plants as well.

BACKGROUND

- Arabinogalactans belong to a group of carbohydrates called *polysaccharides*. Most commercial preparations of arabinogalactan come from the wood of the larch tree (*Larix* species) Arabinogalactan is approved for use as a dietary fiber by the U.S. Food and Drug Administration (FDA).
- As a dietary supplement, larch arabinogalactan is taken to stimulate the immune system, to fight cancer, and as a prebiotic (a substance used to improve bacteria in the colon). Early studies suggest that arabinogalactan may help grow beneficial bacteria in the digestive tract. However, clinical studies have not consistently shown that larch arabinogalactan stimulates the immune system when used as a monotherapy.
- Nonetheless, arabinogalactan may potentially improve the effectiveness of certain drugs. Thus, there is some potential for larch arabinogalactan as an adjunct therapy.
- Arabinogalactans are found in the cell walls of plants and bacteria. It is also found in pollens from mugwort and ragweed that causes allergies. Although these arabinogalactans are also included in this monograph, there is no conclusive evidence to suggest that dietary arabinogalactans from larch or other plant species have similar allergenic effects.

EVIDENCE

Uses Based on Scientific Evidence	Grade
High Cholesterol Although arabinogalactan is a dietary fiber, it is unclear how it affects blood lipid levels (including triglycerides) in patients with high cholesterol. Limited early studies have not shown an effect of arabinogalactan in patients with normal cholesterol levels.	C
Hyperglycemia (High Blood Sugar Levels) Arabinogalactan's effects on blood sugar and insulin levels have been studied. In people without diabetes, it has not been shown to affect these levels.	C
Immune Stimulation There is some evidence suggesting immune-stimulating activity in arabinogalactan; however, its effect on immunity in healthy volunteers is not clear.	C
Kidney Disease (Chronic Renal Failure) Although early results of arabinogalactan's effect in patients with chronic kidney failure are promising, more studies are needed.	C

Uses Based on Tradition or Theory

Allergies, anti-inflammatory, antimicrobial, antiviral, anxiety, arthritis, asthma, attention deficit hyperactivity disorder, autism, autoimmune disorders, bipolar disorder, bladder infections, blood thinner, cancer, colitis, common cold, Crohn's disease, depression, digestive tonic, Down's syndrome, dry eyes, ear infections, encephalopathy (brain disease), endometriosis, eye problems (scratches), fatigue, fibromyalgia, flu, gene therapy, gout, learning disabilities, leprosy, liver protection, mood enhancement, multiple sclerosis, parasites (leishmania), sepsis (blood infection caused by endotoxin), skin conditions, stomach problems (gastritis), ulcers, wound healing, yeast infection.

DOSING

Adults (18 Years and Older)

- There is insufficient evidence to recommend a dose for arabinogalactan in adults. A dose of 1.5-50 g of arabinogalactan has been used daily for up to 6 months.

Children (Younger than 18 Years)

- There is insufficient evidence to recommend a dose for arabinogalactan in children, and pediatric use is not recommended.

SAFETY

Allergies

- Avoid with allergy or hypersensitivity to arabinogalactan or larch.

Side Effects and Warnings

- Arabinogalactan may lower blood sugar levels. Caution is advised in patients with diabetes or low blood sugar and in those taking drugs, herbs, or supplements that affect blood sugar. Blood glucose levels may need to be monitored by a qualified health care professional, and medication adjustments may be necessary.
- Arabinogalactan may cause bloating and abdominal discomfort in people with digestive disorders. Use with caution in people who consume a high-fiber or low-galactose diet.
- Arabinogalactan may have an effect on immune function and should be used with caution in people with immune disorders.
- Occupational exposure to larch dust may cause chronic lung, eye, and skin irritation.

Pregnancy and Breastfeeding

- Arabinogalactan is not recommended in pregnant or breastfeeding women due to a lack of available scientific evidence.

INTERACTIONS

Interactions with Drugs

- Arabinogalactan may lower blood sugar levels. Caution is advised when using drugs that may also lower blood sugar.

Patients taking drugs for diabetes by mouth or injection should be monitored closely by a qualified health care professional. Dosing adjustments may be necessary.
- Arabinogalactan may have additive or competing effects when taken with immune modulating, anticancer, cholesterol-lowering, anti-gout, antifungal, and antibiotic drugs, as well as with drugs that are eliminated by the kidney. Arabinogalactan may also interact with amphotericin B, nucleotide analogs, and antituberculosis drugs.

Interactions with Herbs and Dietary Supplements

- Arabinogalactan may lower blood sugar levels. Caution is advised when using herbs or supplements that may also lower blood sugar levels. Blood glucose levels may require monitoring, and doses may need adjustment.
- Arabinogalactan may have additive or competing effects when taken with immune modulating, anticancer, cholesterol-lowering, anti-gout, antifungal, antibiotic, antituberculosis, and antioxidant herbs and supplements, as well as herbs and supplements that are eliminated by the kidney. Arabinogalactan may also interact with echinacea, mugwort, ragweed, prebiotics, and probiotics.

For a complete list of references, please visit www.naturalstandard.com.

Arabinoxylan

RELATED TERMS

- Arabinoxylane, *Arctostaphylos uva-ursi*, AX, BioBran, cinnaman AX, *Cinnamomum cassia*, *Ganoderma lucidum*, *Hyphomycetes mycelia*, kawaratake mushroom, MGN-3, rice bran, shiitake mushroom, suehirotake mushroom.

BACKGROUND

- Altering the outer shell of rice bran using enzymes from Hyphomycetes mycelia mushroom extract produces arabinoxylan compound. The product called *MGN-3* (or Bio-Bran in Japan) is a complex containing arabinoxylan as a major component.
- Arabinoxylan has been found to improve immune reactions in diabetes and cancer patients. MGN-3 may also be of potential value in treating AIDS patients or patients undergoing chemotherapy. However, there is currently a lack of strong human scientific evidence to support the use of arabinoxylan for any indication.
- Although presented by manufacturers as a generally safe substance without side effects at recommended doses, the U.S. Food and Drug Administration (FDA) ordered a permanent court order in 2004 against the manufacturers of MGN-3, charging that it has been inappropriately promoted as a drug treatment for cancer, diabetes, and HIV.

EVIDENCE

Uses Based on Scientific Evidence	Grade
Cancer (Various Types) Arabinoxylan has been studied in the treatment of cancer. However, the evidence thus far has been inconclusive.	C
Diabetes (Type 2) There is currently a lack of scientific evidence investigating the role of arabinoxylan in diabetics.	C

Uses Based on Tradition or Theory
Asthma, cardiovascular disease, chemotherapy adverse effects (adriamycin chemotherapy gastroprotection, cisplatin chemotherapy gastroprotection), chemotherapy-induced leukopenia (abnormally low white blood cell count), chronic fatigue syndrome, hepatitis, herpes zoster, high cholesterol, HIV, hypertension (high blood pressure), immune system deficiencies, insomnia, neurasthenia (nervous exhaustion), poisoning, postherpetic neuralgia (nerve pain), respiratory disease, stress reduction, tonic (kidney), ulcers.

DOSING

Adults (18 Years and Older)

- For general maintenance, 600 mg daily in divided doses has been used. In clinical research, 3 g of MGN-3 has been given daily for up to 6 months to patients with different types of malignancies (such as multiple myeloma, leukemia, and cancers of the prostate, breast, and cervix). Doses of 15, 30, and 45 mg/kg of MGN-3 have also been taken daily for 2 months.
- For diabetes, 1-12 g of arabinoxylan-rich fiber has been used daily.

Children (Younger than 18 Years)

- There is insufficient evidence to recommend a dose for arabinoxylan in children.

SAFETY

Allergies

- Avoid in people with a known allergy or hypersensitivity to arabinoxylan, mushrooms, yeast, or rice bran.
- Users of MGN-3 (BioBran) should be aware of other constituents (e.g., cornstarch, dextrin, tricalcium phosphate, and silicon dioxide). Patients with allergies or hypersensitivities to these constituents should not take MGN-3.

Side Effects and Warnings

- In general, safety data are lacking; however, arabinoxylan has been well tolerated in clinical practice in Japan at recommended doses for short periods of time.
- Arabinoxylan products such as MGN-3 (BioBran) may contain high calcium and phosphorus levels, which may be harmful for patients with compromised renal (kidney) function.
- Because arabinoxylan may lower blood sugar, patients with diabetes and those taking blood sugar–lowering medications should use arabinoxylan cautiously.

Pregnancy and Breastfeeding

- Arabinoxylan is not recommended in pregnant or breastfeeding women due to a lack of available scientific evidence.

INTERACTIONS

Interactions with Drugs

- MGN-3 may be safely and advantageously used with chemotherapy and radiation to increase the cytotoxic effect of the therapy and to decrease adverse side effects. A qualified health care practitioner, including a pharmacist, should be consulted before combining arabinoxylan with other medications or therapies.
- Arabinoxylan may reduce blood sugar levels and could theoretically interact with blood sugar–lowering medications taken by mouth or insulin.
- Arabinoxylan may possess immunostimulatory properties and could theoretically interact with other drugs that alter the immune system. Caution is advised.

Interactions with Herbs and Dietary Supplements

- Preparations of MGN-3 (BioBran) arabinoxylan product contain unclear amounts of calcium and phosphorous.
- Arabinoxylan may reduce blood sugar levels and could theoretically interact with blood sugar–lowering herbs and supplements.
- Arabinoxylan may possess immunostimulatory properties and could theoretically interact with other herbs and supplements that alter the immune system. Caution is advised.

For a complete list of references, please visit www.naturalstandard.com.

Arginine (L-arginine)

RELATED TERMS

- 2-amino-5-guanidinopentanoic acid, Arg, arginine, arginine hydrochloride (intravenous formulation), dipeptide arginyl aspartate, HeartBars, ibuprofen-arginate, L-arg, L-arginine, NG-monomethyl-L-arginine, Sargenor, Spedifen.
- **Note:** Arginine vasopressin is different from arginine/L-arginine and has an entirely different mechanism. NG-monomethyl-L-arginine is different from arginine/L-arginine and functions as an inhibitor of nitric oxide synthesis.

BACKGROUND

- L-Arginine was first isolated in 1886. In 1932, scientists learned that L-arginine is needed to create urea, a waste product that is necessary for toxic ammonia to be removed from the body. In 1939, researchers discovered that L-arginine is also needed to make creatine, which breaks down into creatinine at a constant rate, and it is cleared from the body by the kidneys.
- Arginine is considered a semi-essential amino acid because even though the body normally makes enough of it, supplementation is sometimes needed. For example, people with protein malnutrition, excessive ammonia production, excessive lysine intake, burns, infections, peritoneal dialysis, rapid growth, urea synthesis disorders, or sepsis may not have enough arginine. Symptoms of arginine deficiency include poor wound healing, hair loss, skin rash, constipation, and fatty liver.
- Arginine changes into nitric oxide, which causes blood vessel relaxation (vasodilation). There is some evidence suggesting that arginine may help treat medical conditions that improve with vasodilation, such as chest pain, clogged arteries (atherosclerosis), coronary artery disease, erectile dysfunction, heart failure, intermittent claudication/peripheral vascular disease, and blood vessel swelling that causes headaches (vascular headaches). Arginine also triggers the body to make protein and has been studied for wound healing, bodybuilding, enhancement of sperm production (spermatogenesis), and prevention of wasting in people with critical illnesses.
- Arginine hydrochloride has a high chloride content and has been used to treat metabolic alkalosis. This use should be under the supervision of a qualified health care professional.
- In general, most people do not need to take arginine supplements because the body usually produces sufficient quantities.

EVIDENCE

Uses Based on Scientific Evidence	Grade
Growth Hormone Reserve Test/Pituitary Disorder Diagnosis Arginine can be injected to measure growth hormone levels in people who might have growth hormone imbalances, such as panhypopituitarism, gigantism, acromegaly, or pituitary adenoma. The U.S. Food and Drug Administration (FDA) has approved this use.	A
Inborn Errors of Urea Synthesis In patients with inborn errors of urea synthesis, high ammonia levels in the blood and metabolic alkalosis may occur, particularly among patients with ornithine carbamoyl transferase (OCT) deficiencies or carbamoyl phosphate synthetase (CPS) deficiencies. Arginine may help treatment by shifting the way the body processes nitrogen. Arginine should be avoided in patients with hyperargininemia (high arginine levels). Other drugs, such as citrulline, sodium benzoate, or sodium phenylbutyrate, may have similar benefits. However, dialysis may be needed at first. This use of arginine should be supervised by a qualified health care professional.	A
Coronary Artery Disease/Angina Early evidence from several studies suggests that arginine taken by mouth or injection may improve exercise tolerance and blood flow in the arteries of the heart. Benefits have been shown in some patients with coronary artery disease and chest pain (angina). However, more research is needed to confirm these findings and to develop safe and effective doses.	B
Critical Illness Some studies suggest that arginine may be beneficial for people with critical or life-threatening illnesses when it is added to nutritional supplements. However, it is unclear what the specific role of arginine is in recovery. Because of the potential for toxicity, large doses of arginine should be avoided.	B
Heart Failure Studies using arginine in patients with chronic heart failure have shown mixed results. Some studies report improved exercise tolerance.	B
Migraine Headache Early studies suggest that adding arginine to ibuprofen (e.g., Motrin or Advil) therapy may decrease migraine headache pain.	B
Peripheral Vascular Disease/Claudication Intermittent claudication causes leg pain and tiredness because cholesterol plaques or clots develop in leg arteries and block blood flow. A small number of studies report that arginine therapy may improve walking distance in patients with claudication.	B
Adrenoleukodystrophy (ALD) Adrenoleukodystrophy (ALD) is a rare inherited metabolic disorder that is characterized by the loss of fatty coverings (myelin sheaths) on nerve fibers in the brain and progressive destruction of the adrenal glands. This condition results in dementia and	C

(Continued)

Uses Based on Scientific Evidence	Grade
adrenal failure. Arginine injections may help manage this disorder, although most study results are inconclusive. Further research is needed to clarify the effects of arginine in ALD.	
Anal Fissures There is some evidence suggesting that arginine may help treat chronic anal fissures, which are small tears that develop in the anus.	C
Autonomic Failure Arginine has been studied in autonomic failure, a condition that may include low blood pressure, but the effect is unclear. Well-designed studies will help clarify this relationship.	C
Breast Cancer It is unclear if arginine can help treat breast cancer patients. Results from early human studies are mixed.	C
Burns Arginine may improve immune function and protein function in burn patients; however, further evidence is needed before arginine can be recommended as a treatment for burn victims.	C
Chemotherapy Adjuvant Clinical studies suggest that arginine supplements may be beneficial for patients undergoing chemotherapy. Larger, high-quality studies are warranted.	C
Chest Pain (Non-Cardiac) Small studies in humans suggest that arginine taken by mouth (not injected) may improve non-cardiac chest pain associated with esophageal motor disorders.	C
Circulation Problems (Critical Limb Ischemia) There is some clinical evidence suggesting that intravenous arginine may increase blood flow in patients with critical limb ischemia. This condition occurs when blood flow to the arms and/or legs is blocked.	C
Dental Pain (Ibuprofen Arginate) Some research suggests that ibuprofen-arginate (Spedifen) may reduce pain after dental surgery faster or more effectively than ibuprofen (e.g., Motrin or Advil) alone.	C
Diabetes (Type 1/Type 2) Early studies in humans suggest that arginine supplements may decrease the severity of diabetes.	C
Diabetic Complications Early studies in humans suggest that arginine supplements may help the body fight some long-term	C

complications of diabetes, including heart disease and nerve damage.

Erectile Dysfunction Early studies have shown that arginine supplements may help treat erectile dysfunction (ED) in men with low nitrate levels in their blood or urine. A combination of ʟ-arginine, glutamate, and yohimbine hydrochloride has been used to treat ED. However, because a combination product was used and yohimbine hydrochloride is an FDA-approved therapy for this condition, the effects of arginine alone are unknown. More research using arginine monotherapy is warranted.	C
Gastrointestinal Cancer Surgery A combination of arginine and omega-3 fatty acids may reduce the length of hospital stays and infections after surgery in gastrointestinal cancer patients. Other research suggests that arginine, omega-3 fatty acids, and glutamine may boost the immune system and reduce inflammation after surgery. More research with arginine alone is needed.	C
Heart Protection during Coronary Artery Bypass Grafting (CABG) Arginine-supplemented "blood cardioplegic solution" may help protect the heart, although this remains inconclusive.	C
High Blood Pressure Some clinical evidence suggests that arginine taken by mouth may help widen the arteries and temporarily reduce blood pressure in patients with high blood pressure and type 2 diabetes. Further clinical evidence is warranted.	C
High Cholesterol Some research suggests that arginine may help treat or prevent high cholesterol.	C
Immunomodulator There is some evidence suggesting that arginine supplementation may boost the immune response elicited by the pneumonia vaccine in older adults. More studies are needed to confirm these results.	C
Intrauterine Growth Retardation Some studies in pregnant women suggest that arginine supplements may improve growth in fetuses that are smaller than average. Additional studies are needed.	C
Kidney Disease or Failure Study results are mixed as to whether arginine as a therapy alone directly helps certain kidney diseases or failure. Arginine may be a helpful adjunct for kidney disease–related conditions such as anemia in older adults.	C

Uses Based on Scientific Evidence	Grade
MELAS Syndrome Some studies have found that long-term supplementation with L-arginine significantly improves endothelial function in patients with MELAS syndrome (mitochondrial myopathy, encephalopathy, lactic acidosis, and stroke).	C
Myocardial Infarction (Heart Attack) Study results of arginine supplementation after myocardial infarction (heart attack) are mixed. Further research is needed before a recommendation can be made. A cardiologist and a pharmacist should be consulted before arginine supplements are taken.	C
Preeclampsia (High Blood Pressure in Pregnancy) Early studies suggest that long-term supplementation with L-arginine may decrease high blood pressure in pregnant women. Arginine may also improve fetal health and growth during preeclampsia. Further research is needed to confirm these results.	C
Pressure Ulcers Studies of arginine for pressure ulcers show mixed results.	C
Prevention of Restenosis after Coronary Angioplasty (PTCA) Arginine has been injected in patients who had stents surgically inserted into arteries in order to widen them. Early research suggests that this therapy may help prevent the arteries from becoming narrow again (called *restenosis*). Additional studies are needed.	C
Raynaud's Phenomenon Early studies in humans have considered the effect of arginine on blood vessel activity in Raynaud's phenomenon, a condition that causes the blood vessels in the fingers, toes, nose, and ears to narrow in response to cold temperatures or stress. However, the effects of arginine remain unclear.	C
Recovery after Surgery Some evidence suggests that arginine may be beneficial when used as a supplement after surgery. However, the role of arginine in this condition is unclear.	C
Respiratory Infections Some studies suggest that arginine supplements may decrease the risk of respiratory (lung) infections.	C
Senile Dementia There is not enough information available to make conclusions about the use of arginine in senile dementia.	C
Transplants Dietary supplementation with L-arginine and canola oil has been associated with decreased rejection rates after the first month in kidney transplant patients. Because it may reduce the risk of heart problems, long-term benefits for patient survival may be particularly important.	C
Wound Healing Arginine has been suggested to improve the rate of wound healing in older adults. Research has shown that an enteral diet supplemented with arginine and fiber improved wound healing after surgery in patients with head and neck cancer. Arginine has also been applied to the skin in order to improve wound healing.	C
Altitude Sickness Based on early research, L-arginine supplementation is not an effective therapy to prevent acute mountain sickness (AMS).	D
Cyclosporine Toxicity Animal studies report that arginine blocks the poisonous (toxic) effects of cyclosporine, a drug used to prevent organ transplant rejection. However, results from human studies have not found that arginine offers any protection from cyclosporine-induced toxicity.	D
Exercise Performance Overall, current available study results conclude that arginine supplementation does not improve exercise performance.	D
Infertility Although there are several studies in this area, it is not clear what effect arginine has on improving the likelihood of getting pregnant. Evidence thus far does not support the use of arginine as a fertility treatment in women who are undergoing *in vitro* fertilization or in men with abnormal sperm.	D
Interstitial Cystitis Arginine has been proposed as a treatment for interstitial cystitis or inflammation of the bladder. However, most human studies have not found that arginine improves symptoms such as urinary frequency or urgency.	D
Kidney Protection during Angiography The contrast media, or dye, used during angiography to map a patient's arteries (or during some CT scans) can be poisonous (toxic) to the kidneys, especially among people with kidney disease. Researchers have studied L-arginine as a way to protect the kidneys in patients with long-term kidney failure who were undergoing angiography. The authors found no evidence that injections of L-arginine protect the kidney from damage due to contrast.	D

(Continued)

Uses Based on Scientific Evidence	Grade
Asthma Although it has been suggested that arginine may treat asthma, human studies have actually found that arginine *worsens* inflammation in the lungs and *contributes* to asthma symptoms. Therefore, taking arginine by mouth or by inhalation is not recommended in people with asthma.	F

Uses Based on Tradition or Theory

AIDS/HIV (prevention of wasting), ammonia toxicity, anti-aging, anti-inflammatory, antiplatelet agent, anxiety, beta-hemoglobinopathies, cancer, chronic pain, cirrhosis, cold prevention, cystic fibrosis, endocrine disorders (metabolic syndrome), glaucoma, hemolytic uremic syndrome (HUS), hepatic encephalopathy, increased muscle mass, infantile necrotizing enterocolitis, infection, inflammatory bowel disease (IBD), ischemic stroke, liver disease, lower esophageal sphincter relaxation, metabolic acidosis, obesity, osteoporosis, pain, peritonitis, preterm labor contractions, sepsis, sexual arousal, sexual function in women, sickle cell anemia, stress, stomach motility disorders, stomach ulcers, supplementation of a low-protein diet, thrombotic thrombocytopenic purpura (TTP), trauma (recovery), tumors, ulcerative colitis.

DOSING
Dietary Sources of Arginine

- Walnuts, filberts (hazelnuts), pecans, Brazil nuts, sesame and sunflower seeds, brown rice, raisins, coconut, gelatin, buckwheat, almonds, barley, cashews, cereals, chicken, chocolate, corn, dairy products, meats, oats, and peanuts.

Adults (18 Years and Older)

- There is a lack of standard or well-established doses of arginine, and many different doses have been used and studied. A common dose is 2-3 g taken by mouth three times daily. In studies, 0.5-16 g of arginine has been taken daily by mouth for up to 6 months. Arginine has been applied to the skin in order to improve wound healing.
- Doses of arginine used intravenously depend on specific institutional dosing guidelines and should be given under the supervision of a health care provider.

Children (Younger than 18 Years)

- There is insufficient evidence to recommend a dose for arginine in children. Pediatric supplementation is not recommended due to potential toxicity.

SAFETY
Allergies

- A severe allergic reaction called *anaphylaxis* has occurred after arginine injections. People with allergies should avoid arginine. Signs of allergy may include rash, itching, or shortness of breath.

Side Effects and Warnings

- Arginine has been well tolerated by most people in studies lasting for up to six months, although there is a possibility of serious side effects (including toxicity) in some people.
- Stomach discomfort, including nausea, stomach cramps, or an increased number of stools, may occur. If arginine is inhaled, people with asthma may experience a worsening of symptoms that may be related to allergy.
- Other potential side effects include low blood pressure and changes in numerous chemicals and electrolytes in the blood. Examples include high potassium, high chloride, low sodium, low phosphate, high blood urea nitrogen, and high creatinine levels. People with liver or kidney diseases may be especially sensitive to these complications and should avoid using arginine except under medical supervision. After injections of arginine, low back pain, flushing, headache, numbness, restless legs, venous irritation, and death of surrounding tissues have been reported.
- In theory, arginine may increase the risk of bleeding. Patients using anticoagulants (blood thinners) or antiplatelet drugs or those with underlying bleeding disorders should speak with their qualified health care providers before using arginine and should be monitored.
- Arginine may increase blood sugar levels. Caution is advised in patients taking prescription drugs to control sugar levels.
- Arginine may increase potassium levels, especially in patients with liver disease.
- L-Arginine may worsen symptoms of sickle cell disease.

Pregnancy and Breastfeeding

- There is insufficient evidence to recommend arginine supplemention during pregnancy or breastfeeding.
- L-Arginine has been used in pregnant women with high blood pressure (preeclampsia) until 10 days after birth, but it should not be used without supervision of an OB/GYN and a pharmacist.

INTERACTIONS
Interactions with Drugs

- Because arginine can increase the activity of some hormones in the body, many possible drug interactions may occur. The prescription drugs aminophylline and the sweetening agent xylitol may decrease the effect that arginine has on glucagon.
- Estrogens (found in birth control pills and hormone replacement therapies) may increase the effects of arginine on growth hormone, glucagon, and insulin. In contrast, progestins (also found in birth control pills and some hormone replacement therapies) may decrease the responsiveness of growth hormone to arginine.
- When used with arginine, some diuretics, such as spironolactone (Aldactone), or ACE-inhibitor blood pressure drugs, such as enalapril (Vasotec), may cause high potassium levels in the blood. Monitoring of blood potassium levels may be required.
- Arginine should be used carefully with drugs such as nitroglycerin or sildenafil (Viagra), because blood pressure may fall too low. Other side effects, such as headache and flushing, may occur when arginine is used with these drugs.
- Because arginine may cause the stomach to make more acid, it may reduce the effectiveness of drugs that block stomach acid such as ranitidine (Zantac) or esomeprazole (Nexium).
- In theory, arginine may increase the risk of bleeding when used with anticoagulants (blood thinners) or antiplatelet drugs. Examples include warfarin (Coumadin), heparin, and clopidogrel (Plavix). Some pain relievers may also increase the risk of bleeding if used with arginine. Examples

include aspirin, ibuprofen (Motrin, Advil), and naproxen (Naprosyn, Aleve, Anaprox).

- It is also possible that arginine may raise blood sugar levels. Patients taking oral or injected drugs for diabetes should be monitored closely by their health care providers while using arginine. Dosing adjustments may be necessary.
- Studies suggest that a combination of ibuprofen and arginine (ibuprofen-arginate/Spedifen) has a faster onset of pain relief than ibuprofen alone. Use of other ibuprofen-based pain relievers, such as Motrin or Advil, with ibuprofen-arginate may increase the risk of toxic effects. Patients should consult their health care providers before combining these medications.

Interactions with Herbs and Dietary Supplements

- Arginine may block the benefits of lysine in treating cold sores. It may increase the activity of growth hormone if used with ornithine.

- In theory, arginine may increase the risk of bleeding when taken with herbs and supplements that are believed to increase the risk of bleeding. Multiple cases of bleeding have been reported with the use of *Ginkgo biloba,* and fewer cases with garlic and saw palmetto. Numerous other agents may theoretically increase the risk of bleeding, although this has not been proven in most cases.
- Arginine may raise blood sugar levels. People using other herbs or supplements that may raise blood sugar levels should be monitored closely by their health care providers while using arginine. Dosing adjustments may be necessary.
- Arginine should be used cautiously in patients taking potassium supplements because of possible additive effects.

For a complete list of references, please visit www.naturalstandard.com.

Arnica

(Arnica spp.)*

RELATED TERMS

- 6-methoxykaempferol, *Aconitum napellus*, alisma, American arnica, *Arnica augustifolia*, *Arnica chamissonis*, *Arnica cordifolia*, arnica da serra, arnica flower, *Arnica fulgens*, *Arnica latifolia*, *Arnica lonchophylla*, *Arnica montana*, arnica root, *Arnica sororia*, arnica spray, *Arnicae flos*, arnicaid, arniflora, arnika, Arnikablüten, Asteraceae (family), bergwohlverleih, bétoine des montagnes, betuletol, bilmes herb, *Caltha alpina*, chamissonolid, common arnica, Compositae (family), donnerblume, engel trank, European arnica, fallherb, fallkraut, flavonoids, fleurs d'arnica, guldblomme, helenalin, herbe aux chutes, hispidulin, jaceosidin, kraftwurz, leopard's bane, lignans, monkshood, mountain arnica, mountain daisy, mountain snuff, mountain tobacco, pectolinarigenin, polmonaria di montagna, prickherb, sesquiterpene lactones, SinEcch, smokeherb, sneezewort, snuffplant, souci des alpes, Spanish flower heads, St. John's strength flower, strengthwort, tabac des Vosges, tabaco de montana, thunderwort, waldblume, wellbestow, wolfesgelega, wolf's bane, wolf's eye, wolf's yellow, wolfsbane, wolfsblume, wolfstoterin, woundherb, wundkraut.
- **Note:** This monograph does not include Mexican arnica (*Heterotheca incloides*).

BACKGROUND

- *Arnica montana* is commonly used in herbal ointments and oils applied on the skin as an anti-inflammatory and pain-relieving agent for aches, bruises, and sprains on unbroken skin. Highly diluted homeopathic preparations are considered safe and are widely used for the treatment of injuries. However, the mechanism of action remains unclear, as homeopathic preparations contain little to no active ingredients. However, full doses of arnica may be toxic when taken by mouth. Arnica may also be damaging to the heart, resulting in high blood pressure.
- The U.S. Food and Drug Administration (FDA) has declared arnica an unsafe herb due to adverse effects reported when taken by mouth. In contrast, the German market offers over 100 preparations of arnica to its consumers. In Canada, arnica is not allowed for use as a non-medicinal oral ingredient.

EVIDENCE

Uses Based on Scientific Evidence	Grade
Bruising Homeopathic and topical (on the skin) arnica is widely used to prevent or treat hemorrhages (heavy bleeding), hematomas (bruises). Effectiveness is unclear.	C
Coagulation (Blood Clotting) Homeopathic arnica does not seem to affect bleeding time or platelet count.	C
Diabetic Retinopathy Homeopathic arnica has been used for improving retinal microcirculation, thereby slowing the progression of damage to the retina of the eye in diabetics.	C
Diarrhea in Children (Acute) Arnica has not been well studied for its effects on diarrhea, but there is some inconclusive evidence that homeopathic arnica may decrease the duration of diarrhea in children.	C
Ileus (Postoperative) Postoperative ileus is characterized by a temporary impairment of gastrointestinal motility. Symptoms may include abdominal pain, nausea and vomiting, reduced desire to eat, and an inability to pass gas or stool. There is early evidence that homeopathic arnica treatment may reduce the duration of ileus after abdominal or gynecologic surgery.	C
Osteoarthritis Arnica gel has been used on the skin for osteoarthritis pain and stiffness, due to its anti-inflammatory constituents. Although there is some promising evidence, additional studies are needed.	C
Pain (Postoperative) Some patients use homeopathic arnica to relieve pain after an operation. However, arnica is often used with other pain-relieving agents. It is unclear how effective arnica is alone for the treatment of pain.	C
Stroke Homeopathic arnica has been used in stroke recovery, though the effectiveness remains uncertain.	C
Trauma Many patients use arnica to relieve pain postoperatively. Further studies are needed to define the effectiveness of arnica in postoperative pain.	C
Muscle Soreness Homeopaths believe that arnica may be effective in relieving pain due to delayed-onset muscle soreness, which is defined by exercise to which people are unaccustomed. Currently, it is not recommended to give arnica for this indication, although it appears to be safe for use.	D

Uses Based on Tradition or Theory
Abortifacient (inducing abortion), abscess (homeopathy), acne, alopecia (hair loss), angina pectoris (chest pain), antibacterial, antifungal, antihistamine, antiseptic, aphrodisiac, aphthous ulcers,

Uses Based on Tradition or Theory—Cont'd

asthma, atherosclerosis, back pain, bad breath, bed sores, blindness, blood loss (postpartum), boils (topical), breast tenderness, bronchitis, burns (post-laser treatment), cancer, canker sores, cardiac abnormalities, cardiotonic, carpal tunnel syndrome, chapped lips, chilblains (cold blisters), chronic venous insufficiency, concussions, contusions, corns, coronary artery disease, cough (smoker's cough), cramps, decongestant, dental caries, diabetes, diaphoretic (induces sweating), diarrhea, dislocations (topical), diuretic (increases urine flow), dysentery (severe diarrhea), exercise performance, exhaustion, eye strain/fatigue, fever (intermittent or traumatic), fibromyalgia, fractures, furunculosis (skin disease), gallstones, gingivitis, gonarthrosis (chronic wear of cartilage in knee joints), hepatitis, hyperlipidemia (high cholesterol), immunostimulant, inflammation, influenza, insect bites, irritated mucous membranes (nostrils), joint pain (topical), kidney problems, liver disorders, mastitis (breast infection/inflammation), miscarriage, musculoskeletal injury, myocarditis/ endocarditis (heart infections), nerve pain, paralysis (spinal), perineal trauma, pharyngitis (sore throat), pleural effusions, pulmonary embolism, respiratory problems, rheumatoid arthritis, sore throat, stimulant, surgical uses, swelling, tender feet, thirst, thrombophlebitis, tumors, varicose veins, whooping cough, wound healing.

DOSING

Adults (18 Years and Older)

- Arnica is toxic if taken internally except when diluted into homeopathic preparations. Homeopathic treatment is usually tailored specifically to the patient's symptoms. Typical homeopathic dosing uses either 5-c or 30-c potency tablets sublingually (under the tongue) three times a day. Doses can be taken for 24 hours or up to 6 months, although a qualified health care practitioner, including a pharmacist, should be consulted before making decisions about dosing.
- Other forms of arnica dosing include tinctures taken by mouth, and ointments or fresh plant gel applied on the skin. There is insufficient evidence to recommend dosing for these forms.

Children (Younger than 18 Years)

- There is insufficient evidence to recommend arnica in children.

SAFETY

Allergies

- Avoid in individuals with a known allergy or hypersensitivity to arnica or any member of the Asteraceae or Compositae families. Possible cross-sensitivity can occur in those allergic to the Asteraceae or Compositae family (*Achillea millefolium, Ambrosia* species, *Anthemis cotula* asters, calendula, chamomile, chrysanthemum, dahlia, daisy, dandelion, dog fennel chicory, *Matricaria chamomilla,* mugwort, marigold, May weed, sunflower, tansy, and yarrow).

Side Effects and Warnings

- Arnica is likely safe when used short-term in oral or sublingual (under tongue) homeopathic doses. It is possibly safe when applied topically/externally to unbroken skin for short-term use. Arnica is likely unsafe when taken by mouth in doses higher than homeopathic dilutions. It may also be unsafe when used topically (on the skin) long term. Using full strength tinctures on hypersensitive or broken skin is potentially toxic and not recommended.
- Ingestion of arnica extracts has been known to increase heartbeat and increase bleeding time.
- Allergic reactions may occur when taking arnica in full strength preparations or when handling the plant. Reactions including Sweet's syndrome; facial eczema; oral lesions (mouth wounds); itchy erythema (reddening of the skin) of the legs, trunk (torso), and face; and dermatitis.
- Taking arnica-containing extracts by mouth has caused severe gastroenteritis (inflammation of the stomach), including gastrointestinal problems due to mucosal irritation, nervousness, nausea, and vomiting.
- Arnica may also cause muscle weakness, collapse, and death. High doses may impair urine flow and damage the kidneys and liver. There is also the potential for organ damage, coma, and death with the internal use of arnica.

Pregnancy and Breastfeeding

- Internal use of arnica is not recommended in pregnant women due to the potential for uterine stimulation and toxicity. Avoid if breastfeeding.

INTERACTIONS

Interactions with Drugs

- Arnica may interact with anesthetic (pain-reducing) drugs, corticosteroids, or anti-inflammatories; reduce the effectiveness of blood pressure–lowering drugs; and/or enhance bleeding if taken with other anticoagulants (blood thinners). Caution is advised.
- Arnica applied to the skin may increase the analgesic effects of hydroxyethyl salicylate.
- Certain constituents found in arnica may lower serum lipids. Caution is advised in patients taking cholesterol-lowering medications.

Interactions with Herbs and Dietary Supplements

- Arnica may interact with herb or supplements with anesthetic (pain-reducing), steroid, or anti-inflammatory effects.
- Arnica may increase the risk of bleeding when taken with drugs that increase the risk of bleeding. Multiple cases of bleeding have been reported with the use of *Ginkgo biloba,* and fewer cases with garlic and saw palmetto.
- Arnica use may reduce the effectiveness of blood pressure–lowering herbs and supplements.
- Arnica used with daisy *(Bellis perennis)* may reduce postpartum blood loss. A qualified health care practitioner, including a pharmacist, should be consulted before combining herbs and supplements.

For a complete list of references, please visit www.naturalstandard.com.

Arrowroot
(*Maranta arundinacea*)

RELATED TERMS

- Albumen, araruta, arrowroot cookie, arrowroot starch, ash, bamboo tuber, Bermuda arrowroot, East Indian arrowroot, *Maranta arundinacea*, Marantaceae (family), obedience plant, reed arrowroot, St. Vincent arrowroot, true arrowroot, West Indian arrowroot.
- **Note:** This plant should not be confused with arrowhead (*Sagittaria* spp.) or Japanese arrowroot *(Pueraria montana)*.

BACKGROUND

- Arrowroot refers to any plant of the genus *Maranta*, but the term is most commonly used to describe the easily digestible starch obtained from the rhizomes of *Maranta arundinacea*. Other plants that produce similar starches include East Indian arrowroot *(Curcuma angustifolia)*, Queensland arrowroot (Cannaceae family), Brazilian arrowroot (Euphorbiaceae family), and Florida arrowroot (*Zamia pumila* or *Zamia integrifolia*). This monograph addresses only true arrowroot, *Maranta arundinacea*.
- The popular name *arrowroot* may be a corruption of the Aru-root of the Aruac Indians of South America or derived from its legendary use as an antidote for poison-tipped arrow toxins. The name may also come from the native Caribbean Arawak people's aru-aru (meal of meals), for whom the plant was a dietary staple.
- Arrowroot powder is prepared from the milky liquid extracted from the grated plant rhizome. Arrowroot has been studied as a remedy for diarrhea, possibly due to its high starch content. Arrowroot has also been taken by mouth as a dietary aid in gastrointestinal disorders and applied on the skin to soothe painful, irritated, or inflamed mucous membranes.

EVIDENCE

Uses Based on Scientific Evidence	Grade
Diarrhea Arrowroot is an edible starch with proposed demulcent (soothing) effects and is a well-known traditional remedy for diarrhea. Some evidence suggests that it may have a beneficial effect in the treatment of diarrhea in irritable bowel syndrome patients. Further evidence is warranted.	C

Uses Based on Tradition or Theory
Antibacterial, antidote to poisons (vegetable poisons, poison-tipped arrows), cholera, dehydration, demulcent, food uses, gangrene, gastrointestinal disorders, inflammation (mucous membranes), insect and spider bites, teething, weight loss.

DOSING

Adults (18 Years and Older)

- Two 5-mL spoonfuls of powdered arrowroot (Thornton & Ross UK Pharmaceutical Company) three times a day with, or as part of, meals for 1 month has been taken by mouth.

Children (Younger than 18 Years)

- There is insufficient evidence to recommend a dose for arrowroot in children.

SAFETY

Allergies

- Patients with a known allergy or hypersensitivity to arrowroot (*Marantana arundinacea*), its constituents, or members of the Marantaceae family should avoid arrowroot.

Side Effects and Warnings

- There is limited available scientific evidence on the side effect profile of arrowroot. Arrowroot is likely safe when used in amounts commonly found in foods, for a short term, or when used as a substitute for wheat or other gluten-containing grains in allergic patients.
- The most common adverse effect of arrowroot is constipation. Upset stomach (dyspepsia) has also been reported.

Pregnancy and Breastfeeding

- Medicinal amounts of arrowroot are not recommended due to lack of scientific evidence.

INTERACTIONS

Interactions with Drugs

- Arrowroot may reduce diarrhea and even cause constipation. Caution is advised when used with antidiarrheal or laxative medications.

Interactions with Herbs and Dietary Supplements

- Arrowroot may reduce diarrhea and even cause constipation. Caution is advised when used with antidiarrheal or laxative herbs and supplements.

For a complete list of references, please visit www.naturalstandard.com.

Ashwagandha
(Withania somnifera)

RELATED TERMS

- Ajagandha, amangura, amukkirag, asan, asgand, asgandh, asgandha, ashagandha, ashvagandha, ashwagada, ashwaganda, ashwagandholine, asoda, asundha, asvagandha, aswagandha, avarada, ayurvedic ainseng, clustered wintercherry, ghoda asoda, Indian ginseng, kanaje Hindi, kuthmithi, samm al ferakh, Solanaceae (family), winter cherry, withania, *Withania coagulans*, *Withania somnifera*, *Withania somniferum*, *Withania somnifera* Dunal, *Withania somnifera* glycowithanolides, *Withania somnifera* Kaul, withanolide A (WL-A).

EVIDENCE

Uses Based on Scientific Evidence	Grade
Diabetes (Type 2) Based on early studies, ashwagandha may decrease blood sugar levels. Additional evidence is required in this area before ashwagandha can be recommended for diabetes.	C
Diuretic Increases in urine volume have been reported with ashwagandha use. Additional evidence is required in this area before ashwagandha can be recommended as a diuretic.	C
High Cholesterol Decreases in serum total cholesterol levels, triglycerides, low-density lipoprotein (LDL), and very low density lipoproteins (VLDL) have been reported with ashwagandha use. Further research is needed before a strong recommendation can be made.	C
Longevity/Anti-Aging The use of ashwagandha as an anti-aging agent is based on traditional use in Indian Ayurvedic medicine to promote physical and mental health, improve resistance to disease, and promote longevity. Human research is lacking in this area, and currently there is insufficient evidence to draw a firm conclusion.	C
Osteoarthritis The use of ashwagandha in osteoarthritis has been suggested based on its reported anti-inflammatory and anti-arthritic properties. Well-designed human research is needed to confirm these results.	C
Parkinson's Disease There is insufficient scientific evidence to recommend the use of ashwagandha in the management of Parkinson's disease.	C

Uses Based on Tradition or Theory

Activity stimulant, adaptogen, allergic reactions, Alzheimer's disease, anaphylaxis, antibacterial, antifungal, antioxidant, anti-tumor, anxiety, aphrodisiac, asthma, astringent, atherosclerosis/hyperlipidemia (lipid peroxidation), back pain, boils, bronchitis, cancer, carbuncles, cardiovascular disease, chemotherapy, cognitive improvement, depression, emaciation, emmenagogue (menstrual blood flow stimulant), endocrine conditions, exercise performance, fatigue, fibrosarcoma, hay fever, hemiplegia, hematopoesis, hiccups, HIV, immunostimulant, infertility, insomnia, kidney protection, liver conditions, lung conditions, lymphoma, memory improvement, menstrual disorders, mood stabilization, nervous exhaustion, neurodegenerative diseases, neurological disorders, parasitic infections (ringworm), radiosensitization, rejuvenation, senile dementia, skin pigmentation disorders (leukoderma), skin ulcerations, stress, stroke, tardive dyskinesia, testicular development, tonic, toxicity (genotoxicity), tuberculosis, ulcers.

DOSING

Adults (18 Years and Older)

- There is insufficient evidence to recommend a dose for ashwagandha in adults. Various preparations are commercially available, including capsules, powders, teas, tinctures, decoctions, and multi-herb formulas.
- In capsule form, daily doses of whole herb is 1-6 g. As a powder, 3 g may be taken two times daily in boiled warm milk. A tea may be made by simmering/boiling 1 part root in 10 parts water for 15-30 minutes and taken twice daily in the amount of ½-1 oz at a time. Tea made from 1-6 g of the whole herb in tea form has been used daily. Tinctures or fluid extracts have been dosed at 2-4 mL, taken three times daily. Tinctures may contain high concentrations of alcohol. As a milk decoction, 5 tsp of dried herb in 1 cup boiling liquid, taken as 2-3 cups with raw sugar or honey, has been used daily. As multi-herb formulas, 3-12 g have been used in combination with other herbs.
- Injected use is not recommended as human data are lacking.

Children (Younger than 18 Years)

- Overall, there is insufficient evidence available to recommend use of ashwagandha in children. Children 8-12 years old have been given 2 g in milk daily for 60 days with no toxicity reported in one trial. In Ayurveda, ashwagandha is considered acceptable to give to debilitated children; however, data from clinical trials are lacking.

SAFETY

Allergies

- Avoid if sensitive or allergic to ashwagandha products or any of their ingredients. Dermatitis (allergic skin rash) was reported in 3 of 42 patients in one ashwagandha trial.

Side Effects and Warnings

- There are few reports of adverse effects associated with ashwagandha; however, there are scant human trials using ashwagandha, and most do not report the doses or standardization/preparation used.
- Ashwagandha may cause sedation, possible life-threatening respiratory depression, decrease in blood pressure, and abnormal heart rhythms. Ashwagandha may cause diarrhea. Nausea and abdominal pain have also been reported. Theoretically, irritation of mucous and serous membranes may occur, and ashwagandha should be avoided in people with peptic ulcer disease.
- Ashwagandha may lower blood sugar levels, based on limited human research (in patients with type 2 diabetes) and therefore may interact with diabetic medications, although the mechanism is unknown.
- Ashwagandha has been reported to possess diuretic properties, and kidney lesions may occur. Ashwagandha may stimulate thyroid function and increase T4 levels, possibly increasing the risk of hyperthyroidism. Ashwagandha may also possess androgenic (testosterone-like) properties, based on rat evidence of increased testicular weight and spermatogenesis, as well as decreased serum follicle-stimulating hormone (FSH) and testosterone levels.
- Ashwagandha may stimulate red and white blood cell production and may increase platelet count, although there is limited study in these areas and the mechanism is unknown. Ashwagandha is rich in iron.
- Ashwagandha may possess immunomodulatory and anti-inflammatory effects.

Pregnancy and Breastfeeding

- Ashwagandha is not recommended due to a lack of available scientific evidence. Ashwagandha may cause abortions.

INTERACTIONS

Interactions with Drugs

- In theory, ashwagandha may increase the effects of amphetamines.
- Ashwagandha may possess androgenic (testosterone-like) properties based on experiments showing increased testicular weight and spermatogenesis in rats.
- Ashwagandha has been reported to significantly increase coagulation time, although the significance in humans is not clear. In theory, effects may be additive with anticoagulants.
- Based on limited human research (in patients with type 2 diabetes), ashwagandha may lower blood sugar levels and therefore may interact with diabetic medications, although the mechanism is unknown.
- Ashwagandha may lower systolic and diastolic blood pressure, and may therefore alter the effects of blood pressure–lowering drugs.
- Ashwagandha has been associated with cholinesterase inhibition, and caution is warranted when taken with cholinesterase-inhibiting medications. Examples of cholinesterase inhibitors include donepezil (Aricept), rivastigmine (Exelon), galantamine (Reminyl), tacrine (Cognex), neostigmine (Prostigmin), edrophonium chloride (Tensilon), and pyridostigmine bromide.

- Ashwagandha extract may reduce cyclophosphamide-induced immunosuppression/leukopenia and urotoxicity. Caution is advised when taking ashwagandha with cyclophosphamide or immunomodulating drugs.
- Although not well studied in humans, ashwagandha may increase paclitaxel's effectiveness on lung cancer. Repeated administration of ashwagandha may attenuate the development of tolerance to narcotics. Ashwagandha may also improve tardive dyskinesia symptoms caused by haloperidol (Haldol).
- Ashwagandha may cause sedation and possible life-threatening respiratory depression, and it may interact with sedatives, hypnotics, or other central nervous system depressants. In early research, ashwagandha was reported to increase the effects of barbiturates and ethanol.
- Ashwagandha may cause hyperthyroidism based on data suggesting thyroid stimulation and increased T4 serum levels, and therefore may interact with drugs for hyperthyroidism or hypothyroidism.
- Ashwagandha may also interact with diuretics (water pills) or chemotherapy agents.

Interactions with Herbs and Supplements

- Ashwagandha may reduce 5-HTP (5-hydroxytryptophan) levels.
- Although not well studied in humans, ashwagandha has been reported to stimulate thyroid function, including increased serum T4 concentrations.
- Ashwagandha has been reported to significantly increase coagulation (blood clotting) time, although the significance in humans is not clear. In theory, the effects of anticoagulant agents and the risk of bleeding may be increased.
- Based on limited human research (in patients with type 2 diabetes), ashwagandha may lower blood sugar levels and therefore may interact with diabetic agents, although the mechanism is unknown.
- Ashwagandha may lower systolic and diastolic blood pressure, and may therefore alter the effects of other agents that lower blood pressure.
- Ashwagandha is rich in iron. It also contains arginine and may therefore add to the total dose and effects when taken with arginine supplements.
- Ashwagandha contains ornithine and may therefore add to the total dose and effects when taken with ornithine.
- Ashwagandha may possess androgenic (testosterone-like) properties, based on rat evidence of increased testicular weight and spermatogenesis. Saw palmetto possesses 5-alpha reductase properties similar to finasteride (Proscar) and may antagonize the potential androgenic effects of ashwagandha.
- Ashwagandha may cause sedation and possible life-threatening respiratory depression, and it may interact with sedatives, hypnotics, or other central nervous system depressants.
- Ashwagandha may also interact with diuretics (water pills).

For a complete list of references, please visit www.naturalstandard.com.

Asparagus
(Asparagus officinalis)

RELATED TERMS

- Asparagamine A, *Asparagus africanus, Asparagus gobicus, Asparagus officinalis, Asparagus racemosus,* edible asparagus, gobicusin A, gobicusin B, iso-agatharesinol, Liliaceae (family), racemofuran, racemosol, Shatavari, sparagrass, Spargel (German), sparrow grass, sperage.

BACKGROUND

- In its wild form in Ancient Greece and Rome, asparagus was used as a diuretic (increasing urine flow) to flush out the kidneys and prevent the formation of kidney stones. In Asian medicine, asparagus root is given for cough, diarrhea, and nervous problems. Asparagus roots and leaves are used in Ayurvedic medicine for female infertility.
- Today, asparagus is most often used as a food. There is very limited research in humans on the medicinal uses of asparagus.

EVIDENCE

Uses Based on Scientific Evidence	Grade
Dyspepsia (Upset Stomach) *Asparagus racemosus* (Shatavari) is used in Ayurveda for dyspepsia (upset stomach). Additional study is needed before a firm conclusion can be made.	C
Galactagogue (Promotes Secretion of Milk) Asparagus may help promote the secretion of milk in women. There is insufficient evidence showing efficacy for this use.	C

Uses Based on Tradition or Theory
Antimicrobial, antioxidant, antispasmodic, antitumor, anxiety, aphrodisiac, blood cleanser, bronchial congestion, cough, demulcent (soothing action on inflammation), diabetes, diarrhea, digestive, diuretic (increasing urine flow), dysentery, food uses, gastric ulcers, hepatoprotection (liver protection), immunostimulation, improving resistance to disease, infertility, inflammation, joint pain and stiffness, kidney stones, liver disease, neurological disorders, rheumatism, soap, tonic, urinary tract inflammation.

DOSING

Adults (18 Years and Older)

- There is insufficient evidence to recommend a dose for asparagus. Traditional dosing has used infusions, fluid extracts, and alcoholic extracts for the treatment of urinary tract inflammation and kidney stones. A typical infusion involves 45-60 g of cut herb in 150 mL of water and is taken daily by mouth. Fluid extract (45-60 mL) has been taken daily by mouth. Alcoholic extract has been taken daily at a dose of 225-300 mL (1:5 g/mL).

Children (Younger than 18 Years)

- There is insufficient evidence to recommend a dose for asparagus in children.

SAFETY

Allergies

- Known allergy/hypersensitivity to asparagus or other members of the Liliaceae family.
- Allergic reactions have been documented for asparagus, including itchy conjunctivitis (inflammation of the eye), runny nose, tightness of the throat, coughing, acute urticaria (hives), inflammation of the skin, and occupational asthma caused by asparagus inhalation.

Side Effects and Warnings

- Asparagus is likely safe when consumed as a food. The primary adverse effects for asparagus are dermatological (skin reactions) and pulmonary (lung) allergic reactions.
- Allergic reactions that have been documented include itchy conjunctivitis (inflammation of the eye), runny nose, worsening of asthma symptoms, tightness of the throat, coughing, acute urticaria (hives), and inflammation of the skin.
- Intestinal obstruction due to inhibition of bowel motility (ileus) of the small intestine has been caused by a high-fiber diet including canned asparagus.
- Patients should not take asparagus if allergic to asparagus. Patients with edema due to impaired kidney or heart function should use cautiously and should consult with a qualified health care professional, including a pharmacist, before starting any new therapies.

Pregnancy and Breastfeeding

- There is insufficient evidence to recommend asparagus during pregnancy and breastfeeding.

INTERACTIONS

Interactions with Drugs

- Asparagus may have diuretic effects (increases urine flow) and may interact with diuretic drugs such as chlorothiazide (Diuril). Caution is advised.

Interactions with Herbs and Dietary Supplements

- Asparagus may have diuretic effects and may interact with other diuretic herbs and supplements.

For a complete list of references, please visit www.naturalstandard.com.

RELATED TERMS

- Alpha-carotene, Antarctic krill, AST, Astacarox, astaxanthin–amino acid conjugate, astaxanthin diester, astaxanthin dilysinate tetrahydrochloride, ASX, Atlantic salmon, basidiomycete yeast, beta-carotene, BioAstin, canthaxanthin, canthoxanthin, Cardax, carotenoid, crayfish, crustaceans, DDA, disodium disuccinate astaxanthin, E161j, *Euphausia superba,* gamma-tocopherol, green microalgae, *Haematococcus* algae extract, *Haematococcus pluvialis,* krill, lutein, lycopene, meso-astaxanthin, microalgae, non-esterified astaxanthin, non-provitamin A carotenoid, ovoester, *Phaffia rhodozyma,* red carotenoid, retinoid, salmon, shrimp, sockeye salmon, tetrahydrochloride dilysine astaxanthin salt, tomato, trout, wild salmon, *Xanthophyllomyces dendrorhous,* xanthophylls.

BACKGROUND

- Astaxanthin is classified as a xanthophyll, which is a carotenoid pigment, and is produced by microalgae, yeast, salmon, trout, krill, shrimp, crayfish, crustaceans, and the feathers of some birds. *Haematococcus pluvialis,* a green microalga and one of the richest sources of natural astaxanthin, was reviewed and cleared for marketing by the U.S. Food and Drug Administration (FDA) in August 1999 as a new dietary ingredient by way of the Dietary Supplement Health and Education Act (DSHEA) (21 CRF part 190.6).

- Astaxanthin is most commonly used for its antioxidant properties. It may be beneficial in decreasing the risks of certain chronic diseases, such as cancer and cardiovascular diseases. It has also been used as an experimental treatment for carpal tunnel syndrome, rheumatoid arthritis, muscle strength and endurance, high cholesterol (LDL oxidation), musculoskeletal injuries, and male infertility.

- Astaxanthin is commonly used as a feed supplement and food coloring additive for salmon, crabs, shrimp, and chickens. According to the Code of Federal Regulations, astaxanthin has a "generally recognized as safe" (GRAS) status when used in salmon foods as a color additive to obtain the desired pink to orange-red color.

EVIDENCE

Uses Based on Scientific Evidence	Grade
Carpal Tunnel Syndrome There is insufficient evidence to recommend for or against the use of astaxanthin for carpal tunnel syndrome.	C
High Cholesterol (LDL Oxidation) There is insufficient evidence to recommend the use of astaxanthin for LDL oxidation prevention.	C
Male Infertility There is insufficient evidence to recommend the use of astaxanthin for male fertility.	C
Muscle Strength Astaxanthin may have positive effects on muscle strength. However, better-quality trials are needed before a recommendation can be made.	C
Musculoskeletal Injuries Astaxanthin does not appear to be effective for muscle injury prevention, although additional research is needed.	C
Rheumatoid Arthritis There is insufficient evidence to recommend the use of astaxanthin for rheumatoid arthritis.	C

Uses Based on Tradition or Theory
Antiandrogen, antibacterial, antihypertensive (lowers high blood pressure), anti-inflammatory, antimicrobial, antiviral, asthma, atherosclerosis (prevention), autoimmune diseases, back pain (chronic), benign prostate hyperplasia, cancer, canker sores, cardiovascular disease (prevention and treatment), central nervous system disorders, dementia (vascular), diabetes, dyspepsia (upset stomach), exercise capacity improvement, eye problems, *Helicobacter pylori* infection, immune stimulant, neurodegenerative diseases (Parkinson's and Alzheimer's diseases), stroke, ultraviolet light skin damage protection, weight loss.

DOSING

Adults (18 Years and Older)

- In general, manufacturers have reported that 3 gelcaps of BioAstin astaxanthin (6 mg) by mouth at each meal for eight weeks was safe in adults. Similarly, no toxicity or side effects were noted when taking up to 19.25 mg of AstaFactor by mouth for 29 days.

- Recommended doses typically range from 2-12 mg daily for 2 weeks to 6 months. BioAstin has been used for carpal tunnel syndrome, rheumatoid arthritis, musculoskeletal injury, and sunburn. For male infertility, an experimental dose was 16 mg (AstaCarox) daily by mouth for 3 months. Safety and effectiveness have not been demonstrated.

- Various seafoods contains astaxanthin as a color-enhancing pigment. A standard serving portion of 4 ounces of Atlantic salmon contains from 0.5-1.1 mg of astaxanthin, whereas the same amount of sockeye salmon may contain 4.5 mg of astaxanthin.

Children (Younger than 18 Years)

- There is insufficient evidence to recommend a dose of astaxanthin in children.

SAFETY

Allergies

- Patients with a known allergy or hypersensitivity to astaxanthin or related carotenoids, including canthaxanthin, or those with hypersensitivity to an astaxanthin algal source, such as *Haematococcus pluvialis,* should not take astaxanthin preparations.

Side Effects and Warnings

- According to the Code of Federal Regulations, astaxanthin has a "generally recognized as safe" (GRAS) status when used as a color additive in various foods. Astaxanthin is likely safe when used as an antioxidant and as adjunctive support in cancer treatment, cardiovascular disease treatment, and ocular health promotion.
- Side effects of astaxanthin use may include decreases in blood pressure, increases in skin pigmentation and hair growth, hormonal changes, lowered calcium levels in the blood, altered blood counts, decreased libido, and enlargement of the breasts (in men).
- Astaxanthin should be used cautiously in patients with hypertension, asthma, parathyroid disorders, or osteoporosis. Avoid use in patients with known allergies to astaxanthin, hormone-sensitive conditions, or immune disorders.

Pregnancy and Breastfeeding

- Astaxanthin is not recommended for use during pregnancy or breastfeeding. Astaxanthin may be unsafe in pregnant women, as it may affect reproductive hormones.
- Astaxanthin has been studied as an agent to treat male infertility, although results were not conclusive or of any benefit.

INTERACTIONS

Interactions with Drugs

- Astaxanthin may decrease blood pressure. Patients currently taking blood pressure–lowering medications should consult with a qualified health care professional, including a pharmacist.
- Astaxanthin may have similar effects as the antihistamines etirizine dihydrochloride and azelastine. Caution is advised when using asthma medications.
- Astaxanthin may interfere with the way the body processes certain herbs or supplements using the liver's cytochrome P450 enzyme system. As a result, blood levels of the other drugs may become too high. Astaxanthin may also alter the effects that other drugs possibly have on the P450 system.
- Astaxanthin may inhibit *Helicobacter pylori* growth and have an additive effect when taken with other medications that have a similar effect.
- Astaxanthin may have hormonal effects and may interact with other hormone-altering medications, such as medications taken for menopause or birth control pills. It may also interact with immunomodulating medications.
- Astaxanthin may lower calcium levels in the blood. In theory, it may interact with parathyroid medications; caution is advised with concomittant use.
- Astaxanthin may decrease low density lipoprotein (LDL) oxidation and may interact with other cholesterol-lowering medications, such asrofecoxib (Vioxx). Patients taking any medications should consult with a qualified health care professional, including a pharmacist.

Interactions with Herbs and Dietary Supplements

- Astaxanthin may have hormonal effects and may interact with other hormone-altering herbs and supplements, such as saw palmetto or black cohosh.
- Astaxanthin may decrease blood pressure. Patients currently taking blood pressure–lowering herbs and supplements should consult with a qualified health care professional, including a pharmacist.
- Astaxanthin may lower calcium levels in the blood. In theory, it may interact with herbs and supplements that alter parathyroid function; caution is advised with concomittant use.
- Concomitant use of astaxanthin with other carotenoids (beta-carotene, lutein, canthaxanthin, and lycopene) may decrease the absorption of astaxanthin due to competitive absorption in the gastrointestinal tract. Caution is advised.
- Astaxanthin may interfere with the way the body processes certain herbs or supplements using the liver's cytochrome P450 enzyme system. As a result, the levels of other herbs or supplements may become too high in the blood. It may also alter the effects that other herbs or supplements possibly have on the P450 system.
- Astaxanthin may inhibit *Helicobacter pylori* growth and have an additive effect when taken with other herbs and supplements that have a similar effect. It may also interact with immunomodulating herbs and supplements.
- Astaxanthin may decrease low density lipoprotein (LDL) oxidation and may interact with other cholesterol-lowering herbs and supplements, such as red yeast rice. Caution is advised.

For a complete list of references, please visit www.naturalstandard.com.

Astragalus
(Astragalus membranaceus)

RELATED TERMS

- *Astragalus gummifera, Astragalus lentiginosus, Astragalus mollissimus, Astragalus mongholicus, Astragalus trigonus*, astragel, baak kei, beg kei, bei qi, buck qi, Fabacea (family), goat's horn, goat's thorn, green dragon, gum dragon, gum tragacanthae, gummi tragacanthae, hoang ky, hog gum, huang-chi, Huang Qi, huangoi, huangqi, hwanggi, ji cao, Leguminosae (family), locoweed, membranous milk vetch, milk vetch, Mongolian milk, Mongolian milk vetch, neimeng hhuangqi, ogi, ougi, radix astragali, spino santo, Syrian tragacanth, tai shen, tragacanth, wong kei, yellow vetch, Zhongfengnaomitong.

BACKGROUND

- Astragalus products are derived from the roots of *Astragalus membranaceus* or related species in the genus *Astragalus*, which are native to China. In traditional Chinese medicine, astragalus is commonly found in mixtures with other herbs and is used in the treatment of numerous ailments, including heart, liver, and kidney diseases, as well as cancer, viral infections, and immune system disorders. Western herbalists began using astragalus in the 1800s as an ingredient in various tonics. The popularity of astragalus increased in the 1980s based on theories about anti-cancer properties, although these proposed effects have not been clearly demonstrated in reliable human studies.
- Some medicinal uses of astragalus are based on its proposed immune stimulatory properties, reported in preliminary laboratory and animal experiments, but not conclusively demonstrated in humans. Most astragalus research has been conducted in China, and has not been well designed or reported.
- Gummy sap (tragacanth) from astragalus is used as a thickener in ice cream, an emulsifier, a denture adhesive, and an anti-diarrheal agent.

EVIDENCE

Uses Based on Scientific Evidence	Grade
Aplastic Anemia Astragalus-containing herbal combination formulas may have beneficial effects in aplastic anemia, although this has not been shown conclusively.	C
Burns Few clinical trials have investigated astragalus in burn patients.	C
Chemotherapy Side Effects In Chinese medicine, astragalus-containing herbal mixtures are sometimes used with the intention to reduce side effects of cancer treatments. However, rigorous research is lacking.	C
Coronary Artery Disease In Chinese medicine, herbal mixtures containing astragalus have been used to treat heart diseases. However, clinical evidence is thus far insufficient.	C
Diabetes There is some evidence, though not definitive, that astragalus can improve the effectiveness of conventional diabetes therapies.	C
Heart Failure There is some evidence, though not definitive, that astragalus may offer symptomatic improvement for chronic heart failure.	C
Hepatitis Research suggests that astragalus may have anti-hepatitis effects; however, effectiveness has not been proven.	C
Herpes Some studies suggest that astragalus may inhibit herpes viruses. Further research is warranted.	C
HIV Antiviral effects have been reported in early studies. Additional studies are warranted.	C
Immune Stimulation Several small studies report that astragalus may stimulate and improve immune system function in conditions such as the common cold, blood disorders, cancer, and HIV/AIDS.	C
Kidney Failure Research suggests that astragalus may be effective in renal disease. However, there is insufficient evidence to support this claim.	C
Liver Disease Research suggests that astragalus may be effective in cirrhosis. Further research is required before a recommendation can be made.	C
Mental Performance Limited clinical evidence suggests that astragalus may aid in mental performance of children with low IQ. Further well-designed clinical trials are required.	C
Myocarditis/Endocarditis (Heart Infections) Several studies suggest that astragalus may improve symptoms of viral myocarditis. However, these studies are small and poorly designed. Larger, higher-quality studies are needed in this area.	C

Uses Based on Scientific Evidence	Grade
Smoking Cessation Astragalus has been used traditionally to aid in smoking cessation. However, this is insufficient evidence to support this use.	C
Tuberculosis Limited clinical evidence suggests the potential for benefit of astragalus in patients with tuberculosis.	C
Upper Respiratory Tract Infection Astragalus is often used in Chinese medicine as a part of herbal mixtures to prevent or treat upper respiratory tract infections. However, supportive clinical evidence is lacking.	C

Uses Based on Tradition or Theory

Adaptogen, adrenal insufficiency (Addison's disease), aging, AIDS/HIV, allergies, Alzheimer's disease, anemia, angina, ankylosing spondylitis, anorexia, antifungal, anti-inflammatory, antimicrobial, antioxidant, asthma, astringent, blood thinner, blood vessel disorders (vascular endothelial cell proliferation), bone loss, bone marrow production, brain damage (minimal brain dysfunction), bronchitis, cardiac ischemia, cardiomyopathy (hypertrophic), cervicitis, chi deficiency (fatigue, weakness, loss of appetite), childbirth (preterm labor), chronic fatigue syndrome, cleanser, colitis (in children; rotovirus enterocolitis), cytomegalovirus, dementia, demulcent, denture adhesive (astragalus sap), dermatitis, diabetic foot ulcers, diabetic neuropathy, diarrhea, digestion enhancement, diuretic (urination stimulant), ear infection, edema, expectorant, fatigue, fever, gangrene, gastrointestinal disorders, graft-versus-host disease, hearing damage, hemorrhage, hemorrhoids, high blood pressure, high cholesterol, hyperthyroidism, infections, insomnia, joint pain, laxative, leprosy, leukemia, low blood platelets, lung cancer, male fertility (sperm motility), memory, menstrual disorders, metabolic disorders, multiple sclerosis, myalgia (muscle pain), myasthenia gravis, nephritis, neuroprotective, night sweats, pain, palpitations, pelvic congestion syndrome, postpartum fever, postpartum urinary retention, prostatitis, psoriasis, rectal prolapse, respiratory infections (infantile), shortness of breath, stamina/strength enhancer, stomach disorders, stomach ulcer, stress, stroke, sweating (excessive), systemic lupus erythematosus (SLE), tissue oxygenation, tonic, uterine bleeding, uterine prolapse, weight loss, wound healing.

DOSING
Adults (18 Years and Older)

- In Chinese medicine, astragalus is used in soups, teas, extracts, and pills. In practice and in most scientific studies, astragalus is one component of multi-herb mixtures. Therefore, precise dosing of astragalus alone is not clear. Safety and effectiveness are not clearly established for any particular dose. Various doses of astragalus have been used or studied, including 250-500 mg of extract taken four times daily; 1-30 g of dried root taken daily (doses as high as 60 g have been reported); or 500-1,000 mg of root capsules taken three times daily. Dosing of tinctures or fluid extracts depends on the strength of the preparations. Various tincture doses have been used, including (1:5) of 3-6 mL three times daily by mouth, or 15-30 drops twice daily by mouth. Note that tinctures may have a high alcohol content.
- For herpes simplex keratitis, 0.5 mL astragalus (1:1 extract) for 3 weeks has been used on the skin. For wound healing, a 10% astragalus ointment has been applied to wound surfaces. According to secondary sources, the maximum dose is 1.3% when used topically in lotions, denture creams, toothpastes, and cosmetics.
- For non–small cell lung cancer, 60 mL has been given intravenously per day. Injections should only be given under the supervision of a qualified health care professional.
- **Note:** In theory, consumption of the tragacanth (gummy sap derived from astragalus) may reduce the absorption of drugs taken by mouth, and they should be taken at separate times.

Children (Younger than 18 Years)

- There is insufficient evidence to recommend a dose of astragalus for children.

SAFETY
Allergies

- In theory, patients with allergies to members of the Leguminosae (pea) family may react to astragalus. Cross-reactivity with quillaja bark (soapbark) has been reported for astragalus gum tragacanth.

Side Effects and Warnings

- Some species of astragalus have caused poisoning in livestock, although these types are usually not used in human preparations, which primarily include *Astragalus membranaceus*. Livestock toxicity, referred to as *locoweed poisoning*, has occurred with species that contain swainsonine (*Astragalus lentiginosus, Astragalus mollissimus, Astragalus nothrosys, Astragalus pubentissimus, Astragalus thuseri*, and *Astragalus wootoni*) or species that accumulate selenium (*Astragalus bisulcatus, Astragalus flavus, Astragalus praelongus, Astragalus saurinus*, and *Astragalus tenellus*). Ingestion of certain toxic astragalus plants may cause neurological syndromes, some of which are irreversible.
- Overall, it is difficult to determine the side effects or toxicity of astragalus because it is most commonly used in combination with other herbs. There are numerous reports of side effects ranging from mild to deadly in the U.S. Food and Drug Administration (FDA) computer database. However, most of these side effects are with multi-ingredient products, and they cannot be attributed to astragalus specifically. Side effects reported in people using combination products that contain astragalus include heart palpitations, abdominal discomfort, diarrhea, and aspiration pneumonia.
- Astragalus is considered traditionally to be safe when used alone and in recommended doses, although safety is not well studied. The most common side effects appear to be mild stomach upset and allergic reactions. In the United States, according to the Code of Federal Regulations, tragacanth (astragalus gummy sap) has "generally recognized as safe" (GRAS) status for food use, but astragalus does not have GRAS status.
- Based on preliminary animal studies and limited human research, astragalus may decrease blood sugar levels. Caution is advised in patients with diabetes or hypoglycemia, and in those taking drugs, herbs, or supplements that affect

blood sugar. Serum glucose levels may need to be monitored by health care professionals, and medication adjustments may be necessary.

- Based on anecdotal reports and preliminary laboratory research, astragalus may increase the risk of bleeding. Caution is advised in patients with bleeding disorders or those taking drugs that may increase the risk of bleeding. Dosing adjustments may be necessary.

- Preliminary reports of human use in China have noted decreased blood pressure at lower doses and increased blood pressure at higher doses. Animal research suggests possible blood pressure–lowering effects. Due to a lack of well-designed studies, no firm conclusions can be drawn. Nonetheless, people with abnormal blood pressure or those taking blood pressure medications should use caution and be monitored by a qualified health care professional. Palpitations have been noted in human reports in China.

- Based on animal research, astragalus may act as a diuretic and increase urination. In theory, this may lead to dehydration or metabolic abnormalities. There is one report of pneumonia in an infant after breathing in an herbal medicine powder including *Astragalus sarcocolla*.

- Because astragalus may stimulate the immune system, individuals with autoimmune diseases or organ transplants should consult a health care professional before starting therapy. Astragalus is not recommended for people with acute inflammation or acute illness with fever.

- Astragalus may increase growth hormone levels.

Pregnancy and Breastfeeding

- Astragalus is not recommended during pregnancy or breastfeeding due to harmful effects seen in animals.

- Many tinctures contain high levels of alcohol and should be avoided during pregnancy.

INTERACTIONS
Interactions with Drugs

- Based on preliminary animal studies and limited human research, astragalus may decrease blood sugar levels. Caution is advised in patients with diabetes or hypoglycemia and in those taking drugs that affect blood sugar. Serum glucose levels may need to be monitored by a health care provider, and medication adjustments may be necessary.

- Preliminary reports of human use in China have noted decreased blood pressure at lower doses and increased blood pressure at higher doses of astragalus. Animal research suggests possible blood pressure–lowering effects. Although well-designed studies are not available, people taking drugs that affect blood pressure should use caution and be monitored by a qualified health care professional. It has been suggested that beta-blocker drugs such as propranolol (Inderal) or atenolol (Tenormin) may reduce the effects on the heart of astragalus, although this has not been well studied.

- Based on anecdotal reports, astragalus may increase the risk of bleeding when taken with drugs that increase the risk of bleeding. Some examples include aspirin, anticoagulants (blood thinners) such as warfarin (Coumadin) or heparin, anti-platelet drugs such as clopidogrel (Plavix), and nonsteroidal anti-inflammatory drugs such as ibuprofen (Motrin, Advil) or naproxen (Naprosyn, Aleve).

- Based on animal research and traditional use, astragalus may act as a diuretic and increase urination. In theory, this may lead to dehydration or metabolic abnormalities (low blood sodium or potassium), particularly when used in combination with diuretics such as furosemide (Lasix), chlorothiazide (Diuril), or spironolactone (Aldactone).

- Based on laboratory and animal studies, astragalus may possess immune-stimulating properties, although research in humans is not conclusive. Some research suggests that astragalus may interfere with the effects of drugs that suppress the immune system, such as steroids or agents used in organ transplants.

- Some sources suggest other potential drug interactions, although there is no reliable scientific evidence in these areas. These include reduced effects of astragalus when used with sedative agents such as phenobarbital or hypnotic agents such as chloral hydrate; increased effects of astragalus when taken with colchicine; increased effects of paralytics such as pancuronium or succinylcholine when used with astragalus; increased effects of stimulants such as ephedrine or epinephrine; increased side effects of dopamine antagonists such as haloperidol (Haldol); and increased side effects of the cancer drug procarbazine when used with astragalus.

- In theory, consumption of the tragacanth (gummy sap derived from astragalus) may reduce absorption of drugs taken by mouth and should be taken at separate times.

- Based on laboratory study, astragalus may be additive to ribavirin, acyclovir, or other antiviral agents.

- Activity of lipid-lowering (cholesterol-lowering) medication may be potentiated.

- Based on human studies, activity of recombinant interferon 1 may be potentiated by astragalus.

- Astragalus may also interact with antibiotics.

Interactions with Herbs and Dietary Supplements

- Based on preliminary animal studies and limited human research, astragalus may decrease blood sugar levels. Caution is advised in patients with diabetes or hypoglycemia, and in those taking herbs or supplements that affect blood sugar. People using other herbs or supplements that may alter blood sugar levels should be monitored closely by a health care professional while using astragalus. Dosing adjustments may be necessary.

- Preliminary reports of human use in China have noted decreased blood pressure at lower doses and increased of blood pressure at higher doses astragalus. Animal research suggests possible blood pressure–lowering effects. Although well-designed studies are not available, people taking herbs or supplements that affect blood pressure should use caution and be monitored by a qualified health care professional.

- Based on anecdotal reports, astragalus may increase the risk of bleeding when taken with herbs or supplements that increase the risk of bleeding. Examples include *Ginkgo biloba* and garlic *(Allium sativum)*.

- Based on animal research and traditional use, astragalus may act as a diuretic and increase urination. In theory, this may lead to dehydration or metabolic abnormalities (low blood sodium or potassium), particularly when used in combination with herbs or supplements that may possess diuretic properties.

- Based on laboratory and animal studies, astragalus may possess immune-stimulating properties, although research in humans is not conclusive. It is not known if astragalus interacts with other agents that are proposed to affect the immune system.

- In theory, consumption of tragacanth (gummy sap derived from astragalus) may reduce the absorption of herbs or supplements taken by mouth and should be taken at separate times.
- Based on laboratory studies, astragalus may inhibit the actions of immunosuppressants and potentiate the effects of immunostimulant herbs such as echinacea or *Panax ginseng*.

- Activity of lipid-lowering (cholesterol-lowering) herbs may be potentiated.
- Astragalus may interact with antibacterial herbs and supplements, CNS stimulants, hypnotics, hormonal herbs and supplements, licorice, rauwolfia alkaloids, and sedatives.

For a complete list of references, please visit www. naturalstandard.com.

Avocado
(Persea americana)

RELATED TERMS

- Abokado, aguacate, ahuacate, ahuacatl, alligator pear, avocado pear, avocato, *Persea americana*, *Persea americana* var. drymifolia Blake, *Persea gratissima*, *Persea leiogyna*, *Persea nubigena* var. *guatamalensis* L., *Persea persea*, *Laurus persea*.

BACKGROUND

- Avocados are fruits that contain 60% more potassium than bananas; they are also sodium and cholesterol free. An avocado has a higher fat content (5 g per serving) than most other fruits, but the fat is monounsaturated, which is considered healthy when consumed in moderation. Diets rich in monounsaturated fatty acids can reduce total cholesterol levels in the blood and increase the ratio of high-density lipoprotein (HDL, "good" cholesterol) to low-density lipoprotein (LDL, "bad" cholesterol).
- Avocado has been taken by mouth to treat osteoarthritis. Its oils have been used topically to treat wounds, infections, arthritis, and to stimulate hair growth. The seeds, leaves, and bark have been used for dysentery and diarrhea. It is also used in topical creams for regular skincare. Historically the Amazonian natives used avocado to treat gout, and the Mayan people believed it could keep joints and muscles in good condition, avoiding arthritis and rheumatism.
- The most promising use for avocado is in a combination product, avocado/soybean unsaponifiables (ASU), which is a combination of avocado oil and soybean oil.
- Caution is advised when taking Mexican avocado due to the constituents, estragole and anethole, which may be hepatotoxic and carcinogenic.

EVIDENCE

Uses Based on Scientific Evidence	Grade
High Cholesterol Avocados added to the diet may lower total cholesterol, LDL ("bad" cholesterol), HDL ("good" cholesterol), and triglycerides.	B
Osteoarthritis (Knee and Hip) A combination of avocado/soybean unsaponifiables (ASU) has been found beneficial in osteoarthritis of the knee and hip.	B
Psoriasis Early scientific studies showed promising effects using avocado in a cream for psoriasis.	C

Uses Based on Tradition or Theory
Aphrodisiac, arthritis, atherosclerosis, cancer, chemoprotectant, connective tissue disorders, dermatitis, diarrhea, dysentery, eczema, gingivitis, gout, hair growth, inflammation (oral), menstrual flow stimulant, neuralgia (nerve pain), periodontitis/gingivitis, scleroderma, sexual arousal, skin care, toothache, wound healing.

DOSING

Adults (18 Years and Older)

- The avocado fruit is typically used for medicinal purposes, although the oil has also been studied. To reduce high cholesterol, ½-1½ avocado, or 300 g, has been consumed daily for 2-4 weeks. Studies have also used avocado-enriched diets, with 75% of the fat coming from the avocado, for 2-4 weeks.

Children (Younger than 18 Years)

- There is insufficient evidence to recommend a dose for avocado in children. Medicinal use should be monitored by a qualified health care professional.

SAFETY

Allergies

- Patients with a known allergy or hypersensitivity to avocado should avoid avocado and avocado products. An association between allergy to latex, chestnut, banana and/or avocado has been reported. Symptoms of allergy may include anaphylaxis, hives, vomiting, intestinal spasms, or bronchial asthma.

Side Effects and Warnings

- In general, it appears that avocado is well tolerated and is likely safe when consumed in amounts commonly found in foods. Caution should be taken when used in people with hypersensitivity to latex.
- Most skin adverse effects are due to allergy, and symptoms may include reddening of the skin, itching, hives, or eczema.
- Adverse effects due to ASU include flulike symptoms, paralysis, gastrointestinal disorders, nausea, gastralgia (stomach pain), vomiting, inflammation of the intestine, migraine headache with fever, headache, drowsiness, bronchial asthma, or vomiting.
- Certain types of avocado oil may cause liver damage. Caution is advised when taking Mexican avocado due to the constituents, estragole and anethole, which may be liver damaging and cancer causing. Caution is advised in patients with compromised liver function.

Pregnancy and Breastfeeding

- Taking avocado in medicinal amounts is not recommended during pregnancy or breastfeeding.
- Some varieties of avocado may be unsafe during breastfeeding. The Guatemalan variety of avocado may cause mammary gland damage and reduce milk production.

INTERACTIONS

Interactions with Drugs

- Avocado may decrease the effect of blood thinning or anti-inflammatory medications. Some examples include aspirin, anticoagulants (blood thinners) such as warfarin (Coumadin) or heparin, anti-platelet drugs such as clopidogel (Plavix), and non-steroidal anti-inflammatory drugs such as ibuprofen (Motrin, Advil) or naproxen (Naprosyn, Aleve). Avocado may also interact with other types of anti-inflammatories.

- Avocado may add to the effects of cholesterol-lowering medications. Patients taking these medications should consult with a qualified health care professional, including a pharmacist.
- Avocado contains moderate amounts of tyramine and may increase the risk of high blood pressure when taken with monoamine oxidase inhibitors (MAOIs). Examples of MAOIs include isocarboxazid (Marplan), phenelzine (Nardil), and tranylcypromine (Parnate). Caution is advised.

Interactions with Herbs and Dietary Supplements

- Avocado may reduce the blood-thinning effect of certain herbs and supplements, such as garlic or *Ginkgo biloba*. It may also interact with herbs and supplements that have anti-inflammatory effects.
- Avocado may add to the effects of cholesterol-lowering agents such as fish oil, garlic, guggul, red yeast, and niacin.
- Avocado contains moderate amounts of tyramine and may increase the risk of high blood pressure when taken with herbs and supplements that have monoamine oxidase inhibitor (MAOI) activity.
- Avocado is rich in beta-sitosterol. Consuming avocado concurrently with other supplements, including beta-sitosterol, could potentially lead to increased side effects.

For a complete list of references, please visit www.naturalstandard.com.

Babassu
(Orbignya phalerata)

RELATED TERMS

- Amid, Arecaceae (family), babacu mesocarp, babassu coconut, babassu mesocarp, babassu oil, babassu palm trees, Brazilian babassu coconut oil, coconut babacu, glucan, mesocarp, MP1, *Orbignya oleifera*, *Orbignya phalerata*, *Orbignya phalerata* Mart., *Orbignya phalerata* Martius, polysaccharide.

BACKGROUND

- Babassu *(Orbignya phalerata)* is a native tree of the Arecaceae (Palmae) family from northern Brazil. Babassu coconut extract has been widely used as a food source. It is used medicinally for wound healing, fever-reducing, blood thinning, thyroid-regulating, and anti-inflammatory properties.
- Babassu coconut (mesocarp) has been widely used to treat pain, fever, constipation, obesity, leukemia, rheumatism, ulcerations, tumors, wounds, and inflammation.

EVIDENCE

Uses Based on Scientific Evidence

No available studies qualify for inclusion in the evidence table.

Uses Based on Tradition or Theory

Anti-inflammatory, antithrombotic (blood thinning), constipation, fever, food uses, hyperthyroidism (overactive thyroid), immunomodulation, insect repellent, leukemia, obesity, pain, promoting healing, rheumatism, skin ulcerations, tumors, wound healing.

DOSING

Adults (18 Years and Older)

- There is insufficient evidence to recommend a dose for babassu in adults.

Children (Younger than 18 Years)

- There is insufficient evidence to recommend a dose for babassu in children.

SAFETY

Allergies

- Avoid in people with a known allergy or hypersensitivity to babassu *(Orbignya phalerata)* or its constituents.

Side Effects and Warnings

- Babassu is likely safe when used in food amounts in people who are not allergic or hypersensitive to babassu or any of its constituents.
- It should be used cautiously in patients taking blood thinners and in patients taking antithyroid (thyroid-regulating) agents.

Pregnancy and Breastfeeding

- Babassu is not recommended in pregnant or breastfeeding women due to a lack of available scientific evidence.

INTERACTIONS

Interactions with Drugs

- Babassu may exhibit anti-inflammatory activity. Caution is advised in patients taking anti-inflammatory agents due to potential interactions.
- Consumption of babassu may exert antithyroid (thyroid-regulating) effects. Caution is advised in patients with thyroid disorders or those taking medications to treat such conditions.
- Babassu may have antithrombotic effects and therefore may increase the risk of bleeding when taken with other antithrombotic drugs. Some examples include aspirin, anticoagulants (blood thinners) such as warfarin (Coumadin) or heparin, anti-platelet drugs such as clopidogrel (Plavix), and non-steroidal anti-inflammatory drugs (NSAIDs) such as ibuprofen (Motrin, Advil) or naproxen (Naprosyn, Aleve).

Interactions with Herbs and Dietary Supplements

- Babassu may have antithrombotic effects and therefore may increase the risk of bleeding when taken with other antithrombotic herbs and supplements.
- Babassu may exhibit anti-inflammatory activity. Caution is advised in patients taking herbs or supplements that also have anti-inflammatory activity due to potential interactions.
- Consumption of babassu may exert antithyroid effects. Caution is advised in patients with thyroid disorders or taking any herbs or supplements to treat such conditions.

For a complete list of references, please visit www.naturalstandard.com.

Bacopa
(Bacopa monnieri)

RELATED TERMS

- *Bacopa monniera* Linn., *Bacopa monniera* Wettst., *Bacopa monnieri*, *Bacopa monnieri* L., bacopasapponin, bacopasaponin C, bacoside, bacoside A, bacoside A3, bacoside B, bacosine, betulinic acid, brahmi, *Herpestis moniera* cuneifolia, *Herpestis monniera*, Jalanimba, Jalnaveri, medhya rasayana, *Moniera cuneifolia*, oroxindin, sambrani chettu, Scrophulariaceae (family), thyme-leaved gratiola, water hyssop, wogonin.

BACKGROUND

- Bacopa *(Bacopa monnieri)* leaf extract is called *brahmi* in Ayurvedic medicine and is widely used in India, especially for enhancing memory, analgesia (pain relief), and epilepsy. Bacopa has traditionally been used to treat asthma, hoarseness, and mental disorders; to help improve mental performance; as a nerve tonic, cardiotonic (heart tonic), and diuretic (increases urine flow); and for the treatment of epilepsy. Bacopa was prominently mentioned in Indian texts as early as the sixth century.
- Most research on bacopa has focused on its effects on learning. Bacopa may also be helpful in managing pediatric attention deficit hyperactivity disorder (ADHD), but clinical evidence is lacking.

EVIDENCE

Uses Based on Scientific Evidence	Grade
Cognition Although bacopa is traditionally used in Ayurvedic medicine to enhance cognition, current evidence is lacking in this area. More research is needed before bacopa can be recommended for enhancing brain function in adults or children.	B
Anxiety (Clinical) Bacopa has traditionally been used in Ayurvedic medicine to treat anxiety. Although early evidence is promising, more study is needed.	C
Epilepsy Although bacopa is traditionally used in Ayurvedic medicine for epilepsy, there is insufficient evidence to support its effectiveness for this indication.	C
Irritable Bowel Syndrome (IBS) Preliminary evidence suggests that bacopa and bael fruit used in combination may treat irritable bowel syndrome (IBS); however, further studies are warranted.	C
Memory Although bacopa is traditionally used in Ayurvedic medicine to enhance memory, there is insufficient evidence to support its effectiveness for this indication.	C

Uses Based on Tradition or Theory

Analgesia, anti-aging, anti-inflammatory, antimicrobial, antioxidant, antipyretic (fever reducer), asthma, attention deficit hyperactivity disorder (ADHD), back pain, bronchitis, cardiotonic, cardiovascular (heart) disease, diuretic (increases urine flow), fatigue, gastric ulcers, *Helicobacter pylori*, hoarseness of voice, immunomodulation, insomnia, laryngitis, learning, mental disorders, mental illness, nerve disorders, rheumatism, sedative, sexual dysfunction, stress.

DOSING

Adults (18 Years and Older)

- There is insufficient evidence to recommend a dose for bacopa in adults. A traditional dose is 50-150 mg two or three times daily by mouth. For anxiety, a traditional dose is 30 mL of bacopa syrup daily in two divided doses (representing 12 g of dry crude drug) for 4 weeks. Other doses include 2 oz of crude aqueous extract taken daily for up to 5 months, or 2-4 mg/kg of defatted alcoholic bacopa extract daily for up to 5 months.

Children (Younger than 18 Years)

- There is insufficient evidence to recommend a dose for bacopa in children. Nevertheless, based on traditional use, 350 mg/tsp of dried plant extracted in a syrup has been taken three times daily for 3 months in children ages 6-8.

SAFETY

Allergies

- Avoid in individuals with a known allergy or hypersensitivity to *Bacopa monnieri*, its constituents, or any member of the Scrophulariaceae (figwort) family.

Side Effects and Warnings

- Side effects of bacopa may include nausea, dry mouth, thirst, and fatigue. Bacopa has been reported to cause palpitations (irregular heartbeats); patients with heart problems should use with caution.
- Use cautiously in patients taking drugs or herbs that are metabolized by cytochrome P450 enzymes, as bacopa may negatively affect these enzymes.
- Use cautiously in patients taking thyroid drugs, as bacopa may increase thyroid hormones.
- Use cautiously in patients taking calcium-blocking drugs, as bacopa may additively interact with them.
- Use cautiously in patients taking sedatives, as bacopa may additively interact with them.

Pregnancy and Breastfeeding

- Bacopa is not recommended in pregnant or breastfeeding women due to a lack of available scientific evidence.

INTERACTIONS

Interactions with Drugs

- Bacopa may additively interact with calcium blocking drugs.

- Bacopa may negatively affect cytochrome P450 enzymes and may interfere with the way the body processes certain drugs. As a result, the levels of these drugs may be altered in the blood. Patients taking any medications should check the package insert and consult with a qualified health care professional, including a pharmacist, about possible interactions.
- Bacopa may increase thyroid hormones and may interact with hypothyroid medicine.
- Bacopa, when taken concomitantly with phenytoin, may reverse phenytoin-induced cognitive impairment. Consult with a qualified health care professional, including a pharmacist, to check for interactions.

Interactions with Herbs and Dietary Supplements

- Bacopa may negatively affect cytochrome P450 enzymes and interfere with the way the body processes certain herbs or supplements. As a result, the levels of other herbs or supplements may become too high in the blood. It may also alter the effects that other herbs or supplements possibly have on the P450 system.

For a complete list of references, please visit www. naturalstandard.com.

Bael Fruit

RELATED TERMS

- Aegelenine, aegeline, *Aegle marmelos*, allocryptopine, alloimperatorin methyl ether, aurapten, -sitosterol, bael, bael tree, bel, beli, Bengal quince, betulinic acid, bilva, bilwa, butyl p-tolyl sulfide, butylated hydroxyanisole, dimethoxy coumarin, essential oil, ethyl phosphonic acid diethyl ester, hexachloro ethane, Indian bael, lupeol, luvangetin, marmelide, marmelosin, marmenol, marmesin, methyl linoleate, montanine, palmitic acid, praealtin D, psoralen, rues, Rutaceae (family), rutacées, rutaretin, rutin, scopoletin, Shivadume, shivaphala, skimmianine, sripal, tannic acid, tannins (condensed), trans-cinnamic acid, umbelliferone, valencic acid, vilvam, wood apple, xanthotoxin, xanthotoxol.

BACKGROUND

- Bael, a native plant of India, can be found over wide areas of southeast Asia. The ripe fruit and unripe fruit, as well as the roots, leaves, and branches have all been used in traditional medicine. In Ayurveda, the ripe fruit has been used for chronic diarrhea and dysentery, as a tonic for the heart and brain, and as adjuvant treatment for dysentery. A decoction of the roots has been used to treat depression, intermittent fevers, and palpitations; the roots are a main ingredient of the Ayurvedic medicine, *dashmool*. The leaves have been given as a febrifuge and as a poultice for treating ulcers and eye disorders. Administration of fresh leaves has been used for weakness of the heart, dropsy, and beriberi.
- Ayurveda practitioners use Indian bael as an ingredient in respective herbal formulations for boils, dysentery, earaches, discharge from the ears, and fever/cold.
- There is little clinical research using bael fruit for any condition; however, Indian bael has been studied in animals and laboratory studies.

EVIDENCE

Uses Based on Scientific Evidence	Grade
Dysentery (Shigellosis) Indian bael has traditionally been used as a treatment for diarrhea. However, capsules of dried powder of the unripe fruit have not shown effectiveness in treating diarrhea in patients with shigellosis.	F

Uses Based on Tradition or Theory
Abortifacient (induces abortion), angina pectoris (chest pain), antifertility agent in women, antifungal, antispasmodic, aphrodisiac, appetite stimulant, asthma, astringent, beriberi, boils, cardiac conditions (pericarditis), cardiotonic, catarrh (inflammation of mucous membrane), cholera, colds, constipation, convulsions, deafness, demulcent (soothes inflamed tissue), depressive disorder (major), diabetes, digestive, digestive complaints, dropsy (edema), ear discharge, earache, expectorant, eye diseases, eye disorders, fever, heart disorders, hemorrhage, hyperlipidemia (high cholesterol), inflammation, laxative, malaria, mental illnesses, nausea, ophthalmia (inflammation of eye), oral hygiene, pain, palpitations, radioprotection, rectal complaints (procititis and pruritus), restorative, scurvy, sexual dysfunction (seminal weakness), snake venom antidote, sores, stomachache, stomachic, swelling, thirst, thyroid disorders, tonic, tumors, ulcers, upper respiratory tract infections, vomiting.

DOSING

Adults (18 Years and Older)

- There is insufficient evidence to recommend a dose for bael fruit. Traditionally, individuals have taken 2-12 g of the fruit powder, 28-56 mL of a bael decoction, or 12-20 mL of an infusion by mouth.

Children (Younger than 18 Years)

- There is insufficient evidence to recommend a dose for bael fruit for children, and use is not recommended.

SAFETY

Allergies

- Avoid in people with a known allergy or hypersensitivity to Indian bael.

Side Effects and Warnings

- In general, there is a lack of safety information on Indian bael. Based on traditional use, Indian bael may be safe when used in the traditional manner and the fresh, ripe fruit is taken by mouth or when preparations of the pulp are taken in a drink (e.g., nectar, squash) or jam. Avoid dosages that exceed those used in traditional medicine.
- Although not well studied in humans, large quantities of Indian bael may result in digestive complaints and constipation. It may also lower blood sugar. Patients taking thyroid hormones, herbs for thyroid disorders, or herbs that may exacerbate or induce hyperthyroidism, should use caution.

Pregnancy and Breastfeeding

- Indian bael is not recommended in pregnant or breastfeeding women due to a lack of available scientific evidence. Indian bael leaves have been traditionally used to induce abortion and to sterilize women.

INTERACTIONS

Interactions with Drugs

- Indian bael, as extracts of the leaves or seeds, may lower blood sugar levels. Caution is advised when using medications that may also lower blood sugar. Patients taking drugs for diabetes by mouth or insulin should be monitored closely by a qualified health care professional, including a pharmacist. Medication adjustments may be necessary.
- Although not well studied in humans, Indian bael may interact with thyroid hormones or anti-thyroid drugs.

Interactions with Herbs and Dietary Supplements

- Indian bael, as extracts of the leaves or seeds, may lower blood sugar levels. Caution is advised when using herbs or supplements that may also lower blood sugar. Blood glucose levels may require monitoring, and doses may need adjustment.

- Although not well studied in humans, Indian bael may interact with thyroid extracts or anti-thyroid herbs or supplements.

For a complete list of references, please visit www.naturalstandard.com.

Bamboo

RELATED TERMS

- Arrow bamboo, *Arundinaria japonica*, bambusa, Dendrocalamus, Fargesia, Himalayacalamus, Indocalamus, Otatea, *Phyllostachys edulis*, Pleioblastus, *Pseudosasa japonica*, Sasaella, *Sasa japonica*, Semiarundinaria, Shibatea, Thamnocallamus.

BACKGROUND

- Bamboo is the hard woody stems of bamboo plants. In ancient China, bamboo cups were used in cupping therapy, or the "horn method." Today, the Chinese still use cupping therapy to stimulate circulation through the tissues, manage pain, and enhance healing.
- In China, people identify bamboo as a symbol of desirable personality characteristics; it represents elasticity, endurance, and perseverance. The stem bends and does not break.
- In folk medicine, the leaves have been used to treat blood diseases and inflammation. Tabashir, which can be found as a hardened material inside bamboo, has been used for tuberculosis, asthma, and leprosy. In Chinese diet therapy, a soup of bamboo shoots and carp is used to treat measles. The tips of the branches have been used in India for uterine disorders. The shoots are said to be an appetite stimulant and digestion aid. The root has been used for ringworm. The juice from the flowers has been used for earache and deafness.
- Cane and bamboo may be alternative basic construction materials for orthotic and prosthetic appliances. Bamboo night splints and upper limb splints are believed to be effective, and bamboo walkers, crutches and wheelchairs are remarkably useful, inexpensive, and lightweight.
- Bamboo shoots are commonly used as food; they have some anti-thyroidal effects, anti-oxidant activity, and pro-oxidant activity. Bamboo may be an alternative bone substitute, although study is lacking in this area. At this time, there is a lack of clinical evidence supporting the use of bamboo for any indication.

EVIDENCE

Uses Based on Scientific Evidence

No available studies qualify for inclusion in the evidence table.

Uses Based on Tradition or Theory

Acupuncture, antioxidant, appetite stimulant, asthma, blood disorders, bone substitute, cancer prevention, cough, cupping therapy, dandruff, deafness, diabetes, digestive aid, earache, gallbladder disorders, gum disease prevention, headache, human immunodeficiency virus (HIV), hypertension (high blood pressure), hyperthyroid, inflammation, leprosy, measles, orthotic/prosthetic appliances, pain, porphyrin photosensitizers, post-natal depression, pro-oxidant, rehabilitation aid, ringworm, sinusitis, toothache, tuberculosis, uterine disorders, wound healing.

DOSING

Adults (18 Years and Older)

- There is insufficient evidence to recommend a dose of bamboo in adults.

Children (Younger than 18 Years)

- There is insufficient evidence to recommend a dose of bamboo in children.

SAFETY

Allergies

- Patients with a known allergy or sensitivity to bamboo products or any of their ingredients should avoid bamboo products. Contact dermatitis of unclear origin has been reported.

Side Effects and Warnings

- In general, there are limited reports of adverse effects associated with bamboo, although it appears likely safe when prepared and manufactured correctly. The shoots of bamboo are edible and usually safe to ingest. Bamboo shoots should be peeled or boiled before consumption.
- In March 2006, a botulism outbreak (from bamboo shoots) occurred in northern Thailand. Symptoms included respiratory failure, abdominal pain, nausea and/or vomiting, diarrhea, dysphagia (difficulty swallowing) and/or dysarthria (impaired speech), ptosis (droopy eyelid), double vision, generalized weakness, urinary retention, and respiratory failure. Most patients exhibited fluctuating pulse and blood pressure. *Melanosis coli* has also been reported after the ingestion of bamboo leaf extract.
- Caution is advised when ingesting home-canned bamboo shoots that are not properly sterilized or canned. Inadequately cooking bamboo shoots, the anaerobic condition in the can, and lack of an acidifier may produce toxins in the food.
- Many cases of penetration injury have been reported from products made of bamboo materials. It was reported that an illegal abortion performed by inserting foreign objects vaginally into the uterus resulted in a septic abortion.
- Caution is advised in patients with thyroid disorders due to theoretical thyroid suppressant properties.

Pregnancy and Breastfeeding

- Bamboo is not recommended in pregnant or breastfeeding women due to a lack of available scientific evidence.

INTERACTIONS

Interactions with Drugs

- Bamboo has been found to have anti-thyroidal activity.
- Theoretically, bamboo may interact with drugs for thyroid disorders. Patients taking any thyroid medications should consult with a qualified health care professional, including a pharmacist.

Interactions with Herbs and Dietary Supplements

- Theoretically, bamboo may interact with herbs and supplements for thyroid disorder. Bamboo has been found to have anti-thyroidal activity. Caution is advised.

For a complete list of references, please visit www.naturalstandard.com.

Banaba
(Lagerstroemia speciosa)

RELATED TERMS

- Banaba extract, banglang (Vietnam), bang-lang (Cambodia), bungor (Malaya, Sabah), Byers wonderful white crape-myrtle, crape myrtle, crepe myrtle, corosolic acid, ellagitannins (flosin B, reginin A, lagerstroemin), flos-reginae Retz, Glucosol, glucosal, intanin (Thailand), jarul (India), Lagerstroemia, *Lagerstroemia indica*, *Lagerstroemia parviflora*, *Lagerstroemia speciosa*, lasubine, Lythraceae (family), lythraceae alkaloids, *Munchausia speciosa*, Pride-of-India, pyinma, Queen's crape myrtle, Queens flower.

BACKGROUND

- Banaba is a medicinal plant that grows in India, Southeast Asia, and the Philippines. Banaba has been used for blood sugar control. The hypoglycemic (blood sugar–lowering) effect of banaba leaf extract is similar to that of insulin, which induces glucose transport from the blood into body cells.
- Currently, research suggests that taking banaba extract, standardized to 1% corosolic acid, by mouth may lower blood sugar in people with type 2 diabetes; however, further evidence is needed before a firm conclusion can be made.

EVIDENCE

Uses Based on Scientific Evidence	Grade
Diabetes Preliminary research investigating the effects of banaba on diabetes reports promising results. However, additional research is necessary before a firm conclusion can be made.	C

Uses Based on Tradition or Theory
Antibacterial, anti-obesity, antitumor, antitussive, dyspepsia (upset stomach), hyperlipidemia (high cholesterol), hypertriglyceridemia (elevated fatty acid compounds in the blood).

DOSING

Adults (18 Years and Older)

- As a treatment for diabetes, 32 and 48 mg/day for 2 weeks have been used.

Children (Younger than 18 Years)

- There is insufficient evidence to recommend a dose of banaba in children.

SAFETY

Allergies

- Avoid in people with a known allergy or hypersensitivity to banaba or its constituents.

Side Effects and Warnings

- Banaba is generally considered to be safe when taken by mouth for up to 15 days for the treatment of type 2 diabetes. No adverse effects have been noted in the available research. Use cautiously in patients with diabetes because banaba may lower blood sugar.

Pregnancy and Breastfeeding

- Banaba is not recommended in pregnant or breastfeeding women due to a lack of available scientific evidence.

INTERACTIONS

Interactions with Drugs

- *Lagerstroemia indica* has been shown to produce antithrombin activity. Caution is advised in patients with bleeding disorders or those taking drugs that may increase the risk of bleeding. Dosing adjustments may be necessary.
- Theoretically, banaba has been shown to produce insulin-like actions and therefore may have additive effects when taken concomitantly with diabetic drugs. Medication adjustments may be necessary.
- Caution is advised when taking concomitantly with xanthine oxidases.

Interactions with Herbs and Dietary Supplements

- The related crepe myrtle *(Lagerstroemia indica)* has been shown to produce antithrombin activity. Caution is advised in patients with bleeding disorders or those taking herbs or supplements that may increase the risk of bleeding. Multiple cases of bleeding have been reported with the use of *Ginkgo biloba* and fewer cases with garlic and saw palmetto. Numerous other agents may theoretically increase the risk of bleeding, although this has not been proven in most cases.
- Banaba may lower blood sugar levels. Caution is advised when taking banaba with other herbs or supplements that may potentially alter blood sugar, such as fenugreek, garlic, or horse chestnut. Blood glucose levels may require monitoring, and doses may need adjustment.

For a complete list of references, please visit www.naturalstandard.com.

Barberry

RELATED TERMS

- Agrecejo, almindelig berberis (Danish), alvo (Spanish), berbamine, Berberidaceae (family), berberidis cortex, berberine *Berberis aristata*, *Berberis dumetorum*, berberidis radicis cortex, *Berberis thunbergii*, berberine bisulfate, berberitze, berberrubine, berberry, bervulcine, columbamine, crespino (Italian), curcuma, epine-vinette (French), European barberry, isotetrandine, jatorrhizine, jaundice berry, Lebanon barberry, mountain grape, oxyacanthine, palmatine, pipperidge bush, piprage, red barberry, sauerdorn (German), sowberry, uva-espin (Portuguese), vinettier, vulcracine.

BACKGROUND

- Barberry has been used in Indian folk medicine for centuries, and the Chinese have used berberine, a constituent of barberry, since ancient times. The first available documented use of berberine was in 1933 for trachoma (infectious eye disease).
- Historically, barberry was commonly used for its antidiarrheal and antibiotic properties. Barberry is considered tonic, purgative, and antiseptic. As a bitter stomachic tonic, it has been used as remedy for dyspepsia and liver dysfunction because of its purported digestive powers. If given in larger doses, it acts as a mild purgative and removes constipation. Traditionally, it is used in cases of jaundice, general debility and biliousness (gastric distress), and diarrhea.
- Of most interest throughout history is berberine, an alkaloid found in barberry as well as goldenseal, tree turmeric, and Oregon grape. The use of berberine is most commonly used for the management of diarrhea related to cholera and for treating trachomas.
- Berberine has promising anti-inflammatory, antineoplastic (anti-cancer), hypoglycemic (blood sugar–lowering), and immunomodulating effects. Current investigations into berberine continue. However, the use of barberry as a whole plant has been relatively unexplored.

EVIDENCE

Uses Based on Scientific Evidence

No available studies qualify for inclusion in the evidence table.

Uses Based on Tradition or Theory

Antifungal, antihelminthic (expels worms), antihistamine, anti-inflammatory, antimicrobial, antimutagenic, antioxidant (free radical scavenging), antiprotozoal (kills protozoa), antiseptic, antiviral, appetite stimulant, arrhythmia (abnormal heart rates), arthritis, back pain (mid and low), cancer, cardiovascular disease, cholecystitis (inflammation of the gall bladder), cholera, cholagogue (bile flow stimulant), congestive heart failure, constipation, diarrhea, diabetes, eye infections, fever (typhus), gallbladder disorders, gallstones, gout (foot inflammation), heartburn, *Helicobacter pylori* infection, hemorrhoids, hepatoprotection (against acetaminophen toxicity), hypertension (high blood pressure), indigestion, infections (*Escherichia coli*), jaundice, liver cirrhosis (hypertyraminemia), malaria, osteoporosis, parasitic infections (leishmania), psoriasis, respiratory disorders, rheumatism, scurvy, sexually transmitted disease (chlamydia), skin graft healing, sore throat, spleen disorders, stomach cramps, stomatitis (mouth sores), thrombocytopenia (low platelet count), tonic, tuberculosis, urinary tract disorders, wound healing.

DOSING

Adults (18 Years and Older)

- There is insufficient evidence to recommend a dose for barberry in adults. The root bark is typically used as a tincture (1:10) in a dose of 20-40 drops daily. A dry extract of 250-500 mg three times daily has also been used. For sore throats, bladder infections, bronchitis, and yeast infections, a typical dose is 1 cup of tea, prepared by steeping 1-2 tsp of whole or squashed berries in 150 mL of boiling water for 10-15 minutes, and strain or steep 2 g of root bark in 250 mL of boiling water for 5-10 minutes.
- A 10% extract of barberry in ointment has been applied to the skin three times daily.

Children (Younger than 18 Years)

- There is insufficient evidence to recommend a dose for barberry in children. Pediatric use is not recommended.

SAFETY

Allergies

- Barberry should be avoided in patients with a known allergy or hypersensitivity to barberry or its constituents.

Side Effects and Warnings

- In general, most herbal experts purport that barberry is generally well tolerated in recommended doses. However, there is little available scientific evidence regarding the safety of barberry, and many adverse effects have been reported following administration of berberine (a constituent found in barberry, goldenseal, and other herbs). Berberine has been reported to cause nausea, vomiting, abdominal discomfort, headache, hypertension, hypotension, (increases and decreases in blood pressure), bradycardia (slowed heart rate), leukopenia (low white blood cell count), respiratory failure, giddiness, skin irritation, paresthesias (abnormal sensations), decreases in blood glucose, and delays in the small intestinal transit time. Berberine has been used as an abortifacient (to induce abortion) and antifertility agent. Although not well studied in humans, berberine may also inhibit osteoclast-like cells or cause excess levels of bilirubin in the blood.
- High doses of berberine may cause diarrhea, cardiac damage, cardiac arrest, nosebleed, hemorrhagic nephritis, kidney irritation, dyspnea (difficulty breathing), respiratory spasms, lethargy, eye irritation, or death. When injected subcutaneously (under the skin), berberine may cause permanent hyperpigmentation.

- Berberine should be used cautiously in patients with diabetes, cardiovascular disease, hypotension (low blood pressure), gastrointestinal disorders, liver dysfunction, or renal (kidney) dysfunction.

Pregnancy and Breastfeeding

- Barberry is not recommended in pregnant or breastfeeding women due to lack of available scientific evidence. Barberry has exhibited uterine stimulant properties, and berberine has been shown to have anti-fertility activity.

INTERACTIONS
Interactions with Drugs

- Concurrent administration of barberry and anti-arrhythmic medication is not recommended due to the unpredictable results of combining two anti-arrhythmic therapies.
- Theoretically, the concomitant use of barberry may decrease tetracycline effectiveness.
- Barberry has displayed anticholinergic activity. Theoretically, combination use of barberry with anticholinergic agents may potentiate these effects. Examples include acetophenenazine, atropine, belladonna, dicyclomine, diphenhydramine, hyosciamine, prochlorperazine, promethazine, scopolamine, trifluoperazine, triflupromazine, and trihexyphenidyl.
- Berberine may increase platelet formation. Caution is advised when using medications that may have competing effects. Examples include aspirin, anticoagulants (blood thinners) such as warfarin (Coumadin) or heparin, anti-platelet drugs such as clopidogrel (Plavix), and non-steroidal anti-inflammatory drugs such as ibuprofen (Motrin, Advil) or naproxen (Naprosyn, Aleve).
- Although not well studied in humans, barberry may have antihistamine effects. Theoretically, barberry may interact with antihistamines.
- There may be additive hypotensive (blood pressure lowering) effects and bradycardia (slowed heart rate) when combining barberry with blood pressure–lowering medications, such as beta-blockers and calcium channel blockers. Caution is advised.
- Although not well studied in humans, barberry's constituent, berberine, and berberine sulfate have anti-inflammatory effects and may interact with COX-2 inhibitors. COX-2 inhibitor drugs include celecoxib (Celebrex) and rofecoxib (Vioxx).
- Barberry contains vitamin C and may have a mild diuretic effect due to its acidity. Theoretically, barberry may interact with other diuretic agents. Caution is advised.
- Preliminary evidence shows that barberry may interfere with the way the body processes certain drugs using the liver's cytochrome P450 enzyme system. As a result, levels of these drugs may be altered in the blood and may cause different effects or potentially serious adverse reactions.
- Barberry has been shown to decrease blood sugar levels. Patients taking diabetes medications by mouth or insulin should consult with a qualified health care professional, including a pharmacist, to check for interactions.

- Theoretically, concomitant use of berberine may have additional effects with other sedative agents. Berberine may cause sedation and motor impairment. Caution is advised when using in combination with other medications that have sedative effects.
- Berberine, an alkaloid purported to be an active ingredient of barberry, may interact with yohimbine. Berberine may also interact additively with L-phenylephrine. Caution is advised.

Interactions with Herbs and Dietary Supplements

- The concurrent use of berberine (a constituent of barberry) and antibiotics may have additive effects. Consult with a qualified health care professional, including a pharmacist, before combining therapies.
- Barberry has displayed anticholinergic activity. Theoretically, combination use of barberry with anticholinergic agents may increase these effects. Examples of anticholinergic herbs include bittersweet (Solanum dulcamara), henbane (Hyoscyamus niger), and Jimson weed (Datura stramonium).
- Berberine may increase platelet formation therefore, caution is advised when using herbs or supplements that may have competing effects.
- Berberine has been shown to decrease blood pressure. Patients taking blood pressure–lowering medications should consult with a qualified health care professional, including a pharmacist.
- Use with other herbs containing berberine may increase the risk of berberine toxicity. Examples of berberine-containing herbs include bloodroot, goldenseal, and celandine.
- Barberry contains vitamin C and may have a mild diuretic effect due to the acid content. Theoretically, barberry may increase the effects of other herbs with potential diuretic effects. Caution is advised.
- Preliminary evidence shows that barberry may interfere with the way the body processes certain drugs using the liver's cytochrome P450 enzyme system. As a result, levels of these drugs may be altered in the blood and may cause different effects or potentially serious adverse reactions.
- Berberine may lower blood sugar levels. Caution is advised when combining with other herbs and supplements that may also lower blood sugar.
- Theoretically, concomitant use of berberine may have additional effects with other sedative agents. Berberine may cause drowsiness and motor impairment. Caution is advised when using in combination with other herbs or supplements that have sedative effects, such as chamomile.
- Yohimbine (a constituent of yohimbe) and barberry competitively interact for binding sites. In addition, the purported anti-fertility properties of berberine may theoretically antagonize the purported pro-fertility effects of yohimbe.
- Berberine may decrease the metabolism of vitamin B, and caution is advised when taking these two agents concurrently.

For a complete list of references, please visit www.naturalstandard.com.

Barley
(Hordeum vulgare)

RELATED TERMS

- Barley flour, barley malt, barley oil, beta-glucan brewers spent grain, dietary fiber, germinated barley foodstuff (GBF), high-protein barley flour (HPBF), Gramineae (family), high-fiber barley, hordenine, hordeum, *Hordeum dislichon, Hordeum distychum, Hordeum murinum, Hordeum vulgare* var Himalaya 292, *Hordeum vulgare* ssp *spontaneium, Hordeum vulgare* ssp *spontaneum*, lunasin, Mai Ya, pearl barley, Poaceae (family), pot barley, prowashonupana (Prowash), scotch barley, tocols, tocopherols, tocotrienols, vitamin E, wild barley, wild barley grass.
- **Note:** Most scientific studies have used foods containing barley rather than barley supplements.

BACKGROUND

- Barley is a grain used as a staple food in many countries. It is commonly used as an ingredient in baked products and soups in Europe and the United States. Barley malt is used to make beer and as a natural sweetener called *malt sugar* or *barley jelly sugar*.
- There is promising evidence that barley may reduce total cholesterol and low-density lipoprotein (LDL, or "bad cholesterol") in mildly hyperlipidemic patients. Barley has a high fiber content.
- Germinated barley foodstuff (GBF) may play a role in the management of ulcerative colitis and mild constipation.

EVIDENCE

Uses Based on Scientific Evidence	Grade
Coronary Heart Disease (CHD) The Food and Drug Administration (FDA) has announced that whole grain barley and barley-containing products are allowed to claim that they reduce the risk of coronary heart disease (CHD). To qualify for the health claim, the barley-containing foods must provide at least 0.75 g of soluble fiber per serving of the food.	B
Constipation Due to its high fiber content, barley has been used traditionally as a treatment for constipation. However, there is limited scientific evidence in this area. Further research is necessary in order to establish safety and dosing recommendations.	C
High Blood Sugar/Glucose Intolerance Early evidence suggests that barley meal may improve glucose tolerance. Better research is necessary before a firm conclusion can be drawn.	C
Ulcerative Colitis Germinated barley foodstuff (GBF), which comes from maturing barley, may be helpful in patients with ulcerative colitis. Scientific evidence in this area is limited,	C
and further research is needed before GBF can be recommended for ulcerative colitis.	
Weight Loss Increasing whole grain foods containing high amounts of soluble or insoluble fiber may help to control weight. Barley has a high fiber content, but studies regarding whether barley promotes weight loss are limited.	C

Uses Based on Tradition or Theory

Antimicrobial, antioxidant, appetite suppressant, asthma, boils, bowel/intestinal disorders, bronchitis, bronchodilation, cancer, celiac disease, colon cancer, diabetes, diarrhea, flavoring agent (sweetener), gastrointestinal inflammation, hair growth stimulant, high blood pressure, improved blood circulation, immunomodulator, irritable bowel syndrome, kidney disease, nutritional supplement, stamina/strength enhancer, stomach upset, weight loss.

DOSING

Adults (18 Years and Older)

- For constipation, limited research has used 9 g of germinated barley foodstuff (GBF) daily for up to 20 days. The U.S. Food and Drug Administration (FDA) allows whole grain barley and barley-containing products to claim that they reduce the risk of coronary heart disease (CHD). To qualify for the health claim, the barley-containing foods must provide at least 0.75 g of soluble fiber per serving.
- For high cholesterol, 1.5 mL of barley oil twice daily or 30 g of barley bran flour daily by mouth has been used in studies. Also, for ulcerative colitis (mild to moderate), 10 g germinated barley foodstuff (GBF) taken three times daily has been studied and reported as well tolerated.
- For hyperglycemia, studies have used 90 g of barley carbohydrates, either alone or enriched with beta-glucan.

Children (Younger than 18 Years)

- There is not enough scientific information to recommend barley for use in children.

SAFETY

Allergies

- Individuals with known allergy or hypersensitivity to barley flour or beer should avoid barley products. Severe allergic reactions (anaphylaxis) and skin rashes have been reported from drinking beer made with malted barley. Patients with allergy/hypersensitivity to gluten, grass pollens, rice, rye, oats, or wheat may also react to barley, especially due to possible cross-contamination with other grain products.
- "Bakers' asthma" is an allergic response from breathing in cereal flours among workers of the baking and milling

industries and can occur due to barley flour exposure. If an individual is allergic to one grain (e.g., barley), there is a possibility that other grains may cause similar symptoms.

Side Effects and Warnings

- Barley appears to be well tolerated in non-allergic healthy adults in recommended doses for short periods of time, as a grain or in the form of beer. Individuals with celiac disease (wheat allergy) may have a higher tendency to develop gastrointestinal (stomach) upset with barley products. Barley may cause a feeling of "fullness."
- Theoretically, eating large amounts of barley may lower blood sugar levels. Caution is advised in patients with diabetes or hypoglycemia, and in those taking drugs, herbs, or supplements that affect blood sugar. Serum glucose levels may need to be monitored by a health care provider, and medication adjustments may be necessary. Hordenine, a chemical in the root of developing barley, may stimulate the sympathetic nervous system. The effect of hordenine from barley on humans is not clear, although it may increase heart rate or wakefulness.
- Eye, nasal, and sinus irritation or asthmatic reactions can occur from exposure to barley dust. Some individuals may experience itching, inflammation, or irritation of the skin, eyelids, arms, or legs. Contact with the malt in beer may cause skin rash.
- Fungal contamination of barley with *Trichothecium roseum* has occurred and may cause a serious condition in which bones break down. Another contaminant that has been found in barley is ochratoxin A.

Pregnancy and Breastfeeding

- Traditionally, women have been advised against eating large amounts of barley sprouts during pregnancy. Infants fed with a formula containing barley water, whole milk, and corn syrup developed malnutrition and anemia, possibly due to vitamin deficiencies.

INTERACTIONS

Interactions with Drugs

- Fiber in barley may decrease the absorption of medications taken by mouth and prevent full beneficial effects. In general, prescription drugs should be taken 1 hour before or 2 hours after barley because the fiber content may reduce the effectiveness of many drugs, vitamins, and minerals.
- Eating barley in large quantities may lower blood sugar concentrations. Caution is advised when using medications that may also lower blood sugar. Patients taking drugs for diabetes by mouth or insulin should be monitored closely by a qualified health care professional. Medication adjustments may be necessary.
- Barley has been associated with decreased total cholesterol and low-density lipoprotein (LDL) concentrations, and may act additively with other cholesterol-lowering agents. Barley may also lower blood pressure and should be used with caution if blood pressure–lowering drugs are also taken.
- Animal data suggest that consuming barley may interfere with the absorption of anthelmintics, which are drugs taken for parasitic worms.

Interactions with Herbs and Dietary Supplements

- Fiber in barley may decrease the absorption of medications taken by mouth and prevent full beneficial effects. In general, prescription drugs should be taken 1 hour before or 2 hours after barley because barley may reduce the effectiveness of many drugs, vitamins, and minerals.
- In theory, barley may lower blood sugar levels. Caution is advised when using herbs or supplements that may also lower blood sugar. Blood glucose levels may require monitoring, and doses may need adjustment.
- Animal data suggest that consuming barley may interfere with the absorption of anthelminthics, which are agents taken to rid the body of parasitic worms.

For a complete list of references, please visit www.naturalstandard.com.

RELATED TERMS

- Alpha-methylene-gamma-butyrolactone moiety, bay laurel, bay tree, costunolide, daphne, dehydrocostus lactone, Grecian laurel, guaianolides, Lauraceae (family), laurel, laurel oil, Laurus, *Laurus nobilis* L., Mediterranean bay, Mediterranean laurel, noble laurel, p-menthane hydroperoxide, reynosin, Roman laurel, santamarine, sesquiterpenes, sweet bay, sweet laurel, true bay, trypanocidal terpenoids, zaluzanin D.
- **Note:** Bay leaf *(Laurus nobilis)* may be confused with California bay leaf *(Umbellularia californica)*, also known as California laurel, Oregon myrtle, or Indian bay leaf (*Cinnamoma tamala*). This monograph only covers bay leaf *(Laurus nobilis)*.

BACKGROUND

- Bay leaf is primarily used to flavor foods, and it is used by chefs of ethnic cuisines, from Italian to Thai. It is also frequently used in salt-free seasonings.
- Bay leaf is thought to be useful for gastric ulcers, high blood sugar, migraines, and infections. Bay leaves and berries have been used for their astringent, diaphoretic (promotes sweating), carminative (promotes digestion), digestive, and stomachic (tones and strengthens the stomach) properties. In the Middle Ages bay leaf was believed to induce abortions. Traditionally, the berries of the bay tree were used to treat furuncles. The leaf essential oil of *Laurus nobilis* has been used as an antiepileptic remedy in Iranian traditional medicine.
- Currently, there is not enough scientific evidence to draw any firm conclusions about the medicinal safety, effectiveness, or dosing of bay leaf.

EVIDENCE

Uses Based on Scientific Evidence

No available studies qualify for inclusion in the evidence table.

Uses Based on Tradition or Theory

Abortifacient (inducing abortion), amenorrhea (absence of menstruation), analgesic (pain-reliever), antibacterial, anticonvulsant, antifungal, anti-inflammatory, antimicrobial, antioxidant, antiseptic, appetite stimulant, arthritis, astringent, bile flow stimulant, bronchitis, cancer, carminative (promotes digestion), colic, dandruff, diabetes, diaphoretic (promotes sweating), digestive, diuretic, ear pain, emetic (induces vomiting), emmenagogue (promotes menstruation), food uses, furuncles (skin boils), hysteria, influenza, insecticide, leukemia, migraine headaches, narcotic, nightmares, rheumatism, sprains, stimulant, stomach ulcers, wound healing.

DOSING

Adults (18 Years and Older)

- There is not enough scientific evidence to recommend dose for bay leaf in adults.

Children (Younger than 18 Years)

- There is not enough scientific evidence to recommend a dose for bay leaf in children.

SAFETY

Allergies

- People with a known allergy to bay leaf *(Laurus nobilis)*, its constituents, and related plants in the Lauraceae family as well as the Compositae/Asteraceae family should not use bay leaf. Contact dermatitis and occupational asthma have been reported.

Side Effects and Warnings

- Overall, bay leaf has few reported effects and is likely safe when used as a flavouring agent in foods. However, it may cause contact dermatitis and occupational asthma. Bay leaves may become lodged in the gastrointestinal tract, causing tears or blockages. These impacted leaves may also obstruct breathing.
- Other reported side effects include hand and face eczema and airborne contact dermatitis.

Pregnancy and Breastfeeding

- Bay leaf is not recommended in pregnant or breastfeeding women due to lack of available scientific evidence.

INTERACTIONS

Interactions with Drugs

- Alcohol extracts of bay leaf may interact with angiotensin-converting enzyme (ACE)–inhibiting agents.
- Bay leaf essential oil may have anticonvulsant effects. Individuals using bay leaf with other medications with anticonvulsant effects should consult with a qualified health care professional, including a pharmacist.
- Bay leaf essential oil may cause sedation and motor impairment. Caution is advised when using in combination with other medications that have sedative effects, such as chamomile.

Interactions with Herbs and Dietary Supplements

- Bay leaf essential oil may have anticonvulsant effects. People using bay leaf with other herbs and supplements with anticonvulsant effects should consult with a qualified health care professional, including a pharmacist.
- Bay leaf essential oil may cause sedation and motor impairment. Caution is advised when using in combination with other herbs and supplements that have sedative effects, such as chamomile.

For a complete list of references, please visit www.naturalstandard.com.

Bear's Garlic
(Allium ursinum)

RELATED TERMS

- Ajoenes, Alliaceae (family) *Allium ursinum,* buckrams, flavonoid glycosides, lectins, ramsons, thiosulfinates, wild garlic, wood garlic.

BACKGROUND

- Bear's garlic, so named because brown bears in Europe tend to eat it, is a wild relative of the chive that is popularly used as a flavoring or dietary vegetable in Central European cuisine. It grows in swampy fields and wooded areas in slightly acidic soil and is often used as a vegetable in salads and cooked dishes.
- Bear's garlic has been confused with lily of the valley and autumn crocus, especially in the spring before flowering. Several cases of colchicine poisoning due to consumption of autumn crocus mistaken for bear's garlic have been reported in recent years. Colchine is a toxic alkaloid that can lead to gastroenterocolitis, followed by multiple organ failure, and sometimes death.
- Although there is a lack of clinical evidence describing the use of bear's garlic for any indication, it may have inhibitory effects on human platelet aggregation. Bear's garlic is not listed on the U.S. Food and Drug Administration's "generally recommended as safe" (GRAS) list.

EVIDENCE

Uses Based on Scientific Evidence

No available studies qualify for inclusion in the evidence table.

Uses Based on Tradition or Theory

Antiplatelet (blood thinner), food use.

DOSING

Adults (18 Years and Older)

- There is insufficient evidence to recommend a dose for bear's garlic in adults.

Children (Younger than 18 Years)

- There is insufficient evidence to recommend a dose for bear's garlic in children.

SAFETY

Allergies

- Avoid in people with a known allergy or hypersensitivity to bear's garlic or other members of the Alliaceae family such as garlic, leeks, shallots, or onions.

Side Effects and Warnings

- Bear's garlic is likely safe when consumed in food amounts.
- Although there are no known toxicities associated with consumption of bear's garlic, several reports of colchicine poisoning, resulting in gastroenterocolitis and sometimes fatal multiple organ failure, have been reported in people who mistakenly consumed autumn crocus instead of bear's garlic. Toxic effects appear to be more severe when autumn crocus leaves are eaten after being cooked and when eaten by people ages 65 and older.
- Bear's garlic is not listed on the U.S. Food and Drug Administration's (FDA's) "generally recommended as safe" (GRAS) list.

Pregnancy and Breastfeeding

- Bear's garlic is not recommended in pregnant or breastfeeding women due to a lack of available scientific evidence.

INTERACTIONS

Interactions with Drugs

- Bear's garlic has demonstrated anti-inflammatory activity and may compete with the effects of non-steroidal anti-inflammatory drugs (NSAIDs).
- Bear's garlic may increase the risk of bleeding when taken with drugs that increase the risk of bleeding. Caution is advised in patients with bleeding disorders; dosing adjustments may be necessary.

Interactions with Herbs and Dietary Supplements

- Bear's garlic may increase the risk of bleeding when taken with herbs or supplements that are believed to increase the risk of bleeding. Multiple cases of bleeding have been reported with the use of *Ginkgo biloba,* and fewer cases with garlic and saw palmetto.
- Bear's garlic may increase the activity of herbs with anti-inflammatory activity.

For a complete list of references, please visit www.naturalstandard.com.

RELATED TERMS

- Anemophilous pollen, apiary products, Asteraceae, bee bread, bee pollen extract, Boraginaceae, *Brassia campestres* L., buckwheat pollen, *Bursera simaruba*, *Cecropia peltata*, cernilton, cernitin pollen extract, Compositae, Convolvulaceae, dandelion pollen (Compositae), dark blue bee pollen, *Echium vulgare* (Boraginaceae), Entomophilous pollen, Eragrostis, Eugenia, *Eupatorium albicaule*, Euphorbiaceae, Fabaceae, floral honey, floral pollen honey, honeybee pollen, Lonchocarpus, maize pollen, mesquite pollen, *Metopium brownei*, *Mimosa bahamensis*, Myrtaceae, pine pollen, Poaceae, pollen, pollen d'abeille, pouteria, propolis, pyrrolizidine alkaloid, rape pollen, Sapindaceae, Sapotaceae, songhuuafen, Spanish bee pollen, *Thouinia canesceras*, Tiliaceae, *Trema micrantha*, *Viguiera dentata*.

BACKGROUND

- Bee pollen is considered a highly nutritious food because it is a rich source of vitamins, minerals, carbohydrates, fats, enzymes, and essential amino acids. Pollen comes from various plants, including buckwheat, maize, pine (songhaufen), rape, and typha (puhuang). Avoid confusion with bee venom, honey, and royal jelly. Bees use propolis, a resinous substance, to construct their hives. Royal jelly is secreted from the salivary glands of bees.

- The lay public probably uses it more often than is prescribed in clinical practice. Typically, bee pollen is used as a dietary supplement. It is also used to enhance athletic stamina and strength and to assist in recovery from illness. Bee pollen is often used as an antidote during allergy season, and it is thought of aid in respiratory complaints such as bronchitis, sinus congestion, and common rhinitis. In the support of hormonal disorders, bee pollen is thought to balance the endocrine system with specific benefits in menstrual and prostate disorders. In Chinese medicine, bee pollen is used for building blood, for reducing cravings for sweets and alcohol, for radioprotection, and as an anticancer treatment. Topically it is used for eczema, skin eruptions, and diaper rash. There is insufficient evidence to support its use for these indications.

EVIDENCE

Uses Based on Scientific Evidence	Grade
Athletic Performance Enhancement It is unclear if bee pollen enhances athletic performance.	C
Cancer Treatment Side Effects Bee pollen may reduce some adverse effects of cancer treatment; however, this remains unclear.	C

Uses Based on Tradition or Theory

Aging, allergies, amenorrhea (absence of menstruation), antibacterial, antifungal, antioxidant, appetite stimulant, arthritis, benign prostatic hypertrophy (BPH), bleeding, bronchitis, chronic renal insufficiency, colitis (inflammation of colon), constipation, cough (bloody), diarrhea, diuretic, dysentery (bloody diarrhea), dysmenorrheal (painful menstruation), eczema, enteritis (inflammation of bowels), growth, hay fever, hemorrhage (cerebral), hemorrhoids, high cholesterol (hyperlipidemia), immunomodulator, infertility, liver dysfunction, memory, menstrual problems, mouth sores, multiple sclerosis, nosebleed, nutrition, pregnancy nutritional supplement, prostatitis (inflammation of prostate), radioprotection, rash, renal impairment, rheumatism, sexual performance, Sjogren's syndrome, skin care, skin eruptions, tonic, vomiting (blood), weight loss.

DOSING

Adults (18 Years and Older)

- Safety, efficacy, and dosing have not been systematically studied. In general, 1/8-1/4 tsp has been taken by mouth once per day. The dosage may be gradually increased to 1-2 tsp one to three times per day.

Children (Younger than 18 Years)

- Safety, efficacy, and dosing have not been systematically studied. Use in children should be supervised by a qualified health care professional.

SAFETY

Allergies

- Avoid in people with a known allergy or hypersensitivity to pollen, especially pollen included in commercial preparations. Allergic reactions may include itching, swelling, shortness of breath, lightheadedness, gastrointestinal upset, rash, asthma, hay fever, nausea, abdominal cramps, diarrhea, vomiting, and anaphylaxis.

Side Effects and Warnings

- In general, most of the adverse effects appear to arise from hypersensitivity or allergy to pollen. Symptoms may include gastrointestinal upset, rash, erythema (reddening of the skin), asthma, hay fever, nausea, respiratory reactions, hives, diarrhea, vomiting, sensitivity to light, hypereosinophilia (increased white blood cell counts in the blood), anorexia, abdominal pain, generalized malaise, headache, itching, and decreased memory. Most symptoms appear to resolve after discontinuing the use of bee pollen.

- There have also been multiple cases of acute hepatitis associated with bee pollen combination products. In these cases, it is not known if bee pollen or another herb might have caused the adverse event.

- Avoid using in patients with blood disorders or liver disease.

Pregnancy and Breastfeeding

- Bee pollen is not recommended during pregnancy or breast-feeding due to a lack of available scientific information.

INTERACTIONS
Interactions with Drugs

- Currently, there is a lack of available scientific evidence describing drug interactions with bee pollen.

Interactions with Herbs and Dietary Supplements

- Currently, there is a lack of available scientific evidence describing herb and supplement interactions with bee pollen.

For a complete list of references, please visit www.naturalstandard.com.

Belladonna
(*Atropa* spp.)

RELATED TERMS

- *Atropa belladonna,* atropa belladonna-AE, beladona, bella-done, belladonnae herbae pulvis standardisatus, belladonna herbum, Belladonna Homaccord, Belladonna Injeel, Belladonna Injeel Forte, belladonna leaf, belladonna pulvis normatus, belladonnae folium, belladonna radix, belladonne, deadly nightshade, deadly nightshade leaf, devil's cherries, devil's herb, die belladonna, die tollkirsche, divale, dwale, dwayberry, galnebaer, great morel, herba belladonna, hoja de belladonna, naughty man's cherries, poison black cherries, powdered belladonna, Solanaceae (family), solanum mortale, solanum somniferum, strygium, stryshon, tollekirsche, tollkirschenblatter.

BACKGROUND

- Belladonna is an herb that has been used for centuries for a variety of indications, including headache, menstrual symptoms, peptic ulcer disease, inflammation, and motion sickness. Belladonna is known to contain active agents with anticholinergic properties, such as the tropane alkaloids atropine, hyoscine (scopolamine), and hyoscyamine.
- There are few available studies of belladonna alone for any indication. Most research has evaluated belladonna in combination with other agents (such as ergot alkaloids or barbiturates) or in highly dilute homeopathic preparations. Preliminary evidence suggests possible efficacy in combination with barbiturates for the management of symptoms associated with irritable bowel syndrome. However, there is currently insufficient scientific evidence regarding the use of belladonna for this or any other indication.
- Common adverse effects include dry mouth, urinary retention, flushing, pupillary dilation, constipation, confusion, and delirium. Many of these effects may occur at therapeutic doses.

EVIDENCE

Uses Based on Scientific Evidence	Grade
Airway Obstruction Belladonna can cause relaxation of the airway and reduce the amount of mucus produced. However, there is a lack of high-quality human research in this area.	C
Ear Infection Little reliable research is available on the use of belladonna for ear infections. Other therapies have been shown to be effective and are recommended for this condition.	C
Headache The available studies of belladonna in the treatment of headache thus far do not show a clear benefit. More studies are needed to test the ability of belladonna alone (not in multi-ingredient products) to treat or prevent headache.	C
Irritable Bowel Syndrome Belladonna has been used historically for the treatment of irritable bowel, and in theory its mechanism of action should be effective for some of the symptoms. However, in the few studies that are available, it is unclear whether belladonna alone (not as part of a mixed product) provides this effect.	C
Menopausal Symptoms Bellergal (a combination of phenobarbital, ergot, and belladonna) has been used historically to treat hot flashes. However, belladonna supplements have not shown clear benefits in clinical studies.	C
Nervous System Disorders The autonomic nervous system, which helps control basic body functions such as sweating and blood flow, is affected in several disorders. To date, clinical studies using belladonna have shown uncertain benefits in treating these disorders.	C
Premenstrual Syndrome (PMS) Bellergal (a combination of phenobarbital, ergot, and belladonna) has been used to treat PMS symptoms. However, there is insufficient evidence supporting this use.	C
Radiation Therapy Rash (Radiation Burn) There is insufficient evidence to recommend belladonna as a treatment for rash after radiation therapy.	C
Sweating (Excessive) There is insufficient evidence to recommend belladonna as a treatment for excessive sweating (hyperhidrosis).	C

Uses Based on Tradition or Theory

Abnormal menstrual periods, acute infections, acute inflammation, anesthetic, antispasmodic, anxiety, arthritis, asthma, bedwetting, bowel disorders, chicken pox, colds, colitis, conjunctivitis (inflamed eyes), dental conditions, diarrhea, diuretic (use as a "water pill"), diverticulitis, earache, encephalitis (inflammation of the brain), eye disorders (dilation of the pupils), fever, flu, glaucoma, gout, hay fever, hemorrhoids, hyperkinesis, inflammation, kidney stones, measles, motion sickness, mumps, muscle and joint pain, muscle spasms, nausea and vomiting during pregnancy, organophosphate poisoning, neuropathy (nerve pain), Parkinson's disease, pancreatitis, peritonitis, rash, scarlet fever, sciatica (back and leg pain), sedative, sore throat, stomach ulcers, teething, toothache, ulcerative colitis, urinary tract disorders (difficulty passing urine), warts, whooping cough.

DOSING
Adults (18 Years and Older)

- A traditional dose of belladonna leaf powder is 50-100 mg taken by mouth, with a maximum single dose of 200 mg (0.6 mg of total alkaloids, calculated as the ingredient hyoscyamine) and a maximum daily dose of 600 mg. A traditional dose of belladonna root is 50 mg, with a maximum single dose of 100 mg (0.5 mg of total alkaloids, calculated as hyoscyamine) and a maximum daily dose of 300 mg. A traditional dose of belladonna extract is 10 mg, with a maximum single dose of 100 mg (0.5 mg of total alkaloids, calculated as hyoscyamine) and a maximum daily dose of 150 mg. The expert German panel, the Commission E, suggests these doses mainly for the treatment of "gastrointestinal spasm." For tincture of belladonna (composed of 27-33 mg of belladonna leaf alkaloids in 100 mL of alcohol), secondary sources suggest either a total dose of 1.5 mg daily (divided into three doses with a double dose at bedtime) or a dose of 0.6-1 mL (0.18-0.3 mg of belladonna leaf alkaloids) taken 3-4 times daily.

- For headache, the combination product Bellergal (40 mg phenobarbital, 0.6 mg ergotamine tartrate, 0.2 mg levorotatory alkaloids of belladonna) has been taken by mouth twice daily.

- Homeopathic doses often depend on the symptom being treated and the style of the prescribing provider. Dosing practices may therefore vary widely. Usually, a homeopathic product is diluted several times. For example, belladonna may be diluted by 100 (1 tsp belladonna added to 99 tsp water) and resulting mixture further diluted 1-100 for 30 or more serial dilutions.

- A belladonna plaster produced by Cuxson Gerrard (England) containing 0.25% belladonna alkaloids (hyoscine 2%, atropine 1%) has been used topically (applied to the skin) for muscle and bone aches. Long-term use may cause a rash at the site of the plaster.

Children (Younger than 18 Years)

- Informal reports suggest a typical dose of 0.03 mL for each kilogram of body weight, taken by mouth three times daily. Another dose that has been used is 0.8 mL for each square meter of body surface area, taken by mouth three times daily (27-33 mg of belladonna leaf alkaloids in 100 mL). The maximum dose is reported as 3.5 mL/day. Safety and effectiveness have not been clearly demonstrated.

- Death in children may occur at 0.2 mg of atropine for each kilogram of a child's weight. Because 2 mg of atropine are often found in one fruit, just two fruits may be deadly for a small child.

- Homeopathic doses often depend on the symptom being treated and the style of the prescribing provider. Dosing practices may therefore vary widely.

SAFETY
Allergies

- Belladonna should be avoided in people who have had significant reactions to belladonna or anticholinergic drugs, or who are allergic to belladonna or other members of the Solanaceae (nightshade) family such as bell peppers, potatoes, and eggplants. Long-term use of belladonna on the skin can lead to allergic rashes.

Side Effects and Warnings

- In smaller doses, belladonna is traditionally thought to be safe, but may cause frequent side effects such as dilated pupils, blushing of the skin, dry mouth, rapid heartbeat, confusion, nervousness, and hallucinations. Based on animal study, belladonna alkaloids may inhibit cognitive function and gastrointestinal motility. High doses can cause death.

- In children, death can be caused by a small amount of belladonna. Several reports of accidental belladonna overdose and death are reported. Belladonna overdose can also occur when it is applied to the skin. Belladonna overdose is highly dangerous and should be treated by qualified medical professionals. Because belladonna can slow the movement of food and drugs through the stomach and gut, the side effects may go on long after the belladonna is swallowed.

- Belladonna may cause redness of the skin, flushing, dry skin, sun sensitivity, hives, and allergic rashes, even at dilute concentrations. A very serious, potentially life-threatening rash called Stevens-Johnson syndrome has been reported. Other side effects reported are headache, hyperactivity, nervousness, dizziness, lightheadedness, drowsiness or sedation, unsteady walking, confusion, slurred speech, exaggerated reflexes, or convulsions. The eyes may be sensitive to light, and vision may be blurry. If pieces of belladonna are put into the eye, the pupils may be dilated permanently.

- Cases report hyperventilation, coma with the loss of breathing, and severe high blood pressure. Others report abdominal fullness, difficult urination, decreased perspiration, slow release of breast milk while nursing, muscle cramps or spasms, and tremors. Belladonna should be avoided in those with difficulty passing urine, enlarged prostate, kidney stones, dry mouth, Sjögren's syndrome, dry eyes, or glaucoma. Belladonna should be used cautiously with a fever. People with myasthenia gravis (a disorder of nerves and muscles) or Down's syndrome may be especially sensitive to belladonna.

- Older adults and children should avoid belladonna, as there are many reports of serious adverse effects in these age groups. Belladonna should not be combined with prescribed anticholinergic agents. People who have had heart disease or a heart attack, fluid in the lungs, high blood pressure, or abnormal heart rhythms should avoid belladonna. Because belladonna can affect the activity of the stomach and intestines, people who have had ulcers, reflux, hiatal hernia, bowel obstruction, poor movement of the intestines, constipation, colitis, or an ileostomy or colostomy after surgery should avoid belladonna.

Pregnancy and Breastfeeding

- Belladonna is not recommended in pregnancy and breastfeeding because of the risks of side effects and poisoning. Belladonna is listed under category C according to the U.S. Food and Drug Administration (FDA) (category C includes drugs for which no thorough studies have been published). In nursing women who use belladonna, belladonna ingredients are found in breast milk, therefore endangering infants.

INTERACTIONS
Interactions with Drugs

- Belladonna may slow the movement of food and medication through the gut, and therefore some medications may be absorbed more slowly. Many prescribed medications can interact with anticholinergic drugs that have similar effects to belladonna. A qualified health care professional, including a pharmacist, should be consulted prior to taking belladonna.

- Atropine is an ingredient in belladonna. Theoretically, drugs that interact with atropine may also interact with belladonna. Some antidepressant medications (tricyclic drugs) can interact with belladonna. The effects of the drug cisapride, used to increase the movement of food through the stomach, may be blocked. Medications that can increase heart rate, especially procainamide, can cause an exaggerated increase in heart rate if given with belladonna. The use of alcohol with belladonna can cause extreme slowing of brain function.
- Belladonna may also interact with alkaloids, atropine, ergot derivatives, hormonal agents, drugs that increase sun sensitivity, drugs cleared by the kidney, scopolamine, and tacrine (Cognex).

Interactions with Herbs and Dietary Supplements

- Belladonna may slow the movement of food and medication through the gut, and therefore some supplements may be absorbed more slowly. The use of belladonna with supplements that have anticholinergic activity, such as Jimson weed *(Datura stramonium)*, may compound its effects (including adverse effects).
- Belladonna may also interact with alcohol, alkaloids, ergot derivatives, hormonal agents, and herbs and supplements that increase sun sensitivity or are cleared by the kidneys.

For a complete list of references, please visit www.naturalstandard.com.

Berberine

RELATED TERMS

- Acetone, berberine, barberry, benzophenanthridine alkaloid, berberin, berberin hydrochloride, berberine alkaloid, berberine bisulfate, berberine chloride, berberine complex, berberine hydrochloride, berberine iodide, berberine sulfate, berberine tannate, *Berberis aquifolium, Berberis aristata, Berberis vulgaris, Coptis chinensis,* coptis, goldenthread, goldenseal, *Hydrastis canadensis,* jiang tang san, Oregon grape, protoberberine, protoberberinium salts, tree turmeric.

BACKGROUND

- Berberine is a bitter-tasting yellow plant alkaloid with a long history of medicinal use in Chinese and Ayurvedic medicine. Berberine is present in the roots, rhizomes, and stem bark of various plants, including goldenseal, (*Hydrastis canadensis*), coptis or goldenthread (*Coptis chinensis*), Oregon grape (*Berberis aquifolium*), barberry (*Berberis vulgaris*), and tree tumeric (*Berberis aristata*). Berberine has also been traditionally used as a dye due for its yellow color.
- Clinical trials have been conducted using berberine. There is some evidence to support its use in the treatment of trachomas (eye infections), bacterial diarrhea, and leishmaniasis (parasitic disease). Berberine also exhibits antimicrobial activity against bacteria, viruses, fungi, protozoans, helminths (worms), and chlamydia (STD). More clinical research is warranted in these areas, as well as cardiovascular disease, skin disorders, and liver disorders.
- Berberine has been shown to be safe in the majority of clinical trials. However, there is a potential for interaction between berberine and many prescription medications, and berberine should not be used by pregnant or breastfeeding women because of potential for adverse effects in the newborn.

EVIDENCE

Uses Based on Scientific Evidence	Grade
Heart Failure Preliminary research suggests that berberine, in addition to a standard prescription drug regimen for chronic congestive heart failure (CHF), may improve quality of life and heart function, and improve mortality. Further research is necessary before a firm conclusion can be drawn in this area.	B
Chloroquine-resistant Malaria One trial has assessed the use of berberine in combination with pyrimethamine in the treatment of chloroquine-resistant malaria. Well-designed clinical trials are still required in this field.	C
Diabetes (Type 2) Historically, berberine has been suggested to aid in glycemic regulation. The safety and effectiveness of berberine for this indication remains unclear. More research is needed in this area.	C
Glaucoma Preliminary study indicates that berberine does not reduce intraocular pressure in patients with glaucoma. The safety and effectiveness of berberine for this indication remains unclear. Additional studies are needed in this area.	C
***H. pylori* Infection** Berberine has been compared with antibacterial drugs and ranitidine in stimulation of ulcer healing and *Helicobacter pylori* clearance. Berberine was suggested to be less effective at ulcer healing than ranitidine, but potentially more effective at *Helicobacter pylori* clearance. Additional studies are needed in this area.	C
Hypercholesterolemia (High Cholesterol) Berberine may reduce triglycerides, serum cholesterol, and LDL cholesterol. Higher-quality trials are needed before berberine's cholesterol-lowering effect can be established.	C
Infectious Diarrhea Berberine has been evaluated as a treatment for infectious diarrhea, including choleric diarrhea, although the data is conflicting. Therefore, there is currently insufficient evidence regarding the efficacy of berberine in the management of infectious diarrhea.	C
Parasitic Infection (*Leishmania*) The benefits of berberine in the treatment of leishmaniasis are widely accepted. Berberine is thought to be equally efficacious as the standard drug treatment of cutaneous leishmaniasis, antimonite (sulfide mineral), although evidence supporting this treatment may preclude its widespread use.	C
Thrombocytopenia (Low Platelet Count) Berberine has been shown to significantly increase platelet production in people with thrombocytopenia both as monotherapy and adjunctive therapy. Additional human studies are needed to confirm these results.	C
Trachoma (Eye Disease) Berberine has been found to possess antimicrobial properties, and there is limited evidence of anti-inflammatory properties as well. Preliminary evidence suggests that berberine eye preparations may be beneficial for trachoma. However, the safety and efficacy of berberine for this indication remains unclear.	C

Uses Based on Tradition or Theory

Alcoholic liver disease, antibacterial, anticonvulsant, antifungal, anti-inflammatory, antimicrobial (typanosomes), antioxidant, antiviral, arthritis, bile secretion, burns, cancer, cardiovascular disease,

Uses Based on Tradition or Theory—Cont'd

dental conditions (root canal), dental hygiene, eye infections (general), fatigue, fever, headaches, high blood pressure, immunostimulant, irritable bowel syndrome (IBS), leukemia, leukopenia, liver disease (alcoholic), osteoporosis, respiratory disorders, sedative, skin infections, urinary tract infection, ventricular tachyarrhythmias, yeast infections.

DOSING

Adults (18 Years and Older)

- A wide range of doses has been studied for berberine, although there is insufficient evidence to support any dose. Berberine is possibly safe when taken by mouth in doses up to 2 g daily for eight weeks. For hypercholesterolemia (high cholesterol), 0.5 g of berberine twice daily for three months has been used. For infectious diarrhea, berberine sulfate 400 mg as a single dose has been used. For thrombocytopenia, berberine bisulfate 5 mg three times daily (20 minutes before meals) for 15 days has been used.
- As an injection into the vein, berberine has been infused at a rate of 0.2 mg/kg per minute for 30 minutes. Injections should be given only under the supervision of a qualified healthcare professional, including a pharmacist.
- For trachoma, 0.2% berberine eye drops for eight weeks have been studied.

Children (Younger than 18 Years)

- There is insufficient evidence to recommend a dose for berberine in children. Nonetheless, berberine is possibly safe when used in otherwise healthy children, as young as two months, at recommended doses for treatment of diarrhea up to six days.

SAFETY

Allergies

- Avoid in people with a known allergy or hypersensitivity to berberine, to plants that contain berberine [*Hydrastis canadensis* (goldenseal), *Coptis chinensis* (coptis or goldenthread), *Berberis aquifolium* (Oregon grape), *Berberis vulgaris* (barberry), and *Berberis aristata* (tree turmeric)], or to members of the Berberidaceae family. Allergic reactions have been reported, with symptoms of vomiting, itching, and a feeling of faintness.

Side Effects and Warnings

- Berberine has been reported to cause nausea, vomiting, hypertension (high blood pressure), respiratory failure, and paresthesias (abnormal sensations such as numbness or tingling); however, clinical evidence of such adverse effects is not prominent in the literature. Rare adverse effects including headache, skin irritation, facial flushing, headache, and bradycardia (slowed heart rate) have also been reported with the use of berberine. Use cautiously when taking berberine for longer than eight weeks because of theoretical changes in bacterial gut flora.
- Use cautiously in people with diabetes, as both human and animal studies indicate that berberine may decrease blood sugar levels. Also use cautiously in people with hypotension (low blood pressure), as berberine may have antihypertensive effects.

- Patients with cardiovascular disease should also use caution, as berberine has been associated with the development of ventricular arrhythmias in subjects with congestive heart failure.
- Berberine may also theoretically cause delays in small intestinal transit time or increase the risk of bleeding.
- Berberine may cause abortion, eye or kidney irritation, nephritis (inflamed kidneys), dyspnea (difficulty breathing), flulike symptoms, giddiness, lethargy, or liver toxicity.
- Patients with leukopenia (abnormally low white blood cell count) should use cautiously because of the potential for development of leukopenia symptoms.
- When injected under the skin, berberine may cause hyperpigmentation in the arm. Use berberine cautiously in people with high exposure to sunlight or artificial light because of potential for adverse phototoxic reactions.
- Avoid in newborns because of the potential for increase in free bilirubin, jaundice, and development of kernicterus (brain damage caused by severe newborn jaundice). Use berberine cautiously in children because of a lack of safety information.

Pregnancy and Breastfeeding

- Berberine is not recommended in pregnant or breastfeeding women because of a lack of available scientific evidence. Although not well studied in humans, berberine has been suggested to have antifertility, abortifacient (abortion inducing), and uterine stimulant activity.
- Berberine may cause kernicterus (brain damage) when used in newborn jaundiced babies, such as bilirubin encephalopathy (degenerative brain disease).

INTERACTIONS

Interactions with Drugs

- Berberine may counter or prevent irregular heartbeat. Caution is advised when taking berberine with other agents that alter heart rate.
- Berberine may decrease the efficacy of tetracycline; in theory, berberine may decrease the efficacy of other agents with antibacterial activity.
- Berberine bisulfate may stimulate platelet formation, and berberine may have an antiheparin action. Thus, berberine may interact with certain drugs that increase the risk of bleeding, and reduce their effectiveness. Some examples include aspirin, anticoagulants (blood thinners) such as warfarin (Coumadin) or heparin, anti-platelet drugs such as clopidogrel (Plavix), and non-steroidal anti-inflammatory drugs (NSAIDS) such as ibuprofen (Motrin, Advil) or naproxen (Naprosyn, Aleve). However, berberine may be hepatoprotective (liver protective) when administered before toxic doses of acetaminophen.
- Berberine may lower blood sugar levels. Caution is advised when using medications that may also lower blood sugar. Patients taking drugs for diabetes by mouth or insulin should be monitored closely by a qualified healthcare professional, including a pharmacist. Medication adjustments may be necessary.
- Berberine may decrease total and LDL cholesterol, as well as triglycerides. Caution is advised in patients taking any cholesterol-lowering agents.
- There may be additive hypotensive (blood pressure lowering) effects and bradycardia (slowed heart rate) when combining berberine with agents that lower blood pressure. Caution is advised.

- Berberine may modulate the expression and function of PGP-170 in hepatoma cells. In theory, berberine may interact with antineoplastic agents.
- Berberine and berberine sulfate have anti-inflammatory effects and may interact with COX-2 inhibitors. COX-2 inhibitor drugs include celecoxib (Celebrex) and rofecoxib (Vioxx).
- Berberine may elevate the blood concentration of cyclosporin A. Caution is advised.
- Berberine may interfere with the way the body processes certain drugs using the liver's "cytochrome P450" enzyme system. As a result, levels of these drugs may be increased in the blood and may cause increased effects or potentially serious adverse reactions. Patients using any medications should check the package insert, and speak with a qualified healthcare professional, including a pharmacist, about possible interactions.
- Although not well studied in humans, there may be a potential for synergism between berberine chloride and fluconazole. Berberine and L-phenylephrine may have additive effects when administered concurrently. Furthermore, berberine may reverse the secretory properties of neostigmine (Prostigmin).
- Berberine and 1,3-bis (2-chloroethyl)-1-nitosurea (BCNU) may have additive effects.
- Berberine may increase sensitization to acetylcholine's hypotensive (blood pressure lowering) effects.
- P-glycoprotein may contribute to the poor intestinal absorption of berberine.
- It is been purported that berberine may have sedative effects. Although human study is lacking, caution is advised.
- Berberine may competitively inhibit the binding of yohimbine to platelets. Patients taking yohimbine should consult with a qualified healthcare professional, including a pharmacist, to check for interactions.

Interactions with Herbs and Dietary Supplements

- Berberine may counter or prevent irregular heartbeat. Caution is advised when taking berberine with other herbs that alter heart rate.
- Berberine may decrease the efficacy of tetracycline; thus, in theory, berberine may decrease the efficacy of herbs with antibacterial activity.
- Berberine bisulfate may stimulate platelet formation, and berberine may have an antiheparin action. Thus, berberine may interact with certain herbs that increase the risk of bleeding and reduce their effectiveness. Multiple cases of bleeding have been reported with the use of *Ginkgo biloba*, and fewer cases with garlic and saw palmetto. Numerous other agents may theoretically increase the risk of bleeding, although this has not been proven in most cases.
- There may be additive hypotensive (blood pressure lowering) effects and bradycardia (slowed heart rate) when combining berberine with herbs that lower blood pressure. Caution is advised.
- Berberine may lower blood sugar levels. Caution is advised when using herbs or supplements that may also lower blood sugar. Blood glucose levels may require monitoring, and doses may need adjustment.
- Berberine may decrease total and LDL cholesterol, as well as triglycerides. Caution is advised in patients taking herbs or supplements with cholesterol-lowering effects, such as red yeast rice.
- Concomitant use of berberine-containing herbs may increase the risk of berberine toxicity. Berberine-containing herbs include: bloodroot, goldenseal, celandine, Chinese goldthread, goldthread, Oregon grape (*Mahonia* species), amur cork tree, and Chinese corktree.
- Berberine may interfere with the way the body processes certain herbs or supplements using the liver's "cytochrome P450" enzyme system. As a result, levels of other herbs or supplements may become too high in the blood. It may also alter the effects that other herbs or supplements possibly have on the P450 system.
- Although not well studied in humans, berberine may have sedative effects.
- Based on clinical study, tyramine-containing foods, such as wine, cheese, and chocolate, may have an interaction with berberine due to berberine's effect on decreasing levels of tyramine.
- Berberine may competitively inhibit the binding of yohimbine to platelets. In addition, due to the antifertility properties of berberine, use of yohimbine for fertility may not be effective.
- Berberine may decrease the metabolism of vitamin B; therefore, the concomitant use of berberine with vitamin B should be avoided.

For a complete list of references, please visit www.naturalstandard.com.

RELATED TERMS

- A-beta-carotene, alpha carotene, beta carotene, beta-cryptoxanthin, carotene, carotenoids, dry beta carotene, eyebright, gamma carotene, green leafy vegetables, palm oil, provitamin A, red palm oil, sunflower oil, synthetic all-trans beta-carotene, retinol.

BACKGROUND

- The name *carotene* was first coined in the early nineteenth century by the scientist Wachenroder after he crystallized the compound from carrot roots. Beta-carotene is a member of the carotenoids, which are highly pigmented (red, orange, yellow), fat-soluble compounds naturally present in many fruits, grains, oils, and vegetables (green plants, carrots, sweet potatoes, squash, spinach, apricots, and green peppers). Alpha, beta, and gamma carotene are considered provitamins because they can be converted to active vitamin A.
- The carotenes possess antioxidant properties. Vitamin A serves several biologic functions including involvement in the synthesis of certain glycoproteins. Vitamin A deficiency leads to abnormal bone development, disorders of the reproductive system, xerophthalmia (a drying condition of the cornea of the eye), and ultimately death.
- Commercially available beta-carotene is produced synthetically or from palm oil, algae, or fungi. Beta-carotene is converted to retinol, which is essential for vision and is subsequently converted to retinoic acid, which is used for processes involving growth and cell differentiation.

EVIDENCE

Uses Based on Scientific Evidence	Grade
Erythropoietic Protoporphyria Erythropoietic protoporphyria is a rare inherited genetic disorder of porphyrin-heme metabolism that has skin and systemic manifestations, including photosensitivity (painful skin sensitivity to sunlight), as well as gallstones and liver dysfunction. It is usually recognized during childhood. The over-the-counter synthetic beta-carotene product Lumitene has been approved by the U.S. Food and Drug Administration (FDA) for photoprotection in this disease. Antihistamines may also be used to reduce symptoms.	A
Carotenoid Deficiency Although consuming of provitamin A carotenoids (alpha-carotene, beta-carotene, and beta-cryptoxanthin) may prevent vitamin A deficiency, no overt deficiency symptoms have been identified in people consuming low-carotenoid diets if they consume adequate vitamin A. After reviewing the published scientific research, the Food and Nutrition Board of the Institute of Medicine (IOM) concluded that the existing evidence in 2000 was insufficient to establish a recommended dietary allowance (RDA) or adequate intake (AI) for carotenoids.	C
Cataract Prevention Study results of beta-carotene supplementation for cataract prevention are conflicting.	C
Chemotherapy Toxicity Observational research suggests that greater dietary intake of beta-carotene may lower the incidence of adverse effects in children undergoing chemotherapy for lymphoblastic leukemia. However, in theory, high-dose antioxidants may interfere with the activity of some chemotherapy drugs or radiation therapy. Therefore, people undergoing cancer treatment should speak with their oncologist if they are taking or considering the use of high-dose antioxidants.	C
Chronic Obstructive Pulmonary Disease (COPD) The prevalence of bronchitis and shortness of breath in male smokers with chronic obstructive pulmonary disorder (COPD) seems to be lower in patients who consume a diet containing high amounts of beta-carotene. However, beta-carotene supplements have not been proven to benefit COPD and may actually increase cancer rates in smokers.	C
Cognitive Performance Antioxidants such as beta-carotene may be helpful for increasing cognition and memory. Long term, but not short-term, beta-carotene supplementation appears to benefit cognition.	C
Cystic Fibrosis Individuals with cystic fibrosis may be deficient in beta-carotene and vitamin E, and it has been suggested that they may be more susceptible to oxidative damage. Theoretically, these patients may benefit from beta-carotene supplementation.	C
Exercise-Induced Asthma Prevention Based on preliminary evidence, taking a mixture of beta-carotene isomers orally may prevent exercise-induced asthma. However, because synthetic beta-carotene has not been well tested for this indication, the difference between the activities of the two supplements cannot be deduced.	C
Immune System Enhancement Preliminary research of beta-carotene for immune system maintenance or stimulation shows mixed results.	C
Oral Leukoplakia Taking beta-carotene orally seems to induce remission in patients with oral leukoplakia. Further research is needed to confirm these results.	C
Osteoarthritis Beta-carotene supplementation does not appear to prevent osteoarthritis, but it might slow progression	C

(Continued)

Uses Based on Scientific Evidence	Grade
of the disease. Well-designed clinical trials are needed before a conclusion can be drawn.	
Polymorphous Light Eruption (PLE) Beta-carotene has been used for polymorphous light eruption (PLE). Additional studies are needed in this area.	C
Pregnancy-Related Complications All-trans beta-carotene (synthetic beta-carotene) taken weekly before, during, and after pregnancy may reduce pregnancy-related mortality, night blindness, postpartum diarrhea, and fever. A regular intake of a micronutrient supplement at a nutritional dose may be sufficient to improve micronutrient status of apparently healthy pregnant women and could prevent low birth weight in newborns. However, further research is necessary to consolidate the evidence in this area before a recommendation can be made.	C
UV-induced Erythema Prevention/Sunburn A combination of antioxidants may help protect the skin against irradiation. Long-term supplementation with beta-carotene may reduce UV-induced erythema and appears to modestly reduce the risk of sunburn in individuals who are sensitive to sun exposure. However, beta-carotene is unlikely to have much effect on sunburn risk in most people.	C
Abdominal Aortic Aneurysm (AAA) Prevention Long-term supplementation with alpha-tocopherol or beta-carotene has been shown not to have a protective or preventive effect in male smokers with large AAAs.	D
Alzheimer's Disease Intake of dietary or supplemental beta-carotene has been shown not to have an effect on Alzheimer's disease risk.	D
Angioplasty There is some concern that when antioxidant vitamins, including beta-carotene, are used together they might have harmful effects in patients after angioplasty. Additional research is needed to determine the effect of beta-carotene specifically. Supplements containing these vitamins should be avoided immediately before and following angioplasty without the recommendation of a qualified healthcare professional.	D
Birthmark/Mole (Dysplastic Nevi) Prevention Beta-carotene has been shown not to reduce the development of new moles in patients with numerous atypical moles.	D
Cancer While diets high in fruits and vegetables rich in beta-carotene have been shown to potentially reduce the incidence of certain cancers, results from randomized	D

controlled trials with oral supplements do not support this claim.

There is some concern that beta-carotene metabolites with pharmacologic activity can accumulate and potentially have carcinogenic effects. A higher, statistically significant incidence of lung cancer in male smokers who took beta-carotene supplements has been discovered. Beta-carotene/vitamin A supplements may have an adverse effect on the incidence of lung cancer and on the risk of death in smokers and asbestos-exposed people or in those who ingest significant amounts of alcohol. In addition, high-dose antioxidants theoretically may interfere with the activity of some chemotherapy drugs or radiation therapy. Therefore, individuals undergoing cancer treatment should speak with their oncologist if they are taking or considering the use of high dose antioxidants.

Beta-carotene in the amounts normally found in food does not appear to have this adverse effect.

	Grade
Cardiovascular Disease Although several studies suggest that diets high in fruits and vegetables containing beta-carotene appear to reduce the risk of cardiovascular disease, most randomized controlled trials with oral supplements of beta-carotene have not supported these claims. A Science Advisory from the American Heart Association states that the evidence does not justify the use of antioxidants such as beta-carotene for reducing the risk of cardiovascular disease.	D
***Helicobacter pylori* Bacteria Eradication** Infection with *Helicobacter pylori* bacteria in the gut can lead to gastric ulcers. Dietary supplementation with beta-carotene has been found not to be effective for this indication.	D
Macular Degeneration Taking beta-carotene and other antioxidants has been proposed to help prevent or delay progression of age-related macular degeneration. However, long-term studies have not shown strong evidence that beta-carotene supplementation can prevent age-related eye disorders.	D
Mortality Reduction Patients given beta-carotene supplements show no reduction in relative mortality rates from all causes based on most available data.	D
Postoperative Tissue Injury Prevention Study results conclude that perioperative supplementation with antioxidant micronutrients has limited effects on strength and physical function following major elective surgery.	D
Stroke Taking all-trans beta-carotene (synthetic beta-carotene) orally has been reported to have no effect on	D

Uses Based on Scientific Evidence	Grade
the overall incidence of stroke in male smokers. Additionally, there is some evidence that beta-carotene actually increases the risk of intracerebral hemorrhage by 62% in patients who also drink alcohol.	

Uses Based on Tradition or Theory
Acute respiratory infections, anemia, angina pectoris (chest pain), asbestosis (chronic lung disease), benign breast diseases, bone marrow transplantation, bronchial asthma, bronchopulmonary dysplasia in premature infants, diabetes, gastritis, glioblastoma, Graves' disease, high cholesterol, HIV, infections (sepsis), iron deficiency (prevention), leukemia (chronic myeloid), low birth weight (prevention), lung function (improving), nasal polyposis, nutrition supplementation (during alcohol rehabilitation), Streptococcal infections (group A), weight loss (HIV, postpartum).

DOSING
General

- **Formulations**: Beta-carotene supplements are available in both oil matrix gelatin capsules and water-miscible forms. Some clinical trials have used water-miscible beta-carotene (10%) beadlets. The water-miscible form seems to produce a significantly higher response in plasma beta-carotene (approximately 47% to 50%) than oil matrix gelatin capsules. Oral dosage is available in capsules (United States and Canada), tablets (United States and Canada), and chewable tablets (Canada).
- **Dietary intake**: Consuming 5 servings of fruit and vegetables daily provides 6 to 8 mg of beta-carotene. Beta-carotene requires some dietary fat for absorption, but supplemental beta-carotene is similarly absorbed when taken with high-fat or low-fat meals. 1,800 micrograms of beta-carotene has been reported to maintain adequate vitamin A levels.
- **Consensus recommendations**: The American Heart Association recommends obtaining antioxidants, including beta-carotene, from a diet high in fruits, vegetables, and whole grains rather than through supplements, until more information is available from randomized clinical trials. Similar statements have been released by the American Cancer Society, the World Cancer Research Institute in association with the American Institute for Cancer Research, and the World Health Organization's International Agency for Research on Cancer. The Institute of Medicine has reviewed beta-carotene but has not made a recommendation for daily intake, citing lack of sufficient evidence. Routine use of beta-carotene supplements is not considered necessary in the general population.

Adults (18 Years and Older)

- 15 to 180 mg taken by mouth of supplemental beta-carotene has been studied for various indications.

Children (Younger than 18 Years)

- There is insufficient available data to recommend high-dose oral supplementation in children.

SAFETY
Allergies

- People who are sensitive to beta-carotene, vitamin A, or any other ingredients in beta-carotene products should avoid supplemental use.

Side Effects and Warnings

- Supplemental beta-carotene in children should be limited to specific medical indications. There is insufficient reliable information available about the safety of large doses of beta-carotene in pregnant or breastfeeding women.
- Supplemental beta-carotene may increase the risk of lung cancer, prostate cancer, intracerebral hemorrhage, and cardiovascular and total mortality in people who smoke cigarettes or have a history of high-level exposure to asbestos. Beta-carotene from foods does not seem to have this effect.
- In people who smoke, beta-carotene may increase cardiovascular mortality. In men who smoke and have had a prior myocardial infarction (MI or heart attack), the risk of fatal coronary heart disease increases by as much as 43% with low doses of beta-carotene. There is some evidence that beta-carotene in combination with selenium, vitamin C, and vitamin E might lower high-density lipoprotein 2 (HDL2) cholesterol levels. HDL levels are protective, so this is considered to be a negative effect. Dizziness and reversible yellowing of palms, hands, soles of feet, and to a lesser extent the face (called *carotenoderma*), can occur with high doses of beta-carotene. Loose stools, diarrhea, unusual bleeding or bruising, and joint pain have been reported.

Pregnancy and Breastfeeding

- U.S. Food and Drug Administration (FDA) Pregnancy Risk Factor C.
- Insufficient data are available on larger oral doses of beta-carotene in pregnant and breastfeeding woman.

INTERACTIONS
Interactions with Drugs

- Preliminary studies in animals indicate that beta-carotene supplementation, when combined with heavy alcohol consumption, may increase liver toxicity and promote cancer.
- Cigarette smoking decreases serum concentrations of beta-carotene and other carotenoids and depletes body stores of beta-carotene. However, oral beta-carotene supplementation should not be recommended in smokers because supplemental beta-carotene in certain doses is associated with a significantly higher risk of lung and prostate cancer in smokers. Smokers and people with a history of asbestos exposure should avoid taking beta-carotene supplements.
- Cholestyramine (Questran) and colestipol (Colestid) can reduce the absorption of fat-soluble vitamins, including beta-carotene. Serum levels of beta-carotene can be reduced, but this is probably only in proportion to the lowering of cholesterol (on which beta-carotene is transported). Supplements are not usually necessary.
- Colchicine can cause disruption of intestinal mucosal function, resulting in malabsorption of beta-carotene.
- Taking beta-carotene in combination with selenium, vitamin C, and vitamin E appears to decrease the effectiveness of the combination of simvastatin (Zocor) and niacin. Theoretically, beta-carotene could reduce the effectiveness of other HMG-CoA reductase inhibitors (statins) such as

atorvastatin (Lipitor), fluvastatin (Lescol), lovastatin (Mevacor), and pravastatin (Pravachol).

- Mineral oil reduces absorption of fat-soluble vitamins, including beta-carotene.
- Oral neomycin sulfate can reduce beta-carotene absorption, but short-term use is unlikely to have a significant effect.
- Orlistat (Xenical) can decrease the absorption of beta-carotene and other fat-soluble vitamins. It is recommended that patients take a multivitamin supplement and separate the dosing time by at least 2 hours before or after taking orlistat.
- Loss of stomach acid can reduce the absorption of a single dose of beta-carotene. Examples of proton pump inhibitors (PPIs) include esomeprazole (Nexium), lansoprazole (Prevacid), omeprazole (Prilosec, Losec), rabeprazole (Aciphex), and pantoprazole (Protonix, Pantoloc).

Interactions with Herbs and Dietary Supplements

- Consumption of a natural carotenoid mixture has been shown to lower the increase in oxidative stress induced by the fish oil. This carotenoid mixture may also enhance the plasma triglyceride-lowering effect of the fish oil.
- Iron supplementation in infants with marginal vitamin A status has led to lower plasma vitamin A concentrations and greater vitamin A liver stores. Some researchers recommend that iron supplementation in infants be accompanied by measures to improve vitamin A status.
- Beta-carotene supplementation has been shown to lower serum lutein concentrations. Lutein from food sources does not seem to result in the decrease in beta-carotene concentrations that accompanies administration of lutein supplements.
- Plant sterols have been shown to reduce beta-carotene bioavailability in some studies and not to have a significant effect in others. The effects on cholesterol levels are also unproven.
- Supplementation of beta-carotene may decrease the vitamin E concentration in tissues.

For a complete list of references, please visit www.naturalstandard.com.

Beta-glucan

B

RELATED TERMS

- Amylodextrins, baker's yeast, barley, beta-glucans, beta glycans, beta-glycans, d-fraction, GD, grifolan, griton-d(r), GRN, lentinan, maitake mushroom, PGG glucan, PGG-glucan, oat beta-glucan, oat fiber, oat fibre, oat gum, *Plantago major* L., poria cocos sclerotium, *Saccharomyces cerevisiae*, schizophyllan (SPG), *Sparassis crispa*, SSG, yeast-derived beta-glucan.

BACKGROUND

- Beta-glucan is a soluble fiber derived from the cell walls of algae, bacteria, fungi, yeasts, and plants. It is commonly used for its cholesterol-lowering effects. Beta-glucans have also been used to treat diabetes and for weight loss.
- Concentrated yeast-derived beta-glucan is more easily incorporated into food products than grain beta-glucans, which are found in cereal grains such as oats and barley. Yeast-derived beta-glucan is also more palatable than oats because it is not soluble in water and does not become viscous in water as beta-glucan from oats does. However, oat-derived beta-glucan may have a higher therapeutic benefit potential.
- The use of beta-glucan is a relatively new practice. Practitioners have used beta-glucan as an immunostimulant or as an adjunct to cancer treatment. Beta-glucan is also used for its cholesterol-lowering effects and glycemic (blood sugar) control. In 1997, the U.S. Food and Drug Administration (FDA) passed a ruling that allowed oat bran to be registered as the first cholesterol-reducing food at an amount of 3 g of beta-glucan daily.

EVIDENCE

Uses Based on Scientific Evidence	Grade
Hyperlipidemia Numerous trials have examined the effects of oral beta-glucan on cholesterol. Small reductions in total and LDL cholesterol ("bad" cholesterol) have been reported. Little to no significant changes have been noted to occur on triglyceride levels or HDL ("good" cholesterol) levels. The sum of existing positive evidence is suggestive and not definitive.	A
Diabetes There are several human trials supporting the use of beta-glucan for glycemic (blood sugar) control. Although early evidence is promising, additional studies are needed before a firm recommendation can be made.	B
Antioxidant In patients with high blood pressure, foods containing oat beta-glucan did not appear to have antioxidant effects. More research is needed before a conclusion can be made.	C
Burns Beta-glucan collagen matrix, which combines the carbohydrate beta-glucan with collagen, has been used as a temporary coverage for partial thickness burns, with good results. Beta-glucan collagen matrix may help reduce pain, improve healing, and lessen scar appearance. However, further studies are needed to confirm these results.	C
Cancer Treatment with a beta-glucan, called *lentinan*, plus chemotherapy (S-1) may help prolong the lives of patients with gastric cancer that has returned or is inoperable. More research is needed in this area.	C
Cardiovascular Disease Evidence suggests that reductions in endothelial function induced by a high-fat meal may be prevented when a high-fat meal is taken along with a beta-glucan–containing cereal or vitamin E. Diabetes, hyperlipidemia (high cholesterol), and hypertension (high blood pressure) data are also promising. Further study is needed in this area.	
Diagnostic Procedure Early research suggests that the amount of beta-glucan detected in the body may help doctors diagnose and monitor candidiasis fungal infections.	C
Heart Protection during Coronary Artery Bypass Grafting (CABG) Early research suggests that treatment with beta-glucan before coronary artery bypass grafting (CABG) heart surgery may help protect against heart damage. More research is needed in this area.	C
High Blood Pressure There is insufficient evidence to recommend for or against the use of beta-glucan for high blood pressure. Better study is needed to determine a relationship.	C
Immune Stimulation Beta-glucan may boost the immune system. Therefore, it has been studied as a possible way to increase the effectiveness of cancer treatments. Although early research is promising, more studies are needed to determine if beta-glucan can help treat breast cancer patients.	C
Infections PGG-glucan, an immunomodulator, has been studied in patients undergoing surgery, particularly abdominal surgery. Currently, PGG-glucan appears to have positive results in decreasing postoperative infection. More study is warranted to make a firm recommendation.	C

(Continued)

107

Uses Based on Scientific Evidence	Grade
Weight Loss Researchers suggest that different types of fiber may have an effect on satiety and energy intake. Short-term use of fermentable fiber or nonfermentable fiber supplements does not appear to promote weight loss. More studies are needed to confirm these findings.	C

Uses Based on Tradition or Theory

Allergies, anti-aging, antibacterial, antiparasitic, antiviral, asthma, atherosclerosis (hardening of the arteries), bedsores, bladder sphincter disorders (sphincter deficiency), colorectal adenocarcinomas, common cold, constipation, Crohn's disease, dermatitis, diabetic ulcers, diarrhea, diverticulitis (colon), ear infections, eczema, fibromyalgia, hepatitis, HIV/AIDS, immunomodulator, immunostimulant, influenza, lung tumor, Lyme disease, multiple sclerosis (MS), radiation burns, respiratory infections, rheumatoid arthritis, shock, skin care, skin conditions, ulcerative colitis, wounds, wrinkle prevention.

DOSING
Adults (18 Years and Older)

- Beta-glucan has been taken by mouth for a variety of conditions. Cereals containing beta-glucan or concentrates containing fiber (typically 8 to 15 grams of beta-glucan) are the most common forms. For hyperlipidemia, 3 to 16 grams of beta-glucan daily have been studied and found moderately effective in reducing LDL ("bad" cholesterol) levels. For high blood pressure, 5.52 grams of beta-glucan daily have been studied. For cardiovascular disease, 4 servings daily of two dietary fibers, beta-glucan (0.75 g per serving) and psyllium (1.78 g per serving), have been studied. For diabetes, 50 to 90 g carbohydrate portions of barley grain with meals have been studied for up to 12 weeks. Higher amounts of fiber and beta-glucan may result in a stronger effect. In addition, 10 g of a barley beta-glucan fiber supplement (Cerogen) that contained 6.31 g of beta-glucan has been added to foods and drinks. For breast cancer, patients have taken beta-glucan daily for 15 days. For heart protection during coronary artery bypass grafting (CABG), 700 mg or 1,400 mg of beta-1,3/1,6-glucan has been taken for five consecutive days before surgery.
- Beta-glucan has also been applied to burns on the skin as a collagen matrix for 24 hours.
- Injections of beta-glucan forms have also been studied, and these should be given only under the guidance of a qualified healthcare professional, including a pharmacist.

Children (Younger than 18 Years)

- There is insufficient evidence to recommend a dose for beta-glucan in children, and use is not recommended.

SAFETY
Allergies

- Avoid in people with a known allergy or hypersensitivity to beta-glucan.

Side Effects and Warnings

- Taken by mouth, both yeast and fungal beta-glucans seem to be well tolerated, with minimal adverse effects. Beta-glucan has Generally Recognized as Safe (GRAS) status in the United States. Lentinan and schizophyllan have been safely used in studies. Although not well studied in humans, the co-administration of aspirin and/or non-steroidal anti-inflammatory drugs (NSAIDs) with beta-glucan can lead to severe gastrointestinal damage resulting in enteric-induced bacterial peritonitis.
- There is insufficient information regarding the safety of beta-glucans when used topically (applied on the skin) or subcutaneously (injected under the skin).
- Most studies that have evaluated the parenteral use of beta-glucans have used specific forms including PGG-glucan from a proprietary strain of *Saccharomyces cerevisiae* and certain fungal-derived forms called *lentinan* and *schizophyllan (SPG)*. PGG-glucan has been safely used in studies when given at appropriate times under the guidance of a qualified healthcare professional.
- When given intravenously, beta-glucans may cause dizziness, headaches, nausea, vomiting, diarrhea, constipation, hives, flushing, rash, high or low blood pressure, and excessive urination.
- Beta-glucan has also been associated with inflammatory airway disease and lung inflammation.
- Particulate beta-glucan may not be safe. Preliminary evidence suggests that intravenous beta-glucans in the microparticulate form may cause serious side effects such as hepatosplenomegaly, granuloma formation, and microembolization.
- Use cautiously in AIDS or AIDS-related complex (ARC) patients. Keratoderma of the palms and soles may develop in patients who are receiving yeast beta-glucans. The condition may begin during the first two weeks of therapy and resolve 2 to 4 weeks after discontinuation of beta-glucans.

Pregnancy and Breastfeeding

- Beta-glucan is not recommended in pregnant or breastfeeding women because of a lack of available scientific evidence.

INTERACTIONS
Interactions with Drugs

- Lentinan may interfere with the way the body processes certain drugs using the liver's "cytochrome P450" enzyme system. As a result, the levels of these drugs may be increased in the blood and may cause increased effects or potentially serious adverse reactions. Patients using any medications should check the package insert and speak with a qualified healthcare professional, including a pharmacist, about possible interactions.
- For wound healing after surgery, evidence suggests that beta-glucans may reduce inflammation and speed the repair of surgical wounds. Severe gastrointestinal damage has been associated with intake of beta-glucan and most non-steroidal anti-inflammatory drugs, such as ibuprofen (Motrin, Advil) and aspirin.
- Preliminary studies suggest that a BCNU/beta-glucan combination may help to improve current chemotherapy treatment efficacy.
- Barley may lower blood sugar levels. Beta-glucan from other sources may alter blood glucose levels. Caution is

advised when using medications that may also lower blood sugar levels. Patients taking drugs for diabetes by mouth or insulin should be monitored closely by a qualified healthcare provider. Medication adjustments may be necessary.

- Theoretically, beta-glucans may decrease the effects of immunosuppressants because of purported immunostimulant effects.
- Beta-glucan–containing sources have been used to treat hyperlipidemia and may act additively with other cholesterol-lowering agents.
- Although not well studied in humans, beta-glucan may alter blood pressure. Caution is advised in patients with low blood pressure or those taking medications for high blood pressure. Consult with a qualified healthcare professional, including a pharmacist, before combining therapies.
- Fiber may affect the absorption of other oral agents by reducing gastrointestinal transit time.
- Hordenine, a chemical in the root of germinating barley, is a sympathomimetic. Therefore, combination use may theoretically result in additive effects. Sympathomimetic effects include increased heart rate, sweating, and increased blood pressure. Check with a qualified healthcare professional, including a pharmacist, before combining therapies.

Interactions with Herbs and Dietary Supplements

- Lentinan may interfere with the way the body processes certain herbs or supplements using the liver's "cytochrome P450" enzyme system. As a result, levels of other herbs or supplements may become too high in the blood. Lentinan may also alter the effects that other herbs or supplements have on the P450 system.
- Beta-glucan–containing sources have been used to treat hyperlipidemia and may act additively with other cholesterol-lowering herbs and supplements, such as red yeast rice. The cholesterol-lowering effects of beta-glucan may increase when taken with plant stanol esters.
- Beta-glucan may reduce inflammation and speed the repair of surgical wounds. Severe gastrointestinal damage has been associated with intake of beta-glucan and most nonsteroidal anti-inflammatory drugs (NSAIDs) or aspirin. Caution is advised when taking anti-inflammatory herbs and supplements in combination with beta-glucan.
- Barley may lower blood sugar levels. Beta-glucan from other sources may alter blood glucose levels. Caution is advised when using herbs or supplements that may also lower blood sugar levels. Blood glucose levels may require monitoring, and doses may need adjustment.
- Fiber may affect the absorption of other oral agents by reducing gastrointestinal transit time.
- Quercetin; selenium; vitamins A, C, and E; or alpha lipoic acid may enhance the antiviral qualities of beta-glucan.
- Although not well studied in humans, beta-glucan may alter blood pressure. Caution is advised in patients taking herbs or supplements for high blood pressure or those with low blood pressure. Consult with a qualified healthcare professional, including a pharmacist, before combining therapies.

For a complete list of references, please visit www.naturalstandard.com.

Betaine anhydrous

RELATED TERMS

- Abromine, alpha-earleine, betaine, betaine glucuronate, BetaPure, Cystadane, glycine, glycine betaine, glycocoll betaine, glycylbetaine, hydroxide, inner salt, lycine, inner salt, oxyneurine, TMG, trimethylammonioacetate trimethylbetaine, trimethylglycine, trimethylglycocoll.
- **Note:** This monograph covers betaine anhydrous, which should not be confused with betaine hydrochloride.

BACKGROUND

- Betaine is found in most microorganisms, plants, and marine animals. Its main physiologic functions are to protect cells under stress and as a source of methyl groups needed for many biochemical pathways. Betaine is also found naturally in many foods and is most highly concentrated in beets, spinach, grain, and shellfish.
- Betaine supplementation has historically been used in the treatment of homocysteinuria resulting from deficiencies in the cystathione beta synthase and methylenetetrahydrofolate reductase genes.
- Betaine supplementation may reduce circulating levels of homocysteine, a potential risk factor for heart disease, stroke, cancer, and Alzheimer's disease.
- Betaine supplementation has been proposed to improve hepatic steatosis, from both alcoholic and nonalcoholic etiologies. While many animal studies have provided plausible mechanisms, data from human studies are limited.
- Betaine in the form of cocamidopropylbetaine has been identified as a cause of contact allergy in some skin care products. In this same form, betaine has been studied as a potential replacement for sodium lauryl sulfate in toothpastes to reduce dry mouth, ulcers, and other mucosal irritations.
- Since the 1980s, betaine has been used as a treatment option for people who have homocystenuria due to a genetic defect in the cystathione beta-synthase (CBS) gene. Pyridoxine (vitamin B6) was beneficial in only 50% of CBS patients, and betaine was a therapeutic option for homocysteine reduction in these unresponsive patients. Benefit was also seen among pyridoxine-responsive patients.
- Early anecdotal reports showed that among CBS variants, treatment with betaine, in addition to B6 and methionine restriction, prevented or delayed clinical complications of the disease, including cardiovascular disease before age 30.

EVIDENCE

Uses Based on Scientific Evidence	Grade
Cardiovascular Disease (in Homocysteinuric Patients) Homocystinuria is a severe form of hyperhomocysteinemia caused by genetic defects in homocysteine-metabolizing genes, most commonly the cystathionine beta-synthase (CBS) gene. Patients with severely elevated homocysteine due to a genetic deficiency can use betaine in combination with other vitamins and diet restrictions to reduce the risk of vascular events. More studies are needed to determine whether betaine supplementation can lower cardiovascular risk within the general population.	B
Hyperhomocysteinemia Overall, betaine supplementation has shown significant reductions in both fasting and postmethionine load homocysteine. However, additional studies are needed to make a strong recommendation.	B
Hyperhomocysteinemia (in Chronic Renal Failure Patients) Hyperhomocysteinemia is a complication found in 80% of end-stage renal failure patients and may contribute to the progression of atherosclerosis among them. The effect of betaine supplementation on reducing homocysteine concentrations within this population has been studied only in addition to folic acid. Additional studies investigating betaine alone are needed to make a firm recommendation.	B
Steatohepatitis (Nonalcoholic) Betaine raises S-adenosylmethionine (SAM) levels that may in turn play a role in decreasing hepatic steatosis. Additional studies are needed to confirm these results.	B
Cholesterol Levels Limited evidence from human trials suggests betaine supplementation increases total cholesterol, LDL, HDL, and triglycerides, which may offset any benefit in CHD risk received through homocysteine lowering. However, the increase in cholesterol appears to be relatively small and of unclear clinical significance.	C
Weight Loss There is currently insufficient available evidence supporting betaine for weight loss.	B

Uses Based on Tradition or Theory

Alzheimer's disease, angina (chest pain), appetite stimulant, arthritis, asthma, atherosclerosis (hardening of the arteries), cognitive improvement, congestive heart failure (CHF), digestion enhancement, dyspnea (shortness of breath), erectile dysfunction, fatigue, high blood sugar/glucose intolerance, hormone-related problems, immune stimulation, kidney function, libido improvement, memory improvement, physical endurance.

DOSING

Adults (18 Years and Older)

- Currently, there is no recommended daily allowance (RDA) set by the United States Food and Nutrition Board for betaine. Manufacturers recommend that betaine powder be dissolved in water, juice, milk, or formula prior to administration and be administered in two doses of 3 g each. For cardiovascular disease (hyperhomocysteinemics), 2 to 15 g daily for up to 17 years has been used. For hyperhomocysteinemia, 1 to 6 g daily of betaine for up to six weeks has been used. For nonalcoholic steatohepatitis, Cystadane has been used at doses up to 20 g daily for up to one year.

Children (Younger than 18 Years)

- Children ages 6 to 14 with cystathionine beta-synthase deficiency, have taken 250 mg/kg daily for three to six months.

SAFETY

Allergies

- Avoid in people with a known allergy or hypersensitivity to betaine anhydrous or cocamidopropylbetaine, a form of betaine.

Side Effects and Warnings

- In the majority of clinical trials among healthy volunteers and renal disease patients, no adverse effects have been reported. In other studies, reported adverse effects are primarily gastrointestinal, such as diarrhea, stomach upset, gastrointestinal irritation, and nausea. However, these transitory events were not severe enough to require discontinuation of betaine use during clinical trials.

- Betaine may also cause mental changes or body odor. Use cautiously in patients with psychiatric conditions.
- Use cautiously in patients with renal disease or those who are obese, as betaine may increase total cholesterol, LDL, HDL, and triglyceride levels when it is taken with folic acid and vitamin B6.

Pregnancy and Breastfeeding

- Betaine is not recommended in pregnant or breastfeeding women because of a lack of available scientific evidence.

INTERACTIONS

Interactions with Drugs

- Although not well studied in humans, betaine supplementation may lower homocysteine concentrations that are elevated by alcohol use.
- Patients with renal disease may experience increases in total cholesterol, LDL, HDL, and triglycerides when betaine is taken with folic acid and vitamin B6. Betaine may increase total cholesterol and LDL cholesterol in obese patients. Caution is advised in patients with high cholesterol or those taking cholesterol-lowering medications.

Interactions with Herbs and Dietary Supplements

- Patients with renal disease may experience increases in total cholesterol, LDL, HDL, and triglycerides when betaine is taken with folic acid and vitamin B6. Betaine may increase total cholesterol and LDL cholesterol in obese patients. Caution is advised in patients with high cholesterol or those taking cholesterol-lowering herbs or supplements, such as red yeast rice.

For a complete list of references, please visit www.naturalstandard.com.

Betel nut
(Areca catechu)

RELATED TERMS

- Amaska, *Areca catechu*, areca quid, areca nut, arecoline, arequier, betal, betel quid, betelnusspalme, chavica etal, gutkha, hmarg, maag, marg, mava, mawa, paan, Palmaceae (family), pan, pan masala, pan parag, pinang, pinlang, *Piper betel* Linn. (leaf of vine used to wrap betel nuts), pugua, ripe areca nut without husk, quid, Sting (Tantric Corporation), supai, ugam.

BACKGROUND

- Betel nut use refers to a combination of three ingredients: the nut of the betel palm *(Areca catechu)*, part of the *Piper betel* vine, and lime. Anecdotal reports have indicated that small doses generally lead to euphoria and increased flow of energy while large doses often result in sedation. Although all three ingredients may contribute to these effects, most experts attribute the psychoactive effects to the alkaloids found in betel nuts.
- Betel nut is reportedly used by a substantial portion of the world's population as a recreational drug due to its stimulant activity. Found originally in tropical southern Asia, betel nut has been introduced to the communities of east Africa, Madagascar, and the West Indies. There is little evidence to support the clinical use of betel nut, but the constituents have demonstrated pharmacologic actions. The main active component, the alkaloid arecoline, has potent cholinergic activity.
- Constituents of betel nut are potentially carcinogenic. Long-term use has been associated with oral submucous fibrosis (OSF), precancerous oral lesions (mouth wounds), and squamous cell carcinoma (cancer). Acute effects of betel nut chewing include worsening of asthma, low blood pressure, and rapid heartbeat.

EVIDENCE

Uses Based on Scientific Evidence	Grade
Anemia Early poor-quality research reports that betel nut chewing may lessen anemia in pregnant women. Reasons for this finding are not clear, and betel nut chewing may be unsafe during pregnancy.	C
Dental Cavities Due to the known toxicities of betel nut use and the availability of other proven products for dental hygiene, the risks of betel nut may outweigh any potential benefits.	C
Saliva Stimulant Betel nut chewing may increase salivation. However, it is not clear if this is helpful for any specific health condition. Due to known toxicities from betel nut use, the risks may outweigh any potential benefits.	C
Schizophrenia Preliminary poor-quality studies in humans suggest improvements in symptoms of schizophrenia with betel nut chewing. However, side effects such as tremors and stiffness have been reported. More research is necessary before a firm conclusion can be drawn.	C
Stimulant Betel nut use refers to a combination of three ingredients: the nut of the betel palm *(Areca catechu)*, part of the *Piper betel* vine, and lime. It is believed that small doses can lead to stimulant and euphoric effects, and betel nut chewing is popular because of these effects. Chronic use of betel nut may increase the risk of some cancers, and immediate effects can include worsening of asthma, high or low blood pressure, and abnormal heart rate. Based on the known toxicities of betel nut use, the risks may outweigh any potential benefits.	C
Stroke Recovery Several poor-quality studies report the use of betel nut taken by mouth in patients recovering from stroke. In light of the potential toxicities of betel nut, additional evidence is needed in this area before a recommendation can be made.	C
Ulcerative Colitis Currently, there is a lack of satisfactory evidence to recommend the use of betel nut for ulcerative colitis. Based on the known toxicities of betel nut use, the risks may outweigh any potential benefits.	C

Uses Based on Tradition or Theory

Alcoholism, aphrodisiac, appetite stimulant, appetite suppressant, asthma, blindness from methanol poisoning, cough, dermatitis (used on the skin), digestive aid, diphtheria, diuretic, ear infection, excessive menstrual flow, excessive thirst, fainting, gas, glaucoma, impotence, intestinal worms, joint pain/swelling, leprosy, respiratory stimulant, toothache, veterinary uses (intestinal worms).

DOSING

Adults (18 Years and Older)

- Betel nut can be chewed alone, but it is often chewed in combination with other ingredients (called a *quid*) including calcium hydroxide, water, catechu gum, cardamom, cloves, anise seeds, cinnamon, tobacco, nutmeg, and gold or silver metal. These ingredients may be wrapped in a betel leaf, followed by sucking the combination in the side of the mouth. It is reported that ingestion of 8 to 30 g of areca nut may be deadly.

Children (Younger than 18 Years)

- Betel nut is not recommended in children because of risks of toxicity, including worsening symptoms of asthma, effects on the heart, and cancer.

SAFETY
Allergies

- Breathing problems with betel nut use have been reported, although no allergic reactions are noted in the available scientific literature. Caution is warranted in people with allergies to other members of the Palmaceae family.

Side Effects and Warnings

- Betel nut cannot be considered safe for human use by mouth. This is due to toxic effects associated with short- or long-term chewing or eating of betel nut.
- Betel nut and the chemicals in betel leaves may cause skin color changes, dilated pupils, blurred vision, wheezing/difficulty breathing, and increased breathing rate. Tremors, slow movements, and stiffness have been reported in people also taking antipsychotic medications. Worsening of spasmodic movements has occurred in patients with Huntington's disease. Seizure has been reported with high doses.
- Cholinergic toxicity symptoms from betel nut use may include salivation, increased tearing, incontinence (lack of urinary control), sweating, diarrhea, and fever. Other problems may include confusion, problems with eye movement, psychosis, amnesia, stimulant effects, and a feeling of euphoria. Long-term users may form a dependence on the effects of betel nut, and discontinuing use may cause signs of withdrawal, such as anxiety or memory lapse.
- Chewing betel nuts can also cause nausea, vomiting, diarrhea, stomach cramps, chest pain, high or low blood pressure, and irregular heartbeat. Heart attack has been associated with betel nut use.
- Betel nut chewing has been shown to have a harmful effect on the gums. The nut may cause the teeth, mouth, lips, and stool to become red-stained. Burning and dryness of mouth may occur.
- Studies of Asian populations have linked precancerous conditions of the mouth and esophagus (oral submucous fibrosis) to betel nut use. There may be a higher risk of cancers of the liver, mouth, stomach, prostate, cervix, and lung with regular betel nut use.
- In animals, a chemical in betel nut alters blood sugar levels. Although human study is lacking in this area, caution is advised in people with diabetes or glucose intolerance, and in those taking drugs, herbs, or supplements that affect blood sugar. Serum glucose levels may need to be monitored, by a healthcare provider, and medication adjustments may be necessary. Betel nut chewers may have a higher risk of developing type 2 diabetes. Animal studies show mixed effects on thyroid function and increased skin temperature. Other problems can include increased blood calcium levels and kidney disease (milk alkali syndrome), possibly due to the calcium carbonate paste sometimes used for preparing betel nuts for chewing.
- Some betel nuts may be contaminated with harmful substances, including aflatoxin (a toxin produced by mold) or lead. Betel nut may cause metabolic syndrome, immunosuppression, and liver toxicity.

Pregnancy and Breastfeeding

- Betel nut is not recommended during pregnancy and breastfeeding because of the risk of birth defects or spontaneous abortion.

INTERACTIONS
Interactions with Drugs

- The effects of anticholinergic drugs may decrease when used in combination with betel nut or its constituent arecoline. Use with cholinergic drugs may cause toxicity (salivation, increased tearing, incontinence, sweating, diarrhea, vomiting, or fever). Betel nut may slow or raise the heart rate and could alter the effects of drugs that slow the heart, such as beta-blockers, calcium channel blockers, or digoxin.
- Betel nut may alter blood sugar levels. Caution is advised when using medications that may also alter blood sugar. Patients taking drugs for diabetes by mouth or using insulin should be monitored closely by a qualified healthcare provider. Medication adjustments may be necessary.
- Betel nut may increase the effects of monoamine oxidase inhibitors (MAOIs), angiotensin-converting enzyme (ACE) inhibitors, phenothiazines, cholesterol-lowering drugs, stimulant drugs, and thyroid drugs. Betel nut may increase or decrease the effects of anti-glaucoma eye drops. Reliable human studies are lacking in these areas.
- Other medications that betel nut may interact with include antibiotics, medications that alter blood pressure, anti-inflammatory medications, or medications taken for cancer or immunosuppression. Patients taking antipsychotic drugs should use cautiously due to reports of increased side effects. Based on the metabolism of betel nut, there may be interactions when taken with muscarinic antagonists. Furthermore, chronic use of betel nut and alcohol may lead to an increased risk of oral cancer.

Interactions with Herbs and Dietary Supplements

- Taking betel nut with other cholinergic herbs may cause toxicity (salivation, tearing, urinary incontinence, sweating, diarrhea, vomiting, facial flushing, and fever) because of the chemical arecoline. Examples of cholinergic herbs include American hellebore, jaborandi, lobelia, pulsatilla, and snakeroot. Betel nut may reduce the effects of herbs with possible anticholinergic properties, such as belladonna, henbane, hyoscyamine, and *Swertia japonica* Makino.
- Betel nut may alter blood sugar levels. Caution is advised when using herbs or supplements that may also alter blood sugar. Blood glucose levels may require monitoring, and doses may need adjustment.
- Betel nut may inhibit monoamine oxidase and therefore may increase the effects of herbs and supplements that may also inhibit monoamine oxidase. Betel nut may also interact with cardioactive agents, such as hawthorn or oleander, or agents that effect thyroid levels, such as bladderwrack.
- Betel nut extracts may lower blood cholesterol levels and may increase the effects of agents that lower cholesterol levels, such as fish oil, garlic, guggul, and niacin.
- Betel nut may cause stimulant and euphoric effects and may add to the effects of stimulants such as caffeine, guarana, or ephedra (ma huang).
- Betel nut has been reported to deplete an essential vitamin (thiamine) and theoretically may cause neurologic damage

including Wernicke-Korsakoff syndrome (confusion, poor muscle coordination, eye movement problems, and amnesia). Based on human studies, chewing betel nut may aggravate the effects of vitamin D deficiency. Theoretically, simultaneous long-term use of betel nut and alcohol may lead to an increased risk of mouth cancer.

- Other herbs or supplements that betel nut may interact with include antibacterials, agents that alter blood pressure, anti-inflammatory agents, or agents taken for cancer or immunosuppression. Patients taking herbs with antipsychotic effects should use these cautiously because of reports of increased side effects. Based on the metabolism of betel nut, there may be interactions when taken with herbs with muscarinic antagonists effects as well.

For a complete list of references, please visit www.naturalstandard.com.

Betony
(*Stachys* spp.)

RELATED TERMS

- Alkaloids, Betoine (French), betonica (Spanish, Italian), *Betonica officinalis*, betonicolide, betonicosides A-D, Betonien (German), betulinic acid, bishopswort, bishop wort, D-camphor, delphinidin, diterpenoid, glycosides, heal-all, hedgenettle, hedge nettles, hyperoside, Labiatae (family), Lamiaceae (family), lousewort, manganese, oleanolic acid, purple betony, rosmarinic acid, rutin, self-heal, stachydrine, *Stachys atherocalyx* C., *Stachys betonica*, *Stachys bombycina*, *Stachys byzanthina* C. Koch, *Stachys byzantina*, *Stachys candida*, *Stachys chrysantha*, *Stachys grandidentata*, *Stachys inflata*, *Stachys lavandulifolia*, *Stachys officinalis*, *Stachys palustris* L., *Stachys parviflora*, *Stachys persica* Gmel., *Stachys plumose*, *Stachys recta*, *Stachys riederi*, *Stachys sieboldii*, *Stachys sieboldii* (Miq.), tannins, ursolic acid, wood betony, woundwort.

BACKGROUND

- The term *betony* is frequently used for many species of *Stachys*. Betony should not be confused with Canada lousewort *(Pedicularis canadensis)*, which is also called wood betony.
- Betony has been regarded as a cure-all by many societies including those from Greece, Italy, Spain, and Britain, as far back as 2000 years ago. Its constituents include tannins, alkaloids, and glycosides, which are typically the active ingredients in herbal remedies.
- Its most commonly reported use is as a nervine (sedative or relaxing agent); the validity of this application has not been confirmed with clinical research.
- Laboratory study has shown that betony may function as an antiinflammatory, although this effect has not been confirmed. At this time, there are no clinical human trials supporting the use of betony for any indication.

EVIDENCE

Uses Based on Scientific Evidence

No available studies qualify for inclusion in the evidence table.

Uses Based on Tradition or Theory

Amenorrhea, anthelmintic (expels worms), antiinflammatory, antimicrobial, antioxidant, antipyretic (fever reducer), antiseptic, antispasmodic, anxiety, asthma, astringent, bronchitis, carminative (digestive aid), colds, diarrhea, diuretic, epilepsy, expectorant, gall bladder disorders, gout (foot inflammation), headache, heartburn, *Helicobacter pylori* infection, hepatitis, hyperglycemia (high blood sugar), hypertension (high blood pressure), kidney stones, liver health, nephritis (kidney inflammation), nervousness, neuralgia (nerve pain), pain, respiratory disorders, rheumatism, sedative, stimulation of digestion, stress, tension, tonic, urolithiasis (kidney/urinary tract stones), vertigo, vulnerary (wound healing).

DOSING

Adults (18 Years and Older)

- There is no proven safe or effective dose for betony in adults. As an infusion, 2-4 g dried herb infused in 1 cup of boiling water for 10-15 minutes and ingested three times daily has been used traditionally. As a liquid extract (1:1 in 25% ethanol), 2-4 mL three times per day has been used. Also, 2-6 mL of tincture (1:5 in 45% ethanol) has been taken one to four times per day in water.

Children (Younger than 18 Years)

- There is no proven safe or effective dose for betony in children.

SAFETY

Allergies

- Avoid in individuals with a known allergy or hypersensitivity to betony or its constituents.

Side Effects and Warnings

- There are currently no high quality studies on the medicinal applications of betony. Based on traditional use and expert opinion, use betony cautiously in patients with hypertension (high blood pressure) or hypotension (low blood pressure) because of potential hypotensive effects. Also use cautiously in patients with diabetes and hypoglycemia because of potential hypoglycemic (blood sugar–lowering) effects.
- Use cautiously in patients with gastrointestinal ulcers because of potential gastrointestinal irritation from betony's tannins.
- Avoid in patients who are pregnant or who are planning to become pregnant because of the traditional use of betony for uterine stimulation.

Pregnancy and Breastfeeding

- Betony should not be used during pregnancy because of a traditional use indication for uterine stimulation (amenorrhea), which suggests a possibility of premature birth or miscarriage. Betony is not recommended in breastfeeding women because of a lack of available scientific evidence.

INTERACTIONS

Interactions with Drugs

- Although not well studied in humans, *Stachys lavandulifolia* has anxiolytic activity. Caution is advised when taking betony with other anxiolytics or sedatives.
- Betony may alter blood sugar levels. Caution is advised when medications that may also alter blood sugar are used. Patients taking drugs for diabetes by mouth or using insulin should be monitored closely by a qualified health care professional, including a pharmacist. Medication adjustments may be necessary.
- Betony contains glycosides and may have hypotensive activity. Caution is advised in patients taking blood pressure–lowering agents.

Interactions with Herbs and Dietary Supplements

- Although not well studied in humans, *Stachys lavandulifolia* has anxiolytic activity. Caution is advised when taking betony with other herbs with potential antianxiety or sedative effects.
- Betony may lower blood sugar levels. Caution is advised when herbs or supplements that may also lower blood sugar are used. Blood glucose levels may require monitoring, and doses may need adjustment.
- Betony may alter blood pressure. Caution is advised in patients taking herbs or supplements that may also alter blood pressure.

For a complete list of references, please visit www.naturalstandard.com.

Bilberry
(*Vaccinium myrtillus*)

RELATED TERMS

- Airelle, anthocyanins, Bickbeere (German), bilberry leaf, black whortle, Blaubeere (Dutch), blaubessen, bleaberry, blueberry, bogberry, bog bilberry, burren myrtle, cranberry, dwarf bilberry, dyeberry, Ericaceae (family), European blueberry, Heidelbeere (Dutch), Heidelbeereblatter, heidelberry, huckleberry, hurtleberry, lingonberry, lowbush blueberry, Mirtillo nero (Italian), *Myrtilli folium*, *Myrtilli fructus*, *Myrtilus niger* Gilib., Optiberry, resveratrol, sambubiosides, trackleberry, *Vaccinium angulosum* Dulac, *Vaccinium montanum* Salibs., *Vaccinium myrtillus* anthocyanoside extract, VMA extract, VME, whortleberry, wineberry.

BACKGROUND

- Bilberry, a close relative of blueberry, has a long history of medicinal use. The dried fruit has been popular for the symptomatic treatment of diarrhea, for topical relief of minor mucus membrane inflammation, and for a variety of eye disorders, including poor night vision, eyestrain, and myopia.
- Bilberry fruit and its extracts contain a number of biologically active components, including a class of compounds called anthocyanosides. These have been the focus of recent research in Europe.
- Bilberry extract has been evaluated for efficacy as an antioxidant, mucostimulant, hypoglycemic, antiinflammatory, "vasoprotectant," and lipid-lowering agent. Although preclinical studies have been promising, human data are limited and largely of poor quality. At this time, there is not sufficient evidence in support of (or against) the use of bilberry for most indications. Notably, the evidence suggests a lack of benefit of bilberry for the improvement of night vision.
- Bilberry is commonly used to make jams, pies, cobblers, syrups, and alcoholic/nonalcoholic beverages. Fruit extracts are used as a coloring agent in wines.

EVIDENCE

Uses Based on Scientific Evidence	Grade
Atherosclerosis ("Hardening" of the Arteries), Peripheral Vascular Disease Bilberry has been used traditionally to treat heart disease and atherosclerosis. There is some laboratory research in this area, but there is a lack of clear information in humans.	C
Cataracts Bilberry extract has been used for a number of eye problems, including the prevention of cataract worsening. Supportive evidence is limited.	C
Chronic Venous Insufficiency Chronic venous insufficiency is a condition that is more commonly diagnosed in Europe than in the United States, and it may include leg swelling, varicose veins, leg pain, itching, and skin ulcers. A standardized extract of bilberry called *Vaccinium myrtillus* anthocyanoside (VMA) is popular in Europe for the treatment of chronic venous insufficiency. However, the research is preliminary and not yet conclusive.	C
Diabetes Mellitus Bilberry has been used traditionally in the treatment of diabetes, and animal research suggests that bilberry leaf extract can lower blood sugar levels. Clinical evidence is lacking.	C
Diarrhea Bilberry is used traditionally to treat diarrhea, but there is a lack of reliable research in this area.	C
Fibrocystic Breast Disease There is limited research suggesting a possible benefit of bilberry in the treatment of fibrocystic disease of the breast.	C
Glaucoma High intraocular pressure is considered a risk factor for glaucoma development. Products containing bilberry may reduce the risk of glaucoma development.	C
Painful Menstruation (Dysmenorrhea) Preliminary evidence suggests that bilberry may be helpful for the relief of menstrual pain, although the evidence thus far is inconclusive.	C
Retinopathy Based on animal research and several small human studies, bilberry may be useful in the treatment of retinopathy in patients with diabetes or high blood pressure. However, it remains unclear whether bilberry is beneficial for this condition.	C
Stomach Ulcers (Peptic Ulcer Disease) Bilberry extract has been suggested to promote stomach ulcer healing. There is some support for this use from laboratory and animal studies, but there is a lack of reliable clinical evidence.	C
Night Vision Traditional use and several unclear studies from the 1960s and 1970s suggest possible benefits of bilberry for night vision. However, more recent well-designed	D

(Continued)

Uses Based on Scientific Evidence	Grade
studies report no benefits. Based on this evidence, it does not appear that bilberry is helpful for improving night vision.	

Uses Based on Tradition or Theory
Age-related macular degeneration, angina (chest pain), angiogenesis (blood vessel formation), antifungal, antimicrobial, antioxidant, antiseptic, antiviral, arthritis, bleeding gums, burns, cancer, cardiovascular disease, chemoprotectant, chronic fatigue syndrome, common cold, cough, dermatitis, dysentery (severe diarrhea), edema (swelling), encephalitis (tick-borne), eye disorders, fevers, gout (painful inflammation), heart disease, hematuria (blood in the urine), hemorrhoids, high blood pressure, high cholesterol level, kidney disease, lactation suppression, laxative (fresh berries), leukemia, liver disease, macular degeneration, oral ulcers, pharyngitis, poor circulation, retinitis pigmentosa, scurvy, skin infections, sore throat, stomach upset, tonic, urine (bloody), urinary tract infection, varicose veins of pregnancy, vision improvement.

DOSING

Adults (18 Years and Older)

- Fresh berries, 55-115 g three times daily or 80-480 mg of aqueous extract three times daily by mouth (standardized to 25% anthocyanosides), have been used traditionally.
- The following have been used traditionally: dried fruit, 4-8 g by mouth with water two times per day; decoction of dried fruit by mouth three times per day (made by boiling 5-10 g of crushed dried fruit in 150 mL of water for 10 minutes and straining while hot); or cold macerate of dried fruit by mouth three times per day (made by soaking dried crushed fruit in 150 mL of water for several hours). Experts have warned that patients should use dried bilberry preparations because the fresh fruit may actually worsen diarrhea.
- Some experts recommend using a mouthwash gargle of 10% dried fruit decoction as needed for mucus membrane inflammation.

Children (Younger than 18 Years)

- There is not enough scientific evidence to recommend the use of bilberry in children.

SAFETY

Allergies

- People with allergies to plants in the Ericaceae family or to anthocyanosides may have reactions to bilberry. However, there is a lack of reliable published cases of serious allergic reactions to bilberry.

Side Effects and Warnings

- Bilberry is generally believed to be safe in recommended doses for short periods of time, based on its history as a foodstuff. There is a lack of known reports of serious toxicity or side effects, although if it is taken in large doses, there is an increased risk of bleeding, upset stomach, or hydroquinone poisoning.

- Based on human use, bilberry fresh fruit may cause diarrhea or have a laxative effect. Based on animal studies, bilberry may cause low blood sugar levels. Caution is therefore advised in patients with diabetes or hypoglycemia and in those taking drugs, herbs, or supplements that affect blood sugar. Serum glucose levels may need to be monitored by a health care provider, and medication adjustments may be necessary.
- In theory, bilberry may decrease blood pressure, based on laboratory studies.
- With the use of bilberry leaf extract, there is a theoretical increased bleeding risk, although there are no reliable published human reports of bleeding. Caution is advised in patients with bleeding disorders, in patients taking drugs that may increase the risk of bleeding, or before some surgeries and dental procedures.

Pregnancy and Breastfeeding

- There is not enough scientific evidence to recommend the safe use of bilberry during pregnancy or breastfeeding, although eating bilberry fruit is believed to be safe based on its history of use as a foodstuff. One study used bilberry extract to treat pregnancy-induced leg swelling (edema), and no adverse effects were reported.

INTERACTIONS

Interactions with Drugs

- Bilberry may lower blood sugar levels, although there is a lack of reliable human studies in this area. Caution is advised when medications that may also lower blood sugar are used. Patients taking drugs for diabetes by mouth or insulin should be monitored closely by a qualified health care provider. Medication adjustments may be necessary.
- Based on human use, bilberry may increase diarrhea when taken with drugs that cause or worsen diarrhea, such as laxatives or some antibiotics. Bilberry theoretically may increase the risk of bleeding when taken with drugs that increase the risk of bleeding. Some examples include aspirin, anticoagulants ("blood thinners") such as warfarin (Coumadin) or heparin, antiplatelet drugs such as clopidogrel (Plavix), and nonsteroidal antiinflammatory drugs such as ibuprofen (Motrin, Advil) or naproxen (Naprosyn, Aleve). There are no reliable published human reports of bleeding with the use of bilberry. Based on theory, bilberry may further lower blood pressure when taken with drugs that decrease blood pressure.
- Based on early laboratory study, berry extracts have been shown to inhibit *Helicobacter pylori*, an ulcer-producing bacteria, and enhance the effects of the prescription drug clarithromycin (Biaxin).
- Bilberry may also interact with anticancer agents, liver-damaging agents, and estrogen-containing medications. Consult with a qualified health care professional, including a pharmacist, to check for interactions.

Interactions with Herbs and Dietary Supplements

- Based on animal research, bilberry may lower blood sugar levels. Although there is a lack of reliable human study in this area, caution is advised when herbs or supplements that may also lower blood sugar are used. Blood glucose levels may require monitoring, and doses may need adjustment.

- Based on theory, bilberry may lower blood pressure further when taken with herbs or supplements that decrease blood pressure.
- Based on theory, bilberry may increase the risk of bleeding when taken with herbs and supplements that are believed to increase the risk of bleeding. Multiple cases of bleeding have been reported with the use of *Ginkgo biloba*, and fewer cases have been reported with garlic and saw palmetto. Numerous other agents may theoretically increase the risk of bleeding, although this has not been proven in most cases.
- Based on traditional use, bilberry may increase diarrhea or laxative effects when taken with herbs and supplements that are also believed to have laxative effects.

- Consuming bilberry with quercetin supplements may result in additive effects. Cooking bilberries with water and sugar to make soup may decrease the amount of quercetin by 40%. Berries contain resveratrol, which has been studied as an antioxidant for cardiovascular disease and for cancer, and may have additive effects when taken with supplements like grape seed.
- Bilberry may also interact with anticancer agents, antioxidants, liver-damaging agents, and herbs or supplements with hormonal properties. Consult with a qualified health care professional, including a pharmacist, to check for interactions.

For a complete list of references, please visit www.naturalstandard.com.

Biotin
(Vitamin H)

RELATED TERMS

- ARP [N-(Aminooxyacetyl)-N′-(D-biotinoyl) hydrazine], biocytin, biotin-alkaline phosphate, biotin cadaverine, biotin nitrilotriacetic acid, biotin NTA, biotin-PEO$_4$-amine, Biotin-PEO$_2$-PPO$_2$-amine, biotin-PEO$_3$-maleimide, biotin-PEO$_4$-propionate succinimidyl ester, biotinidase, coenzyme R, D-biotincis-hexahydro-2-oxo-1H-thieno[3,4-d]-imidazole-4-valeric acid, dUTP biotin, factor alpha, tripotassium salt (BNTA), vitamin Bw, vitamin H, W factor.
- **Note:** This review does not cover the use of biotin in radioimmunotherapy (radioactive therapy) or radiolabeling for diagnostic procedures.

BACKGROUND

- Biotin is an essential water-soluble B vitamin. The name *biotin* is taken from the Greek word *bios*, meaning "life." Without biotin, certain enzymes do not work properly and various complications can occur involving the skin, intestinal tract, and nervous system. Metabolic problems including very low blood sugar levels between meals, high blood ammonia, or acidic blood (acidosis) can occur. Death is theoretically possible, although no clear cases have been reported. Recent studies suggest that biotin is also necessary for processes on the genetic level in cells (DNA replication and gene expression).
- Biotin deficiency is extremely rare. This is because daily biotin requirements are relatively small, biotin is found in many foods, and the body is able to recycle much of the biotin it has already used. Significant toxicity has not been reported in the available literature with biotin intake.

EVIDENCE

Uses Based on Scientific Evidence	Grade
Biotin Deficiency Biotin deficiency is extremely rare. Some potential causes of biotin deficiency are long-term use of certain antiseizure medications, prolonged oral antibiotic use, intestinal malabsorption (e.g., short gut syndrome), intravenous feeding (total parenteral nutrition [TPN]) without added biotin, and eating raw egg whites on a regular basis. Supplementing with biotin appears helpful for the treatment of this deficiency.	A
Biotin-Responsive Inborn Errors of Metabolism Disorders such as multiple carboxylase deficiency can cause inborn errors of metabolism that cause a "functional" biotin deficiency. High-dose biotin is used to treat these disorders. Management should be under strict medical supervision.	A
Brittle Fingernails Biotin has been suggested as a treatment for brittle fingernails, particularly in women. There is not sufficient scientific evidence to form a clear conclusion.	C
Cardiovascular Disease Risk (in Diabetes) A combination of biotin and chromium may help lower cholesterol and decrease the risk of developing clogged arteries (called atherosclerosis) in diabetics. However, other research on biotin alone found that biotin did not affect cholesterol, glucose, or insulin levels but did decrease triglyceride levels.	C
Diabetes Mellitus (type 2) In early research, biotin has been reported to decrease insulin resistance and improve glucose tolerance, which are both properties that may be beneficial in patients with type 2 (adult-onset) diabetes. Other research suggests that a combination of biotin and chromium may help improve blood sugar control. However, clinical evidence is limited.	C
Hepatitis (in Alcoholics) Antioxidant therapy with biotin, vitamins A-E, selenium, zinc, manganese, copper, magnesium, folic acid, and coenzyme Q10 did not improve survival rates in alcoholics with hepatitis. The isolated effects of biotin are unclear.	C
Pregnancy Supplementation Marginal biotin deficiency has been found to commonly occur during pregnancy. Biotin supplementation during pregnancy is not currently standard practice, and prenatal vitamins generally do not contain biotin. However, individual patients may be considered for biotin supplementation by health care practitioners on a case-by-case basis.	C
Total Parenteral Nutrition (TPN) Intravenous feeding solutions (TPN) should contain biotin so that biotin deficiency in recipient patients is avoided. This applies for patients in whom TPN is the sole source of nutrition.	C

Uses Based on Tradition or Theory
Alopecia areata (hair loss), antioxidant, basal ganglia disease, cancer, Crohn's disease, exercise capacity improvement, hyperlipidemia, metabolic disorders (3-methylcrotonylglycinuria), Parkinson's disease, peripheral neuropathy, Rett syndrome, seborrheic dermatitis, uncombable hair syndrome, vaginal candidiasis, wound healing (periodontal).

DOSING
Adults (18 Years and Older)

- The U.S. Food and Nutrition Board of the National Academy of Science's Institute of Medicine recommends a daily adequate intake (AI) of 30 mcg in adults 19 years and older (a daily AI of 25 mcg is recommended in those ages 14-18 years old). In pregnant women older than 14 years, an AI of 30 mcg is recommended. During breastfeeding, a daily AI of 35 mcg is recommended. Most healthy nonpregnant individuals with regular diets obtain these amounts of biotin through dietary consumption.

- The U.S. Recommended Dietary Allowance (RDA) for biotin is 300 mcg daily. This is the dose used in many dietary supplements. Toxicity with biotin intake has not been reported in the available literature, and doses as high as 200 mg daily have been used in patients with inborn errors of metabolism without significant reported toxicity.

- Biotin is available as capsules and tablets in various doses as lozenges. Treatment for biotin deficiency should be under strict medical supervision. There is disagreement among experts about the proper dose. In adults, intramuscular (injected into the muscle) doses as low as 150-300 mcg daily have been suggested. Higher doses between 10 and 40 mg of biotin daily have also been recommended (given by mouth, injected into the muscle, or injected into the veins).

Children (Younger than 18 Years)

- The U.S. Food and Nutrition Board of the National Academy of Science's Institute of Medicine recommends a daily adequate intake (AI) of 5 mcg daily (~0.7 mcg/kg) in infants ages 0-6 months old; 6 mcg daily (~0.7 mcg/kg) in infants ages 7-12 months old; 8 mcg daily in children ages 1-3 years old; 12 mcg daily in children ages 4-8 years old; 20 mcg daily in children ages 9-13 years old; and 25 mcg in adolescents ages 14-18 years old.

- Treatment for biotin deficiency and biotin-responsive inborn errors of metabolism should be under strict medical supervision. There is disagreement among experts about the proper dose.

SAFETY
Allergies

- Individuals with hypersensitivity to constituents of biotin supplements should avoid these products.

Side Effects and Warnings

- Significant toxicity with biotin intake has not been reported in the available literature, and very high doses have been used in patients with inborn errors of metabolism without reported toxicity. However, doses higher than the U.S. Food and Nutrition Board's recommended daily AI should not be exceeded in healthy individuals unless under medical supervision.

Pregnancy and Breastfeeding

- Marginal biotin deficiency has been found to commonly occur during pregnancy. Serious concern has been focused on this finding because biotin deficiency is teratogenic (causes birth defects) in many animals. It has been suggested by some experts that biotin supplements should be considered for widespread use in pregnant women, although there is not enough available scientific information to make this recommendation.

- The recommended daily AI by the U.S. Food and Nutrition Board should not be exceeded unless under medical supervision.

INTERACTIONS
Interactions with Drugs

- Antiseizure medications, such as phenytoin (Dilantin), primidone (Mysoline), carbamazepine (Tegretol), phenobarbital (Solfoton), and possibly valproic acid, have been associated with reduced blood levels of biotin. Patients using these medications should consult with a qualified health care professional, including a pharmacist, to see whether biotin supplementation may be necessary.

- Broad-spectrum antibiotics such as sulfa drugs can alter the normal intestinal bacteria (flora) that make biotin. Biotin supplementation may be necessary if deficiency is found.

- Isotretinoin (Accutane) may reduce biotinidase activity. It is not clear whether biotin supplementation may be warranted during long-term use.

- Biotin may increase the effects of lipid-lowering medications.

Interactions with Herbs and Supplements

- High-doses of pantothenic acid can lead to malabsorption of biotin in the gut and can lower levels of biotin in the body. Caution is advised.

- Biotin may increase the effects of lipid-lowering herbs or supplements.

- Eating raw egg whites on a regular basis increases the risk of biotin deficiency.

For a complete list of references, please visit www.naturalstandard.com.

Bitter Almond and Laetrile
(*Prunus dulcis*, syn. *Prunus amygdalus*)

RELATED TERMS

- Aci badem, almendra amara, amande amere, amendoa amarga, *amygdala amara*, amygdalus dulcis amara, bitter almond oil, bittere amandel, bittermandel, gorkiy mindal, karvasmanteli, keseru mandula, ku wei bian tao, ku xing ren, lawz murr, mandorla amara, *Prunus amygdalus amara, Prunus communis amara, Prunus dulcis* (Mill.) D.A. Webb var. *amara* (DC.) H.E. Moore, Rosaceae (family), volatile almond oil.
- **Note:** Bitter almond should not be confused with "sweet almond." Sweet almond seeds do not contain amygdalin and can be eaten, whereas bitter almonds can be toxic.

BACKGROUND

- The almond is closely related to the peach, apricot, and cherry (all classified as drupes in the genus *Prunus*). Unlike the others, however, the outer layer of the almond is not edible. The edible portion of the almond is the seed. Sweet almonds and bitter almonds belong to the same species; a compound called amygdalin differentiates the bitter almond from the sweet almond. In the presence of water (hydrolysis), amygdalin yields glucose and the chemicals benzaldehyde and hydrocyanic acid (HCN). HCN, the salts of which are known as cyanide, is poisonous. To be used in food or as a flavoring agent, the bitter almond oil must have the HCN removed. Once it is removed, the oil is called volatile almond oil and is considered to be almost pure benzaldehyde. Volatile almond oil can still be toxic in large amounts.

EVIDENCE

Uses Based on Scientific Evidence	Grade
Cancer (Laetrile) "Laetrile" is an alternative cancer drug marketed in Mexico and other countries outside the United States. Laetrile is derived from amygdalin, found in the pits of fruits and nuts such as the bitter almond. Early evidence suggests that laetrile is not beneficial in the treatment of cancer. In 1982, the U.S. National Cancer Institute concluded that laetrile was not effective for cancer therapy. Nonetheless, many people still travel to use this therapy outside the United States. Multiple cases of cyanide poisoning, including deaths, have been associated with laetrile therapy.	D

Uses Based on Tradition or Theory
Antibacterial, antiinflammatory, antiitch, antispasmodic, cough suppressant, expectorant, hyperoxia (lack of oxygen), local anesthetic, mental health (neuropsychometric symptoms in AIDS patients), muscle relaxant, pain suppressant, psoriasis, sedative.

DOSING

Adults (18 Years and Older)

- Because of potential toxicity, there is no widely accepted standard dose for bitter almond.

Children (Younger than 18 Years)

- Because of potential toxicity, bitter almond products should be avoided in children.

SAFETY

Allergies

- Allergies to almonds are common and have led to severe reactions, including throat swelling that interferes with breathing. Those allergic to other nuts should also avoid almonds.

Side Effects and Warnings

- Laetrile, derived from the amygdalin found in the pits of fruits and nuts such as the bitter almond, is considered unsafe in any form because of its potential for causing cyanide toxicity. Reactions are more severe when laetrile is taken by mouth than when injected into a vein or muscle. Some of the side effects have included dilated pupils, dizziness, drooping eyelids, drowsiness, headache, increased breathing, muscle weakness, nausea, stomach pain, and vomiting. High doses of bitter almond or laetrile may lead to a slowing of brain functions or breathing. Several cases of cyanide poisoning (some fatal) have been reported.
- Drowsiness or sedation may occur with bitter almond. Use cautiously if driving or operating heavy machinery.

Pregnancy and Breastfeeding

- Bitter almonds are not recommended in pregnant or breastfeeding women because of insufficient available data and potential risk of birth defects.

INTERACTIONS

Interactions with Drugs

- In theory, bitter almond may increase the amount of drowsiness caused by some drugs. Examples include benzodiazepines such as lorazepam (Ativan) or diazepam (Valium), barbiturates such as phenobarbital, narcotics such as codeine, some antidepressants, and alcohol. Caution is advised while driving or operating machinery. The use of alcohol with almond oil should be avoided because the combination was shown in mice to cause a toxic reaction (nausea, vomiting, increased breathing, sweating).
- Amygdalin, bitter almond, and laetrile may also interact with analgesics (pain relievers), central nervous system (CNS) depressants, agents that suppress or stimulate the immune system, and agents that are excreted through the kidneys. However, evidence in humans is lacking.

Interactions with Herbs and Dietary Supplements

- Bitter almond may increase the amount of drowsiness caused by some herbs or supplements. Caution is advised while driving or operating machinery.
- Amygdalin, bitter almond, and laetrile may also interact with analgesics (pain relievers), CNS depressants, agents that suppress or stimulate the immune system, and agents that are excreted through the kidneys. However, human evidence is lacking.

For a complete list of references, please visit www.naturalstandard.com.

B

Bitter Melon
(Momordica charantia and MAP30)*

RELATED TERMS

- African cucumber, alpha-momorcharin, ampalaya, balsam-apple, Balsambirne (German), balsam pear, balsambirne, balsamo, beta-momorcharin, bitter apple, bitter cucumber, bitter gourd, bittergurke, bitter melon capsules, bitter melon extract, bitter melon juice, bitter melon malt vinegar, bitter melon seed oil, carilla gourd, cerasse, charantin, chinli-chih, cundeamor, Cucurbitaceae (family), fructus momordica grosvenori, GlyMordica, goya, kakara, karavella, karela, kareli, kathilla, kerala, Koimidori bitter melon, kuguazi, K'u-kua, Lai margose, MAP30, *Momordica charantia*, momordique, pavakkachedi, pepino montero, P'ut'ao, sorosi, sushavi, vegetable insulin, wild cucumber.

BACKGROUND

- Bitter melon (*Momordica charantia*) belongs to the melon family and has traditionally been used as a remedy for lowering blood sugar in patients with diabetes. Preliminary data exists on bitter melon use in human immunodeficiency virus (HIV) and cancer. Extracts and powdered formulations of the fruit are most frequently used, although teas made from the stems and leaves are sometimes recommended.
- Bitter melon is also consumed as a foodstuff and is found as an ingredient in some south Asian curries. The raw fruit is available in specialty Asian markets, where it is commonly known as *karela*.

EVIDENCE

Uses Based on Scientific Evidence	Grade
Cancer MAP30, a protein isolated from bitter melon extract, has been reported to possess anticancer activity, although potential anticancer effects have not been studied in humans. Additional study is needed before a strong recommendation can be made.	C
Diabetes Mellitus (Hypoglycemic Agent) Preliminary research suggests that bitter melon may decrease serum glucose levels; however, reports are mixed. Because safety and efficacy have not been established, bitter melon should be avoided in patients with diabetes except under the strict supervision of a qualified health care professional, including a pharmacist, with careful monitoring of blood sugar levels.	C
Human Immunodeficiency Virus (HIV) There is some evidence that a protein in bitter melon called MAP30 may have antiviral activity, but this is not supported by sufficient clinical evidence.	C

DOSING
Adults (18 years and Older)

- Because of the wide variations in preparation techniques of bitter melon, the proper dosing cannot be determined at the present time. Bitter melon has sometimes been administered as a fruit juice in doses of 50 mL or 100 mL in diabetic patients. Juice formulations have been reported to have more potent effects on blood sugar and laboratory values than the powder of the sun-dried fruit. However, safety and efficacy have not been established for any specific dose(s) of bitter melon.
- Subcutaneous administration of bitter melon has been studied in humans, although safety, efficacy, and dosing have not been clearly established.

Children (Younger than 18 Years)

- There are not enough scientific data to recommend bitter melon for use in children. Caution is advised, based on two case reports of hypoglycemic coma in children after the ingestion of bitter melon tea.

SAFETY
Allergies

- Individuals with allergies to plants related to the bitter melon or members of the Curcurbitaceae (gourd or melon) family, including Persian melon, honeydew, casaba, muskmelon, and cantaloupe, may have cross-sensitivity to bitter melon.

Side Effects and Warnings

- Headaches have been reported after the ingestion of bitter melon seeds. However, details regarding severity and duration of headaches are limited. Considerable increases in liver enzyme levels have been observed in animals after drinking bitter melon fruit juice and seed extract. These effects, however, have not been associated with significant damage or changes in the liver. The clinical relevance in humans has not been studied, so caution is advised, particularly in patients with underlying liver disease. The seeds and outer rind of bitter melon contain a toxic chemical (lectin), which inhibits protein synthesis in the intestinal wall. Although this has not been correlated with signs or symptoms in humans, ingestion of bitter melon seeds or outer rind should be avoided because of potential adverse effects.

- Bitter melon may lower blood sugar levels. Caution is advised in patients with diabetes or hypoglycemia (low blood sugar) and in those taking drugs, herbs, or supplements that affect blood sugar. Serum glucose levels may need to be monitored by a health care provider, and medication adjustments may be necessary. Two case reports have documented hypoglycemic coma and convulsions in children after the administration of a bitter melon tea.
- Ingestion of bitter melon (or bitter melon seeds) should be avoided in patients with glucose-6-phosphate dehydrogenase (G6PDH) deficiency because of the risk of hemolytic reaction and "favism." Favism is the onset of hemolytic anemia with symptoms including headache, fever, stomach pain, and coma. G6PDH deficiency and favism are most common in people from the Mediterranean area and the Middle East.
- The fertility rate of mice that were fed with daily bitter melon juice dropped from 90% to 20% in one study. Sperm production was inhibited in dogs that were fed a bitter melon fruit extract for 60 days. However, laboratory studies of a protein isolated from bitter melon seeds, called MAP30, have found that they do not affect sperm motility.

Pregnancy and Breastfeeding

- Bitter melon is not recommended during pregnancy; two proteins isolated from the raw fruit possess properties that may cause an abortion in animals. Lowered fertility rates are also possible.

INTERACTIONS
Interactions with Drugs

- Bitter melon may lower blood sugar levels. Caution is advised when medications that may also lower blood sugar are used. Patients taking drugs for diabetes by mouth or using insulin should be monitored closely by a qualified health care professional, including a pharmacist.
- Elevations in liver enzyme levels have been reported. Theoretically, bitter melon may interact with drugs metabolized by or affecting the liver.
- The antiviral protein of bitter melon may enhance the therapies of the HIV antagonist dexamethasone and indomethacin.

Bitter melon may have antiviral and immunomodulating effects and therefore may have additive effects with other drugs with similar activity.

- Bitter melon leaf extracts have been observed to reverse chemotherapy drug resistance.
- Bitter melon may lower triglyceride levels and therefore may have additive effects with other drugs with similar activity.
- Absorption, distribution, metabolism, and elimination (pharmacokinetics) of other drugs may be altered by bitter melon.
- Bitter melon may induce abortion, reduce fertility rates, or inhibit production of sperm. Caution is advised in patients taking fertility agents or antifertility agents.
- In theory, bitter melon may interact with medications used to treat parasites (anthelmintics).

Interactions with Herbs and Dietary Supplements

- Bitter melon may lower blood sugar levels. Caution is advised when herbs or supplements that may also lower blood sugar are used. Blood sugar levels may require monitoring, and doses may need adjustment.
- Elevations in liver enzyme levels have been reported. Theoretically, bitter melon may interact with drugs metabolized by or affecting the liver.
- Bitter melon leaf extracts have been observed to reverse chemotherapy drug resistance.
- Bitter melon may lower triglyceride levels and therefore may have additive effects with other drugs with similar activity.
- Absorption, distribution, metabolism, and elimination (pharmacokinetics) of other drugs may be altered by bitter melon.
- Bitter melon may induce abortion, reduce fertility rates, or inhibit production of sperm. Caution is advised in patients taking herbs or supplements with proposed fertility or antifertility effects.
- In theory, bitter melon may also interact with herbs or supplements that suppress or enhance the immune system. Furthermore, bitter melon may interact with medications used to treat parasites (anthelmintics), although human evidence is lacking in this area.

For a complete list of references, please visit www.naturalstandard.com.

Bitter Orange
(*Citrus aurantium*)

RELATED TERMS

- Aurantii pericarpium, auraptene, bergamot aromatherapy oil, bergamot orange, bergapten, beta-daucosterol (XI), beta-sitosterol, bigaradier, chisil, *Citri aurantii* fructus (CAF), *Citri grandis* pericarpium (CGP), *Citrus amara, Citrus aurantium, Citrus aurantium dulcis, Citrus aurantium* extract (CAE), *Citrus aurantium* L., *Citrus aurantium* L. var. *amara, Citrus aurantium sinensis* (CAS), *Citrus aurantium* ssp. *bergamia, Citrus aurantium* var. *amara, Citrus aurantium* var. *dulcis* (sweet orange), *Citrus bigaradia*, citrus essential oils (EOs), citrus extract, Citrus L. Rutaceae, citrus peel extract, *Citrus silension* (CS), *Citrus vulgaris, Citrus xaurantium*, corteza de naranja amarga (Spanish), *Citrus aurantium*, var. Cyathifera Y. Tanaka, Daidai, *Fructus aurantii*, Goutou orange, Goutou sour orange, green orange, hesperidin, Kijitsu, limonene, marmalade, marmin, m-synephrine, naranja amarga, naringin, N-methyltyramine, neohesperidin, neroli oil, nobiretin, nonvolatile fraction, octopamine, oil of bergamot, oxedrine, oxypeucedanin, pericarps of *Citrus grandis*, phenylephrine, pomeranze, *Poncirus trifoliata* x *C. aurantium*, Rutaceae (family), Seville orange, Shangzhou Zhiqiao, sour orange, sour orange flower, sour orange leaf, sweet orange, synephrine, tangeretin, volatile oil, Xiangcheng, Xiucheng, Zhiqino, Zhi Qiao, Zhi Shi.

BACKGROUND

- Bitter orange *(Citrus aurantium)* comes from a flowering, fruit-bearing evergreen tree native to tropical Asia but is now widely cultivated in the Mediterranean region and elsewhere. Bitter orange contains synephrine, an alkaloid with similarities to ephedrine.
- Over the centuries, bitter oranges were highly valued for their food and medicinal properties. In ancient China, unripe bitter oranges were used to make zhi shi, an herbal extract used to treat constipation, improve energy (chi), and calm nerves in cases of insomnia and shock. In the Amazon rainforest, indigenous tribes used bitter orange tea as a laxative and to relieve nausea, stomach pains, indigestion, gas, and constipation.
- It is claimed that bitter orange is an effective weight loss aid and a safe alternative to ephedra. However, evidence shows some increase in heart rate and short-term calorie burn, and it may raise blood pressure and exacerbate existing heart problems. Weight loss benefits are unproven, and safety questions remain. The U.S. Food and Drug Administration (FDA) banned the sale of ephedrine-containing dietary supplements. Some products previously containing ephedrine have been reformulated to include *Citrus aurantium*.

EVIDENCE

Uses Based on Scientific Evidence	Grade
Aging There is inconclusive evidence that a combination product including immature bitter orange may improve symptoms of aging.	C
Fungal Infections Preliminary research shows potential antifungal effects of bitter orange oil. Clinical evidence is insufficient.	C
Weight Loss Since the ban on ephedra, some weight loss products previously containing ephedrine have been reformulated to include bitter orange. Although bitter orange is popularly used for weight loss, the effects of bitter orange are largely unknown.	C
Dementia (Behavior Challenges) Bitter orange has been used in aromatherapy, although it does not appear to reduce combative, resistive behaviors in individuals with dementia. Currently, there is no evidence supporting the use of bitter orange for dementia and behavioral challenges.	D

Uses Based on Tradition or Theory

Analgesic (pain reliever), anemia, antioxidant, anxiety, appetite stimulant, aromatherapy, bed sores, blood purification, bruises, cancer, circulation, cleansing impurities from the body, constipation, cosmetic, diabetes, duodenal ulcers, dyspepsia (upset stomach), energy enhancement, epilepsy, exhaustion, eye inflammation, flatulence (gas), flavoring agent, frostbite, functional conditions, gastrointestinal disorders, headache, heart disorders, indigestion, insecticide, insomnia, kidney and bladder disorders, laxative, leukemia, muscular pain, nasal congestion, nausea, neuralgia (nerve pain), prolapsed uterus, rheumatic pain, sedative, tonic, viral infections (Rotavirus, Peste des petits ruminants).

DOSING

Adults (18 Years and Older)

- There is insufficient evidence to recommend a dose for bitter orange as a medicinal agent. However, bitter orange has "generally recognized as safe" (GRAS) status for the use in foods in the United States.

Children (Younger than 18 Years)

- There is insufficient evidence to recommend a dose for bitter orange in children.

SAFETY

Allergies

- Avoid in individuals with a known allergy or hypersensitivity to bitter orange or the Rutaceae family.

Side Effects and Warnings

- Bitter orange has GRAS status for the use in foods in the United States. Despite the lack of systematic study on the safety and efficacy of bitter orange, there are several theoretical side effects that may occur from the use of bitter orange. For instance, bitter orange may cause adverse cardiovascular effects in otherwise healthy individuals; avoid in patients with preexisting cardiovascular (heart) disease. Theoretically, bitter orange may worsen narrow-angle glaucoma. It may also trigger migraine or cluster headaches. Use cautiously in patients with hyperthyroidism (overactive thyroid gland). Bitter orange may worsen the condition because of its synephrine content.

- Because of its potential photosensitizing effects, use topical bitter orange preparations cautiously in patients with fair skin.
- Avoid using in patients with intestinal colic, based on reports of convulsion and death in children who consume large amounts of bitter orange peel. Also avoid using in patients taking QT interval–prolonging drugs or with long QT interval syndrome. Theoretically, bitter orange might increase the risk of ventricular arrhythmias (irregular heart rhythms).
- Avoid using with drugs or dietary supplements with stimulant properties. Concurrent use might increase the risk of hypertension (high blood pressure) and adverse cardiovascular effects.

Pregnancy and Breastfeeding

- Bitter orange is not recommended in pregnant or breast-feeding women because of a lack of available scientific evidence.

INTERACTIONS
Interactions with Drugs

- Theoretically, bitter orange might be antagonized by alpha blocking agents. Caution is advised.
- Theoretically, concomitant use of bitter orange and beta blockers might cause acute hypertension (high blood pressure).
- Large amounts of caffeine might increase the risk of hypertension and adverse cardiovascular effects with bitter orange because of its synephrine content.
- Theoretically, concurrent use of monoamine oxidase inhibitors (MAOIs) with synephrine-containing bitter orange preparations might increase the blood pressure–raising effects of synephrine and potentially cause a hypertensive crisis. Bitter orange contains tyramine, octopamine, and synephrine, which are MAO substrates. Caution is advised when bitter orange is taken with other MAOIs.
- Bitter orange juice may interfere with the way the body processes certain drugs using the liver's cytochrome P450 enzyme system. As a result, the levels of these drugs may be decreased in the blood and this may reduce the intended effects. Patients taking any medications should check the package insert and speak with a qualified health care professional, including a pharmacist, about possible interactions.
- Oil of bergamot, which comes from *Citrus aurantium* ssp. *bergamia*, may cause hyperpigmentation or dermatitis or make a patient more sensitive to laser treatment. Caution is advised when bitter orange is taken with other photosensitizing agents.

- Bitter orange might prolong the QT interval in some patients, especially when in combination with other stimulants such as caffeine. Theoretically, bitter orange could have an additive effect when combined with drugs that prolong the QT interval and potentially increase the risk of ventricular arrhythmias (irregular heartbeats). Use of bitter orange with other cardioactive agents may also increase this risk.
- Theoretically, drugs with central nervous system (CNS) stimulant properties, such as phenylpropanolamine and pseudoephedrine, might increase the risk of hypertension and adverse cardiovascular effects of bitter orange because of its synephrine content.
- Theoretically, bitter orange may interact with thyroid medications or worsen hyperthyroidism because of its synephrine content.

Interactions with Herbs and Dietary Supplements

- Theoretically, antiadrenergic herbs or supplements might antagonize bitter orange. Caution is advised.
- Honey reduces the absorption of naringin, a flavone glycoside of bitter orange.
- Theoretically, concurrent use of herbs with MAOI activity with synephrine-containing bitter orange preparations might increase the blood pressure–raising effects of synephrine and potentially cause a hypertensive crisis. Bitter orange contains tyramine, octopamine, and synephrine, which are MAO substrates. Caution is advised when bitter orange is taken with other herbs with MAOI effects.
- Bitter orange may interfere with the way the body processes certain herbs or supplements using the liver's "cytochrome P450" enzyme system. As a result, the levels of other herbs or supplements may become too high in the blood. It may also alter the effects that other herbs or supplements possibly have on the P450 system.
- Theoretically, *Panax ginseng* might prolong the QT interval on an electrocardiogram (ECG). Thus, combining *Panax ginseng* and bitter orange might have an additive effect on the QT interval and increase the risk for arrhythmias (irregular heart beats). Use of bitter orange with other cardioactive herbs or supplements may also increase this risk.
- Oil of bergamot, which comes from *Citrus aurantium* subsp. *bergamia*, may cause hyperpigmentation or dermatitis and may make a patient more sensitive to laser treatment. Caution is advised when bitter orange is taken with other photosensitizing herbs.
- Theoretically, herbs and supplements with stimulant properties, such as ephedra, guarana, and mate, might increase the risk of hypertension (high blood pressure) and adverse cardiovascular effects with bitter orange because of its synephrine content.
- Theoretically, bitter orange may interact with herbs affecting the thyroid or worsen hyperthyroidism because of its synephrine content.

For a complete list of references, please visit www.naturalstandard.com.

Blackberry

(Rubus fruticosus)

RELATED TERMS

- Anthocyanins, chickasaw blackberry, marionberry, olallieberry, Rosaceae (family), Rubus, *Rubus fruticosus, Rubus villosus*, wild blackberry.

BACKGROUND

- Blackberry is a rambling vine with thumb-sized black composite berries. The plant grows easily in temperate climates and is often found in recently cleared areas. Laboratory studies have found blackberries to be high in antioxidants, although no benefits were observed in one clinical trial. More research is needed in this area before a potential therapeutic recommendation can be made.
- Because of the tannins in the blackberry plant's root bark and leaves, blackberry has been used as an astringent and tonic and for dysentery (severe diarrhea) and diarrhea. A tea of the root bark has also been used for whooping cough.

EVIDENCE

Uses Based on Scientific Evidence	Grade
Antioxidant Several laboratory studies indicate that blackberry fruit is high in antioxidants, which may be due to the berries' anthocyanin content. However, more research is needed in this area to determine its effects on antioxidant levels in humans.	C

Uses Based on Tradition or Theory
Astringent, boils, cancer, diarrhea, dysentery (severe diarrhea), gout (foot inflammation), skin conditions (scaldhead), tonic, whooping cough.

DOSING

Adults (18 Years and Older)

- There is insufficient evidence to recommend a dose for blackberry.

Children (Younger than 18 Years)

- There is insufficient evidence to recommend a dose for blackberry.

SAFETY

Allergies

- Avoid in individuals with a known allergy or hypersensitivity to blackberry (*Rubus fruticosus*) or its constituents. There is a case report of severe food-precipitated anaphylaxis associated with antiphospholipid syndrome in a patient allergic to blackberry.

Side Effects and Warnings

- Blackberry is likely safe when used in food amounts in healthy patients. There are few reports in the available literature of adverse effects related to blackberries. There is a case report of sporotrichosis (a chronic fungal infection of the skin and lymph nodes) possibly due to picking blackberries, and one study found that fresh, incubated blackberries were contaminated with mold.

Pregnancy and Breastfeeding

- Based on traditional use, blackberry is likely safe in food amounts in pregnant or breastfeeding women. However, other uses are not recommended because of a lack of sufficient data.

INTERACTIONS

Interactions with Drugs

- Blackberry fruit is high in antioxidants, although early evidence does not suggest that ingestion of blackberry affects antioxidant levels in humans.
- Although not well studied in humans, blackberry may have anticancer activity. Caution is advised when combining blackberry with other anticancer agents.

Interactions with Herbs and Dietary Supplements

- Blackberry fruit is high in antioxidants, although early evidence does not suggest that ingestion of blackberry affects antioxidant levels in humans.
- Although not well studied in humans, blackberry may have anticancer activity. Caution is advised when combining blackberry with other anticancer herbs or supplements.

For a complete list of references, please visit www.naturalstandard.com.

Black Cohosh
(*Actaea racemosa*, formerly *Cimicifuga racemosa*)

RELATED TERMS

- *Actaea macrotys*, *Actaea racemosa* L., actee a grappes (French), amerikanisches Wanzenkraut (German), baneberry, BCE, black cohosh roots, black snakeroot, botrophis serpentaria, bugwort, cimicifuga, *Cimicifugae racemosa* rhizoma, cimicifugawurzelstock (German), cohosh bugbane, ethanolic aqueous extract, herbe au punaise (French), hydroxytyrosol, isoferulic acid, isopropanolic black cohosh extract, macrotys, *Macrotys actaeoides*, phytoestrogen, Ranunculaceae (family), rattle root, rattle snakeroot, rattle top, rattle weed, rhizoma actaeae richweed, rhizome of black cohosh, rich weed, schwarze Schlangenwurzel, snakeroot, solvlys, squaw root, squawroot, *Thalictroides racemosa*, Traubensilberkerze, Wanzenkraut (German).
- **Note:** Do not confuse black cohosh with blue cohosh (*Caulophyllum thalictroides*), which contains chemicals that may damage the heart and raise blood pressure. Do not confuse black cohosh with *Cimicifuga foetida*, bugbane, fairy candles, or sheng ma; these are species from the same family (Ranunculaceae) with different effects.

BACKGROUND

- Black cohosh is popular as an alternative to hormonal therapy for treating menopausal (climacteric) symptoms such as hot flashes, mood disturbances, diaphoresis, palpitations, and vaginal dryness. Several studies have shown black cohosh to improve menopausal symptoms for up to 6 months, although the most current evidence is mixed.
- The mechanism of action of black cohosh remains unclear, and the effects on estrogen receptors or hormonal levels (if any) are not definitively known. Recent evidence suggest that there may be no direct effects on estrogen receptors, although this is an area of active controversy. Safety and efficacy beyond 6 months have not been proven, although recent reports suggest safety of short-term use, including in women experiencing menopausal symptoms for whom estrogen replacement therapy is contraindicated. Nonetheless, caution is advisable until better quality safety data are available. Use of black cohosh in high-risk populations (such as in women with a history of breast cancer) should be supervised by a licensed health care professional.

EVIDENCE

Uses Based on Scientific Evidence	Grade
Arthritis Pain (Rheumatoid Arthritis, Osteoarthritis) There is not enough human research to make a clear recommendation regarding the use of black cohosh for painful joints in rheumatoid arthritis or osteoarthritis.	C
Breast Cancer There is not enough human research to make a clear recommendation regarding the use of black cohosh for breast cancer.	C
Menopausal Symptoms Black cohosh is a popular alternative to prescription hormonal therapy for the treatment of menopausal symptoms such as migraine headaches, sleep disturbances, hot flashes, mood problems, perspiration, heart palpitations, and vaginal dryness. Initial human research suggests that black cohosh may improve some of these symptoms for up to 6 months. However, the current evidence is mixed, and more studies are needed to make a strong recommendation.	C
Migraine (Menstrual) Approximately 30% of women afflicted with migraines have menstrual-related migraines. Black cohosh may be a potential treatment for these migraines, although additional study of black cohosh alone is needed to make a strong recommendation.	C

Uses Based on Tradition or Theory

Abortifacient (induces abortion), AIDS, antiinflammatory, antioxidant, antispasmodic, anxiety, aphrodisiac (increases sexual desire), appetite stimulant, asthma, back pain, bone diseases, breast cysts, breast pain/inflammation (mastitis), bronchitis, cancer, cervical dysplasia (abnormal pap smear), chemotherapy-induced premature menopause, child birth (labor induction), chorea, cough remedy, decreased blood platelets, depression, diarrhea, dizziness, dyspareunia (painful sexual intercourse), edema (swelling), emmenagogue (promotes menstruation), endometriosis, estrogenic agent, fever, gall bladder disorders, gingivitis, headache, heart disease/palpitations, high blood pressure, infertility, inflammation, insect repellent, itchiness, joint pain, kidney inflammation, leukorrhea (abnormal vaginal discharge), liver disease, malaria, measles, menstrual period problems, miscarriage, muscle pain, muscle spasms, nerve pain, ovarian cysts, pain, pancreatitis (inflamed pancreas), perimenopausal symptoms, perspiration, pertussis (whooping cough), polycystic breast disease, polycystic ovarian syndrome, premenstrual syndrome (PMS), rash, rheumatism, ringing in the ears, sleep disorders, snakebites, sore throat, tamoxifen-related hot flashes, urinary disorders, urogenital atrophy (tissues of the vagina and bladder become thinner, often resulting in pain and infection), uterine diseases and bleeding, wrinkle prevention, yellow fever.

DOSING
Adults (18 Years and Older)

- There is no proven effective dose for black cohosh. The British Herbal Compendium recommends 40-200 mg of dried rhizome daily in divided doses, although traditional doses have been as high as 1 g three times daily. As a tincture/liquid, the British Herbal Compendium recommends 0.4-2 mL of a (1:10) 60% ethanol tincture daily. For menopausal symptoms, studies have used 20 mg or 40 mg Remifemin tablets (containing 1 or 2 mg of 27-deoxyactein) twice daily or 40 drops of a liquid extract. Some clinical studies have used 20 mg taken twice daily. Isopropanolic black cohosh has been taken at a dose of 40 mg/day for 12 weeks.

Children (Younger than 18 Years)

- There is not enough scientific information to recommend black cohosh in children.

SAFETY
Allergies

- Avoid if allergic to black cohosh or other members of the Ranunculaceae (buttercup or crowfoot) family. In nature, black cohosh contains small amounts of salicylic acid (which is found in aspirin), but it is not clear how much (if any) is present in commercially available products. Black cohosh should be used cautiously in people allergic to aspirin or to other salicylates.

Side Effects and Warnings

- Black cohosh is generally well tolerated in recommended doses and has been studied for up to 6 months. High doses of black cohosh may cause frontal headache, dizziness, perspiration, or visual disturbances. Several side effects have been noted in studies including constipation, intestinal discomfort, loss of bone mass (leading to osteoporosis), irregular or slow heartbeat, low blood pressure, muscle damage, nausea, and vomiting. Dysphoria and "heaviness in the legs" may occur.
- It is not clear whether black cohosh is safe in individuals with hormone-sensitive conditions such as breast cancer, uterine cancer, or endometriosis. There is controversy as to whether black cohosh is similar to estrogen in its mechanism, although recent studies suggest that it may not be. The influence of black cohosh on antiestrogen drugs (like tamoxifen) or hormone replacement therapy is not clear. It is not known whether black cohosh possesses the beneficial effects that estrogen is believed to have on bone mass or the potential harmful effects such as increased risk of stroke or hormone-sensitive cancers.
- A few gynecological organ–related adverse events have been reported including vaginal bleeding and miscarriage; however, the effects of black cohosh in these events are unclear.
- Hepatitis (liver damage) and liver failure have been reported with the use of black cohosh–containing products. Liver transplantation has been required in some patients. These reports are concerning, although the cases have been criticized by some as not being adequately substantiated. Nonetheless, patients with liver disease should consult a licensed health care professional before using black cohosh.
- Black cohosh should also be used cautiously in patients with a history of blood clots, seizure disorder, or high blood pressure.

Pregnancy and Breastfeeding

- Safety during pregnancy and breastfeeding has not been established. Black cohosh may relax the muscular wall of the uterus and some nurse–midwives in the United States use black cohosh to stimulate labor. Black cohosh may also have hormonal effects, and caution is advised during breastfeeding. There is one report of severe multiorgan damage in a child delivered with the aid of both black cohosh and blue cohosh (*Caulophyllum thalictroides*) who was not breathing at the time of birth. The child survived with permanent brain damage. However, blue cohosh is known to have effects on the heart and blood vessels and may have been responsible for these effects.
- Tinctures may be ill-advised during pregnancy because of potentially high alcohol content.

INTERACTIONS
Interactions with Drugs

- The potential estrogen-like effects of black cohosh continue to be debated, and the active chemical contents of black cohosh have not been clearly identified. Although recent studies suggest no significant effects of black cohosh on estrogen receptors in the body, caution is warranted in people taking both black cohosh and estrogens because of unknown effects. The influence of black cohosh in combination with tamoxifen is not clear in studies, and it is not known whether tamoxifen counteracts the effects of black cohosh. Drugs like raloxifene may also interact.
- Black cohosh may lower blood pressure and therefore should be used cautiously with other hypotensive agents such as beta-blockers like metoprolol (Lopressor, Toprol) or propranolol (Inderal) and calcium-channel blockers like diltiazem (Cardizem, Tiazac) or verapamil (Isoptin, Calan). Black cohosh may contain small amounts of salicylic acid and may increase the antiplatelet effects of other agents such as aspirin.
- Black cohosh may alter the way the liver breaks down or metabolizes certain drugs. In theory, because of possible alcohol content in some tinctures of black cohosh, combination with disulfiram (Antabuse) or metronidazole (Flagyl) may cause nausea and vomiting.
- Although not well studied in humans, black cohosh may potentially interact with antidepressants and antihistamines. It may also interact with agents taken for the treatment of cancer and osteoporosis. Other potential interactions include pain relievers, anesthetics, antiinflammatory drugs, cholesterol-lowering drugs, and antiseizure drugs.

Interactions with Herbs and Dietary Supplements

- Black cohosh should be used cautiously in people taking herbs with possible hormonal effects. This is a theoretical concern, and it is not clear whether the amounts of salicylates present in commercial or processed black cohosh products have significant effects in humans.
- Seizures were reported in a woman taking a combination of black cohosh, chaste tree (berries and seeds), and evening primrose oil for 4 months who also consumed alcohol. The cause of her seizures is not clear.
- Both black cohosh and blue cohosh (*Caulophyllum thalictroides*) are used by nurse–midwives in the United States to assist birth. There is one report of severe multiorgan damage in a child delivered with the aid of both black cohosh and blue cohosh who was not breathing at the time

of birth. The child survived with permanent brain damage. However, blue cohosh is known to have effects on the heart and blood vessels and may have been responsible for these effects. Pennyroyal and black cohosh should not be used together, as there is a possibility of increased toxicity and death.

- Black cohosh may lower blood pressure and therefore interact with other herbs or supplements that also affect blood pressure.
- In theory, black cohosh may increase the risk of bleeding when taken with herbs and supplements that are believed to increase the risk of bleeding. Multiple cases of bleeding have been reported with the use of *Ginkgo biloba*, garlic, and saw palmetto. Numerous other agents may theoretically increase the risk of bleeding, although this has not been proven in most cases.
- Black cohosh may alter the way the liver breaks down or metabolizes certain herbs and supplements.
- Although not well studied in humans, black cohosh may potentially interact with herbs and supplements with antidepressant, antihistamine, or antioxidant effects. It may also interact with herbs or supplements taken for the treatment of cancer and osteoporosis. Interactions with pain relievers, anesthetics, antiinflammatory drugs, cholesterol-lowering therapies, and St. John's wort are also possible.

For a complete list of references, please visit www.naturalstandard.com.

Black Currant
(Ribes nigrum)

RELATED TERMS

- Alpha-linolenic acid, (18:3n3), anthocyanidin glycosides, anthocyanin, anthocyanoside, astragalin, BCA, BCSO, black currant, black currant berry, black currant juice, black currant powder, black currant seed oil, cassis (French, Spanish), cassitee (German), European black currant, Feuilles de Cassis (French), gamma-linolenic acid (18:3n6, GLA), Gichtbeerblaetter (German), groselha preta (Portuguese), groselheira preta (f) (Bot.), Grossulariaceae (family), isoquercitrin, kurokarin extract, linoleic acid, (18:2n6), omega-3 fatty acids, omega-6 fatty acid, phenolic compounds, polyphenolic antioxidants, proanthocyanidins, prodelphinidins, quercetin, Quinsy berries, red currant, *Ribes nero*, Ribes nigri folium, *Ribes nigrum*, *Ribes rubrum*, Ribis nigri folium, Rob, rutin, Saxifragaceae (family), schwarze Johannisbeerblaetter (German), schwarze Johannisbeere (German), Squinancy berries, solbaerbusk (Danish), stearidonic acid, svart vinbar (Swedish).

BACKGROUND

- The black currant shrub is native to Europe and parts of Asia and is particularly popular in Eastern Europe and Russia. Traditional herbalists uphold that black currant has diuretic (increases urine flow), diaphoretic (promotes sweating), and antipyretic (fever reducer) properties. In Europe, it has been used topically (applied to the skin) to treat skin disorders, such as atopic dermatitis, and as part of gargles to treat sore throats. Black currant juice has been boiled down into a sugary extract, called Rob, to treat sore throat inflammation, colds, the flu, and febrile (fever) illness. A mixture made from black currant bark has been used to treat calculus (hardened plaque), edema (swelling), and hemorrhoids.
- With a vitamin C content estimated to be five times that of oranges (2000 mg/kg), black currant has potential dietary benefits. Black currant is also rich in rutin and other flavonoids, which are known antioxidants. Because of black currant's high essential fatty acid content, researchers believe that it may be effective in the treatment of inflammatory conditions and pain management, as well as in regulating the circulatory system and increasing immunity.
- As a medicinal treatment, black currant seed oil is the most commonly used part of the plant and is available in capsule form. The effectiveness of black currant seed oil is mixed, and safety concerns seem to be minor in nonallergic people.

EVIDENCE

Uses Based on Scientific Evidence	Grade
Antioxidant There is currently a lack of information in humans on the effectiveness of black currant juice as an antioxidant.	C
Chronic Venous Insufficiency (a Blood Flow Disorder) Chronic venous insufficiency is a condition in which damaged valves in the veins or a blood clot in the	C

leg may cause ongoing swelling or blood pooling in the legs. Black currant treatment may benefit those with blood flow disorders, such as chronic venous insufficiency, although this remains inconclusive.

Hypertension (High Blood Pressure) Patients with hypertension have blood pressure above the normal range. Black currant seed oil supplementation may lower blood pressure, although this remains inconclusive.	C
Immunomodulation There is currently a lack of information in humans on the effectiveness of black currant seed oil in changing immune system function.	C
Musculoskeletal Conditions (Stiffness) Results are conflicting.	C
Night Vision Anthocyanosides in black currant in theory may be helpful for improving night vision. However, strong evidence is lacking.	C
Nutritional Supplementation (Phenylketonuria) There is currently a lack of information in humans on the effectiveness of black currant seed oil for nutritional supplementation in phenylketonuric patients.	C
Rheumatoid Arthritis There is some promising evidence that black currant seed oil may reduce the signs and symptoms of rheumatoid arthritis. However, additional research is needed to confirm these findings.	C
Stress There is currently a lack of information in humans on the effectiveness of black currant seed oil for stress.	C

Uses Based on Tradition or Theory

Alcoholism, antiinflammatory, antithrombotic (blood thinner), atopic dermatitis, bladder stones, breast tenderness, calculus (hardened plaque), cardioprotective, cardiovascular disease (heart disease), chronic inflammatory conditions, cleansing (tea), colds, colic, convulsions, coughs, cramps, depression, diaphoretic (promotes sweating), diarrhea, diuretic, dropsy, dysmenorrhea (painful periods), edema, gout (foot inflammation), *Helicobacter pylori* infection, hemorrhoids, hepatitis, herpes, herpes simplex virus type 1, herpes simplex virus type 2, influenza, insect bites, liver and gallbladder complaints, menopausal symptoms, menstrual disorders, osteoarthritis, pain, prevention of upper respiratory tract infections, respiratory problems, rheumatism, skin disorders, sore throat, tumors (hemorrhoidal), weight loss, whooping cough, wounds.

DOSING
Adults (18 Years and Older)

- As a dietary supplement, black currant is available in 500 mg and 1000 mg capsules that typically contain black currant seed oil, vegetable glycerine, and gelatin. Black currant is likely safe at 1000 mg daily. Black currant juice is also commercially available and has been taken in doses up to 1.5 L daily, when mixed with apple juice. Maximum doses of black currant seed oil used in clinical trials range from 4.5-6 g daily up to 8 weeks, although safety and effectiveness have not been established. Black currant anthocyanins have been taken in doses of 7.7-50 mg daily for up to 2 months. Based on some herbal textbooks, toxicity is not a significant concern when black currant is consumed as food or ingested in 500 mg tablets three times daily.

Children (Younger than 18 Years)

- There is insufficient evidence to recommend a dose for black currant in children.

SAFETY
Allergies

- Avoid in individuals with a known allergy or hypersensitivity to black currant, its constituents, or plants in the Saxifragaceae family.

Side Effects and Warnings

- In general, there is a lack of safety information about black currant. Anecdotal information indicates that black currant seed oil may cause diarrhea. Furthermore, some people are not able to tolerate black currant seed oil in capsule form, which results in diarrhea and other mild gastrointestinal symptoms. The gamma-linolenic acid in black currant may alter blood pressure. Use cautiously in patients with high blood pressure or those taking blood pressure medication.
- Avoid in patients with hemophilia or those taking anticoagulants (blood thinners) unless otherwise recommended by a qualified health care provider, as black currant may enhance the effects of anticoagulants.
- Use cautiously in pregnant and breastfeeding women and in children and the elderly, as their immunity and bodily functions are compromised or underdeveloped.
- Use cautiously in patients taking monoamine oxidase inhibitors (MAOIs) or vitamin C supplements or in patients with epilepsy.
- Use cautiously in those with venous disorders, as black currant may increase peripheral blood flow and circulation.

Pregnancy and Breastfeeding

- Black currant is not recommended in pregnant or breastfeeding women because of a lack of available scientific evidence; therefore, pregnant women and breastfeeding mothers should avoid the use of black currant seed oil, unless a qualified health care provider recommends otherwise.

INTERACTIONS
Interactions with Drugs

- Black currant seed oil may have antibacterial activity; use cautiously with antibiotics and antiulcer medications.
- Black currant may increase the risk of bleeding when taken with drugs that increase the risk of bleeding, such as warfarin (Coumadin), clopidogrel (Plavix), aspirin (Bayer, Ecotrin, St John), enoxaparin (Lovenox), and dalteparin (Fragmin).
- Black currant may alter blood pressure; use cautiously with blood pressure medications because of possible additive effects.
- Black currant may have antioxidant effects. Patients taking other antioxidants should use black currant with caution.
- Black currant may have MAOI effects. Use cautiously with antidepressant medications, such as MAOIs, because of possible additive effects.
- Black currant may interact with antiviral agents. Consult a qualified health care professional, including a pharmacist, to check for interactions.
- Black currant seed oil may have immune-enhancing effects in the elderly and should be used cautiously with other agents that affect the immune system.
- Black currant may interact with nonsteroidal antiinflammatory agents (NSAIDS) and COX-2 inhibitors; use cautiously.

Interactions with Herbs and Dietary Supplements

- Black currant may increase the risk of bleeding when taken with herbs and supplements that are believed to increase the risk of bleeding. Multiple cases of bleeding have been reported with the use of *Ginkgo biloba*, and fewer cases have been reported with garlic and saw palmetto.
- Black currant may have MAOI effects. Use cautiously with herbs and supplements with antidepressant activity.
- Black currant may interact with antiinflammatory herbs and supplements; use cautiously because of possible additive effects.
- Black currant anthocyanins have antioxidant effects, and caution is advised when black currant is taken with other agents with antioxidant effects.
- Black currant may interact with antiviral agents. Consult a qualified health care professional, including a pharmacist, to check for interactions.
- Blackcurrant seed oil (BSO), a rich source of gamma-linolenic acid, may alter blood pressure. Use cautiously with herbs and supplements that may also alter blood pressure because of possible additive effects.
- Black currant seed oil may have immune-enhancing effects in the elderly and should be used cautiously with other agents that affect the immune system.
- Black currant fruit and juice contain rutin and other flavonoids. The flavonoids found in black currant belong to one of two classes: the anthocyanin class or the proanthocyanidin class. Caution is advised when black currant is taken with other herbs or supplements containing these flavonoids because of additive effects.
- Black currant fruit has a high vitamin C content. Use cautiously with other vitamin C supplements or multivitamin preparations.

For a complete list of references, please visit www.naturalstandard.com.

Black Horehound
(Ballota nigra)

RELATED TERMS

- Alpha-humulene, alpha-pinene, alpha-tocopherol, alyssonoside, angoroside A, arenarioside, ballonigrin, Ballota, *Ballota antalyense, Ballota glandulosissima, Ballota larendana, Ballota macrodonta, Ballota nigra, Ballota nigra* subsp. *anatolica, Ballota pseudodictamnus, Ballota rotundifolia, Ballota saxatilis*, ballotenol, ballotetroside, ballotinone, beta-pinene, black horehound, black stinking horehound, caffeoyl-L-malic acid, caffeoyl malic acid, caryophyllene, copaene, delta-cadinene, diterpene, forsythoside B, germacrene-D, gout, lactoylate flavonoids, Lamiaceae (family), lavandulifolioside, linalool, marrubiin, phenylpropanoid, phenylpropanoid glycosides, polyphenols, sabinene, verbascoside.
- **Note:** Black horehound should not be confused with white horehound (*Marrubium vulgare* L.) or water horehound (*Lycopus americanus*, also known as bugleweed).

BACKGROUND

- Black horehound (*Ballota nigra*) is a three-foot, perennial herb of the family Lamiaceae. It is native to the Mediterranean and central Asia and can be found throughout Europe and the eastern United States. Black horehound has a very strong smell and can be recognized by its clusters of hairy, reddish-purple flowers. The aerial parts of the plant are used medicinally, either alone or in combination with other herbs. Usually, the aerial parts are prepared as an herbal extract.
- Black horehound has been used in traditional European herbalism for nervous dyspepsia (upset stomach), traveling sickness, morning sickness in pregnancy, arthritis, gout (foot inflammation), menstrual disorders, and bronchial complaints.
- Black horehound has been used for nausea and vomiting and as a mild sedative. However, its popularity has waned because of the plant's extremely foul odor. Although clinical data are lacking, laboratory studies indicate that black horehound may have some sedative, antioxidant, and antibiotic properties.

EVIDENCE

Uses Based on Scientific Evidence

No available studies qualify for inclusion in the evidence table.

Uses Based on Tradition or Theory

Animal bites (dog), antibacterial, antioxidant, antispasmodic, anxiety, arthritis, astringent, blood purifier, bronchial irritation, cleansing, convulsions, depression, diuretic, emmenagogue (stimulates menstruation), expectorant, genital warts, gout (foot inflammation), high cholesterol level, hysteria, insect bites, insomnia, intestinal worms, menopause, menstrual disorders, motion sickness, nausea and vomiting, nervous disorders, nervous stomach, nutrition, resolvent, scrapes, sedative, snake bite, stimulant, stomach disorders, sunburn, travel sickness, uterotonic.

DOSING

Adults (18 Years and Older)

- There is insufficient evidence to recommend a dose for black horehound. Traditionally, black horehound has been taken as a dried herb, tea, syrup, or tincture. For instance, 2-4 g of dried herb has been taken three times daily; 3 cups of tea (prepared with the use of 2 oz. fresh horehound leaves per 2.5 cups of fresh, nonchlorinated water) has been taken daily; 1 teaspoonful of syrup has been taken three times a day, or every 2 hours, for acute illness; and 10-15 drops of tincture (1:10, 45% ethanol) has also been taken three times daily.

Children (Younger than 18 Years)

- There is insufficient evidence to recommend a dose for black horehound in children.

SAFETY

Allergies

- Avoid in individuals with a known allergy or hypersensitivity to black horehound, its constituents, or related members of the Lamiaceae family.

Side Effects and Warnings

- Adverse effects information is based on traditional health practice patterns and expert opinion; there are no available reliable human trials demonstrating safety or efficacy of black horehound. Overdose may result in death.
- Black horehound is possibly unsafe when used in pregnant or breastfeeding women, children, and patients taking iron supplements or sedating agents. It is also theoretically unsafe when used in patients with Parkinson's disease, as black horehound may block the effects of dopamine in the brain.

Pregnancy and Breastfeeding

- Black horehound is not recommended in pregnant or breastfeeding women because of a lack of available scientific evidence.

INTERACTIONS

Interactions with Drugs

- Although not well studied in humans, black horehound may have antibiotic (antibacterial) and antioxidant effects. Use cautiously when taking black horehound with other agents with similar effects because of possible additive effects.
- Black horehound may inhibit low-density lipoprotein (LDL) oxidation. Caution is advised when it is taken concomitantly with other cholesterol-lowering agents, including statins.
- Black horehound may decrease the efficacy of dopamine agonists.
- Black horehound may also have neurosedative effects and may increase the amount of drowsiness caused by some

drugs. Examples include benzodiazepines such as lorazepam (Ativan) or diazepam (Valium), barbiturates such as phenobarbital, narcotics such as codeine, some antidepressants, and alcohol. Use caution while driving or operating machinery.

Interactions with Herbs and Dietary Supplements

- Although not well studied in humans, black horehound may have antibiotic (antibacterial) and antioxidant effects. Use cautiously when taking black horehound with other herbs or supplements with similar effects because of possible additive effects.

- Black horehound may inhibit LDL oxidation. Use caution when taking concomitantly with other cholesterol-lowering agents, such as red yeast rice.
- Black horehound may decrease the efficacy of dopamine agonists.
- When black horehound is taken internally, it may interfere with the absorption of iron and other minerals.
- Black horehound may also have neurosedative effects and may increase the amount of drowsiness caused by some herbs or supplements.

For a complete list of references, please visit www.naturalstandard.com.

Black Pepper

(*Piper nigrum*)

RELATED TERMS

- Bisalkaloids, black pepper oil, Brazilian black pepper, dipiperamide D, dipiperamide E, green pepper, pink pepper, Piperaceae (family), piperine, piptigrine, red pepper, white pepper, wisanine.
- **Note:** Black pepper, white pepper, green pepper, pink pepper, and red pepper are all differently preserved berries or seeds of the *Piper nigrum* plant.

BACKGROUND

- Black pepper (*Piper nigrum*) is native to India and other southeast Asian countries. Although black pepper has been used as a spice for millennia, it has also traditionally been used in India to treat diarrhea. In the Ayurvedic tradition, a preparation called Trikatu (black pepper, long pepper, and ginger) is prescribed routinely for a variety of diseases.
- Recent laboratory studies indicate that black pepper may also be beneficial in pain and Alzheimer's disease. In clinical trials, inhalation of black pepper oil improved withdrawal symptoms of cigarette smoking and the ability to swallow in poststroke patients.
- Ingestion of black pepper may cause dyspepsia (upset stomach) and other gastrointestinal adverse effects. Inhalation of black pepper has caused respiratory irritation, edema, and even respiratory arrest, severe anoxia, and death. There may also be a link between ingestion of black pepper and nasopharyngeal or esophageal cancer.
- The U.S. Food and Drug Administration (FDA) has approved black pepper, black pepper oil, black pepper oleoresin, piperidine, and piperine as "generally recognized as safe" (GRAS) for use in foods in the United States.

EVIDENCE

Uses Based on Scientific Evidence	Grade
Smoking Cessation Sensory cues associated with cigarette smoking can suppress certain smoking withdrawal symptoms, including the craving for cigarettes. Inhalation of black pepper essential oil may reduce cravings and physical symptoms associated with cigarette smoking withdrawal.	C
Stroke Recovery (Difficulty Swallowing) Nasal inhalation of volatile black pepper oil in poststroke patients may improve swallowing dysfunction symptoms. However, more research is needed in this area.	C

Uses Based on Tradition or Theory
Allergic rhinitis, Alzheimer's disease, antibacterial, antiinflammatory, antioxidant, diarrhea, food uses, *Helicobacter pylori* infection, insecticidal, measles, obesity, pain, positive energy balance.

DOSING

Adults (18 Years and Older)

- There is insufficient evidence to recommend a dose for black pepper in adults. However, nasal inhalation of volatile black pepper oil for 1 minute for up to 1 month has been studied to help with difficulty swallowing during stroke recovery.

Children (Younger than 18 Years)

- There is insufficient evidence to recommend a dose for black pepper in children.

SAFETY

Allergies

- Avoid in individuals with a known allergy or hypersensitivity to black pepper.

Side Effects and Warnings

- Black pepper is likely safe when consumed in food amounts. The U.S. FDA has approved black pepper, black pepper oil, black pepper oleoresin, piperidine, and piperine as GRAS for use in foods in the United States.
- Patients taking cholinergic agonists, cyclosporin A, digoxin, cytochrome P450 metabolized agents, herbs or drugs by mouth, phenytoin, propranolol, rifampicin (rifampin), or theophylline should use black pepper cautiously.
- Possible side effects of taking black pepper in medicinal amounts by mouth may include stomach upset or other gastrointestinal adverse effects. Use cautiously in patients with gastrointestinal disorders.
- Inhaling black pepper may cause respiratory irritation, edema (swelling), and even respiratory arrest, severe anoxia (lack of oxygen), and death.
- There may also be a link between ingestion of black pepper and nasopharyngeal or esophageal cancer, although there is controversy in this area.
- Avoid in patients with a known allergy or hypersensitivity to black pepper (*Piper nigrum*), its constituents, or members of the Piperaceae family.

Pregnancy and Breastfeeding

- Black pepper is not recommended in pregnant or breastfeeding women in amounts greater than those found in foods because of a lack of available scientific evidence.

INTERACTIONS

Interactions with Drugs

- Inhalation of black pepper may cause respiratory irritation and edema (swelling). Piperine, a constituent of black pepper, may increase the bioavailability of theophylline (an agent used for asthma). Caution is advised in patients with respiratory conditions or in those taking asthma medications.
- Although not well studied in humans, a link may exist between ingestion of black pepper and certain types of cancer. Patients taking anticancer medications should use black pepper with caution.

- Black pepper may have antiinflammatory, antioxidant, and pain-relieving effects; use cautiously with drugs that have similar effects.
- Extracts of black pepper seeds may inhibit acetylcholinesterase. Use cautiously with cholinergic agonists. Consult a qualified health care professional, including a pharmacist, to check for interactions.
- Constituents isolated from black pepper may interfere with the way the body processes certain drugs using the liver's "cytochrome P450" enzyme system. As a result, the levels of these drugs may be increased in the blood and may cause increased effects or potentially serious adverse reactions. Patients using any medications should check the package insert and speak with a qualified health care professional, including a pharmacist, about possible interactions.
- Piperine may alter the transport of certain agents (cyclosporine, digoxin) in intestinal cells. Cyclosporine is often prescribed to reduce the risk of rejection of organ and bone marrow transplants, and digoxin is a heart medication. Consult with a qualified health care professional, including a pharmacist, as dosing may need adjustment.
- Use cautiously with drugs taken by mouth, as black pepper may alter the transit time of other agents in the body and may change the effectiveness of these agents.
- Piperine from black pepper may enhance the bioavailability of phenytoin significantly, possibly by increasing its absorption. Phenytoin sodium (Dilantin, Epanutin) is a commonly used antiepileptic (seizure medication). Use black pepper cautiously with other antiepileptics because of possible additive effects.
- Piperine may increase the bioavailability of propranolol (Inderal), a nonselective beta blocker that is used in the treatment of high blood pressure, prevention of migraines, controlling tremors, suppressing the symptoms of hyperthyroidism (fast heart rate, tremor), lowering portal pressure in portal high blood pressure when this has led to esophageal varices, as well as in the management of anxiety and panic disorders.
- Piperine may increase plasma concentrations of rifampicin (rifampin), which belongs to a class of antibiotics. Caution is advised when black pepper is combined with other antibiotic medications.

Interactions with Herbs and Dietary Supplements

- Inhalation of black pepper may cause respiratory irritation and edema (swelling). Piperine, a constituent of black pepper, may increase the bioavailability of theophylline (an agent used for asthma). Caution is advised in patients with respiratory conditions or in those taking herbs and supplements to manage asthma.
- Although not well studied in humans, a link may exist between ingestion of black pepper and certain types of cancer. Patients taking anticancer herbs or supplements should use black pepper with caution.
- Black pepper may have antiinflammatory, antioxidant, and pain-relieving effects; use cautiously with herbs or supplements that have similar effects.
- Extracts of black pepper seeds may inhibit acetylcholinesterase. Use cautiously with cholinergic agonists. Consult a qualified health care professional, including a pharmacist, to check for interactions.
- Constituents isolated from black pepper may interfere with the way the body processes certain herbs or supplements using the liver's cytochrome P450 enzyme system. As a result, the levels of other herbs or supplements may become too high in the blood. It may also alter the effects that other herbs or supplements possibly have on the P450 system.
- Piperine may alter the transport of certain agents (cyclosporine, digoxin) in intestinal cells. Cyclosporine is often prescribed to reduce the risk of rejection of organ and bone marrow transplants, and digoxin is a heart medication. Caution is advised when black pepper is taken with other herbs or supplements used for these conditions. Consult with a qualified health care professional, including a pharmacist, as dosing may need adjustment.
- Piperine from black pepper may enhance the bioavailability of epigallocatechin gallate (EGCG), a polyphenol constituent from green tea (*Camellia sinensis*).
- Use cautiously with herbs or supplements taken by mouth, as black pepper may alter the transit time of other agents in the body and may change the effectiveness of these agents.
- Piperine from black pepper may enhance the bioavailability of phenytoin, possibly by increasing its absorption. Phenytoin sodium (Dilantin, Epanutin) is a commonly used antiepileptic (seizure medication). Use black pepper cautiously with other antiepileptics because of possible additive effects.
- Piperine may increase the bioavailability of propranolol (Inderal), a nonselective beta blocker that is used in the treatment of high blood pressure, prevention of migraines, controlling tremors, suppressing the symptoms of hyperthyroidism (fast heart rate, tremor), lowering portal pressure in portal high blood pressure when this has led to esophageal varices, as well as in the management of anxiety and panic disorders. Caution is advised when black pepper is taken with any herbs or supplements used for the above conditions because of possible altered effects.
- Piperine may increase plasma concentrations of rifampicin (rifampin), which belongs to a class of antibiotics. Caution is advised when black pepper is combined with other antibacterial herbs or supplements.

For a complete list of references, please visit www.naturalstandard.com.

Black Seed
(Nigella sativa)

RELATED TERMS

- Ajenuz, alanine, alkaloids, alpha-hederin, alpha-spinasterol, arachidonic acid protein, aranuel, arginine, ascorbic acid, asparagine, Baraka, beta-sitosterol, black caraway, black cumin, black cumin seed, black onion seed, blackseed, blessed seed, calcium, campesterol, carvacrol, carvone, charnushka (Russian), citronellol, cominho negro, cominho-negro dicotyledon, copper, corek otu (Turkish), cymene, crude fiber, crystalline nigellone, cymene, cystine, d-limonene, dehydroascorbic acid, dihomolinoleic acid, dithymoquinone, eicosadienoic acid, fennel flower, fennel-flower, fitch, folacin, glucose, glutamic acid, glycine, habbah Albarakah, Habbatul Baraka, hazak (Hebrew), iron, isoleucine, kalonji (Hindi), leucine, linoleic acid, linolenic acid, lipase, love in the mist, lysine, melanin, methionine, myristic acid, nigella, *Nigella damascena* L., *Nigella sativa*, *Nigella suava* L., Nigelle de Crete, nigellicin, nigellidin, nigellimin, nigellimin-N-oxide, nigellin, nigellone, niacin, nutmeg flower, nutmeg-flower, oleic acid, palmitic acid, palmitoleic acid, pentacyclic triterpene, phenylalanine, phosphorus, phytosterols, potassium, pyridoxine, Ranunculaceae (family), riboflavin, Roman coriander, saponin, Schwarzkummel, seeds of blessing, siyah daneh (Persian), sodium, stearic acid, stigmasterol, tannin, terpine, terpineol, threonine, thymohydroquinone (TQ), thymol, thymoquinone, toute epice, tryptophan, tyrosine, zinc.

BACKGROUND

- Black seed *(Nigella sativa)* is an annual flowering plant, native to southwest Asia, that has been used primarily in candies and liquors, as well as medicinally. In many Arabian, Asian, and African countries, black seed oil is used as a natural remedy for a wide range of diseases.
- Black seed has been studied clinically for reducing allergies. Black seed has also been studied for use in cancer, immune disorders, inflammation, stomach and respiratory conditions, and for women's health.

EVIDENCE

Uses Based on Scientific Evidence	Grade
Allergies There is limited clinical evidence suggesting that black seed may decrease allergies. Further research is needed to confirm these results.	C

Uses Based on Tradition or Theory
Abdominal pain, abortion inducing, abscesses, antibacterial, antifungal, antiinflammatory, antioxidant, anxiety, arthritis, asthma, boils, breast cancer, breast milk stimulant, bronchitis, bruises, cancer, colon cancer, colorectal cancer, congestion, constipation, contraceptive, cough, diabetes, diarrhea, digestive tonic, diuretic, dysentery, earache, edema, eye infections, fever, flu, genital area infections, hair loss, headache, hemorrhoids, high blood pressure, immune function, inflammation, intestinal inflammation, laxative, lipid-lowering effects, liver cancer, liver conditions, lung cancer, lung conditions, malnutrition, menstrual flow stimulant, muscle soreness, nasal congestion, neurological disorders, pancreatic cancer, paralysis, parasites, respiratory problems, sinus infection, skin disorders, snakebites, stimulant, stomach cancer, stomach disorders, stomach ulcer, sweating, throat cancer, tonic, warts.

DOSING

Adults (18 Years and Older)

- Black seed capsules at a dose of 40-80 mg/kg have been used daily for the treatment of allergies.
- Black seed oil has been taken by mouth and used on the skin for the treatment of allergies, arthritis, anxiety, bruises, cold symptoms, diarrhea, headache, high blood pressure, flu, muscle soreness, rheumatic disease, sinus infection, and stomach disorders.
- Black seed oil has been used on the scalp for hair loss, on the skin for the treatment of fungal infections, rubbed on the back and chest for asthma and cough, massaged on the abdomen for colic, dripped in the ear for earache, and rubbed on the forehead and surrounding facial areas for treatment of headache.
- The vapor of black seed oil has been inhaled for the treatment of acne, asthma, cough, and sinusitis.

Children (Younger than 18 Years)

- There is no proven safe or effective dose for black seed and use in children is not recommended.

SAFETY

Allergies

- Avoid in individuals with a known allergy or sensitivity to black seed. Skin irritation may occur after the use of black seed or black seed oil applied to the skin.

Side Effects and Warnings

- Black seed is generally safe when taken by mouth in amounts found in foods.
- Use cautiously in patients with immune disorders because of its effects on the immune system.
- Avoid in patients who are trying to conceive or who are pregnant, as black seed may prevent uterine contractions and conception.

Pregnancy and Breastfeeding

- Avoid in patients who are pregnant or breastfeeding or trying to conceive.

INTERACTIONS

Interactions with Drugs

- Black seed may inhibit conception and uterine contractions. Caution is advised in patients taking drugs used for fertility or to induce labor.

- Black seed may have additive effects with antibiotics, drugs used to reduce inflammation, drugs used for parasites, drugs used for asthma, lipid-lowering drugs, anticancer drugs, and drugs that affect the immune system.

Interactions with Herbs and Dietary Supplements

- Black seed may inhibit conception and uterine contractions. Caution is advised in patients taking herbs or supplements used for fertility or to induce labor.

- Black seed may have additive effects with antioxidants, antibiotics, herbs and supplements used to reduce inflammation, herbs and supplements used for parasites, herbs and supplements used for asthma, lipid-lowering herbs and supplements, anticancer herbs and supplements, and herbs and supplements that affect the immune system.

For a complete list of references, please visit www.naturalstandard.com.

Black Tea
(*Camellia sinensis*)

RELATED TERMS

- Caffeine, camellia, *Camellia assamica*, camellia tea, *Camellia sinensis*, catechin, Chinese tea, green tea, oolong tea, tea for America, *Thea bohea*, *Thea sinensis*, *Thea viridis*, theifers.

BACKGROUND

- Black tea is made from the dried leaves of *Camellia sinensis*, a perennial evergreen shrub. Black tea has a long history of use dating back to China approximately 5000 years ago. Green tea, black tea, and oolong tea are all derived from the same plant and produced through different processes.
- Black tea, like other teas derived from *Camellia sinensis*, is a source of caffeine, a methylxanthine that stimulates the central nervous system, relaxes smooth muscle in the airways to the lungs (bronchioles), stimulates the heart, and acts on the kidney as a diuretic (increasing urine). One cup of tea contains about 50 mg of caffeine, depending on the strength and size of the cup (as compared with coffee, which contains 65 to 175 mg of caffeine per cup). Tea also contains polyphenols (catechins, anthocyanins, phenolic acids), tannin, trace elements, and vitamins.
- The tea plant is native to Southeast Asia and can grow up to a height of 40 feet but is usually maintained at a height of 2 to 3 feet by regular pruning. The first spring leaf buds, called the *first flush*, are considered the highest quality leaves. When the first flush leaf bud is picked, another one grows, which is called the *second flush*, and this continues until an *autumn flush*. The older leaves picked farther down the stems are considered to be of poorer quality.
- Tea varieties reflect the growing region (e.g., Ceylon or Assam), the district (e.g., Darjeeling), the form (e.g., pekoe is cut, gunpowder is rolled), and the processing method (e.g., black, green, or oolong). India and Sri Lanka are the major producers of black tea.
- Historically, tea has been served as a part of various ceremonies and has been used to stay alert during long meditations. A legend in India describes the story of Prince Siddhartha Gautama, the founder of Buddhism, who tore off his eyelids in frustration at his inability to stay awake during meditation while journeying through China. A tea plant is said to have sprouted from the spot where his eyelids fell, providing him with the ability to stay awake, meditate, and reach enlightenment. Turkish traders reportedly introduced tea to Western cultures in the sixth century. By the eighteenth century, tea was commonly consumed in England, where it became customary to drink tea at 5 PM.
- Black tea reached the Americas with the first European settlers in 1492. Black tea gained notoriety in the United States in 1773 when colonists tossed black tea into Boston Harbor during the Boston Tea Party. This symbolic gesture was an early event in the Revolutionary War.

EVIDENCE

Uses Based on Scientific Evidence	Grade
Asthma Research has shown caffeine to cause improvements in airflow to the lungs (bronchodilation). However, it is not clear whether caffeine or tea use has significant clinical benefits in people with asthma.	C
Cancer Prevention Several studies have explored a possible association between regular consumption of black tea and rates of cancer in populations. This research has yielded conflicting results, with some studies suggesting benefits and others reporting no effects. Laboratory and animal studies report that components of tea, such as polyphenols, have antioxidant properties and effects against tumors. However, effects in humans remain unclear, and these components may be more common in green tea rather than in black tea. Some animal and laboratory research suggests that components of black tea may be carcinogenic, although effects in humans are not clear. Overall, the relationship of black tea consumption and human cancer remains undetermined.	C
Colorectal Cancer Although there is strong evidence from animal and laboratory studies that black tea may help prevent colon cancer, clinical studies are limited.	C
Dental Cavity Prevention There is limited research using black tea as a mouthwash for the prevention of dental cavities (caries) or plaque. It is not clear whether this is a beneficial therapy.	C
Diabetes Black tea may lower blood sugar levels. A combination of black tea–green tea extract did not lower blood sugar levels in patients with type 2 diabetes. However, black tea alone did lower blood sugar and increase insulin levels in healthy patients. The isolated effects of black tea are not clear.	C
Heart Attack Prevention/Cardiovascular Risk There is conflicting evidence from a small number of studies examining the relationship of tea intake with the risk of heart attack. Tea may reduce the risk of platelet aggregation or endothelial dysfunction, proposed to be beneficial against blocked arteries	C

Uses Based on Scientific Evidence	Grade
in the heart. The long-term effects of tea consumption on cardiovascular risk factors, such as cholesterol levels and atherosclerosis, are not fully understood. Other research suggests that drinking black tea regularly does not affect plasma homocysteine levels or blood pressure. Black tea may increase heart rate.	
Memory Enhancement Several preliminary studies have examined the effects of caffeine, tea, or coffee use on short- and long-term memory. It remains unclear whether tea is beneficial for this use.	C
Mental Performance/Alertness Limited, low-quality research reports that the use of black tea may improve cognition and a sense of alertness. Black tea contains caffeine, which is a stimulant.	C
Metabolic Enhancement Additional research is needed to understand exactly how black tea may affect human metabolism.	C
Methicillin-Resistant *Staphylococcus aureus* (MRSA) Infection There is limited evidence that inhaled tea catechin is temporarily effective in the reduction of MRSA and shortening of hospitalization in elderly patients with MRSA-infected sputum. Additional research is needed to further explore these results.	C
Oral Leukoplakia/Carcinoma Early studies report that black tea may lead to clinical improvement in oral leukoplakia and therefore prevent oral carcinoma. Further research is needed to confirm these results.	C
Osteoporosis Prevention Preliminary research suggests that chronic use of black tea may improve bone mineral density (BMD) in older women. Better research is needed in this area before a conclusion can be drawn.	C
Stress Based on early research, black tea may reduce stress and help patients feel more relaxed. More research is needed to confirm these findings. It should be noted that high doses of caffeine have been linked to anxiety.	C
Weight Loss Black tea has been used as part of a combination supplement to help patients lose weight. Although patients in the study lost weight, the effects of black tea alone are unclear.	C

Uses Based on Tradition or Theory

Acute pharyngitis, antioxidant, anxiety, cancer multidrug resistance, circulatory/blood flow disorders, cleansing, Crohn's disease, diarrhea, diuretic (increasing urine flow), gum disease, headache, hyperactivity (children), immune enhancement/improving resistance to disease, influenza, joint pain, kidney stone prevention, melanoma, obesity, osteoarthritis, pain, prostate cancer, stomach disorders, toxin/alcohol elimination from the body, trigeminal neuralgia, vomiting.

DOSING
Adults (18 Years and Older)
- Black tea has not been proven as an effective therapy for any condition and benefits of specific doses are not established. A maximum of eight cups of black tea daily has been suggested. One cup of tea contains approximately 50 mg of caffeine, depending on the strength of the tea and the size of the cup.

Children (Younger than 18 Years)
- There is a lack of available information about the safety or effectiveness of black tea in children. Because of the caffeine content, caution is advised.

SAFETY
Allergies
- People with known allergy/hypersensitivity to caffeine or tannin should avoid black tea. Skin rash and hives have been reported with caffeine ingestion.

Side Effects and Warnings
- Studies of the side effects of black tea specifically are limited. However, black tea is a source of caffeine, for which multiple reactions are reported.
- Caffeine is a stimulant of the central nervous system and may cause insomnia in adults, children, and infants (including nursing infants of mothers taking caffeine). Caffeine acts on the kidneys as a diuretic (increasing urine and urine sodium/potassium levels and potentially decreasing blood sodium/potassium levels) and may worsen incontinence. Caffeine-containing beverages may increase the production of stomach acid and may worsen ulcer symptoms. Tannin in tea can cause constipation. Caffeine in certain doses can increase heart rate and blood pressure, although people who consume caffeine regularly do not seem to experience these effects in the long-term.
- An increase in blood sugar levels may occur after drinking black tea containing high levels of caffeine. Other early studies suggest that green tea may lower blood sugar levels and increase insulin levels. Caffeine-containing beverages such as black tea should be used cautiously in patients with diabetes. People with severe liver disease should use caffeine cautiously, as levels of caffeine in the blood may build up and last longer. Skin rashes have been associated with caffeine ingestion. In laboratory and animal studies, caffeine has been found to affect blood clotting, although effects

in humans are not known. It is unclear whether black tea with or without caffeine would have similar effects. Black tea may stain teeth.

- Caffeine toxicity/high doses: High doses of caffeine may cause symptoms of anxiety, delirium, agitation, psychosis, or detrussor instability (unstable bladder). Conception may be delayed in women who consume large amounts of caffeine. Seizure, muscle spasm, life-threatening muscle breakdown (rhabdomyolysis), and life-threatening abnormal heart rhythms have been reported with caffeine overdose. Extremely high doses may be fatal.
- Caffeine withdrawal: Chronic use can result in tolerance, psychological dependence, and may be habit forming. Abrupt discontinuation may result in withdrawal symptoms such as headache, irritation, nervousness, anxiety, tremor, or dizziness. In people with psychiatric disorders such as affective disorder or schizoaffective disorder, caffeine withdrawal may worsen symptoms or cause confusion, disorientation, excitement, restlessness, violent behavior, or mania.
- Chronic effects: Several population studies initially suggested a possible association between caffeine use and fibrocystic breast disease, although more recent research has not found this connection. Limited research reports a possible relationship between caffeine use and multiple sclerosis, although evidence is not definitive in this area. Animal research reports that tannin fractions from tea plants may increase the risk of cancer, although it is not clear that the tannin present in black tea has significant carcinogenic effects in humans.
- Drinking tannin-containing beverages, such as black tea, may contribute to iron deficiency. In infants, black tea has been associated with impaired iron metabolism and microcytic anemia.

Pregnancy and Breastfeeding

- Large amounts of black tea should be used cautiously in pregnant women, as caffeine crosses the placenta and has been associated with spontaneous abortion, intrauterine growth retardation, and low birth weight. Heavy caffeine intake during pregnancy may increase the risk of later developing sudden infant death syndrome (SIDS). Very high doses of caffeine have been associated with birth defects, including limb and palate malformations.
- Caffeine is readily transferred into breast milk. Caffeine ingestion by infants can lead to sleep disturbances/insomnia. Infants nursing from mothers consuming high levels of caffeine daily have been reported to experience tremors and heart rhythm abnormalities. Components present in breast milk may reduce infants' ability to metabolize caffeine, resulting in higher than expected caffeine levels. Tea consumption by infants has been associated with anemia, reductions in iron metabolism, and irritability.

INTERACTIONS
Interactions with Drugs

- Studies of the interactions of black tea with drugs are limited. However, black tea is a source of caffeine, for which multiple interactions have been documented.
- Black tea may increase the effects of drugs that cause the blood vessels to narrow (called vasopressors).
- The combination of caffeine with ephedrine, an ephedra alkaloid, has been implicated in numerous severe or life-threatening cardiovascular events such as very high blood pressure, stroke, or heart attack. This combination is commonly used in over-the-counter weight loss products and may also be associated with other adverse effects, including abnormal heart rhythms, insomnia, anxiety, headache, irritability, poor concentration, blurred vision, and dizziness. Stroke has also been reported after the nasal ingestion of caffeine with amphetamine.

- Caffeine may add to the effects and side effects of other stimulants including nicotine, beta-adrenergic agonists such as albuterol (Ventolin), or other methylxanthines such as theophylline. Conversely, caffeine can counteract drowsy effects and mental slowness caused by benzodiazepines like lorazepam (Ativan) or diazepam (Valium). Phenylpropanolamine and caffeine should not be used together because of reports of numerous potentially serious adverse effects, although forms of phenylpropanolamine taken by mouth have been removed from the U.S. market because of reports of bleeding into the head.
- When taken with caffeine, a number of drugs may increase caffeine blood levels or the length of time caffeine acts on the body, including disulfiram (Antabuse), oral contraceptives (OCPs) or hormone replacement therapy (HRT), ciprofloxacin (Cipro), norfloxacin, fluvoxamine (Luvox), cimetidine (Tagamet), verapamil, and mexiletine. Caffeine levels may be lowered by taking dexamethasone (Decadron). The metabolism of caffeine by the liver may be affected by multiple drugs, although the effects in humans are not clear.
- Caffeine may lengthen the effects of carbamazepine or increase the effects of clozapine (Clozaril) and dipyridamole. Caffeine may affect serum lithium levels, and abrupt cessation of caffeine use by regular caffeine users taking lithium may result in high levels of lithium or lithium toxicity. Levels of aspirin or phenobarbital may be lowered in the body, although clinical effects in humans are not clear.
- Although caffeine by itself does not appear to have pain-relieving properties, it is used in combination with ergotamine tartrate in the treatment of migraine or cluster headaches (e.g., Cafergot). It has been shown to increase the headache-relieving effects of other pain relievers such as acetaminophen and aspirin (e.g., Excedrin). Caffeine may also increase the pain-relieving effects of codeine or ibuprofen (Advil, Motrin).
- As a diuretic, caffeine increases urine and sodium losses through the kidney and may add to the effects of other diuretics such as furosemide (Lasix).
- There is controversy as to how black tea and caffeine affect blood clotting. Black tea may contain vitamin K, which when used in large quantities can reduce the blood-thinning effects of warfarin (Coumadin), a phenomenon that has been reported in a human case. However, black tea may also increase the risk of bleeding when taken with anticoagulants or antiplatelet therapies. Caution is advised.
- Based on preliminary data, theanine, a specific glutamate derivative in green tea (which is the same species as black tea), may reduce the adverse reactions caused to the heart and liver by the prescription cancer drug doxorubicin. Further research is needed to confirm these results.
- Based on preliminary data, ingestion of green tea may decrease low-density lipoprotein (LDL) cholesterol and thus may theoretically interact with other cholesterol-lowering drugs.
- Other potential interactions may include drugs such as adenosine, alcohol, antidiabetics, antipsychotics, fluconazole, hydrocortisone, levodopa, MAOI antidepressants, phenytoin, proton pump inhibitors (PPIs), riluzole, and timolol.

Interactions with Herbs and Dietary Supplements

- Studies of black tea interactions with herbs and supplements are limited. However, black tea is a source of caffeine for which multiple interactions have been documented.
- There is controversy as to how black tea and caffeine affect blood clotting. Caution is advised when herbs or supplements that affect blood clotting are used.
- Black tea may increase the effects of herbs or supplements that cause the blood vessels to narrow (called vasoconstrictors).
- Black tea may increase or decrease the effects of antidiabetic agents.
- Caffeine may add to the effects and side effects of other stimulants. The combination of caffeine with ephedrine, which is present in ephedra (ma huang), has been implicated in numerous severe or life-threatening cardiovascular events such as very high blood pressure, stroke, or heart attack. This combination is commonly used in over-the-counter weight loss products and may also be associated with other adverse effects including abnormal heart rhythms, insomnia, anxiety, headache, irritability, poor concentration, blurred vision, and dizziness.
- Cola nut, guarana (*Paullina cupana*), and yerba mate (*Ilex paraguayensis*) are also sources of caffeine and may add to the effects and side effects of caffeine in black tea. A combination product containing caffeine, yerba mate (*Ilex paraguayensis*), and damiana (*Turnera diffusa*) has been reported to cause weight loss, slowing of the gastrointestinal tract, and a feeling of stomach fullness.
- As a diuretic, caffeine increases urine and sodium losses through the kidney and may add to the effects of other diuretic agents.
- Based on preliminary data, ingestion of black tea may lower LDL cholesterol and thus may theoretically interact with other cholesterol-lowering herbs and supplements.
- Bitter orange, calcium, iron, MAOIs, and tannin-containing herbs and supplements may also interact.
- Black tea may increase the effects of antioxidants.

For a complete list of references, please visit www.naturalstandard.com.

Black Walnut
(*Juglans nigra*)

RELATED TERMS

- American walnut, ellagic acid, Juglandaceae (family), *Juglans nigra*, juglone, methyl 2-benzimidazolylcarbamate, nogal americano, noguerira-preta, noyer noir, plumbagin, quinones, sesquiterpenes, Schwarze Walnuss (German), tannins.

BACKGROUND

- Black walnut (*Juglans nigra*) is a large tree known for its high-quality wood and edible nut, which is commonly used as a food ingredient.
- The U.S. Food and Drug Administration (FDA) announced a health claim stating that eating 1.5 oz per day of walnuts as part of a diet low in fat may reduce the risk of heart disease.
- Black walnut contains tannins, which may help with irritation and may improve tissue firmness. Traditionally, it has been used to relieve constipation and diarrhea.

EVIDENCE

Uses Based on Scientific Evidence

No available studies qualify for inclusion in the evidence table.

Uses Based on Tradition or Theory

Acne, antibacterial, anti-inflammatory, antioxidant, antiviral, astringent, cancer, colic, constipation, cosmetic uses (hair dye), diarrhea, eczema, headache, heart disease, herpes, high blood pressure, hyperglycemia (high blood sugar levels), indigestion, insect bites, mood enhancement, mouth sores, parasitic worm infections, skin disinfectant/sterilization, sore throat, syphilis, toothache, warts, wound care.

DOSING

Adults (18 Years and Older)

- Black walnut powder has been taken by mouth as a capsule or tablet and has also been used on the skin.

Children (Younger than 18 Years)

- There is insufficient evidence to recommend a dose for black walnut in children.

SAFETY

Allergies

- Avoid in patients with known allergy or sensitivity to black walnut, its constituents, including black walnut tree pollen, or to members of the Juglandaceae family. Patients allergic to other nuts may also be allergic to black walnut. Black walnut may irritate the skin.

Side Effects and Warnings

- Black walnut may irritate the skin and may cause stomach upset. When taken for a long time, black walnut may cause mouth or stomach cancer or liver or kidney damage. Use cautiously in patients with stomach disorders or liver or kidney conditions.
- Black walnut may alter blood pressure or affect blood vessels. Caution is advised in patients taking drugs, herbs, or supplements that alter blood pressure or compress blood vessels.

Pregnancy and Breastfeeding

- Black walnut is not recommended for pregnant or breast-feeding women because of lack of sufficient data.

INTERACTIONS

Interactions with Drugs

- Black walnut may bind with other drugs when taken at the same time. It is recommended to wait at least 2 hours before taking any drugs after black walnut.
- Black walnut may alter blood pressure or affect blood vessels. Caution is advised in patients taking drugs that alter blood pressure or compress blood vessels.
- Black walnut may have additive effects with laxatives, antimicrobials, drugs used for the stomach, nausea, inflammation, or cancer, or drugs that harm the liver or kidney.

Interactions with Herbs and Dietary Supplements

- Black walnut may bind with other herbs or supplements when taken at the same time. It is recommended to wait at least 2 hours before taking any herbs or supplements after black walnut.
- Black walnut may alter blood pressure or affect blood vessels. Caution is advised in patients taking herbs or supplements that alter blood pressure or compress blood vessels.
- Black walnut may have additive effects with laxatives, antimicrobials, herbs or supplements used for the stomach, nausea, inflammation, or cancer, herbs or supplements that harm the liver or kidney, or herbs or supplements that contain chemicals called tannins.

For a complete list of references, please visit www.naturalstandard.com.

Blessed Thistle
(*Cnicus benedictus*)

RELATED TERMS

- Bitter thistle, *Carbenia benedicta*, cardin, Cardo Santo, Carduus benedictus, Chardon Benit, *Cnici benedicti herba*, cnicus, holy thistle, Kardo-benedictenkraut, St. Benedict thistle, salonitenolide, spotted thistle.
- **Note:** Blessed thistle should not be mistaken for milk thistle (*Silybum marianum*) or other members of the thistle family.

BACKGROUND

- Blessed thistle leaves, stems, and flowers have traditionally been used in "bitter" tonic drinks and in other preparations taken by mouth to enhance appetite and digestion. Blessed thistle may also be included in the unproven anticancer herbal remedy Essiac. This herb has been tested in laboratory studies for its properties against infections, cancer, and inflammation with promising results. However, high-quality trials showing benefits in humans are lacking.

EVIDENCE

Uses Based on Scientific Evidence	Grade
Bacterial Infections Laboratory studies report that blessed thistle (and chemicals in blessed thistle such as cnicin and polyacetylene) has activity against several types of bacteria and no effects on some types. Reliable human study is lacking.	C
Indigestion and Flatulence (Gas) Blessed thistle is traditionally believed to stimulate stomach acid secretion and has been used as a treatment for indigestion or gas. However, there is limited scientific evidence in these areas.	C
Viral Infections Laboratory studies report no activity of blessed thistle against herpes viruses, influenza, or poliovirus. Effects of blessed thistle (or chemicals in blessed thistle called lignans) against human immunodeficiency virus (HIV) are not clear. There is insufficient evidence to recommend blessed thistle as a treatment for viral infections.	C

Uses Based on Tradition or Theory
Abortifacient, anorexia, appetite stimulant, astringent, bleeding, blood purifier, boils, breast milk stimulant, bubonic plague, cancer, cervical dysplasia, choleretic (bile flow stimulant), colds, contraceptive (birth control), diaphoretic (sweat stimulant), diarrhea, digestion enhancement, diuretic (increases urine), expectorant, fever reducer, gallbladder disease, inflammation, jaundice, liver disorders, malaria, memory improvement, menstrual disorders, menstrual flow stimulant, painful menstruation, rabies, salivation stimulant, skin ulcers, wound healing, yeast infections.

DOSING

Adults (18 Years and Older)

- Tea, tinctures, and liquid extracts are available. Traditional doses include 1.5-3 g of dried blessed thistle flowering tops steeped in 150 mL of boiling water taken three times daily or 1-3 teaspoons of dried blessed thistle herb in 1 cup of boiling water for 5-15 minutes taken three times daily (sometimes recommended to be used 30 minutes before meals). In addition, 1.5-10 mL of other preparations have been taken by mouth up to three times daily. It may be bitter in taste.

Children (Younger than 18 Years)

- Blessed thistle is not recommended for use in children because of a lack of reliable safety data.

SAFETY

Allergies

- Allergic reactions to blessed thistle including rash may occur, as well as cross-sensitivity to mugwort and *Echinacea*. Cross-reactivity may also occur with bitter weed, blanket flower, chrysanthemum, coltsfoot, daisy, dandelion, dwarf sunflower, goldenrod, marigold, prairie sage, ragweed, and other plants in the Asteraceae/Compositae family.

Side Effects and Warnings

- Blessed thistle is generally considered to be safe when used by mouth in recommended doses for short periods of time, with few reported side effects. Direct contact with blessed thistle can cause skin and eye irritation.
- Blessed thistle taken in high doses may cause stomach irritation and vomiting. Blessed thistle is traditionally believed to increase stomach acid secretion and may be inadvisable in patients with stomach ulcers, reflux disease (heartburn), hiatal hernia, or Barrett's esophagus.
- Blessed thistle contains tannins. Long-term ingestion of plants containing tannins may cause gastrointestinal upset, liver disease, kidney toxicity, or increased risk of developing esophageal or nasal cancer. The effects of blessed thistle tannins in humans are not known.
- Laboratory studies suggest that blessed thistle may increase the risk of bleeding, although effects in humans are not known. Caution is advised in patients with bleeding disorders or in those taking agents that may increase the risk of bleeding. Dosing adjustments may be necessary.
- Many tinctures contain high levels of alcohol and should be avoided when an individual is driving or operating heavy machinery.

Pregnancy and Breastfeeding

- Blessed thistle has been used traditionally to stimulate menstruation and abortion and therefore should be avoided during pregnancy. Although blessed thistle has been used historically to stimulate breast milk flow, it is not recommended during breastfeeding because of limited safety information. Reliable research is lacking in these areas.

- Many tinctures contain high levels of alcohol and should be avoided during pregnancy.

INTERACTIONS

Interactions with Drugs

- Traditionally, blessed thistle is believed to stimulate stomach acid secretion and it may reduce the effectiveness of drugs such as cimetidine (Tagamet), famotidine (Pepcid), nizatidine (Axid), or ranitidine (Zantac).
- Based on laboratory studies, blessed thistle may increase the risk of bleeding when taken with drugs that also increase the risk of bleeding (although effects in humans are not known). Some examples include aspirin, anticoagulants ("blood thinners") such as warfarin (Coumadin) or heparin, antiplatelet drugs such as clopidogrel (Plavix), and nonsteroidal antiinflammatory drugs (NSAIDs) such as ibuprofen (Motrin, Advil) or naproxen (Naprosyn, Aleve).

- Many tinctures contain high levels of alcohol and may cause nausea or vomiting when taken with metronidazole (Flagyl) or disulfiram (Antabuse).

Interactions with Herbs and Dietary Supplements

- Based on laboratory studies, blessed thistle may increase the risk of bleeding when taken with herbs or supplements that are believed to increase the risk of bleeding (although effects in humans are not known). Multiple cases of bleeding have been reported with the use of *Ginkgo biloba*, and fewer cases have been reported with garlic and saw palmetto. Numerous other agents may theoretically increase the risk of bleeding, although this has not been proven in most cases.

For a complete list of references, please visit www.naturalstandard.com.

Bloodroot
(*Sanguinaria canadensis*)

RELATED TERMS

- Alkaloids, beta-homochelidonine, benzylisoquinoline alkaloids, berbine, blood root, chelerythrine, chelilutine, chelirubine, coon root, Papaveraceae (family), paucon, pauson, protopine, pseudochelerythrine, puccoon, puccoon-root, red Indian paint, red puccoon, red resin, red root, redroot, SaE, Sangrovit, sanguilutine, *Sanguinaria canadensis*, sanguinaria dentifrice, sanguinaria extract, sanguinarin, sanguinarine, sanguinarine chloride, sanguinarine hydroxide, sanguinarine nitrate, sanguinarine sulfate, sanguinarium, sanguiritrin, sanguirubine, sangvinarin, snakebite, sweet slumber, tetterwort, white puccoon.
- **Note:** This monograph also discusses sanguinarine, an alkaloid of bloodroot, which is also found in other plants such as Mexican prickly poppy (*Argemone mexicana*), *Chelidonium majus*, and *Macleaya cordata*. However, Mexican sanguinaria extract (*Polygonum aviculare*) is not included, as it is not known to contain sanguinarine or other major constituents of bloodroot.

BACKGROUND

- Bloodroot (*Sanguinaria canadensis*) has been used historically by some Native American tribes as a medicinal agent to stimulate the digestive system and induce vomiting. It has also been used as an antimicrobial. More recently, the main active constituent of bloodroot, sanguinarine, has been added to dentifrices (used to clean teeth) to reduce plaque and treat gingivitis and periodontal disease. More research is needed in this area to determine sanguinarine's efficacy for these conditions, although there is some concern that chronic oral use of sanguinarine may cause leukoplakia (precancerous white patches in the mouth) and oral dysplastic lesions (abnormal mouth wounds).
- In a report from 2003, the U.S. Food and Drug Administration (FDA) Dental Plaque Subcommittee of the Nonprescription Drugs Advisory Committee concluded "…that sanguinaria extract at 0.03-0.075% concentration is safe, but there are insufficient data available to permit final classification of its effectiveness in an oral rinse or dentifrice dosage form as an [over the counter] antigingivitis/antiplaque active ingredient." However, expert opinion considers bloodroot unsafe when used internally. In 2005, legal action was taken against an unlicensed practitioner for prescribing bloodroot to several women with breast cancer who suffered disfigurement and tissue damage after topically using the cream.

EVIDENCE

Uses Based on Scientific Evidence	Grade
Plaque/Gingivitis Gingivitis is a bacterially elicited inflammation of the marginal gingiva, and bloodroot has traditionally been associated with antimicrobial activity. Sanguinarine, a constituent of bloodroot, has been used as a toothpaste or mouthrinse ingredient. The results of these studies are mixed.	B
Periodontal Disease Periodontal disease is a bacterially elicited inflammation of the gingiva and periodontal tissue. Preliminary study has not suggested a benefit of sanguinarine for this condition, although results are mixed.	C

Uses Based on Tradition or Theory

Analgesic (pain reliever), anesthesia, antibacterial, antifungal, antiinflammatory, antimicrobial, antioxidant, antiseptic, asthma, athlete's foot, bacterial skin infections, bronchitis, burn wound healing, cancer, cough, croup, diuretic, dysentery (severe diarrhea), dyspepsia (upset stomach), eczema, edema, emetic (induces vomiting), emmenagogue (induces menstruation), expectorant, gastrointestinal conditions, halitosis (bad breath), heart disease, hypotension (low blood pressure), insect repellent, leprosy, liver tonic, migraine headaches, mouth and throat infections, muscle weakness, palpitations, parasites, pesticide, respiratory stimulant, rheumatic pain, ringworm, sedative, skin disorders, sore throat, tonic (gastrointestinal), tuberculosis, varicose ulcers.

DOSING
Adults (18 Years and Older)

- There is insufficient evidence to recommend a dose for bloodroot in adults. For gingivitis prevention, oral rinses containing 300 µg/mL of sanguinaria extract have been used twice daily for up to 6 months. For periodontal disease, oral rinses containing 0.01% sanguinarine have been used daily for up to 6 weeks to reduce plaque formation in patients with established and developing plaque and periodontal disease.

Children (Younger than 18 Years)

- There is insufficient evidence to recommend a dose for bloodroot in children.

SAFETY
Allergies

- Avoid in individuals with a known allergy or hypersensitivity to bloodroot (*Sanguinaria canadensis*) or its constituents.

Side Effects and Warnings

- In a report from 2003, the U.S. FDA Dental Plaque Subcommittee of the Nonprescription Drugs Advisory Committee concluded "…that sanguinaria extract at 0.03%-0.075% concentration is safe, but there are insufficient data available to permit final classification of its effectiveness in an oral rinse or dentifrice dosage form as an [over the counter] antigingivitis/antiplaque active ingredient." However, expert opinion considers bloodroot unsafe when used internally. In 2005, legal action was taken against an unlicensed practitioner for prescribing bloodroot to several women with breast cancer who suffered disfigurement and tissue damage after topically using the cream. Bloodroot can be toxic even at low doses.

- Use cautiously in patients taking anti–*Helicobacter pylori* or antimicrobial agents.
- Use cautiously in patients taking opioids or central nervous system (CNS) depressants, as sanguinarine is a morphine-like alkaloid that may cause sedation, faintness, vertigo, and possibly impair decision making and increase response time.
- Use sanguinarine-containing dentifrices cautiously in patients using tobacco products as sanguinarine may cause leukoplakia (precancerous white patches in the mouth) or dysplastic lesions (abnormal mouth wounds).
- Avoid sanguinarine-containing dentifrices in patients with oral lesions (wounds in the mouth), as sanguinarine may irritate or cause oral lesions.

Pregnancy and Breastfeeding

- Traditionally, bloodroot was used to stimulate menstruation and should therefore not be used during pregnancy. Bloodroot is not recommended in breastfeeding women because of a lack of available scientific evidence.

INTERACTIONS
Interactions with Drugs

- Methanol extracts of *Sanguinaria canadensis* rhizomes may inhibit the growth of *Helicobacter pylori*. Sanguinarine may also have antibacterial, antifungal, and antiprotozoal activity. Caution is advised when bloodroot is taken with any agents with similar effects.
- Bloodroot contains sanguinarine, a morphine-like alkaloid that may cause sedation, faintness, vertigo, and possibly impair decision making and increase response time. These effects may be more pronounced when bloodroot is used with agents that act similarly.
- Sanguinarine may interfere with the way the body processes certain drugs using the liver's cytochrome P450 enzyme system. As a result, the levels of these drugs may be increased in the blood and may cause increased effects or potentially serious adverse reactions. Patients using any medications should check the package insert and speak with a qualified health care professional, including a pharmacist, about possible interactions.

- Bloodroot may interact with hormonal agents.
- Large doses of bloodroot may cause nausea, vomiting, CNS sedation, low blood pressure, shock, coma, and death. Caution is advised when agents that may contribute to these adverse effects are taken, such as sedatives or blood pressure–lowering agents.
- Bloodroot may cause tissue damage when applied to the skin, which may cause other topical medications used at the same time to be absorbed systemically, possibly resulting in unwanted adverse effects. Caution is advised when bloodroot is used on the skin along with other topical agents.

Interactions with Herbs and Dietary Supplements

- Methanol extracts of *Sanguinaria canadensis* rhizomes may inhibit the growth of *Helicobacter pylori*. Sanguinarine may also have antibacterial, antifungal, and antiprotozoal activity. Caution is advised when bloodroot is taken with any herbs or supplements with similar effects.
- Sanguinarine may interfere with the way the body processes certain herbs or supplements using the liver's cytochrome P450 enzyme system. As a result, the levels of other herbs or supplements may become too high in the blood. It may also alter the effects that other herbs or supplements possibly have on the P450 system.
- Bloodroot may interact with hormonal agents.
- Bloodroot contains sanguinarine, a morphine-like alkaloid that may cause sedation, faintness, vertigo, and possibly impair decision making and increase response time. These effects may be more pronounced when bloodroot is used with herbs or supplements that act similarly, such as opioids or CNS-depressing herbs or supplements.
- Large doses of bloodroot may cause nausea, vomiting, CNS sedation, low blood pressure, shock, coma, and death. Caution is advised when herbs and supplements that may contribute to these adverse effects are taken, such as herbs with sedative effects or blood pressure–lowering effects.
- Bloodroot may cause tissue damage when applied to the skin, which may cause other topical medications used at the same time to be absorbed systemically, possibly resulting in unwanted adverse effects. Caution is advised when bloodroot is used on the skin along with other topical herbs or supplements.

For a complete list of references, please visit www.naturalstandard.com.

Blue Cohosh
(*Caulophyllum thalictroides*)

RELATED TERMS

- Alkaloid, alpha-isolupanine, anagyrine, aporphine, baptifoline, beechdrops, Berberidaceae (family), blue cohosh root, blue ginseng, blueberry, caulophylline, *Caulophyllum*, *Caulophyllum thalictroides* Mich., *Leontice thalictroides* (L.), lupanine, magnoflorine, Mastodynon, N-methylcytosine, papoose root, quinolizidine alkaloids, saponins, sparteine, squaw root, taspine, thalictroidine, triterpene saponins, yellow ginseng.
- **Note:** Blue cohosh (*Caulophyllum thalictroides*) should not be confused with black cohosh (*Cimicifuga racemosa*), an over-the-counter herbal supplement sold as a menopausal and menstrual remedy.

BACKGROUND

- Blue cohosh has been used for hundreds of years by Native American women to facilitate labor. Today, the herb is most commonly used to stimulate labor and to ease the effects of childbirth.
- Modern herbalists often recommend blue cohosh as an emmenagogue to induce menstruation and as a uterine stimulant and antispasmodic. It is also frequently used as a diuretic to eliminate excess fluids, as an expectorant to treat congestion, and as a diaphoretic to eliminate toxins by inducing sweating. Traditional herbalists will often combine blue cohosh and black cohosh to effect a more balanced treatment for nerves and to enhance the herbs' antispasmodic effects. Blue cohosh is combined with other herbs to promote their effects in treating bronchitis, nervous disorders, urinary tract ailments, and rheumatism. Blue cohosh is also thought to help pelvic inflammatory disease, endometriosis, erratic menstruation, and retained placenta. In addition, the herb is also believed to relieve ovarian neuralgia (nerve pain).
- Although blue cohosh has been indicated for many conditions, all indications lack sufficient scientific data to support their efficacy and safety at this time. More research is needed in these areas before firm conclusions can be drawn.

EVIDENCE

Uses Based on Scientific Evidence

No available studies qualify for inclusion in the evidence table.

Uses Based on Tradition or Theory

Abortifacient (induces abortion), amenorrhea (absence of menstruation), antiinflammatory, antipyretic (reduces fever), antispasmodic, arthritis, bronchitis, cervical dysplasia (abnormal, possible precancerous cells), colic in children, contraception, cramps, demulcent (soothes inflammation), deobstruent, diaphoretic (induces sweating), diuretic, earache, endometriosis, epilepsy, expectorant (expels phlegm), gastric disorders, genitourinary disorders, hormonal imbalances, inflammatory conditions, labor induction, labor pain, laxative, leukorrhea (vaginal discharge), liver cancer, menstruation irregularities, muscle weakness, nervous disorders, neuralgia (nerve pain), pain (pregnancy), pelvic inflammatory disease, pregnancy, rheumatic pain, sexually transmitted disease (chlamydia), uterine inflammation, uterine stimulant, vaginitis (inflammation of vagina).

DOSING

Adults (18 Years and Older)

- Based on available scientific evidence, there is no proven safe or effective dose for blue cohosh. As a decoction, 4 g twice daily or 1-3 g every 3-4 hours has been used. As a fluid extract, 0.5-1.0 mL (1:1 in 70% alcohol) three times daily as a preparation for pregnancy has been used. As an infusion/tea, 2-4 fl oz (1 oz root to 1 pint boiling water) two to four times daily has been used. Also, 300-1000 mg of the dried whole herb up to three times daily has been used.

Children (Younger than 18 Years)

- There is not enough scientific evidence to safely recommend the use of blue cohosh in children.

SAFETY

Allergies

- Avoid in individuals with a known allergy or sensitivity to blue cohosh (*Caulophyllum thalictroides*), any of its constituents, or members of the Berberidaceae family.

Side Effects and Warnings

- One commonly reported effect of blue cohosh is its uterine-stimulating effects, which may be viewed as a desirable effect when used to induce labor but an adverse effect when used for other purposes during pregnancy.
- Other adverse effects of blue cohosh may include nausea, vomiting, abdominal pain, and cardiotoxic effects on the fetus (when used in pregnant women). Myocardial infarction (heart attack), congestive heart failure, shock, and myocardial toxicity have also been reported.
- Strokes and seizures have been documented in infants whose mothers ingested blue cohosh during pregnancy.
- Because of nicotinic effects of the constituent N-methylcytosine, blue cohosh could cause dilated pupils, hyperventilation, nystagmus (involuntary, alternating, rapid and slow movements of the eyeballs), thirst, hyperthermia, seizures, hypertension or hypotension (high or low blood pressure), chest pain, tachycardia (fast heart rate), irregular pulse, or coma.
- Blue cohosh may cause hyperglycemia (increased blood sugar levels) and anemia in infants following maternal use.
- Patients who smoke or who are quitting smoking and those with diabetes should use blue cohosh cautiously and consult with a qualified health care professional, including a pharmacist.

Pregnancy and Breastfeeding

- Pregnancy: Although there is conflicting evidence about the use of blue cohosh during pregnancy, it has traditionally been used to induce labor or abortion. The use of blue cohosh to induce abortion has been associated with adverse effects in the mother and/or fetus. There have been reports of cardiotoxicity in the newborn infants of the mothers who ingested blue cohosh; the resulting adverse effects included congestive heart failure, myocardial infarction (heart attack) or toxicity, stroke, and shock. Use of blue cohosh during pregnancy to stimulate the uterus to ease the effects of labor should be used only under medical supervision.

- Breastfeeding: Blue cohosh is not recommended in breastfeeding women because of a lack of available scientific evidence.

INTERACTIONS
Interactions with Drugs

- Blue cohosh may increase blood glucose levels. Caution is advised when medications that may lower blood sugar are used. Patients taking drugs for diabetes by mouth or using insulin should be monitored closely by a qualified health care professional. Medication adjustments may be necessary.

- Blue cohosh may have antispasmodic effects. Individuals using blue cohosh with other drugs with antispasmodic effects should consult with a qualified health care professional, including a pharmacist.

- Blue cohosh may cause coronary vasoconstriction (decreased blood flow due to constriction of blood vessels), tachycardia (increased heart rate), and possible increases in blood pressure. Individuals taking medications that affect heart rate or blood pressure should consult with a qualified health care professional, including a pharmacist.

- A constituent of blue cohosh, methylcytosine, is similar to nicotine and may lead to nicotinic toxicity. Caution is advised in patients who smoke or use other products containing nicotine.

- Blue cohosh may induce labor and should not be used with oxytocin (Pitocin).

Interactions with Herbs and Dietary Supplements

- Blue cohosh may have antispasmodic effects. Individuals using blue cohosh with other herbs or supplements with antispasmodic effects should consult with a qualified health care professional, including a pharmacist.

- Blue cohosh may cause coronary vasoconstriction, tachycardia, and possible increases in blood pressure. Individuals taking herbs and supplements that affect heart rate or blood pressure should consult with a qualified health care professional, including a pharmacist.

- Blue cohosh may increase blood glucose levels. Caution is advised when herbs or supplements that may alter blood sugar are used.

- Blue cohosh may induce labor, and caution is advised when blue cohosh is taken with other herbs and supplements that have labor-inducing effects.

- A constituent of blue cohosh, methylcytosine, is similar to nicotine and may lead to nicotinic toxicity. Caution is advised in patients who smoke or use other products containing nicotine.

For a complete list of references, please visit www.naturalstandard.com.

Boldo
(*Peumus boldus*)

RELATED TERMS

- Ascaridole, asymmetric monoterpene endoperoxide, baldina, *Boldea fragrans*, boldina, boldine ([s]-2,9-dihydroxy-1, 10-dimethoxyaporphine), boldine houde, boldoa, *Boldoa fragrans*, boldoak boldea, boldo-do-Chile, boldo folium, boldoglucin, boldu, *Boldu boldus*, boldus, boldus boldus, bolldin, bornyl-acetate, Chilean boldo tree, coclaurine, coumarin, cuminaldehyde, diethylphthalate, eugenol, farnesol, fenchone, gamma terpinene, isoboldine, kaempferols, laurolitsine, laurotetanine, molina, Monimiaceae (family), norboldine, norisocorydine, pachycarpine, P-cymene, P-cymol, *Peumus boldus*, *Peumus boldus* Mol., *Peumus fragrans*, pronuciferine, qian-hu, reticuline, rhamnosides, sabinene, sinoacutine, tannins, terpinoline, thymol, trans-verbenol.

BACKGROUND

- Boldo is an evergreen shrub found in the Andean regions of Chile and Peru and also is native to parts of Morocco. Boldo was employed in Chilean and Peruvian folk medicine and recognized as an herbal remedy in a number of pharmacopoeias, mainly for the treatment of liver ailments.
- Boldine, a major alkaloidal constituent found in the leaves and bark of the boldo tree, has been shown to possess antioxidant and antiinflammatory activity. The German Commission E has approved boldo leaf as treatment for mild dyspepsia (upset stomach) and spastic gastrointestinal complaints. Well-designed human studies on the efficacy of boldo are lacking.

EVIDENCE

Uses Based on Scientific Evidence

No available studies qualify for inclusion in the evidence table.

Uses Based on Tradition or Theory

Anthelmintic (expels worms), anticoagulant (blood thinner), antiinflammatory, antioxidant (free radical scavenging), antipyretic (fever reducer), antiseptic, appetite stimulant, chemoprotective, cholagogue (increases bile flow), choleretic (stimulates bile formation), congestion, cystitis (bladder infection), digestion, diuretic, dyspepsia (upset stomach), earache, food uses, gallstones, gastrointestinal disorders, gonorrhea (STD), headache, hepatic (liver) disorders, hepatoprotection (liver protection), hypertension (high blood pressure), hypnotic, laxative, menstrual pain, nausea, neuromuscular blockade, pain, radioprotection, rheumatism, sedative, sunscreen, syphilis, urinary tract infection (UTI).

DOSING
Adults (18 Years and Older)

- There is insufficient evidence to recommend a dose for boldo in adults. A common dose of the liquid extract, 1:1 in 45% alcohol, is 0.1-0.3 mL three times daily. Traditional doses are 60-200 mg of the dried leaf three times daily or as a tea three times daily. The tea is prepared by steeping 1 g of the dried leaf in 150 mL boiling water for 5-10 minutes and then straining. The average daily dose of the boldo leaf by infusion is 3 g. A tincture, 1:10 in 60% alcohol, is usually given as 0.5-2 mL three times daily.

Children (Younger than 18 Years)

- There is insufficient evidence to recommed a dose for boldo in children.

SAFETY
Allergies

- Avoid in individuals with a known allergy or hypersensitivity to boldo (*Peumus boldus*) or its constituents. Boldo intake has also been linked to one case of IgE-mediated anaphylactic allergic reaction.

Side Effects and Warnings

- Boldo has "generally recognized as safe" (GRAS) status for use in foods in the United States. However, there is limited information regarding the side effects of boldo.
- Use cautiously in patients taking anticoagulant or antiplatelet (blood-thinning) agents. Boldo may increase the risk of bleeding.
- Use cautiously in patients taking hepatotoxic (liver-damaging) agents. Boldo may cause hepatotoxicity, and theoretically, concurrent use of boldo with hepatotoxic drugs may increase the risk of liver damage.
- Use cautiously in patients taking diuretic drugs. Historically, boldo has been used as a diuretic and therefore may cause an additive effect when used with diuretic agents.
- Use cautiously in patients with bile duct obstruction. Boldo is thought to stimulate bile flow, and theoretically, it may exacerbate bile duct obstruction.
- Use cautiously in patients who drink alcohol. Boldo may cause hepatotoxicity (liver damage), and theoretically, concurrent use of boldo with alcohol may increase the risk of liver damage. Avoid in patients with liver disease.

Pregnancy and Breastfeeding

- Boldo is not recommended in pregnant or breastfeeding women. Pregnant rats taking 800 mg/kg of crude extract of boldo and boldine by mouth demonstrated anatomical alterations in the fetus. However, the German Commission E notes no contraindications to the use of ascaridole-free boldo preparations in pregnancy and breastfeeding.

INTERACTIONS
Interactions with Drugs

- Concomitant use of boldo and anticoagulant or antiplatelet (blood-thinning) drugs may increase the risk of bleeding. Some examples of drugs that may increase the risk of bleeding include aspirin, anticoagulants such as warfarin (Coumadin) or heparin, antiplatelet drugs such as clopidogrel (Plavix), and nonsteroidal antiinflammatory drugs (NSAIDs) such as ibuprofen (Motrin, Advil) or naproxen (Naprosyn, Aleve).

- Boldo may have antiinflammatory effects, although this has not been well studied in humans. Caution is advised when boldo is used with other antiinflammatory agents.
- Historically, boldo has been used as a diuretic and therefore may cause an additive effect when used with diuretic drugs. Boldo oil may also act as an irritant.
- Boldo may cause hepatotoxicity. Theoretically, concomitant use of boldo with hepatotoxic drugs (e.g., ketoconazole, ritonavir, and valproic acid) may increase the risk of liver damage.

Interactions with Herbs and Dietary Supplements

- Concomitant use of boldo and anticoagulant or antiplatelet (blood-thinning) herbs and supplements may increase the risk of bleeding. Multiple cases of bleeding have been reported with the use of *Ginkgo biloba*, and fewer cases have been reported with garlic and saw palmetto. Numerous other agents may theoretically increase the risk of bleeding, although this has not been proven in most cases.
- Boldo may have antiinflammatory effects, although this has not been well studied in humans. Use of other antiinflammatory herbs or supplements may have additive effects.
- Historically, boldo has been used as a diuretic and therefore may cause an additive effect when used with other diuretic herbs and supplements. Boldo oil may also act as an irritant.
- Boldo may cause hepatotoxicity (liver damage). Theoretically, concomitant use of boldo with other hepatotoxic herbs and supplements (e.g., chaparral, comfrey, and pennyroyal oil) may increase the risk of liver damage.

For a complete list of references, please visit www.naturalstandard.com.

Boneset
(*Eupatorium perfoliatum*)

RELATED TERMS

- Agueweed, Asteraceae (family), astragalin, common boneset, Compositae (family), crosswort, dendroidinic acid, eucannabinolide, eufoliatin, eufoliatorin, eupafolin, eupatorin, *Eupatorium connatum* Michx., *Eupatorium perfoliatum*, *Eupatorium perfoliatum* D2, euperfolide, euperfolitin, feverwort, flavonoids, gravelroot, hebenolide, helenalin, hyperoside, Indian sage, kaempferol, quercetin, rutin, sesquiterpene lactones, snakeroot, sterols, sweat plant, sweating plant, tearal, teasel, thoroughwax, thoroughwort, thorough-stem, vegetable antimony, wild Isaac, wild sage, wood boneset.
- **Note:** Avoid confusion with gravel root (*Eupatorium purpureum*), which is also known as boneset. Snakeroot is a common name used for poisonous *Eupatorium* species, but boneset should not be confused with *Ageratina* spp., which are more commonly known as snakeroot.

BACKGROUND

- Boneset (*Eupatorium perfoliatum*) is native to eastern North America and was used by Native Americans to treat fevers, including dengue fever and malaria. Today, boneset is used primarily in homeopathic medicine for fevers, influenza (flu), digestive problems, and liver disorders. However, the use of boneset is limited because other drugs generally are more effective.
- Boneset may be effective when taken by mouth as an immunostimulant and an antiinflammatory agent. However, there is insufficient reliable information available about the effectiveness of boneset for its other uses.
- Products containing boneset have been placed in the "Herbs of Undefined Safety" category by the U.S. Food and Drug Administration (FDA).

EVIDENCE

Uses Based on Scientific Evidence	Grade
Colds/Flu Traditionally, boneset has been used to treat fevers and infectious diseases, such as colds and influenza. Preliminary evidence suggests that boneset may treat cold symptoms. However, this remains equivocal.	C

Uses Based on Tradition or Theory
Animal bite (reptile), antiinflammatory, antipyretic (fever reducer), antispasmodic, antiviral, arthritis, astringent, bitter tonic, broken bones, bronchitis (acute), carminative (digestive aid), catarrh (inflammation of mucous membrane), cathartic (relieves constipation), cholagogue (stimulates bile flow), constipation, coughs, dengue (fever), diaphoretic (promotes sweating), diuretic, dysentery (severe diarrhea), dyspepsia (upset stomach), edema (swelling), emetic (induces vomiting), emmenagogue (stimulates menstruation), fevers (chronic), gastrointestinal distress, headache, HIV/AIDS, immunomodulator, jaundice, laxative, liver disease, malaria, migraine, muscle weakness, musculoskeletal pain, nasal inflammation, night sweats, parasites and worms, pneumonia, respiratory congestion, rheumatism, skin conditions, stimulant, tonic, typhoid, yellow fever.

DOSING

Adults (18 Years and Older)

- There is insufficient evidence to recommend a dose for boneset. Boneset is used in the dried form and is available commercially as dried flowers and leaves, as a tincture (an alcohol solution), and in tablets and capsules. Boneset is usually taken as an infusion (tea) or tincture. Some sources state that boneset should not be taken for longer than 2 weeks at a time. Others say that continual use of boneset should be limited to a few weeks, at the most. No form of boneset is recommended for chronic use that lasts longer than 6 months. High-quality scientific evidence is lacking in this area.

Children (Younger than 18 Years)

- There is insufficient evidence to recommend a dose for boneset in children.

SAFETY

Allergies

- Avoid in individuals with a known allergy or hypersensitivity to boneset (*Eupatorium perfoliatum*), any of its constituents, or related members of the Asteraceae/Compositae family such as dandelion, goldenrod, ragweed, sunflower, and daisies.

Side Effects and Warnings

- There are currently no high-quality studies on the medicinal applications of boneset, and the following information is based on traditional use and expert opinion. Boneset may cause nausea, vomiting, and diarrhea in large doses and may even cause coma or death. Boneset may also contain hepatotoxic (liver-damaging) unsaturated pyrrolizidine alkaloids. Products containing boneset have been placed in the "Herbs of Undefined Safety" category by the U.S. FDA.
- Use cautiously, as boneset is known to cause both vomiting and diarrhea, which may increase the chance of dehydration in small children, elderly individuals, or individuals suffering from a chronic condition.
- Use cautiously in patients sensitive to boneset or Asteracae/Compositae plants, such as dandelion, goldenrod, ragweed, sunflower, and daisies, as boneset may cause contact dermatitis.
- Use cautiously even in the amounts recommended by manufacturers, as boneset may promote sweating, the production of urine, and catharsis. All of these effects could cause excessive fluid loss from the body, possibly also decreasing the body's potassium supplies. Low potassium levels can result in muscle weakness and potentially dangerous changes in heart rhythm.

- Avoid in patients with known liver or kidney conditions and patients who ingest moderate to large amounts of alcohol, as boneset may contain hepatotoxic (liver-damaging) pyrrolizidine alkaloids.

Pregnancy and Breastfeeding

- Although not well studied in humans, boneset may be toxic and long term use by pregnant or breastfeeding women should be avoided. Fresh boneset contains tremerol, a toxic chemical that can cause nausea, vomiting, weakness, muscle tremors, and increased respiration. Higher doses can cause coma and death. Dried boneset is not thought to contain tremerol.

INTERACTIONS

Interactions with Drugs

- Although not well studied in humans, boneset may have weak antibacterial and antiinflammatory effects. Caution is advised in patients taking agents that have similar effects.
- Homeopathic boneset may have antiviral effects. Caution is advised in patients taking other antiviral agents or immunomodulators.
- Boneset may cause excessive fluid loss from the body, possibly also decreasing the body's potassium supplies. Low potassium levels can result in muscle weakness and potentially dangerous changes in heart rhythm.

- Unsaturated pyrrolizidine alkaloids are common in the genus of boneset and might also be found in boneset. Caution is advised when agents are taken that are potentially liver damaging, as the combination may increase the risk of liver damage.

Interactions with Herbs and Dietary Supplements

- Although not well studied in humans, boneset may have weak antibacterial and antiinflammatory effects. Caution is advised in patients taking herbs or supplements that have similar effects.
- Homeopathic boneset may have antiviral effects. Caution is advised in patients taking other antiviral agents or immunomodulators.
- Boneset may cause excessive fluid loss from the body, possibly also decreasing the body's potassium supplies. Low potassium levels can result in muscle weakness and potentially dangerous changes in heart rhythm. Caution is advised in patients taking potassium or any herbs or supplements with diuretic effects.
- Unsaturated pyrrolizidine alkaloids are common in the genus of boneset and might also be found in boneset. Caution is advised when herbs or supplements are taken that are potentially liver damaging, as the combination may increase the risk of liver damage.

For a complete list of references, please visit www.naturalstandard.com.

Borage
(*Borago officinalis*)

RELATED TERMS

- Borage, borage oil, borage seed, *Borago officinalis*, gamma-linolenic acid (GLA), Glandol, n-6 polyunsaturated fatty acids (PUFA), n-6 PUFA, starflower, starflower oil.

BACKGROUND

- Borage *(Borago officinalis)* is an herb native to Syria that has spread throughout the Middle East and Mediterranean. Borage flowers and leaves may be eaten, and borage seeds are often pressed to produce oil very high in GLA.
- Borage is popularly used for premenstrual syndrome (PMS) and menopausal symptoms. Borage is also a popular supplement among elderly women. Borage is known for its antiinflammatory properties and has been studied for the treatment of gum disease, rheumatoid arthritis, and asthma.
- There is currently controversy about the safety of borage. Consumers should use caution when taking borage, as there have been cases of poisoning after confusion with foxglove.

EVIDENCE

Uses Based on Scientific Evidence	Grade
Acute Respiratory Distress Syndrome Acute respiratory distress syndrome occurs when the lung malfunctions because of injury to the small air sacs and the capillaries of the lungs. Borage may improve heart and lung function and reduce lung inflammation in acute respiratory distress syndrome.	B
Periodontitis/Gingivitis Preliminary evidence suggests that borage has antiinflammatory effects that may make it beneficial in treating periodontitis (gum disease). Additional research is needed to determine the best dosing and administration of borage oil.	B
Rheumatoid Arthritis Preliminary evidence suggests that gamma linolenic acid (GLA) has known antiinflammatory effects that may make it beneficial in treating rheumatoid arthritis.	B
Alcohol-Induced Hangover Borage oil may help treat or prevent alcohol-induced hangovers, although the effectiveness is uncertain.	C
Asthma Preliminary evidence suggests that GLA may have some immunosuppressant activity that may be helpful in reducing asthma symptoms.	C
Atopic Dermatitis Atopic dermatitis is a skin disorder that is characterized by itching, scaling, and thickening of the skin and is usually located on the face, elbows, knees, and arms. The evidence for borage oil in the treatment of atopic dermatitis is mixed.	
Cystic fibrosis Cystic fibrosis is a genetic disorder affecting the mucus lining of the lungs leading to breathing problems and other difficulties. Preliminary evidence indicates that borage oil may have some benefits in cystic fibrosis patients.	C
Hyperlipidemia Hyperlipidemia is an excess level of fats in the blood. These fats can be triglycerides or cholesterol. Hyperlipidemia is often associated with increased risk of heart disease and strokes. GLA may decrease plasma triglyceride levels and increase HDL cholesterol concentration. However, more research is needed to define borage's effects on lipid levels in the blood.	C
Infant Development/Neonatal Care (in Preterm Infants) Preterm infants may need essential fatty acid supplementation. GLA supplementation may increase cognitive development, weight gain, and length gain, particularly in boys.	C
Malnutrition (Inflammation Complex Syndrome) Currently, there is insufficient available evidence evaluating the effectiveness of borage in the treatment of malnutrition.	C
Seborrheic Dermatitis (Infantile) Seborrheic dermatitis is a type of inflammatory skin rash. Currently, there is insufficient evidence to support borage in the treatment of seborrheic dermatitis.	C
Stress Borage oil may decrease heart changes to acute stress. However, clinical evidence is limited.	C
Supplementation in Preterm and very Low Birth Weight Iinfants (Fatty Acids) A borage oil–containing formula does not appear to affect preterm and very low birth weight infants.	C

Uses Based on Tradition or Theory

Anti-inflammatory, antioxidant, autoimmune disorders, cancer, *Helicobacter pylori* infection, immune function, menopausal symptoms, premenstrual syndrome (PMS), seborrheic dermatitis (adults).

DOSING
Adults (18 Years and Older)

- Borage is likely safe when used in food or spice amounts or when 1-3 g is used daily in healthy adults for up to 24 weeks.
- There is insufficient evidence to recommend a dose for borage. However, 2-3 g daily GLA (borage oil) for 24 weeks to 12 months has been used for asthma. For atopic eczema studies have used 500-3000 mg of borage oil–containing capsules daily for 12-24 weeks.

Children (Younger than 18 Years)

- There is insufficient evidence to recommend a dose for borage in children. Nonetheless, two capsules of borage oil twice daily for 12 weeks has been used. For prevention of atopic dermatitis, patients have taken a borage oil supplement containing 100 mg GLA daily for the first 6 months of life.

SAFETY
Allergies

- Avoid in individuals with a known allergy or hypersensitivity to borage or its constituents.

Side Effects and Warnings

- Borage has been confused with foxglove, and ingestion of foxglove leaves has caused accidental poisoning.
- Borage may lower the seizure threshold. Use cautiously in patients with epilepsy or in those taking anticonvulsants.
- When used in combination with other herbs and supplements, borage may lower blood sugar levels.
- Use cautiously in patients with bleeding disorders or in those taking warfarin, other anticoagulants, or antiplatelet agents, as borage seed oil may increase the risk of bleeding or potentiate the effects of warfarin therapy.
- Avoid in patients with compromised immune systems or similar immunological conditions.

Pregnancy and Breastfeeding

- Borage is not recommended in pregnant or breastfeeding women due to a lack of available scientific evidence. One pregnant woman using borage seed oil complained of mild intestinal gas. Gamma linolenic acid, which is found in borage, may alter breast milk production.

INTERACTIONS
Interactions with Drugs

- Borage may have antibacterial effects against *Helicobacter pylori*. Use cautiously with antibiotics and antiulcer medications because of possible additive effects.
- Borage may increase the risk of bleeding, especially when taken with drugs that increase the risk of bleeding, such as warfarin therapy.
- Preliminary evidence suggests that borage may lower the seizure threshold. Use cautiously in patients with seizures or in those taking anticonvulsant medications.
- Preliminary evidence suggests that borage oil may have antiinflammatory properties. Use cautiously with antiinflammatory medications because of possible additive effects.
- Although not well studied in humans, GLA may decrease plasma triglyceride levels and may increase high-density lipoprotein (HDL) cholesterol concentrations. Use cautiously in patients taking cholesterol-lowering medications because of possible additive effects.
- Borage oil may alter heart function. Use cautiously in patients with heart conditions or in those taking cardiovascular medications.
- Preliminary evidence suggests that GLA may alter immune responses. Use cautiously with other immunomodulators.
- Concomitant nonsteroidal antiinflammatory (NSAID) drug use may undermine borage oil effects; use cautiously.

Interactions with Herbs and Dietary Supplements

- Although not well studied in humans, borage may have antibacterial effects against *Helicobacter pylori*. Use cautiously with herbs and supplement that may have antibacterial or antiulcer activity.
- Preliminary evidence suggests that borage seed oil may potentially increase the risk of bleeding or potentiate the effects of warfarin therapy. Use cautiously with bleeding disorders or with herbs and supplements that are believed to increase the risk of bleeding. Multiple cases of bleeding have been reported with the use of *Ginkgo biloba*, and fewer cases have been reported with garlic and saw palmetto.
- Preliminary evidence suggests that borage may lower the seizure threshold. Use cautiously in patients with seizures or in those taking anticonvulsant herbs or supplements.
- Preliminary evidence suggests that borage oil may have antiinflammatory properties. Use cautiously with antiinflammatory herbs or supplements because of possible additive effects.
- Although not well studied in humans, GLA may decrease plasma triglyceride levels and may increase HDL cholesterol concentrations. Use cautiously in patients taking cholesterol-lowering herbs, such as red yeast rice, because of possible additive effects.
- Borage oil may alter heart function. Use cautiously in patients with heart conditions or in those taking cardiovascular herbs or supplements.
- Preliminary evidence suggests that GLA may alter immune responses. Use cautiously with other immunomodulators.

For a complete list of references, please visit www.naturalstandard.com.

RELATED TERMS

- 1-Amino-3-[(dihydroxyboryl)methyl]-cyclobutanecarboxylic acid, 2-APB (2-aminoethoxydiphenyl borate), 3-[3-(7-NH(3)(+)-nido-m-carboran-1-yl)propan-1-yl] thymidine, 3-carboranyl thymidine analogs (3CTA), 3-carboranylalkyl thymidine analogs, 3-[(closo-o-carboranyl)methyl] thymidine, 4-META/MMA-TBBO, 10B (pure isotope), 11B (pure isotope), 12-dicarba-closo-dodecaboranel-carboxylate (BCH), alanin-boric compound acid, amine-boranes, amorphous boron (impure boron), AN-2690, Arc Dia TPX, atomic number 5, B, BCH (12-dicarba-closo-dodecaboranel-carboxylate), BF$_2$ (borondifluoride), BF$_3$ (borontrifluoride), bisphenylboronate, boracic acid [B(OH)$_3$], boracite, boracium, boranophosphate, borate transporter, borates, borax [Na$_2$B$_4$O$_5$(OH)$_4$•8H$_2$O], Borax, bore, boric acid, boric anhydride, boron 10 (pure isotope), boron 11 (pure isotope), boron aspartate, boron citrate, boron-enriched cathode, boron fluoride, boron glycinate, boron hydroxide [B(OH)$_3$], boron neutron capture therapy (BNCT), boron nitride, boron oxide [B$_2$O$_3$], boron sesquioxide, boronated aminocyclobutanecarboxylic acid, boronic acid, boron-ophenylalanine (BPA), burah [Na$_2$B$_4$O$_5$(OH)$_4$•8H$_2$O], buraq [Na$_2$B$_4$O$_5$(OH)$_4$•8H$_2$O], C&B Metabond, carborane (a carbon–boron compound), closo-dodecarborate, colemanite, crystalline boron (99% pure boron), decaborane, dicarba-closo-dodecaborane, dipyrrylmethene-BF2, Dobill's Solution, Drug Vitrum Osteomag, furan boron ethers, kernite [Na$_2$B$_4$O$_5$(OH)$_4$•2H$_2$O], magnesium perborate, metaboric acid, rasorite [Na$_2$B$_4$O$_5$(OH)$_4$•2H$_2$O], MMA-TBB (methyl methacrylate tri-n-butylborane), mono-phenylboronate, NH(2)-closo-m-carborane, NH(3)(+)-nido-m-carborane-substituted thymidine analogues, orthoboric acid, ortho-carborane derivative, sassolite, sodium biborate, sodium borate, sodium borocaptate, sodium metaborate, sodium perborate, sodium pyroborate, sodium tetraborate [Na$_2$B$_4$O$_5$(OH)$_4$•8H$_2$O], sal sedativum [B(OH)$_3$], sodium tetraborate, Superbond C&B, Tincal, TBB (tri-n-butylborane), TBBO (tri-n-butylborane partial oxide), tetracarboranylketone 4, thermal water, tincal [Na$_2$B$_4$O$_5$(OH)$_4$•8H$_2$O], tribromide, tributylborane (TBB), trifluoride-methanol [BF$_3$-MeOH], tri-n-butylborane partial oxide (TBBO), ulexite [CaB$_4$O$_7$*NaBO$_2$*8H$_2$O], zwitterionic 3-carboranyl thymidine analogues.

BACKGROUND

- Boron is a trace element that is found throughout the environment. It has been suggested for numerous medicinal purposes, but there is a lack of strong evidence for any specific use. Preliminary studies report that boron may not be helpful for enhancing bodybuilding, reducing menopausal symptoms, or treating psoriasis.

EVIDENCE

Uses Based on Scientific Evidence	Grade
Hormone Regulation Boron may increase hormone (estrogen) levels in women, reducing vaginal discomfort after menopause. However, strong supportive clinical evidence is lacking.	C
Improving Cognitive Function Preliminary clinical evidence suggests better performance on tasks of eye-hand coordination, attention, perception, short-term memory, and long-term memory with boron supplementation.	C
Osteoarthritis Based on human population research, in a boron-rich environment, people appear to have fewer joint disorders. It has also been proposed that boron deficiency may contribute to the development of osteoarthritis. However, there is insufficient clinical evidence that supplementation with boron is beneficial as prevention against or as a treatment for osteoarthritis.	C
Osteoporosis Animal and preliminary human studies report that boron may play a role in mineral metabolism, with effects on calcium, phosphorus, and vitamin D. However, research of bone mineral density in women taking boron supplements does not clearly demonstrate benefits in osteoporosis.	C
Vaginitis Inorganic boron (boric acid, borax) has been used as an antiseptic based on proposed antibacterial and antifungal properties. It is proposed that boric acid may have effects against candidal and noncandidal vulvovaginitis. There is weak evidence that boric acid capsules used in the vagina may be effective for vaginitis.	C
Bodybuilding Aid (Increasing Testosterone) There is preliminary negative evidence for the use of boron for improving performance in bodybuilding by increasing testosterone. Although boron is suggested to raise testosterone levels, in early human research, total lean body mass has not been affected by boron supplementation in bodybuilders.	D

(Continued)

Uses Based on Scientific Evidence	Grade
Menopausal Symptoms It has been proposed that boron affects estrogen levels in postmenopausal women. However, preliminary studies have found no changes in menopausal symptoms.	D
Prevention of Blood Clotting (Coagulation Effects) It has been proposed that boron may affect the activity of certain blood clotting factors. Study results conflict. There is not enough evidence in this area to form a clear conclusion.	D
Psoriasis (Boric Acid Ointment) Preliminary clinical evidence suggests that an ointment including boric acid does not report significant benefits in psoriasis.	D

Uses Based on Tradition or Theory

Antiinflammatory, antiseptic, antiviral, bone healing, breast cancer, cancer, diabetes, diaper rash (avoid because of case reports of death in infants from absorbing boron through skin or when taken by mouth), eye cleansing, high cholesterol levels, hypersensitivity to temperature, increasing lifespan, leukemia, onychomycosis (fungal infection), pain, prostate cancer, rheumatoid arthritis, vitamin D deficiency, wound care.

DOSING
Adults (18 Years and Older)

- The average reported boron intake in the American diet is 1.17 mg per day for men, 0.96 mg per day for women, and 1.29-1.47 mg per day for vegetarians. High boron content foods include peanut butter, wine, grapes, beans, and peaches. In addition, 2.5-6 mg have been taken by mouth in studies.
- For psoriasis, 1.5% boric acid with 3% zinc oxide ointment applied to the skin as needed has been studied. Boric acid powder capsules administered vaginally daily have also been studied. Safety and effectiveness have not been well established.

Children (Younger than 18 Years)

- There is insufficient evidence to recommend a dose of boron in children. Case reports exist of death in infants following the use of boron (taken by mouth or placed on the skin).

SAFETY
Allergies

- Boron should be avoided in patients who have a history of reactions to boron, boric acid, borax, citrate, aspartate, or glycinate.

Side Effects and Warnings

- Boron is potentially toxic, although humans tend to rapidly excrete it; therefore, boron does not usually accumulate in high levels. In adults, it is believed that adverse reactions associated with low doses of boron per day are less likely to occur, and there are few reports of toxicity. Large doses may result in acute poisoning. There are fatal case reports of infants who have been exposed to boron by mouth or on the skin. Historically, a honey and borax solution was used to clean infant pacifiers, and topical boric acid powder was used to prevent diaper rash. However, these practices were associated with several infant deaths.

- Boron toxicity may cause skin rash, nausea, vomiting (may be blue-green color), diarrhea (may be blue-green color), abdominal pain, and headache. Low blood pressure and metabolic changes in the blood (acidosis) have been reported. Agitation and irritability or the opposite reaction (weakness, lethargy, depression) may occur. Fever, hyperthermia, tremors, and seizure have been reported. Based on animal study, excess amounts of boron ingestion have been shown to cause testicular toxicity, decreased sperm motility, and reduced fertility. Hair loss has been reported with boron poisoning. Chronic boron exposure may cause dehydration, seizures, low red blood cell count, as well as kidney or liver damage.

- Boron is proposed to increase blood levels of estrogen and testosterone, with mixed results of research. Boron may be associated with reduced blood levels of calcitonin, insulin, or phosphorus and with increased levels of vitamin D_2, calcium, copper, magnesium, or thyroxine. Exposure to boric acid or boron oxide dust can cause eye irritation, dryness of the mouth or nose, sore throat, and productive cough.

Pregnancy and Breastfeeding

- There is not enough scientific evidence to recommend the safe use of boron during pregnancy or breastfeeding. There is a trace amount of boron distributed to human milk. Excessive amounts of boron taken by mouth may cause toxicity in male fertility.

INTERACTIONS
Interactions with Drugs

- Magnesium may interfere with the effects of boron in the body. Sources of magnesium may include antacids containing magnesium oxide or magnesium sulfate (milk of magnesia, Maalox).
- In theory, use of boron with estrogen-active drugs such as birth control pills or hormone replacement therapy may result in increased estrogen effects. Use of boron with testosterone-active drugs such as Testoderm may result in increased testosterone effects.
- Supplemental boron may decrease insulin levels in the blood. It may also alter thyroid hormone levels.
- Alzheimer's drugs, analgesics (pain relievers), androgens, antiinflammatory agents, antilipemics (cholesterol-lowering), antineoplastic agents, antiviral agents, arthritis agents, dopamine agonists, dopamine antagonists, drugs that damage the liver, osteoporosis agents, and drugs eliminated by the kidney may interact with boron.

Interactions with Herbs and Dietary Supplements

- Boron supplementation may result in increased calcium levels in the blood and may add to the effects of calcium or vitamin D supplementation. Boron may interact with herbs or supplements that have effects similar to antacids.
- Supplemental boron may decrease phosphorous levels in the blood.
- In theory, use of boron with estrogen-active herbs or supplements may result in increased estrogen effects.

- Supplemental boron may decrease insulin levels in the blood. It may also alter thyroid hormone levels.
- Alzheimer's agents, analgesics (pain relievers), androgens, antiinflammatory agents, antilipemics (cholesterol-lowering), antineoplastics, antivirals, arthritis agents, dopamine agonists, dopamine antagonists, herbs and supplements that damage the liver, osteoporosis agents, phytoestrogens, and herbs and supplements cleared by the kidneys may interact with boron.

For a complete list of references, please visit www.naturalstandard.com.

Boswellia
(Boswellia serrata)

RELATED TERMS

- 11-Keto β-boswellic acid, acetyl-11-keto β-boswellic acid (AKBA), African elemi (*Boswellia frereana*), Arabian incense (Bakhour), Bibe incense (*Boswellia carterii*), birdwood, *Boswellia, Boswellia carterii, Boswellia dalzielii, Boswellia frereana, Boswellia ovalifoliolata, Boswellia papyrifera, Boswellia sacra, Boswellia serrata, Boswellia serrata* gum resins, BSB108, Burseraceae (family), carterii, dhup, frankincense, guggals, H15, indish incense, Mexican bursera, Nopane (*Boswellia*), oleogum resins, oleo-resin, olibanum, pentacyclic triterpenoid, S-compound, sacra, salai guggal, sallai guggul, Sallaki.

BACKGROUND

- Resin extracts from the *Boswellia serrata* tree have been found to have antiinflammatory effects. Animal and laboratory studies suggest possible efficacy for inflammatory conditions such as inflammatory bowel disease, rheumatoid arthritis, and osteoarthritis, although high-quality human data are lacking. Initial human evidence suggests the efficacy of boswellia as a chronic therapy for asthma (but not for the relief of acute asthma exacerbations). Further studies are warranted in this area.

- As opposed to nonsteroidal antiinflammatory drugs (NSAIDs), long-term use of boswellia has not been shown to cause gastrointestinal irritation or ulceration, although adverse effects have not been well studied in humans.

EVIDENCE

Uses Based on Scientific Evidence	Grade
Asthma (Chronic Therapy) Boswellia has been proposed as a potential chronic asthma therapy. Future studies are needed to assess the long-term efficacy and safety of boswellia and to compare the efficacy of boswellia to standard therapies. Boswellia should not be used for the relief of acute asthma exacerbations.	B
Brain Tumors Boswellia has been used as a cancer treatment, but there are not enough human data to support this use over standard therapies. Cancer should be treated by a medical oncologist.	B
Crohn's Disease Boswellia has been noted to possess antiinflammatory properties. However, limited human data exist, and there is inadequate evidence for or against the use of boswellia in the treatment of Crohn's disease.	C
Osteoarthritis Because of boswellia's potential antiinflammatory properties, boswellia has been suggested as a potential treatment for osteoarthritis.	C
Rheumatoid Arthritis Because of boswellia's potential antiinflammatory properties, boswellia has been suggested as a potential treatment for rheumatoid arthritis (RA). However, data are conflicting and combination products have sometimes been used. Therefore, there is currently insufficient evidence to recommend for or against the use of boswellia for RA.	C
Ulcerative Colitis Because of boswellia's potential antiinflammatory properties, boswellia has been suggested as a potential treatment for ulcerative colitis. At this time, however, only a limited number of human trials have evaluated this use of boswellia, with inconclusive results. Therefore, there is inadequate evidence for or against this use of boswellia.	C

Uses Based on Tradition or Theory

Acne, amenorrhea (lack of a menstrual period), analgesic (pain reliever), antibacterial, antifungal, antiinflammatory, antioxidant, antiseptic, astringent, autoimmune diseases (encephalomyelitis), belching, bladder inflammation, blood purification, boils, breast cysts, bruises, bursitis, cancer, carminative (digestion aid), cervical spondylosis, chemopreventive, chronic obstructive pulmonary disease (COPD), cicatrizant (scar formation), cystitis, digestive, diuretic, dyspepsia (upset stomach), emmenagogue (induces menstruation), expectorant, gas, genital area infections, hepatitis (hepatitis C), hyperlipidemia (high cholesterol), immunostimulant, infections, insomnia, leukemia, multiple sclerosis, nephritis, parasitic infections (trypanosomiasis), pain, peptic ulcer disease, pimples, sedative, sexually transmitted diseases (STDs), skin ulcers/sores, stomach ulcers, syphilis, tendonitis, toxin-induced liver damage, tumors (meningioma), upper respiratory infections, uterine infections, varicose veins, wound healing, wrinkle prevention.

DOSING

Adults (18 Years and Older)

- There is insufficient evidence to recommend a dose for boswellia. For asthma, 300 mg three times a day of boswellia powdered gum resin capsules (S-compound) taken by mouth has been used. Another dose that has been taken is 400 mg three times daily (extract standardized to 37.5% boswellic acids per dose). For Crohn's disease, 1200 mg three times daily of standardized *Boswellia serrata* gum resin H15 has been taken by mouth for up to 8 weeks. For rheumatoid arthritis, 400 mg three times daily of standardized *Boswellia serrata* gum resin H15 has been taken by mouth. For ulcerative colitis, 350-400 mg three times daily (extract standardized to 37.5% boswellic acids per dose) has been taken by mouth.

Children (Younger than 18 Years)

- There is insufficient evidence to recommend a dose of boswellia in children. Some experts believe that regular use of boswellia may mask the symptoms of asthma in children and may delay diagnosis. Use in children should be supervised by a qualified health care professional.

SAFETY
Allergies

- Avoid in individuals with a known allergy to boswellia, its constituents, or members in the Burseraveae family. Allergic contact dermatitis has been associated with the use of a naturopathic cream containing *Boswellia serrata* extract.

Side Effects and Warnings

- Boswellia is generally believed to be safe when used as directed, although safety and toxicity have not been well studied in humans. The most common complaints in trials have been nausea and acid reflux. A qualified health care professional, including a pharmacist, should be consulted before use.
- Dermatitis (itchy, inflamed skin) has been reported in clinical trials using Articulin-F, a combination product containing gum resin from *Boswellia serrata* as well as *Withania somnifera* (ashwagandha), *Curcuma longa* (turmeric), and zinc complex. However, it is not clear whether boswellia alone would cause these effects.
- Boswellia extract has been associated with mild gastrointestinal upset, abdominal fullness, epigastric pain, gastroesophageal reflux symptoms, diarrhea, and nausea. It is not clear to what extent these symptoms were related to the patients' underlying colitis or the boswellia specifically in some cases because of the use of a combination product.

Pregnancy and Breastfeeding

- Reports in the Indian literature suggest that resin from boswellia is an emmenagogue (promotes menstruation) and may induce abortion. Safety of boswellia during pregnancy has not been systematically studied and therefore cannot be recommended.

INTERACTIONS
Interactions with Drugs

- Boswellia may potentiate the actions of pharmaceutical leukotriene inhibitors such as zafirlukast (Accolate) and montelukast (Singulair), which are used in the treatment of asthma.
- Theoretically, use with other antiproliferative agents may increase effects or toxicity of boswellia.
- The gum of boswellia may lower cholesterol and triglyceride levels and may increase the effects of lipid-lowering agents. It may also bind to/impair absorption of lipid-soluble agents.
- Nonsteroidal antiinflammatory drugs may interfere with the proposed benefits of boswellia in arthritis.
- Boswellia may increase the effects of antifungals.
- Boswellia may interact with immunomodulators, drugs broken down by the liver, antibiotics, fat soluble drugs, and sedatives.

Interactions with Herbs and Supplements

- Boswellia may act additively with agents used in the treatment of osteoarthritis, such as glucosamine and chondroitin.
- Theoretically, use with other antiproliferative agents may increase effects or toxicity of boswellia.
- Boswellia may increase the effects of antifungals.
- The gum of boswellia has been reported to lower cholesterol and triglyceride levels in rats and may increase the effects of lipid-lowering agents, such as garlic.
- Boswellia may interact with immunomodulators, herbs and supplements broken down by the liver, antibiotics, fat soluble drugs, chondroitin, glycosaminoglycans (GAGS), and sedatives.

For a complete list of references, please visit www.naturalstandard.com.

Bovine Colostrum

RELATED TERMS

- Adult bovine serum, affinity purified bovine colostrum antibodies, albumin, BioEnergy, Bioenervi, bovine, bovine casein, bovine colostral globulins, bovine colostrum-containing oral hygiene products, bovine colostrum cystatin, breast milk, butanol-extractable iodine, calcium, casein, cell growth factor, chromium, colostral antibodies (hyperimmune and natural), colostral fractions, colostral whey, colostrinin, colostrokinin, colostrum inhibitory factor (CIF), colostrum lozenges, colostrum, complement 3 and 4 (C3 & C4), concentrated bovine colostrum protein, cow colostrum, dynamic colostrum, epidermal growth factor, fibroblast growth factor, fibronectin, first milking colostrum, folic acid, gamma globulin, glutamic acid, glycine, glycoconjugates, glycogen, glycoprotein, growth factors, growth hormone, haemopexin, haptoglobulin, heat-denatured bovine immunoglobulin, human colostra, hyperimmune bovine colostrum, hyperimmune cow colostrum-immunized bovine colostrum, immunoglobulins, isoleucine, kappa casein, lactalbumin, *Lactobacillus acidophilus*, *Lactobacillus bifidobacterium*, *Lactobacillus bifidus*, lactobin (LIG), lactobin-R, lactoferrin, lactoperoxidase, leucine, liquid gold, Mega Bovine Colostrum, Mega-Colostabs, methionine, native bovine, oral bovine immunoglobulin milk concentrate, orosomucoids, orotic acid, osteoprotegerin (OPG), pantothenic acid, passive antibody immunotherapy platelet-derived growth factor, polychlorinated biphenyls, potassium, prealbumin, prolactin, proline, proline-rich polypeptide, purified bovine apolactoferrin, retinoic acid, ribonuclease II-1, super milk, Symbiotics Colostrum PLUS, transforming growth factor, ultrafiltrate fraction (UF) of bovine colostrum, Viable AC-2, whey proteins, xanthine oxidase enzyme.

BACKGROUND

- Bovine colostrum is the premilk fluid produced by cow mammary glands during the first 2-4 days after giving birth. Bovine colostrum delivers growth, nutrient, and immune factors to the offspring.
- Traditional uses of bovine colostrum have been for eye conditions, oral health, and respiratory tract infections. The investigation of clinical effects of bovine colostrum in humans began in the late 1980s and continues today.
- Bovine colostrum may be useful for exercise performance enhancement and gastrointestinal injury due to bowel disease and nonsteroidal antiinflammatory drugs (NSAIDs). Although early evidence looks promising, additional study is still needed to determine the safety and effectiveness of bovine colostrum.
- Hyperimmune bovine colostrum is also commercially available, and some evidence exists for its use, as well as the use of isolated immunoglobulins (antibodies). Most evidence is in support of its use for diarrhea associated with certain types of bacterial and viral infections or immune system deficiencies.

EVIDENCE

Uses Based on Scientific Evidence	Grade
Colitis Preliminary evidence suggests that bovine colostrum may be effective for improving gastrointestinal health.	C
Diarrhea Bovine colostrum may be effective for improving gastrointestinal health. Preliminary evidence suggests that colostrum inhibits the adhesion or activity of certain bacteria to intestinal cells, which may help in the treatment of diarrhea.	C
Exercise Performance Enhancement Although human study is currently conflicting, bovine colostrum may be effective for improving exercise performance.	C
Helicobacter pylori **Infection** Based on preliminary study, use of bovine colostrum did not appear to be of benefit in *Helicobacter pylori* infection.	C
Immune Function Bovine colostrum contains immunoglobulins or antibodies that are released into the bloodstream in response to infections. These immunoglobulins may help improve immune system functions.	C
Immune System Deficiencies (Cryptosporidiosis) *Cryptosporidium parvum* is a parasite that may cause severe, debilitating diarrhea in patients with acquired immunodeficiency syndrome (AIDS). Preliminary evidence suggests a potential benefit of bovine colostrum in this area.	C
Infections (Rotavirus) Bovine colostrum that is high in antibodies to certain viruses, such as rotavirus, may help prevent rotavirus-associated diarrhea.	C
Multiple Sclerosis Bovine colostrum has been used for multiple sclerosis, although early results do not indicate any benefit.	C
Oral Hygiene Bovine colostrum has shown potential for immune stimulation and may be useful in oral hygiene products. Currently, there is insufficient available evidence to recommend for or against colostrum for this use.	C

Uses Based on Scientific Evidence	Grade
Sore Throat Bovine colostrum has shown potential for immune stimulation and may be helpful in treating sore throat. Currently, there is insufficient available evidence to recommend for or against colostrum for this use.	C
Surgery (Recovery from) Bovine colostrum has been studied in individuals undergoing coronary bypass operations, but no benefit was found.	C
Upper Respiratory Tract Infection Bovine colostrum has shown potential for immune stimulation. However, early evidence has not shown any benefit for treating upper respiratory tract infection duration, although bovine colostrum may reduce symptoms.	C

Uses Based on Tradition or Theory

Aging, antibacterial, antiinflammatory, antimicrobial, antioxidant, antiviral, bodybuilding, bowel health, cancer, cognitive function, depression, diabetes, fat burning, fracture healing, gastrointestinal conditions, gastrointestinal distress (NSAID-induced), healing time reduction, hyperglycemia (high blood sugar), inflammatory bowel disease (IBD), keratitis (eye inflammation), longevity, measles, mood stimulant, mucositis from cancer treatment, nerve damage, osteoporosis, rheumatoid arthritis, skin conditions, xerostomia (dry mouth).

DOSING
Adults (18 Years and Older)

- There is insufficient evidence to recommend a dose of bovine colostrum. The dose amount and dosage formulations vary. Doses of 400-5000 mg taken 1-3 times per day in tablet, powder, or solution form for up to 10 days have been reported.

Children (Younger than 18 Years)

- There is insufficient evidence to recommend a dose of bovine colostrum in children. Various doses and preparations have been studied that are generally well tolerated with minor side effects. A common dosing range is 7-20 g of bovine colostrum per day in divided doses for up to 14 days. Hyperimmune milk concentrate (20 g daily) has also been administered for 5 days in children experiencing diarrhea as a result of shigella infection. Other studies have studied purified immunoglobulins (antibodies) from bovine colostrum for up to 1 month, but no benefit was found.

SAFETY
Allergies

- Avoid in individuals with a known allergy or hypersensitivity to dairy products.

Side Effects and Warnings

- Adverse reactions to bovine colostrum supplements are mainly gastrointestinal and may include nausea and vomiting, bloating, and diarrhea. In general, bovine colostrum is generally well tolerated. However, bovine colostrum is a potential source of environmental contaminants, such as pesticides.
- Heat-denatured bovine immunoglobulin may be a risk factor for atherosclerosis (hardening of the arteries). However, it is not clear how use of bovine colostrum relates to this risk. Use cautiously in patients with atherosclerosis.
- Bovine colostrum is a source of insulin-like growth factor-1 (IGF-1), which has been found to correlate with the risk of prostate cancer and colorectal cancer in men, premenopausal breast cancer in women, and lung cancer in both men and women. Not all studies agree with these findings, and it is not clear how this relates to the use of bovine colostrum. Avoid in patients with, or at risk of, cancer because of the potential for IGF-1-induced increased risk for certain types of cancer.
- Avoid in pregnant and breastfeeding women because of a lack of information.
- Use cautiously in individuals with immune system disorders because of the potential for immune system effects of bovine colostrum.
- Use cautiously in individuals taking medications, such as antidiarrhea agents (e.g., loperamide [Imodium]), insulin, and central nervous system agents (amphetamines, caffeine) because of the potential for reduced or increased efficacy.

Pregnancy and Breastfeeding

- Bovine colostrum is not recommended in pregnant or breastfeeding women because of a lack of available scientific evidence. Bovine colostrum is a potential source of environmental contaminants, such as pesticides.

INTERACTIONS
Interactions with Drugs

- In general, there are no reported drug interactions associated with bovine colostrum. However, the number of compounds in bovine colostrum is large, although levels may be small, and each may have unknown effects or interactions with other drugs.
- Preliminary studies have indicated bovine colostrum's antimicrobial effects. Thus, bovine colostrum may have additive effects when taken with antibiotics, and caution is advised.
- Preliminary evidence suggests that the presence of insulin in bovine colostrum is at least partially responsible for some of its effects. Thus, using insulin in combination with bovine colostrum may have additive effects. Patients taking drugs for diabetes by mouth or using insulin should be monitored closely by a qualified health care professional, including a pharmacist. Medication adjustments may be necessary.
- Because of the antidiarrheal effects of bovine colostrum, caution is advised when bovine colostrum is combined with other antidiarrheal agents; the combination may have additive effects.
- Bovine colostrum is a source of IGF-1. Several studies have found that IGF-1 levels correlate with the risk of prostate cancer and colorectal cancer in men, premenopausal breast cancer in women, and lung cancer in both men and women.

Not all studies agree with these findings, and it is not clear how this relates to the use of bovine colostrum. Nevertheless, caution is advised in patients taking anticancer agents and bovine colostrum because of unknown effects.

- Human colostrum is a rich source of the antioxidant CoQ10. It is not known whether bovine colostrum also contains CoQ10. Caution is advised in patients taking antioxidant agents because of possible additive effects.
- Bovine colostrum may have antiviral activity. Caution is advised in patients taking antiviral agents because of possible additive effects.
- Bovine colostrum may affect the brain's mood-regulating chemicals (serotonin and dopamine). Thus, combined use with other agents that affect the central nervous system, such as amphetamines or caffeine, may have additive or contradictory effects.
- There are conflicting data regarding the use of bovine colostrum for exercise performance enhancement. It is unclear whether bovine colostrum would interact with other exercise performance enhancers in humans.
- Colostrum may have effects on the immune system, although the clinical significance in humans is unknown. Use cautiously with other immunomodulators.
- Caution is also advised in patients taking NSAIDS because of possible additive effects.

Interactions with Herbs and Dietary Supplements

- Preliminary studies have indicated bovine colostrum's antimicrobial effects. Thus, bovine colostrum may have additive effects when taken with herbs and supplements with antibacterial effects, and caution is advised.
- Because of the antidiarrheal effects of bovine colostrum, caution is advised when bovine colostrum is combined with other antidiarrheal agents; the combination may have additive effects.
- In theory, colostrum may alter the effects of herbs with antiinflammatory effects.

- Bovine colostrum is a source of IGF-1. Several studies have found that IGF-1 levels correlate with the risk of prostate cancer and colorectal cancer in men, premenopausal breast cancer in women, and lung cancer in both men and women. Not all studies agree with these findings, and it is not clear how this relates to the use of bovine colostrum. Caution is advised in patients with or at risk of cancer or taking herbs or supplements with anticancer effects.
- Preliminary evidence suggests that bovine colostrum may have antiviral activity, and caution is advised in patients taking herbs or supplements with antiviral activity because of possible additive effects.
- Bovine colostrum may affect the brain's mood-regulating chemicals (serotonin and dopamine). Thus, combined use with other herbs that affect the central nervous system may have additive or contradictory effects.
- Human colostrum contains CoQ10. Thus, it is likely that bovine colostrum also contains CoQ10. Combined use with CoQ10 supplements or herbs or supplements with antioxidant activity may have additive effects.
- There are conflicting data regarding the use of bovine colostrum for exercise performance enhancement. It is unclear whether bovine colostrum would interact with other exercise performance enhancers in humans.
- Results from in vitro studies suggest that the presence of insulin in bovine colostrum is at least partially responsible for some of its effects. Thus, using herbs or supplements with hypoglycemic (blood sugar–lowering) effects in combination with bovine colostrum may have additive effects.
- Colostrum may have effects on the immune system, although the clinical significance is unknown. Use cautiously with other immunomodulator herbs or supplements.

For a complete list of references, please visit www.naturalstandard.com.

Boxwood
(Buxus sempervirens)

RELATED TERMS

- Benzenemethanethiol, Buxaceae (family), buxozine-C, *Buxus balearica*, *Buxus sempervirens* L., *Buxus sempervirens* var. *bullata*, common box, European box, Flu Guard, SPV30, SPV-30, volatile thiol.

BACKGROUND

- Boxwood is an evergreen shrub native to southern Europe, western Asia, and northern Africa.
- An extract of boxwood, SPV-30 (Arkopharma, France), has been studied for its potential effects in human immunodeficiency virus (HIV) and acquired immunodeficiency syndrome (AIDS); however, available clinical evidence is inconclusive. Product claims for SPV-30 have been controversial.
- There is currently insufficient available evidence in humans to support the use of boxwood for any medical indication.

EVIDENCE

Uses Based on Scientific Evidence	Grade
HIV/AIDS Trials have been conducted for SPV30 (extract of boxwood, Arkopharma, France). However, rigorous clinical study is needed to confirm results of SPV30 for HIV infection and AIDS.	C

Uses Based on Tradition or Theory
Aromatic, fatigue, sense of well-being.

DOSING

Adults (18 Years and Older)

- There is insufficient evidence to recommend a dose for boxwood in adults.

Children (Younger than 18 Years)

- There is insufficient evidence to recommend a dose for boxwood in children.

SAFETY

Allergies

- Avoid in individuals with a known allergy or hypersensitivity to boxwood or its constituents.
- Skin rash is possible.

Side Effects and Warnings

- There are few reports available of adverse effects associated with boxwood. However, skin rash has been reported.
- Use cautiously in patients with HIV/AIDS or high blood pressure.

Pregnancy and Breastfeeding

- Boxwood is not recommended in pregnant or breastfeeding women because of a lack of available scientific evidence.

INTERACTIONS

Interactions with Drugs

- Boxwood may alter blood pressure and interact with heart medications.
- Boxwood may interact with cholinergic drugs or antivirals.
- Boxwood may increase the effects of steroids; caution is advised.

Interactions with Herbs and Dietary Supplements

- Boxwood may alter blood pressure and interact with herbs and supplements that affect the heart.
- Boxwood may interact with cholinergic agents or antivirals.
- Boxwood may increase the effects of steroidal agents; caution is advised.

For a complete list of references, please visit www.naturalstandard.com.

Bromelain

(Ananas comosus, Ananas sativus)

RELATED TERMS

- *Ananas comosus, Ananas sativus*, Ananase, Bromelain-POS, Bromelainum, Bromeliaceae (family), Bromelin, Bromelins, Debridase, Phlogenzym (rutosid, bromelain, and trypsin), enzyme-rutosid combination, ERC (rutosid, bromelain, trypsin), plant protease concentrate, pineapple, pineapple extract, rutosid, Traumanase, trypsin.

BACKGROUND

- Bromelain is a sulfur-containing proteolytic digestive enzyme that is extracted from the stem and the fruit of the pineapple plant (*Ananas comosus*, family Bromeliaceae).
- When taken with meals, bromelain is believed to assist in the digestion of proteins. When taken on an empty stomach, it is believed to act medicinally as an antiinflammatory agent.
- The expert panel, the German Commission E, approved bromelain for the treatment of swelling/inflammation of the nose and sinuses caused by injuries and surgery in 1993.

EVIDENCE

Uses Based on Scientific Evidence	Grade
Inflammation Several preliminary studies suggest that when taken by mouth, bromelain can reduce inflammation or pain caused by inflammation.	B
Sinusitis (Sinus Inflammation) It is proposed that bromelain may be a useful addition to other therapies used for sinusitis (such as antibiotics) because of its ability to reduce inflammation/swelling. Studies report mixed results, although overall bromelain appears to be beneficial for reducing swelling and improving breathing.	B
Burn Debridement A bromelain-derived debriding agent, Debridase, has been studied on deep second-degree and third-degree burns with positive preliminary results.	C
Cancer There is not enough information to recommend for or against the use of bromelain in the treatment of cancer, either alone or in addition to other therapies.	C
Chronic Obstructive Pulmonary Disease (COPD) There is not enough information to recommend for or against the use of bromelain in COPD.	C
Digestive Enzyme/Pancreatic Insufficiency Bromelain is an enzyme with the ability to digest proteins. However, there is little reliable scientific research on whether bromelain is helpful as a digestive aid.	C

Knee Pain Bromelain may reduce mild acute knee pain in a dose-dependent manner.	C
Muscle Soreness The effects of bromelain on muscle soreness following intense exercise are unclear.	C
Nutrition Supplementation There is not enough information to recommend for or against the use of bromelain as a nutritional supplement.	C
Osteoarthritis of the Knee There is conflicting evidence on the effectiveness of bromelain to treat osteoarthritis.	C
Rash Bromelain may help treat skin rash. This treatment may be effective because bromelain has been shown to decrease inflammation, regulate the immune system, and have antiviral effects.	C
Rheumatoid Arthritis (RA) There is not enough information to recommend for or against the use of bromelain in RA.	C
Steatorrhea (Fatty Stools due to Poor Digestion) There is not enough information to recommend for or against the use of bromelain in the treatment of steatorrhea.	C
Urinary tract infection (UTI) There is not enough information to recommend for or against the use of bromelain in UTIs.	C

Uses Based on Tradition or Theory

Acquired immunodeficiency syndrome (AIDS), acute lateral ankle sprain, allergic rhinitis (hay fever), amyloidosis (deposits of amyloid proteins causing disease), angina (chest pain), antibiotic absorption problems in the gut, appetite suppressant, atherosclerosis ("hardening" of the arteries), autoimmune disorders, back pain, blood clot treatment, bronchitis, bruises, bursitis, cancer prevention, carpal tunnel syndrome, colitis, common cold, cough, diarrhea, epididymitis (painful inflammation of the epididymis), episiotomy pain (after childbirth), food allergies, frostbite, gout, heart disease, hemorrhoids, immune system regulation, infections, injuries, joint disease, "leaky gut" syndrome, menstrual pain, pain, parasites, Peyronie's disease, pneumonia, poor blood circulation in the legs, ciatica, scleroderma, shingles pain/postherpetic neuralgia, shortening of labor, skin infections, smooth muscle relaxation, sports or other physical injuries, staphylococcal bacterial infections, stomach ulcer/stomach ulcer prevention, swelling (after surgery or injury), tendonitis, treatment of scar tissue, ulcerative colitis, upper respiratory tract infection, varicose veins, wound healing.

DOSING

Adults (18 years and older)

- A variety of doses have been used and studied. Research in the 1960s and 1970s used 120-240 mg of bromelain concentrate tablets daily (Traumanase or Ananase; 2500 Rorer units per mg) in three to four divided doses for up to 1 week to treat inflammation. The German expert panel, the Commission E, has recommended 80-320 mg (200-800 FIP units) taken two to three times daily. Some authors recommend 500-1000 mg of bromelain to be taken three times daily, and many manufacturers sell products standardized to 2000 GDU in 500-mg tablets. Effects of bromelain may occur at lower doses, and treatment may be started at a low dose and increased as needed.
- Cream containing 35% bromelain in an oil-containing base has been applied to the skin to clean wounds.

Children (younger than 18 years)

- There is not enough scientific research to recommend safe use of bromelain in children.

SAFETY

Allergies

- There are multiple reports of allergic and asthmatic reactions to bromelain products, including throat swelling and difficulty breathing. Allergic reactions to bromelain may occur in individuals allergic to pineapples or other members of the Bromeliaceae family, and in people who are sensitive/allergic to honeybee venom, latex, birch pollen, carrot, celery, fennel, cypress pollen, grass pollen, papain, rye flour, or wheat flour.

Side Effects and Warnings

- Few serious side effects have been reported with the use of bromelain. The most common side effects reported are stomach upset and diarrhea. Other reported reactions include increased heart rate, nausea, vomiting, irritation of mucus membranes, and menstrual problems.
- In theory, bromelain may increase the risk of bleeding. Caution is advised in people who have bleeding disorders or who are taking drugs that increase the risk of bleeding. Dosing adjustments may be necessary. Bromelain should be used with caution in people with stomach ulcers, active bleeding, a history of bleeding, or taking medications that thin the blood or before some dental or surgical procedures.
- Bromelain may increase heart rate at higher doses and should be used cautiously in people with heart disease. Some experts warn against bromelain use by people with liver or kidney disease, although there is limited scientific information in these areas. Bromelain may cause abnormal uterine bleeding or heavy/prolonged menstruation.

Pregnancy and Breastfeeding

- Bromelain is not recommended during pregnancy or breastfeeding, as little safety information is available. Bromelain may cause abnormal uterine bleeding.

INTERACTIONS

Interactions with Drugs

- In theory, bromelain may increase the risk of bleeding when taken with drugs that increase the risk of bleeding. Some examples include aspirin, anticoagulants ("blood thinners") such as warfarin (Coumadin) or heparin, antiplatelet drugs such as clopidogrel (Plavix), and nonsteroidal antiinflammatory drugs (NSAIDs) such as ibuprofen (Motrin, Advil) or naproxen (Naprosyn, Aleve). In addition, bromelain theoretically may add to the antiinflammatory effects of NSAIDs.
- Human studies suggest that bromelain may increase the absorption of some antibiotics, notably amoxicillin and tetracycline, and increase the levels of these drugs in the body. Bromelain may increase the actions of the chemotherapy (anticancer) drugs 5-fluorouracil and vincristine, although reliable scientific research in this area is lacking. In theory, use of bromelain with blood pressure medications in the angiotensin-converting enzyme (ACE) inhibitor class, such as captopril (Capoten) or lisinopril (Zestril), may cause larger drops in blood pressure than expected.
- Some experts suggest that bromelain may cause drowsiness or sedation and may increase the amount of drowsiness caused by some drugs. Examples include benzodiazepines such as lorazepam (Ativan) or diazepam (Valium), barbiturates such as phenobarbital, narcotics such as codeine, some antidepressants, and alcohol. Use caution while driving or operating machinery.
- Bromelain may also interact with heartbeat-regulating medications, magnesium, and nicotine.

Interactions with Herbs and Dietary Supplements

- In theory, bromelain may increase the risk of bleeding when taken with herbs and supplements that are believed to increase the risk of bleeding. Multiple cases of bleeding have been reported with the use of *Ginkgo biloba*, and fewer cases have been reported with garlic and saw palmetto. Numerous other agents may theoretically increase the risk of bleeding, although this has not been proven in most cases.
- Bromelain and the enzyme trypsin are suggested to have stronger antiinflammatory effects when combined, based on preliminary animal research. It has been suggested that zinc might block the effects of bromelain in the body whereas magnesium may increase the effects, although scientific research in these areas is lacking.
- Bromelain may also interact with herbs and supplements that effect the heart, antibacterials, soy, sedatives, and tobacco.

For a complete list of references, please visit www.naturalstandard.com.

Buchu

(Agathosma betulina)

RELATED TERMS

- *Agathosma betulina, Agathosma crenulata, Agathosma serratifolia, Barosma betulina,* barosma camphor, *Barosma crenulata, Barosma serratifolia,* barosmae folium, boegoe (Afrikaans), boochoo, bookoo, bucco, buchu brandy, buchu camphor, bucku, diosma, diosmin, hesperidin, ibuchu (Xhosa), long buchu, oil of buchu, oval buchu, ovate buchu, round buchu, round-leaf buchu, Rutaceae (family), short buchu, shortbroad buchu, true buchu.
- **Note:** This monograph does not include Indian buchu (*Myrtus communi*), which is an unrelated plant.

BACKGROUND

- Buchu (*Agathosma betulina*) leaves and oil of buchu were used by the indigenous people of the Cape area of South Africa for hundreds of years. Although its original use is unclear, it appears to have been applied topically on the skin, possibly as an insect repellant, and also used internally for stomach problems, rheumatism, and bladder problems. Buchu's original genus *Barosma* was changed to *Agathosma*.
- Buchu contains both diosmin and hesperidin, which indicates it may have antiinflammatory, hypolipidemic (blood cholesterol–lowering), and vasoprotective actions.
- Most of the plants are still grown in South Africa where the government exercises strict control over the gathering of the leaves to prevent destruction of wild plants.

EVIDENCE

Uses Based on Scientific Evidence

No available studies qualify for inclusion in the evidence table.

Uses Based on Tradition or Theory

Abortifacient (induces abortion), acquired immunodeficiency syndrome (AIDS), antiinflammatory, antimicrobial, antiseptic (antibacterial), antispasmodic, appetite stimulant, astringent, bloody urine, bruises, carminative (reduces gas), cholera, colds, colon inflammation, congestive heart failure, cough, cystitis (bladder infection), diabetes, diaphoretic (promotes sweating), digestive, diuretic, edema, flavoring agent, fragrance, gout (foot inflammation), gum inflammation, hangovers, hypertension (high blood pressure), improving urine flow, incontinence, influenza, insect repellent, kidney function, kidney infection, kidney stones, muscle aches, nephritis (kidney inflammation), premenstrual syndrome, prostate disorders, respiratory disorders, rheumatism, sexually transmitted diseases, sinus problems, sprains and strains, stimulant, stomachache, tonic, urethritis (inflamed uretha), urinary tract tonic, urolithiasis (kidney stones), uterine stimulant, vaginal irritation.

DOSING

Adults (18 Years and Older)

- There is insufficient evidence to recommend a dose for buchu. Historically, dried buchu leaf 1-2 g has been taken in capsules three times daily. As a fluid extract, 0.125-0.25 fl oz has been used. Also, 1-2 teaspoons of buchu leaves may be infused for 5-10 minutes in a cup of boiling water (leaves should not be boiled) and ingested two or three times daily. A tincture of 1-4 mL may be given three times daily or 10-20 drops of tincture in water three times daily after meals.

Children (Younger than 18 Years)

- There is insufficient evidence to recommend a dose for buchu in children, and use is not recommended.

SAFETY

Allergies

- Avoid in individuals with a known allergy or hypersensitivity to buchu.

Side Effects and Warnings

- There are little available data on the safety of buchu. In general, buchu may cause upset stomach, diarrhea, or kidney irritation. Traditional experts recommend monitoring liver function when buchu is used because of its potentially hepatotoxic (liver-damaging) effects.
- Buchu may increase the risk of bleeding. Caution is advised in patients with bleeding disorders or taking drugs that may increase the risk of bleeding. Dosing adjustments may be necessary.
- Although not well studied in humans, high concentrations of buchu oil appear to block calcium channels, which could lead to cardiac arrest. Buchu may also increase menstrual flow and may also induce abortion.
- Use cautiously in patients with seizure disorders, as buchu might cause spasmogenic action followed by spasmolysis.

Pregnancy and Breastfeeding

- Buchu is not recommended in pregnant or breastfeeding women because of a lack of available scientific evidence. According to traditional use, buchu may be an abortifacient (induce abortion) and may stimulate uterine contractions.

INTERACTIONS

Interactions with Drugs

- Buchu may increase the risk of bleeding when taken with drugs that increase the risk of bleeding. Some examples include aspirin, anticoagulants ("blood thinners") such as warfarin (Coumadin) or heparin, antiplatelet drugs such as clopidogrel (Plavix), and nonsteroidal antiinflammatory drugs such as ibuprofen (Motrin, Advil) or naproxen (Naprosyn, Aleve).

- High concentrations of buchu oil may block calcium channels. Patients taking calcium channel blocker medications should consult with a qualified health care professional, including a pharmacist.
- Buchu may additively interact with cardiac glycoside drugs.
- Buchu may also interact additively with diuretic (increasing urine flow) drugs, such as chlorothiazide (Diuril) or bumetanide (Bumex). Caution is advised.

Interactions with Herbs and Dietary Supplements

- Buchu may increase the risk of bleeding when taken with herbs and supplements that are believed to increase the risk of bleeding. Multiple cases of bleeding have been reported with the use of *Ginkgo biloba*, and fewer cases have been reported with garlic and saw palmetto. Numerous other agents may theoretically increase the risk of bleeding, although this has not been proven in most cases.
- Buchu may interact additively with diuretic herbs or cardiac glycoside herbs such as foxglove.

For a complete list of references, please visit www.naturalstandard.com.

Buckshorn Plantain
(*Plantago coronopus*)

RELATED TERMS
- Plantaginaceae (family), *Plantago coronopus, Plantago coronopus* L.
- **Note:** This monograph only covers *Plantago coronopus*; however, other species of *Plantago* have been referred to as buckhorn plantain (not buckshorn), such as *Plantago lanceolata.*

BACKGROUND
- Buckshorn plantain is found in Europe, western Asia, and northern Africa. The leaves are sometimes used in an Italian salad called misticanza, which means *wild greens.* In the Canary Islands, buckshorn plantain has been used to treat kidney and urinary disorders. However, there is insufficient available evidence in humans to support the use of buckshorn plantain for any indication.

EVIDENCE

Uses Based on Scientific Evidence

No available studies qualify for inclusion in the evidence table.

Uses Based on Tradition or Theory

Antibacterial, kidney diseases, laxative, leukemia, malaria, urinary disorders.

DOSING
Adults (18 Years and Older)
- There is insufficient evidence to recommend a dose for buckshorn plantain in adults.

Children (Younger than 18 Years)
- There is insufficient evidence to recommend a dose for buckshorn plantain in children.

SAFETY
Allergies
- Avoid in individuals with a known allergy or hypersensitivity to buckshorn plantain (*Plantago coronopus*) or its constituents.

Side Effects and Warnings
- Insufficient evidence is available.

Pregnancy and Breastfeeding
- Buckshorn plantain is not recommended in pregnant or breastfeeding women because of a lack of available scientific evidence.

INTERACTIONS
Interactions with Drugs
- Insufficient evidence is available.

Interactions with Herbs and Dietary Supplements
- Insufficient evidence is available.

For a complete list of references, please visit www.naturalstandard.com.

Bupleurum
(Bupleurum spp.)

RELATED TERMS

- Apiaceae (family), bei chai hu, beichaihu, bupleuran 2IIc, *Bupleurum chinese* D.C., *Bupleurum exaltatum, Bupleurum falcatum, Bupleurum falcatum* L. var. *scorzonerifolium, Bupleurum fruticescens, Bupleurum fruticosum* L., *Bupleurum ginghausenii, Bupleurum longifolium, Bupleurum multinerve, Bupleurum octoradiatum,* bupleuri radix (Latin), bupleuri radix saponins, bupleurum root, *Bupleurum rotundifolium* L., *Bupleurum scorzonerifolium Willd., Bupleurum stewartianum,* chai hu, chaifu, chaihu (Chinese), chai hu chaiku-saiko, Chinese thoroughwax root, echinocystic acid 3-O-sulfate, hare's ear root (English), He Jie Decoction, hydroxysaikosaponins, isochaihulactone, juk-siho, kara-saiko, Minor Bupleurum Decoction, mishima-saiko, nanchaihu, northern Chinese thorowax root, phenylpropanoids, radix bupleur, saiko (Japanese), saikosaponins, segl-hareore (Danish), shi ho, sho-saiko-to, shoku-saiko, shrubby hare's-ear, sickle-leaf hare's-ear, siho (Korean), thorowax, thoroughwax, TJ-9, triterpene saponins, Umbelliferae (family), wa-saiko, xiao chai hu tang, yamasaiko.

BACKGROUND

- Bupleurum has been widely used for over 2000 years in Asia and is used today in Japan and China for hepatitis, cirrhosis, and other conditions associated with inflammation. Other traditional uses that are not supported by human scientific studies include the treatment of deafness, dizziness, diabetes, wounds, and vomiting. Bupleurum root is an important ingredient in *xiao-chai-hu-tan/sho-saiko-to,* also known as Minor Bupleurum Decoction, a combination of nine herbs, including ginseng, ginger, and licorice, that is used in traditional Chinese and Japanese herbal medicine for hepatitis and cirrhosis.
- Clinical studies have suggested that this combination may be effective in the treatment of hepatitis B and in the prevention of hepatocellular carcinoma. The mixture has also shown some promise as a liver-protecting agent and as an adjuvant in the treatment of human immunodeficiency virus (HIV) infection. The effect of bupleurum is inseparable from the effects of the other ingredients in *xiao-chai-hu-tan/sho-saiko-to;* thus, it is difficult to make any firm conclusions based on studies of this combination product. However, because there is some promising early clinical evidence of efficacy for these formulae in the treatment and prevention of hepatitis-associated liver disease, a number of the studies of the combination preparations are included in this review.

EVIDENCE

Uses Based on Scientific Evidence	Grade
Brain Damage (Minimal, in Children) An herbal combination formula containing bupleurum has been used as a treatment for children with minimal brain dysfunction. Early study is inconclusive, and additional study is needed to make a firm recommendation.	C
Fever Chinese studies have suggested that bupleurum may be helpful for reducing fever. However, additional study is needed to draw a firm conclusion about safety and effectiveness. In traditional Chinese medicine, bupleurum is often used in combination with other herbs.	C
Hepatitis Traditional use from China, as well as preliminary human study, seems to suggest that bupleurum and/or herbal combination formulas containing bupleurum may be helpful in the treatment of chronic hepatitis. Further research is warranted to make a firm recommendation.	C
Hepatocellular Carcinoma (Prevention) Hepatocellular carcinoma (HCC) arises predominantly in patients with cirrhosis, both hepatitis-associated and non–hepatitis-associated. *Sho-saiko-to,* the Japanese version of the classical bupleurum-based formula, has been examined for a possible role in preventing the development of HCC in patients with cirrhosis. Early study suggests that this formula may help prevent progression to HCC in patients with cirrhosis, although more study is needed for a strong recommendation.	C
Thrombocytopenic Purpura Primary thrombocytopenic purpura may respond in some cases to treatment with bupleurum-containing herbal formulas. However, currently there is insufficient available evidence for or against the use of bupleurum for this indication.	C

Uses Based on Tradition or Theory

Adrenal insufficiency (stimulation), amenorrhea (absence of menstruation), analgesia (pain relief), angina (chest pain), anorexia, antibacterial, antifungal, antiinflammatory, antioxidant, antipseudomonal, antiseptic, antitussive, antiviral, asthma, bronchitis, cancer, cirrhosis (liver disease), common cold, constipation, contraceptive, deafness, dementia, depression, diabetes, diaphoresis (excessive sweating), diarrhea, dizziness, dysmenorrhea (painful menstruation), epilepsy, fatigue, fever, gastric ulcer, headache, hemorrhoids, hepatoprotection (liver protection), herpes simplex virus infection, HIV, hot flashes, hypercholesterolemia (high blood cholesterol levels), hyperlipidemia (high blood lipid levels), immune system enhancement, immunosuppression, indigestion, influenza, kidney disease, kidney protection, liver disease (chronic), liver health, lung cancer, lung congestion, malaria, melanoma, menstrual irregularities, muscle cramps, myalgia (muscle pain), nausea, pain, pain (epigastric), pancreatitis (inflammation of the pancreas), Parkinson's disease, premenstrual syndrome (PMS), pulmonary edema, rectal prolapse, rheumatoid arthritis, sedation, spleen disorders (liver stagnation and spleen deficiency

(Continued)

syndrome [LSSDS]), solid tumors, systemic lupus erythematosis (SLE), tinnitus, tuberculosis (pulmonary), ulcers, upper respiratory tract infection, uterine prolapse, vertigo, viral infections (poliovirus), vomiting, wounds.

DOSING
Adults (18 Years and Older)

- There is insufficient evidence to recommend a dose for bupleurum. Bupleurum is typically taken in combination formulas with other herbs and has not been well studied alone. Traditionally, 1.5-9 g of bupleurum root have been used daily. Also, 1.5-3 mL of a fluid extract may be given daily. For hepatitis, doses of 5.4 g of combination therapy sho-saiko-to daily have been studied for 12 weeks. For prevention of hepatocellular carcinoma, sho-saiko-to has been administered at a dose of 7.5 g daily in combination with conventional treatment.

Children (Younger than 18 Years)

- There is insufficient evidence to recommend a dose for bupleurum in children, and use is not recommended. Bupleurum is typically taken in combination formulas with other herbs and has not been well studied alone.

SAFETY
Allergies

- Avoid in individuals with a known allergy or hypersensitivity to Bupleurum species, any of its constituents, the Apiaceae or Umbelliferae (carrot) families, snakeroot, cow parsnip, or poison hemlock. There are some reports that mention allergic reactions occurring in patients given intramuscular injections of bupleurum.

Side Effects and Warnings

- In recommended doses, many practitioners agree that bupleurum is well tolerated. However, available safety data are lacking. Reports of adverse effects are largely theoretical and based on side effects from combination therapy; it is difficult to attribute the adverse effects to bupleurum alone.
- Reported side effects include decreased appetite, nausea, reflux, abdominal distension, gas, and increased bowel movements following large doses of bupleurum. Rare instances of nausea, loss of appetite, and abdominal fullness have been reported following treatment with the combination therapy sho-saiko-to. Combinations containing bupleurum have been associated with eosinophilic pneumonia, pulmonary edema, and multiple cases of pneumonitis (inflammation of the lungs). Use cautiously in patients with hypertension (high blood pressure), diabetes, or edema because of the possibility of adrenal stimulation.
- There have been unverified reports of sedation, drowsiness, and lethargy, which are noted as frequent side effects. Rare instances of fatigue and paresthesia (abnormal sensations) were noted in one study that investigated the combination therapy sho-saiko-to. Use cautiously in patients operating motor vehicles or hazardous machinery because of a possible risk of sedation.
- Although not well studied in humans, bupleurum may increase the risk of bleeding. Caution is advised in patients

with bleeding disorders or taking drugs that may increase the risk of bleeding. Dosing adjustments may be necessary.
- Use cautiously in patients with diabetes. Saikosaponins, constituents of Bupleurum, may increase blood sugar levels.

Pregnancy and Breastfeeding

- Bupleurum is not recommended in pregnant or breastfeeding women because of a lack of available scientific evidence.

INTERACTIONS
Interactions with Drugs

- Bupleurum may increase the risk of bleeding when taken with drugs that increase the risk of bleeding. Some examples include aspirin, anticoagulants ("blood thinners") such as warfarin (Coumadin) or heparin, antiplatelet drugs such as clopidogrel (Plavix), and nonsteroidal antiinflammatory drugs such as ibuprofen (Motrin, Advil) or naproxen (Naprosyn, Aleve).
- Saikosaponins, constituents of Bupleurum, may increase blood sugar levels. Caution is advised when medications that may alter blood sugar levels are used. Patients taking drugs for diabetes by mouth or using insulin should be monitored closely by a qualified health care professional, including a pharmacist. Medication adjustments may be necessary.
- Bupleurum may stimulate the adrenals and may decrease the effects of antihypertensives (drugs for high blood pressure). Patients taking blood pressure medications, including beta-blockers or angiotensin-converting enzyme (ACE) inhibitors, should use bupleurum cautiously.
- Although not well-studied in humans, bupleurum may reduce cholesterol levels. Caution is advised in patients taking cholesterol-lowering agents.
- Because of the possibility of adrenal stimulation, bupleurum may decrease the effects of diuretics or increase the effects of corticosteroids (steroids).
- Bupleurum may have immune inhibitory effects and might additively or synergistically enhance immunosuppressant effects.
- Sho-saiko-to, a combination herbal formula that contains bupleurum, was found to enhance the anti-HIV-1 activity of lamivudine in laboratory study. Consult a qualified health care professional, including a pharmacist, before combining bupleurum or combination formulas containing bupleurum with antiviral or hepatitis B agents.
- Bupleurum may increase the amount of drowsiness caused by some drugs. Examples include benzodiazepines such as lorazepam (Ativan) or diazepam (Valium), barbiturates such as phenobarbital, narcotics such as codeine, some antidepressants, and alcohol. The use of bupleurum in combination with alcohol might additively or synergistically enhance sedation. Use caution while driving or operating machinery.
- In theory, bupleurum may interact with medications metabolized by the liver. There are mixed reports of bupleurum acting as both a protective agent for the liver and an agent that has toxic effects on the liver. Additionally, combination products containing bupleurum may interact with any medication taken by mouth and may alter the way medications are absorbed in the body.
- Although human evidence is lacking, bupleurum may also interact with Alzheimer's disease medications, antibiotics, anticancer medications, or HIV medications (antiretrovirals). Consult with a qualified health care professional, including a pharmacist, to check for interactions.

B

Interactions with Herbs and Dietary Supplements

- Bupleurum may increase the risk of bleeding when taken with herbs and supplements that are believed to increase the risk of bleeding. Multiple cases of bleeding have been reported with the use of *Ginkgo biloba*, and fewer cases have been reported with garlic and saw palmetto. Numerous other agents may theoretically increase the risk of bleeding, although this has not been proven in most cases.
- Saikosaponins, constituents of bupleurum, may increase blood sugar levels. Caution is advised when herbs or supplements that may alter blood sugar levels are used. Patients should be monitored closely by a qualified health care professional, including a pharmacist. Medication adjustments may be necessary.
- *Sho-saiko-to*, a combination herbal formula that contains bupleurum, was found to enhance the anti-HIV-1 activity of lamivudine in laboratory study. Consult a qualified health care professional, including a pharmacist, before combining bupleurum or combination formulas containing bupleurum with antiviral herbs or supplements.
- Saikosaponins, constituents of bupleurum, may decrease triglyceride concentrations or decrease the effects of blood pressure–lowering agents. Caution is advised in patients taking cholesterol-lowering herbs or supplements, such as red yeast rice, or herbs or supplements that lower blood pressure. Consult with a qualified health care professional, including a pharmacist, to check for interactions.
- Bupleurum may stimulate the adrenals and may have additive effects with corticosteroids (steroids) or decrease the effects of diuretics (agents that increase urine flow).
- Bupleurum may have immune inhibitory effects and may additively or synergistically enhance immunosuppressant effects.
- Bupleurum may increase the amount of drowsiness caused by some herbs or supplements.
- In theory, bupleurum may interact with herbs or supplements metabolized by the liver. There are mixed reports of bupleurum acting as both a protective agent for the liver and an agent that has toxic effects on the liver. Additionally, combination products containing bupleurum may interact with any medication taken by mouth and may alter the way medications are absorbed in the body.
- Although human evidence is lacking, bupleurum may interact with herbs and supplements taken for Alzheimer's disease, cancer, or HIV. Bupleurum may also interact with herbs or supplements with antibacterial effects. Consult with a qualified health care professional, including a pharmacist, to check for interactions.

For a complete list of references, please visit www. naturalstandard.com.

Burdock
(*Arctium lappa*)

RELATED TERMS

- Akujitsu, anthraxivore, arctii, *Arctium lappa* Linne, *Arctium minus*, *Arctium tomentosa*, *Arctium tomentosum* Mill., Asteraceae (family), bardana, Bardanae radix, bardane, bardane grande (French), beggar's buttons, burdock root, burr, burr seed, chin, clot-burr, clotbur, cocklebur, cockle button, cocklebuttons, Compositae (family), cuckold, daiki kishi, edible burdock, fox's clote, grass burdock, great bur, great burdock, great burdocks, gobo (Japan), Grosse klette (German), happy major, hardock, hare burr, hurrburr, Kletterwurzel (German), lampazo (Spanish), lappola, love leaves, niu bang zi, oil of lappa, personata, Philanthropium, thorny burr, turkey burrseed, woo-bang-ja, wild gobo.

BACKGROUND

- Burdock has historically been used to treat a wide variety of ailments, including arthritis, diabetes, and hair loss. It is a principal herbal ingredient in the popular cancer remedies Essiac (rhubarb, sorrel, slippery elm) and Hoxsey formula (red clover, poke, prickly ash, bloodroot, barberry).
- Burdock fruit has been found to lower blood sugar levels in animals, and early human studies have examined burdock root in diabetes. Laboratory and animal studies have explored the use of burdock for bacterial infections, cancer, human immunodeficiency virus (HIV), and kidney stones. However, there is currently insufficient human evidence regarding the efficacy of burdock for any indication.

EVIDENCE

Uses Based on Scientific Evidence	Grade
Diabetes Animal research and initial human studies suggest possible blood sugar–lowering effects of burdock root or fruit. However, the available human research has not been well designed, and the evidence is unclear.	C
Quality of Life in Cancer Patients (Breast Cancer) Burdock is an ingredient in the popular purported cancer remedy, Essiac. Preliminary evidence suggests that burdock may have anticancer effects and increase quality of life in cancer patients.	C

Uses Based on Tradition or Theory

Abscesses, acne, anorexia nervosa, aphrodisiac, arthritis, back pain, bacterial infections, bladder disorders, blood thinner, boils, burns, cancer, canker sores, catarrh, common cold, cosmetic uses, dandruff, detoxification, diuretic (increases urine flow), eczema, fever, fungal infections, gout, hair loss, headache, hemorrhoids, HIV, hives, hormonal effects, ichthyosis (skin disorder), impotence, inflammation, kidney diseases, kidney stones, laxative, lice, liver disease, liver protection, measles, pain, pneumonia, psoriasis, respiratory infections, rheumatoid arthritis, ringworm, sciatica, scurvy, seborrhea (overactivity of sebaceous skin glands), skin disorders, skin moisturizer, sores, sterility, syphilis, tonsillitis, ulcers, urinary tract infections, venereal diseases, warts, wound healing.

DOSING

Adults (18 Years and Older)

- There is insufficient evidence to recommend a dose for burdock, although a range of doses and types of preparations have been used. It is available as a dried root, tablets/capsules, decoctions, tinctures, fluid extract, and root teas. Burdock has been used as a diuretic (to increase urine flow) with preparations made from powdered burdock seeds into a yellow product called oil of lappa.
- Burdock has been used on the skin as a compress or plaster for eczema, psoriasis, baldness, and warts.

Children (Younger than 18 Years)

- There is insufficient evidence to recommend a dose for burdock for children.

SAFETY

Allergies

- Allergy to burdock may occur in individuals with allergy to members of the Asteraceae/Compositae family, including ragweed, chrysanthemums, marigolds, and daisies. Severe allergic reactions (anaphylaxis) have been associated with burdock. Allergic skin reactions have been associated with the use of burdock plasters on the skin. Caution should be used in patients with allergies or intolerance to pectin because certain parts of the burdock plant contain different levels of pectin complex.

Side Effects and Warnings

- Based on traditional use, burdock is generally believed to be safe when taken by mouth in recommended doses for short periods of time. Handling the plant or using preparations on the skin (such as plasters) has occasionally been reported to cause allergic skin reactions. Diuretic effects (increased urine flow) and estrogen-like effects have been reported with oral burdock use in patients with HIV. Although reports of symptoms such as dry mouth and slow heart rate have been noted in people taking burdock products, it is believed that contamination with belladonna may be responsible for these reactions. Contamination may occur during harvesting.
- In theory, tannins present in burdock may be toxic, although toxicity has not been reported in animal studies. Tannins can cause stomach upset and in high concentrations may result in kidney or liver damage. Long-term use of tannins may increase the risk of head and neck cancers, although this has not been seen in humans. Based on animal research and limited human study, burdock may cause increases or reductions in blood sugar levels. Caution is advised in patients with diabetes or hypoglycemia and in those taking drugs, herbs, or supplements that affect blood sugar.

Blood sugar levels may need monitoring by a qualified health care provider, and medication adjustments might be necessary. In theory, burdock may also cause electrolyte imbalances (e.g., changes in potassium or sodium levels in the blood) due to diuretic effects (increased urine flow).

- Several case reports of burdock root tea poisoning exist along with cases of burdock ophthalmia (eye inflammation). There have been several reports of stomatitis (mouth sores) present in dogs that have come in contact with burdock, burs, and bristles.

Pregnancy and Breastfeeding

- Based on animal studies that show components of burdock to cause uterine stimulation, burdock is sometimes recommended to be avoided during pregnancy. Because of limited scientific study, burdock cannot be considered safe during pregnancy or breastfeeding.

INTERACTIONS
Interactions with Drugs

- Based on animal research and limited human study, burdock may either lower or raise blood sugar levels. Caution is advised when medications that may also affect blood sugar are used. Patients taking drugs for diabetes by mouth or using insulin should be monitored closely by a qualified health care provider. Medication adjustments may be necessary. Burdock has been associated with diuretic effects (increased urine flow) in one human report and in theory may cause excess fluid loss (dehydration) or electrolyte imbalances (e.g., changes in potassium or sodium levels in the blood). These effects may be increased when burdock is taken at the same time as diuretic drugs such as chlorothiazide (Diuril), furosemide (Lasix), hydrochlorothiazide (HCTZ), or spironolactone (Aldactone). Based on limited human evidence that is not entirely clear, burdock may have estrogen-like properties and may act to increase the effects of estrogenic agents including hormone replacement therapies such as Premarin or birth control pills.

- Based on animal research, burdock may increase the risk of bleeding when taken with drugs that increase the risk of bleeding (although human research is lacking). Some examples include aspirin, anticoagulants ("blood thinners") such as warfarin (Coumadin) or heparin, antiplatelet drugs such as clopidogrel (Plavix), and nonsteroidal antiinflammatory drugs such as ibuprofen (Motrin, Advil) or naproxen (Naprosyn, Aleve). Tinctures of burdock may contain high concentrations of alcohol (ethanol) and may lead to vomiting if used with disulfiram (Antabuse) or metronidazole (Flagyl).

- Medications taken to treat gout, cancer, or HIV may interact with burdock. There is also a possible interaction with antibiotics.

Interactions with Herbs and Dietary Supplements

- Based on animal research and limited human study, burdock may either lower or raise blood sugar levels. Caution is advised when herbs or supplements that can also alter blood sugar are used. Blood glucose levels may require monitoring, and doses may need adjustment.

- Burdock has been associated with diuretic effects (increased urine flow) in one human report and, in theory, may cause excess fluid loss (dehydration) or electrolyte imbalances (e.g., changes in potassium or sodium levels in the blood) when used with other diuretic herbs or supplements.

- Based on animal research, burdock may increase the risk of bleeding when taken with herbs and supplements that are believed to increase the risk of bleeding. Multiple cases of bleeding have been reported with the use of *Ginkgo biloba*, fewer cases with garlic, and two cases with saw palmetto. Numerous other agents may theoretically increase the risk of bleeding, although this has not been proven in most cases.

- Herbs or supplements taken to treat gout, cancer, or HIV may interact with burdock. There is also a possible interaction with herbs with antibacterial, antioxidant, or antiinflammatory effects (such as ginger).

For a complete list of references, please visit www.naturalstandard.com.

Butterbur
(Petasites hybridus)

RELATED TERMS

- Blatterdock, bog rhubarb, bogshorns, butcher's rhubarb, butterbur coltsfoot, butterburr, butter-dock, butterdock, butterfly dock, capdockin, coughwort, donnhove, European pestroot, exwort, flapper-bags, flapperdock, fuki, horsehoof, langwort, paddy's rhubarb, pestwurz, Petadolex, Petadolor H, Petaforce, petasites, petasites flower, petasites leaf, petasites rhizome, *Petasites hybridus*, *Petasites officinalis*, *Petasites ovatus*, *Petasites vulgaris*, petasitidis folium (flower), petasitidis rhizoma (rhizome), plaguewort, purple butterbur, sweet coltsfoot, Tesalin, *Tussilago farfara*, *Tussilago hybrida*, *Tussilago petasites*, umbrella leaves, umbrella plant, western coltsfoot, wild rhubarb, ZE 339.

BACKGROUND

- Butterbur is a perennial shrub, found throughout Europe as well as parts of Asia and North America. It is usually found in wet, marshy ground, in damp forests, and adjacent to rivers or streams. The leaves of the plant are responsible for its botanical and common names. The common name is attributed to the large leaves being used to wrap butter during warm weather.
- Butterbur has been traditionally used as an antispasmodic and analgesic (pain reliever), specifically for conditions afflicting the stomach, bile ducts, and duodenum (part of small intestine). Butterbur is believed to help strengthen digestion and improve obstructed bile flow. Butterbur has also been given for inflammation of the urinary tract and cramps. There is compelling initial evidence from clinical trials to suggest benefits in prevention of migraine headache. Evidence in support of use for allergic rhinitis prevention is also promising. Benefits have not been demonstrated scientifically for any other condition.
- Use should be limited to commercially available products free of pyrrolizidine alkaloids that are generally believed to be well tolerated.

EVIDENCE

Uses Based on Scientific Evidence	Grade
Allergic Rhinitis Prevention Comparisons of butterbur to prescription drugs such as fexofenadine (Allegra) and cetirizine (Zyrtec) have reported similar efficacy. These results suggest benefits of butterbur for prevention of allergic rhinitis. Additional study is warranted before a strong recommendation can be made.	B
Migraine Prophylaxis Pain relief and headache prevention are traditional uses of butterbur. Current, available evidence is compelling enough to suggest benefits of butterbur for migraine prevention, although additional evidence is necessary before a strong recommendation can be made. Comparisons to other agents used for this purpose such as beta-blockers or feverfew have not been conducted.	B

Allergic Skin Disease	C
There is limited human evidence in this area, although preliminary research suggests that butterbur may not suppress allergic skin reactions when compared with the prescription drug fexofenadine (Allegra), which does suppress these reactions. Additional study is needed.	

Asthma	C
Butterbur was used historically to treat asthma, and initial human research suggests possible benefits. However, additional study is needed to make a firm recommendation.	

Uses Based on Tradition or Theory

Antispasmodic, anxiety, appetite stimulant, cardiovascular conditions, chills, chronic cough, colds, cramps, diuretic (increases urine flow), fever, gastric ulcers, headache treatment, indigestion, insomnia, irritable bladder, ocular allergy, pain, plague, urinary complaints, urinary tract spasm, whooping cough, wound/skin healing.

DOSING

Adults (18 Years and Older)

- Studies have reported safety and good tolerability of commercially available butterbur products (which are free of potentially carcinogenic pyrrolizidine alkaloid constituents), when used orally in recommended doses for up to 12-16 weeks.
- For allergic rhinitis, 50 mg of standardized butterbur (Petadolex, standardized to contain 7.5 mg of petasin and isopetasin per 50-mg tablet) has been used twice daily. A large study used one tablet of carbon dioxide extract standardized to 8.0 mg of total petasin per tablet (Tesalin), taken four times daily, while a smaller study reported that two standardized tablets taken three times daily was effective.
- Dosing for asthma is undefined because of a lack of evidence. However, 50 mg of standardized butterbur (Petaforce), administered in two divided daily doses, in patients maintained on inhaled corticosteroids has been used. Petadolex, 150 mg daily in three divided doses for 2-4 months, has also been studied.
- For migraine prophylaxis, 50-75 mg Petadolex twice daily for up to 4 months has been studied. One study suggested that the 75-mg dose but not the 50-mg dose is effective.

Children (Younger than 18 Years)

- For asthma, 50-150 mg daily (depending on age) of a pyrrolizidine-free butterbur rhizome extract standardized to 7.5 mg of petasin and isopetasin per 50-mg tablet (Petadolex) may be effective. However, because of a lack of safety and efficacy data, butterbur cannot be recommended for this or any other use in children at this time.

SAFETY
Allergies

- Avoid in individuals with a known allergy or hypersensitivity to *Petasites hybridus* or other plants from the Asteraceae/Compositae family such as ragweed, marigolds, daisies, and chrysanthemums.

Side Effects and Warnings

- Studies have reported safety and good tolerability of commercially available butterbur products (which are free of potentially carcinogenic pyrrolizidine alkaloid constituents), when used orally in recommended doses in the short-term. Raw, unprocessed butterbur plant should not be ingested because of the potential hepatotoxic (liver-damaging) effects of pyrrolizidine alkaloids with long-term use (specifically, concern of venoocclusive disease). This includes any teas, capsules of raw herb, or unprocessed tinctures or extracts. Use should be limited to commercially available products that are free of pyrrolizidine alkaloids. The plant's pyrrolizidine alkaloids are also thought to be carcinogenic (cancer causing), mutagenic, and nephrotoxic (kidney damaging).
- When taken by mouth, butterbur may cause headache, drowsiness, fatigue, itchy eyes, eye discoloration, breathing difficulties, skin discoloration, or pruritis (severe itching).
- Butterbur taken by mouth may also cause sustained constipation, discoloration of stool, dysphagia (difficulty swallowing), severe nausea, vomiting, diarrhea, or stomach upset. Butterbur may increase liver enzyme levels.

Pregnancy and Breastfeeding

- Butterbur (*Petasites hybridus*) is not recommended in women who are pregnant or breastfeeding because of a lack of safety studies.

INTERACTIONS
Interactions with Drugs

- Administration of butterbur with anticholinergics may not be advisable. Numerous drugs and drug classes may interact with anticholinergic agents. Examples include acetophenazine, amantadine, amitriptyline, atropine, benztropine, bethanechol, biperiden, brompheniramine, carbinoxamine, chlorpromazine, clemastine, clidinium, clozapine, cyclopentolate, cyproheptadine, dicyclomine, diphenhydramine, dixyrazine, ethopropazine, fenoterol, fluphenazine, haloperidol, homatropine, hyoscyamine, ipratropium, loxapine, mesoridazine, methdilazine, methotrimeprazine, olanzapine, oxybutynin, perazine, periciazine, perphenazine, pimozide, pipotiazine, prochlorperazine, procyclidine, promazine, promethazine, propiomazine, quinidine, scopolamine, thiethylperazine, thioridazine, thiothixene, trifluoperazine, triflupromazine, trihexyphenidyl, trimeprazine, triprolidine. Consult with a qualified health care professional, including a pharmacist, before taking butterbur preparations.

Interactions with Herbs and Dietary Supplements

- Raw, unprocessed butterbur may contain toxic pyrrolizidine alkaloids, although commercially available products should be free of pyrrolizidine alkaloids. Nonetheless, concomitant use of other agents containing pyrrolizidine alkaloids should be avoided because of the potential for additive toxicity.
- Combination use with anticholinergic agents may potentiate therapeutic and adverse effects. Examples of anticholinergic herbs include belladonna, bittersweet (*Solanum dulcamara*), henbane (*Hyoscyamus niger*), and Jimson weed (*Datura stramonium*).

For a complete list of references, please visit www.naturalstandard.com.

Cajeput
(Melaleuca quinquenervia)

RELATED TERMS

- Alloaromadendrene, alpha-terpineol, betulinaldehyde, betulinic acid, cajeput, cajeput essential oil, castalin, dendra, ellagic acid, flavonoids, gallic acid, grandinin, ledene, ledol, linalool, *Melaleuca*, *Melaleuca cajuputi*, *Melaleuca decora*, *Melaleuca* leaves, *Melaleuca leucadendra* (L), *Melaleuca leucadendron*, *Melaleuca leucadendron* leaf, *Melaleuca* pollen, *Melaleuca quinquenervia* leaves, *Melaleuca quinquenervia* tree, *Melaleuca* tree, *Melaleuca* tree pollen, Myrtaceae (family), niaouli, oxyresveratrol, palustrol, paper bark tree, phytol, piceatannol, platanic acid, polyphenols, punk tree, roseoside, squalene, ursolic acid, Vietnamese cajeput oil, viridiflorol.
- **Note:** Cajeput oil should not be confused with tea tree oil, although the plants are part of the same genus. According to the U.S. Department of Agriculture, *Melaleuca leucadendron* and *Melaleuca quinquenervia* refer to the same plant and this monograph may use these terms interchangeably.

BACKGROUND

- According to the U.S. Department of Agriculture, *Melaleuca leucadendron* and *Melaleuca quinquenervia* refer to the same plant.
- Cajeput (*Melaleuca quinquenervia leucadendron*, *Melaleuca leucadendron*) is a tree native to Australia. Cajeput oil is extracted from the leaves and twigs of the plant. Cajeput leaves may be useful for high blood pressure, herpes simplex, and *Helicobacter pylori* inhibition. They may also have hypoglycemic effects and may be able to lower blood sugar levels. However, currently there is not enough scientific evidence in humans to support the use of cajeput oil for any indication.

EVIDENCE

Uses Based on Scientific Evidence

No available studies qualify for inclusion in the evidence table.

Uses Based on Tradition or Theory

Anesthetic (pain blocker), antibacterial, antihistamine, antioxidant, diabetes, *Helicobacter pylori* gastric infection, herpes simplex, hypertension (high blood pressure), mosquito repellent.

DOSING
Adults (18 Years and Older)

- There is insufficient evidence to recommend a dose for cajeput oil in adults.

Children (Younger than 18 Years)

- There is insufficient evidence to recommend a dose for cajeput oil in children.

SAFETY
Allergies

- Avoid in individuals with a known allergy or hypersensitivity to cajeput. Cajeput pollen is a known allergen and may cause positive skin test reactions. In addition, there is a high cross-sensitivity between cajeput, *Paspalum notatum*, and *Callistemon citrinus* pollen.

Side Effects and Warnings

- There are very few reported adverse effects associated with cajeput. Nonetheless, use cautiously in patients with diabetes, hypoglycemia (low blood sugar levels), or high or low blood pressure. Leaves harvested from certain areas of the world may contain carcinogenic (cancer-causing) chemicals.

Pregnancy and Breastfeeding

- Cajeput oil is not recommended in pregnant or breastfeeding women because of a lack of available scientific evidence.

INTERACTIONS
Interactions with Drugs

- In theory, cajeput oil may intensify local anesthetic power when combined with other anesthetics.
- Although not well studied in humans, cajeput may have potential interactions with antibiotics, antihistamines, antioxidants, or mosquito repellent agents. Consult a qualified health care professional, including a pharmacist, to check for interactions.
- Cajeput oil may lower blood sugar levels. Caution is advised in patients with diabetes or hypoglycemia (low blood sugar levels) and in those taking drugs that affect blood sugar. Serum glucose levels may need to be monitored by a qualified health care professional, including a pharmacist, and medication adjustments may be necessary.
- Cajeput may inhibit the growth of *Helicobacter pylori*. Use cautiously with ulcer medications. Cajeput fruit may also inhibit herpes simplex 1, and an interaction is possible when it is taken in combination with other antiviral agents. In addition, early evidence suggests that cajeput leaves may alter blood pressure. Use cautiously in patients taking blood pressure medications.
- Cajeput may interfere with the way the body processes certain drugs using the liver's cytochrome P450 enzyme system. As a result, the levels of these drugs may be increased in the blood and may cause increased effects or potentially serious adverse reactions. Patients using any medications should check the package insert and speak with a qualified health care professional, including a pharmacist, about possible interactions.

Interactions with Herbs and Dietary Supplements

- In theory, cajeput oil may intensify local anesthetic power when combined with other anesthetic herbs or supplements.
- Although not well studied in humans, cajeput may have potential interactions with antibiotics, antihistamines,

antioxidants, or mosquito repellent herbs or supplements. Consult a qualified health care professional, including a pharmacist, to check for interactions.

- Cajeput oil may lower blood sugar levels. Caution is advised when herbs or supplements that may also lower blood sugar are used. Blood glucose levels may require monitoring, and doses may need adjustment.
- Cajeput may inhibit the growth of *Helicobacter pylori*. Use cautiously with herbs and supplements used to manage ulcers. Cajeput fruit may also inhibit herpes simplex 1, and an interaction is possible when it is taken in combination with other antiviral herbs and supplements. In addition, early evidence suggests that cajeput leaves may alter blood pressure. Use cautiously in patients taking blood pressure–altering herbs and supplements.
- Cajeput may interfere with the way the body processes certain herbs or supplements using the liver's cytochrome P450 enzyme system. As a result, the levels of other herbs or supplements may become too high in the blood. It may also alter the effects that other herbs or supplements possibly have on the P450 system.

For a complete list of references, please visit www. naturalstandard.com.

Calamus
(Acorus calamus)

RELATED TERMS

- Acoraceae (family), acorenone, Acori graminei rhizoma, acorone, *Acorus calamus* L., *Acorus calamus* L. essential oils, *Acorus calamus* Linn. var. *angustatus Bess*, *Acorus calamus* var. *angustatus Bess*, *Acorus gramineus* Sol. ex Aiton, *Acorus gramineus* Soland, *Acorus tatarinowii*, *Acorus tatarinowii* Schott, alkaloids, Araceae (family), aromatic calamus, asarone, bach, bicyclogermacrene, bornyl acetate, calamendiol, calamenone, *Calamus aromaticus*, calamus rhizome, calarene, camphene, camphor, caryophyllene, cedrol, changpo, changpo oil, cinnamon sedge, flagroot, flavonoids, germacrene A, gladdon, grass myrtle, gums, kamseh-chang, khusiol, lectins, limonene, linalool, lin-ne, methyl linoleate, mucilage, myrcene, myrtle flag, myrtle sedge, phenols, prezizaene, quinone, rat root, rattan palm, Romanian *Acorus calamus* L., sabinene, saponins, shi chang pu, shuichangpu, squamulosone, sweet calamus, sweet cane, sweet flag, sweet grass, sweet myrtle, sweet root, sweet rush, sweet sedge, sweetflag, sweetflag oil, tannins, terpinolene, torilenol, triterpenes, ugragandha, vacha, vaj, vekhand.

BACKGROUND

- *Acorus calamus* L. (family Araceae/Acoraceae) has long, narrow leaves and an aromatic rootstock. It is similar to the iris in appearance and can be found in moist habitats such as the banks of ponds or streams and swamps in North America, Europe, and Asia.
- Traditional medicine includes use of the rhizome, and the herb's main traditional uses include therapy for colic, dyspepsia (upset stomach), and flatulence (gas). In Ayurveda there is major use of calamus for diseases of the kidney and liver, eczema, rheumatism, and enhancement of memory. Currently, traditional uses lack substantiation in the available medical literature. Vomiting was the primary toxicity reported following use of the root for assumed production of euphoria.

EVIDENCE

Uses Based on Scientific Evidence

No available studies qualify for inclusion in the evidence table.

Uses Based on Tradition or Theory

Alveolitis, antiaging, antibacterial, anticonvulsive, antifungal, antiinflammatory, antimicrobial, antioxidant, antispasmodic, anxiety (neurosis), aphrodisiac, arrhythmia (irregular heartbeat), blood flow disorders (ischemia), brighten dreams, bronchitis, cancer, cognitive improvement (old age), colic, convulsions, cough, diabetes, diarrhea, digestive, drug addiction (nicotine), epilepsy, fever (remittent), flavoring (tea), general health maintenance, gout, heavy metal/lead toxicity (nickel), hemorrhoids, hyperlipidemia (high cholesterol levels), hysteria, immunomodulation, indigestion, inflammation, insect repellant, insecticide, insomnia, learning, memory loss, mental disorders, myiasis (infestation of tissue by fly larvae), neural protective, neuropathy (numbness), sedation, skin diseases, sleep aid, spasmolytic (for spasms), stress reduction, systemic sclerosis (chronic disease characterized by excessive deposits of collagen), tranquilizer, tuberculosis (bacterial infection of the lungs), tumors, ulcer, vitality problems.

DOSING

Adults (18 Years and Older)

- There is insufficient evidence to recommend a dose for calamus.

Children (Younger than 18 Years)

- There is insufficient evidence to recommend a dose for calamus in children.

SAFETY

Allergies

- Avoid in individuals with a known allergy or hypersensitivity to calamus.

Side Effects and Warnings

- Calamus may cause stomach upset. Use cautiously for relief of stomach complaints in children.
- Skin rash may occur with the oil.

Pregnancy and Breastfeeding

- Calamus is not recommended in pregnant or breastfeeding women because of a lack of available scientific evidence.

INTERACTIONS

Interactions with Drugs

- Use cautiously in cancer patients or patients taking antineoplastic agents as the effects of calamus on cancer are controversial.
- Calamus may increase constipation from calcium channel blockers.
- Calamus may affect heart rhythm and interact with heart medications, such as digoxin. Thus, use cautiously in patients with heart problems or taking heart medications.
- Calamus may also interact with immunostimulating agents, hypnotics (i.e., barbiturates), antispasmodic agents, antifungals, antibiotics, amphetamines, cholesterol-lowering agents, antiinflammatory agents, anticholinergics, or antioxidant agents. Consult with a qualified health care professional, including a pharmacist, to check for interactions.

Interactions with Herbs and Dietary Supplements

- Use cautiously in cancer patients or patients taking herbs or supplements with anticancer effects as the effects of calamus on cancer are controversial.

- Calamus may affect heart rhythm and interact with herbs and supplements that alter the heart, such as foxglove.
- Calamus may also interact with immunostimulating herbs and supplements, hypnotics (i.e., barbiturates), antispasmodic herbs and supplements, antifungals, antibacterials, amphetamines, cholesterol-lowering herbs and supplements, antiinflammatory agents, anticholinergics, or antioxidant herbs and supplements. Consult with a qualified health care professional, including a pharmacist, to check for interactions.

For a complete list of references, please visit www.naturalstandard.com.

Calcium

RELATED TERMS

- AdvaCAL, Alka-Mints, Apo-Cal, atomic number 20, Bica, Bo-Ne-Ca, bone meal, bovine cartilage, Ca, Cal-100, Calcanate, Calcefor, Calci Aid, Calci-Fresh, Calcigamma, Calcilos, Calcimax, Calcit, calcitonin, Calcitridin, calcitriol, calcium acetate, calcium aspartate, calcium carbonate, calcium chelate, calcium chloride, calcium citrate, calcium citrate malate, Calcium Dago (Germany), calcium formate, calcium gluceptate, calcium gluconate, Calcium Klopfer (Austria), calcium lactate, calcium lactate gluconate, calcium lactogluconate, calcium orotate, calcium oxalate, Calcium Pharmavit (Hungary), calcium phosphate, calcium pyruvate, Calcium-Sandoz Forte (Bulgaria), Calcuren (Finland), Caldoral (Colombia), Calmate 500 (Philippines), CalMax, Calmicid, Cal-Quick, Calsan (Mexico, Peru, Philippines), Calsup, Cal-Sup (New Zealand), Caltab (Thailand), Caltrate, Cantacid (Korea), Cartilade, CC-Nefro 500 (Germany), Chooz, Chooz Antacid Gum 500 (Israel), Citrical, coral calcium, dairy products (milk, cheese, yogurt, etc.), dicalcium phosphate, Dimacid, dolomite, Estroven, Fixical (France), Gaviscon, heated oyster shell-seaweed calcium, hydroxyapatite, (oral 44Ca and intravenous 42Ca), isotopically enriched milk, LeanBalance, Living Calcium, Maalox, Maalox Quick Dissolve (Canada), magnesium, Netra (Israel), Neutralin, Noacid (Uruguay), nonfat milk, Orocal (France), Os-Cal, Ospur Ca 500 (Germany), Osteocal 500 (France), osteocalcin, osteocalcin concentration, Osteomin (Mexico), OsteoPrime, Osteo Wisdom, oyster shell calcium, oyster shell electrolysate (OSE), Pepcid Complete, Pluscal (Argentina), Posture-D, Renacal (Germany), Rocaltrol, Rolaids, salmon calcitonin, Sandocal, shark cartilage, tricalcium phosphate, Tums, Tzarevet X (Israel), Viactiv.

BACKGROUND

- The Romans used lime (calcium oxide), slacked lime (calcium hydroxide), and hydraulic cement in construction works. Calcium (Latin *calx*, meaning *lime*) was first isolated in its metallic form by Sir Humphrey Davy in 1808 through the electrolysis of a mixture of calcium oxide and mercury oxide.
- Chelated calcium refers to the way in which calcium is chemically combined with another substance. Calcium citrate is an example of such a chelated preparation. Calcium may also be combined with other substances to form preparations such as calcium lactate or calcium gluconate. Calcium carbonate can be refined from limestone, natural elements of the earth, or from shell sources, such as oyster. Shell sources are often described on the label as a "natural" source. Calcium carbonate from oyster shells is not "refined" and can contain variable amounts of lead.
- Calcium is the most abundant mineral in the human body and has several important functions. More than 99% of total body calcium is stored in the bones and teeth, where it supports the structure. The remaining 1% is found throughout the body in blood, muscle, and the intracellular fluid. Calcium is needed for muscle contraction, blood vessel constriction and relaxation, the secretion of hormones and enzymes, and nervous system signaling. A constant level of calcium is maintained in body fluid and tissues so that these vital body processes function efficiently.
- The body gets the calcium it needs in two ways. One method is dietary intake of calcium-rich foods including dairy products, which have the highest concentration per serving of highly absorbable calcium, and dark, leafy greens or dried beans, which have varying amounts of absorbable calcium. Calcium is an essential nutrient required in substantial amounts, but many diets are deficient in calcium.
- The other way the body obtains calcium is by extracting it from bones. This happens when blood levels of calcium drop too low and dietary calcium is not sufficient. Ideally, the calcium that is taken from the bones will be replaced when calcium levels are replenished. However, simply eating more calcium-rich foods does not necessarily replace lost bone calcium, which leads to weakened bone structure.
- Hypocalcemia is defined as a low level of calcium in the blood. Symptoms of this condition include sensations of tingling, numbness, and muscle twitches. In severe cases, tetany (muscle spasms) may occur. Hypocalcemia is more likely to be due to a hormonal imbalance that regulates calcium levels rather than a dietary deficiency. Excess calcium in the blood can cause nausea, vomiting, and calcium deposition in the heart and kidneys. This usually results from excessive doses of vitamin D and can be fatal in infants.
- The Surgeon General's 2004 report "Bone Health and Osteoporosis" stated that calcium has been singled out as a major public health concern today because it is critically important to bone health and the average American consumes levels of calcium that are far below the amount recommended. Vitamin D is important for good bone health because it aids in the absorption and utilization of calcium. There is a high prevalence of vitamin D insufficiency in nursing home residents, hospitalized patients, and adults with hip fractures.
- Calcium supplements are widely used to reduce bone resorption in osteoporosis, and many studies support this use. Calcium supplementation is also used for colorectal neoplasia and in pregnancy.

EVIDENCE

Uses Based on Scientific evidence	Grade
Antacid (Calcium Carbonate) Calcium carbonate is a U.S. Food and Drug Administration (FDA)–approved over-the-counter (OTC) drug used to treat gastric hyperacidity (high acid levels in the stomach).	A
Bone Loss (Prevention) Multiple studies of calcium supplementation in the elderly and postmenopausal women have found that high calcium intakes can help reduce the loss of bone	A

Uses Based on Scientific evidence	Grade
density. Studies have indicated that bone loss could be prevented in many areas, including ankles, hips, and spine.	
Cardiopulmonary Resuscitation (CPR) Calcium chloride may be given intravenously (IV) by a qualified health care professional in cardiac resuscitation, particularly after open-heart surgery, when epinephrine fails to improve weak or ineffective myocardial contractions. Calcium chloride is contraindicated for cardiac resuscitation in the presence of ventricular fibrillation. CPR with calcium chloride should only be done under the supervision of a qualified health care professional.	A
Deficiency (Calcium) Calcium gluconate is used to treat conditions arising from calcium deficiencies such as hypocalcemia (low blood calcium), tetany (muscle spasms), hypocalcemia related to hypoparathyroidism (low levels of the parathyroid hormone), and hypocalcemia due to rapid growth or pregnancy. It is also used for the treatment of hypocalcemia for conditions requiring a prompt increase in plasma calcium levels (e.g., tetany in newborns and tetany due to parathyroid deficiency, vitamin D deficiency, and alkalosis) and for the prevention of hypocalcemia during exchange transfusions. Treatment of hypocalcemia should only be done under supervision of a qualified health care professional.	A
High Blood Phosphorous Level Hyperphosphatemia (high phosphate level in the blood) is associated with increased cardiovascular mortality in adult dialysis patients. Calcium carbonate or acetate can be used effectively as phosphate binders. Use may increase calcium phosphate products in blood. Treatment of high blood phosphorous levels should only be done under supervision of a qualified health care professional.	A
Osteoporosis Osteoporosis is a disorder of the skeleton in which bone strength is reduced, resulting in an increased risk of fracture. Although osteoporosis is most commonly diagnosed in white postmenopausal women, women of other racial groups and ages, men, and children may also develop osteoporosis. Calcium is the nutrient consistently found to be the most important for attaining peak bone mass and preventing osteoporosis. Adequate vitamin D intake is required for optimal calcium absorption. Adequate calcium and vitamin D are deemed essential for the prevention of osteoporosis in general, including postmenopausal osteoporosis. Although calcium and vitamin D alone are not recommended as the sole treatment of osteoporosis, they are necessary additions to pharmaceutical treatments. The vast majority of clinical trials investigating the efficacy of	A
pharmaceutical treatments for osteoporosis have investigated these agents in combination with calcium and vitamin D. So, although calcium alone is unlikely to have an effect on the rate of bone loss following menopause, osteoporosis cannot be treated in the absence of calcium. Treatment of postmenopausal osteoporosis should only be done under supervision of a qualified health care professional.	
Toxicity (Magnesium) Calcium gluconate is used in the treatment of hypermagnesemia (high levels of magnesium in the blood). Case studies suggest intravenous calcium can aid in the improvement of symptoms. Treatment of magnesium toxicity should only be done under supervision of a qualified health care professional.	A
Black Widow Spider Bite Calcium supplementation is used in the treatment of black widow spider bites to relieve muscle cramping in combination with antiserum, analgesics (pain relievers), and muscle relaxants. Treatment of a black widow spider bite should only be done under the supervision of a qualified health care professional.	B
High Blood Potassium Level Calcium gluconate may aid in antagonizing the cardiac toxicity and arrhythmia (abnormal heart rhythm) associated with hyperkalemia (high blood potassium), provided the patient is not receiving digitalis drug therapy. Treatment of hyperkalemia should only be done under supervision of a qualified health care professional.	B
High Blood Pressure Several studies have found that introducing calcium to the system can have hypotensive (blood pressure–lowering) effects. These studies indicate that high calcium levels lead to sodium loss in the urine and lowered parathyroid hormone (PTH) levels, both of which result in the lowering of blood pressure. However, one study found that these results did not hold true for middle-aged patients with mild to moderate essential hypertension. In the DASH (Dietary Approaches to Stop Hypertension) study, three servings per day of calcium-enriched low-fat dairy products reduced systolic and diastolic blood pressure. This research indicates that a calcium intake at the recommended level may be helpful in preventing and treating moderate hypertension. Treatment of high blood pressure should only be done under supervision of a qualified health care professional.	B
Premenstrual Syndrome (PMS) There is a link between lower dietary intake of calcium and symptoms of premenstrual syndrome. Calcium supplementation has been suggested in various clinical trials to decrease overall symptoms associated with PMS, such as depressed mood, water retention, and pain.	B

(Continued)

Uses Based on Scientific evidence	Grade
Bone Stress Injury Prevention Calcium supplementation above normal daily dietary intake did not reduce stress fractures in men. Thus calcium supplementation may not be effective in preventing stress fractures, but further studies must be done to validate these results.	C
Colorectal Cancer Colorectal cancer is the most common gastrointestinal cancer and the second leading cause of cancer deaths in the United States. Colorectal cancer is caused by a combination of genetic and environmental factors, but the degree to which these two factors influence the risk of colon cancer in individuals varies. Most large prospective studies have found increased calcium intake to be only weakly associated with a decreased risk of colorectal cancer. Further studies are needed to verify these results. Treatment of colorectal cancer should only be done under the supervision of a qualified health care professional.	C
Growth (Mineral Metabolism in Very Low Birth Weight Infants) Growth of very low birth weight infants correlates with calcium intake and retention in the body. It is possible that human milk fortifiers commonly used may have inadequate levels of calcium for infants of very low birth weight. Bone mineralization is also lower in very low birth weight infants at theoretical term than in infants born at term. Use of a formula containing higher levels of calcium has been suggested to allow improved bone mineralization in these infants.	C
High Blood Pressure (Pregnancy-Induced) For the general population, meeting current recommendations for calcium intake during pregnancy may help prevent pregnancy-induced high blood pressure (PIH). Further research is required to determine whether women at high risk of PIH would benefit from calcium supplementation above the current recommendations. Treatment of PIH should only be done under supervision of a qualified health care professional.	C
Hyperparathyroidism (Secondary) In patients undergoing hemodialysis, calcium supplementation may reduce secondary hyperparathyroidism (high blood levels of parathyroid hormone caused by another medical condition or treatment). Treatment of hyperparathyroidism should only be done under the supervision of a qualified health care professional.	C
Lead Toxicity (Acute Symptom Management) A chelating treatment of calcium has been suggested to reduce blood levels of lead in cases of lead toxicity. Reduced symptoms have been observed in most, but not all, patient case reports and case histories. Adequate	C

calcium intake appears to be protective against lead toxicity. Treatment of lead toxicity should only be done under the supervision of a qualified health care professional.

Osteomalacia/Rickets Rickets and osteomalacia (bone softening) are commonly thought of as diseases caused by vitamin D deficiency; however, calcium deficiency may also be another cause in sunny areas of the world where vitamin D deficiency would not be expected. Calcium gluconate is used as an adjuvant in the treatment of rickets and osteomalacia, as well as a single therapeutic agent in non–vitamin D deficient rickets. Research continues into the importance of calcium alone in the treatment and prevention of rickets and osteomalacia. Treatment of rickets and osteomalacia should only be done under the supervision of a qualified health care professional.	C
Osteoporosis Prevention (Steroid-Induced) Calcium supplementation in patients taking long-term, high-dose inhaled steroids for asthma may reduce bone loss resulting from steroid intake. Treatment with the use of the prescription drug pamidronate with calcium has been shown to be superior to calcium alone in the prevention of corticosteroid-induced osteoporosis. Inhaled steroids have been reported to disturb normal bone metabolism, and they are associated with a decrease in bone mineral density. Results suggest that long-term administration of high-dose inhaled steroids induces bone loss that is preventable with calcium supplementation with or without the prescription drug etidronate. Long-term studies involving more patients should be done to confirm these preliminary findings.	C
Prostate Cancer (Increased Risk) The lack of agreement among studies suggests complex interactions among risk factors for prostate cancer. Until the relationship between calcium and prostate cancer is clarified, it is reasonable for men to consume recommended intakes as per the Food and Nutrition Board of the Institute of Medicine. Treatment of prostate cancer should only be done under the supervision of a qualified health care professional.	C
Weight Loss Diets with higher calcium density (high levels of calcium per total calories) have been associated with a reduced incidence of being overweight or obese in several studies. Although more research is needed to understand the relationships between calcium intake and body fat, these findings emphasize the importance of maintaining adequate calcium intake while attempting to diet or lose weight.	C
Vaginal Disorders (Atrophy, Wasting, or Thinning of the Vaginal Tissue) Stopping treatment with topical hormone replacement therapy and switching to treatment with	D

Uses Based on Scientific evidence	Grade
calcium plus vitamin D made vaginal atrophy worse in one study. Increases in painful or difficult intercourse and urinary leaks were reported. Menopausal complaints of hot flashes and night sweats were also worse than before calcium plus vitamin D therapy.	

Uses Based on Tradition or Theory

Bone density improvement (lactating women), bone loss, carcinoma, cardiac arrest, diarrhea, high cholesterol levels, intestinal disorders, ischemic stroke (prevention), leg cramps (pregnancy), medullary thyroid cancer (diagnosis), multiple sclerosis, neuromuscular blockade (antagonism), psoriasis, reducing fluoride levels (children), Zollinger-Ellison (diagnosis).

DOSING
General

- A good food source of calcium contains a substantial amount of calcium in relation to its calorie content and contributes at least 10% of the U.S. recommended dietary allowance (RDA) for calcium in a selected serving size. The RDA for calcium is 1000 mg/day for adults (except pregnant or lactating women) and children older than 4 years and is used as the standard in nutrition labeling of foods. This allowance is based on the 1968 RDA for 24 sex-age categories set by the Food and Nutrition Board of the National Academy of Sciences. Adequate intake (AI) recommendations published in August 1997 were set at 1000 mg for men and women aged 19-50 and 1200 mg for individuals older than 50 years.

Adults (18 Years and Older)

- Doses ranging from 400-3000 mg daily of a calcium supplement have been taken by mouth in several studies. Note that there are many forms available. Different conditions may require unique dosing and should be discussed with a qualified health care provider. Intravenous (through the vein) calcium may be given by a qualified health care provider.

Children (Younger than 18 Years)

- Healthy adolescents have received a calcium supplement containing 1000 mg daily as calcium citrate malate for 14 days or 1000 mg effervescent calcium tablet daily. A dose of 850 mg daily calcium has also been given orally to prepubescent boys in food products. Special dosing may be recommended by a qualified health care provider for certain indications.

SAFETY
Allergies

- Avoid in individuals with a known allergy or hypersensitivity to calcium supplements or any of their ingredients. Some people are lactose intolerant. Dairy products contain lactose, and dairy products are a common food source of calcium. Lactose intolerance can cause cramping, bloating, gas, and diarrhea. Lactose intolerance affects the population in varying degrees.

- Avoid calcium supplementation in those who are very sensitive to any component of a calcium-containing supplement or who have hypercalcemia (high levels of calcium in the blood). Conditions causing hypercalcemia include sarcoidosis (inflammation in the lymph nodes and other organs), hyperparathyroidism (high levels of parathyroid hormone), and hypervitaminosis D (high levels of vitamin D).

Side Effects and Warnings

- Calcium supplementation is likely safe when used orally and intravenously, as recommended by a qualified health care professional. It is also likely safe when used orally and appropriately in pregnancy and lactation, as recommended by a qualified health care professional. Routine dietary intake and supplementation in recommended doses are not associated with significant adverse effects.

- Avoid calcium supplements made from dolomite, oyster shells, or bone meal because such compounds may contain unacceptable levels of lead. Avoid in patients with hypercalcemia (high blood levels of calcium), hypercalciuria (high levels of calcium in urine), hyperparathyroidism (high levels of parathyroid hormone), bone tumors, digitalis toxicity, ventricular fibrillation (ventricles of the heart contract in unsynchronized rhythm), kidney stones (renal calculi), kidney disease or disorders, and sarcoidosis (inflammation of lymph nodes and various other tissues).

- Excretion of abnormally large amounts of calcium in the urine is a well-established side effect of administration.

- Low levels of calcium in the blood and tissues can cause sensations of tingling, numbness, muscle twitches, and muscle spasms (tetany). This condition is more likely to be due to a hormonal imbalance in the regulation of calcium rather than a dietary deficiency.

- Excess calcium in the blood can be without symptoms or it can cause loss of appetite, nausea, vomiting, constipation, abdominal pain, dry mouth, thirst, frequent urination, and calcium deposition in the heart and kidneys. More severe hypercalcemia may result in confusion, delirium, coma, and, if not treated, death. Hypercalcemia has been reported only with the consumption of large quantities of calcium supplements usually in combination with antacids, particularly in the past when peptic ulcers were treated with large quantities of milk, calcium carbonate (antacid), and sodium bicarbonate (absorbable alkali).

- Avoid high doses of calcium without food in those who are prone to the formation of calcium-containing kidney stones, as calcium supplementation in the absence of food may be associated with an increased risk of calcium oxalate stone formation. Consult a qualified health care professional if you are prone to kidney stones before using calcium supplements.

- Use cautiously in those with achlorhydria (absence of hydrochloric acid [HCl] in gastric juices) as low levels of gastric acid during digestion reduces urinary phosphate and calcium excretion. It may be advisable to take calcium carbonate with food to stimulate gastric acid production. Consult a qualified health care provider.

- Avoid cigarette smoking, as this decreases intestinal calcium absorption and may lead to decreased bone mineral density.

- Use cautiously in those taking large amounts of vitamin D. Excess calcium in the blood (hypercalcemia) can cause nausea, vomiting and calcium deposition in the heart and kidneys. This usually results from excessive doses of vitamin D and can be fatal in infants. Consult a qualified health care provider.

- Use cautiously in individuals with heart arrhythmias and ventricular fibrillation (irregular heart beating). Large fluctuations in free calcium during intravenous calcium infusion can cause the heart to slow down or beat too rapidly. Although calcium appears to have benefits for bone density and osteoporosis, calcium should be used cautiously in postmenopausal women because of an increased possibility of cardiovascular side effects. Consult a qualified health care provider.

Pregnancy and Breastfeeding

- The Standing Committee on the Scientific Evaluation of Dietary Reference Intakes, Food, and Nutrition Board suggests that current calcium recommendations for nonpregnant women are also sufficient for pregnant women because intestinal calcium absorption increases during pregnancy.
- Pregnant women are especially vulnerable to accelerated bone turnover because of the physiological stress of pregnancy and lactation. Studies indicate that pregnant women should take calcium supplements to prevent bone density loss. The National Academy of Sciences recommends that women who are pregnant or breastfeeding consume calcium each day. For pregnant teens, the recommended intake is higher.
- Consult a qualified health care professional to determine dosing during pregnancy and breastfeeding.

INTERACTIONS
Interactions with Drugs

- Intestinal aluminum absorption is increased in healthy and kidney failure patients taking even small amounts of calcium citrate. As a result, all citrate-containing preparations are contraindicated in chronic renal failure patients taking aluminum-containing compounds.
- Anticonvulsants decrease calcium absorption by increasing the metabolism of vitamin D. Anticonvulsant intake can lead to hypocalcemia (low blood calcium) and softening of the bones (osteomalacia).
- Intake of a bisphosphonate and calcium may decrease the absorption of the bisphosphonate. Patients should take bisphosphonates at least 30 minutes before calcium. Optimally, the two would be consumed at different times of the day.
- Caffeine may increase urinary calcium excretion and has been implicated in osteoporosis; however, research is still conflicting. Caffeine has a small effect on calcium absorption.
- Calcitriol is a form of vitamin D that is used to treat and prevent low levels of calcium in the blood of patients whose kidneys or parathyroid glands (glands in the neck that release natural substances to control the amount of calcium in the blood) are not working normally.
- When given intravenously, calcium can reverse the effects of calcium channel blockers (commonly used for high blood pressure). Calcium channel blockers include nifedipine (Adalat, Procardia), verapamil (Calan, Isopin, Verelan), diltiazem (Cardizem), isradipine (DynaCirc), felodipine (Plendil), and amlodipine (Norvasc).
- Cholestyramine (commonly used for high cholesterol) can reduce the absorption of vitamin D, which, in turn, reduces the absorption of calcium.

- Corticosteroids (commonly used for inflammation) can cause significant bone loss (osteoporosis) if the recommended level of calcium and vitamin D intake is not met.
- Calcium levels should be monitored if the heart rhythm medication digoxin is taken because of the potential for interaction with high blood levels of calcium and the need for adequate blood levels of calcium. Patients taking digoxin should consult with a qualified health care professional before using calcium supplements.
- Alcohol can affect calcium status by reducing the intestinal absorption of calcium. It can also inhibit enzymes in the liver that help convert vitamin D to its active form, which in turn reduces calcium absorption. However, the amount of alcohol required to affect calcium absorption is unknown. Evidence is currently conflicting on whether moderate alcohol consumption is helpful or harmful to bone.
- Fluoroquinolone antibiotics form complexes with calcium in the gastrointestinal tract, which can lead to reduced absorption of both if taken at the same time.
- Use of H_2 blockers (commonly used to treat acid reflux), such as ranitidine, at the same time as calcium carbonate or calcium phosphate may interfere with the absorption of these calcium salts.
- Hormone replacement therapy (HRT) alone may be associated with a fall in calcium absorption efficiency. However, the bone-preserving effects of estrogen treatment are increased by calcium supplementation. Estrogen increases supplemental calcium absorption in postmenopausal women.
- Use of inositol hexaphosphate (phytic acid) and calcium may decrease the absorption of calcium.
- Mineral oil or stimulant laxatives (cascara, senna, and bisacodyl), when used for prolonged periods, can reduce dietary calcium and vitamin D absorption, often causing osteomalacia (bone softening).
- Intake of levothyroxine (Synthroid, Levothroid, Levoxyl) at the same time as calcium carbonate has been found to reduce levothyroxine absorption and to increase serum thyrotropin levels. Levothyroxine may adsorb (stick) to calcium carbonate in an acidic environment, which may block its absorption.
- Loop diuretics, including furosemide (Lasix), bumetanide (Bumex), ethacrynic acid (Edecrin), and torsemide (Demadex), at high doses may reduce serum calcium levels because they increase urinary calcium excretion.
- Orlistat (Xenical) has been shown to induce a relative increase in bone turnover (increased resorption or bone loss), which may be due to the malabsorption of vitamin D and/or calcium.
- The effect of dietary phosphorus on calcium is minimal. Some researchers speculate that the detrimental effects of consuming foods high in phosphate such as carbonated soft drinks is due to the replacement of milk with soda rather than the phosphate level itself.
- Increasing dietary potassium intake in the presence of a low sodium diet may help decrease calcium excretion, particularly in postmenopausal women.
- Use of proton pump inhibitors (to treat ulcers), such as esomeprazole, and calcium carbonate or calcium phosphate at the same time can cause decreased absorption of these calcium salts.
- Typically, dietary sodium and protein increase calcium excretion as their intake is increased. However, if a high-

protein, high-sodium food also contains calcium, this may help counteract the loss of calcium.

- Calcium may form complexes with sotalol (a beta-blocker drug used to treat irregular heartbeats), which reduces its absorption. A physician should be contacted to determine optimal timing of doses. Patients taking sotalol should consult a qualified health care professional before using calcium supplements.
- Intake of a tetracycline and calcium may decrease the absorption of the tetracycline, including doxycycline, minocycline, and tetracycline. Allow 2-4 hours between the intake of tetracyclines and calcium supplements.
- Thiazides are diuretics that reduce calcium excretion by the kidneys. These diuretics include chlorothiazide (Diuril), hydrochlorothiazide (HydroDIURIL, Esidrix), indapamide (Lozol), metolazone (Zaroxolyn), and chlorthalidone (Hygroton).
- An interaction between levothyroxine (a thyroid hormone) and calcium carbonate is also possible.

Interactions with Herbs and Dietary Supplements

- Calcium carbonate and aluminum hydroxide taken together have produced a significant rise in serum and urine aluminum levels.
- Combined use of inositol hexaphosphate (phytic acid) and calcium may decrease the absorption of calcium.
- Inulin, found in fresh cheese, does not appear to acutely affect serum ionized calcium concentrations.
- Stimulant laxatives (cascara, senna, and bisacodyl) when used for prolonged periods can reduce dietary calcium and vitamin D absorption, often causing osteomalacia (bone softening).
- Combining calcium salts may increase absorption or alter efficacy.
- Large doses of magnesium salts can cause hypocalcemia (low levels of blood calcium). Oral magnesium supplements do not affect calcium absorption.
- Combined use of iron and calcium may not inhibit the absorption of iron over long periods of time. Combined use of fluoride, magnesium, or zinc and calcium may decrease the absorption of these minerals. However, these possible mineral interactions have not been shown to be of clinical significance.
- Mineral oil can interfere with calcium utilization and retention by reducing the absorption of calcium and vitamin D.
- Combined use of nondigestible fructooligosaccharides or inulin and calcium may increase the absorption of calcium in the colon.
- Calcium taken orally can bind with phosphate in the gut, which prevents its absorption and reduce the hyperphosphatemia (high levels of phosphate in the blood) associated with renal failure. Calcium carbonate or calcium acetate is used for this purpose, whereas calcium citrate is not recommended because it increases aluminum absorption.
- Although the effects of high phosphorus intakes on calcium balance and bone health are presently unclear, the substitution of large quantities of soft drinks for milk or other sources of dietary calcium is cause for concern with respect to bone health in adolescents and adults. The effect of dietary phosphorus on calcium is minimal.
- Reports show that increased sodium intake results in increased loss of calcium in the urine, which suggests that an effect of reducing bone loss by increasing calcium supplementation can also be achieved by reducing sodium intake.
- Intake of sodium alginate and calcium may decrease the absorption of calcium.
- Excessive vitamin A use has also been found to alter bone turnover. Too much preformed vitamin A can promote fractures. Avoid vitamin supplements that have large amounts of vitamin A as preformed vitamin A, unless prescribed by a doctor. Vitamin A in the form of beta-carotene does not appear to increase one's fracture risk.
- Use of vitamin D and calcium increases the absorption of calcium. Vitamin D is important and recommended for optimal calcium absorption.

For a complete list of references, please visit www.naturalstandard.com.

Calendula
(Calendula officinalis)

RELATED TERMS

- Alloocimene, Asteraceae (family), bride of the sun, bull flower, butterwort, *Calendula arvensis* L., *Calendula micrantha*, *Calendula officinalis*, calendula flower, calendula herb, *Calendulae flos*, *Calendulae herba*, *Caltha officinalis*, Calypso Orange Florensis, cis-tagetone, claveton (Spanish), Compositae (family), cowbloom, death-flower, dihydrotagetone, drunkard gold, Fiesta Gitana Gelb, fior d'ogni (Italian), flaminquillo (Spanish), fleurs de tous les mois (French), gauche-fer (French), gold bloom, goldblume (German), golden flower of Mary, goulans, gouls, holligold, holygold, husband's dial, kingscup, Laser Activated Calendula Extract (LACE), limonene, lutein, maravilla, marybud, marigold, marigold dye, marigold flowers, May Orange Florensis, marygold, mejorana (Spanish), methyl chavicol, patuletin, patulitrin, piperitenone, piperitone, poet's marigold, pot marigold, publican and sinner, Ringelblume (German), ruddles, Scotch marigold, shining herb, solsequia, souci (French), souci des champs (French), souci des jardins (French), summer's bride, sun's bride, water dragon, yolk of egg.
- **Note:** Calendula or marigold should not be confused with the common garden or French marigold (*Tagetes* spp.).

BACKGROUND

- Calendula, also known as marigold, has been widely used on the skin to treat minor wounds, skin infections, burns, bee stings, sunburn, warts, and cancer. Most scientific evidence regarding its effectiveness as a wound-healing agent is based on animal and laboratory study, while human research is virtually lacking.
- One study in breast cancer patients receiving radiation therapy suggests that calendula ointment may be helpful in preventing skin dermatitis (irritation, redness, and pain).

EVIDENCE

Uses Based on Scientific Evidence	Grade
Radiation Skin Protection Women receiving radiation therapy to the breast for breast cancer, when using calendula ointment applied to the skin at least twice daily during treatment, have reduced dermatitis (skin irritation, redness, pain). However, this evidence cannot be considered conclusive because of limitations of its design. Based on this evidence, however, calendula may be considered in patients who experience radiation dermatitis that cannot be controlled with other therapies.	B
Ear Infection Calendula has been studied for reducing pain caused by ear infections, although the effectiveness is uncertain. Some human studies suggest that calendula may possess mild anesthetic (pain-relieving)	C
properties equal to those of similar nonherbal eardrop preparations.	
Skin Inflammation Limited animal research suggests that calendula extracts may reduce inflammation when applied to the skin. Human studies are lacking in this area.	C
Venous Leg Ulcers Calendula has been suggested as a possible treatment for venous leg ulcers; however, supportive evidence is insufficient.	C
Wound and Burn Healing Calendula is commonly used on the skin to treat minor skin wounds; however, supportive evidence is insufficient.	C

Uses Based on Tradition or Theory

Abscesses, acne, anemia, antiinflammatory, antioxidant, antiviral, anxiety, appetite stimulant, atherosclerosis (clogged arteries), athlete's foot, bacterial infections, benign prostatic hypertrophy, bladder irritation, blood purification, blood vessel clots, bowel irritation, bruises, cancer, cholera, circulation problems, conjunctivitis, constipation, contact dermatitis, cosmetic, cough, cramps, detoxification (purging agent), diabetes, diaper rash, diaphoresis (sweating), diarrhea, diuretic, dizziness, dystrophic nervous disturbances, eczema, edema, epididymitis, eye inflammation, fatigue, fever, frostbite, fungal infections, gastrointestinal inflammation, gastrointestinal tract disorders, gingivitis, gout, gum disease prevention, headache, heart disease, hemorrhoids, herpes keratitis, herpes simplex virus infections, high cholesterol levels, human immunodeficiency virus (HIV), immune system stimulant, immunomodulation, indigestion, influenza, insomnia, jaundice, kidney or bladder stones, liver cancer, liver dysfunction, liver–gallbladder function stimulator, menstrual period abnormalities, metabolic disorders, migraine, mosquito repellant, mouth and throat infections, muscle spasms, muscle wasting, nausea, nervous disorders (iatrogenic disability), nervous system disorders, nosebleed, oral hygiene (oral cavity irrigation), pain, parasite infection, prostatitis, ringing in the ears, skin cancer, sore throat, spleen disorders, syphilis, toothache, tuberculosis, ulcerative colitis, ulcers (peptic ulcer disease), urinary retention, uterus problems, varicose veins, venous disorders (phlebitis, thrombophlebitis), vitamin deficiencies (lutein or beta-carotene), warts, yeast infections.

DOSING
Adults (18 Years and Older)

- For ear infections, the combination herbal product Otikon Otic (which includes calendula) has been used in a dose of 5 drops placed in the affected ear three times daily. Five drops of NHED solution (which contains garlic [*Allium sativum*], *Verbascum thapsus*, *Calendula flores*, St. John's wort [*Hypericum perfoliatum*], lavender [*Lavandula angustifolia*], and vitamin E in olive oil) have been instilled into an affected ear three times daily.

- Two European expert panels, the German Commission E and the European Scientific Cooperative on Phytotherapy (ESCOP), recommend a 2% to 5% ointment applied three to four times daily as needed.
- A 1:1 tincture in 40% alcohol or a 1:5 tincture in 90% alcohol, diluted at least 1:3 with freshly boiled water, has been applied to the skin as a compress three to four times daily.

Children (Younger than 18 Years)

- There is insufficient evidence to recommend a dose of calendula in children.

SAFETY
Allergies

- People with allergies to plants in the Aster/Compositae family, such as ragweed, chrysanthemums, marigolds, and daisies, are more likely to have an allergic reaction to calendula. There is one case of a severe allergic reaction (anaphylactic shock) after gargling with a calendula preparation.

Side Effects and Warnings

- Aside from allergic reactions, few severe reactions have been found in published reports. In one small animal study, calendula was associated with a fatal reduction in blood glucose levels, accompanied by decreased levels of serum lipids and protein. Skin (atopic dermatitis) and eye irritation have been reported.

Pregnancy and Breastfeeding

- It is not clear whether calendula is safe for use during pregnancy or breastfeeding. In animal studies, calendula has had effects on the uterus, and calendula has traditionally been thought to have harmful effects on sperm and to cause abortions. However, it is not clear whether these effects occur with the use of calendula on the skin.

INTERACTIONS
Interactions with Drugs

- In early animal studies, high doses of calendula were reported to cause drowsiness. It is not clear whether the use of calendula on the skin of humans has this effect. In theory, the use of calendula in combination with sedative drugs may lead to increased drowsiness. Examples include benzodiazepines such as lorazepam (Ativan) or diazepam (Valium), barbiturates such as phenobarbital, narcotics such as codeine, some antidepressants, and alcohol. Use caution while driving or operating machinery.
- In early animal studies, high doses of calendula preparations were reported to lower blood pressure. It is not clear whether the use of calendula on the skin of humans has this effect. In theory, the use of calendula in combination with drugs that lower blood pressure may lead to increased effects.
- Calendula may also increase the effects of antispasmodics, which are drugs that help stop muscle spasms.
- Use cautiously if taking drugs that can damage the liver or kidneys because calendula may increase the risk of organ damage.
- Other possible interactions include increases in the activity of hypoglycemic (diabetic) medications or insulin, antifungal medications, or agents that decrease levels of lipids and triglycerides (cholesterol-lowering drugs.)

Interactions with Herbs and Dietary Supplements

- In animals, high doses of calendula were reported to cause drowsiness. It is not clear whether the use of calendula on the skin of humans has this effect. Use of calendula in combination with herbs or supplements that have possible sedative effects may lead to increased drowsiness. Use caution while driving or operating machinery.
- In animals, high doses of calendula preparations were reported to lower blood pressure. It is not clear whether the use of calendula on the skin of humans has this effect. In theory, the use of calendula in combination with herbs that may lower blood pressure may lead to increased effects.
- Other possible interactions include increases in the activity of hypoglycemic (diabetic) medications or insulin, antifungals, or agents that decrease levels of lipids and triglycerides (cholesterol-lowering agents).
- Calendula may also increase the effects of herbs or supplements that help stop muscle spasms (called antispasmodics).
- Use cautiously if taking herbs or supplements that can damage the liver or kidneys because calendula may increase the risk of organ damage.
- Because the stem and leaves of calendula contain lutein and beta-carotene, a possible supplement interaction exists with products that contain these ingredients.

For a complete list of references, please visit www.naturalstandard.com.

California Poppy
(*Eschscholzia californica*)

RELATED TERMS
- *Eschscholzia californica*, Papaveraceae (family).

BACKGROUND
- Historically, California poppy has been used as a sedative to relieve insomnia and nervousness.
- California poppy may bind with the same receptors as monoamine oxidase inhibitors (MAOIs) and selective serotonin reuptake inhibitors (SSRIs). Caution should be used in patients taking these agents.
- There is insufficient evidence in humans to support the use of California poppy for any indication.
- Native Americans used California poppy medicinally.

EVIDENCE

Uses Based on Scientific Evidence

No available studies qualify for inclusion in the evidence table.

Uses Based on Tradition or Theory

Insomnia, nervousness, sedative.

DOSING
Adults (18 Years and Older)
- There is insufficient evidence to recommend a dose for California poppy in adults.

Children (Younger than 18 Years)
- There is insufficient evidence to recommend a dose for California poppy in children.

SAFETY
Allergies
- Avoid in individuals with a known allergy or hypersensitivity to California poppy (*Eschscholzia californica*) or its constituents.

Side Effects and Warnings
- There is insufficient evidence available on the medicinal applications of California poppy. California poppy is possibly unsafe when used in patients taking SSRIs or MAOIs.

Pregnancy and Breastfeeding
- California poppy is not recommended in pregnant or breastfeeding women because of a lack of available scientific evidence.

INTERACTIONS
Interactions with Drugs
- Although not well studied in humans, California poppy (*Eschscholzia californica*) may interact with antidepressant agents, including MAOIs and SSRIs. Caution is advised in patients taking antidepressants.
- California poppy may have hypotensive (blood pressure–lowering) effects. Caution is advised in patients with hypertension or hypotension and in those taking blood pressure–altering drugs.
- California poppy may increase the amount of drowsiness caused by some drugs. Examples include benzodiazepines such as lorazepam (Ativan) or diazepam (Valium), barbiturates such as phenobarbital, narcotics such as codeine, some antidepressants, and alcohol. Use caution while driving or operating machinery.

Interactions with Herbs and Dietary Supplements
- Although not well studied in humans, California poppy (*Eschscholzia californica*) may interact with antidepressant herbs or supplements, including MAOIs and SSRIs. Caution is advised in patients taking herbs and supplements with possible antidepressant or MAOI effects such as 5-hydroxytryptophan (5-HTP), ephedra, hops, St. John's wort, and vitamin B_6.
- California poppy may have hypotensive (blood pressure–lowering) effects. Caution is advised in patients with hypertension or hypotension and in those taking blood pressure–altering herbs or supplements. Herbs and supplements with hypotensive effects include black cohosh, flaxseed, garlic, ginger, and ginkgo, among others.
- California poppy may increase the amount of drowsiness caused by some herbs or supplements. Examples may include 5-HTP, celery, hops, lavender aromatherapy, sage, Siberian ginseng, and St. John's wort. Use caution while driving or operating machinery.

For a complete list of references, please visit www.naturalstandard.com.

Caper
(*Capparis spinosa*)

RELATED TERMS

- Alcaparra (Portuguese), alcaparro (Spanish), caparra (Spanish), caper, caperberry, caperbush, cappariloside, cappero (Italian), capperone (Italian), capres (French), caprier (French), fabagelle (French), glucocapperin, hydroxycinnamic acids, kabarra (Punjabi), kabra (Bengali), kaempferol glycoside, kapernstrauch (German), kapersy (Russian), kappar (Estonian), kapper (German), kappertjes (Dutch), kapricserje (Hungarian), kapris (Swedish and Finnish), kiari (Hindi), kobra (Hindi), lussef (Egyptian), mustard oil (methyl isothiocyanate), quercetin glycoside, rutin, tapana (French), torkav (Estonian).

BACKGROUND

- Caper (*Capparis spinosa*) traditionally has been used for gas, liver function, heart disease, kidney disorders, parasitic worm infections, anemia, arthritis, gout, and as a tonic. Caper has also been used for low blood sugar levels. Preliminary evidence suggests antioxidant, liver protective, antiinflammatory, antimicrobial, and sun-protective properties.
- The combination therapy Liv-52 (Himalaya Herbals, India), which contains ferric oxide, caper, and several other herbal ingredients, may be an effective treatment for cirrhosis. The efficacy of caper alone for cirrhosis or other conditions remains unproven.

EVIDENCE

Uses Based on Scientific Evidence	Grade
Cirrhosis There is limited evidence of the effect of capers alone on cirrhosis.	C

Uses Based on Tradition or Theory
Anemia, antioxidant, antispasmodic, antiviral, diabetes, diuretic, dropsy, gas, gout, heart disease, herpes simplex virus, high blood pressure, immune system regulation, inflammatory conditions, kidney disease (kidney disinfectant), painful urination, parasitic worm infections, rheumatism, sun protection, tonic.

DOSING
Adults (18 Years and Older)

- Three tablets daily of Liv-52 (a combination product from Himalaya Herbals, India) has been used for 6 months for cirrhosis.

Children (Younger than 18 Years)

- There is insufficient evidence to recommend a dose for caper, and use in children is not recommended.

SAFETY
Allergies

- Avoid in individuals with a known allergy or hypersensitivity to caper. Cross-sensitivity with mustard oil may be possible.

Side Effects and Warnings

- There is limited evidence of adverse effects with the use of caper. Cross-sensitivity with mustard oil may be possible. Rash has been reported when caper was applied to the skin in a wet compress.
- Caper may lower blood sugar levels. Caution is advised in patients with diabetes or hypoglycemia and in those taking drugs, herbs, or supplements that affect blood sugar. Blood glucose levels may need to be monitored by a qualified health care professional, including a pharmacist, and medication adjustments may be necessary.
- Caper may cause low blood pressure. Caution is advised in patients taking herbs or supplements that lower blood pressure.
- Use with caution in patients taking diuretics. Use with caution in patients who are prone to iron overload as the combination product Liv-52 (Himalaya Herbals, India) contains iron.

Pregnancy and Breastfeeding

- Caper is not recommended in pregnant or breastfeeding women because of a lack of available scientific evidence.

INTERACTIONS
Interactions with Drugs

- Caper may lower blood sugar levels. Caution is advised when medications that may also lower blood sugar are used. Patients taking drugs for diabetes by mouth or injection should be monitored closely by a qualified health care professional. Medication adjustment may be necessary.
- Caper may lower blood pressure. Caution is advised in patients taking medications that lower blood pressure.
- Caper may have additive effects when used with sun-protective, immune system–modulating, diuretic, antiviral, antiinflammatory, antimicrobial, antifungal, antioxidant, and iron-containing drugs. Caper may counter the effects of nonsteroidal antiinflammatory agents (NSAIDs) and cyclooxygenase-2 (COX-2) inhibitors.

Interactions with Herbs and Dietary Supplements

- Caper may lower blood sugar levels. Caution is advised when herbs or supplements that may also lower blood sugar are used. Blood glucose levels may require monitoring, and doses may need adjustment.
- Caper may lower blood pressure. Caution is advised in patients taking herbs or supplements that may also lower blood pressure.
- Caper may have additive effects when used with antifungal, antiinflammatory, antimicrobial, antioxidant, antiviral, diuretic, immune system–modulating, sun-protective, and iron-containing herbs or supplements.

For a complete list of references, please visit www.naturalstandard.com.

Caprylic Acid
(Octanoic Acid)

RELATED TERMS

- Alpha-hydroxy caprylic acid, medium-chain fatty acid, medium chain triglyceride (MCT), monocaprylin, octanoic acid, suberic acid.

BACKGROUND

- Caprylic acid is an eight-carbon fatty acid naturally found in palm and coconut oil and in the milk of humans and bovines (cows). Caprylic acid is classified as a medium-chain fatty acid and is chemically known as octanoic acid. The U.S. Food and Drug Administration (FDA) has approved caprylic acid with "generally recognizable as safe" (GRAS) status. It is used as parenteral nutrition in patients who require nutrition supplementation, as well as in some drugs, foods, and cosmetics.
- Nutritionists often recommend caprylic acid for use in treating candidiasis (yeast infection) and bacterial infections. However, there are insufficient clinical data available to support the use of caprylic acid for any claimed therapeutic indications.

EVIDENCE

Uses Based on Scientific Evidence	Grade
Epilepsy (Children) Some forms of epilepsy respond to diets that are high in fat and low in carbohydrates. Currently, the effects of caprylic acid alone to treat epilepsy in children are unclear.	C

Uses Based on Tradition or Theory
Antibacterial, antifungal, chylothorax, dialysis (hypoalbuminemia in maintenance hemodialysis), digestive disorders (dysbiosis), malabsorption (lipid), nutritional supplementation.

DOSING

Adults (18 Years and Older)

- There is insufficient evidence to recommend a dose for caprylic acid. In general, 300-1200 mg daily, preferably 30 minutes before meals, has been ingested.

Children (Younger than 18 Years)

- There is insufficient evidence to recommend a dose for caprylic acid, and use in children is not recommended.

SAFETY

Allergies

- Avoid in individuals with a known allergy or hypersensitivity to caprylic acid and its derivatives, such as caprylate salts.

Side Effects and Warnings

- The most common side effects associated with high fatty acid intake are nausea, bloating, constipation, vomiting, abdominal pain, and diarrhea. These side effects can range from mild to severe. Patients taking large amounts of triglycerides may also experience belching, heartburn, and indigestion. Otherwise, caprylic acid appears well tolerated at doses appropriate for nutritional supplementation. It is also possibly safe when used under the guidance of a physician for intractable seizures.
- Although not well studied in humans, caprylic acid may increase susceptibility to carbaryl exposure and decrease the body's ability to clear carbaryl, a highly toxic insecticide.
- Hypocalcemia (low calcium blood level), drowsiness, lethargy, kidney stones, hypouricemia (low uric acid), acidosis, growth retardation, and increased rate of infection have been reported in human studies using a ketogenic diet to treat epilepsy. The effects of caprylic acid alone are not well understood in this diet. Avoid in patients with kidney stones or a tendency of developing kidney stones. Use cautiously in infants, children, pregnant women, breastfeeding mothers, and those prone to upset stomachs.

Pregnancy and Breastfeeding

- Caprylic acid is not recommended in pregnant or breastfeeding women because of a lack of available scientific evidence.

INTERACTIONS

Interactions with Drugs

- Caprylic acid may alter the effects of drugs that are highly bound to albumin. Patients taking any medications should check the package insert and consult with a qualified health care professional, including a pharmacist.
- Theoretically, caprylic acid may increase susceptibility to carbaryl exposure and decrease the body's ability to clear carbaryl, a highly toxic insecticide. Caution is advised.
- Indomethacin can inhibit the cardiovascular effects of octanoic acid. Patients taking cardiovascular medications should consult with a qualified health care professional, including a pharmacist, about interactions.
- Although not well studied in humans, caprylic acid may also interact with inotropic agents, nimodipine, phenylbutazone, warfarin, and nonsteroidal antiinflammatory drugs (NSAIDs).

Interactions with Herbs and Dietary Supplements

- Octanoic acid may alter the effects of nonsteroidal antiinflammatory agents. Caution is advised in patients taking herbs and supplements that have similar effects as nonsteroidal antiinflammatory agents.

For a complete list of references, please visit www.naturalstandard.com.

Cardamom
(Elettaria cardamomum)

RELATED TERMS

- *Aframomum, Amomum, Amomum cardamomum, Amomum subulatum* Roxb., amooman, bai dou kou, Bari Ilaichi, bastard cardamom, buah pelaga (Malay), cardamom oil, cardamome (French), cardamomo (Italian, Spanish), cardamon, cardamone (Italian), cardamomi fructus, chhoti elachi (Indian), elaichi, e(e)lachie (Indian), ela(i)chi (Indian), *Elettaria cardamomum, Elettaria cardamomum* Maton var. *Miniscula Burkill*, elam (Tamil), enasal (Sinhalese), grains of paradise, grawahn (Thai), greater cardamom, Heel kalan, illaichi (Indian), Indian cardamom, kapulaga (Indonesian), Kardamom (German), Kardamomma (Iceland), kravan (Thai), large cardamom, lesser cardamom, Nepal cardamom, Malabar cardamom, Mysore cardamom, phalazee (Burmese), protocatechualdehyde, protocatechuic acid, Siam cardamom, true cardamom, ts'ao-k'ou (Chinese), Unmadnashak Ghrita, winged Java cardamom, Zingiberaceae (family).

BACKGROUND

- Cardamom is the dried, unripened fruit of the perennial *Elettaria cardamomum*. Enclosed in the fruit pods are tiny, brown, aromatic seeds, which are both pungent and sweet to the taste. Cardamom pods are generally green but are also available in bleached white pod form. It is available both in the whole pod and as decorticated seeds with the outer hull removed.
- The spice known as cardamom is the fruit of several plants of the *Elettaria, Aframomum,* and *Amomum* genera in Zingiberaceae, or ginger family. In general, *Aframomum* is used as a spice. *Elettaria* is used both as a spice and as medicine, and *Amomum* is used as an ingredient in several traditional medicines in China, India, Korea, and Vietnam.
- Cardamom has been used traditionally as a digestive aid, stimulant, breath freshener, and aphrodisiac. Current research has implicated cardamom's potential therapeutic value as an inhibitor of human platelet aggregation.

EVIDENCE

Uses Based on Scientific Evidence

No available studies qualify for inclusion in the evidence table.

Uses Based on Tradition or Theory

Allergic skin reactions (contact dermatitis), antacid, anticonvulsant, antiinflammatory, antimutagenic, antipyretic (fever reducer), antiseptic (pulmonary), aphrodisiac, appetite stimulant, asthma, breath freshener, bronchitis, cardiac conditions, carminative (digestive aid), colds, colon cancer, constipation, cough, depression, digestion, dyspepsia (upset stomach), enhanced vision, flatulence (gas), food flavoring, food uses, gastrointestinal disorders, immunostimulant, infections (teeth and gum), inflammation (eyelids), intestinal spasm, irritable bowel syndrome (IBS), laxative, liver and gallbladder complaints, loss of appetite, lung congestion, mouth and throat inflammation, nausea, nutritional intolerance in children (grains), sedative, skin conditions, snake bites, sore throats, stimulant, stings (scorpion), stress, tuberculosis, urinary tract infection, weight loss.

DOSING

Adults (18 Years and Older)

- There is insufficient evidence to recommend a dose of cardamom. Traditionally, the typical dose of cardamom is 1.5 g of the ground seeds per day. As a digestive, a tea prepared from 1 teaspoon of freshly crushed cardamom seeds infused in 1 cup boiled water for 10-15 minutes has been used.

Children (Younger than 18 Years)

- There is insufficient evidence to recommend a dose of cardamom, and use in children is not recommended.

SAFETY

Allergies

- Avoid in individuals with a known allergy or hypersensitivity to cardamom. Chronic contact dermatitis has occurred with repeated exposure to cardamom.

Side Effects and Warnings

- Very few adverse effects have been reported with cardamom. Primarily, the seeds may cause allergic contact dermatitis. The cardamom seed may trigger gallstone colic (spasmodic pain) and is not recommended for self-medication in patients with gallstones. Although not well studied, cardamom may increase the risk of bleeding. Caution is advised in patients taking medications that also increase the risk of bleeding.

Pregnancy and Breastfeeding

- Cardamom is not recommended in pregnant or breastfeeding women because of a lack of available scientific evidence. Avoid using amounts greater than those found in food.

INTERACTIONS

Interactions with Drugs

- Cardamom may increase the risk of bleeding when taken with drugs that also increase the risk of bleeding. Examples include aspirin, anticoagulants ("blood thinners") such as warfarin (Coumadin) or heparin, antiplatelet drugs such as clopidogrel (Plavix), and nonsteroidal antiinflammatory drugs such as ibuprofen (Motrin, Advil) or naproxen (Naprosyn, Aleve).
- Cardamom may interfere with the way the body processes many drugs using the liver's cytochrome P450 enzyme system. As a result, the levels of these drugs may be increased in the blood in the short-term (causing increased effects or potentially serious adverse reactions) and/or decreased in the blood in the long-term (which can reduce the intended effects). Examples of medications that may be affected by cardamom in this manner

include carbamazepine, cyclosporin, irinotecan, midazolam, nifedipine, birth control pills, simvastatin, theophylline, tricyclic antidepressants, warfarin, or human immunodeficiency virus (HIV) drugs such as nonnucleoside reverse transcriptase inhibitors (NNRTIs) or protease inhibitors (PIs).

- Cardamom may have antispasmodic effects. Patients taking antispasmodic drugs or muscarinic agents should use cardamom with caution. Although not well studied, cardamom may also interact with indomethacin.

Interactions with Herbs and Dietary Supplements

- Cardamom may increase the risk of bleeding. In theory, this risk may be further increased when cardamom is taken with other herbs or supplements that also increase the risk of bleeding. Multiple cases of bleeding have been reported with the use of *Ginkgo biloba*, and two cases have been reported with saw palmetto. Numerous other agents may theoretically increase the risk of bleeding, although this has not been proven in most cases.
- Cardamom may interfere with the way the body processes certain herbs and supplements using the liver's cytochrome P450 enzyme system. As a result, the levels of these drugs may be increased in the blood in the short-term, causing increased effects or potentially serious adverse reactions, or decreased in the blood in the long-term, which can reduce the intended effects.
- Cardamom may have antispasmodic effects. Patients taking antispasmodic herbs and supplements or muscarinic agents should use cardamom with caution.

For a complete list of references, please visit www.naturalstandard.com.

Carob
(Ceratonia siliqua)

RELATED TERMS

- Alanine, algaroba, arobon, Caesalpinioideae (subfamily), carob bean gum, carob flour, carob gum, Carobel, caruba, cellulose, ceratonia gum, *Ceratonia siliqua*, cheshire gum, China-Eisenwein, cinnamic acid, Fabaceae (family), flavonoids, free gallic acid, fructose, galactomannan, gallic acid, gallotannins, glucose, glycine, goma de garrofin, gomme de caroube, gumilk, hemicellulose, Leguminosae (family), leucine, locust bean, locust bean gum, maltose, methyl gallate, Pomana A, phenolic antioxidants, phenylalanine, praline, St. John's bread, sucrose, tannins, Thiacyl au Caroube, tyrosine, valine.

BACKGROUND

- Carob (*Ceratonia siliqua*) is a leguminous evergreen tree of the family Leguminosae (pulse family). Although it was originally native to Mediterranean regions, it is now cultivated in many warm climates, including Florida and California. The pods may be ground into a powder, which is often used as a cocoa substitute because it has a somewhat similar taste to chocolate and one third of the calories.
- Carob has been used to treat infantile diarrhea, and carob bean gum has been used to control hyperlipidemia (high cholesterol) and as a dietary adjunct to elevated plasma cholesterol management.
- There are conflicting data on the effect of carob bean gum as a formula thickener and its effect on regurgitation frequency. The use of soluble dietary fibers, such as carob bean gum, has been shown to alter food structure, texture and viscosity, the rate of starch degradation during digestion, and the regulation of postprandial blood sugar and insulin levels.
- As a food, the U.S. Food and Drug Administration (FDA) has given carob "generally recognized as safe" (GRAS) status.

EVIDENCE

Uses Based on Scientific Evidence	Grade
Hypercholesterolemia (High Cholesterol) Fiber, such as oat fiber, has been shown to reduce serum cholesterol levels. Carob pod fiber or carob bean gum may also have this ability, although additional research is needed to confirm these findings.	B
Diarrhea in Children Traditionally, carob has been used for the treatment of gastrointestinal conditions, especially diarrhea. Preliminary research used different types of carob products as an adjunct to oral rehydrating solution and showed promising results.	C
Gastroesophageal Reflux Disease (in Infants) Locust bean gum is a common food thickener and may prove helpful in infantile gastroesophageal reflux. However, the effectiveness has not been shown conclusively.	C

Uses Based on Tradition or Theory

Anthelmintic (expels worms), antioxidant, antiviral, cancer, celiac disease, cough (retching, in infants), demulcent (soothing agent), diabetes, diarrhea (in adults), digestive disorders, dyspepsia (upset stomach), eye infections, flavoring agent, food uses, improvement in eyesight, laxative, nausea and vomiting during pregnancy, nutritional deficiencies, obesity, stomach pain, vomiting (in infants).

DOSING

Adults (18 Years and Older)

- There is insufficient evidence to recommend a dose for carob. Traditionally, 20 g carob has been used daily with plenty of water. As a powder, 20-30 g added to water, tea, or milk has been taken once daily.

Children (Younger than 18 Years)

- There is insufficient evidence to recommend a dose for carob in children, and use is not recommended.

SAFETY

Allergies

- Avoid in individuals with a known allergy or hypersensitivity to carob (*Ceratonia siliqua*), its constituents, or any plants in the Fabaceae family, including tamarind. Pollen from the carob tree has been reported as an important inhalant allergen. Asthma and rhinitis to carob bean flour have been reported. Explosive vomiting, urticaria (hives), and a rash have also been reported following allergy to an antiregurgitation milk formula containing carob bean gum in an infant. Individuals allergic to peanuts may also have cross-sensitivity to raw carob pulp.

Side Effects and Warnings

- There is a lack of reports of serious adverse effects related to the consumption of carob. The consumption in designated therapeutic doses can be generally considered as safe, although side effects may include a feeling of fullness. Carob is likely safe when consumed in amounts usually found in foods; in the United States carob has GRAS status.
- Carob is possibly unsafe when used in infants with gastroesophageal reflux in pregnant women or in patients with anemia, diabetes, hyperlipidemia (high cholesterol), hypouricemia (low uric acid), known allergies to members of the Fabaceae family, peanuts, or other nuts, or who have experienced previous complications with powdered, bulk-forming laxative drinks. Carob is also possibly safe when used by patients taking herbs or drugs by mouth, as carob bean gum may decrease bowel transit time. Use cautiously in patients with diabetes, as locust bean gum may decrease the glucose response and glycemic index.
- In patients with renal (kidney) failure, ingestion of locust bean gum showed laxative effects, decreased high blood

pressure and caused a fall in serum urea, creatinine, and phosphorus levels.

- A 5-month-old child who was allergic to an antiregurgitation milk formula containing carob bean gum experienced urticaria (hives) and a rash within 30 minutes of administration of the formula. Thickening milk feeds (Carobel) may cause necrotizing enterocolitis (a serious intestinal illness in babies that may cause tissue damage to the intestines) in low birth-weight infants.
- Avoid in patients with a chromium, cobalt, copper, iron, or zinc disorder or deficiency, as carob bean gum may reduce absorption of these minerals. Use cautiously in patients with anemia (red blood cell deficiency) as carob bean gum may reduce the absorption of iron. Avoid in patients with metabolic disorders or acute diarrhea or in underweight infants.

Pregnancy and Breastfeeding

- Carob is not recommended in pregnant or breastfeeding women because of a lack of available scientific data.

INTERACTIONS
Interactions with Drugs

- Carob may alter blood sugar levels. Caution is advised when medications that may also affect blood sugar are used. Patients taking drugs for diabetes by mouth or insulin should be monitored closely by a qualified health care provider. Medication adjustments may be necessary.
- Carob bean gum may reduce hyperlipidemia (high cholesterol) in adults and low-density lipoprotein (LDL; "bad") cholesterol levels in children and adolescents with elevated plasma LDL cholesterol levels. Caution is advised in patients taking cholesterol-lowering agents because of additive effects.
- Although not well studied in humans, carob bean gum polysaccharides may block a step in rubella virus replication subsequent to virus attachment and may interact with antiviral agents. Consult with a qualified health care professional, including a pharmacist, before combining therapies.

- Carob leaf extracts may act as chemopreventive agents. Use caution when taking with other drugs with similar effects.
- Carob bean gum may decrease bowel transit time or increase fecal weight. It may also reduce the adherence of *Escherichia coli* on intestinal epithelial. Thus, it may interact with laxatives or other agents taken by mouth, and caution is advised.
- In children and infants with acute diarrhea, carob bean juice or carob pod powder may reduce the symptoms of infectious diarrhea. Caution is advised when carob is taken with other agents that have similar effects.

Interactions with Herbs and Dietary Supplements

- Based on a laboratory study, carob may reduce the adherence of *Escherichia coli* on intestinal epithelial.
- Carob may lower blood sugar levels. Caution is advised when herbs or supplements that can also alter blood sugar are used. Blood glucose levels may require monitoring, and doses may need adjustment.
- Carob bean gum may reduce hyperlipidemia (high cholesterol) in adults and LDL ("bad") cholesterol levels in children and adolescents with elevated plasma LDL cholesterol levels. Caution is advised in patients taking cholesterol-lowering herbs, such as red yeast rice, because of additive effects.
- Carob bean gum polysaccharides may block a step in rubella virus replication subsequent to virus attachment. Caution is advised in patients taking herbs with antiviral effects because of possible additive effects.
- Carob leaf extracts may act as chemopreventive agents. Caution is advised when taking with other herbs with similar effects.
- Although not well studied in humans, carob bean gum may reduce the absorption of zinc, iron, copper, chromium, and cobalt. Carob bean gum may decrease bowel transit time or increase fecal weight, and caution is advised when laxative herbs, such as psyllium, are also used.

For a complete list of references, please visit www.naturalstandard.com.

Carrageenan
(*Chondrus crispus*)

RELATED TERMS

- Algae, algal polysaccharides, anhydrogalactose, bejin behan (Breton), bejin gwenn (Breton), *Betaphycus gelatinum,* blomkalstang (Danish), botelho crespo (Portuguese), bouch (Breton), bouch farad youd (Breton), bo.uch gad (Breton), bouch gwenn (Breton), bouchounoù (Breton), cairgin (Gaelic), *Callophyllis hombroniana,* caragaen, caragahen, carragaheen, carrageen, carrageen moss, carrageenin, carrageentang (Danish), carragheen, carrahèen (French), carragheenan, Carraguard, carraigín (Irish), carrapucho (Galician), *Chondrus crispus,* chondrus extract, *Chondrus mamillosus,* clúimhín cait (Irish), clúimhín caitcarraigín (Irish), cottonii, creba (Galician), curly gristle moss, curly moss, Dorset weed, Dragendorff, driesflik (Norwegian), *Eucheuma cottonii, Eucheuma denticulatum, Eucheuma gelatinae, Eucheuma* spp., *Eucheuma spinosum,* fiadháin (Irish), fjörugrös (Icelandic), folha de alface (Portuguese), folhina (Portuguese), fuco carageo, fuco crispo (Italian), *Fucus crispus* Linné, galactopyranose, galactose 4-sulfate, gelatintang (Norwegian), *Gigartina acicularis, Gigartina canaliculata, Gigartina mamillosa, Gigartina pistillata, Gigartina skottsbergii, Gigartina stellata,* Gigartinaceae (family), Gigartinales, goémon blanc (French), goémon fries (French), goémon rouge (French), hirakotoji (Japanese), *Hypnea musciformis,* Iers mos (Dutch), iota carrageenan, *Iridaea ciliata, Iridaea laminaroides,* Irish moss extract, Irländischer Perltang (German), Irländisches Moos (German), Irlandsk mos (Danish), jargod (Breton), jelly moss, Kallymeniaceae, kappa carrageenan, *Kappaphycus alvarezii, Kappaphycus cottonii, Kappaphycus striatum,* karragaheen (German), karrageentari (Faroese), karragen (Turkish), karragenalg (Swedish), karragentang (Swedish), Killeen, knorpeltang (German), krusflik (Norwegian), lambda carrageenan, lambda-carrageenan, Lamouroux, lichen, liken ruz (Breton), liquen (Spanish), marine algae, *Mastocarpus mamillosus* Kützing, *Mastocarpus stellatus,* mathair an diulisg (Gaelic), *Mazzaella laminaroides,* mousse d'irlande, mousse marine perlée (French), mousse perlée (French), mu carrageenan, muschio irlandese (Italian), musco d'Irlanda (Italian), musgo de Irlanda (Spanish), musgo gordo (Portuguese), musgo marino (Spanish), musgo marino perlado (Spanish), musgo perlado (Spanish), mwsog Iwerddon (Welsh), nu carrageenan, ouca riza (Galician), ougnachou-ru (Breton), pata de galiña (Galician), PC 213, PC-503, pearl moss, perimoos, perlmoos (German), petit goémon (French), *Phacelocarpus peperocarpos,* pigwiacis, pioka (Breton), poligeenan, red algae, red seaweed, Rhodophyceae, *Rhodophyta, Sarcothalia crispate,* sea moss, seamuisin, seaweed, seaweed extract, *Sphaerococcus crispus* Agardh, *Sphaerococcus mamillosus* Agardh, spinosum, stackhouse, teil piko (Breton), teles (Breton), theta carrageenan, tilez (Breton), tochaka (Japanese), tsunomata (Japanese), upsilon carrageenan, vaginal gel, white wrack.

BACKGROUND

- Carrageenans are carbohydrates extracted from red seaweeds (such as Irish moss) and other sources. Irish moss grows around Ireland, as well as other coasts in Europe, and the Atlantic coasts of the United States. The Irish moss popularly used as a ground cover (*Sagina subulata*) is not the same as the Irish moss discussed in this monograph (*Chondrus crispus*).
- Traditionally, carrageenan has been taken by mouth to soothe mucous membranes and as a laxative. Extracts of carrageenan have been used as food additives for hundreds of years. Carrageenan is currently used as a thickener and stabilizer for a wide range of foods and is also used in personal hygiene products and drugs.
- Carrageenan may lower lipid (cholesterol and triglyceride) and blood sugar levels. Although not well studied in humans, carrageenan-based gels may help prevent human immunodeficiency virus (HIV) transmission.

EVIDENCE

Uses Based on Scientific Evidence	Grade
HIV Infection (Prevention) Although not well studied in humans, carrageenan-based gels may prevent HIV transmission during sexual intercourse. Overall, studies suggest that carrageenan may be safe for use by males and females. High-quality clinical study is needed to confirm these early results.	C
Lipid-Lowering (Cholesterol and Triglycerides) In clinical study, a diet containing carrageenan-enriched foods lowered cholesterol and triglyceride levels. Further clinical trials are required before carrageenan can be recommended for its lipid-lowering effects.	C

Uses Based on Tradition or Theory
Anorectal lesions, antiinflammatory, antimicrobial, antioxidant, bladder disorders, bronchitis, cancer, cough, demulcent, diabetes, diarrhea, food uses, gastrointestinal disorders, heart disease, herpes simplex virus, high blood pressure, human papillomavirus, immune function, kidney disorders, laxative, obesity, rickets, sexually transmitted diseases (STDs), tuberculosis, ulcers.

DOSING

Adults (18 Years and Older)

- Traditionally, carrageenan is taken by mouth as a tea after it is boiled and flavored.
- For lipid lowering, carrageenan-enriched foods have been taken for 8 weeks.
- For HIV prevention, 5 mL of carrageenan gel has been applied inside the vagina for 7 days; one application a minimum of three times per week has also been used.

Children (Younger than 18 Years)

- There is insufficient evidence to recommend a dose for carrageenan in children.

SAFETY
Allergies

- Avoid in individuals with a known allergy or hypersensitivity to seaweed, algae, or carrageenan.

Side Effects and Warnings

- Carrageenan is generally safe and well-tolerated when used by mouth at levels found in foods. Carrageenan is possibly unsafe when taken by mouth in degraded, poligeenan form, or when taken by infants. The fiber in carrageenan may impair the absorption of drugs, herbs, or supplements taken by mouth.
- Carrageenan may increase the risk of bleeding. Caution is advised in patients with bleeding disorders or taking drugs, herbs, or supplements that may increase the risk of bleeding. Dosing adjustments may be necessary.
- Carrageenan may lower blood sugar levels. Caution is advised in patients with diabetes or hypoglycemia and in those taking drugs, herbs, or supplements that affect blood sugar. Blood glucose levels may need to be monitored by a qualified health care professional, including a pharmacist, and medication adjustments may be necessary.
- Carrageenan may cause low blood pressure. Caution is advised in patients with blood pressure disorders or in those taking drugs, herbs, or supplements that lower blood pressure.
- Carrageenan may have negative effects on the immune system that may result in increased inflammation or infection. Caution is advised in patients with immune or inflammatory disorders or in those using drugs, herbs, or supplements for these disorders.
- Carrageenan may cause cramping, diarrhea, and possibly an increased risk of stomach cancer or stomach ulcers. Caution is advised in patients with stomach or intestinal disorders or with or at risk of cancer.
- Carrageenan gel applied to the vagina may cause bladder fullness, difficulty urinating, genital warmth, lower abdominal pain, vaginal itching and burning, and abnormal vaginal discharge.

Pregnancy and Breastfeeding

- Carrageenan is not recommended for pregnant or breastfeeding women because of lack of sufficient data. Carrageenan may be unsafe in infants.

INTERACTIONS
Interactions with Drugs

- Carrageenan may impair absorption of drugs taken by mouth.
- Carrageenan may lower blood sugar levels. Caution is advised when medications that may also lower blood sugar are used. Patients taking drugs for diabetes by mouth or insulin should be monitored closely by a qualified health care professional, including a pharmacist. Medication adjustments may be necessary.
- Carrageenan may increase the risk of bleeding when taken with drugs that increase the risk of bleeding. Some examples include aspirin, anticoagulants ("blood thinners") such as warfarin (Coumadin) or heparin, antiplatelet drugs such as clopidogrel (Plavix), and nonsteroidal antiinflammatory drugs such as ibuprofen (Motrin, Advil) or naproxen (Naprosyn, Aleve).
- Carrageenan may cause low blood pressure. Caution is advised in patients taking drugs that lower blood pressure.
- Carrageenan may increase inflammation or affect the immune system. Caution is advised in patients taking drugs that stimulate or suppress the immune system.
- Carrageenan applied vaginally may increase side effects of other vaginal drugs.
- Carrageenan may add to the effects of cholesterol-lowering agents, anticancer agents, HIV drugs, antiviral drugs, eye medications, azoxymethane, nitrosomethylurea, and azido-deoxythymidine (AZT).

Interactions with Herbs and Dietary Supplements

- Carrageenan may impair absorption of herbs or supplements taken by mouth.
- Carrageenan may lower blood sugar levels. Caution is advised when herbs or supplements that may also lower blood sugar are used. Blood glucose levels may require monitoring, and doses may need adjustment.
- Carrageenan may increase the risk of bleeding when taken with herbs and supplements that are believed to increase the risk of bleeding. Multiple cases of bleeding have been reported with the use of *Ginkgo biloba*, and fewer cases have been reported with garlic and saw palmetto. Numerous other agents may theoretically increase the risk of bleeding, although this has not been proven in most cases.
- Carrageenan may cause low blood pressure. Caution is advised in patients taking herbs or supplements that lower blood pressure.
- Carrageenan may increase inflammation or affect the immune system. Caution is advised in patients taking herbs or supplements that stimulate or suppress the immune system.
- Carrageenan applied vaginally may increase side effects of other vaginal herbs or supplements.
- Carrageenan may add to the effects of antiviral herbs or supplements, antioxidants, herbs or supplements used to lower cholesterol levels, or herbs or supplements used for cancer, HIV, or for the eye.

For a complete list of references, please visit www.naturalstandard.com.

Carrot
(Daucus carota)

RELATED TERMS

- Alpha-carotene, anthocyanins, beta-carotene, carotenoid, carotenoids, carrot cake, carrot jam, carrot juice, carrot puree, carrot soup, *Daucus carota*, dietary fiber, grated carrots, lycopene, lycopene red carrots, myristicin, purple carrots, red carrots, Umbelliferae (family), vitamin A, white carrots.

BACKGROUND

- Carrot (*Daucus carota*) is a well-known root vegetable. The thick tap root's color can range from white to orange to red or purple. This change in color represents the nutrients in the carrot because some pigments, such as beta-carotene and lycopene, are also nutrients.

- Carrot probably originated around Afghanistan, where there is the greatest variety of carrots today. Usually only the root is consumed, although the leaves are also edible. Although primarily used as a food source, carrots have also traditionally been used to treat infantile diarrhea. Carrot roots have been used to treat digestive problems, intestinal parasites, and tonsillitis. Other potential uses include vitamin A deficiency, antioxidant activity, constipation, and anemia. More research is needed in all of these areas, as the currently available research is of low quality.

EVIDENCE

Uses Based on Scientific Evidence	Grade
Acute Diarrhea A carrot-rice–based rehydration solution may decrease the duration of diarrhea when compared with two conventional rehydration solutions. However, more research is needed.	C
Antioxidant Carrot ingestion may have antioxidant activity, although more research is needed in this area.	C
Vitamin A Deficiency Carrot jam may improve growth in young children with vitamin A deficiency. Although the results seem promising, more research is needed.	C

Uses Based on Tradition or Theory
Anemia (red blood cell deficiency), cancer, constipation, deficiency (vitamin C, zinc), diabetes, fertility, fibromyalgia, gastrointestinal disorders, immunomodulation, intestinal parasites, menopausal symptoms, tonsillitis.

DOSING

Adults (18 Years and Older)

- There is insufficient evidence to recommend a dose for carrots. However, 100 g of grated carrots daily for 60 days has been used to improve vitamin A status in breastfeeding women in one study.

Children (Younger than 18 Years)

- There is insufficient evidence to recommend a dose for carrots in children.

SAFETY

Allergies

- Avoid in individuals with a known allergy or hypersensitivity to carrot. Carrot pollen contains an allergen that is similar to the birch pollen allergens. Because of this similarity, patients allergic to birch pollen may also have allergic reactions to carrot. Several other plants also have similar allergens, including apples, stone fruits, celery, nuts, orange, lychee fruit, strawberry, persimmon, zucchini, mugwort (*Artemisia vulgaris*), pear, potato, spices, nuts, mustard, Leguminoseae vegetables, and soybeans. Food allergy symptoms include hives, swelling, skin rashes, asthma, diarrhea, or anaphylactic reactions.

Side Effects and Warnings

- Carrot is likely safe when taken in food amounts, but carrot products should not be used excessively in nursing bottles for small children as they are likely unsafe.
- Carrot food allergy symptoms include hives, swelling, skin rashes, asthma, diarrhea, or anaphylactic reactions.
- Compulsive carrot eating is a rare condition in which the patient craves carrots. Withdrawal symptoms include nervousness, cravings, insomnia, water brash, and irritability.
- Use cautiously in patients with hypoglycemia (low blood sugar), diabetes, hormone-sensitive conditions, or bowel obstruction.

Pregnancy and Breastfeeding

- Carrot, as an herbal medicine, is not recommended in pregnant or breastfeeding women because of a lack of scientific research. Carrot juice may alter the flavor of breast milk. Eating grated carrots may improve vitamin A and iron levels in the blood of breastfeeding mothers at risk of deficiency.

INTERACTIONS

Interactions with Drugs

- Consumption of processed and cooked carrots may alter blood sugar levels. Caution is advised in patients with diabetes or in those taking blood sugar–altering medications.
- A carrot–rice-based rehydration solution may cause diarrhea in children. Caution is advised in patients taking antidiarrheal medications because of conflicting effects.
- Several studies in humans suggest that carrot juice may interact with antioxidants. Caution is advised in patients taking antioxidant medications because of possible additive effects.
- Although not well studied in humans, carrot extracts may have hormonal effects. Caution is advised in patients taking hormones because of possible additive effects.
- Preliminary evidence suggests that consumption of carrots may increase fecal bulking/weight and dry matter. Caution

is advised in patients taking laxatives because of possible additive effects.

- Preliminary evidence suggests that consumption of carrots may increase gastrointestinal transit time. Caution is advised in patients taking any medications by mouth.

Interactions with Herbs and Dietary Supplements

- A carrot–rice-based solution may cause diarrhea in children; therefore, caution is advised in patients taking antidiarrheal herbs or supplements because of conflicting effects.
- Several studies in humans suggest that carrot juice may interact with antioxidants. Caution is advised in patients taking other herbs or supplements with antioxidant activity because of possible additive effects.
- Consumption of processed and cooked carrots may alter blood sugar levels. Caution is advised in patients taking blood sugar–altering herbs or supplements.

- Preliminary evidence suggests that consumption of carrots may increase fecal bulking/weight and dry matter. Caution is advised in patients taking laxative herbs or supplements because of possible additive effects.
- Ingestion of grated carrots may increase iron, zinc, vitamin A, and vitamin C levels in the blood. Combined use with iron supplements or multivitamins may have additive effects.
- Preliminary evidence suggests that consumption of carrots may increase gastrointestinal transit time. Caution is advised in patients taking herbs or supplements by mouth.
- Although not well studied in humans, carrot extracts may have hormonal effects. Caution is advised in patients taking hormone therapy or hormonal supplements.
- Based on a clinical study in breastfeeding women, ingestion of grated carrots may increase serum levels of vitamin A and iron.

For a complete list of references, please visit www.naturalstandard.com.

Cascara
(*Rhamnus purshiana*)

RELATED TERMS

- Aloe, aloe-emodin, amerikanische faulbaumrinde, amerikanische faulbaum, anthracene glycosides, anthranoid, anthraquinone, anthroid, anthrone C-glycosides, *Artemisia scoparia*, ayapin, bearberry bark, bearwood, bitter bark, California buckthorn, carminic acid, casanthranol, cascara buckthorn, cascara fluid extract aromatic, cascara liquid extract, cascararinde, cascara sagrada, cascara sagrada (dried bark), cascara sagrada extract, cascara sagrada fluid extract (bitter cascara), cascarosides, cassia, cassia senna, chittem bark, coffee tree, dihydroxy-anthraquinones, dihydroxy-anthrones, dihydroxy-dianthrones, dogwood bark, emodin, fimbriatone, *Frangula purshiana*, nepodin, parietin, Persian bark, phytoestrogens, Polygonaceae, purshiana bark, pursh's buckthorn, Rhamnaceae (family), Rhamni purshianae cortex, *Rhamnus purshiana*, rhein, rheum, sacred bark, sagrada bark, Sagradafaulbaum (German), vegetable laxatives, wahoo plant, *Xanthoria elegans*, yellow bark.

BACKGROUND

- Cascara is obtained from the dried bark of *Rhamnus purshiana* (Rhamnaceae), both a medicinal and poisonous plant. It is found in Europe, western Asia, and in North America from northern Idaho to the Pacific coast in mountainous areas. In Spanish, cascara sagrada means *sacred bark*, perhaps because this woody shrub has provided relief for constipation. Cascara has been used as a tree bark laxative by Native American tribes and Spanish and Mexican priests since the 1800s. The cascara sagrada bark is aged for a year so that the active principles become milder, as freshly dried bark produces too strong a laxative for safe use.

- Cascara possesses purgative, toxic, therapeutic, and tonic activity. It is most commonly used as an anthraquinone stimulant laxative for bowel cleansing. Stimulant and cathartic laxatives are the most commonly abused laxatives and have the potential for causing long-term damage.

EVIDENCE

Uses Based on Scientific Evidence	Grade
Bowel Cleansing Early studies have examined the use of cascara for bowel preparation. Evidence is insufficient to suggest effectiveness over conventional treatments for this indication.	C
Constipation Cascara sagrada is widely accepted as a mild and effective treatment for chronic constipation. However, the available scientific evidence is limited.	C

Uses Based on Tradition or Theory

Abdominal pain, anal fissures, analgesic (pain reliever), antibacterial, antiparasitic, antiviral (herpes simplex virus II and vaccinia virus), cholagogue (promotes bile flow), dyspepsia (upset stomach), emetic (induces vomiting), flavoring agent, gallstones, hemorrhoids, immunosuppression, leukemia, liver disease, spleen problems, sunscreen, urinary stones.

DOSING

Adults (18 Years and Older)

- There is insufficient evidence to recommend a dose for cascara. A traditional dose is 20-30 mg daily of the active ingredient, hydroxyanthracene derivatives. This is calculated as cascaroside A, from the cut bark, powder, or extracts. Doses of 300-1000 mg dried bark have also been given at bedtime for constipation. The cascara liquid extract is often given in a dose of 2-5 mL three times daily. Traditionally, 4-6 mL of aromatic fluid extract have been administered at bedtime for constipation. As a tea, cascara has been given for constipation; a dose is 1 cup of tea, which can be made by steeping 2 g of finely chopped bark in 150 mL of boiling water for 5-10 minutes, then straining. The appropriate amount of cascara is the smallest dose that is necessary to maintain soft stools.

Children (Younger than 18 Years)

- There is insufficient evidence for cascara in children, and use is not recommended. Traditionally, 1-3 mL of aromatic fluid extract (typically one half of the adult dose) has been given daily to children 2 years and older. For the dried bark preparation, 150-500 mg daily has been used.

SAFETY

Allergies

- Avoid in individuals with a known allergy or hypersensitivity to cascara or the Rhamnaceae family. Cascara sagrada exposure has resulted in occupational asthma and rhinitis. Symptoms of allergy may include contact urticaria ("hives") or rash.

Side Effects and Warnings

- Cascara was formerly approved by the U.S. Food and Drug Administration (FDA) as safe and effective, but this designation was removed in 2002 because of a lack of supporting evidence. When taken by mouth, cascara can commonly cause mild abdominal discomfort, colic, and cramps. Long-term use may lead to potassium depletion, albuminuria (albumin in the urine above a specified level indicating potential kidney damage), hematuria (blood in the urine), disturbed heart function, muscle weakness, finger clubbing (enlargement), and cachexia (extreme weight loss). It is purported that the bark of cascara must be aged for 1 year or heat-treated to remove harsh constituents, which may produce severe vomiting, intestinal cramping, and/or spasms.

- Cascara sagrada bark is noted in the German Commission E Monographs to be associated with potassium loss. Patients taking cascara sagrada bark for more than 1-2 weeks may experience hypokalemia. Signs and symptoms include lethargy, muscle cramps, headaches, paresthesias, tetany (painful muscular spasms and tremors), peripheral edema, polyuria (excessive urination), breathlessness, and hypertension (high blood pressure). Use cautiously in children because of the risk of electrolyte loss, specifically potassium.
- Mild abdominal discomfort, colic, gastric melanosis (abnormal deposits of melanin), cholestatic hepatitis, ascites (fluid in the abdomen), portal hypertension (high blood pressure), cramps, nausea, vomiting, diarrhea, and cathartic (produces bowel movement) colon have been reported with chronic use of cascara and other anthraquinone laxatives. In some cases, chronic use may also cause pseudomelanosis coli. Pseudomelanosis coli (pigment spots in the lining of the large intestine) is believed to be harmless, usually reverses with discontinuation, and is not directly associated with an increased risk of developing colorectal adenoma or carcinoma.
- Cascara may increase the risk of bleeding. Caution is advised in patients with bleeding disorders or in those taking drugs that may increase the risk of bleeding. Dosing adjustments may be necessary.
- Use cascara cautiously in elderly patients. Weakness, discoordination, and orthostatic hypotension (low blood pressure when standing) may be exacerbated in elderly patients as a result of significant electrolyte loss when stimulant laxatives are used repeatedly to evacuate the colon. Be aware that cascara may hasten the passage of all oral medications through the gut, thereby inhibiting their action.
- Avoid using cascara in people with nausea or vomiting, inflammatory bowel disease, appendicitis, intestinal obstruction, or acute intestinal inflammation. This includes people with Crohn's disease, ulcerative colitis, and appendicitis. It is also contraindicated for people who have ulcers, and abdominal pain of unknown origin. Be aware that prolonged use of cascara may lead to dependence on laxatives for stools and tolerance.

Pregnancy and Breastfeeding

- Cascara is thought to be excreted into breast milk and may cause diarrhea. Avoid use in pregnant and breastfeeding women.

INTERACTIONS

Interactions with Drugs

- Cascara may increase the risk of bleeding when taken with drugs that increase the risk of bleeding. Some examples include aspirin, anticoagulants ("blood thinners") such as warfarin (Coumadin) or heparin, antiplatelet drugs such as clopidogrel (Plavix), and nonsteroidal antiinflammatory drugs (NSAIDs) such as ibuprofen (Motrin, Advil) or naproxen (Naprosyn, Aleve).
- Cascara may inhibit the absorption of digitalis glycosides, such as digoxin, and decrease their effects on the heart. Consult with a qualified health care professional, including a pharmacist, before combining therapies.
- Cascara has been used as a laxative, and laxative-induced diarrhea may result in decreased absorption of isoniazid or sulfisoxazole.
- Use of cascara with other laxatives may theoretically cause electrolyte and fluid depletion. Theoretically, concomitant use of cascara with diuretics (agents that increase urine flow), corticosteroids (steroids), or potassium-depleting drugs may cause excessive loss of potassium.

Interactions with Herbs and Dietary Supplements

- Cascara may increase the risk of bleeding when taken with herbs and supplements that are believed to increase the risk of bleeding. Multiple cases of bleeding have been reported with the use of *Ginkgo biloba*, and fewer cases have been reported with garlic and saw palmetto. Numerous other agents may theoretically increase the risk of bleeding, although this has not been proven in most cases.
- Theoretically, concomitant use of cascara with diuretic herbs and supplements may cause excessive loss of potassium. Caution is advised in patients taking herbs or supplements that increase the flow of urine or that have diuretic effects.
- Cascara may inhibit the absorption of digitalis glycosides, such as foxglove, and decrease their cardiac (heart) action. Cascara may also interact with squill. Consult with a qualified health care professional, including a pharmacist, before combining therapies.
- Theoretically, concomitant use of cascara along with potassium-depleting herbs, such as horsetail, may increase the risk of potassium depletion. Use of stimulant laxatives or licorice with cascara may also increase the risk of potassium depletion.
- Cascara induces increased speed of intestinal emptying, which theoretically may result in decreased absorption of vitamin K.

For a complete list of references, please visit www.naturalstandard.com.

Cat's Claw
(*Uncaria* spp.)

RELATED TERMS

- Ammonia-treated quinic acid (QAA), ancajsillo, Ancajsillo, ancayacu, aublet, auri huasca, bejuco de agua, cat's claw inner bark extract, C-Med-100, deixa paraguayo, gambir, garabato, garabato amarillo, garabato blanco, garbato casha, garbato colorado, garbato gavilán, garra gavilán, geissoschizine methyl ether, Gou-Teng, griffe du chat, hawk's claw, jijyuwamyúho, jipotatsa, Krallendorn, kugkuukjagki, life-giving vine of Peru, misho-mentis, mitraphylline, nature's aspirin, *Nauclea aculeata*, *Nauclea tomentosa*, *Ourouparia guianensis*, *Ourouparia tomentosa*, paotati-mösha, paraguaya, Peruvian cat's claw, pale catechu, popokainangra, quinic acid (QA), radix Uncariae tomentosae (Willd.), rangayo, Rubiaceae (family), samento, tambor hausca, tomcat's claw, torõn, tsachik, tua juncara, uña de gato, uña de gato de altura, uña de gato del bajo, uña de gavilán, uña a huasca, *Uncaria guianensis*, *Uncaria tomentosa*, unganangi, unganangui, un huasca, UT extract, UTE, vegicaps.
- There are 34 *Uncaria* species other than *Uncaria tomentosa*.

BACKGROUND

- Cat's claw (*Uncaria tomentosa*) was originally found in Peru, and its use has been said to date back to the Inca civilization, possibly as far back as 2000 years. It has been used for birth control, as an antiinflammatory, as an immunostimulant, for cancer, and as an antiviral. The Peruvian Ashaninka priests considered cat's claw (*Uncaria tomentosa*) to have great powers and life-giving properties and therefore used it to ward off disease.
- Multiple plant species are marketed under the name cat's claw, the most common being *Uncaria tomentosa* and *Uncaria guianensis*. Both are used to treat the same indications, although supposedly the former may be a more efficacious immunostimulant.
- Cat's claw (*Uncaria tomentosa*) may be contaminated with other *Uncaria* species, including *Uncaria rhynchophylla* (used in Chinese herbal preparations under the name Gou-Teng), which purportedly may lower blood pressure, lower heart rate, or act as a neuroinhibitor. Reports exist of a potentially toxic Texan-grown plant, *Acacia gregii*, being substituted for cat's claw in commercial preparations.
- In Germany and Austria, cat's claw is a registered pharmaceutical and can be dispensed with only a prescription. Today, cat's claw is widely used and is one of the top herbal remedies sold in the United States, despite a lack of high-quality human evidence.

EVIDENCE

Uses Based on Scientific Evidence	Grade
Allergies There is insufficient evidence to recommend cat's claw for allergic respiratory diseases at this time. Early studies have been conducted in Europe assessing the effects of cat's claw in patients with allergic respiratory diseases; a 10-year follow-up revealed that some patients experienced improvements.	C
Antiinflammatory Cat's claw may reduce inflammation, and this has led to research of cat's claw for conditions such as rheumatoid arthritis. Large, high-quality human studies are needed that compare the effects of cat's claw monotherapy vs. placebo.	C
Cancer Preliminary evidence suggests that cat's claw may slow tumor growth. However, this research is preliminary and has not identified specific types of cancer that may benefit; the results are not clear.	C
Immune Stimulant A few early studies suggest that cat's claw may boost the immune system, including that in patients with HIV. However, results from different studies have been conflicting.	C
Knee Pain from Osteoarthritis Preliminary research suggests that cat's claw may reduce pain from knee osteoarthritis.	C

Uses Based on Tradition or Theory

Abscesses, acne, aging, allergies, Alzheimer's disease, amnesia, antibacterial, anticonvulsive, antifungal, antihistamine, antimicrobial, antioxidant, antiparasitic, antiviral, appetite stimulant, arrhythmia, asthma, atopic dermatitis, birth control, bowel disease, bursitis, candidal infection, cervical dysplasia, chemical sensitivities, chemotherapy-induced leukopenia, childbirth (recovery), chronic fatigue syndrome, cirrhosis, colds, colitis, contraception, Crohn's disease, cysts, dementia, depression, diabetes, diarrhea, digestive problems, diverticulitis, dysentery, edema, endometriosis, fever, fibromyalgia, fistulas, gastritis, gastrointestinal disorders, genetic damage (enhances DNA repair), gingivitis, gonorrhea, gout, heart disease, hemorrhage, hemorrhoids, hepatoprotection, herpes, high blood pressure, high cholesterol levels, HIV, inflammatory bowel disease (IBD), influenza, kidney cleanser, kidney disease, leaky gut syndrome, leukemia, leukopenia, liver disease, long-term debility, lung inflammation, lupus, menstrual irregularity, multidrug resistance of tumor cells, multiple sclerosis (MS), nerve pain, neuroprotection, pain (including bone pain), premenstrual syndrome, prostate problems, radiation burns, radiation side effects, sexually transmitted diseases, shingles, sinusitis, skin disorders, sore throats, stimulant, stomach pain, stomach ulcers, stroke, sunscreen, tonic, tumors, ulcers, urinary tract infections, urinary tract inflammation, vasorelaxant, viral infection, weakness, wound healing.

DOSING
Adults (18 Years and Older)

- There is insufficient evidence to recommend a dose for cat's claw. Capsules, extracts, tinctures, decoctions, and teas are commercially available. Anecdotal evidence suggests that 20 mg to 25 g may be given in divided does.
- Cat's claw is also available in preparations for the skin, but there is insufficient evidence to recommend dosing for this form.

Children (Younger than 18 Years)

- There is insufficient evidence to recommend a dose for cat's claw in children.

SAFETY
Allergies

- People with allergies to plants in the Rubiaceae family or any species of *Uncaria* may be more likely to have allergic reactions to cat's claw. A typical allergic reaction may be itching or severe rash. Allergic inflammation of the kidneys has been reported.

Side Effects and Warnings

- Few side effects have been reported from using cat's claw at recommended doses. Most side effects are believed to be rare, and some side effects are theoretical and have not been reported in humans. Examples of possible side effects include stomach discomfort, nausea, diarrhea, slow heartbeats or altered rhythm of heartbeats, kidney disease, acute kidney failure, neuropathy, decreases in estrogen or progesterone levels, and an increased risk of bleeding. Because cat's claw theoretically may increase the risk of bleeding, patients may need to stop taking cat's claw before some surgeries, and this needs to be discussed with a qualified health care provider. Caution is advised in patients with bleeding disorders or in those taking drugs that may increase the risk of bleeding. Dosing adjustments may be necessary.
- Some natural medicine experts discourage the use of cat's claw in people with conditions affecting the immune system, such as acquired immunodeficiency syndrome (AIDS) or human immunodeficiency virus (HIV), some types of cancer, multiple sclerosis, tuberculosis, and rheumatological diseases (rheumatoid arthritis, lupus, etc.). However, there are no specific studies or reports in this area, and the risks of cat's claw use in people with these conditions are not clear.
- Many tinctures contain high levels of alcohol; driving or operating heavy machinery should be avoided.

Pregnancy and Breastfeeding

- Cat's claw cannot be recommended during pregnancy or breastfeeding. Historically, cat's claw has been used to prevent pregnancy and to induce abortion. Women who are pregnant or wish to become pregnant should not take cat's claw. Many tinctures contain high levels of alcohol and should be avoided during pregnancy.

INTERACTIONS
Interactions with Drugs

- In theory, cat's claw may increase the risk of bleeding when taken with drugs that increase the risk of bleeding. Some examples include aspirin, anticoagulants ("blood thinners") such as warfarin (Coumadin) or heparin, antiplatelet drugs such as clopidogrel (Plavix), and nonsteroidal antiinflammatory drugs (NSAIDs) such as ibuprofen (Motrin, Advil) or naproxen (Naprosyn, Aleve).
- In theory, cat's claw may interfere with the way the body processes certain drugs using the liver's "cytochrome P450" enzyme system. As a result, the levels of these drugs may be increased in the blood and may cause increased effects or potentially serious adverse reactions.
- Because one component in cat's claw may alter the rhythm of the heart (e.g., it may slow heartbeats) or lower blood pressure, cat's claw should be used cautiously by people who take drugs to treat irregular heart rhythms, such as amiodarone (Cordarone) or digoxin (Lanoxin), or drugs to lower blood pressure, such as verapamil (Calan).
- Because cat's claw is believed to affect the immune system, people taking immunosuppressants such as corticosteroids, drugs for rheumatological diseases (rheumatoid arthritis, lupus, etc.), or drugs to prevent rejection of transplanted organs should consult a health care provider and pharmacist before using cat's claw. Examples of such drugs are azathioprine, cyclosporine, and prednisone.
- Cat's claw may interact with hormonal agents, cholesterol-lowering agents, diuretics, and agents that affect the kidneys.
- Although not well studied in humans, cat's claw may interact with drugs that increase sensitivity to light, analgesics, anesthetics, antibiotics, antihistamines, antiinflammatory agents, and antiviral agents. Cat's claw may also interact with drugs used to treat cancer.
- Many tinctures contain high levels of alcohol and may cause nausea or vomiting when taken with metronidazole (Flagyl) or disulfiram (Antabuse).

Interactions with Herbs and Supplements

- Very few interactions between cat's claw and herbs or supplements have been reported. In theory, cat's claw may interfere with the way the body processes certain herbs or supplements using the liver's cytochrome P450 enzyme system. As a result, the levels of other herbs or supplements may become too high in the blood. It may also alter the effects that other herbs or supplements possibly have on the P450 system.
- It is possible that cat's claw may lower blood pressure. Additive effects may be seen with black cohosh, curcumin, or ginger, for example.
- Cat's claw may alter the rhythm of heartbeats. As a result, cat's claw should be used carefully if also taken with other herbs that affect the heart, such as foxglove/digitalis.
- In theory, cat's claw may increase the risk of bleeding when taken with herbs and supplements that are believed to increase the risk of bleeding. Multiple cases of bleeding have been reported with the use of *Ginkgo biloba,* and fewer cases have been reported with garlic and saw palmetto. Numerous other agents may theoretically increase the risk of bleeding, although this has not been proven in most cases.
- Cat's claw may decrease estrogen levels; therefore, the effects of other agents believed to have estrogen-like properties may be altered.
- Cat's claw may decrease the effectiveness of iron supplements and interact with cholesterol-lowering herbs and supplements, diuretics, mushrooms, or herbs that affect the kidneys.

- Although not well studied in humans, cat's claw may interact with herbs or supplements that increase sensitivity to light. Other potential interactions are with pain relievers, anesthetics, antibiotics, antihistamines, antiinflammatory agents, antioxidants, and antiviral agents. Cat's claw may also interact with herbs used to treat cancer.

For a complete list of references, please visit www.naturalstandard.com.

C

Cedar
(*Cedrus* spp.)

RELATED TERMS

- Cedar of Lebanon, cedars of Lebanon, cedarwood, cedarwood oil, *Cedrus deodara*, *Cedrus libani*, Coniferales, essential oils, *Juniperus ashei*, Pinaceae (family), Pinales, plicatic acid.
- **Note:** Cedar (*Cedrus* spp.) should not be confused with *Cryptomeria japonica* (Japanese cedar), *Thuja occidentalis* (northern white cedar or eastern white cedar), *Thuja plicata* (western red cedar), or *Juniperus* spp. (mountain cedar or eastern red cedar) as they are not closely related. This monograph only includes information on *Cedrus* spp.

BACKGROUND

- Cedar is native to the mountains of the western Himalayan and the Mediterranean regions. Because moths and other insects are repelled by the scent of the wood and oil, cedar wood has been used in closets and chests to preserve fabrics and textiles. In one clinical study, patients with alopecia areata who were massaged with a combination of cedarwood oil, other aromatic oils, and carrier oils had significantly improved symptoms. However, there are currently no further well-designed studies in humans available to support the use of cedar for any condition.
- In atopic patients, cedar pollen may cause allergic symptoms, including asthma. Occupational exposure to cedar wood dust may have irritant, allergenic, or carcinogenic effects.

EVIDENCE

Uses Based on Scientific Evidence	Grade
Alopecia Areata (Hair Loss) Alopecia areata, a disorder in which the immune system attacks the hair follicles causing loss of hair on the scalp, face, and other parts of the body, is a difficult condition to treat. Massage with cedarwood in carrier oils may improve the symptoms of alopecia areata. However, the evidence is insufficient to make a recommendation.	C

Uses Based on Tradition or Theory
Insect repellent.

DOSING

Adults (18 Years and Older)

- There is insufficient evidence to recommend a dose for cedar in adults.

Children (Younger than 18 Years)

- There is insufficient evidence to recommend a dose for cedar in children.

SAFETY

Allergies

- Avoid in individuals with a known allergy or hypersensitivity to cedar, its pollen, its constituents, wood dust, or members of the Pinaceae family.
- Atopic populations may experience allergic symptoms, including asthma, after exposure to cedar pollen. Occupational exposure to wood dust may also have irritant and allergenic effects, including bronchial asthma, rhinitis (hay fever), inflammation in the lungs caused by inhaling dust, organic dust toxic syndrome (ODTS), bronchitis, allergic dermatitis, and conjunctivitis (pinkeye).

Side Effects and Warnings

- There is currently insufficient available evidence to assess the safety of taking cedar by mouth. Cedar is likely safe when cedarwood oil in carrier oils is applied to the skin. However, in sensitive patients, cedar pollen may cause allergic symptoms, including asthma. Occupational exposure to cedar wood dust may have irritant, allergenic, or carcinogenic effects and may increase the risk of Hodgkin's disease. There may also be a possible increased risk of lung cancer. Microorganisms in the wood may cause alveolitis allergica and ODTS, aspergillomycosis (fungus infections), bronchial asthma, and rhinitis.

Pregnancy and Breastfeeding

- Cedar is not recommended in pregnant or breastfeeding women because of a lack of available scientific evidence.

INTERACTIONS

Interactions with Drugs

- Insufficient evidence is available.

Interactions with Herbs and Dietary Supplements

- Insufficient evidence is available.

For a complete list of references, please visit www.naturalstandard.com.

Celery

(Apium graveolens)

RELATED TERMS

- 5-Methoxypsoralen, alpha-methylene gamma-butyrolactone group, Apiaceae (family), *Apium graveolens*, *Apium graveolens* L., celeriac, celery extract, celery juice, celery profilin, celery root, celery seed, celery seed oil, celery soup, celery spice, celery tuber, cross-reactive carbohydrate determinants, crude celery, furocoumarins, immunogenic food, methoxsalen (8-methoxypsoralen), phthalide, profilin, psoralen, raw celery, sedanolide, Umbelliferae (family).

BACKGROUND

- Wild celery can be found throughout Europe, the Mediterranean, and parts of Asia. The leaves, stalks, root, and seeds can be eaten. In western cuisine, the stalks of its domesticated cousin are commonly used in cooking and may be eaten raw, alone or in salads, or as a cooked ingredient in various recipes. Celery seed has also been used as a diuretic (increases urine flow) and to treat gout (foot inflammation). However, there is insufficient evidence in humans to support the use of celery for any indication.
- Allergy to celery is fairly common, as celery contains an allergen similar to the birch pollen allergen. Both raw and cooked celery can cause reactions that range from contact dermatitis to anaphylactic shock.
- The ancient Greeks and Egyptians cultivated celery, which was probably originally used as a medicine. Some Egyptian tombs also contained celery leaves and flowers.

EVIDENCE

Uses Based on Scientific Evidence	Grade
Mosquito Repellent Celery extract may be an effective mosquito repellent. Preliminary evidence is promising.	C

Uses Based on Tradition or Theory
Antioxidant, arthritis, cancer, inflammatory joint diseases (rheumatoid arthritis, osteoarthritis), larvicide (insecticide), tonic.

DOSING
Adults (18 Years and Older)

- There is insufficient evidence to recommend a dose for celery in adults. Celery is likely safe in food amounts.

Children (Younger than 18 Years)

- There is insufficient evidence to recommend a dose for celery in children. Celery is likely safe in food amounts.

SAFETY
Allergies

- Avoid in individuals with a known allergy or hypersensitivity to celery (*Apium graveolens*) or its constituents. Allergy to celery is fairly common, especially among those with sensitivity to birch pollen–related allergens. Raw celery, cooked celery, and celery juice can all cause allergic reactions. Reactions range from contact dermatitis to anaphylactic shock. In addition, celery ingestion or contact and subsequent exposure to ultraviolet radiation can cause phytophotodermatitis. Symptoms of celery allergy have included laryngeal edema, celery-dependent exercise-induced anaphylaxis, and anaphylactic shock.

Side Effects and Warnings

- Celery is likely safe when used in food amounts in nonallergic individuals.
- Allergy to celery is fairly common, especially among those with sensitivity to birch pollen–related allergens. Avoid in patients eating large amounts of psoralen-containing foods or herbs, such as limes, lemons, parsley, figs, parsnip, carrots, certain oranges, some natural grasses, and dill.
- Use cautiously in patients with bile secretion disorders.
- Avoid high celery intake in pregnant patients.

Pregnancy and Breastfeeding

- Celery is not recommended in pregnant or breastfeeding women because of a lack of available scientific evidence. High celery intake may increase the risk of sensitization against food allergens.

INTERACTIONS
Interactions with Drugs

- Patients hypersensitive to celery who take celery and certain agents, such as conversion enzyme inhibitors (ACE inhibitors), alcohol, aspirin, or beta-blockers, may increase the likelihood of developing food-induced anaphylactic shock.
- Celery may increase the risk of bleeding when taken with drugs that increase the risk of bleeding. Some examples include aspirin, anticoagulants ("blood thinners") such as warfarin (Coumadin) or heparin, antiplatelet drugs such as clopidogrel (Plavix), and nonsteroidal antiinflammatory drugs (NSAIDS) such as ibuprofen (Motrin, Advil) or naproxen (Naprosyn, Aleve).
- Although not well studied in humans, celery may lower blood pressure. Caution is advised in patients taking blood pressure medications because of possible additive effects.
- Although not well studied in humans, celery may alter cholesterol levels. Caution is advised in patients taking cholesterol medications because of possible additive effects.
- Celery may have antispasmodic activity. Caution is advised in patients taking seizure medications because of possible additive effects.
- Celery may interfere with the way the body processes certain drugs using the liver's "cytochrome P450" enzyme system. As a result, the levels of these drugs may be increased in the blood and may cause increased effects or potentially serious adverse reactions. Patients using any medications should check the package insert and speak with a qualified health care professional, including a pharmacist, about possible interactions.
- Celery may have diuretic (increased urine flow) properties. Caution is advised in patients taking other diuretics because of possible additive effects.

- Although not well studied in humans, celery may increase the amount of drowsiness caused by some drugs. Examples include benzodiazepines (tranquilizers) such as lorazepam (Ativan) or diazepam (Valium), barbiturates such as phenobarbital, narcotics such as codeine, some antidepressants, and alcohol. Use caution while driving or operating machinery.

Interactions with Herbs and Dietary Supplements

- Celery may increase the risk of bleeding when taken with herbs and supplements that are believed to increase the risk of bleeding. Multiple cases of bleeding have been reported with the use of *Ginkgo biloba*, and fewer cases have been reported with garlic and saw palmetto.
- Although not well studied in humans, celery may lower blood pressure. Caution is advised in patients taking other herbs or supplements with blood pressure-altering activity because of possible additive effects.
- Celery may alter cholesterol levels. Caution is advised in patients taking herbs or supplements with cholesterol-altering activity, such as red yeast rice, because of possible additive effects.

- Celery may have antispasmodic activity. Caution is advised in patients taking other antispasmodic herbs or supplements because of possible additive effects.
- Celery may interfere with the way the body processes certain herbs or supplements using the liver's cytochrome P450 enzyme system. As a result, the levels of other herbs or supplements may become too high in the blood. It may also alter the effects that other herbs or supplements possibly have on the P450 system.
- Celery may have diuretic (increased urine flow) properties. Caution is advised in patients taking other diuretic herbs or supplements because of possible additive effects.
- Celery may increase the amount of drowsiness caused by some herbs or supplements. Use caution while driving or operating machinery.
- In theory, patients hypersensitive to celery who take celery and willow bark may increase the likelihood of developing food-induced anaphylactic shock.

For a complete list of references, please visit www.naturalstandard.com.

Chamomile

(*Matricaria recutita*, syn. *Matricaria suaveolens, Matricaria chamomilla, Anthemis nobilis, Chamaemelum nobile, Chamomilla chamomilla, Chamomilla recutita*)

RELATED TERMS

- *Anthemis arvensis, Anthemis cotula, Anthemis nobile, Anthemis nobilis, Anthemis xylopoda,* apigenin, Asteraceae/Compositae (family), baboonig, babuna, babunah, babunah camomile, babunj, bunga kamil, camamila, camamilla, camomile, camomile sauvage, camomilla, Camomille Allemande, Campomilla, Ulbricht chamaemeloside, *Chamaemelum nobile* L., chamomile flowers, *Chamomilla, Chamomilla recutita,* chamomillae ramane flos, chamomille commune, classic chamomile, common chamomile, double chamomile, Echte Kamille (Dutch), English chamomile, feldkamille (German), fleur de chamomile (French), fleurs de petite camomille (French), Flores Anthemidis, flos chamomillae, garden chamomile, German chamomile, Grosse Kamille, Grote Kamille, ground apple, Hungarian chamomile, Kamille, Kamillen, kamitsure, kamiture, Kleine, kleme kamille, lawn chamomile, low chamomile, manzanilla, manzanilla chiquita, manzilla comun, manzanilla dulce, matricaire, *Matricaria chamomilla, Matricaria maritima* (L.), *Matricaria recutita, Matricaria suaveolens,* matricariae flos, matricariae flowers, may-then, Nervine, pin heads, rauschert, Romaine, romaine manzanilla, Roman chamomile, Romische Kamille, single chamomile, STW 5 (containing *Iberis*, peppermint, chamomile), sweet chamomile, sweet false chamomile, sweet feverfew, true chamomile, whig-plant, wild chamomile.

BACKGROUND

- Chamomile has been used medicinally for thousands of years and is widely used in Europe. It is a popular treatment for numerous ailments, including sleep disorders, anxiety, digestion/intestinal conditions, skin infections/inflammation (including eczema), wound healing, infantile colic, teething pains, and diaper rash. In the United States, chamomile is best known as an ingredient in herbal tea preparations advertised for mild sedating effects.
- German chamomile (*Matricaria recutita*) and Roman chamomile (*Chamaemelum nobile*) are the two major types of chamomile used for health conditions. They are believed to have similar effects on the body, although German chamomile may be slightly stronger. Most research has used German chamomile, which is more commonly used everywhere except for England, where Roman chamomile is more common.
- Although chamomile is widely used, there is not enough reliable research in humans to support its use for any condition. Despite its reputation as a gentle medicinal plant, there are many reports of allergic reactions in people after eating or coming into contact with chamomile preparations, including life-threatening anaphylaxis.

EVIDENCE

Uses Based on Scientific Evidence	Grade
Cardiovascular Conditions Chamomile is not well-known for its cardiac effects, and there is little research in this area.	C
Common Cold There is limited evidence that inhaling steam with chamomile may help common cold symptoms.	C
Diarrhea in Children There is limited evidence that chamomile with apple pectin may reduce the length of time that children experience diarrhea.	C
Eczema The German Commission E authorizes the use of topical chamomile for diseases of the skin. However, little research has been done on topical chamomile for eczema.	C
Gastrointestinal Conditions Chamomile is used traditionally for numerous gastrointestinal conditions, including digestion disorders, "spasm" or colic, upset stomach, flatulence (gas), ulcers, and gastrointestinal irritation. However, currently there is a lack of reliable human research available in any of these areas.	C
Hemorrhagic Cystitis (Bladder Irritation with Bleeding) There is limited evidence that the combination of chamomile baths plus chamomile bladder washes and antibiotics is superior to antibiotics alone for hemorrhagic cystitis.	C
Hemorrhoids There is limited evidence that chamomile ointment may improve hemorrhoids.	C
Infantile Colic Chamomile is reputed to have antispasmodic activity, but there is little research to substantiate this claim.	C
Mucositis from Cancer Treatment (Mouth Ulcers/Irritation) Poor-quality studies have used chamomile mouthwash for the prevention or treatment of mouth mucositis caused by radiation therapy or cancer chemotherapy. Results are conflicting, and it remains unclear whether chamomile is helpful in this situation.	C
Quality of Life in Cancer Patients A small amount of research suggests that massage using chamomile essential oil may improve anxiety and quality of life in cancer patients. However, this evidence is not conclusive.	C
Skin Inflammation Topical chamomile preparations have traditionally been used to soothe skin inflammation. The existing	C

(Continued)

209

Uses Based on Scientific Evidence

Uses Based on Scientific Evidence	Grade
clinical evidence shows that chamomile may be of little if any benefit while animal studies support its antiinflammatory action.	
Sleep Aid/Sedation Traditionally, chamomile preparations, such as tea and essential oil aromatherapy, have been used for insomnia and sedation (calming effects). However, there is insufficient evidence to support this use.	C
Vaginitis (Inflammation of the Vagina) Vaginitis may involve itching, discharge, or pain with urination. Chamomile douche may improve symptoms of vaginitis with few side effects. Because infection (including sexually transmitted diseases), poor hygiene, or nutritional deficiencies can cause vaginitis, medical attention should be sought by people with this condition.	C
Wound Healing There is promising preliminary evidence supporting the topical use of chamomile for wound healing. However, the available literature is not adequate to support a recommendation either for or against this use.	C
Postoperative Sore Throat/Hoarseness due to Intubation Chamomile spray has not been found to prevent postoperative sore throat and hoarseness any more than normal saline.	D

Uses Based on Tradition or Theory

Abdominal bloating, abortifacient, abrasions, abscesses, acne, anorexia, antibacterial, anticoagulant, antifungal, antioxidant, antipruritic, antiseptic, antispasmodic, anxiety, aromatic, arthritis, asthma, back pain, bedsores, bladder disorders, blood purification, bruises, burns, cancer, canker sores, carpal tunnel syndrome, catarrh, chicken pox, constipation, contact dermatitis, cough, Crohn's disease, croup, delirium tremens (DTs), diaper rash, diaphoretic, diuretic (increases urination), diverticulitis, dry skin, dysmenorrhea (painful menstruation), ear infections, eye disorders (blocked tear ducts), eye infections, fatty liver, fever, fistula healing, frostbite, gallstones, gingivitis, gout, hay fever, headaches, heartburn, hives, hypoglycemia (low blood sugar), hysteria, impetigo, inflammatory conditions, insect bites, insomnia, intestinal cramps, irregular menstrual cycles, irritable bowel syndrome, kidney disorders, leg ulcers, liver disorders, low back pain, malaria, mastitis (breast inflammation), menopause, menstrual cramps, menstrual disorders, morphine withdrawal, motion sickness, muscle strength, nasal inflammation, nausea, nervous stomach, neuralgia (nerve pain), nightmares, oral hygiene (mouthwash), osteoporosis, parasites/worms, peptic ulcers, perineal trauma, poison ivy, postnatal depression, psoriasis, rash (heat), respiratory inflammation, restlessness, rheumatism, Roemheld syndrome, sciatica, seizure disorder, sinusitis, stomach cramps, sunburn, sunstroke, teething pain (mouth rinse), tension, tics, toothache, travel sickness, tuberculosis, ulcerative colitis, ulcers, uterine disorders, uterine stimulant, uterine tonic, vaginal infections, viral infection (flu-like symptoms or polio), vomiting, vomiting/nausea during pregnancy.

DOSING

Adults (18 Years and Older)

- Capsules/tablets containing 400-1600 mg in divided doses have been taken by daily mouth. As a liquid extract (1:1 in 45% alcohol), 1-4 mL daily three times has been taken by mouth. A tincture (1:5 in alcohol) has been taken as a 15-mL dose three-four times daily. As a mouth rinse, a 1% fluid extract or 5% tincture has been used.
- Chamomile is frequently consumed as tea, and 1-4 cups of chamomile tea is commonly taken daily.
- There are no standard doses for chamomile used on the skin. Some natural medicine publications have recommended paste, plaster, or ointment containing 3% to 10% chamomile flower heads. Chamomile has also been used as a bath additive and as a douche.

Children (Younger than 18 Years)

- There is insufficient evidence to recommend the safe use of chamomile products in children.

SAFETY

Allergies

- There are multiple reports of serious allergic reactions to chamomile taken by mouth or as an enema, including anaphylaxis, throat swelling, and shortness of breath. Skin allergic reactions have been frequently reported, including dermatitis and eczema. Chamomile eyewash can cause allergic conjunctivitis (pinkeye).
- People with allergies to other plants in the Asteraceae (Compositae) family should avoid chamomile. Examples include aster, chrysanthemum, mugwort, ragweed, and ragwort. Cross-reactions may occur with celery, chrysanthemum, feverfew, tansy, and birch pollen. Individuals with allergies to these plants should avoid chamomile. Contact skin allergy has been reported.

Side Effects

- Impurities (adulterants) in chamomile products are common and may cause adverse effects. Atopic dermatitis (skin rash) has been reported.
- Chamomile in various forms may cause drowsiness or sedation. Use caution when driving or operating heavy machinery. In large doses, chamomile can cause vomiting. Because of its coumarin content, chamomile may theoretically increase the risk of bleeding. Caution is advised in patients with bleeding disorders or in those taking drugs that may increase the risk of bleeding. Dosing adjustments may be necessary. Increases in blood pressure are possible.

Pregnancy and Breastfeeding

- In theory, chamomile may act as a uterine stimulant or lead to abortion. It therefore should be avoided during pregnancy. There are not enough scientific data to recommend the safe use of chamomile while breastfeeding.

INTERACTIONS
Interactions with Drugs

- Chamomile interactions are not well studied scientifically.
- Chamomile may increase the amount of drowsiness caused by some drugs. Examples include benzodiazepines such as lorazepam (Ativan) or diazepam (Valium), barbiturates such as phenobarbital, narcotics such as codeine, some antidepressants, and alcohol. Use caution while driving or operating machinery.
- In theory, chamomile may increase the risk of bleeding when used with anticoagulants or antiplatelet drugs. Some examples include aspirin, anticoagulants ("blood thinners") such as warfarin (Coumadin) or heparin, antiplatelet drugs such as clopidogrel (Plavix), and nonsteroidal antiinflammatory drugs (NSAIDs) such as ibuprofen (Motrin, Advil) or naproxen (Naprosyn, Aleve).
- Chamomile may interfere with the way the body processes certain drugs using the liver's "cytochrome P450" enzyme system. As a result, the levels of these drugs may be increased in the blood and may cause increased effects or potentially serious adverse reactions. Patients using any medications should check the package insert and speak with a health care professional, including a pharmacist, about possible interactions.
- Be aware that many tinctures contain high levels of alcohol and may cause vomiting when taken with metronidazole (Flagyl) or disulfiram (Antabuse).
- An extract containing *Matricaria chamomilla*, *Sideritis euboea*, *Sideritis clandestina*, and *Pimpinella anisum* was associated with selective estrogen receptor modulator (SERM) properties against osteoporosis. Theoretically, chamomile may interact with SERM drugs like raloxifene (prescription drug used for osteoporosis) or tamoxifen (a prescription drug used for cancer).
- Constituents in chamomile may alter blood sugar or blood pressure. Patients taking medications that affect blood sugar or blood pressure should be cautious.
- Chamomile may have antiinflammatory effects. Theoretically, use of chamomile with other antiinflammatory drugs, such as NSAIDs or ibuprofen, may have additive effects.
- Chamomile may interact with medications that act as cardiac depressants, central nervous system depressants, calcium channel blockers, cardiac glycosides, and respiratory depressants.

- Chamomile may also interact with antibiotics, antifungals, antihistamines, diuretics, as well as drugs for high cholesterol, ulcers, diarrhea, or gastrointestinal disorders.

Interactions with Herbs and Dietary Supplements

- Chamomile may increase the amount of drowsiness caused by some herbs or supplements. Use caution while driving or operating machinery.
- In theory, chamomile may increase the risk of bleeding when taken with other products that are believed to increase the risk of bleeding. Multiple cases of bleeding have been reported with the use of *Ginkgo biloba*, and fewer cases have been reported with garlic and saw palmetto. Numerous other agents may theoretically increase the risk of bleeding, although this has not been proven in most cases.
- Chamomile may interfere with the way the body processes certain drugs using the liver's cytochrome P450 enzyme system. As a result, the levels of other herbs or supplements may become too high in the blood. It may also alter the effects that other herbs or supplements possibly have on the P450 system. Patients using any medications should check the package insert and speak with a health care professional, including a pharmacist, about possible interactions.
- Chamomile may have antiestrogenic effects and interact with herbs and supplements like red clover or soy.
- Based on preliminary study, constituents in chamomile may alter blood sugar or blood pressure. Patients taking herbs or supplements that affect blood sugar or blood pressure should be cautious.
- Chamomile may have antiinflammatory effects. Theoretically, the use of chamomile with other antiinflammatory herbs and supplements may have additive effects.
- Chamomile may interact with herbs and supplements that act as cardiac depressants, cardiac glycosides, respiratory depressants, or spasmolytics.
- Chamomile may also interact with antibacterial, antifungal, antihistamine, or diuretic herbs and supplements, as well as herbs and supplements used for high cholesterol, ulcers, diarrhea, or gastrointestinal disorders.

For a complete list of references, please visit www.naturalstandard.com.

Chaparral and Nordihydroguaiaretic Acid (NDGA)

(*Larrea tridentata, Larrea divaricata*)

RELATED TERMS

- 1-Aryl tetralin lignans, chaparral taxa, chaparral tea, chaparro, creosote, creosote bush, dwarf evergreen oak, el gobernadora (Spanish), falsa alcaparra (Spanish), flavonoids, furanoid lignans, geroop, gobernadora, greasewood, guaiaretic acid, guamis, gumis, hediondilla, hideonodo, hydrocarbons, jarillo, kovanau, kreosotstrauch, larrea, *Larrea divaricata, Larrea glutiosa, Larrea mexicana, Larrea mexicana* Moric, *Larrea tridentate, Larrea tridentata* (DC) Coville, lignans, maltose-M3N, M4N, NDGA, nordihydroguaiaretic acid, Nordy, palo ondo (Spanish), sapogenins, shoegoi, sonora covillea, sterols, tasago, triterpenes, volatile oils, wax esters, ya-tmep, yah-temp, Zygophyllaceae (family).

BACKGROUND

- Chaparral is a shrub found in the desert regions of southwestern United States and Mexico. It was used by Native American populations for indications including chickenpox (varicella), colds, diarrhea, menstrual cramps, pain, rheumatic diseases, skin disorders, snake bites, and as an emetic. Chaparral tea was also used for purported effects of removing lysergic acid diethylamide (LSD) residue, thereby preventing recurrent hallucinations. Chaparral leaves have also been used externally for bruises, scratches, wounds, and hair growth.
- The chaparral component NDGA has been evaluated as a treatment for cancer, but because of risk of toxicity, it is considered unsafe and not recommended for use.

EVIDENCE

Uses Based on Scientific Evidence	Grade
Cancer Chaparral and one of its components called nordihydroguaiaretic acid (NDGA) have antioxidant ("free-radical scavenging") properties and have been proposed as cancer treatments. However, chaparral and NDGA have been linked with cases of kidney and liver failure, liver cirrhosis, kidney cysts, and kidney cancer in humans. In response to these reports, the U.S. Food and Drug Administration (FDA) removed chaparral from its "generally recognized as safe"" (GRAS) list in 1970. Chaparral and NDGA are generally considered unsafe and are not recommended for use.	C

Uses Based on Tradition or Theory
Abdominal cramps, abortion inducing, abrasions, acne, actinic keratosis (a skin condition), alcohol withdrawal, allergies, antibacterial, antiinflammatory, antioxidant, antiparasitic, antiseptic, antiviral, arthritis, autoimmune disorders, blood purifier, bowel cramps, breathing problems, bronchitis, bruises, burns, bursitis, cavities (preventive mouthwash), central nervous system disorders, chickenpox, cold sores, colds, coughs, cytomegalovirus, dandruff, decomposition, diabetes, diarrhea, diuretic (increases urine flow), dysentery, enteritis, Epstein-Barr virus, fertility, flu, food additive, gas, gastrointestinal disorders, genitourinary infections, hair tonic, hallucinations (including those due to LSD ingestion), heartburn, herpes simplex virus (cold sores), herpes zoster virus, immune function stimulation, immune system disorders, impetigo, indigestion, intestinal problems, Kaposi's sarcoma, kidney or bladder stones, leukemia, liver cleanser, liver metabolic function, melanoma, menstrual cramps, menstrual disorders, multidrug resistance (trastuzumab), neuritis, nutritional supplement, pain, painful joints, premenstrual syndrome (PMS), preservative, psoriasis, respiratory tract infections, rheumatic diseases, sciatica, skin disorders, skin infections, snakebite pain, stomach ulcer, tuberculosis, urinary tract infections, venereal disease, vomiting, wound healing (poultice).

DOSING

Adults (18 Years and Older)

- Safety has not been established for any dose. Small doses of tea have been used; for example, 1 teaspoon of chaparral leaves and flowers steeped in 1 pint of water for 15 minutes, consumed 1-3 cups daily for up to a maximum of several days. Chaparral tea has also been made by steeping 7-8 g of crumbled dried leaves, stems, and twigs in 1 quart of hot water. As a water extract, chaparral might be consumed in the amount of 1-3 cups of chaparral tea per day for a period of 2-3 weeks, although this is not recommended.
- A tincture has also been used; for example, 20 drops up to three times daily. These preparations may be associated with less toxicity and possibly contain fewer allergenic compounds than capsules or tablets. Oil or powder forms of chaparral have also been used, applied to an affected area of skin several times daily.
- Capsules or tablets may deliver large doses leading to toxicity and are not recommended. Exposure to lignans, which may yield toxicity, appears to be greater from capsules or tablets than from chaparral tea.

Children (Younger than 18 Years)

- Chaparral is not recommended for use in children because of lack of scientific data and potential toxicity.

SAFETY

Allergies

- People with allergy or hypersensitivity to chaparral or any of its components including NDGA, nor-isoguaiasin, dihydroguaiaretic acid, partially demethylated dihydroguaiaretic acid, and demethoxyisoguaiasin may have allergic reactions to chaparral.
- There are human case reports of allergic hypersensitivity (contact dermatitis) to chaparral and to its resin.

Side Effects and Warnings

- Chaparral has been associated with multiple serious and potentially fatal adverse effects in animals and humans. Animals given the chaparral component NDGA developed kidney or gastrointestinal cysts and liver cell death. In humans, chaparral has been associated with kidney and liver failure, liver cirrhosis, kidney cysts, and kidney cancer. Human case reports note rash and fever with use of chaparral. Nausea, vomiting, diarrhea, abdominal cramps, and mouth inflammation have also been reported in people consuming chaparral. Exposure to lignans, which may yield toxicity, appears to be greater from capsule or tablets than from decoctions of chaparral tea. The U.S. Food and Drug Administration (FDA) removed chaparral from the "generally recognized as safe" (GRAS) list in 1970 and considers chaparral to be unsafe. Elevations of liver enzymes or altered kidney function tests (serum creatinine) may occur with chaparral.

- Based on an animal study, chaparral may lower blood sugar levels. Caution is advised in patients with diabetes or hypoglycemia and in those taking drugs, herbs, or supplements that affect blood sugar. Serum glucose levels should be monitored closely, and medication adjustments may be necessary. Aggravation of hypothyroidism may occur.
- In theory, chaparral may also increase the risk of bleeding and may add to the effects of anticoagulants (blood thinners) or antiplatelet drugs. Use of chaparral with any of these drugs should be discussed with a health care professional.

Pregnancy and Breastfeeding

- Chaparral cannot be recommended during pregnancy or breastfeeding because of the risk of birth defects or spontaneous abortion.
- Chaparral may inhibit ovulation and decrease the chance that women will become pregnant.

INTERACTIONS
Interactions with Drugs

- Based on animal studies and human case reports, chaparral has been associated with kidney damage, cysts, cancer, and kidney failure. Theoretically, use of chaparral with other agents known to alter kidney function or induce toxicity should be avoided, including sulfa antibiotics, aminoglycoside antibiotics, cyclooxygenase-2 (COX-2) inhibitors, nonsteroidal anti-inflammatory drugs (NSAIDs), and a number of other drugs. Patients who are using other medications and who are considering chaparral should consult with a qualified health care professional, including a pharmacist. Based on animal study and human case reports, chaparral has also been associated with liver damage. Theoretically, the use of chaparral with other agents known to induce liver toxicity should be avoided; these include amiodarone, carmustine, or danazol.
- Based on animal study, chaparral may lower blood sugar levels. Caution is advised when medications that may also lower blood sugar are used. Patients taking drugs for diabetes by mouth or injection should be monitored closely by a qualified health care professional. Medication adjustments may be necessary. Based on human research, chaparral may increase the risk of bleeding when taken with drugs that also increase the risk of bleeding. Some examples include aspirin, anticoagulants ("blood thinners") such as warfarin (Coumadin) or heparin, antiplatelet drugs such as clopidogrel (Plavix), and NSAIDs such as ibuprofen (Motrin, Advil) or naproxen (Naprosyn, Aleve).
- Based on animal research, chaparral may interfere with the way the body processes certain drugs using the liver's cytochrome P450 enzyme system. As a result, the levels of these drugs may be increased in the blood and may cause increased effects or potentially serious adverse reactions.

Patients using any medications should check the package insert and speak with a qualified health care professional or pharmacist about possible interactions. Based on historical use, chaparral may interact with monoamine oxidase inhibitors (MAOIs), such as isocarboxazid (Marplan), phenelzine (Nardil), and tranylcypromine (Parnate). There is also the possibility that blood pressure may become dangerously high if chaparral is taken with MAOIs, although there is limited research supporting this.

- Chaparral may aggravate indomethacin-induced gastric ulcers and inhibit the metabolism of barbiturate drugs such as phenobarbital. Effects of thyroid medications may be altered, although this is unproven.
- Chaparral may also interact with cancer, antiviral, gastrointestinal, immunosuppressant, thyroid, and abortion-inducing drugs.

Interactions with Herbs and Dietary Supplements

- Based on animal studies and human case reports, chaparral has been associated with kidney damage, cysts, cancer, and kidney failure. Theoretically, the use of chaparral with other herbs or supplements known to alter kidney function or induce toxicity should be avoided; these include agents with high levels of tannins. Chaparral may increase the risk of high blood pressure if used with other herbs with this effect. Based on animal research and human case reports, chaparral has also been associated with liver damage. Theoretically, the use of chaparral with other herbs or supplements known to induce liver toxicity should be avoided.
- Based on animal research, chaparral may lower blood sugar levels. Caution is advised when herbs or supplements that may also lower blood sugar are used. Blood glucose levels may require monitoring, and doses may need adjustment.
- Based on clinical evidence, chaparral may increase the risk of bleeding when taken with herbs and supplements that are believed to increase the risk of bleeding. Multiple cases of bleeding have been reported with the use of *Ginkgo biloba*, and fewer cases have been reported with garlic and saw palmetto. Numerous other agents may theoretically increase the risk of bleeding, although this has not been proven in most cases. Chaparral may also interact with vitamin K, which is necessary for blood clotting. By working against the action of vitamin K, chaparral may increase the risk of bleeding.
- Based on animal research, chaparral may interfere with the way the body processes certain herbs or supplements using the liver's cytochrome P450 enzyme system. As a result, the levels of other herbs or supplements may become too high in the blood. It may also alter the effects that other herbs or supplements may have on the P450 system. Patients using any medications should check the package insert and speak with a health care professional or pharmacist about possible interactions.
- Based on historical use, chaparral may interact with herbs or supplements with possible MAOI effects, such as 5-hydroxytryptophan (5-HTP) or dehydroepiandrosterone (DHEA). Chaparral may also interact with anticancer, antioxidant, antiviral, gastrointestinal, immunostimulant, immunosuppressant, and abortion-inducing herbs and supplements.
- Effects of thyroid-active agents may be altered, although this is unproven.

For a complete list of references, please visit www.naturalstandard.com.

Chasteberry
(*Vitex agnus-castus*)

RELATED TERMS

- Abraham's balm, Abrahams-strauch, Agneau chaste (French), Agni casti fructus (Latin), Agnocasto, agnus castus, agnus-castus, chaste berry, chaste tree, chaste tree berry, chastetree, gattilier (French), hemp tree, Keuschlammfruchte (German), kyskhedstrae (Danish), monk's pepper, Moenchspfeffer (German), petit poivre (French), Verbenaceae (family), vitex.

BACKGROUND

- The chaste tree is native to the Mediterranean and central Asia. Its berries have long been used for a variety of abnormalities including "corpus luteum deficiency," mastalgia (breast pain), and menstrual abnormalities.
- Chasteberry has been shown to inhibit prolactin secretion by competitively binding to dopamine receptors. Available evidence suggests that chasteberry may be an effective treatment option for hyperprolactinemic (elevated serum prolactin levels) conditions, and premenstrual syndrome (PMS). Chasteberry does not appear to affect levels of luteinizing hormone or follicle-stimulating hormone.
- Currently, clinical trials have found that treatment with chasteberry has been well tolerated with minimal side effects.
- The dried fruit of chasteberry plants has been used for thousands of years as a means of treating various ailments, ranging from impotence to breast pain. It was popular in ancient Greece and Rome to help promote celibacy. More recently, chasteberry has gained recognition for its success in alleviating some signs and symptoms of hyperprolactinemia and premenstrual syndrome. It is thought to have a normalizing effect on the menstrual cycle and has been used successfully to treat both amenorrhea (absence of menstruation) and menorrhagia (heavy menstruation).

EVIDENCE

Uses Based on Scientific Evidence	Grade
Hyperprolactinemia (Excessive Prolactin in the Blood) Chasteberry may inhibit prolactin secretion and thus has been suggested as a potential therapy in hyperprolactinemia, a condition characterized by elevated serum prolactin levels.	B
Corpus Luteum Deficiency/Luteal Phase Deficiency *Corpus luteum deficiency* (CLD) is a term more commonly used in Europe than in the United States and refers to irregular development of the corpus luteum after ovulation that results in abnormal progesterone secretion and incomplete endometrial differentiation. The term *luteal phase deficiency* (LPD) has also been used in this setting and has been implicated both in infertility and recurrent pregnancy loss. The use of chasteberry for this condition remains controversial.	C

Cyclic Mastalgia (Breast Pain) Despite preliminary promising results, it remains unclear whether chasteberry is an effective treatment in the management of cyclic mastalgia.	C
Irregular Menstrual Cycles It remains unclear whether chasteberry is an effective therapy in the management of irregular menses.	C
Premenstrual Dysphoric Disorder (PMDD) There is limited controlled trial evidence suggesting possible benefits of chasteberry in the alleviation of symptoms of PMDD.	C
Premenstrual Syndrome (PMS) Most studies evaluating chasteberry in PMS have been of poor study design, although one recent trial demonstrating benefit is of high quality.	C

Uses Based on Tradition or Theory

Acne, amenorrhea (absence of menstruation), antifungal, antiinflammatory, anxiety, benign prostatic hypertrophy (BPH, enlarged prostate), chastity, constipation, cystic endometrial hyperplasia (abnormal thickening of the inner lining of the uterus), dementia, depression due to menopause, diarrhea, dysmenorrhea (painful periods), dyspepsia (upset stomach), endometriosis (growth of endometrial tissue outside the uterus), epilepsy, expulsion of the placenta, female infertility, fevers, fibrocystic breasts, flatulence (gas), fluid retention, follicular ovarian cysts, hangovers, hot flashes, hypogonadism (underactive sex organs), impotence, inflammation, lactation, libido, menopause, menorrhagia (heavy menstruation), menstrual dermatoses, "menstrual neuroses," metrorrhagia (from functional causes, continuous or noncyclical uterine bleeding), mouth ulcers, nervousness, oligomenorrhea (lengthened cycle), orofacial herpes simplex, overactive libido, polymenorrhea (shortened cycle), postpartum bleeding, premenstrual aphthous ulcerative stomatitis (mouth sores), prevention of miscarriage in patients with progesterone insufficiency, reducing sexual desire, rheumatic conditions, secondary amenorrhea, snake bite, upper respiratory tract infections, vaginal dryness.

DOSING

Adults (18 Years and Older)

- Some experts recommend taking chasteberry on an empty stomach in the morning for maximal benefits. However, no studies have confirmed this finding. Various doses of chasteberry have been used in studies and practice. Traditional doses have ranged from 3.5-4.5 mg of dried extract to 600 mg of dried fruit daily. Other traditional doses include aqueous alcoholic extract (derived from 30-40 mg of dried fruit) daily in 50%-70% alcohol (v/v); 0.03-0.04 mL daily of fluid extract (1:1 g/mL); 0.15-0.2 mL daily of tincture (1:5 g/mL); 2.6-4.2 mg daily of a dried extract (9.5-11.5:1 w/w); or 0.5-1.0 g of dried fruit three times daily.

Children (Younger than 18 Years)

- There is insufficient evidence to recommend a dose for chasteberry in children.

SAFETY
Allergies

- Avoid in individuals with a known allergy or hypersensitivity to members of the *Vitex* (Verbenaceae) family or any chasteberry components. Mild skin reactions have been reported in clinical trials including eczema, itching, rash, skin eruptions, urticaria (hives) and allergic exanthema.

Side Effects and Warnings

- Chasteberry is likely safe when used orally in otherwise healthy adults using appropriate doses for the short-term alleviation of signs and symptoms associated with PMS or hyperprolactinemia (elevated serum prolactin levels). Chasteberry appears to be generally well tolerated with few adverse events reported. In an observational trial of 551 patients, approximately 5% experienced side effects, which were primarily mild. However, there are currently no available studies evaluating the long-term effects of chasteberry.
- Rare occurrences of the following side effects have been reported: acne, alopecia (hair loss), eczema, itching, rash, skin eruptions, urticaria (hives), headache, vertigo, seizure, drowsiness, agitation, fatigue, sweating and dry mouth, depressed mood, increased intraocular pressure, tachycardia (fast heart rate), palpitations, circulatory disorders, pulmonary edema (lung swelling), diarrhea, nausea, gas/flatulence, heartburn, vomiting, altered gonadotropin and ovarian hormone levels, hot flashes, mastalgia (breast pain), cycle changes, fibroid growth and weight gain, polyuria (frequent urination), menstrual bleeding, vaginitis (inflamed vagina), pelvic disease, and nosebleed.
- Nevertheless, use cautiously in patients taking oral contraceptives or hormone replacement therapy.
- Use cautiously in patients taking dopamine agonists or antagonists. Additionally, caution is advised in patients with Parkinson's disease and other illnesses of the central nervous system because medications used for these conditions often affect dopamine and taking them with chasteberry may increase effects and side effects.

- Avoid using in patients with hormone-sensitive cancers or conditions, those who are pregnant or breastfeeding, and in women undergoing in vitro fertilization.

Pregnancy and Breastfeeding

- Except under strict medical supervision, chasteberry should not be used in pregnancy because of potential uterine stimulatory properties. Some clinicians have used chasteberry in progesterone-deficient women during their first trimester to prevent miscarriage, but it is not known whether chasteberry is helpful or safe for this indication.
- Chasteberry is not recommended in breastfeeding women because of a lack of available scientific evidence. Chasteberry competitively binds to dopamine receptors and has been shown to affect prolactin secretion, possibly resulting in decreased breast milk production. However, some clinicians actually use low doses to stimulate milk production with some reported benefits.

INTERACTIONS
Interactions with Drugs

- Chasteberry has been shown to bind to D-2 receptors and therefore may alter dopaminergic effects. Caution is advised in patients with Parkinson's disease and other illnesses of the central nervous system because medications used for these conditions often affect dopamine and taking them with chasteberry may increase effects and side effects.
- Chasteberry may increase plasma levels of estrogens and progesterone. Caution is advised in patients taking birth control pills or other agents that alter hormones, such as hormone replacement therapy.

Interactions with Herbs and Dietary Supplements

- Chasteberry has been shown to bind to D-2 receptors and therefore may alter dopaminergic effects. Caution is advised in patients with Parkinson's disease and other illnesses of the central nervous system because medications used for these conditions often affect dopamine and taking them with chasteberry may increase effects and side effects.
- Chasteberry may increase plasma levels of estrogens and progesterone. Caution is advised in patients taking herbs or supplements that may also alter hormone levels because of possible adverse effects.

For a complete list of references, please visit www.naturalstandard.com.

Cherry

(Prunus africana, Prunus avium, Prunus emarginata, Prunus serotina, various Prunus spp.)

RELATED TERMS

- African cherry, anthocyanins, antioxidants, Balaton tart cherry, Bet v1, bing sweet cherries, cherry bezoar, cherry-brandy, cherry extract, cherry jam, cherry juice, cherry pip bezoars, cherry pit, cherry stalk, cherry stone, cherry wood, choke cherries, choke-cherry, cyanide, cyanidin, makore, nitrates, nitrites, phenolic compounds, polyphenolic compounds, Pru av 1, Pru av 2, Pru av 3, Pru av 4, Prunoideae (sub-family), *Prunus africana*, *Prunus avium*, *Prunus cerasus*, *Prunus emarginata*, *Prunus padus*, *Prunus serotina*, Rosaceae (family), rPru av 1, rPru av 3, rPru av 4, sour cherry, sweet cherries, tart cherries, tart cherry, wild cherry, wild cherry bark, wild cherry bark extract, wild cherry bezoar, wild cherry extract.
- **Note:** This monograph does not include Indian cherry *(Withania somnifera)*, Barbados cherry *(Malpighia glabra)*, ground cherry *(Physalis* spp.), or the finger cherry tree *(Rhodomyrtus macrocarpa)*.

BACKGROUND

- Cherries have been used as both food and medicine. African cherry *(Prunus africana)* has been used to treat enlarged prostate and other disorders. Cherries contain polyphenols, which may have antioxidant, anticancer, and anti-inflammatory properties. However, there is limited scientific evidence to support these uses.
- Preliminary research suggests that cherry may be able to relieve exercise-induced muscle damage. Cherry has also been used historically to relieve the symptoms of gout. The available clinical evidence is insufficient to support these uses.
- Cherries appear to be highly allergenic. There are many reports of sensitivity to cherries and cross-reactivity with other plants. People who are allergic to birch pollen may also be sensitive to cherries.

EVIDENCE

Uses Based on Scientific Evidence	Grade
Muscle Strains/Pain (Exercise-Induced Muscle Damage Prevention) Preliminary research suggests that cherry juice may prevent damage to muscles caused by exercise. More evidence is needed.	B

Uses Based on Tradition or Theory
Age-related nerve damage, anti-inflammatory, antioxidant, bladder cancer, breathing problems, cancer, colds, colon cancer, degenerative diseases, fever, flavoring, gout, gynecologic disorders, heart disease, malnutrition, prostate enlargement, sore throat.

DOSING

Adults (18 Years and Older)

- There is insufficient evidence to recommend a dose for cherry. Twelve fluid ounces of a tart cherry juice blend has been used twice daily for 8 days.

Children (Younger than 18 Years)

- There is insufficient evidence to recommend a dose for cherry in children.

SAFETY

Allergies

- Avoid in people with a known allergy or sensitivity to cherry, birch pollens, apples, grapes, plums, peaches, apricots, soy, peanuts, or mungbeans. Allergic reactions may range from skin rash to anaphylaxis.

Side Effects and Warnings

- Cherry may alter the absorption of oral drugs, herbs, or supplements. Cherry may stimulate gastrointestinal function following peptic ulcer surgery. Consuming cherry pits or other parts of the cherry plant may cause pain and gastrointestinal problems.

Pregnancy and Breastfeeding

- Cherry is likely safe in nonallergenic pregnant or breastfeeding women in reasonable food quantities. Supplemental use is not recommended because of a lack of available scientific evidence.

INTERACTIONS

Interactions with Drugs

- Cherry consumption may alter the absorption of drugs taken by mouth. Cherries may add to the effects of anti-inflammatory, anticancer, and gastrointestinal drugs.

Interactions with Herbs and Dietary Supplements

- Cherry consumption may alter the absorption of herbs and supplements taken by mouth. Cherries may add to the effects of anti-inflammatory, anticancer, gastrointestinal, and antioxidant herbs and supplements.

For a complete list of references, please visit www.naturalstandard.com.

Chia
(*Salvia hispanica*)

RELATED TERMS

- Chia, chia fresca, cryptotanshinone, dan shen (Chinese), danshen (Chinese), golden chia, ilepesh (Chumas), Lamiaceae (family), Mexican chia, miltionone, pashi (Native American), running food, Salba, SalbaMune, *Salvia columbariae*, *Salvia columbariae* Benth., *Salvia hispanica* L., *Salvia miltiorrhiza*, tanshinone, white Salba.

BACKGROUND

- Chia (*Salvia hispanica*) is a plant that belongs to the Lamiaceae (mint) family. Chia is believed to have come from Central America, where the chia seed was considered a staple in the ancient Aztec diet. Native Americans in the southwestern United States used the seeds of a related plant, "golden chia" or *Salvia columbariae*. People in China and other countries use the roots of another relative, "dan shen" or *Salvia miltiorrhiza*, for medicinal purposes.
- Chia is promoted for its high omega-3, omega-6, and omega-9 content. Animal studies suggest that chia may lower blood cholesterol, LDL (low-density lipoproteins or "bad" cholesterol) and triglycerides, while increasing HDL (high-density lipoproteins or "good" cholesterol). Chia may also have anticancer activity. Studies in humans are limited.
- The oval-shaped seeds of *Salvia hispanica* are approximately 1 mm in diameter and are dark-brown to grayish-white in color. The white seed color is a recessive trait that has apparently been selected for by some cultivators; for example, the brand-name *Salvia hispanica* product Salba (Core Naturals, LLC) consists of seeds that are lighter in color than traditional varieties. Some brands of *Salvia hispanica* are claimed to have a more stable content of omega-3 fatty acids, especially alpha-linoleic acid (ALA), than generic *Salvia hispanica* seeds. Recent clinical studies suggest that Salba may decrease the risk of heart disease in people with type 2 diabetes. *Salvia hispanica* is also promoted as a weight-loss supplement; however, clinical evidence thus far does not support this claim.

EVIDENCE

Uses Based on Scientific Evidence	Grade
Atherosclerosis Research conducted in animals suggest that diets containing chia seed may decrease risk factors for cardiovascular disease (CVD). The available evidence suggests that the benefits of Salba in humans are similar to those of other whole grains. Clinical evidence is conflicting, and it remains unclear if *Salvia hispanica* is superior to other whole grains.	C
Weight Loss Based on the available clinical evidence, supplementation with *Salvia hispanica* does not significantly promote weight loss.	D

Uses Based on Tradition or Theory

Alcoholism, allergies, angina, anticoagulant (blood thinner), antioxidant, antiviral, athletic performance enhancement, cancer, celiac disease, constipation, coronary heart disease (CHD), death and dying, depression, diabetes, heart attack, high blood pressure, high cholesterol levels, hormonal/endocrine disorders, hunger, inflammation, ischemic injury (damage from lack of oxygen to heart), joint pain, kidney disorders, liver disease, metabolic disorders (electrolyte imbalances), nerve disorders, obesity, pancreatitis, skin conditions, stroke, tumors, vasodilatation (dilating veins/lowering blood pressure).

DOSING

Adults (18 Years and Older)

- Chia seeds have been studied for up to 4 weeks at a maximum dose of 10 g. The recommended serving by the manufacturer of Salba is 2 tablespoons (15 g), which reportedly contains more than 3,000 mg of omega-3 fatty acids, 5 g of fiber, and various minerals.
- For the prevention of cardiovascular disease, 33-41 g of Salba has been provided daily for 12 weeks, in ground form or incorporated into bread.

Children (Younger than 18 Years)

- For children ages 4.5-19 years, the average chia consumption may be 1.4 g daily with a maximum daily dose of 4.3 g. The manufacturer of Salba has recommended up to 1 tbsp daily for children.

SAFETY

Allergies

- Avoid in individuals with a known allergy or hypersensitivity to chia, its constituents, or members of the genus *Salvia*. Allergic reactions to chia protein are possible, as are cross-reactivity reactions in people allergic to sesame and mustard seeds.

Side Effects and Warnings

- Although chia seeds and golden chia have been consumed as food for centuries, there are currently limited safety data available on chia or Salba. Gastrointestinal side effects have been reported.
- Chia should be used cautiously in people with low blood pressure or in people taking heart medications because of the risk of additive effects.
- Chia should be avoided in people taking anticoagulants (blood thinners) such as warfarin, because of an increased risk of bleeding.

Pregnancy and Breastfeeding

- Chia cannot be recommended during pregnancy or breastfeeding because of a lack of scientific safety data.

INTERACTIONS

Interactions with Drugs

- In theory, chia may increase the risk of bleeding when taken with anticoagulants (blood thinners) such as warfarin. Salba may lower blood pressure and should be used with caution in those taking heart medications because of the risk of additive effects. Chia may have anticancer activity and may add to the effects of anticancer drugs. Chia may affect the way in which the liver breaks down some drugs.

Interactions with Herbs and Dietary Supplements

- In theory, chia may interact with herbs and supplements that have anticlotting activity, such as ginkgo, garlic, and dong quai. Salba may lower blood pressure and should be used with caution in those taking herbs and supplements that also lower blood pressure or have other effects on the heart. Chia may have anticancer activity and may add to the effects of herbs and supplements with anticancer effects. Chia may affect the way in which the liver breaks down some herbs or supplements.

- Chia contains antioxidants and may therefore add to the activity of other antioxidants, such as vitamins A, C, and E. Chia contains omega-3 fatty acids and may add to the effect of other herbs and supplements that contain omega-3 fatty acids, such as fish oil.

For a complete list of references, please visit www.naturalstandard.com.

Chicory
(*Cichorium intybus*)

RELATED TERMS

- Achicoria, achicoria amarga, almeirao, asparagus, Asteraceae, barbe de capucin, Belgian endive, beta-D-fructofuranosidase, blaue Wegwarte, blue dandelion, blue sailors, Brunswick, cichorii herba, chicon, cichorei, cicoria radicchio, *Cichorium*, *Cichorium bottae*, *Cichorium calvum*, *Cichorium endivia*, *Cichorium intybus*, *Cichorium pumilum*, *Cichorium spinosum*, Chicorii Radix, chicory acids, chicory extracts, chicory fructooligosaccharides, chicory inulin, chicory inulin hydrolysate, chicory roots, cichorium cikoria, cikorie, coffeeweed, common chicory, common chicory root, common endive, Compositae, curly endive, dahlia extract, endive, escarole, FOS, French endive, fructo-oligosaccharides, fructooligosaccharides, garden chicory, Hendibeh, Hindiba, Hinduba, Italian dandelion, inulin hydrolysate, Kasani, Kasni, Kiku-Niga-Na, Magdeburg, oligofructose, oligosaccharides, prebiotic, radichetta, radicchio, sativum, SC-FOS, short chain fructo-oligosaccharides, succory, watcher of the road, wild chicory, wilde cichorei, wild succory, witloof chicory, zikorifa.

BACKGROUND

- Chicory is native to Europe and temperate regions in Asia; it has been naturalized to the United States. Chicory was cultivated as early as 5,000 years ago by Egyptians as a medicinal plant. Traditionally, chicory juice was used as part of a remedy for headaches. The Romans used chicory as a vegetable or in salads. The root was ground and used as a caffeine-free coffee substitute.

- Chicory is still an important salad vegetable in Europe, especially in France, Belgium, and Holland. In the United States, chicory is also grown as a salad green. Preliminary study has investigated chicory for chronic hepatitis; however, at this time there is a lack of high-quality clinical evidence supporting chicory for any indication.

EVIDENCE

Uses Based on Scientific Evidence	Grade
Chronic Hepatitis There is insufficient evidence to recommend for or against the use of chicory for chronic hepatitis.	C

Uses Based on Tradition or Theory
Abortifacient (induces abortion), antibacterial, antiinflammatory, antimalarial, antioxidant, bile flow stimulant, breast cancer, cancer, colon cancer, constipation, diabetes, diuretic, dyspepsia (upset stomach), emmenagogue (promotes menstruation), food additive, gall bladder disorders, gastrointestinal disorders, headache, hypercalcemia (abnormally high calcium in the blood), hyperlipidemia (high cholesterol levels), hypertriglyceridemia (excess of fatty acid compounds in the blood), inflammation (eyes), laxative, liver protection, obesity, osteoporosis, sedative, stimulant, swelling, tachycardia (fast heart rate), tonic, weight loss.

DOSING

Adults (18 Years and Older)

- There is insufficient evidence to recommend a dose for chicory in adults. Common doses that have been traditionally used range from 4-14 g for treating constipation and hypertriglyceridemia and for a probiotic effect. Doses as high as 30 g daily have been taken by mouth to improve bowel function. Chicory tea may be prepared by steeping 2-4 g of the root in 150 mL boiling water for 10 minutes and then straining. A common dose of chicory is 3-6 g of root per day.

Children (Younger than 18 Years)

- There is insufficient evidence to recommend a dose for chicory in children.

SAFETY

Allergies

- Avoid in individuals with a known allergy or hypersensitivity to chicory or members of the Asteraceae or Compositae family, including ragweed, chrysanthemums, marigolds, and daisies. Chicory may cross-react with birch pollen and cause birch pollen–associated allergy syndrome. Occupational asthma has been reported in a chicory grower.

Side Effects and Warnings

- There has been long-standing historical use of chicory with few adverse effects noted anecdotally or in the available scientific literature. Chicory appears to be generally well-tolerated, but skin rash and contact dermatitis have been reported with its use. Weight loss, loss of appetite, and myalgic encephalomyelitis (chronic fatigue syndrome) associated with chicory have also been reported. Chicory is likely safe when consumed as a food additive.

- Skin rash and contact dermatitis associated with chicory use have been reported. The sesquiterpene lactones of the plant may be the allergens. Also, the caffeic acid derivatives from *Cichorium intybus* have displayed vasorelaxant activity.

- Chicory use should be monitored in patients with gallstones because of its bile-stimulating effect. Fructo-oligosaccharides can cause flatulence (gas), belching, abdominal pains, intestinal sounds, and bloating, which occur commonly but are mild.

Pregnancy and Breastfeeding

- Chicory is not recommended in pregnant or breastfeeding women because of a lack of available scientific evidence. When taken by mouth during pregnancy, chicory may induce menstruation or miscarriage.

INTERACTIONS

Interactions with Drugs

- Chicory may interact with drugs metabolized by cytochrome P450. As a result, the levels of these drugs may be decreased in the blood and reduce the intended effects. Patients taking any medications should check the package insert and speak with a qualified health care professional, including a pharmacist, about possible interactions.

Interactions with Herbs and Dietary Supplements

- Chicory extract (inulin) may marginally increase the absorption of dietary calcium.
- Theoretically, chicory may interact with herbs and supplements metabolized by cytochrome P450. As a result, the levels of herbs or supplements may become too high in the blood. It may also alter the effects that other herbs or supplements may possibly have on the P450 system.

For a complete list of references, please visit www.naturalstandard.com.

Chitosan
(Deacetylated Chitin Biopolymer)

RELATED TERMS

- Absorbitol, carboxybutyl chitosan, chitin, chitosan ascorbate, deacetylated chitin biopolymer, deacetylated chitosan, enzymatic polychitosamine hydrolysate, Exofat, Fat Absorb, Fat Blocker, Fat Breaker, Fatsorb, Fat Trapper, Fat Trapper Plus, Fronac N, glucosamine, HEP-30, kitosan, LipoSan Ultra, microcrystalline chitosan, mono-carboxymethylated chitosan, N-acetylated glucosamine, Nofat, Novamic, Somagril, sulfated carboxymethylchitosan, sulfated chitosan, sulfated N-acetylchitosan, trimethyl chitosan chloride.

BACKGROUND

- Chitosan comes from chitin, which is part of the outer shell-like structure of insects, spiders, and crustaceans.
- Chitosan is sold in the United States and other countries as a form of dietary fiber that reduces fat absorption. However, scientific evidence suggests only a small effect of chitosan on fat absorption.
- Chitosan may be effective for lowering levels of blood cholesterol or lipids. It is unclear whether the use of chitosan is equal to or better than other treatments for high cholesterol levels. Evidence suggests that chitosan may help improve cholesterol levels when combined with a low-calorie diet.
- Some evidence indicates that chitosan may be useful for patients undergoing hemodialysis for kidney failure and in the management of dental plaque.

EVIDENCE

Uses Based on Scientific Evidence	Grade
High Cholesterol Study results suggest that chitosan may help improve cholesterol levels when combined with a low-calorie diet.	B
Obesity/Weight Loss While most studies suggest that chitosan is an effective weight loss therapy, others have found it is ineffective.	B
Dental Plaque Some evidence suggests that chitosan has antibacterial properties and may reduce dental plaque.	C
Kidney Failure Limited evidence suggests that chitosan may be useful during long-term hemodialysis.	C
Wound Healing There is limited evidence on the effects of topical chitosan in wound healing.	C

Uses Based on Tradition or Theory

Antacid, antimicrobial, appetite suppressant, arthritis, blood clotting disorders, cancer, chlamydia, diabetes mellitus, heart disease, high blood pressure, human immunodeficiency virus (HIV), immune function, infections, leukemia, nerve regeneration, physical endurance, sleep.

DOSING

Adults (18 Years and Older)

- Doses of chitosan include 1-6 g daily for up to 8 weeks and 450 mg three times daily for up to 12 weeks. Chitosan has been applied to the skin for 3-6 months.

Children (Younger than 18 Years)

- There is insufficient evidence to recommend a dose for chitosan in children.

SAFETY

Allergies

- Avoid in individuals with a known allergy or hypersensitivity to chitosan, its constituents, chitin, or crustaceans. People with shellfish allergies may be allergic to chitosan.

Side Effects and Warnings

- Chitosan may lower blood sugar levels. Caution is advised in patients with diabetes or hypoglycemia and in those taking drugs, herbs, or supplements that affect blood sugar. Serum glucose levels may need to be monitored by a qualified health care professional, and medication adjustments may be necessary.
- Oral chitosan may increase the risk of bleeding, likely by inhibiting vitamin K absorption. Caution is advised in patients with bleeding disorders or in patients taking drugs, herbs, or supplements that may increase the risk of bleeding. Dosing adjustments may be necessary.
- Chitosan may cause stomach discomfort, constipation, gas, diarrhea, nausea, and throat dryness. Chitosan may interfere with fat absorption from the intestine, causing excessive fat to be lost in the stool, and may reduce absorption of the fat-soluble vitamins A, D, E, and K. Chitosan may also cause headache, swollen heels and wrists, and itching of the skin.

Pregnancy and Breastfeeding

- Chitosan is not recommended in pregnant or breastfeeding women because of a lack of available scientific evidence.
- Chitosan may reduce absorption of calcium and vitamin D.

INTERACTIONS

Interactions with Drugs

- Oral chitosan may increase the risk of bleeding, likely by inhibiting vitamin K absorption. Caution is advised in patients with bleeding disorders or in patients taking drugs that may increase the risk of bleeding. Some examples include aspirin, anticoagulants ("blood thinners") such as warfarin (Coumadin) or heparin, antiplatelet drugs such as clopidogrel (Plavix), and nonsteroidal antiinflammatory drugs such as ibuprofen (Motrin, Advil) or naproxen (Naprosyn, Aleve).

- Chitosan may lower blood sugar levels. Caution is advised when medications that may also lower blood sugar are used. Patients taking drugs for diabetes by mouth or injection should be monitored closely by a qualified health care provider. Medication adjustments may be necessary.
- Chitosan may have additive effects when used with cholesterol-lowering, antiobesity, or antibiotic drugs. Chitosan may also slow the absorption of oral contraceptives.

Interactions with Herbs and Dietary Supplements

- Chitosan may lower blood sugar levels. Caution is advised when herbs or supplements that may also lower blood sugar are used. Blood glucose levels may require monitoring, and doses may need adjustment.
- Oral chitosan may increase the risk of bleeding, likely by inhibiting vitamin K absorption. Caution is advised in patients taking herbs or supplements that may increase the risk of bleeding.
- Chitosan may have additive effects when used with cholesterol-lowering, antiobesity, or antibiotic herbs and supplements.
- Use of chitosan may decrease the absorption of calcium, magnesium, selenium, essential fatty acids, fat-soluble vitamins A, D, E, and K, and may also slow the absorption of oral contraceptives. Use of chitosan with vitamin C may decrease fat absorption.

For a complete list of references, please visit www.naturalstandard.com.

Chlorophyll

RELATED TERMS

- ABCG2 substrates, chlorin e6, chlorin p6, chlorophyll a, chlorophyll b, chlorophyll c, chlorophyll d, chlorophyllin, chlorophyllypt, chlorophyll lipiodol, chlorophyll phytol, copper chlorophyll, *Laminaria*, microalgae, nutraceutical, Nullo, peridinin chlorophyll-alpha protein, pheophorbide, pheophorbide a, pheophytin a, photodynamic antimicrobial therapy (PACT), phytanic acid, phytochemicals, porphobilinogen, porphyrin, PPBa, pristanic acid, protochlorophyllide, protoporphyrin IX, purpurin-18, retinoid X receptor (RXR) agonist, uroporphyrinogen-III.

BACKGROUND

- Chlorophyll is a chemoprotein commonly known for its contribution to the green pigmentation in plants and is related to protoheme, the red pigment of blood. It can be obtained from green leafy vegetables (such as broccoli, Brussels sprouts, cabbage, lettuce, and spinach), algae (such as chlorella and spirulina), wheat grass, and numerous herbs (such as alfalfa, damiana, nettle, and parsley).
- Chlorophyll has been used traditionally to improve bad breath and other forms of body odor, including odors of urine, feces, and infected wounds. More recently, chlorophyll has been used to aid in the removal of various toxins via the liver and remains a key compound for improving the function of essential detoxification pathways. Supportive evidence suggests it may be used as an antiinflammatory agent for conditions such as pancreatitis; it also exhibits potent antioxidant and chemoprotective activities. Scientific research has demonstrated it may be an effective therapeutic agent in chemoprevention and in the treatment of herpes simplex, benign breast disease, tuberculosis, and rheumatoid arthritis. Type 2 diabetes and obesity are also being explored as areas where chlorophyll can also be used.

EVIDENCE

Uses Based on Scientific Evidence	Grade
Cancer (Laser Therapy Adjunct) Preliminary evidence suggests that chlorophyll may aid in the reduction of side effects associated with photodynamic therapies such as those used in the management of malignant tumors.	C
Fibrocystic Breast Disease The benefits of chlorophyll in benign breast disease may be attributed to its ability to alter liver enzyme pathways involved in estrogen metabolism. A combination product containing chlorophyll may be beneficial for this condition, but research is preliminary.	C
Herpes (Simplex and Zoster) Chlorophyll may treat herpes simplex and herpes zoster, although research is preliminary.	C
Pancreatitis (Chronic) Chlorophyll-a may reduce the mortality rate of experimental pancreatitis.	C
Pneumonia (Active Destructive) Chlorophyll may help to regulate T-lymphocyte counts in patients with active destructive pneumonia. Further studies are required to further elaborate on the immune-modifying effects of chlorophyll.	C
Poisoning (Reduce Yusho Symptoms) Yusho is poisoning caused by ingestion of rice oil contaminated with polychlorinated biphenyls, specifically polychlorinated dibenzofurans (PCDFs) and polychlorinated biphenyls (PCBs). A chlorophyll-rich diet may increase PCDF and PCB elimination, but further high-quality research is needed.	C
Protection from Aflatoxins Chlorophyll may be of use as a chemopreventive agent because of its ability to inhibit the tumor-promoting effects of carcinogens. Chlorophyll may act to improve the detoxification of toxins involved in cancer promotion.	C
Reduction of Odor from Incontinence/Bladder Catheterization Based on historical use, chlorophyll has been suggested to improve bodily odor in colostomy patients. Despite empirical use, clinical research did not support these findings.	C
Rheumatoid Arthritis Diets high in chlorophyll have been hypothesized to modify intestinal flora, which may result in improved management of immune disorders, including rheumatoid arthritis.	C
Tuberculosis Preliminary evidence suggests that chlorophyll intake during chemotherapy treatment in patients with tuberculosis may improve immune parameters and free radical indices, such as malonic dialdehyde.	C

Uses Based on Tradition or Theory
Anemia, cancer prevention, antioxidant, antiviral, atherosclerosis (hardening of the arteries), bad breath, blood disorders (porphyria), constipation, deodorant, detoxification, diabetes, food uses (colorant), gastrointestinal conditions, hyperlipidemia (high cholesterol level), obesity, wound healing.

DOSING
Adults (18 Years and Older)

- There is insufficient evidence to recommend a dose for chlorophyll. For bad breath, 100 mg has been taken two or three times daily. For colostomy odor, 75 mg has been taken three times daily for up to 100-200 mg daily in divided doses. In addition, 300 mg daily has been used if odor was still not controlled. In a patient who has had an ostomy, 1-2 tablets of 100 mg have been placed in the empty pouch each time it is reused or changed. For protection from aflatoxins, chlorophyllin 100 mg has been administered three times daily for 4 months. For pancreatitis, an infusion of 5-20 mg water-soluble chlorophyll-a has been taken daily for 1-2 weeks followed by intermittent administration thereafter. For pneumonia, infusion of 0.25% chlorophyllypt solution in physiological sodium chloride solution has been administered by intravenous drip.
- Evidence suggests chlorophyll may aid the growth of new tissue when applied topically (on the skin) for burns and wounds.

Children (Younger than 18 Years)

- There is insufficient evidence to recommend dose for chlorophyll in children.

SAFETY
Allergies

- Avoid in individuals with a known allergy or hypersensitivity to chlorophyll or any of its metabolites; contact may result in a photosensitive rash. Copper chlorophyll (E141) could be a pseudoallergen.

Side Effects and Warnings

- It appears that chlorophyll is generally safe and without many side effects or toxicities in nonsensitive people. Adverse effects are usually gastrointestinal or dermatological in nature. Common gastrointestinal complaints may include nausea, diarrhea, green stools, and abdominal cramping. When taken by mouth, chlorophyllin may cause green discoloration of the urine.
- Use cautiously in patients who show signs of photosensitivity, such as a rash, to chlorophyll or any of its metabolites.
- Use cautiously in patients with compromised liver function because of the possibility of the development of jaundice.
- Use cautiously in patients taking immunosuppressant agents as chlorophyll may normalize T-lymphocyte counts.
- Use cautiously in patients with diabetes or in those taking diabetic agents as chlorophyll may have antidiabetic effects.

Pregnancy and Breastfeeding

- Chlorophyll is not recommended in pregnant or breastfeeding women because of a lack of available scientific evidence.

INTERACTIONS
Interactions with Drugs

- The chlorophyll metabolite phytanic acid may have antidiabetic activity. Caution is advised when medications that may lower blood sugar are used. Patients taking drugs for diabetes by mouth or using insulin should be monitored closely by a qualified health care professional, including a pharmacist. Medication adjustments may be necessary.
- Phytanic and pristanic acids are thought to affect catabolic lipid metabolism. Caution is advised when taking chlorophyll with agents that lower cholesterol levels, such as statins.
- Although not well studied in humans, chlorophyll or its metabolites may have antineoplastic (anticancer) properties. Caution is advised in patients taking other anticancer agents.
- The chlorophyll metabolites phytanic and pristanic acids may have antiobesity properties. Caution is advised when chlorophyll is taken with other agents for weight loss.
- Chlorophyll may have antioxidant and antiviral properties. Caution is advised in patients taking drugs with antioxidant and antiviral properties because of possible additive effects.
- Chlorophyll may have detoxifying effects, especially on dioxins, polychlorinated dibenzofurans (PCDFs), and polychlorinated dibenzo-p-dioxins (PCDDs).
- Chlorophyll and some of its synthetically produced derivatives may be photosensitizing. Chlorophyll may cause hyperpigmentation, dermatitis, or make a patient more sensitive to laser treatment.

Interactions with Herbs and Dietary Supplements

- Phytanic and pristanic acids are thought to affect catabolic lipid metabolism. Caution is advised when chlorophyll is taken with herbs or supplements that lower cholesterol levels, such as red yeast rice.
- Although not well studied in humans, chlorophyll or its metabolites may have antineoplastic (anticancer) properties. Caution is advised in patients taking anticancer herbs or supplements.
- Chlorophyll may have antioxidant and antiviral properties. Caution is advised in patients taking herbs or supplements with antioxidant and antiviral properties because of possible additive effects.
- Although not well studied in humans, chlorophyll may have detoxifying effects, especially on dioxins, PCDFs, and PCDDs.
- The chlorophyll metabolite phytanic acid may have antidiabetic activity. Caution is advised when herbs or supplements that may lower blood sugar are used. Blood glucose levels may require monitoring, and doses may need adjustment.
- Chlorophyll and some of its synthetically produced derivatives may be photosensitizing. Chlorophyll may cause hyperpigmentation, dermatitis, or make a patient more sensitive to laser treatment. Beta-carotene or canthaxanthin may prevent or lessen chlorophyll-induced photosensitivity.
- Although not well studied in humans, vitamin C (ascorbic acid) and pantothenic acid may exert preventive effects against photosensitized hemolysis.
- The chlorophyll metabolites phytanic and pristanic acids may have antiobesity properties. Caution is advised when chlorophyll is taken with other herbs or supplements for weight loss.

For a complete list of references, please visit www.naturalstandard.com.

RELATED TERMS

- Beta-hydroxyethyl trimethylammonium hydroxide, CDP-choline, choline bitartrate, choline chloride, choline citrate, citicoline, cytidine 5-diphosphocholine (CDP-choline), intrachol, lecithin, lipotropic factor, PhosChol, phosphatidylcholine, TRI, tricholine citrate (TRI), trimethylethanolamine.
- **Note:** Choline should not be confused with choline salicylate, choline magnesium trisalicylate, choline theophyllinate, or succinylcholine.

BACKGROUND

- Choline is an essential nutrient related to the water-soluble B-complex vitamins, folate, pyridoxine, and B_{12} and to the essential amino acid, methionine. It is synthesized in the body as well as consumed in the diet. The largest dietary source of choline is egg yolk. Choline can also be found in high amounts in liver, peanuts, fish, milk, brewer's yeast, wheat germ, soy beans, bottle gourd fruit, fenugreek leaves, shepherd's purse herb, Brazil nuts, dandelion flowers, poppy seeds, mung beans and other beans, and a variety of meats and vegetables, including cabbage and cauliflower.
- Choline is a major building block of lecithin. Choline is a precursor to acetylcholine, a chemical used to transfer nerve impulses. Therefore, choline is believed to have neurological effects.
- Choline is a product of the breakdown of the muscle relaxant succinylcholine, which is used extensively in anesthesia. Theoretically, choline may exhibit similar muscle-relaxing effects.
- Choline is a constituent of phosphatidylcholine (PC), which is a component of cell walls and membranes. It is involved in fat and cholesterol metabolism and transport. In this form, choline aids in fat metabolism and transport away from the liver.
- Pure choline is rarely used because of its undesirable side effects of fishy odor. Therefore, lecithin or purified phosphatidylcholine is more commonly used.

EVIDENCE

Uses Based on Scientific Evidence	Grade
Asthma Choline is possibly effective when taken by mouth for asthma. Choline supplements seem to decrease the severity of symptoms, number of symptomatic days, and the need to use bronchodilators in asthma patients. There is some evidence that higher daily doses might be more effective than lower daily doses.	B
Fatty Liver (Hepatic Steatosis) Choline, when given intravenously, has orphan drug status for total parenteral nutrition (TPN)–associated hepatic steatosis (fat deposits in the liver).	B
Nutritional Supplement (Infant Formula) Choline is likely effective when used orally as a supplement in infant formulas.	B
Total Parenteral Nutrition (Associated Liver Dysfunction) Choline is likely effective when used intravenously to treat total parenteral nutrition–associated hepatic dysfunction.	B
Acute Viral Hepatitis Many studies have assessed the use of choline for hepatitis, although there is a lack of sufficient evidence to recommend for or against the use of choline in the treatment of acute viral hepatitis.	C
Allergic Rhinitis Oral tricholine citrate (TRI) may effectively relieve allergic rhinitis symptoms. Further research is needed before a strong recommendation can be made.	C
Brain Injuries (Craniocerebral) Early treatment with choline alphoscerate (CA), a substrate of phosphatidylcholine and a carrier of choline, was shown to be safe. When taken as part of complex pharmacotherapy, it has shown beneficial effects on cervical cord injury (CCI) patients. Additional study is needed to confirm these findings.	C
Coma There is a lack of sufficient evidence to recommend for or against the use of choline in coma patients. Available research is limited.	C
Ischemic Stroke Although many studies have found promising results, others have not shown statistical significance when assessing choline for the treatment of acute ischemic stroke. Because of conflicting data, choline therapy cannot be recommended.	C
Muscle Mass/Body Mass There is lack of sufficient evidence for the use of choline for changing body composition, specifically, changing body fat and lean muscle.	C
Parkinson's Disease Data regarding efficacy of choline in the treatment of Parkinson's disease are conflicting and inconclusive.	C
Postsurgical Recovery There is a lack of sufficient evidence to recommend for or against the use of choline in patients recovering from surgery.	C
Alzheimer's Disease/Cognitive Decline Numerous studies have assessed the use of choline in cerebrovascular diseases, memory performance, dementia, and Alzheimer's disease without significant benefit.	D

(Continued)

Uses Based on Scientific Evidence	Grade
Cerebellar Ataxia Choline is possibly ineffective when taken by mouth for treating cerebellar ataxia.	D
Improving Sports Performance (Endurance Sports) Research has shown that choline does not significantly improve performance or delay fatigue during endurance sports.	D
Schizophrenia Choline has been studied in schizophrenia with negative results.	D

Uses Based on Tradition or Theory

Aging, alcoholism, allergy, anesthesia, ataxia, attention deficit hyperactivity disorder (ADHD), autism, bipolar disorder, body building, brain function improvement, brain injuries (cranioencephalic), bronchitis (dust-induced), cancer prevention, cardiovascular health, childhood growth promotion, clogged arteries, cocaine dependence, cognitive disorders, colitis (necrotizing enterocolitis), concussions, digestive disorders, dizziness, edema (cerebral), energy, exercise performance enhancement, fatigue, fetal development, gallbladder stones, glaucoma, growth, hemorrhage (intracerebral), hepatitis, high cholesterol levels, Huntington's chorea/disease, hyperhomocysteinemia, hypoxia (brain), infections, infertility, ischemic injury (focal), jaundice, liver health, liver protection, male tonic, mania, memory loss, mental performance/alertness, nervous system function, reproduction disorders, respiratory distress (newborn syndrome), seizures, tardive dyskinesia, Tourette's syndrome, vascular disorders, vertigo, vision problems (amblyopia), wasting of brain regions (cerebellar), weight loss.

DOSING

Adults (18 Years and Older)

- The "average" diet supplies 400-900 mg of choline daily, which is presumed to be adequate. According to the Institute of Medicine, although the adequate intake (AI) has been set for choline by the Institute of Medicine's Food and Nutrition Board, there are few data to assess whether a dietary supply of choline is needed at all ages, and it may be that the choline requirement can be met by endogenous synthesis at some of these stages.
- The recommended daily intake by the U.S. Food and Nutrition Board of the Institute of Medicine for men 18-70+ years: 550 mg/day, not to exceed 3.5 g/day; for women 19-70+ years: 425 mg/day, not to exceed 3.5 g/day; for women 18 years: 400 mg/day, not to exceed 3 g/day; for pregnant women: 450 mg/day; for breastfeeding women: 550 mg/day.
- Upper intake levels (UL) should not exceed 3.5 g daily for adults and the elderly. Dosages at the upper limit intake levels are contraindicated for persons suffering from trimethylaminuria, kidney disease, liver disease, depression, and Parkinson's disease, as they may be at risk of side effects.

- There is no proven effective dose for Alzheimer's disease, asthma, fatty liver, or seizure; however, choline has been studied for the treatment of these conditions at various doses.

Children (Younger than 18 Years)

- The Committee on Nutrition of the American Academy of Pediatrics recommends the fortification of infant formula to at least 7 mg choline per 100 kilocalories. This quantity corresponds to roughly 9 ± 2 mg/dL of choline present in human breast milk. Children ages 1-8 years should not exceed 1 g daily, children ages 9-13 should not exceed 2 g daily, and children 14-18 years should not exceed 3 g of choline daily.
- Recommended daily intake by the U.S. Food and Nutrition Board of the Institute of Medicine for infants 6-12 months: 150 mg/day; for infants up to 6 months: 125 mg/day; for children 9-13 years: 375 mg/day, not to exceed 2 g/day; for children 4-8 years: 250 mg/day, not to exceed 1 g/day; for children 1-3 years: 200 mg/day, not to exceed 1 g/day; for girls 14-18 years: 400 mg/day, not to exceed 3 g/day; for boys 14-18 years: 550 mg/day, not to exceed 3.5 g/day.
- Upper intake levels (UL) per day should not exceed 1 g daily by mouth for children 1-8 years; 2 g daily by mouth for children 9-13 years; 3 g daily by mouth for adolescents (14-18 years old). Maximum daily choline upper intake levels for infants are not available; choline should only be from formula or breast milk and food.

SAFETY
Allergies

- Avoid in individuals with a known allergy or hypersensitivity to choline, lecithin, or phosphatidylcholine.

Side Effects and Warnings

- Choline is generally regarded as safe and appears to be well tolerated. High intake of choline may cause low blood pressure, steatorrhea (undigested fat in stool), nausea, vomiting, salivation, diarrhea, constipation, anorexia, dizziness (vertigo), sweating, insomnia, and headache. Choline can possibly trigger existing epilepsy. Dosages at the upper limit intake levels (UL) are contraindicated for person suffering from trimethylaminuria, Parkinson's disease, or kidney or liver disease.
- Skin rash has been reported. A cold and cough were noted in patients taking citicoline in a trial. Choline should be used cautiously by people with kidney or liver disorders. Agitation, paranoia, and severe depression have been reported. Use cautiously in patients with a history of depression.
- Because choline is a product of the breakdown of succinylcholine, it may produce similar side effects as the drug, like respiratory depression. A "fishy" odor has been associated with choline. Sweating and stunted growth may occur.

Pregnancy and Breastfeeding

- The Food and Nutrition Board of the Institute of Medicine of the National Academy of Science states that choline is vital in prenatal supplementation. During pregnancy, choline intake of the mother may influence memory and brain development in the growing infant. Studies on choline and lecithin supplementation clearly show an increase in blood choline levels following supplementation.

- Pregnant and lactating women and children may consume choline within the recommended adequate intake (AI) parameters; supplementation outside of dietary intake is usually not necessary if a healthy diet is consumed.

INTERACTIONS
Interactions with Drugs

- Choline supplementation has been associated with decreasing urinary excretion of carnitine in young adult women.
- A study concluded that chronic treatment with lithium enhances the effects of choline in the brain. A preliminary report of magnetic resonance imaging (MRI) studies did not observe a significant positive relationship between increases in brain choline and increases in brain lithium.
- CDP-choline can cause an increase in plasma concentrations of dopa.
- Methotrexate may diminish pools of all choline metabolites. Choline supplementation reverses fatty liver caused by methotrexate administration in rats.
- Pentazocine exhibits neuromuscular blocking effects in part through a depressive action on cholinoceptive sites on the nerve motor end terminals, presenting a possible interaction if administered with choline.

- Although a few studies have linked choline with partially reversing the effects of scopolamine, a later study failed to demonstrate similar effects.
- Choline is a product of the breakdown of succinylcholine. Taking choline with succinylcholine may theoretically intensify effects and/or toxicity.

Interactions with Herbs and Supplements

- Choline supplementation has been associated with decreasing urinary excretion of carnitine in young adult women.
- A study concluded that chronic treatment with lithium enhances the effects of choline in the brain. A preliminary report of MRI studies did not observe a significant positive relationship between increases in brain choline and increases in brain lithium.
- Choline, via its metabolism to betaine, works in concert with vitamins B_6, B_{12}, and folic acid in the metabolism of the potentially atherogenic substance homocysteine.

For a complete list of references, please visit www.naturalstandard.com.

Chondroitin Sulfate

RELATED TERMS

- ACS4-ACS6, ADAMTS7B, aggrecan, agrin, biglycan, biostat, CDS, chondroitin sulfate A, chondroitin sulfate C, chondroitin sulfate proteoglycan, chondroitin sulfates, chondroitin sulfuric acid, chondroitin sulphate, chondroitin sulphate A sodium, chondroitin-4-sulfate, chondroitin-6-sulfate, chondroitinase ABC, chondroprotective agents, chondrosine, chonsurid, CHST11, condroitin, Condrosulf, Condrosulf 400, CS, CS/DS, CSA, CSC, CSPG D-galactosamine, decorin, dentin sialoprotein, DexSol, D-glucuronic acid, disease modifying osteoarthritis drugs (DMOAD), extended chondroitin sulfate/dermatan, fucosylated chondroitin sulfate, GAG, galacotosaminoglucuronoglycan sulfate (Matrix), glucosamine hydrochloride, glucosamine salts, glucosamine sulfate, glucosaminoglycan, Matrix, neurocan, neuroglycan C, NGC, Optisol, perineuronal nets, PNs, sodium chondroitin sulfate 0.2%, sodium chondroitin, Structum, sulphate, symptomatic slow acting drug in osteoarthritis type XV, Syndecan, SYSADOA type XV, Uropol-S, Viscoat.

BACKGROUND

- Chondroitin was first extracted and purified in the 1960s. It is currently manufactured from natural sources (shark/beef cartilage or bovine trachea) or by synthetic means. The consensus of expert and industry opinions supports the use of chondroitin and its common partner agent, glucosamine, for improving symptoms and stopping (or possibly reversing) the degenerative process of osteoarthritis.

EVIDENCE

Uses Based on Scientific Evidence	Grade
Osteoarthritis Multiple controlled clinical trials since the 1980s have examined the use of oral chondroitin in patients with osteoarthritis of the knee and other locations (spine, hips, finger joints). Most of these studies have reported significant benefits in terms of symptoms (such as pain), function (such as mobility), and reduced medication requirements (such as antiinflammatory agents). However, most studies have been brief (6-month duration) with methodological weaknesses. Despite these weaknesses and potential for bias in the available results, the weight of scientific evidence points to a beneficial effect when chondroitin is used for 6-24 months. Longer-term effects are not clear. Preliminary studies of chondroitin applied to the skin have also been conducted. Chondroitin is frequently used with glucosamine. Glucosamine has independently been demonstrated to benefit patients with osteoarthritis (particularly of the knee). It remains unclear whether there is added benefit of using these two agents together compared with using either alone.	A
Bladder Control Several studies have shown promise for using chondroitin for interstitial cystitis, which is a chronic inflammation of the bladder. Chondroitin sulfate may also be helpful in patients with overactive bladder or unstable bladder control.	B
Coronary Artery Disease (Secondary Prevention) Several studies in the early 1970s assessed the use of oral chondroitin for the prevention of subsequent coronary events in patients with a history of heart disease or heart attack. Although favorable results were reported, because of methodological weaknesses in this research and the widespread current availability of more proven drug therapies for patients in this setting, a recommendation cannot be made in this area.	C
Interstitial Cystitis There is preliminary research administering intravesicular chondroitin in patients diagnosed with interstitial cystitis.	C
Iron Absorption Enhancement Early research suggests that taking chondroitin with iron may enhance iron absorption in healthy individuals. It is unclear whether taking chondroitin would help patients with iron deficiencies absorb more iron.	C
Ophthalmological Uses Chondroitin is sometimes used as a component of eye solutions for keratoconjunctivitis, corneal preservation, and intraocular pressure. These solutions should only be used under the supervision of an ophthalmologist.	C
Psoriasis Preliminary research suggests that chondroitin may help treat psoriasis.	C
Muscle Soreness (Delayed Onset) Chondroitin was thought to be beneficial for delayed onset muscle soreness because chondroitin sulfate is often used as an antiinflammatory and pain reliever for osteoarthritis. However, research thus far does not support this use.	D

Uses Based on Tradition or Theory

Aging, allergies, Alzheimer's disease, analgesic, angina (chest pain), anticoagulant (blood thinner), antiinflammatory, antioxidant, antithrombotic, atherosclerosis, bone healing, breast cancer, cardiovascular health, chronic venous ulcers, deep intraosseous defects, gonarthrosis, gum disease, headaches, heart attack

Uses Based on Tradition or Theory—Cont'd

(treatment and prevention), high cholesterol levels, human immunodeficiency virus/acquired immunodeficiency syndrome (HIV/AIDS), hyperglycemia/diabetes, iron deficiency anemia, joint pain, joint problems (cartilage repair, disk degeneration, synovial fluid productions), kidney stones, leukemia, malaria, nerve regeneration, osteoporosis, premature birth prevention, respiratory ailments, rheumatoid arthritis, snoring, soft tissue injury (torn ligaments and tendons), spinal cord injury, sports injuries, venous leg ulcers, wound healing.

DOSING

Adult (18 Years and Older)

- Doses of 200-400 mg by mouth twice to three times daily or 800-1200 mg once daily have been used in studies. Higher doses (up to 2000 mg) appear to have similar efficacy. In the treatment of osteoarthritis, full effects may take several weeks to occur.
- It is not clear what dose is optimal when used in combination with glucosamine or whether the combination is as effective as or more effective than either agent alone.
- For osteoarthritis, 50-100 mg has been administered as a single daily injection or divided into two daily injections. Medical supervision is recommended.

Children (Younger than 18 Years)

- There is insufficient evidence to recommend a dose for chondroitin in children.

SAFETY

Allergies

- Use cautiously if allergic or hypersensitive to chondroitin sulfate products. Use cautiously in patients with shellfish allergy because of the possibility of allergic reaction. Hives, rash, sun skin sensitivity, and worsening of previously well-controlled asthma have been reported.

Side Effects and Warnings

- Chondroitin sulfate appears to be well tolerated for up to 3 years.
- Adverse effects that have been rarely reported or are theoretical include headache, motor uneasiness, euphoria, hives, rash, photosensitivity, hair loss, breathing difficulties, subjective tightness in the throat or chest, exacerbation of previously well-controlled asthma, chest pain, elevated blood pressure, lower extremity edema, gastrointestinal pain/

dyspepsia, nausea, diarrhea, constipation, transaminitis, increased risk of bleeding (theoretical), bone marrow suppression (animal research), and eyelid edema.
- Avoid in individuals with prostate cancer or at increased risk of prostate cancer because of a risk of increased spread or recurrence of prostate cancer.

Pregnancy and Breastfeeding

- Avoid in pregnant or breastfeeding women as effects are unknown, and there is structural similarity to heparin, a blood thinner that is contraindicated during pregnancy.

INTERACTIONS

Interactions with Drugs

- In theory, chondroitin may increase the risk of bleeding when taken with drugs that increase the risk of bleeding. Some examples include aspirin, anticoagulants ("blood thinners") such as warfarin (Coumadin) or heparin, antiplatelet drugs such as clopidogrel (Plavix), and nonsteroidal antiinflammatory drugs such as ibuprofen (Motrin, Advil) or naproxen (Naprosyn, Aleve).
- Use cautiously with hyaluronidase or agents with hydrophilic (attraction to water) properties. Consult with a qualified health care professional, including a pharmacist, to check for interactions.
- Also use cautiously when combining chondroitin with other agents that may cause sun sensitivity, as chondroitin may increase sun sensitivity.

Interactions with Herbs and Dietary Supplements

- In theory, chondroitin may increase the risk of bleeding when taken with herbs and supplements that are believed to increase the risk of bleeding. Multiple cases of bleeding have been reported with the use of *Ginkgo biloba*, and fewer cases have been reported with garlic and saw palmetto. Numerous other agents may theoretically increase the risk of bleeding, although this has not been proven in most cases.
- Based on preliminary data, chondroitin may increase iron absorption. It may also interact with or alter concentrations of calcium, camphor, glucosamine, manganese, peppermint oil, and shark cartilage.
- Use cautiously with herbs or supplements with hydrophilic (attraction to water) properties. Consult with a qualified health care professional, including a pharmacist, to check for interactions. Also use cautiously when combining chondroitin with other agents that may cause sun sensitivity, as chondroitin may increase sun sensitivity.

For a complete list of references, please visit www.naturalstandard.com.

Chromium (Cr)

RELATED TERMS

- Atomic number 24, chromic chloride, chromium (III), chromium 3, chromium 3+, chromium acetate, chromium chloride, chromium III picolinate, chromium nicotinate, chromium picolinate, chromium polynicotinate, chromium trichloride, chromium tripicolinate, chromium yeast, chromium-3+, chromium-enriched yeast, Cr, Cr III, Cr-3, Cr-3+, Cr-III, glucose tolerance factor, glucose tolerance factor-Cr, GTF, GTF-Cr, hexavalent chromium, trivalent chromium.

BACKGROUND

- Chromium is an essential trace element that exists naturally in trivalent and hexavalent states. Trivalent chromium (chromium/Cr III), typically found in foods and supplements, appears to have very low toxicity and a wide margin of safety. Hexavalent chromium (chromic oxide, chromate) is a known toxin, and long-term occupational exposure may lead to skin problems, a perforated nasal septum, and lung cancer.
- Although chromium has been suggested for many conditions, there is not enough information to make any strong recommendations at this time. Chromium is available in several forms, such as chromium-enriched yeast and chromium picolinate. Chromium has been studied for its short-term and long-term effects. Chromium picolinate is the most studied synthetic chromium product that is commonly promoted for weight loss, although there is a lack of research to support this.
- Chromium may alter blood sugar levels, which should be closely monitored in people with diabetes.

EVIDENCE

Uses Based on Scientific Evidence	Grade
Hypoglycemia (Low Blood Sugar) Chromium has been studied in the treatment of diabetes and high blood sugar. It may also help regulate blood sugar in patients with low blood sugar disorders.	B
Polycystic Ovary Syndrome (Glucose Tolerance) Chromium picolinate may help improve glucose tolerance in women with polycystic ovary syndrome. However, chromium does not appear to alter hormones.	B
Bipolar Disorder There is lack of sufficient available evidence to recommend chromium for bipolar disorder.	C
Bone Loss (Postmenopausal Women) There is a lack of evidence for or against the use of chromium for the treatment of bone resorption in postmenopausal women.	C
Cardiovascular Disease An association has been made between high chromium levels in the blood and a lower risk of coronary artery disease (clogged arteries in the heart). Chromium should be used cautiously, however, because of possible increases in blood pressure.	C
Cognitive Function Preliminary research suggests that chromium picolinate may help improve cognitive function in the elderly.	C
Depression Early studies show that chromium picolinate may improve symptoms of depression in people with atypical depression.	C
Diabetes Mellitus Chromium has been studied for sugar abnormalities in people with types 1 and 2 diabetes, as well as at-risk populations. Some studies suggest that taking chromium by mouth may lower blood sugar levels, whereas other studies show no effects. Some research reports that chromium may improve symptoms of hypoglycemia (low blood sugar).	C
High Cholesterol Studies show conflicting results for the use of chromium in treating high cholesterol levels. A few studies show that chromium may lower cholesterol levels, but other studies show no effects. Many natural medicine experts and textbooks do not recommend chromium for treating high cholesterol levels over more proven therapies.	C
Immunosuppression Chromium, in combination with copper, may have potential suppressive effects on immune function. The evidence thus far has not been conclusive.	C
Parkinson's Disease Chromium has been studied for its protective benefits in Parkinson's disease and is included in antioxidant multivitamins. However, clinical evidence is lacking.	C
Schizophrenia Early study shows a lack of effect of chromium supplementation on mental state and body weight in people with schizophrenia.	C
Obesity/Weight Loss Chromium has been studied for its ability to treat obesity, but overall, results have not shown any benefit.	F

Uses Based on Scientific Evidence	Grade
Although chromium may help improve lean body mass (by reducing fat and increasing muscle), it does not appear to show effects in general weight loss.	

Uses Based on Tradition or Theory

Acne, antioxidant, athletic performance, glaucoma, hypothyroidism, migraines, premenstrual syndrome (PMS), psoriasis, Turner's syndrome.

DOSING
Adults (18 Years and Older)

- Chromium is available in several forms, such as trivalent chromium, chromium-enriched yeast, and chromium picolinate. Chromium has been studied short-term and long-term. Although there have been many studies involving chromium, overall, the evidence is mixed. There is no proven effective dose for any type of chromium for any indication. Studies in humans have used doses of 200-1000 mcg of chromium picolinate per day by mouth as capsules or tablets. As chromium-enriched yeast, 150-400 mcg has been commonly studied. As chromium picolinate, lower doses of 200-250 mcg have been used. It should be noted, however, that some natural medicine experts believe that adequate dietary intake of chromium is only 24-45 mcg daily, although others recommend 50-200 mcg daily.

Children (Younger than 18 Years)

- The dosing and safety of chromium have not been studied thoroughly in children and high doses of chromium are generally not recommended. Some practitioners have recommended an adequate chromium intake of 0.2-35 mcg/day, depending on age.

SAFETY
Allergies

- Avoid in patients with a known allergy or hypersensitivity to chromium. People with allergies to chromate or leather may be more likely to have allergic reactions to chromium.
- Allergic reactions from handling chromium or reactions to its use in medical devices (orthopedic prosthesis, dental restorations) may occur.

Side Effects and Warnings

- Chromium, in its trivalent form, appears to be well tolerated with rare or uncommon adverse effects. However, the hexavalent form is not well tolerated and may be toxic. Hexavalent chromium appears to be associated with lung cancers. Long-term occupational exposure to hexavalent chromium may also lead to skin problems and a perforated nasal septum.
- The most common complaints include stomach discomfort and nausea or vomiting. Very rarely, skin rashes, insomnia or sleep disturbances, headaches, mood changes, muscle damage, or anemia may occur.
- It is possible that chromium may lower blood sugar levels. As a result, it should be used cautiously in patients who are taking drugs for diabetes.
- It is possible that chromium may have adverse effects on the heart, blood, kidneys, or liver. There are also rare reports of respiratory effects, such as cough, shortness of breath, wheezing, rhinitis, asthma, and headache, after inhaling chromium.
- Cognitive, perceptual, and motor changes may also occur, although they are unlikely.
- There is some evidence that chromium, in combination with copper, may have potential suppressive effects on the immune system. Caution should be used in those with a suppressed immune system, such as in human immunodeficiency virus (HIV) or transplant patients.

Pregnancy and Breastfeeding

- Many natural medicine experts and textbooks state that chromium is safe if taken by pregnant or breastfeeding women in the amount of 45 μg/day by mouth. However, scientific studies have not clearly proven safety and effectiveness.

INTERACTIONS
Interactions with Drugs

- Chromium may lower blood sugar levels. Caution is advised if drugs that may lower blood sugar levels are taken. Patients taking oral drugs for diabetes or using insulin should be monitored closely by health care professionals while using chromium.
- Lithium and nicotinic acid may also increase the tendency for blood sugar levels to become low. In contrast, when chromium is used with corticosteroids, such as prednisone, increases in blood sugar levels may occur. Dosing adjustments may be necessary.
- Chromium may modify serotonin function in the brain and therefore may interact with prescription antidepressants, such as sertraline (Zoloft) and fluoxetine (Prozac).
- In theory, some drugs may decrease chromium levels in the body and may interfere with chromium's activities. Examples include drugs that reduce acid in the stomach, such as esomeprazole (Nexium), ranitidine (Zantac), antacids, and corticosteroids (e.g., prednisone). In contrast, aspirin and nonsteroidal antiinflammatory drugs, such as ibuprofen (Motrin or Advil) and naproxen (Naprosyn, Aleve, or Anaprox), may increase chromium levels in the body, which could lead to increased side effects.
- Picolinic acid, a component often found with chromium, may alter the metabolism of certain chemicals in the brain. If these chemicals are altered, the doses of some drugs used to treat conditions such as depression or Parkinson's disease may need to be changed.
- Chromium may interact with drugs that alter the body's immune response. Caution is advised in patients with compromised immune systems.
- Corticosteroids may increase the amount of chromium excreted in the urine. This may result in chromium deficiency or increased blood sugar levels.
- Chronic alcohol use may increase the chance of liver and kidney damage when an individual takes or is exposed to a form of chromium called hexavalent chromium.
- Chromium supplementation may increase cholesterol (high-density lipoprotein [HDL]) concentrations among patients taking beta-blockers. Caution is advised in patients taking medications for heart disorders along with chromium.

- Chromium may increase blood pressure. Caution is advised in patients taking medications that alter blood pressure.
- Chromium may interfere with the way the body processes certain drugs using the liver's "cytochrome P450" enzyme system. As a result, the levels of these drugs may be decreased in the blood and the intended effects may be reduced. Patients taking any medications should check the package insert and speak with a qualified health care professional, including a pharmacist, about possible interactions.
- There is insufficient evidence to support the use of chromium in the treatment of weight loss; caution may be warranted with the use of chromium and weight loss agents.

Interactions with Herbs and Dietary Supplements

- Chromium may alter blood sugar levels. People using herbs or other supplements that may alter blood sugar levels, such as bitter melon (*Momordica charantia*), should be monitored closely by health care professionals while using chromium. Dosing adjustments may be necessary.
- Chromium taken with other supplements may alter the amount of chromium in the body. In theory, antiinflammatory herbs and supplements may increase chromium levels in the body, which could lead to a tendency for increased side effects. In theory, zinc may decrease chromium levels in the body and may interfere with chromium's activities. It is possible that vitamin C may also alter chromium levels. Chromium taken with iron may affect the way iron is processed in the body. Chromium picolinate used with biotin may show favorable effects on regulating blood sugar, but additional study is needed in this area.
- Chromium has been shown to decrease serotonin levels and may interact with herbs and supplements that affect serotonin.
- Chromium may interact with herbs or supplements that alter the body's immune response. Caution is advised in patients with compromised immune systems.
- Although not well studied in humans, chromium supplementation may increase cholesterol (HDL) concentrations when taken with other herbs or supplements used for heart disorders. Caution is advised.
- Chromium may increase blood pressure. Caution is advised in patients taking herbs or supplements that alter blood pressure.
- Chromium may interfere with the way the body processes certain herbs or supplements using the liver's cytochrome P450 enzyme system. As a result, the levels of other herbs or supplements may become too high in the blood. It may also alter the effects that other herbs or supplements possibly have on the P450 system.
- There is insufficient evidence to support the use of chromium in the treatment of weight loss. Caution may be warranted with use of chromium and herbs and supplements used for weight loss.

For a complete list of references, please visit www.naturalstandard.com.

Chrysanthemum
(Chrysanthemum spp.)

RELATED TERMS

- Alantolactone, alpha-pinene, alpha-thujone, apigenin, arnidiol, Asteraceae (family), beta-caryophyllene, borenolide, brein, calenduladiol, camphor, chrysancorin, *Chrysanthemum boreale*, *Chrysanthemum boreale* M, *Chrysanthemum boreale* Makino, *Chrysanthemum cinerariaefolium*, *Chrysanthemum coccineum*, *Chrysanthemum coronarium* L., *Chrysanthemum coronarium* var. spatiosum, *Chrysanthemum indicum*, *Chrysanthemum leucanthemum*, *Chrysanthemum morifolium* extract, *Chrysanthemum multiflorum*, *Chrysanthemum parthenium*, *Chrysanthemum viscidehirtum*, *Chrysanthemum x morifolium* Ramat, *Chrysanthemum zawadskii coccineum*, chrysin, cis-chrysanthenol, coflodiol, Compositae family, *Dendranthema*, dicaffeoylquinic acids, erythrodiol, faradiol, faradiol alpha-epoxide, flavonoids, feverfew, glucuronide, Indian standard series, jiangtangkang (Chinese), JTK, linarin, longispinogenin (Chinese), luteolin, maniladiol (Chinese), marguerite, oleananes, ox-eye daisy, parthenolide, PC-SPES, pyrethrins, pyrethroids, pyrethrum, sesquiterpene lactones, sesquiterpenes, *Tanacetum parthenium* (L.) Schultz-Bip, taraxastanes, uvaol, ursanes.
- **Note:** This monograph does not cover tansy (*Tanacetum vulgare*), which is sometimes classified as *Chrysanthemum vulgare*; please see the tansy monograph for more information on this topic. Although *Chrysanthemum* is a component of PC-SPES, this monograph does not cover PC-SPES; please see the PC-SPES monograph for more information on this topic.
- WARNING: PC-SPES HAS BEEN RECALLED FROM THE U.S. MARKET AND SHOULD NOT BE USED.

BACKGROUND

- Chrysanthemum is a genus of over 30 species of flowering plants, which are commonly used for ornamental, food, and insecticidal uses. Pyrethrins (natural organic compounds) extracted from the seed casings of chrysanthemum, such as *Chrysanthemum cinerariifolium* and *Chrysanthemum coccineum*, are used as insecticides and insect repellents. Pyrethrins are known to have a relatively low risk of chronic accumulation, but poisoning may occur from accidental or intentional ingestion or chronic exposure.
- Preliminary laboratory studies suggest that chrysanthemum may be beneficial for the treatment of gout (foot inflammation) and may alter immune function. In clinical trials, chrysanthemum has decreased diabetes symptoms and a combination including chrysanthemum reduced precancerous lesions. Although the studies in these areas seem promising, more research is needed.
- The U.S. Food and Drug Administration (FDA) does not list chrysanthemum on its "generally recognized as safe" (GRAS) list.

EVIDENCE

Uses Based on Scientific Evidence	Grade
Cancer (Precancerous Lesions) Early study indicates that hua-sheng-ping (includes *Chrysanthemum morifolium*, *Glycyrrhiza uralensis*, and *Panax notoginseng*) may be beneficial for patients with precancerous lesions. However, more research is needed.	C
Diabetes A study using a chrysanthemum product, jiangtangkang, indicated that jiangtangkang may be beneficial for patients with non–insulin-dependent diabetes. However, results are mixed, and additional studies are needed before a firm recommendation can be made.	C

Uses Based on Tradition or Theory

Anesthetic (reduces pain), antibacterial, antifungal, antiinflammatory, antioxidant, cancer, Epstein-Barr virus, gout (foot inflammation), herpes simplex virus, HIV, hypertension (high blood pressure), immunomodulation, insecticide, migraine, molluscicide, mosquito repellent.

DOSING
Adults (18 Years and Older)

- There is insufficient evidence to recommend a dose for chrysanthemum in adults. Jiangtangkang (a chrysanthemum product), 8 g, three times daily for 6 months has been used to treat diabetes.

Children (Younger than 18 Years)

- There is insufficient evidence to recommend a dose for chrysanthemum in children.

SAFETY
Allergies

- Avoid in individuals with a known allergy or hypersensitivity to chrysanthemum, its constituents, or members of the Asteraceae/Compositae family, such as dandelion, goldenrod, ragweed, sunflower, and daisies.
- There are numerous case reports and studies showing that allergies to chrysanthemum are very common, and chrysanthemum may be the strongest sensitizer of the cultivated Compositae plants, with an estimated 60% of Europeans being allergic. Patients may be sensitive to pollen, leaves, flowers, stems, the whole plant, and even chrysanthemum oleoresin extract and chrysanthemum oil of turpentine. Occupational exposure is associated with allergy. Symptoms of allergy may include asthma, skin rash, eczema, photosensitivity, hay fever, inflammation of the sinuses, or hives.
- There have also been cases of cross-sensitivity between chrysanthemum and feverfew, tansy, chamomile, *Artemisia vulgaris*, Liliaceae plants, tulip, Easter lily (*Lilium longiflorum*), *Gerbera*, lettuce, *Senecio cruentus*, *Aster*, *Matricaria*, *Solidago*, daisy, dandelion, *Parthenium hysterophorus* L., *Xanthium strumarium* L., *Helianthus annuus* L., *Frullania dilatata*, *Frullania tamarisci*, *Arnica longifolia* Eaton, *Arnica montana* L., primrose,

sunflower, ragweed, the pollen of the Amaryllidaceae family (*Alstroemeria* and *Narcissus*), and mugwort.

Side Effects and Warnings

- Chrysanthemum is likely safe when pesticide- and preservative-free flowers are used in food amounts. There is a lack of information about its use medicinally for any indication.
- Clinical reports suggest that pyrethrins, which are chemicals found in chrysanthemum, may cause skin inflammation or eye disorders, such as corneal (part of the eye) erosion. Poisoning from pyrethrins can occur and is usually due to accidental or intentional ingestion but may also be caused by chronic exposure. Adverse effects are related to toxicity in the nervous system. There is no known antidote for pyrethrin and pyrethroid poisoning; treatment is symptomatic and supportive. Two deaths from acute asthma have been attributed to pyrethrins. Avoid large acute or chronic doses of ingested pyrethrin. Also avoid pyrethrin in patients with compromised liver function, epilepsy, asthma, or who are pregnant or breastfeeding.
- Use chrysanthemum cautiously in patients taking medication for gout (foot inflammation), cancer, or human immunodeficiency virus (HIV).
- Use cautiously in patients with compromised immune systems or taking immunomodulators.
- Avoid in patients with photosensitivity or taking photosensitizers.

Pregnancy and Breastfeeding

- Chrysanthemum is not recommended in pregnant or breastfeeding women because of a lack of available scientific evidence.

INTERACTIONS

Interactions with Drugs

- Chrysanthemum may have anesthetizing (pain-numbing), antibacterial, anticancer, antifungal, antioxidant, and antiinflammatory activity. Caution is advised in patients taking agents with similar effects because of potential additive effects.
- Chrysanthemum may inhibit certain enzymes that play a role in gout (foot inflammation). Use cautiously with medications that treat gout.
- Chrysanthemum may have anti-HIV activity. Use cautiously with antiretroviral medications because of possible additive effects. Chrysanthemum may also interact with immunosuppressants.

- Pyrethrins from *Chrysanthemum cinerariifolium* have been studied in the treatment of the herpes virus. Although there is a lack of information in humans, caution is advised in patients taking herpes agents.
- The chrysanthemum product jiangtangkang may improve fasting blood glucose (sugar) and postmeal blood glucose levels and increase sensitivity to insulin in patients with non–insulin-dependent diabetes. Although there is conflicting evidence in this area, caution is advised in patients taking agents for diabetes or hypoglycemia.
- Chrysanthemum may cause photosensitization, hyperpigmentation, skin inflammation, or make a patient more sensitive to laser treatment. Use cautiously with photosensitizing agents.

Interactions with Herbs & Dietary Supplements

- Chrysanthemum may have anesthetizing (pain-numbing), antibacterial, anticancer, antifungal, antioxidant, and antiinflammatory activity. Caution is advised in patients taking herbs or supplements with similar effects because of potential additive effects.
- Chrysanthemum may inhibit certain enzymes that play a role in gout (foot inflammation). Use cautiously with herbs or supplements used in the treatment of gout.
- Chrysanthemum may have anti-HIV activity. Use cautiously with antiretroviral herbs or supplements because of possible additive effects. Chrysanthemum may also interact with immunosuppressants.
- Pyrethrins from *Chrysanthemum cinerariifolium* have been studied in the treatment of the herpes virus. Although there is a lack of information in humans, caution is advised in patients taking antiherpes, herbs or supplements.
- The chrysanthemum product jiangtangkang may improve fasting blood glucose (sugar) and postmeal blood glucose levels and increase sensitivity to insulin in patients with non–insulin-dependent diabetes. Although there is conflicting evidence in this area, caution is advised in patients taking herbs or supplements for diabetes or hypoglycemia (high or low blood sugar).
- Chrysanthemum may cause photosensitization, hyperpigmentation, dermatitis, or make a patient more sensitive to laser treatment. Use cautiously with herbs and supplements with similar effects.

For a complete list of references, please visit www.naturalstandard.com.

Cinnamon
(*Cinnamomum* spp.)

RELATED TERMS

- American cinnamon, Batavia cassia, Batavia cinnamon, breyne, cannelle (French), cannellier de Ceylan (French), cannellier de Chine (French), cassia, cassia bark, cassia cinnamon, cassia lignea, cassia rou gui, catechins, Ceylon cinnamon, Chinese cinnamon, chinesischer Zimt (German), chinesischer Zimtbaum (German), cinnamaldehyde, cinnamate, cinnamic acid, cinnamon-dhal chini, Cinnamomi cassiae, Cinnamomi cassiae cortex, Cinnamomi ceylanici cortex, Cinnamomi cortex, Cinnamomi flos, Cinnamomi osmophloeum, Cinnamomi ramulus, *Cinnamomum, Cinnamomum aromaticum, Cinnamomum aromaticum* Nees., *Cinnamomum burmannii, Cinnamomum cassia, Cinnamomum cassia* Blume, *Cinnamomum cassia* J. Presl., *Cinnamomum loureiroi, Cinnamomum mairei* Levl., *Cinnamomum migao, Cinnamomum obtusifolium, Cinnamomum osmophloeum* clones (A and B), *Cinnamomum osmophloeum* Kaneh., *Cinnamomum sieboldii, Cinnamomum sieboldii* Meissn, *Cinnamomum tamala, Cinnamomum tejpata, Cinnamomum verum, Cinnamomum verum* J. Presl., *Cinnamomum zeylanicum, Cinnamomum zeylanicum* bark, *Cinnamomum zeylanicum* Blume, *Cinnamomum zeylanicum* Nees, cinnamon bark, cinnamon bark essential oil, cinnamon bark oil, cinnamon cortex, cinnamon essential oil, cinnamon extract, cinnamon flower, cinnamon fruit stalks, cinnamon leaf, cinnamon leaf essential oil, cinnamon leaf oil, cinnamon twig, cinnamon water, cinnamophilin, condensed tannins, cortex cinnamomi, cortex cinnamomum, coumarin, (E)-cinnamaldehyde, echter Kanel (German), eugenol, false cinnamon, gixin, gui, guipi, guirou, guixin, guizhi, guizhi tang, gum, jungui, keishi (Japanese), keychi (Korean), Lauraceae (family), linalool, Malabar leaf, Malabathrum, Malobathrum, monoterpenes, mucilage, mugui, ocotea quixos, Oleum Malabathri, padang cassia, padang cinnamon, phenolic compounds, pinene, proanthocyanidins, ramulus Cinnamomi (*Cinnamomum cassia* Presl), resin, rougui, Saigon cassia, Saigon cinnamon, sesquiterpenes (pinene), Seychelles cinnamon, sweet wood, *trans*-cinnamaldehyde, *trans*-cinnamic acid, true cinnamon, xiao-jian-zhong, xiao-jian-zhong-tang, yin xiang, Zimt (German), Zimtblüten (German), Zimtrinde (German), Zimtrindle (German).
- Traditional Chinese medicine formula examples are as follows: Bai hu jia gui zhi tang, da qing long tang, dang gui si ni tang, ge gen tang, gui zhi fu ling wan, gui zhi tang, ling gui zhu gan tang, ma huang tang, tao he cheng qi tang.
- **Note:** This monograph focuses on cinnamon varieties that are edible and does not include *Cinnamomum camphora* or the camphor tree, which can be very harmful or deadly in humans in large doses, or *Cinnamomum kotoense*, which is an ornamental plant.

BACKGROUND

- Cinnamon has been used as a spice in several cultures for centuries. It was traditionally used to relieve stomach pain and gas; it is still used for these conditions today. The bark of two cinnamon species (*Cinnamomum zeylanicum* and *Cinnamomum cassia*) is used as a spice (cinnamon bark).

- There is a lack of scientific information to support the use of cinnamon for any condition. However, laboratory studies suggest that cinnamon may be useful in the treatment of diabetes (type 2) because of its blood sugar–lowering effects.
- Furthermore, cinnamon and its constituents may have anti-inflammatory, antibacterial, antifungal, and antioxidant properties, and it may prove effective in the supportive treatment of conditions such as cancer or severe virus infections.
- Cinnamon has been granted "generally recognized as safe" (GRAS) status as a food additive by the U.S. Food and Drug Administration (FDA). GRAS substances are considered safe by the experts and not restricted, as is the case with other food additives.

EVIDENCE

Uses Based on Scientific Evidence	Grade
Allergic Rhinitis Cinnamon has demonstrated antiallergic properties in vitro. Based on limited clinical evidence, a combination product including *Cinnamomum zeylanicum, Malpighia glabra*, and *Bidens pilosa* has demonstrated reduced allergic nasal symptoms in patients with allergic rhinitis.	C
Anginia The use of cinnamon for angina has been studied; however, it was used in combination with *Salvia miltiorrhiza, Panax notoginseng*, and *Cinnamomum camphora*. The effectiveness of cinnamon alone is unclear.	C
Antioxidant Cinnamon has been suggested as an antioxidant in various studies and reviews. Based on limited clinical evidence, a dried aqueous extract of cinnamon (Cinnulin PF) has been shown to improve the antioxidant status of overweight or obese individuals with impaired fasting glucose.	C
Bacterial Infection Preliminary evidence suggests that cinnamon may treat bacterial infections, including chronic salmonellosis. The use of cinnamon for bacterial enteric infections has been suggested; however, supportive evidence is not sufficient.	C
Candidiasis (Yeast Infection in the Mouth) There is a lack of available evidence to support the use of cinnamon in humans for this condition.	C
Diabetes (Type 2) There is a lack of available evidence to support the use of cinnamon in humans for type 2 diabetes.	C

(Continued)

Uses Based on Scientific Evidence	Grade
Eye Disorders Preliminary evidence suggests that an herbal eyedrop preparation (OphthaCare) may be useful in the treatment of various ophthalmic disorders including conjunctivitis, conjunctival xerosis (dry eye), acute dacryocystitis, degenerative conditions (pterygium or pinguecula), and disorders in postoperative cataract patients. However, the eyedrop preparation was a combination product containing *Cinnamomum camphora*, in addition to *Carum copticum, Terminalia bellirica, Emblica officinalis, Curcuma longa, Ocimum sanctum, Rosa damascena*, and meldespumapum. The effectiveness of cinnamon alone remains unclear.	
***Helicobacter pylori* Infection** Laboratory studies have found that cinnamon extract does not appear to be effective in curing *Helicobacter pylori* infection, which causes gastrointestinal ulcers.	C
Insect Repellant In lab studies, cassia oil (*Cinnamomum cassia*) sprays reduced dust mites (*Dermatophagoides farinae* and *Dermatophagoides pteronyssinus*). Preliminary clinical evidence suggests that cinnamon may be useful as an insect repellant.	C
Lung Cancer Preliminary evidence suggests that cinnamon may be useful in the treatment of lung cancer. The product used, however, was a combination product containing ginseng, cinnamon bark, Japanese angelica root, astragalus root, peony root, citrus unshiu peel, rehmannia root, polygala root, atractylodes rhizome, schisanda fruit, poria sclerotium, and glycyrrhiza.	C
Metabolic Syndrome (Coronary Heart Disease) Preliminary research suggests that a water-soluble cinnamon extract (Cinnulin PF) may be useful for treating metabolic syndrome in prediabetic subjects.	C

Uses Based on Tradition or Theory

Abdominal pain, abortifacient (induces abortion), abscess, acaricidal (kills mites), acne, analgesic (pain reliever), anesthetic (numbing agent), anthelmintic (expels worms), antibacterial, anticoagulant (blood thinner), antidepressant, antifungal, antiinflammatory, antimicrobial, antioxidant, antiparasitic, antiplatelet (blood thinner), antipyretic (fever reducer), antiseptic, antispasmodic, antitumor, antiviral, arrhythmia (irregular heartbeat), arthritis, asthma, bloating, blood purification, bronchitis, cancer, chest pain, chronic bronchitis, chronic diarrhea, colds/flu, colic, cough, cystitis (bladder inflammation), dental caries, dermatitis, diarrhea, digestive aid, digestive disorders, diuretic (increases urine flow), dyspepsia (upset stomach), eczema, emmenagogue (promotes menstruation), flavoring, food poisoning, food preservation, food uses, gastric ulcer, gastritis (heartburn), gout (foot inflammation), gum disease, gynecological disorders, high blood pressure, high cholesterol

levels, HIV/AIDS, hyperthyroid (overactive thyroid), immunostimulation, inflammatory conditions, insect bites, insect repellent, insecticide, kidney disorders, lice, liver disease, long-term debility, loss of appetite, muscle aches, nausea, neuralgia (nerve pain), neuroprotective (protects the nervous system), premature ejaculation, respiratory tract infection, rheumatism, sciatica (a condition in which pain shoots down a leg or arm as a result of a pinched nerve), sinusitis (inflamed sinuses), skin conditions, snake repellent, sore throat, spermicide, toothache, urethritis (urinary tract inflammation), viral infections, weight gain, wound healing.

DOSING
Adults (18 Years and Older)
- There is insufficient evidence to recommend a dose for cinnamon. Cinnamon is likely safe when taken by mouth short-term (up to 6 weeks) in dosages up to 6 g daily and in amounts commonly found in foods.
- Commercially available cinnamon candy has been taken daily by mouth for 1 week for treating yeast infections in the mouth in human immunodeficiency virus (HIV) patients. For type 2 diabetes, studies have used 1,500 mg to 6 g of cinnamon daily for up to 40 days, but there is conflicting information about effective dosing. In addition, 80 mg of cinnamon extract has been taken daily for 4 weeks, but there is not enough information to recommend this dose in the treatment of *Helicobacter pylori* infection, which causes gastrointestinal ulcers.

Children (Younger than 18 Years)
- There is insufficient evidence to recommend a dose for cinnamon in children.

SAFETY
Allergies
- Avoid in individuals with a known allergy or hypersensitivity to cinnamon, its constituents, members of the Lauraceae family, or Balsam of Peru.

Side Effects and Warnings
- Cinnamon is likely safe when taken by mouth short-term.
- As with any spice or drug, cinnamon can be contaminated by microorganisms during storage. Caution is advised when cinnamon products are chosen.
- Some people may be allergic or sensitive to cinnamon, but this is rare. Skin rash and inflammation, mouth sores, tongue inflammation, gum disease, acne, mouth lesions, and inflammation of the lips have been noted after application of cinnamon (e.g., cinnamon oils, flavored chewing gums, mints, or toothpastes) on the mouth or face. Cinnamaldehyde (the chemical compound that gives cinnamon its spice) may cause swelling of the lips, mouth tissue, and the face, and hives, skin rash, and mouth sores. Prolonged exposure to cinnamon-flavored gum may cause cancer.
- Although not well-studied in humans, cinnamon bark may cause a decrease in platelet counts in the blood after long-term use.
- Asthma and other breathing difficulties were seen in spice-factory workers.
- Use cautiously in patients taking drugs, herbs, or supplements broken down by the liver.

- Cinnamon may lower blood sugar levels. Use cautiously in patients with diabetes or low blood sugar (hypoglycemia).
- Cinnamon may enhance the effect of antibiotics.
- Cinnamon may interact with cardiovascular (heart) agents because of its effects on blood and the cardiovascular system (e.g., antiarrhythmic properties). Use cautiously in people with heart conditions.

Pregnancy and Breastfeeding

- Cinnamon is not recommended in medicinal amounts in pregnant or breastfeeding women because of a lack of available scientific evidence.
- Cinnamon may act as a spermicide, thereby preventing pregnancy by killing sperm; however, it is not recommended as a form of birth control.

INTERACTIONS
Interactions with Drugs

- Cinnamon may have antibacterial activity. Use cautiously with antibiotic medications because of possible additive effects.
- Cinnamon may lower blood sugar levels. Caution is advised when medications that may also lower blood sugar are used. Patients taking drugs for diabetes by mouth or using insulin should be monitored closely by a qualified health care professional, including a pharmacist. Medication adjustments may be necessary.
- Cinnamon may increase the risk of bleeding when taken with drugs that increase the risk of bleeding. Some examples include aspirin, anticoagulants ("blood thinners") such as warfarin (Coumadin) or heparin, antiplatelet drugs such as clopidogrel (Plavix), and nonsteroidal antiinflammatory drugs (NSAIDs) such as ibuprofen (Motrin, Advil) or naproxen (Naprosyn, Aleve).
- The antifungal properties of cinnamon may enhance the effect of commonly used antifungals.
- Cinnamon may have antispasmodic effects. Use cautiously if taking other antispasmodics.
- Cinnamon bark extract may have antiviral effects. Use cautiously if taking antiviral medications because of possible additive effects.
- Cinnamon may affect heart rate and thus may interact with heart agents. Caution is advised in people taking agents for heart conditions.
- Cinnamon may interfere with the way the body processes certain drugs using the liver's cytochrome P450 enzyme system. As a result, the levels of drugs in the blood may

be altered. It may also alter the effects other drugs potentially may have on the P450 system.
- Cinnamon may have effects on the immune system. Use cautiously with other agents that alter the immune system. Consult with a qualified health care professional, including a pharmacist, to check for interactions.

Interactions with Herbs and Dietary Supplements

- Cinnamon may have antibacterial activity. Use cautiously with antibacterial herbs and supplements because of possible additive effects.
- Cinnamon may increase the risk of bleeding when taken with herbs and supplements that are believed to increase the risk of bleeding. Multiple cases of bleeding have been reported with the use of *Ginkgo biloba*, and fewer cases have been reported with garlic and saw palmetto.
- The antifungal properties of cinnamon may enhance the effects of commonly used antifungals.
- Cinnamon bark has been shown to contain very high concentrations of antioxidants. Use cautiously with herbs and supplements that are taken for their antioxidant effects because of possible additive effects.
- Cinnamon may have antispasmodic effects. Use cautiously with other antispasmodics.
- *Cinnamomum cassia* bark extract may have antiviral effects. Use cautiously with antiviral herbs or supplements because of possible additive effects.
- Cinnamon may affect heart rate and thus may interact with heart agents. People taking herbs or supplements that alter heart rate should use cinnamon with caution.
- Cinnamon may interfere with the way the body processes certain herbs or supplements using the liver's cytochrome P450 enzyme system. As a result, the levels of other herbs or supplements in the body may be altered. It may also alter the effects other herbs or supplements potentially may have on the P450 system.
- Cinnamon may lower blood sugar levels. Caution is advised in patients with diabetes or hypoglycemia and in those taking herbs or supplements that affect blood sugar. Serum glucose levels may need to be monitored by a qualified health care professional, including a pharmacist, and doses may need adjustment.
- Cinnamon may have effects on the immune system; use cautiously with herbs and supplements with similar effects.

For a complete list of references, please visit www.naturalstandard.com.

RELATED TERMS

- Akipula, aluminum silicate, anhydrous aluminum silicates, askipula, beidellitic montmorillonite, benditos, bioelectrical minerals, chalk, cipula, clay dirt, clay dust, clay lozenges, clay suspension products, clay tablets, colloidal minerals, colloidal trace minerals, fossil farina, humic shale, Indian healing clay, kaolin, kipula, mountain meal, NovaSil, panito del senor (Spanish), plant-derived liquid minerals, terra sigillata, tirra santa, white clay, white mud.

BACKGROUND

- Clay has been used medicinally for centuries in Africa, India, and China and by Native American groups. Uses have included gastrointestinal disorders and as an antidote for poisoning.
- The practice of eating dirt, clay, or other nonnutritious substances may be referred to as "pica" or "geophagia." This practice is common in early childhood, in mentally handicapped or psychotic patients, and in pregnant women. There is some evidence that mineral deficiencies, such as iron deficiency, may lead to pica, and prevalence is higher in developing countries and in poor communities. Chronic clay ingestion may lead to iron malabsorption and further precipitate this condition.
- There is insufficient scientific evidence to recommend for or against the use of clay for any medical condition. The potential for adverse effects with chronic oral ingestion of clay may outweigh any potential benefits.

EVIDENCE

Uses Based on Scientific Evidence	Grade
Fecal Incontinence Associated with Psychiatric Disorders (Encopresis): Clay Modeling Therapy in Children There is not enough scientific research to support a recommendation for play with modeling clay as an effective therapeutic intervention in children with constipation and encopresis (involuntary bowel movement).	C
Functional Gastrointestinal Disorders There is not enough scientific evidence to recommend the medicinal use of clay by mouth in patients with gastrointestinal disorders. Some clay preparations have been found to be similar to Kaolin and Kaopectate, which are used to treat gastrointestinal disturbances including diarrhea. However, overall, there are significant potential risks that accompany the use of clay, including intestinal blockage and injury as well as lead poisoning.	C
Mercuric Chloride Poisoning Clay lozenges have been used historically in the treatment of mercuric chloride poisoning and were officially mentioned in several European pharmacopoeias, including the Royal College, until the	C

middle nineteenth century. However, there is not enough scientific evidence to recommend the use of clay by mouth for poisoning at this time, as there is a risk that the clay itself may contain contaminants.

Protection from Aflatoxins Aflatoxins are toxic substances from the fungus *Aspergillus flavus*. This fungus infects peanuts, and ingestion of aflatoxins from peanuts and cereals (primarily in warm and humid regions) has been associated with liver cancers in humans and multiple cancers in animals. Phyllosilicate clay has been shown to adhere to aflatoxins in laboratory study, and HSCAS clay in animal diets may diminish or block exposure to aflatoxins. However, the risks of chronic clay exposure likely do not justify the potential benefit.	C

Uses Based on Tradition or Theory

Acidosis (too much acid in the blood), animal bites, blood purification, cancer, constipation, detoxification, diarrhea, dysentery, eye disorders, fevers, heart disorders, menstruation difficulties, nausea and vomiting during pregnancy, nutrition, plague, poisoning, skin fairness, smoking, syphilis, vomiting, water purification, weight loss.

DOSING

Adults (18 Years and Older)

- There is insufficient evidence to recommend the safe use of clay.

Children (Younger than 18 Years)

- There is insufficient evidence to recommend the safe use of clay in children.

SAFETY

Allergies

- There is a lack of clay allergy reports in the available scientific literature. However, in theory, allergy/hypersensitivity to clay, clay products, or constituents of clay may occur.

Side Effects and Warnings

- The practice of eating dirt, clay, or other nonnutritious substances is called *pica* or *geophagia* and may occur in early childhood or in mentally handicapped people. Clay or dirt eating has been associated with lead poisoning in infants, children, and pregnant women, with potential risks such as low red blood cell count and brain damage. Death has occurred related to complications of lead poisoning and brain damage after drinking from a glazed clay pitcher. Clay pots containing candy have been recalled in the United States by the U.S. Food and Drug Administration (FDA) because of high levels of lead in the candy, absorbed from the clay pots. Pica may carry a risk of central nervous system damage. The risk of neurolathyrism, a neurodegenerative, irreversible disorder that causes spastic paraparesis of the body leading to paralysis, was reported to quadruple in a case-control study in Ethiopia when grass pea was cooked with clay utensils.

- Clay products may contain varying amounts of contaminants, including aluminum, arsenic, barium, nickel, and titanium. Elevated levels of 2,3,7,8-tetracholorodibenzo-p-dioxin have been found in fish and eggs from chickens fed a diet including clay. Chronic clay eating has also been associated with imbalances of blood chemistry, such as increased calcium or magnesium and decreased iron and potassium. Myopathy due to severe hypokalemia (low blood potassium levels) has been reported in one case report with large quantities of clay ingestion.

- In the nineteenth century, a condition called *Cachexia Africana* was described and included a swollen appearance, enlarged heart, increased urination, and death. Descriptions of people who chronically ate clay in the nineteenth century noted skin that was initially dry and shiny, and in late stages of disease, especially in children, skin ulcerations occurred over the arms and legs. Chronic clay eating has also been associated with small gonads (testes) and muscle injury.

- Heartburn, gas, loss of appetite, constipation, diarrhea, abdominal pain, bloating, flatulence, and vomiting after meals have been reported with use of clay. Clay eating has also been associated with intestinal blockage and injury, bowel rupture (perforation), formation of stones in the intestine, and enlarged liver/spleen.

- It is reported that children with pica are more likely to develop lung infections. Chronic bronchitis, trouble breathing, and infections have been associated with dust exposure in the heavy clay industry. Hookworm infections may result from eating clay. Tetanus contracted from clay has been described in an infant who ate clay and in a newborn whose umbilical cord was wrapped in clay.

Pregnancy and Breastfeeding

- Use of clay during pregnancy or breastfeeding is not recommended. Eating clay during pregnancy may increase the risk of toxemia or complications at birth.

INTERACTIONS
Interactions with Drugs

- Clay may inhibit the absorption of drugs such as cimetidine (Tagamet) if both are taken together.
- Kaolin has been shown to reduce the bioavailability of quinine in laboratory study.

Interactions with Herbs and Dietary Supplements

- Clay can interfere with iron absorption.

For a complete list of references, please visit www.naturalstandard.com.

Cleavers

(Galium aparine)

RELATED TERMS

- Asperulosidic acid, catchweed, coachweed, clivers, false cleavers, *Galium aparine*, *Galium spurium* L., glucosides, goosegrass, iridoids (family), stickyweed, sticky willy, Tirmanici yogurtotu (Turkish).

BACKGROUND

- Cleavers (*Galium aparine*) is a climbing plant native to North America, Europe, and Asia. In the Anatolia region of Turkey, it is known as Tirmanici yogurtotu. According to some herbalists, cleavers is a good lymphatic and blood-purifying tonic; it is used especially for swollen glands and skin eruptions caused by lymphatic congestion. It has also been recommended as a diuretic for chronic cystitis (inflamed bladder) and prostatitis (enlarged prostate). Currently, there is insufficient evidence in humans to support the use of cleavers for any indication.

EVIDENCE

Uses Based on Scientific Evidence

No available studies qualify for inclusion in the evidence table.

Uses Based on Tradition or Theory

Antiinflammatory, breast tenderness, cancer (bone marrow), choleretic (stimulates the flow of bile), chronic prostatitis (enlarged prostate), cleansing (kidneys and blood), cystitis (chronic, inflamed bladder), deodorant, detoxification (lymphatic system), diuretic, epilepsy, gout (foot inflammation), immunomodulator, menopause, skin eruptions, stomach ailments, swollen glands.

DOSING

Adults (18 Years and Older)

- There is insufficient evidence to recommend a dose for cleavers in adults.

Children (Younger than 18 Years)

- There is insufficient evidence to recommend a dose for cleavers in children.

SAFETY

Allergies

- Avoid in individuals with a known allergy or hypersensitivity to cleavers (*Galium aparine*), its constituents, or members of the Rubiaceae family.

Side Effects and Warnings

- There is insufficient evidence in humans to support the use of cleavers for any indication, and there is a lack of safety information. Cleavers has traditionally been used as a diuretic, and caution is advised in patients taking diuretics or in those with urinary or renal (kidney) disorders.

Pregnancy and Breastfeeding

- Cleavers is not recommended in pregnant or breastfeeding women because of a lack of available scientific evidence.

INTERACTIONS

Interactions with Drugs

- Although not well studied in humans, cleavers may have diuretic properties. Caution is advised when cleavers is taken with other agents that have diuretic effects and increase the flow of urine.

Interactions with Herbs and Dietary Supplements

- Although not well studied in humans, cleavers may have diuretic properties. Caution is advised when cleavers is taken with other herbs or supplements that have diuretic effects and increase the flow of urine.

For a complete list of references, please visit www.naturalstandard.com.

Clove

(Syzygium aromaticum, syn. *Eugenia aromatica)*

RELATED TERMS

- 2-Methoxy-4-(2-propenyl)-phenol, *Caryophylli, Caryophylli aetheroleum* Caryophylli flos, *Caryophyllus aromaticus,* cengke, cengkeh, chiodo di garofano (Italian), choji, chor boghbojh, chor poghpch, cinnamon nails, clau, clavos, clou de girofle (French), clovas de comer, clove, clove bud, clove bud oil, clove cigarettes, clove essential oil, clove leaf, clove oil, craveiro da india, cravinho, cravo, cravo de olor, cuisoare, ding heung, ding xiang, dinh huong, dok chan, dried clove, Eugenia bud, *Eugenia aromatica, Eugenia caryophyllata, Eugenia caryophyllus,* Flores caryophylli, gahn plu, garifallo, garifalo, garifano, garn ploo, Gewurznelken Nagelein (German), gozdzik, gozdzikow korzenny, graambu, ground clove, gvazdikelia, gvozdika, harilik nelgipuu, hrebicek, iltze kanela, jeonghyang, jeonghyong namu, jonghyang, kabsh qarunfil, kala, kalmpir, kan phou, kan phu, karafuu, karamfil, karanfil, kariofilla, kariofilo, khan pluu, khlam puu, klabong pako, klincic, klinceky, klincki, krambu, kreteks, krinfud, kruidnagel, krustnaglinas, kryddernellike, kryddnejlikor, kullobu, kurobu, kvapnusis gvazdikmedis, labanga, labango, laung, lavang, lavanga, lavangalu, lavnagamu, lay hnyin, leoung, ley nyim bwint, mikhak, mikhaki, mixaki, moschokarfi, Myrtaceae (family), nageljnove zbice, nagri, negull, neilikka, nelk, nelke, nellik, nellike, nejlikor, oil of clove, oleum caryophylli, pentogen, qalampir, shriisanjnan, *Syzygium aromaticum, Syzygium aromaticum* (L) Merr. & Perry. (clove), szegfu, szegfuszeg, tropical myrtle, tsiporen.
- **Note:** Do not confuse clove with: baguacu, black plum, *Eugenia cumini, Eugenia edulis, Eugenia jambolana, Eugenia umbelliflora,* Jamun, java apple, java plum, SCE, *Syzygium cordatum, Syzygium cumini, Syzygium samarangense,* water apple, or wax apple.

BACKGROUND

- Clove is widely cultivated in Indonesia, Sri Lanka, Madagascar, Tanzania, and Brazil. It is used in limited amounts in food products as a fragrant flavoring agent and as an antiseptic.
- Clinical trials assessing monotherapy of clove are limited, although the expert panel German Commission E has approved the use of clove as a topical antiseptic and anesthetic. Other uses for clove, such as premature ejaculation, dry socket, and fever reduction, lack reliable human clinical evidence.
- Clove is sometimes added to tobacco in cigarettes, and clove cigarettes ("kreteks") typically contain 60% tobacco and 40% ground cloves.
- Eugenol, a constituent of clove, has been used for analgesic, local anesthetic, antiinflammatory, and antibacterial effects. It is used in the form of a paste or mixture as dental cement, filler, and restorative material.
- Plant oils, including clove, may be used in livestock to inhibit microbial fermentation in waste products. Clove oil may be found in high concentration licorice (glycyrrhizin) products to prevent gel formation in an aqueous solution.

EVIDENCE

Uses Based on Scientific Evidence

Uses Based on Scientific Evidence	Grade
Dental Pain Clove essential oil is commonly used as a dental pain reliever. Early studies have found that a homemade clove gel may be as effective as benzocaine 20% gel. Clove oil combined with zinc oxide paste may be effective for dry socket (inflammation after tooth extraction).	B
Fever Reduction Animal studies suggest that clove can lower fever, but clinical evidence is lacking.	C
Mosquito Repellent In laboratory and field tests, undiluted clove oil repelled multiple species of mosquitoes for up to 2 hours. However, undiluted clove oil may also cause skin rash in sensitive people.	C
Premature Ejaculation Limited clinical evidence suggests that a combination cream with clove and other herbs may be helpful in the treatment of premature ejaculation. The effectiveness of clove alone is unclear.	C

Uses Based on Tradition or Theory

Abdominal pain, acaricidal (an agent that destroys mites), allergies, antibacterial, antifungal, antihistamine, antimicrobial, antimutagenic, antioxidant, antiseptic, antispasmodic, antiviral, aphrodisiac, asthma, atherosclerosis (hardening of the arteries), athlete's foot, bad breath, blood purifier, blood thinner, cancer, cavities, colic, cough, counterirritant, decreased gastric transit time, dental plaque and gingivitis (mouthwash), diabetes, diarrhea, dyspepsia, expectorant, flavoring (for food and cigarettes), food preservative, gout, hernia, herpes simplex virus, hiccups, high blood pressure, inflammation, insecticidal, insulin mimetic, gas, lice, lipid-lowering, mouth and throat inflammation, mouthwash, muscle relaxant, muscle spasm, nausea or vomiting, neurodegeneration, oral candidiasis (thrush), oral edema, pain, parasites, smooth muscle relaxant (clove oil), stomach pain, tooth or gum pain, toxicity (prevention of arsenite-induced toxicity), ulcers, vaginal candidiasis (prevention and treatment), vasorelaxant (clove oil).

DOSING

Adults (18 Years and Older)

- There is insufficient evidence to recommend a specific dose of clove by mouth, on the skin, or by any other route.

Children (Younger than 18 Years)
- There is insufficient evidence to recommend a specific dose of clove by mouth, on the skin, or by any other route.

SAFETY
Allergies
- Allergic reactions to clove or its component eugenol have been reported, including possible severe reactions (anaphylaxis). Signs of allergy may include rash, itching, or shortness of breath. Eugenol or clove can cause allergic rashes when applied to skin or inside the mouth. Hives have been reported in clove cigarette smokers. Individuals with a known allergy to clove, its component eugenol, or to Balsam of Peru should avoid the use of clove by mouth, inhaled from cigarettes, or applied to the skin.

Side Effects and Warnings
- Clove is generally regarded as safe for food use in the United States. However, when clove is taken by mouth in large doses, in its undiluted oil form, or used in clove cigarettes, side effects may occur, including vomiting, sore throat, seizure, sedation, difficulty breathing, fluid in the lungs, vomiting of blood, blood disorders, kidney failure, and liver damage or failure. People with kidney or liver disorders or who have had seizures should avoid clove. Serious side effects are reported more often in young children, even with small doses, and therefore clove supplements should be avoided in children and pregnant or nursing women.
- Clove or clove oil may cause an increased bleeding risk, based largely on laboratory research. Caution is advised in patients with bleeding disorders or taking drugs that may increase the risk of bleeding. Dosing adjustments may be necessary. It is not clear what doses or methods of using clove may increase this risk. Clove use should be stopped before surgery.
- When applied to the skin or inside of the mouth, clove can cause burning, loss of sensation or painful sensation, local tissue damage, dental pulp damage, higher risk of cavities, or sore lips. Undiluted clove oil has a high risk of causing contact dermatitis (rash) and even burns if applied to the skin at full strength. The application of clove combination herbal creams to the penis has been said to cause episodes of difficulty with erection or ejaculation.
- Clove oil taken by mouth may lower blood sugar levels. Caution is advised in patients with diabetes or hypoglycemia and in those taking drugs, herbs, or supplements that affect blood sugar. Serum glucose levels may need to be monitored by a health care provider, and medication adjustments may be necessary.
- Contamination can occur if clove is improperly stored.

Pregnancy and Breastfeeding
- Not enough information about safety is available to recommend the use of clove supplements in pregnant or breastfeeding women.

INTERACTIONS
Interactions with Drugs
- Based on laboratory research, clove theoretically may increase the risk of bleeding when taken with drugs that increase the risk of bleeding. It is not clear what doses or methods of using clove may increase this risk. Some examples of drugs that increase bleeding risk include aspirin, anticoagulants ("blood thinners") such as warfarin (Coumadin) or heparin, antiplatelet drugs such as clopidogrel (Plavix), and nonsteroidal antiinflammatory drugs such as ibuprofen (Motrin, Advil) or naproxen (Naprosyn, Aleve).
- Clove oil taken by mouth may lower blood sugar levels. Caution is advised when medications that may also lower blood sugar are used. Patients taking drugs for diabetes by mouth or using insulin should be monitored closely by a qualified health care provider. Medication adjustments may be necessary.
- When applied to the skin, eugenol, a component of clove, may reduce the ability to feel and react to painful stimulation. Therefore, use of clove products on the skin with other numbing or pain-reducing products such as lidocaine/prilocaine cream (Emla) or as capsaicin cream (Zostrix) theoretically may increase effects.
- Clove may also react with antifungals, antiinflammatory agents, antihistamines, antineoplastics, and drugs taken for cardiovascular conditions. Clove may also affect the way in which the liver breaks down certain drugs.

Interactions with Herbs and Dietary Supplements
- Based on laboratory research, clove may increase the risk of bleeding when taken with herbs and supplements that are believed to increase the risk of bleeding. It is not clear what doses or methods of using clove may increase this risk. Multiple cases of bleeding have been reported with the use of *Ginkgo biloba*, some cases have been reported with garlic, and fewer cases have been reported with saw palmetto. Numerous other agents may theoretically increase the risk of bleeding, although this has not been proven in most cases.
- Clove may lower blood sugar levels. Caution is advised when herbs or supplements that may also lower blood sugar are used. Blood glucose levels may require monitoring, and doses may need adjustment.
- When applied to the skin, eugenol (a component of clove) may reduce the ability to feel and react to painful stimulation. Therefore, use with other numbing or pain-reducing herbal products such as capsaicin (Zostrix) may in theory cause exaggerated effects.
- Clove may also react with antiinflammatory, antifungal, antihistamine, and antineoplastic herbs and herbs taken for cardiovascular conditions. Clove may also affect the way in which the liver breaks down certain herbs.

For a complete list of references, please visit www.naturalstandard.com.

Codonopsis
(*Codonopsis pilosula*)

RELATED TERMS

- Bastard ginseng, bellflower, bonnet bellflower, Campanulaceae (family), chuan dang, codonoposide, condonoposide 1c, *Codonopsis eupolyphaga*, *Codonopsis lanceolata*, *Codonopsis modesta*, *Codonopsis nervosa* var., *Codonopsis ovata* Benth., *Codonopsis philosula*, *Codonopsis pilosula*, *Codonopsis pilosula* (Franch.) Nannf., *Codonopsis pilosula* (Franch.) Nannf. var. volubilis, *Codonopsis pilosula* modesta, *Codonopsis pilosular*, *Codonopsis silvestris*, *Codonopsis tangshen*, *Codonopsis tubulosa*, dangshen, friedelin, poor man's ginseng, radix codonopsis, radix *Codonopsis pilosula*, alpha-spinasterol, tang shen, tang-shen, tangshenoside, tangshenoside I, taraxerol.

BACKGROUND

- Codonopsis is a small perennial native to Asia, which is especially abundant in the Shanxi and Szechuan provinces of China. Codonopsis has been used in China for over 2,000 years as a tonic for the lungs and spleen, and to strengthen and nourish the blood and balance metabolic function.
- Historically, codonopsis is thought to have properties similar to ginseng. The Chinese name for codonopsis, dangshen, indicated that it was ginseng from the Shandang region; *shen* is the key term to describe ginseng or a ginseng-like herb. Like ginseng, codonopsis is referred to as an *adaptogen*, a substance that nonspecifically enhances and regulates the body's ability to withstand stress. Adaptogens increase the body's general performance in ways that help the whole body resist disease. Codonopsis is thought to benefit the entire body by boosting strength, increasing stamina and alertness, rejuvenating the body, strengthening the immune system, aiding recovery from chronic illness, reducing stress, and stimulating the appetite.
- At this time, there is insufficient high-quality evidence in humans to support the use of codonopsis for any indication.

EVIDENCE

Uses Based on Scientific Evidence

No available studies qualify for inclusion in the evidence table.

Uses Based on Tradition or Theory

Anorexia, anoxic brain injury, antioxidant, appetite stimulant, ascites (fluid in the abdomen), asthma, blood circulation, brain damage, cancer, chronic diarrhea, coagulation disorders, contraception, cough, diabetes, dyspnea (difficulty breathing), endurance, gastric cancer, gastric ulcers, HIV, hypertension (high blood pressure), immune function, kidney disorders, liver damage, lowered blood cell counts, memory, metabolic enhancement, motility disorders, myocardial injury, nerve regeneration, obesity, palpitations, senility, solar ultraviolet protection, stress, systemic lupus erythematosus (SLE), thyroid disorders, tonic, uterus contraction, vomiting, weight gain.

DOSING

Adults (18 Years and Older)

- There is insufficient evidence to recommend a dose of codonopsis for adults. Traditionally, 3-9 g of codonopsis decoction has been used; some conditions may require dosages up to 30 g daily.

Children (Younger than 18 Years)

- There is insufficient evidence to recommend a dose of codonopsis for children.

SAFETY

Allergies

- Avoid in people with a known allergy or hypersensitivity to *Codonopsis pilosula*, its constituents, or related species from the Campanulaceae family.

Side Effects and Warnings

- There is insufficient clinical information available regarding the safety of codonopsis. Few adverse effects in humans have been reported for codonopsis.
- Use cautiously in patients with bleeding disorders or those who are taking anticoagulant or antiplatelet agents.
- Use cautiously in patients who are taking laxatives or stool softeners or who have inflamed bowel or appendicitis. Traditionally, codonopsis is used to promote digestion and cleanse the intestinal tract.
- Use cautiously in patients using antacids or gastric reflux medications, as *Codonopsis pilosula* may reduce gastric acid–pepsin secretion.
- Use cautiously in patients using oral medication, as *Codonopsis pilosula* extract may inhibit gastrointestinal movement.
- Avoid using in women who are trying to become pregnant.

Pregnancy and Breastfeeding

- Codonopsis is not recommended in pregnant or breastfeeding women due to a lack of available human scientific evidence.

INTERACTIONS

Interactions with Drugs

- Although not well studied in humans, *Codonopsis pilosula* may reduce gastric acid–pepsin secretion. Caution is advised in patients taking antacid medications due to possible additive effects.
- In humans, codonopsis has been observed to inhibit platelet aggregation. Caution is advised in patients taking drugs that may also increase the risk of bleeding. Some examples include aspirin, anticoagulants (blood thinners) such as warfarin (Coumadin) or heparin, antiplatelet drugs such as clopidogrel (Plavis), and nonsteroidal anti-inflammatory drugs (NSAIDs) such as ibuprofen (Motrin, Advil) or naproxen (Naprosyn, Aleve).
- Codonopsis has exhibited antifertility activity in rats. Caution is advised when taking codonopsis with fertility medications.

- Traditionally, codonopsis is used to promote digestion and cleanse the intestinal tract. Caution is advised in patients taking laxatives due to possible additive effects.
- *Codonopsis pilosula* extract may inhibit gastrointestinal movement. Thus, caution is advised when taking codonopsis with any agents taken by mouth, because the effect of the agents may be altered.

Interactions with Herbs and Dietary Supplements

- Although not well studied in humans, *Codonopsis pilosula* may reduce gastric acid–pepsin secretion. Caution is advised in patients taking herbs or supplements with antacid activity due to possible additive effects.
- In humans, codonopsis has been observed to inhibit platelet aggregation. Caution is advised in patients taking other herbs or supplements thought to increase the risk of bleeding. Multiple cases of bleeding have been reported with the use of *Ginkgo biloba*, and fewer cases with garlic and saw palmetto. Numerous other agents may theoretically increase the risk of bleeding, although this has not been proven in most cases.
- Codonopsis has exhibited antifertility activity in rats. Caution is advised when taking codonopsis with any herbs or supplements with intended fertility effects.
- Traditionally, codonopsis is used to promote digestion and cleanse the intestinal tract. Caution is advised in patients taking other herbs or supplements with laxative activity due to possible additive effects.
- *Codonopsis pilosula* extract may inhibit gastrointestinal movement. Thus, caution is advised when taking codonopsis with any agents taken by mouth, because the effect of the agents may be altered.

For a complete list of references, please visit www.naturalstandard.com.

Coenzyme Q10

RELATED TERMS

- Andelir, CoenzymeQ, Co-enzyme Q10, Coenzyme Q (50), CoQ, CoQ10, CoQ(50), Co-Q10, CoQ-10, 2,3 dimethoxy-5 methyl-6-decaprenyl benzoquinone, Heartcin, idebenone (synthetic analogue), Kaneka Q10, mitoquinone, Neuquinone, Q10, Q-Gel, Solu Q10, Taidecanone, ubidecarenone, ubiquinone, ubiquinone-10, ubiquinone-Q10, Udekinon, vitamin q10, vitamin Q10.

BACKGROUND

- Coenzyme Q10 (CoQ10) is produced by the human body and is necessary for the basic cell functions. CoQ10 levels are reported to decrease with age and to be low in patients with some chronic diseases such as heart conditions, muscular dystrophies, Parkinson's disease, cancer, diabetes, and HIV/AIDS. Some prescription drugs may also lower CoQ10 levels.
- Levels of CoQ10 in the body can be increased by taking CoQ10 supplements, although it is not clear that replacing "low CoQ10" is beneficial.
- CoQ10 has been used, recommended, and studied for numerous conditions, but it remains controversial as a treatment in many areas.

EVIDENCE

Uses Based on Scientific Evidence	Grade
Coenzyme Q10 Deficiency Coenzyme Q10 is normally produced by the human body, although deficiency may occur in patients with impaired CoQ10 biosynthesis due to severe metabolic or mitochondrial disorders, not enough dietary CoQ10 intake, or too much CoQ10 use by the body. Depending on the cause of CoQ10 deficiency, supplementation or increased dietary intake of CoQ10 and the vitamins and minerals needed to produce CoQ10 may be effective.	A
High Blood Pressure (Hypertension) Preliminary research suggests that CoQ10 causes small decreases in blood pressure (systolic and possibly diastolic). Low blood levels of CoQ10 have been found in people with hypertension, although it is not clear if CoQ10 "deficiency" is a cause of high blood pressure. Well-designed long-term research is needed to strengthen this recommendation.	B
Age-Related Macular Degeneration Early studies show that acetyl-L-carnitine, n-3 fatty acids, and Coenzyme Q10 (Phototrop) may help age-related macular degeneration. More research is needed using Coenzyme Q10 alone before a recommendation can be made.	C
Alzheimer's Disease Promising preliminary evidence suggests that CoQ10 supplements may slow down, but not cure, dementia in people with Alzheimer's disease. Additional well-designed studies are needed to confirm these results before a firm recommendation can be made.	C
Angina (Chest Pain from Clogged Heart Arteries) Preliminary small human studies suggest that CoQ10 may reduce angina and improve exercise tolerance in people with clogged heart arteries. Better studies are needed before a firm recommendation can be made.	C
Anthracycline Chemotherapy Heart Toxicity Anthracycline chemotherapy drugs, such as doxorubicin (Adriamycin), are commonly used to treat cancers such as breast cancer or lymphoma. Heart damage (cardiomyopathy) is a major concern with the use of anthracyclines, and CoQ10 has been suggested to protect the heart. However, studies in this area are small and not high quality, and the effects of CoQ10 remain unclear.	C
Asthma CoQ10 may benefit asthma patients when added to other therapies. More research is needed. Asthma should be treated by a qualified health care provider.	C
Breast Cancer Supplementation with CoQ10 has not been proven to reduce cancer and has not been compared to other forms of treatment for breast cancer.	C
Cancer More research is needed to determine if CoQ10 may help cancer when used with other therapies. Cancer should be treated by a qualified health care provider.	C
Cardiomyopathy (Dilated, Hypertrophic) There is conflicting evidence from research on the use of CoQ10 in patients with dilated or hypertrophic cardiomyopathy.	C
Chronic Fatigue Syndrome Preliminary evidence suggests that CoQ10 may improve symptoms of chronic fatigue syndrome.	C
Cocaine Dependence A combination of Coenzyme Q10 and L-carnitine has been studied to reduce cocaine usage, but early studies are inconclusive.	C

(Continued)

Uses Based on Scientific Evidence	Grade
Coronary Heart Disease There is insufficient scientific evidence to recommend the use of CoQ10 in patients with coronary heart disease.	C
Exercise Performance Results are variable, with some research suggesting benefits, and other studies showing no effects. Most trials have not been well designed.	C
Friedreich's Ataxia Preliminary research has produced promising evidence for the use of CoQ10 in the treatment of Friedreich's ataxia. However, the evidence thus far has been insufficient to support this indication.	C
Gum Disease (Periodontitis) Preliminary clinical studies suggest possible benefits of CoQ10 taken by mouth or placed on the skin or gums in the treatment of periodontitis.	C
Heart Attack (Acute Myocardial Infarction) There is preliminary human study of CoQ10 given to patients within 3 days after a heart attack.	C
Heart Conditions (Mitral Valve Prolapse in Children) There is preliminary evidence supporting the use of CoQ10 in children with mitral valve prolapse. Well-designed clinical trials are warranted.	C
Heart Failure The evidence for CoQ10 in the treatment of heart failure is controversial and remains unclear. Different levels of disease severity have been studied (New York Heart Association classes I to IV). Better research is needed in this area studying the effects on quality of life, hospitalization, and death rates before a recommendation can be made.	C
Heart Protection during Surgery Several studies suggest that the function of the heart may be improved after major heart surgeries such as coronary artery bypass graft (CABG) or valve replacement when CoQ10 is given to patients before or during surgery.	C
HIV/AIDS There is limited evidence that natural levels of CoQ10 in the body may be reduced in people with HIV/AIDS. There is a lack of reliable scientific research showing that CoQ10 supplements have any effect on this disease.	C
Hypertriglyceridemia Preliminary studies on CoQ10 for high triglyceride levels in the blood are unclear.	C

	Grade
Increasing Sperm Count (Idiopathic Spermatozoa) There is preliminary evidence that supports the use of CoQ10 in the treatment of increasing sperm count and motility.	C
Kidney Failure There is initial evidence to support the use of CoQ10 in the treatment of renal (kidney) failure.	C
Lipid Lowering (Adjunct to Statin Therapy) Coenzyme Q10 may reduce some adverse effects associated with statin therapy for high cholesterol, including reduced heart function.	C
Migraine There is some evidence to support the use of CoQ10 treatment in migraine prevention or treatment.	C
Mitochondrial Diseases and Kearns-Sayre Syndrome CoQ10 is often recommended for patients with mitochondrial diseases, including myopathies, encephalomyopathies, and Kearns-Sayre syndrome. CoQ10 may help improve function in children with maternally-inherited diabetes and deafness, though the evidence thus far has not been conclusive.	C
Muscular Dystrophies Preliminary studies in patients with muscular dystrophy taking CoQ10 supplements describe improvements in exercise capacity, heart function, and overall quality of life.	C
Myelodysplastic Syndrome Preliminary studies have produced unclear results.	C
Parkinson's Disease There is promising (though preliminary) clinical evidence supporting the use of CoQ10 for treating Parkinson's disease.	C
Postsurgical Recovery (Adjuvant) In patients with stage I and II melanoma with surgically removed lesions, CoQ10 may decrease the rate of recurrence. Although these results are promising, more studies are needed.	C
Prostate Cancer A combination that included CoQ10 did not significantly affect PSA levels in patients with prostate cancer. Although PSA levels may be an indicator of cancer, it is unclear whether CoQ10 would have any effect on cancer treatment of prevention.	C
Tinnitus (Ringing in the Ears) Patients with tinnitus may have low levels of CoQ10; however, it remains unclear whether supplementation will benefit this condition.	C

Uses Based on Scientific Evidence	Grade
Diabetes Available evidence suggests that CoQ10 does not affect blood sugar levels in patients with type 1 or type 2 diabetes, and it does not alter the need for diabetes medications.	D
Huntington's Disease There is negative evidence from studies that used CoQ10 in the treatment of Huntington's disease.	D

Uses Based on Tradition or Theory

Abnormal heart rhythms, amyotrophic lateral sclerosis (ALS), anemia, antioxidant, Bell's palsy, breathing difficulties, cerebellar ataxia, chronic obstructive pulmonary disease (COPD), cognitive performance, deafness, fibromyalgia, gingivitis, hair loss (and hair loss from chemotherapy), hepatitis B, high cholesterol, immune system diseases, infertility, insomnia, ischemia, leg swelling (edema), life extension, liver enlargement or disease, lung disease, MELAS syndrome (mitochondrial myopathy, encephalopathy, lactacidosis, stroke), multiple sclerosis, muscle wasting, neurodegenerative disorders, nutrition, obesity, Papillon-Lefevre syndrome, physical performance, psychiatric disorders, reduction of phenothiazine drug side effects, reduction of tricyclic antidepressant (TCA) drug side effects, speech disorders (Landau-Kleffner syndrome), stomach ulcer.

DOSING

Adults (18 Years and Older)

- A general dose of CoQ10 is 50-1,200 mg taken daily by mouth in divided doses.
- To treat gum disease, 85 mg of CoQ10 per milliliter of soybean oil suspension has been applied to the surface of affected areas once weekly.
- Most studies of CoQ10 for heart protection during bypass surgery have used CoQ10 taken by mouth. One study used intravenous CoQ10, 5 mg/kg of body weight, given 2 hours before surgery. Safety is not clear. Any therapies used close to the time of surgery should be discussed with the surgeon and a pharmacist prior to starting.

Children (Younger than 18 Years)

- There is insufficient evidence to recommend the safe use of CoQ10 in children. A qualified health care provider should be consulted before considering use.

SAFETY

Allergies

- In theory, allergic reactions to supplements containing CoQ10 may occur. Itching or rash has been reported.

Side Effects and Warnings

- There are few serious reported side effects of CoQ10. Side effects are typically mild and brief, stopping without any treatment needed. Reactions may include nausea, vomiting, stomach upset, heartburn, diarrhea, loss of appetite, skin itching, rash, insomnia, headache, dizziness, itching, irritability, increased light sensitivity of the eyes, fatigue, or flu-like symptoms.

- CoQ10 may lower blood sugar levels. Caution is advised in patients with diabetes or hypoglycemia, and in those taking drugs, herbs, or supplements that affect blood sugar. Serum glucose levels may need to be monitored by a health care provider, and medication adjustments may be necessary.
- Low blood platelet number was reported in one person taking CoQ10. However, other factors (viral infection, other medications) may have been responsible. Lowering of platelets may increase the risk of bruising or bleeding, although there is a lack of known reports of bleeding from CoQ10. Caution is advised in people who have bleeding disorders or who are taking drugs that increase the risk of bleeding. Dosing adjustments may be necessary.
- CoQ10 may decrease blood pressure, and caution is advised in patients with low blood pressure or those taking blood pressure medications. Elevations of liver enzymes have been reported rarely, and caution is advised in people with liver disease or those taking medications that may harm the liver. CoQ10 may lower blood levels of cholesterol or triglycerides. Thyroid hormone levels may be altered based on one study.
- Organ damage due to lack of oxygen/blood flow during intense exercise has been reported in a study of patients with heart disease, although the specific role of CoQ10 is not clear. Vigorous exercise is often discouraged in people using CoQ10 supplements.

Pregnancy and Breastfeeding

- There is not enough scientific evidence to support the safe use of CoQ10 during pregnancy or breastfeeding. In men, sperm may be affected.

INTERACTIONS

Interactions with Drugs

- In theory and based on a human case report, CoQ10 may reduce the effectiveness of warfarin (Coumadin) and may limit or prevent effective anticoagulation (blood thinning). CoQ10 may reduce blood pressure or add to the effects of other blood pressure–lowering drugs. In theory, CoQ10 may affect thyroid hormone levels and alter the effects of thyroid drugs such as levothyroxine (Synthroid), although this has not been proven in humans. CoQ10 may also interact with antiretroviral or antiviral drugs.
- Based on theory and human research, a number of drugs may deplete natural levels of CoQ10 in the body. It has not been shown that there are benefits of CoQ10 supplements in people using these agents. Examples include diabetes drugs, tricyclic antidepressants, antipsychotics, beta-blockers, HMG-CoA reductase inhibitors (statins), Alzheimer's drugs, heart drugs, cancer drugs, immune system–altering drugs, and diuretic drugs (water pills).

Interactions with Herbs and Dietary Supplements

- CoQ10 may reduce blood pressure and may result in additive effects when taken with other herbs or supplements that also lower blood pressure. Diuretic herbs, such as licorice and horsetail, may also decrease blood pressure and therefore interact with CoQ10. CoQ10 may also interact with herbs and supplements with antiviral effects. In theory, CoQ10 may affect thyroid hormone levels and alter the effects of herbs or supplements that alter the thyroid.
- Although not well studied in humans, it is possible that some herbs or supplements used to lower cholesterol or

alter blood sugar levels may also decrease the level of CoQ10 in the body.

- Red rice yeast may reduce CoQ10 blood levels. CoQ10 may add to the effects or side effects of L-carnitine. CoQ10 may also interact with vitamin A, C, or E. It may also theoretically reduce the effectiveness of warfarin or other blood-thinning agents, such as garlic (*Allium sativum*), *Ginkgo biloba*, or saw palmetto (*Serenoa repens*).

- Herbs or supplements used for Alzheimer's disease, heart disorders, diabetes, cancer, viral conditions, and immune system altering may interact with CoQ10.

For a complete list of references, please visit www. naturalstandard.com.

Coleus
(*Coleus forskohlii*)

RELATED TERMS

- Coleon U-quinone coleus, coleonol, *Coleus amboinicus* Lour (CA), *Coleus barbatus* Benth, *Coleus blumei*, *Coleus blumei* Benth, *Coleus carnosifolius*, *Coleus galeatus*, *Coleus kilimandschari*, *Coleus parvifolius*, *Coleus scutellarioides*, coleus solenostemon rotundifolius, *Coleus xanthanthus*, colforsin, colforsin daropate hydrochloride, forscolin, forskoditerpenoside A, forskoditerpenoside B, forskolin, forskolin G, forskolin H, HL 362, FSK88, Labiatae (family), Lamiaceae (family), L-75-1362B, NKH477, *Plectranthus barbatus*, *Plectranthus forskohlii*, rosmarinic acid, rosmarinic acid, xanthanthusin E, xanthanthusins F-K.

BACKGROUND

- Coleus species have been used in Asian traditional medicine to treat angina, asthma, bronchitis, epilepsy, insomnia, skin rashes, and a wide range of digestive problems. Since the 1970s, research was predominantly concentrated on forskolin, a root extract of *Coleus forskohlii*. Studies suggest that forskolin may have clinical use in treating heart, lung, and eye conditions.
- Although most studies have used the isolated forskolin extract, it is believed that the whole coleus plant may be more effective, due to the presence of multiple compounds that may act synergistically. Generally, coleus appears to be well tolerated with few adverse effects.

EVIDENCE

Uses Based on Scientific Evidence	Grade
Asthma There is a lack of sufficient data to recommend for or against the use of coleus in the treatment of bronchial asthma.	B
Cardiomyopathy Forskolin may improve heart function in patients with cardiomyopathy though the evidence thus far is limited.	B
Glaucoma Limited evidence suggests that coleus improves glaucoma.	B
Anti-inflammatory Action after Cardiopulmonary Bypass Evidence is insufficient to recommend coleus as an anti-inflammatory to patients recovering after cardiopulmonary bypass.	C
Breast Milk Stimulant Coleus has been used as a breast milk stimulant for hundreds of years; however, the effectiveness has not been well documented and scientific evidence is limited.	C
Breathing Aid for Intubation Pretreatment with coleus before intubation may be beneficial, especially for middle-aged smokers. More research is needed.	C
Depression and Schizophrenia Limited evidence suggests that coleus may be useful in the management of depression or schizophrenia.	C
Erectile Dysfunction Forskolin may enhance smooth muscle relaxation; however, it remains unclear whether it offers therapeutic benefits for erectile dysfunction.	C

Uses Based on Tradition or Theory

Abdominal colic, abdominal cramps, abortion, allergies, angina (chest pain), anti-HIV 1, antioxidant, atherosclerosis (hardening of the arteries), atopic dermatitis, autoimmune diseases, bladder infection, bladder pain, bloating, bronchitis, cancer, cataract, cerebral vascular insufficiency, circulatory tonic, congestive heart failure, convulsions, diabetes, digestion, dysmenorrhea (painful menstruation), eczema, epilepsy, gas, gastric diseases, high blood pressure, hypothyroidism (underactive thyroid), immunostimulant, inflammatory disease, insomnia, irritable bowel syndrome (IBS), ischemic heart disease, liver diseases, malabsorption, menstrual cramps, metastatic cancer, obesity, painful urination, peptic ulcer, poor sperm motility, psoriasis (chronic skin disease), skin rashes, spasmolytic spastic colon, stroke, sunless tanning thrombosis (blood clots), urinary tract infection (UTI), weight loss, worms.

DOSING
Adults (18 Years and Older)

- There is insufficient evidence to recommend a dose for coleus. Many natural medicine experts recommend 50 mg of coleus extract (18% forskolin), taken 1-3 times daily by mouth, although the safety or efficacy of these doses has not been demonstrated. A dose of 250 mg of less-concentrated coleus extract (1% forskolin) is commonly taken 1-3 times daily. As a dried root, 6-12 g daily has been used, and as a fluid extract, 6-12 mL daily has been used.
- Colforsin daropate (0.5-0.75 mcg/kg/min) has been used for its anti-inflammatory action after cardiopulmonary bypass and to aid in airway resistance after tracheal intubation. Although coleus has been studied for depression, schizophrenia, cardiomyopathy, and glaucoma, commercially available products have not been rigorously studied for these uses.

Children (Younger than 18 Years)

- There is insufficient evidence to recommend a dose for coleus in children.

SAFETY
Allergies

- Avoid in people with a known allergy or hypersensitivity to *Coleus forskohlii* and related species. Rash may occur in sensitive people.

Side Effects and Warnings

- Coleus is generally regarded as safe, although long-term safety data are lacking. Inhalation of forskolin may cause sore throat, upper respiratory tract irritation, mild to moderate cough, tremor, or restlessness. Coleus eye drops may produce a milky covering over the eyes.
- Coleus may lower blood sugar and stimulate the thyroid gland. Use cautiously in patients with thyroid disorders. Also use cautiously in diabetic patients. Colenol, a compound isolated from coleus, stimulates insulin release.
- Theoretically, coleus may increase the risk of bleeding. Use cautiously in patients with a history of bleeding, hemostatic disorders, or drug-related hemostatic problems. Discontinue use in patients at least 2 weeks prior to surgical or dental procedure, due to risk of bleeding. Avoid use in patients with active bleeding.
- Use cautiously in patients with low blood pressure or those at risk for hypotension. Also use cautiously in patients with heart disease or asthma.
- Avoid during pregnancy due to possibility of abortifacient (abortion inducing) effects.

Pregnancy and Breastfeeding

- Coleus is not recommended in pregnant or breastfeeding women due to a lack of available scientific evidence. It is unknown if coleus is excreted in the breast milk.

INTERACTIONS
Interactions with Drugs

- When used with other blood-thinning agents, such as aspirin, ibuprofen, and naproxen, coleus may increase the risk of bleeding.
- Although not well studied in humans, forskolin may interact with antidepressants, antihistamines, blood pressure–altering agents, asthma medications, beta-blockers, inotropic agents, or thyroid medications. It may also interact with drugs used for cancer and weight loss, or drugs that are processed through the liver.
- Coleus should be used cautiously when taken concurrently with agents that are dependent on pH and gastric action for breakdown and activation such as newer cephalosporin antibiotics, itraconazole, ketoconazole, and warfarin.
- Although not well studied in humans, topical forskolin may significantly reduce intraocular pressure (IOP). When used with other medications that decrease IOP, it may result in additive effects.
- Colenol, a compound isolated from coleus, stimulates insulin release, and use with blood sugar–lowering agents or exogenous insulin may result in additive effects.

Interactions with Herbs and Dietary Supplements

- When used with other blood-thinning herbs or supplements, such as *Ginkgo biloba* and garlic, coleus may increase the risk of bleeding.
- Although not well studied in humans, forskolin may interact with antidepressants, antihistamines, blood pressure–altering agents, asthma agents, heart agents, inotropic agents, or thyroid medications. It may also interact with herbs or supplements used for cancer and weight loss, or drugs that are processed through the liver.
- Although not well studied in humans, topical forskolin may significantly reduce intraocular pressure (IOP). When used with other herbs or supplements that decrease IOP, it may result in additive effects.
- Colenol, a compound isolated from coleus, stimulates insulin release, and its use with blood sugar–lowering herbs or supplements, such as bitter melon, may result in additive effects.

For a complete list of references, please visit www.naturalstandard.com.

RELATED TERMS

- Argyrol, electro colloidal silver, electro-colloidal silver, ionic silver, ProAg catheter, silver protein, silver protein solution.

BACKGROUND

- Colloidal silver is a suspension of submicroscopic metallic silver particles in a colloidal base. Long-term use of silver preparations can lead to argyria, a permanent condition in which silver salts deposit in the skin, eyes, and internal organs. The skin can often appear ashen-gray due to the deposition of the silver salts. Argyria has been mistaken for cyanotic heart disease.
- Today, colloidal silver is not generally recognized as safe or effective. However, some researchers believe that it has antibacterial properties, which may warrant further studies. Despite the lack of scientific evidence, colloidal silver is most commonly used as a natural antibiotic or healing agent. It is either applied to the skin or ingested as a drink to promote healing or to combat disease.
- The U.S. Food and Drug Administration (FDA) has taken action against several colloidal drug companies, including Web site advertisers, for making unsubstantiated claims for their product. Colloidal silver products are usually marketed as dietary supplements. Therefore, the manufacturers do not need to go through the same rigorous approval processes as drug companies.

EVIDENCE

Uses Based on Scientific Evidence

No available studies qualify for inclusion in the evidence table.

Uses Based on Tradition or Theory

Acne, allergies, antibacterial, antifungal, antiviral, arthritis, athlete's foot, biofilm, bladder inflammation, blood purification, boils, burns, cancer, cholera, colds, colitis, conjunctivitis (pinkeye), dermatitis, diabetes, diarrhea, diphtheria, ear infections, eczema, flu, food poisoning, gastritis, genital herpes, gonorrhea, hepatitis, herpes, HIV/AIDS, impetigo (bacterial skin infection), leprosy, leukemia, lupus, Lyme disease, malaria, meningitis, pneumonia, prostatitis (enlarged prostate), psoriasis (chronic skin disease), rheumatism, ringworm, scarlet fever, shingles, skin cancer, sore throat, stomach ulcers, syphilis, tonsillitis, tuberculosis, typhoid, ulcers, warts, whooping cough, yeast infections.

DOSING

Adults (18 Years and Older)

- There is insufficient evidence to recommend a dose for colloidal silver in adults.

Children (Younger than 18 Years)

- There is insufficient evidence to recommend a dose for colloidal silver in children.

SAFETY

Allergies

- Avoid in individuals with a known allergy or hypersensitivity to silver. Allergy to silver protein has been reported.

Side Effects and Warnings

- Colloidal silver is likely unsafe when taken by mouth or applied to the skin. The U.S. Food and Drug Administration (FDA) issued a final rule in August 1999 establishing that all over-the-counter (OTC) drug products containing colloidal silver ingredients or silver salts for internal or external use are not Generally Recognized as Safe (GRAS) and effective and are misbranded. This rule was issued because colloidal silver has been marketed for many serious disease conditions. Colloidal silver may also cause kidney damage, stomach distress, headaches, fatigue, and skin irritation.

Pregnancy and Breastfeeding

- Colloidal silver is not recommended in pregnant or breastfeeding women due to a lack of available scientific evidence.

INTERACTIONS

Interactions with Drugs

- Insufficient available evidence.

Interactions with Herbs and Dietary Supplements

- Insufficient available evidence.

For a complete list of references, please visit www.naturalstandard.com.

Comfrey
(*Symphytum* spp.)

RELATED TERMS

- 7-Acetylintermedine, acetyllcopsamine, allantoin, allantoin-beta-cyclodextrin, anadoline, asperum polymer, ass ear, assear, asses-ears, Beinwell (German), black root, black wort, blackwort, blue comfrey, bocking 14, boneset, Boraginaceae (family), Borago-Symphytum, borraja, bourrache, bruisewort, bulbous comfrey, buyuk karakafesotu, Caucasian comfrey, comfrey extract, comfrey herb, comfrey root, common comfrey, comphrey, consolida, consolida aspra (Italian), consolidae radix, consolida majoris, consolide maggiore (Italian), consormol, consoude, consoude grande (French), consoude rude (French), consound, consuelda (Spanish), creeping comfrey, Crimean comfrey, echimidine, Extr. Rad. Symphyti, glucofructan, great comfrey, ground comfrey root, gum plant, healing blade, healing herb, heliotrine, hirehari-so, hydroxycinnamate-derived polymer, integerrimine, intermedine, knitback, knitbone, Kytta-Balsam f, Kytta-Plasma f, Kytta-Salbe f, lasiocarpine, liane chique, lithospermic acid, lycopsamine, medicinal comfrey, mucopolysaccharides, navadni gabez (Slovenian), nipbone, okopnik sherohovaty (Russian), oreille d'ane (French), otonecine-pyrrolizidine alkaloids, prickley comfrey, pyrrolizidine alkaloid, Quaker comfrey, radix symphyti, rauher Beinwell (German), rauhe Wallwurz (German), Reinweld (German), retronecine, retrorsine, retrorsine N-oxide, riddelliine, ridelliine N-oxide, rosmarinic acid, rough comfrey, ru kulsukker (Danish), Russian comfrey, ruwe smeerworted (Dutch), salsify, saponins, senecionine, senecionine N-oxide, seneciphylline, senkirkine, simfit (Italian), slippery root, S. x uplandicum, symlandine, symphyti herba, symphyti folium, symphyti radix, symphytine, symphytum alkaloids, *Symphytum asperrimum* Donn, *Symphytum asperum*, *Symphytum asperum* Lepechin, *Symphytum asperum x officinale*, *Symphytum bulbosum*, *Symphytum caucasicum*, *Symphytumcaucasicvum*, Symphytum cream, *Symphytumgrandiflorum*, *Symphytumibericum*, *Symphytum officinale* Linn, *Symphytum orientale*, *Symphytum peregrinum* Lebed, Symphytum radix, *Symphytum* spp., *Symphytum tauricum*, *Symphytum tuberosum*, *Symphytum x uplandicum*, *Symphytum x uplandicum* Nyman, Syrupus de Symphyto (Spanish), tannins, tarharaunioyrtti (Finnish), the great comfrey, tuberous comfrey, 7-uplandine, wallwort, wallwurz (German), white comfrey, yalluc (Saxon), zinzinnici (Italian).

BACKGROUND

- Comfrey (*Symphytum* spp.) is native to both Europe and Asia and has traditionally been used as both a food and forage crop. Three plant species in the genus *Symphytum* are medicinally relevant and include wild or common comfrey (*Symphytum officinale* L.), prickly or rough comfrey (*Symphytum asperum* Lepechin, syn *Symphytum asperrimum* Donn), and Caucasian, Quaker, Russian, or blue comfrey (*Symphytum* x *uplandicum* Nyman [*Symphytum peregrinum* Lebed.]), which originated as a natural hybrid of *Symphytum officinale* L. and *Symphytum asperum* Lepechin.
- Comfrey has traditionally been applied to the skin (topically) for inflammation, pain and wound healing, it has also been taken by mouth (orally) for gastrointestinal, respiratory, and gynecological concerns.
- Although evidence supporting oral use of comfrey is lacking, clinical trials suggest topical comfrey may be advantageous for pain and inflammation associated with injuries.
- Although comfrey has been traditionally used both orally and topically, recent evidence suggesting carcinogenic and hepatotoxic effects has led to withdrawal of oral products from the market in many countries. Warnings to avoid use on open wounds have been issued.

EVIDENCE

Uses Based on Scientific Evidence	Grade
Inflammation Comfrey may have anti-inflammatory effects. Clinical trials investigating topical application of comfrey-containing creams have found significant reductions in inflammation and pain associated with sprains and muscle injuries.	B
Pain Comfrey may have anti-inflammatory effects. Clinical trials investigating topical application of comfrey-containing creams have found significant reductions in inflammation and pain associated with sprains and muscle injuries.	B
Myalgia A comfrey-containing cream has been applied on the skin to reduce pain associated with myalgia. Improvements in pain at rest and in motion were noted. However, the evidence thus far is not conclusive.	C

Uses Based on Tradition or Theory

Acne, aging, analgesic (pain reliever), anemia, angina (chest pain), antifungal, anti-inflammatory, antimicrobial, antioxidant, antipyretic (fever reducer), arthritis, broken bones, bronchitis, bruises, burns, cancer, conjunctivitis (pinkeye), cough, cough (bloody), dermatitis, diaper rash, diarrhea, expectorant (induces cough), eye infections (blepharitis), food uses, gangrene, gastritis, gout (foot inflammation), gum disease, gynecological disorders, hair tonic, hemorrhoids, hernia, high blood pressure, impetigo (pus-filled blisters), inflammatory bowel disease, lupus, mastitis (painful inflammation of breast), otitis (ear infection), pharyngitis, pleurisy (lung inflammation), rash, sexual arousal, sinusitis, skin disorders, sports injuries, sprains, thyroid disorders, tissue healing after surgery, ulcers, urine blood, uterine tonic, varicose veins, vasoprotective, wound healing.

DOSING

Adults (18 Years and Older)

- Due to safety concerns, taking comfrey by mouth is not recommended and oral sources cannot be sold in the United States. Traditional uses of comfrey include ingestion as an herbal tea. The 1990 German Commission E Monographs suggest maximal daily doses of 100 mcg (external) unsaturated pyrrolidine alkaloids. The American Herbal Products Association's Botanical Safety Handbook from 1977 has similar recommendations.
- Traditionally, a cloth or gauze soaked in an infusion (100 g fresh, peeled root simmered in 250 mL water for 10-15 minutes) has been applied to the skin several times daily (duration not noted). For a salve, olive oil and beeswax may be added and cooled.

Children (Younger than 18 Years)

- There is insufficient evidence to recommend data for comfrey in children.

SAFETY

Allergies

- Avoid in people with a known allergy or hypersensitivity to comfrey or its constituents.

Side Effects and Warnings

- Comfrey is possibly safe when used as a cream applied to the skin for short-term (up to 2 weeks) treatment of minor injuries with no open wounds. Alkaloids may also be absorbed through intact skin, so precautions should still be taken. Use caution when using topical creams containing comfrey for extended periods.
- Comfrey is likely unsafe when taken by mouth (orally) due to toxic pyrrolizidine alkaloids in comfrey. The U.S. Food and Drug Administration (FDA) has recommended removal of oral comfrey products from the market. Products made of comfrey root contain high levels of pyrrolizidine alkaloids.
- Possible side effects associated with comfrey use include abdominal pain, acute pneumonitis (inflammation of the lungs), ascites (accumulation of serous fluid in the abdominal cavity), Budd-Chiari syndrome (a rare liver disease in which a blood clot occurs in the large vein leading from the liver called the hepatic vein), cancer, damage to Disse's space, disruption of the sinusoidal wall, dose-dependent liver damage, elevated serum transaminase levels, extravasation of red blood cells, heart problems, hemorrhagic necrosis, hepatic necrosis, hepatic veno-occlusive disease, hepatomegaly, jaundice, liver damage, liver failure, liver tumor induction, loss of definition of hepatocyte cellular membranes, loss of hepatocyte microvilli, loss of sinusoidal lining cells, obstructive ileus, occlusion of sublobular veins, phytobezoar, platelets in areas of bleb formation around hepatocytes, severe portal hypertension, sinusoids filled with debris including cellular debris, hepatocyte organelles and red blood cells, skin redness, small venous radicles of the liver, swelling of hepatocytes, vascular congestion, venous endophlebitis, and zone 3 necrosis of hepatocytes.
- Avoid oral comfrey due to hepatotoxic (liver damaging) and carcinogenic (cancer causing) pyrrolizidine alkaloids; oral use has caused death. Avoid topical comfrey in individuals with or at risk for hepatic disorders, cancer, or immune disorders due to potential for absorption of toxic compounds.

- Use topical (applied to the skin) creams containing comfrey cautiously in patients using anti-inflammatory medications due to potential for additive effects.
- Use cautiously in patients taking cytochrome P450 3A4-inducing agents, which may increase the conversion of compounds in comfrey to toxic metabolites.

Pregnancy and Breastfeeding

- Avoid comfrey during pregnancy and breastfeeding as it may be hepatotoxic (liver damaging). Toxins from comfrey can be found in milk from grazing animals that have consumed comfrey. Thus it is likely that comfrey toxins would also be excreted in human breast milk.

INTERACTIONS

Interactions with Drugs

- Taking comfrey by mouth may increase the activity of the hepatic enzyme, aminopyrine N-demethylase.
- Comfrey applied to the skin may offer anti-inflammatory effects. Caution is advised in patients taking anti-inflammatory medications due to possible additive effects.
- Based on the potential for carcinogenic activity, oral (by mouth) or topically (applied to the skin) absorbed comfrey may have antagonistic effects to chemotherapeutic agents. Caution is advised when taking concurrently with other chemotherapeutic agents.
- Agents that induce CYP3A4 may increase the conversion of compounds in comfrey to toxic metabolites.
- Comfrey taken by mouth or applied to the skin may have additive adverse effects on the liver when used in combination with hepatotoxic (liver damaging) medications.

Interactions with Herbs and Dietary Supplements

- Oral products containing comfrey leaf in combination with other ingredients were found to have lower total levels of alkaloids compared with bulk comfrey root or leaf.
- Oral comfrey (*Symphytum officinale*) may increase the activity of the hepatic enzyme, aminopyrine N-demethylase.
- Based on clinical evidence topical comfrey may offer anti-inflammatory effects. Caution is advised in patients taking anti-inflammatory herbs, such as oral licorice or topical *Ginkgo biloba*, due to possible additive effects.
- Based on the potential for carcinogenic activity, comfrey taken by mouth or applied to the skin may have antagonistic effects to chemotherapeutic agents. Caution is advised when taking concurrently with other herbs or supplements with potential chemotherapeutic effects.
- Agents that induce CYP3A4 may increase the conversion of compounds in comfrey to toxic metabolites.
- Oral or absorbed comfrey may have additive adverse effects on the liver when used in combination with hepatotoxic (liver damaging) herbs, such as kava, or supplements.
- The combination of pokeweed (*Phytolacca americana*) and comfrey may result in additive effects. Although not well studied in humans, both herbs can precipitate human glycoproteins, agglutinate sheep red blood cells (SRBCs), and stimulate lymphocyte adherence to nylon fibers.
- Oral or absorbed comfrey, in combination with other pyrrolizidine alkaloid–containing herbs, may increase total levels of pyrrolizidine alkaloid consumed, which increases the risk for toxicity. Herbs containing pyrrolizidine alkaloids include alkanna, borage, butterbur, coltsfoot, forget-me-not, gravel root, hemp agrimony, hound's tongue, lungwort, and *Senecio* species.

- Rosemary (*Rosmarinus officinalis* L.) or sassafras (*Sassafras albidum* Nutt.) extracts and comfrey extracts may both induce glutathione (GSH) adducts.
- Comfrey may have uterine tonic effects. Other uterine tonic agents include chamomile (*Matricaria chamomilla* L.), pot marigold calendula (*Calendula officinalis* L.), cockscomb (*Celosia cristata* L.), plantain (*Plantago lanceolata* L. and *Plantago major* L.), shepherd's purse (*Capsella bursa pastoris* L.), and St. John's wort (*Hypericum perforatum* L.).

For a complete list of references, please visit www.naturalstandard.com.

Copper

RELATED TERMS

- Copper 7, copper acetate, copper amino acid chelates, copper citrate, copper gluconate, copper glycinate, copper intrauterine device, copper sebecate, copper sulfate, copper T, Cu, Cu IUD, cuivre, cupric oxide, cupric sulfate, cuprum, $CuSO_4$, elemental copper, inorganic copper, organic copper.

BACKGROUND

- Copper is a mineral that occurs naturally in many foods, including vegetables, legumes, nuts, grains, and fruits, as well as shellfish, avocado, and beef (organs such as liver). Because copper is found in the earth's crust, most of the world's surface water and ground water used for drinking purposes contains small amounts of copper.
- Copper is involved in numerous biochemical reactions in human cells. Copper is a component of multiple enzymes and is involved with the regulation of gene expression; mitochondrial function/cellular metabolism; connective tissue formation; as well as the absorption, storage, and metabolism of iron. Copper levels are tightly regulated in the body.
- Copper toxicity is rare in the general population. Wilson's disease is a genetic disorder in which the body cannot rid itself of copper, resulting in deposition in organs and serious consequences such as liver failure and neurological damage. Obstruction of bile flow, contamination of dialysis solution (in patients receiving hemodialysis for kidney failure), Indian childhood cirrhosis, and idiopathic copper toxicosis are other rare causes of potentially dangerous excess copper levels. Such people should be followed closely by a physician and a nutritionist.
- Copper deficiency may occur in infants fed only cow-milk formulas (which are relatively low in copper content) or synthetic low-lactose diets, premature/low-birth-weight infants, infants with prolonged diarrhea or malnutrition, people with malabsorption syndromes (including celiac disease, sprue, or short bowel syndrome), people with cystic fibrosis, older adults, or people receiving intravenous total parenteral nutrition (TPN) or other restrictive diets.
- Medicinal use of copper compounds dates to Hippocrates in 400 B.C. Bacterial growth is inhibited on copper's surface, and hospitals historically installed copper-alloy doorknobs and push-panels as a measure to prevent transmission of infectious disease.

EVIDENCE

Uses Based on Scientific Evidence	Grade
Copper Deficiency Copper deficiency may occur in infants fed only cow-milk formulas (which are relatively low in copper content) or synthetic low-lactose diets, premature/low-birth-weight infants, infants with prolonged	A

diarrhea or malnutrition, people with malabsorption syndromes (including celiac disease, sprue, or short bowel syndrome), people with cystic fibrosis, older adults, or people receiving intravenous total parenteral nutrition (TPN) or other restrictive diets. Such individuals may require supplementation with copper (and other trace elements).

Age-Related Macular Degeneration There is not enough scientific evidence available to determine if copper plays a role in this disorder.	C
Alzheimer's Disease Prevention Conflicting study results report that copper intake may either increase or decrease the risk of developing Alzheimer's disease. Additional research is needed before a recommendation can be made.	C
Arthritis The use of copper bracelets in the treatment of arthritis has a long history of traditional use, with many anecdotal reports of effectiveness. There are research reports suggesting that copper salicylate may reduce arthritis symptoms more effectively than either copper or aspirin alone. More studies are needed before a recommendation can be made.	C
Cancer Preliminary research reports that lowering copper levels theoretically may arrest the progression of cancer by inhibiting blood vessel growth (angiogenesis). Copper intake has not been identified as a risk factor for the development or progression of cancer.	C
Cardiovascular Disease Prevention/ Atherosclerosis The effects of copper intake or blood copper levels on cholesterol, atherosclerosis (cholesterol plaques in arteries), or coronary artery disease remain unclear. Studies in humans are mixed, and further research is needed in this area.	C
Childhood Growth Promotion Severe copper deficiency may retard growth. Adequate intake of micronutrients including copper and other vitamins may promote growth as measured by length gains.	C
Immune System Function Copper is involved in the development of immune cells and immune function in the body. Severe copper deficiency appears to have adverse effects on immune function, although the exact mechanism is not clear.	C

(Continued)

Uses Based on Scientific Evidence	Grade
Marasmus Copper deficiency may occur in this condition, and supplementation with copper may play a role in the nutritional treatment of infants with this condition. Infants with marasmus should be managed by a qualified health care professional.	C
Menkes' Kinky-Hair Disease Menkes' kinky-hair disease is a rare disorder of copper transport/absorption. Copper supplementation may be helpful in this disease, although further research is necessary before a clear management recommendation can be made.	C
Osteoporosis/Osteopenia Osteopenia and other abnormalities of bone development related to copper deficiency may occur in copper-deficient low-birth-weight infants and young children. Supplementation with copper may be helpful in the treatment and/or prevention of osteoporosis, although early human evidence is conflicting. The effects of copper deficiency or copper supplementation on bone metabolism and age-related osteoporosis require further research before clear conclusions can be drawn.	C
Plaque Prevention A preliminary study suggests that rinsing with a copper solution is effective in plaque reduction. Further research is required before recommendations can be made.	C
Schizophrenia Some studies of schizophrenic patients report high blood copper levels with low urinary copper (suggesting that copper is being retained), and low blood zinc levels. In some of these cases, zinc was observed to be helpful as an antianxiety agent. The role of copper supplementation is not clear.	C
Sideroblastic Anemia Copper deficiency is one of the causes of sideroblastic anemia that should be considered when evaluating this condition, particularly when the anemia is unresponsive to iron therapy alone. This anemia appears to be caused by defective iron mobilization due to decreased ceruloplasmin activity.	C
Systemic Lupus Erythematosus (SLE) A preliminary study suggests that copper offers no benefit to individuals with SLE. Further research is required before recommendations can be made.	C
Trimethylaminuria (TMAU) Trimethylaminuria (TMAU) is a metabolic disorder characterized by the inability to oxidize and convert dietary-derived trimethylamine (TMA) to trimethylamine N-oxide (TMAO). Preliminary evidence suggests that the use of copper chlorophyllin results	C

in a reduced urinary free TMA concentration and normalization of TMAO. Further research is required in this field before recommendations can be made.	
Neural-Tube Defect Prevention The risk of neural tube defects is decreased in women who take folic acid and multivitamins during the periconception period. Supplementation with trace elements alone such as copper does not appear to prevent these defects.	D

Uses Based on Tradition or Theory

Aflatoxin toxicity, age-related memory problems, allergies, anemia, antibacterial, antioxidant, athletic performance, bone diseases (growth), bone healing, bronchitis, cancer, cataracts (prevention/progression), cognition, cystic fibrosis, decreasing cadmium absorption, depression, fatigue, fetal development, hematopoiesis (stimulation of blood cell production), Hodgkin's disease, hypercholesterolemia (high cholesterol), hyperactivity, hypertension (high blood pressure), infertility, learning disabilities, muscle ache, muscle cramps, optic nerve damage (ethambutol-induced), oral deodorant, *Pasteurella* infection, phenylketonuria, pneumonia, premenstrual syndrome, psoriasis, rheumatic heart disease, skin problems (stretch marks), stomach ulcer, toxicity (pyrrolizidine alkaloid), vitiligo, weight gain, wound healing.

DOSING
Adults (18 Years and Older)
- The U.S. Recommended Daily Allowance (RDA) is 900 mcg for adults, 1,000 mcg for pregnant women, 1,300 mcg for nursing women, and 890 mcg for adolescents 14-18 years old. Surveys suggest that most Americans consume less than the RDA for copper each day. Up to 10,000 mcg/day appears to be safe for consumption in adults. Vegan diets appear to provide adequate amounts of copper.
- In a number of clinical trials, copper doses of 2-10 mg by mouth were safely used in patients. For plaque inhibition, a 1.1 mM copper rinse has been used for 4 days. The appropriate application of ointment preparations containing copper in concentrations up to 20% has also been studied with no apparent toxic effects.

Children (Younger than 18 Years)
- The U.S. Recommended Daily Allowance (RDA) for children is 890 mcg for adolescents 14-18 years old, 700 mcg for children 9-13 years old, 440 mcg for children 4-8 years old, 340 mcg for children 1-3 years old, 220 mcg for infants 7-12 months old, and 200 mcg for infants 0-6 months old. Surveys suggest that most Americans consume less than the RDA of copper each day. Up to 3,000-5,000 mcg daily appears to be safe for consumption in children.
- Copper deficiency may occur in infants fed only cow-milk formulas (which are relatively low in copper content) or synthetic low-lactose diets, premature/low-birth-weight infants, infants with prolonged diarrhea or malnutrition, people with malabsorption syndromes (including celiac disease, sprue, or short bowel syndrome), people with cystic

fibrosis, older adults, or people receiving total parenteral nutrition (TPN) or other restrictive diets. Such situations may merit copper supplementation (and other trace elements), which should be under the supervision of a healthcare professional. In the United States, copper is not available in infant supplements.

- Management of marasmus should be under the supervision of a healthcare professional, although 20-80 mcg/kg of copper sulfate supplementation daily by mouth has been reported as safe.

SAFETY
Allergies

- There is insufficient available evidence.

Side Effects and Warnings

- Copper toxicity is rare in the general population. Excess copper consumption may lead to liver, kidney, or neurologic damage. Excess dosing may lead to toxic symptoms including weakness, abdominal pain, nausea, vomiting, and diarrhea, with more serious signs of acute toxicity including liver damage, kidney failure, pleural damage, coma, and death. Other medical problems associated with copper toxicity in studies or anecdotally include anxiety, depression, fatigue, learning disabilities, memory lapses, diminished concentration, insomnia, seizure, delirium, stuttering, hyperactivity, arthralgias, myalgias, hypertension, gingivitis, dermatitis, discoloration of skin/hair, preeclampsia, postpartum psychosis, weight gain, or transaminitis. Acute copper poisoning has occurred through the contamination of beverages by storage in copper containing containers as well as from contaminated water supplies. In the U.S., the health-based guideline for a maximum water copper concentration of 1.3 mg/L has been enforced by the Environmental Protection Agency.
- Genetic disorders affecting copper metabolism such as Wilson's disease, Indian childhood cirrhosis, or idiopathic copper toxicosis, place people at risk of adverse effects of chronic copper toxicity at significantly lower intake levels. Trientine is a copper-chelating agent used in the management of Wilson's disease. Penicillamine has also been used to bind copper and enhance its elimination in Wilson's disease. Zinc in therapeutic dosages has been used to inhibit copper absorption in patients with Wilson's disease. Animal research suggests that supplementation with taurine may reduce toxic effects of copper when given in combination, although it is not clear if this is the case in humans.
- Copper-T devices are a type of intrauterine device (IUD) used for birth control that have been linked to the development of anemia and increased risk of pelvic infection in some users. Copper released from the IUDs may cause hormonal changes and alter the menstrual cycle in women. Other common side effects include pain/cramps, abnormal bleeding, and device expulsion. In some cases, pelvic inflammatory disease (PID) or anemia may develop.

Pregnancy and Breastfeeding

- **Pregnancy:** It is unclear if copper supplementation is necessary during pregnancy to maintain adequate levels. Copper is potentially unsafe when used orally in higher doses than the recommended dietary allowances (RDA). Animal studies suggest that trace metal aberrations, including copper, may be related to disturbed fetal growth or teratogenicity, particularly in the setting of diabetic pregnancy.

- **Breastfeeding:** Copper is potentially unsafe when used orally in higher doses than the RDA. Copper is present in breast milk.

INTERACTIONS
Interactions with Drugs

- Antacids may interfere with copper absorption.
- Several human studies indicate that taking certain antipsychotics (haloperidol and risperidone), nifedipine, or oral contraceptives may alter copper levels in the body, although clinical significance is unknown. Copper levels should be monitored by a qualified health care professional.
- Ethambutol (Myambutol) and its metabolite chelate copper, resulting in depleted levels. Copper chelation in the retina may contribute to ethambutol-induced optic neuropathy. Whether supplemental copper can prevent this adverse effect is not clear.
- Penicillamine (Cuprimine, Depen) is used to bind copper and enhance its elimination in Wilson's disease. Because it dramatically increases the urinary excretion of copper, individuals taking penicillamine for reasons other than copper overload may have an increased requirement for copper.
- Trientine (Syprine, Trien) is a copper-chelating agent used in the management of Wilson's disease.
- Levels of copper may be reduced after zidovudine (Retrovir, AZT), although there is some evidence that this may be beneficial in HIV/AIDS patients, and therefore copper supplements may not be advisable.

Interactions with Herbs and Dietary Supplements

- Several herbs and supplements, such as boron, vitamin C, selenium, molybdenum, and manganese may alter (decrease or increase) copper levels in the body. Although copper may increase the concentration of cadmium in tissues based on animal research, cadmium supplementation does not appear to significantly alter copper levels. Calcium or rapeseed oil-meal may alter the metabolism of copper.
- Long-term high copper intake may cause decreases in plasma concentrations of folate.
- Animal studies suggest that low copper levels may result in decreased serum dehydroepiandrosterone (DHEA) levels, although it is unclear if increased copper intake increases DHEA levels.
- Adequate copper nutritional status appears to be necessary for normal iron metabolism, transport, and red blood cell formation. High iron intake may interfere with copper absorption. Copper deficiency is associated with retention of iron in the liver.
- Animal research suggests that supplementation with taurine may reduce toxic effects of copper when given in combination, although it is not clear if this is the case in humans.
- High levels of supplemental zinc intake over extended periods of time may result in decreased copper absorption in the intestines or copper deficiency possibly due to increased synthesis of the intestinal cell protein metallothionein, which binds some metals. This may be the mechanism by which zinc induces sideroblastic anemia. However, some animal research suggests that high dietary zinc may not interfere with tissue or plasma concentrations of copper.

For a complete list of references, please visit www. naturalstandard.com.

Coral
(Anthozoa)

RELATED TERMS

- Anthozoa (class), Bio-Eye hydroxyapatite implant, calcium carbonate matrix, carbonate bone replacement graft (BRG), coral carbonate, coral grafts, coral water, coralline, *Goniopora* species, hydroxyapatite, natural coral, natural coral calcium, NC (porites), sea coral calcite.
- **Note:** This review does not include a detailed description of calcium, a major constituent of coral.

BACKGROUND

- Corals are sea organisms that grow in colonies. Corals are most often found in tropical oceans and are known as reef builders because they secrete calcium carbonate to form a hard skeleton.
- Natural and man-made coral are currently being studied for use in bone grafts. Coral has been shown to increase bone strength when incorporated into surrounding bone.
- Although coral may be useful as a bone graft substitute, researchers state that more long-term information on safety and effectiveness is needed. Coral has been associated with an increased rate of infection and may cause problems in those who have or are prone to kidney stones.

EVIDENCE

Uses Based on Scientific Evidence	Grade
Bone Healing (Reconstructive Surgery and Grafting) Coral may strengthen bone. Natural and man-made coral are currently being studied for use as substitutes for bone grafts.	C

Uses Based on Tradition or Theory
Arthritis, cancer, heart disease.

DOSING

Adults (18 Years and Older)

- There is insufficient evidence to recommend a dose for coral.

Children (Younger than 18 Years)

- There is insufficient evidence to recommend a dose for coral. Use in children is not recommended.

SAFETY

Allergies

- Avoid with allergy or hypersensitivity to coral and other marine products.

Side Effects and Warnings

- Coral should be avoided in people who have or are prone to kidney disease or kidney stones. Coral may increase the risk of infection and wound irritation when used for bone grafting.

Pregnancy and Breastfeeding

- Coral is not recommended in pregnant or breastfeeding women due to a lack of available scientific evidence.

INTERACTIONS

Interactions with Drugs

- Coral, which contains calcium, may theoretically interact with blood pressure medications called *calcium channel blockers* (such as verapamil or diltiazem).

Interactions with Herbs and Dietary Supplements

- Coral contains calcium and may have additive effects when take with other supplements containing calcium, especially in people who have kidney problems or kidney stones.

For a complete list of references, please visit www.naturalstandard.com.

Cordyceps
(Cordyceps sinensis)

RELATED TERMS

- Aweto, caoor, caterpillar fungus, Chinese caterpillar fungus, chongcao, cordycepin, *Cordyceps cicadae, Cordyceps militaris, Cordyceps nipponica, Cordyceps ophioglossoides, Cordyceps pseudomilitaris, Cordyceps sinensis, Cordyceps sinensis* (Berk) Succ., *Cordyceps sinensis* mycelium, *Cordyceps* spp., *Cordyceps tuberbulata,* Cs4, CS-4, deer fungus parasite, dong chong xia cao, dong chong zia cao, dong zhong chang cao, fungus, hsia ts'ao tung ch'uung, jinshuibao, mummio, semitake, shilajit, *Sphaeria sinensis,* summer grass winter worm, summer-plant winter-worm, tochukaso, vegetable caterpillar, yarsha gumba, yertsa gonbu ze-e cordyceps.

BACKGROUND

- *Cordyceps sinensis,* the *Cordyceps* species most widely used as a dietary supplement, naturally grows on the back of the larvae of a caterpillar from the moth *Hepialus armoricanus* Oberthur found mainly in China, Nepal, and Tibet. The mycelium invades the caterpillar and eventually replaces the host tissue. The stroma (fungal fruit body) grows out of the top of the caterpillar. The remaining structures of the caterpillar along with the fungus are dried and sold as the dietary supplement cordyceps.
- Commonly known as "dong chong xia cao" (summer-plant, winter-worm) in Chinese, cordyceps has been used as a tonic food in China and Tibet and has been used as a food supplement and tonic beverage among the rich because of its short supply due to overharvesting. It is also an ingredient in soups and other foods used traditionally in Chinese medicine for thousands of years helping debilitated patients recover from illness.
- Cordyceps is used therapeutically for asthma, bronchitis, chemoprotection, exercise performance, hepatitis B, hepatic cirrhosis, hyperlipidemia (high cholesterol), as an immunosuppressive agent, and in chronic renal failure.
- The fungus became popular in 1993 when two female Chinese athletes, who admitted using cordyceps supplements, beat the world records in the track and field competition at the Stuttgart World Championships for the 1,500-, 3,000-, and 10,000-meter runs. The women were drug tested for any banned substances such as steroids and were negative. Their coach attributed the performance to the cordyceps supplementation.

EVIDENCE

Uses Based on Scientific Evidence	Grade
Hepatitis B Cordyceps may stimulate the immune system and improve serum gamma globulin levels in hepatitis B patients. Currently, there is insufficient evidence to recommend for or against the use of cordyceps for chronic hepatitis B. However, the results are promising. Additional study of cordyceps and current hepatitis treatments is needed.	B
Hyperlipidemia (High Cholesterol) Cordyceps may lower total cholesterol and triglyceride levels, although these changes may not be permanent or long lasting. Longer studies with follow up are needed to determine the long-term effects of cordyceps on hyperlipidemia.	B
Anti-Aging Cordyceps may improve various symptoms related to aging. However, higher quality studies testing specific symptoms of aging are needed before the effects of cordyceps can be described. Currently, there is insufficient evidence to recommend the use of cordyceps for anti-aging.	C
Asthma Cordyceps may reduce some asthma symptoms. Additional studies are needed to make a firm recommendation.	C
Bronchitis There is insufficient evidence from controlled clinical trials to recommend the use of cordyceps for bronchitis. Most studies using cordyceps have found improved symptoms with cordyceps more than the control drugs. Although results are promising, more studies should be performed before a firm recommendation can be made.	C
Chemoprotective There is insufficient evidence to recommend the use of cordyceps as a chemoprotective agent in aminoglycoside toxicity. However, the results are promising.	C
Exercise Performance Enhancement In 1993, two female Chinese athletes, who admitted using cordyceps supplements, beat the world records in the track and field competition at the Stuttgart World Championships for the 1,500-, 3,000-, and 10,000-meter runs. However, there is insufficient evidence from conflicting controlled clinical trials to recommend the use of cordyceps for improving exercise performance. More studies are needed in this area.	C
Immunosuppression Two studies using combination herbal treatments that included cordyceps indicate that these combinations suppressed the immune system in kidney transplant and lupus nephritis patients. However, as these treatments used combination products, the effect of cordyceps cannot be defined. More studies with cordyceps as a monotherapy are needed.	C

(Continued)

259

Uses Based on Scientific Evidence	Grade
Liver Disease (Hepatic Cirrhosis) In traditional Chinese medicine, cordyceps has been used to support and improve liver function. Herbal combinations that included cordyceps have improved liver and immune function. However, the effect of cordyceps alone is unclear.	C
Renal Failure (Chronic) In traditional Chinese medicine, cordyceps is used to strengthen kidney function. Limited evidence indicates that cordyceps may improve renal function in patients with chronic renal failure.	C
Sexual Dysfunction There is not enough available scientific evidence to support this indication.	C

Uses Based on Tradition or Theory

Addiction (opiates), Alzheimer's disease, anemia, anti-inflammatory, antioxidant, arrhythmia (irregular heartbeat), atherosclerosis (hardening of the arteries), bone marrow production, cancer, cardiovascular disease, cough, diabetes, fatigue, fertility, hematopoiesis (formation of blood cells), hemorrhage, hypertension (high blood pressure), longevity, lower backache, memory, menstruation irregularities, mucilage, muscle weakness, nephritis (inflammation of kidneys), neurodegeneration, night sweats, radiation protection, respiratory disease, senility (weakness), systemic lupus erythematosus (SLE), tinnitus, tonic, tranquilizer, tuberculosis, urinary incontinence (nocturia).

DOSING
Adults (18 Years and Older)

- Typical doses of cordyceps are 3-9 g fermented cordyceps (such as Cs-4 extract, CordyMax), given daily for up to 4-8 weeks. These doses have been used for anti-aging, chronic renal failure, hepatitis, and as a chemoprotective or performance enhancer. Lower doses of 999 mg taken in three 333-mg capsules have been studied for hyperlipidemia (high cholesterol).

Children (Younger than 18 Years)

- There is insufficient evidence to recommend a dose for cordyceps in children, and use is not recommended.

SAFETY
Allergies

- Avoid in people with a known allergy or hypersensitivity to cordyceps, mold, or fungi.

Side Effects and Warnings

- Minimal side effects have been reported with the use of cordyceps in humans. Cordyceps is likely safe when used in patients with asthma, bronchitis, hepatitis B, hepatic cirrhosis, hyperlipidemia (high cholesterol), immunosuppression, and chronic renal (kidney) failure. It is also likely safe when used as a chemoprotective agent or an exercise performance enhancer, although the effectiveness remains unclear.

- Cordyceps may cause dry mouth, nausea, loss of appetite, diarrhea, or dizziness. Due to the increasing popularity of *Cordyceps sinesis*, some supplements have been adulterated; some manufacturers substitute other species of cordyceps. The safety of these supplements is not clear.
- When taken by mouth, cordyceps (jin shiubao capsules) may cause tightness in the chest, wheezing, or palpitations. The symptoms may be alleviated after administration of an antihistamine. Skin rashes have also been observed.
- Although not well studied in humans, cordycep's polysaccharides may increase corticosteroid production. Cordyceps may also increase 17-beta-estradiol and progesterone production. It may also inhibit platelet aggregation and increase the risk of bleeding.
- Use cautiously in patients with prostate conditions or in people taking immunosuppressive medications, hormonal replacement therapy, or birth control. Avoid in patients with myelogenous-type cancers based on reports of cordyceps causing proliferation of progenitor red blood cells.

Pregnancy and Breastfeeding

- Cordyceps is not recommended in pregnant or breastfeeding women due to lack of available scientific evidence. Cordyceps may be possibly unsafe in pregnant women, as it may affect steroid hormone levels.

INTERACTIONS
Interactions with Drugs

- Concomitant administration of cordyceps and aminoglycosides may reduce amikacin-induced nephrotoxicity (kidney damage) in older adults.
- Cordyceps may reduce heart rate. Caution is advised in patients with heart disease or those taking antiarrhythmic agents.
- Although not well studied in humans, cordyceps may increase the risk of bleeding when taken with drugs that increase the risk of bleeding. Some examples include aspirin, anticoagulants (blood thinners) such as warfarin (Coumadin) or heparin, antiplatelet drugs such as clopidogrel (Plavix), and nonsteroidal anti-inflammatory drugs (NSAIDs) such as ibuprofen (Motrin, Advil) or naproxen (Naprosyn, Aleve).
- Cordyceps may induce sex steroid–like effects. Patients taking hormonal replacement therapy or birth control pills should use cordyceps with caution.
- Cordyceps may stimulate the immune system and may decrease the efficacy of immunosuppressants such as prednisolone or cyclophosphamide.
- Use of cordyceps with cyclosporin may reduce nephrotoxicity (kidney damage) in kidney-transplanted patients. Furthermore, administration of cordyceps and gentamycin may return blood urea nitrogen (BUN), serum creatinine (SCr), sodium excretion, and urinary nephroaminoglycosidase to more normal ranges during drug-induced nephrotoxicity (kidney toxicity). Concomitant administration of cordyceps with kidney-damaging drugs may reduce amikacin-induced kidney damage in older adults.
- Cordyceps may lower blood sugar levels. Caution is advised when using medications that may also lower blood sugar levels. Patients taking drugs for diabetes by mouth or insulin should be monitored closely by a qualified health care provider. Medication adjustments may be necessary.
- Cordyceps may lower blood pressure. Caution is advised when using medications that may also lower blood

pressure. Patients taking drugs for blood pressure, such as angiotensin-converting enzyme (ACE) inhibitors, should be monitored closely by a qualified health care professional, including a pharmacist.

- Preliminary evidence suggests that cordyceps may have additive effects when used with medications that lower cholesterol. Caution is advised.
- Cordyceps mycelium extracts may inhibit monoamine oxidase type B. Patients taking MAOIs (monoamine oxidase inhibitors, a class of antidepressants) such as isocarboxazid (Marplan), phenelzine (Nardil), or tranylcypromine (Parnate) should consult with a qualified health care professional, including a pharmacist, before combining therapies.

Interactions with Herbs and Dietary Supplements

- Cordyceps may reduce heart rate. Caution is advised in patients with heart disease or those taking antiarrhythmic agents.
- Although not well studied in humans, cordyceps may increase the risk of bleeding when taken with herbs and supplements that are believed to increase the risk of bleeding. Multiple cases of bleeding have been reported with the use of *Ginkgo biloba,* and fewer cases with garlic and saw palmetto. Numerous other agents may theoretically increase the risk of bleeding, although this has not been proven in most cases.

- Cordyceps may induce sex steroid–like effects. Patients taking herbs and supplements with potential hormonal effects, such as black cohosh or St. John's wort, should use cordyceps with caution.
- Cordyceps may lower blood sugar levels. Caution is advised when using herbs or supplements that may also lower blood sugar. Blood glucose levels may require monitoring, and doses may need adjustment.
- Cordyceps may lower blood pressure. Caution is advised when using herbs or supplements that may also lower blood pressure.
- Cordyceps may stimulate the immune system and may decrease the efficacy of immunosuppressants.
- Preliminary evidence suggests that cordyceps may have additive effects when used with herbs or supplements that lower cholesterol, such as red yeast rice. Caution is advised.
- Cordyceps mycelium extracts may inhibit monoamine oxidase type B. Caution is advised in patients taking herbs and supplements with potential MAOI (monoamine oxidase inhibitor, antidepressant) activity. Consult with a qualified health care professional, including a pharmacist, before combining therapies.

For a complete list of references, please visit www.naturalstandard.com.

Coriolus
(Coriolus versicolor)

RELATED TERMS

- A beta-1,4-glucan, basidiomycetes, basidiomycotinae, *Boletus versicolor*, BRM (biological response modifier), cloud mushroom, *Coriolus versicolor*, Kawaratake, Kayken Caps, Krestin, Polyporaceae, *Polyporus versicolor*, polysaccharide K, polysaccharide Kureha, *Polystictus versicolor*, protein-bound B-glucan, proteoglycans, PSK, PSP, *Saru-no-koshikake*, strain CM-101, turkey tail mushroom, *Trametes versicolor*, yun zhi.

BACKGROUND

- Protein-bound polysaccharide (PSK) is obtained from cultured mycelia of *Coriolus versicolor*, a mushroom thought to have antimicrobial, antiviral, and antitumor properties. Coriolus has been used in traditional Chinese medicine (TCM) since the Ming Dynasty of China.
- In the 1980s, the Japanese government approved the use of PSK for treating several types of cancers. By 1984 it ranked nineteenth on the list of the world's most commercially successful drugs, with annual sales of $255 million.
- PSK extracts are available for clinical use in Japan, where it is widely used for cancer immunochemotherapy. In Japan, PSK is currently used as a cancer treatment, in conjunction with surgery, chemotherapy, and/or radiation. Its active ingredient can be administered as a tea or in oral capsule form. In the United States, a similar product is labeled simply *Coriolus versicolor* extract. *Coriolus versicolor* is available in limited supply in U.S. markets. In Japan, PSK is currently the best-selling cancer medicine.

EVIDENCE

Uses Based on Scientific Evidence	Grade
Colorectal Cancer (Adjuvant) PSK in addition to chemotherapy and surgery has been associated with increased disease-free survival rate for patients with colorectal cancer in various clinical trials as opposed to these pharmaceutical drugs alone. Well-designed clinical trials are needed to confirm these results, along with optimal dosing regimens and optimal pharmaceutical combinations. PSK does not seem to affect the cure rate of colon cancer.	C
Esophageal Cancer (Adjuvant) A small number of clinical trials have examined the ability of PSK in conjunction with chemotherapy and radiation to increase survival time in esophageal cancer. However, the available evidence is insufficient to support effectiveness.	C
Gastric Cancer (Adjuvant) Several clinical trials or case studies have investigated the use of PSK in combination with chemotherapy in the treatment of gastric cancer. Results from many of the clinical trials show that PSK administered along with chemotherapy is associated with increased two- to five-year survival rates. However, some trials found no significant effect on survival over this same period of time. No significant increase in survival has been shown in long-term (greater than five years) studies.	C
Leukemia (Adjuvant) There is some preliminary evidence that adjunct PSK therapy may prolong duration of remission and survival time in patients with acute leukemia. In patients with acute nonlymphocytic leukemia, no significant increases in survival were found. It remains unclear if PSK therapy may in fact prolong remission and increase survival time in people with acute leukemia.	C
Liver Cancer (Adjuvant) Study results of PSK as an adjunct therapy for liver cancer yield mixed results. Well-designed clinical trials are needed to determine the role of PSK on survival time and remission in people with liver cancer.	C
Lung Cancer (Adjuvant) PSK has been studied as an adjuvant therapy in lung cancer patients, though supportive evidence is limited.	C
Nasopharyngeal Carcinoma (Adjuvant) In preliminary human studies, PSK, used as adjuvant treatment to radiotherapy, with or without chemotherapy, has been shown to increase the five-year survival rate following treatment.	C
Non-Small Cell Lung Cancer (NSCLC) (Adjuvant) There is limited clinical evidence supporting the use of PSK after radiation therapy in patients with stages I, II, and III NSCLC.	C
Breast Cancer (Adjuvant) The available evidence does not support the use of PSK, in conjunction with hormone therapy, chemotherapy, and/or surgery, to increase survival rates in breast cancer patients.	D

Uses Based on Tradition or Theory

AIDS, antibacterial, antifungal, antineoplastic, antioxidant, antiviral, atherosclerosis, cancer prevention, chemotherapy side effects, hepatic disorders, hepatitis, herpes, HIV, immunomodulator, infections, kidney disease prevention, liver protection, pancreatic cancer, postsurgical recovery, radiation therapy side effects, stamina, strength.

DOSING
Adults (18 Years and Older)

- For antitumor effects, 3 g of PSK has been daily (or every other day) by mouth, either alone or with conventional therapy. PSK has also been administered at a dose of 2 g/m^2 daily in three divided doses for 1 month.

- For gastric cancer (stomach, colorectal, colon), PSK has been taken by mouth in doses of $2\text{-}3 \text{ g/m}^2$ daily for up to 3 years as maintenance treatment.

Children (Younger than 18 Years)

- There is insufficient available evidence to recommend.

SAFETY
Allergies

- Avoid if known allergy/hypersensitivity to PSK, *Coriolus versicolor*, or any of its constituents.

Side Effects and Warnings

- PSK generally seems to have a low incidence of mild and tolerable side effects. In one report, three cases of toxicity were noted, and PSK was discontinued. PSK has been associated with side effects of gastrointestinal upset and darkening of the fingernails, but these effects have been limited and general safety has been demonstrated with daily oral doses for extended periods. Darkening of the fingernails and coughing have been reported during administration of the powdered drug.
- Low blood cell counts such as leukopenia, thrombocytopenia, and albuminuria (protein in the urine) were observed in two clinical trials. It should be noted that patients also received chemotherapy in addition to PSK in these trials, which may have contributed.
- Use cautiously in patients with coronary artery disease due to antiangiogenic properties (inhibition of new blood vessel growth) in the heart.

Pregnancy and Breastfeeding

- Not recommended due to lack of sufficient data.

INTERACTIONS
Interactions with Drugs

- Liver function impairment and toxicity has been reported.
- Antiangiogenic properties (inhibition of new blood vessel growth) have been proposed. In theory, there could be an additive effect when PSK is taken in conjugation with other known antiangiogenic agents such as Leflunomide.

- Thrombocytopenia (low blood platelet count) has been reported. Theoretically, this could increase the risk of bleeding. Leukopenia and albuminuria were also observed in two clinical trials. It should be noted that patients also received chemotherapy in addition to PSK in these trials. These effects may be attributed to either PSK or chemotherapy.
- Numerous animal and human studies have demonstrated that PSK improves survival time in patients with lung cancer, gastric cancer, stomach cancer, colon cancer, or leukemia when used in conjunction with chemotherapy.
- PSK in immunochemotherapy has been used in combination with hormone therapy to treat pancreatic cancer; therefore additive effects are possible.
- Numerous animal and human studies have demonstrated that PSK improves survival time in patients with lung cancer, gastric cancer, stomach cancer, colon cancer, or leukemia when used in conjunction with chemotherapy.

Interactions with Herbs and Dietary Supplements

- Liver function impairment and toxicity have been reported.
- Antiangiogenic properties (inhibition of new blood vessel growth) have been proposed. In theory, there could be an additive effect when PSK is taken in conjunction with other known antiangiogenic herbs and supplements such as shark cartilage, horse chestnut, feverfew, and bilberry.
- Thrombocytopenia (low blood platelet count) has been reported. Theoretically, this could increase the risk of bleeding. Leukopenia and albuminuria were also observed in two clinical trials. It should be noted that patients also received chemotherapy in addition to PSK in these trials. These effects may be attributed to either PSK or chemotherapy.
- PSK in immunochemotherapy has been used in combination with hormone therapy to treat pancreatic cancer; therefore additive effects are possible.
- Theoretically, PSK may have a synergistic effect with other immunotherapeutic herbs and supplements. Numerous animal and human studies have demonstrated that PSK improves survival time in patients with lung cancer, gastric cancer, stomach cancer, colon cancer, or leukemia when used in conjunction with chemotherapy.

For a complete list of references, please visit www.naturalstandard.com.

Corn Poppy
(Papaver rhoeas)

RELATED TERMS

- Alkaloids, anthocyanins, astragaline, coptisine, depsides, field poppy, Flanders poppy, flavonoids, glaudine, glycosides, hyperoside, hypolaetin, isocorydine, isoquercitrine, kaempferol, luteolin, Papaveraceae (family), *Papaver rhoeas*, p-hydroxybenzoic acid, protocatechuic acid, quercetin, red corn poppy, red poppy, rhoeadine, stylopine, wild poppy.

BACKGROUND

- Corn poppy *(Papaver rhoeas)* is well known for its showy red flowers and should not be confused with the opium poppy *(Papaver somniferum)*. In the Mediterranean, corn poppy greens are eaten as a vegetable.
- Corn poppy extracts may reduce morphine withdrawal symptoms. Corn poppy may also have iron-chelating activities and should be used cautiously in patients undergoing chelation therapy or those with thalassemia or anemia. However there is insufficient clinical evidence to support the use of corn poppy for any indication.

EVIDENCE

Uses Based on Scientific Evidence

No available studies qualify for inclusion in the evidence table.

Uses Based on Tradition or Theory

Antioxidant, chelating agent (heavy metals), food uses, gastric ulcers, morphine withdrawal, sedative.

DOSING
Adults (18 Years and Older)

- There is insufficient evidence to recommend a dose for corn poppy in adults.

Children (Younger than 18 Years)

- There is insufficient evidence to recommend a dose for corn poppy in children.

SAFETY
Allergies

- Avoid with a known allergy or hypersensitivity to corn poppy. Corn poppy flowers may cause hives in allergic individuals.

Side Effects and Warnings

- Corn poppy is likely safe when the leaves, petals, and seeds are used in food amounts.
- There is little information currently available about the adverse effects associated with corn poppy. However, there have been reports of contact urticaria (hives) due to the flowers.
- Use cautiously in patients undergoing chelation therapy or those with thalassemia (blood disorders) or anemia (red blood cell deficiency), as corn poppy may have iron-chelating activities.
- Use cautiously in patients taking sedatives, as corn poppy may cause drowsiness.

Pregnancy and Breastfeeding

- Corn poppy is not recommended in pregnant or breastfeeding women due to a lack of available scientific evidence.

INTERACTIONS
Interactions with Drugs

- Corn poppy may have antioxidant properties.
- Corn poppy root may have potent antiulcerogenic effects. Use cautiously with anti-ulcer medications due to possible additive effects.
- Corn poppy greens may possess iron-chelating activities. Use cautiously with heavy metal antagonists, chelating agents, and iron salts.
- Corn poppy extracts may decrease morphine withdrawal symptoms.
- Corn poppy may increase the amount of drowsiness caused by some drugs. Examples include benzodiazepines such as lorazepam (Ativan) or diazepam (Valium), barbiturates such as phenobarbital, narcotics such as codeine, some antidepressants, and alcohol. Caution is advised while driving or operating machinery.

Interactions with Herbs and Dietary Supplements

- Corn poppy may have antioxidant properties.
- Corn poppy root may have potent antiulcerogenic effects. Use cautiously with anti-ulcer herbs and supplements due to possible additive effects.
- Corn poppy greens may possess iron-chelating activities. Use cautiously with heavy metal antagonists, chelating agents, and iron supplements.
- Corn poppy extracts may decrease morphine withdrawal symptoms.
- Corn poppy may increase the amount of drowsiness caused by some herbs or supplements. Caution is advised while driving or operating machinery.

For a complete list of references, please visit www.naturalstandard.com.

Corydalis
(*Corydalis* spp.)

RELATED TERMS

- Alkaloids, berberine, carboxylic acids, Chinese medicinal herb, coptisine, *Corydalis ambigua*, *Corydalis incise*, *Corydalis pallida*, *Corydalis saxicola* Bunting, *Corydalis sempervirens*, *Corydalis stricta* Steph., *Corydalis tubers*, *Corydalis turtschaninovii*, *Corydalis yanhusuo*, corynoline, corynoloxine, cytotoxic activity, dehydroapocavidine, dehydrocavidine, feruloylmethoxytyramine, Fumariaceae (family), isoquinoline alkaloid, L-tetrahydropalmatine (rotundium), oxocorynoline, Papaveraceae (family), protopine, tetradehydroscoulerine, tetrahydropalmatine (THP), traditional Chinese medicine (TCM).

BACKGROUND

- Various types of corydalis have been included in traditional Chinese medicine (TCM) preparations and are most commonly used to treat gastritis-like disorders. Corydalis has been studied for other medical conditions, including pain caused by intense cold, parasitic infections, irregular heart rhythms, chest pain, and bacterial infections (especially from *Helicobacter pylori*). There is currently not enough human evidence to support these or any uses of corydalis.
- Corydalis may interact with certain medications, including sedatives, hypnotics, drugs taken for irregular heart rhythms, some pain relievers, and anticancer drugs and may be unsafe for use during pregnancy.

EVIDENCE

Uses Based on Scientific Evidence	Grade
Angina (Chest Pain) Corydalis may be of benefit in chest pain caused by clogged arteries called angina. However, the available evidence is insufficient to determine effectiveness.	C
Arrhythmia (Abnormal Heart Rhythm) Preliminary evidence suggests certain compounds found in corydalis may help abnormal heart rhythms.	C
***Helicobacter pylori* Infection in Stomach Ulcers** Preliminary evidence suggests that corydalis may be of benefit in bacterial infections with *Helicobacter pylori* in stomach ulcers. However, the effectiveness remains unclear.	C
Pain (Cold-Induced) Preliminary studies suggest that corydalis may have pain-relieving properties. However, the available evidence is insufficient to determine effectiveness.	C
Parasite Infection Corydalis may be helpful in the treatment of infections caused by the parasite *Echinococcus granulosus* caused by the Hydatid worm. However, the available evidence is insufficient to determine effectiveness.	C

Uses Based on Tradition or Theory

Antibacterial, cancer, gastritis, HIV, hypnotic, pain relief, sedation, ulcers.

DOSING

Adults (18 Years and Older)

- Doses of 3.25 g and 6.5 g of raw corydalis extracts have been taken by mouth to treat pain. Rotundium, a component of corydalis, has been used for abnormal heart rhythms.

Children (Younger than 18 Years)

- There is insufficient evidence for corydalis in children.

SAFETY

Allergies

- Avoid in people with known allergy or sensitivity to corydalis.

Side Effects and Warnings

- Corydalis is generally considered to be safe and has been used since ancient times as part of traditional Chinese medicine (TCM) preparations.
- Individuals taking sedatives or hypnotics, drugs that treat abnormal heart rhythms (including bepridil), pain relievers, and anticancer drugs should use corydalis with caution.

Pregnancy and Breastfeeding

- Corydalis is not recommended in pregnant or breastfeeding women due to a lack of available scientific evidence.

INTERACTIONS

Interactions with Drugs

- Corydalis may alter the effects of pain relievers; antibiotics; anticancer drugs; sedative or hypnotic drugs; and drugs taken to treat HIV, abnormal heart rhythms, or chest pain caused by clogged arteries.

Interactions with Herbs and Dietary Supplements

- Corydalis may alter the effects of pain relievers; antibiotics; antivirals; anticancer herbs and supplements; sedatives; and herbs and supplements taken to treat abnormal heart rhythms or chest pain caused by clogged arteries. Corydalis may also interact with herbs and supplements containing tyramine.

For a complete list of references, please visit www.naturalstandard.com.

Couch Grass

(Elytrigia repens, syn. Triticum repens, Agropyron repens, Elymus repens)

RELATED TERMS

- *Agropyron cristatum* L., *Agropyron desertorum, Agropyron elongatum, Agropyron intermedium, Agropyron mongolicum, Agropyron pectiniforme, Agropyron repens* L. *Beauv., Agropyron scabrifolium El Palmar INTA, Agropyron scabrifolium Seleccion Anguil, Agropyron smithii, Agropyron trachycaulum, Agropyron trichophorum,* ayrik, chiendent, common couch, creeping quackgrass, crested wheatgrass, cutch, devil's grass, dog grass, durfa grass, echte quecke, *Elymus repens, Elytrigia repens,* grama, grama de las boticas, grama del norte, gramigna, gramigua, groesrod graminis rhizome, joula, kweek, najm, nejil, pied de poule, quackgrass, quick grass, quitch grass, Scotch quelch, Scotch grass, squaw wein, squaw wijn, triticum, *Triticum repens* L., twitch, twitchgrass, vigne squaw, wheat grass, witch grass.

BACKGROUND

- Couch grass is stated to possess diuretic properties due to the presence of carbohydrates such as mannitol and inulin. It has been traditionally used for urinary tract infections and conditions relating to the kidneys, including kidney stones. The essential oil has been used for its antimicrobial effects, while the extracts of couch grass have been used as a dietary component in patients with diabetes. There is a lack of clinical evidence, however, to support these claims. Literature on couch grass is primarily in journals on botany and genomics.
- Couch grass is listed by the Council of Europe as a natural source of food flavoring. In the United States, it is listed as GRAS (generally recognized as safe).

EVIDENCE

Uses Based on Scientific Evidence

No available studies qualify for inclusion in the evidence table.

Uses Based on Tradition or Theory

Anti-inflammatory, benign prostatic hypertrophy (BPH, enlarged prostate), bladder inflammation, bronchitis, chronic skin disorders, colds, constipation, cough, cystitis, demulcent (locally soothing agent), diabetes, diuretic, emollient (softens skin), expectorant (induces coughing), fever, flavoring, gallbladder stones, gout (foot inflammation), increased sweating, irrigation therapy, kidney disorders, kidney stones, laxative, liver disorders, inflammation (oral), prostatitis (enlarged prostate), rheumatic pain, tonic, urethritis (painful urination), urinary disorders, urinary tract infection (UTI).

DOSING
Adults (18 Years and Older)

- There is insufficient evidence to recommend a dose for couch grass in adults. Traditionally, 4-8 g of dried rhizome has been taken three times daily. As a liquid (1:1 in 25% alcohol) extract, 4-8 mL has been given three times daily. As a tincture (1:5 in 40% alcohol), 5-15 mL has been given three times daily.

Children (Younger than 18 Years)

- There is insufficient evidence to recommend a dose for couch grass in children.

SAFETY
Allergies

- Avoid in people with known allergy or hypersensitivity to any constituent of couch grass, or to other members of the Poaceae/Gramineae family. Inulin may trigger an allergic reaction in some individuals, which may manifest as throat swelling, nasal itching, coughing, or difficulty breathing.

Side Effects and Warnings

- The safety and efficacy of couch grass has not been systematically studied for any indication in available reports. However, traditional use suggests that couch grass is generally well tolerated. Couch grass is accepted in the Indian and Colonial Addendum of the British Pharmacopoeia for use in the Australian, Eastern, and North American colonies, where it is much employed.
- Excessive and prolonged use of couch grass should be avoided due to its reputed diuretic action, as this may result in hypokalemia (abnormally low potassium levels in the blood).
- Caution is advised in patients who have edema (swelling) caused by heart or kidney disease. Based on tradition, couch grass should be taken with plenty of fluids to flush out the urinary tract.

Pregnancy and Breastfeeding

- Couch grass is not recommended in pregnant or breastfeeding women due to lack of available scientific evidence.

INTERACTIONS
Interactions with Drugs

- Due to its mild diuretic property, couch grass may increase the risk for high blood pressure and abnormally low potassium levels in the blood. Caution is advised in patients taking other blood pressure medications due to possible additive effects.
- Theoretically, couch grass may have an additive effect with other diuretic drugs.

Interactions with Herbs and Dietary Supplements

- Theoretically, couch grass may increase the risk for high blood pressure and abnormally low potassium levels in the blood due to its mild diuretic effects. Caution is advised in patients taking other blood pressure–altering herbs or supplements due to possible additive effects.
- Theoretically, couch grass may have an additive effect with other diuretic herbs and supplements.

For a complete list of references, please visit www. naturalstandard.com.

Cowhage
(*Mucuna pruriens*)

RELATED TERMS

- *Dolichos pruriens*, Fabaceae (family), kapikachu, kiwach, *Mucuna birdwoodiana*, *Mucuna pruriens*, *Mucuna sempervirens*, velvet bean.

BACKGROUND

- Cowhage *(Mucuna pruriens)* seeds have been used in traditional Ayurvedic medicine to treat Parkinson's disease. This traditional use is supported by laboratory analysis that shows cowhage contains 3.6%-4.2% levodopa, the same chemical used in several Parkinson's disease drugs that is a precursor to dopamine. In a few clinical trials in Parkinson's disease patients, cowhage treatments yielded positive results. Cowhage seeds have nutritional quality comparable to soybeans and other conventional legumes, but several antinutritional/antiphysiological compounds prevent these seeds from being used as a food source.

EVIDENCE

Uses Based on Scientific Evidence	Grade
Parkinson's Disease Cowhage contains 3.6%-4.2% levodopa, the same chemical used in several Parkinson's disease drugs. Cowhage treatments have yielded positive results in preliminary studies. Further research may yield optimal dosing.	C

Uses Based on Tradition or Theory
Anticoagulant (blood thinner), diabetes, fracture healing, hyperprolactinemia (excessive prolactin in the blood).

DOSING
Adults (18 Years and Older)

- There is insufficient evidence to recommend a dose for cowhage in adults. For Parkinson's disease, 15-30 g of a cowhage preparation has been taken daily by mouth for 1 week. Sachets containing a derivative of cowhage, called *HP-200*, have also been used.

Children (Younger than 18 Years)

- There is insufficient evidence to recommend a dose for cowhage in children.

SAFETY
Allergies

- Avoid in people with a known allergy or hypersensitivity to cowhage *(Mucuna pruriens)* or its constituents. Hairs on cowhage flowers and pods can cause severe pruritus (itching).

Side Effects and Warnings

- Few adverse effects have been reported for cowhage. In one study in Parkinson's disease patients, a derivative of *Mucuna pruriens* caused mild adverse effects that were mainly gastrointestinal in nature. Cowhage has also caused acute toxic psychosis, which may be due to its levodopa content. Use cautiously in patients with Parkinson's disease and/or those taking levodopa, dopamine, dopamine agonists, dopamine antagonists, or dopamine reuptake inhibitors, as cowhage seeds contain the dopamine precursor levodopa.
- Hairs on cowhage flowers and pods can cause severe pruritus (itching), and have also been used to artificially induce pruritus.
- Use cautiously in patients taking monoamine oxidase inhibitors (MAOIs), as the levodopa in cowhage seeds may interact and cause high blood pressure.
- Use cautiously in patients taking anticoagulants (blood thinners) or those with diabetes or hypoglycemia, due to the potential for additive effects.
- Avoid in patients with psychosis or schizophrenia, as cowhage has caused acute toxic psychosis.
- Avoid in pregnant or breastfeeding women, as cowhage may inhibit prolactin secretion.

Pregnancy and Breastfeeding

- Cowhage is not recommended in pregnant or breastfeeding women due to a lack of available scientific evidence. Two early studies indicate that cowhage may inhibit prolactin secretion.

INTERACTIONS
Interactions with Drugs

- The leaves of *Mucuna pruriens* may dose-dependently prolong blood clotting. Caution is advised in patients taking drugs that also increase the risk of bleeding. Some examples include aspirin, anticoagulants (blood thinners) such as warfarin (Coumadin) or heparin, antiplatelet drugs such as clopidogrel (Plavix), and nonsteroidal anti-inflammatory drugs (NSAIDs) such as ibuprofen (Motrin, Advil) or naproxen (Naprosyn, Aleve).
- Use cautiously in patients taking diabetes medications, as cowhage may alter blood sugar levels. Caution is advised when using medications that may also lower blood sugar levels. Patients taking drugs for diabetes by mouth or insulin should be monitored closely by a qualified health care professional, including a pharmacist. Medication adjustments may be necessary.
- Cowhage seeds contain levodopa, which may cause high blood pressure when taken with monoamine oxidase inhibitors (MAOIs). Caution is advised in patients with hypertension (high blood pressure) or those taking medication that alters blood pressure due to possible additive effects.
- In a case report, cowhage caused an outbreak of acute toxic psychosis. Caution is advised in patients with mental illnesses.
- Based on a clinical study in Parkinson's disease patients, cowhage may increase serum levodopa concentrations.

Caution is advised in Parkinson's disease patients taking levodopa, dopamine, dopamine agonists, dopamine antagonists, anticholinergics, and antiparkinsonian agents due to possible additive effects.

Interactions with Herbs and Dietary Supplements

- The leaves of *Mucuna pruriens* may dose-dependently prolong blood clotting. Use cautiously in patients with bleeding disorders or those taking other blood-thinning herbs or supplements due to a possible increase in the risk of bleeding. Multiple cases of bleeding have been reported with the use of *Ginkgo biloba,* and fewer cases with garlic and saw palmetto. Numerous other agents may theoretically increase the risk of bleeding, although this has not been proven in most cases.
- In a case report, cowhage caused an outbreak of acute toxic psychosis. Use cautiously in patients with mental illnesses.
- Ayahuasca *(Banisteriopsiscaapi)* is a known monoamine oxidase inhibitor (MAOI); cowhage seeds contain levodopa, which may cause high blood pressure when taken with MAOIs. Use cautiously in patients with hypertension (high blood pressure) or those taking herbs or supplements, such as ayahuasca, that alter blood pressure.
- Ergot *(Claviceps purpura)* has known dopamine agonist activity; cowhage seeds contain levodopa, which is a precursor to dopamine. Use cautiously in patients with mental illnesses, such as depression, as the combination of cowhage and ergot may result in additive effects.
- Jimson weed *(Datura stramonium)* is a known anticholinergic; cowhage seeds contain levodopa, which may interact with anticholinergics. Use cautiously in patients with Parkinson's disease, as the combination of cowhage and Jimson weed may result in additive effects.
- Fava beans *(Vicia faba)* contain levodopa, as do cowhage seeds. Use cautiously with fava beans due to possible additive effects.
- Cowhage may alter blood sugar levels. Caution is advised in patients with diabetes or hypoglycemia, and those taking herbs or supplements that affect blood sugar. Blood glucose levels may require monitoring, and doses may need adjustment.

For a complete list of references, please visit www.naturalstandard.com.

Cramp Bark
(Viburnum opulus)

RELATED TERMS

- American guelder-rose, Caprifoliaceae (family), common guelder-rose, cranberry tree, European cranberry bush, guelder rose, pembina, proanthocyanidins, snowball tree, *Viburnum opulus, Viburnum opulus* L., *Viburnum prunifolium* L., viopudial.

BACKGROUND

- Cramp bark *(Viburnum opulus)* is native to Europe, northern Africa, and northern Asia. It has been used throughout the world as an ornamental plant. The bark has traditionally been used for cramps, including menstrual cramps and cramping associated with arthritis. Viopudial isolated from *Viburnum opulus* displays antispasmodic effects on smooth muscle. However, there is currently insufficient available evidence in humans to support the use of cramp bark for any indication.

EVIDENCE

Uses Based on Scientific Evidence

No available studies qualify for inclusion in the evidence table.

Uses Based on Tradition or Theory

Allergies, anti-inflammatory, antioxidant, antispasmodic, arthritis, asthma, astringent, cancer, colic, cramps, low blood pressure, menstrual pain, skin disinfectant/sterilization, stomach ulcers, vasodilator.

DOSING
Adults (18 Years and Older)

- There is insufficient evidence to recommend a dose for cramp bark in adults.

Children (Younger than 18 Years)

- There is insufficient evidence to recommend a dose for cramp bark in children.

SAFETY
Allergies

- Avoid in people with a known allergy or hypersensitivity to cramp bark or its constituents.

Side Effects and Warnings

- There is no safety information currently available for cramp bark. Use cautiously in patients taking immunomodulators.

Use cautiously in patients taking blood pressure–altering agents.

Pregnancy and Breastfeeding

- Cramp bark is not recommended in pregnant or breastfeeding women due to a lack of available scientific evidence.

INTERACTIONS
Interactions with Drugs

- Cramp bark may have disinfectant activity. Caution is advised in patients taking antibiotics.
- Cramp bark may have antioxidant activity. Caution is advised in patients taking antioxidant drugs.
- Cramp bark may prevent gastroduodenal mucosal damage. Caution is advised in patients with ulcers or those taking antiulcer medications.
- Cramp bark may have antispasmodic effects on smooth muscle. Caution is advised in patients taking antispasmodic agents.
- Cramp bark extract may have astringent activity. Caution is advised in patients taking astringent agents.
- Cramp bark may lower blood pressure. Caution is advised in patients with hypertension or hypotension and in those taking blood pressure–altering drugs.
- Cramp bark berries may enhance phagocytosis. Caution is advised in patients taking other immunosuppressant agents.

Interactions with Herbs and Dietary Supplements

- Cramp bark may have disinfectant activity. Caution should be used in patients using other antibacterial herbs or supplements.
- Cramp bark may have antioxidant activity. Caution is advised if taking other herbs or supplements with antioxidant activity.
- Cramp bark may have antispasmodic effects on smooth muscle. Caution is advised in patients taking other herbs or supplements with antispasmodic effects.
- Cramp bark extract may have astringent activity. Caution is advised if taking other herbs or supplements with astringent effects.
- Cramp bark may prevent gastroduodenal mucosal damage. Caution is advised in patients taking other herbs or supplements with antiulcer effects.
- Cramp bark may lower blood pressure. Caution is advised in patients with hypertension or hypotension and those taking herbs or supplements with blood pressure–altering effects.
- Cramp bark berries may enhance phagocytosis. Caution is advised in patients taking other immunosuppressant herbs or supplements.

For a complete list of references, please visit www.naturalstandard.com.

Cranberry
(*Vaccinium macrocarpon*)

RELATED TERMS

- American cranberry, Arandano Americano, Arandano trepador, bear berry, black cranberry, bog cranberry, Ericaceae (family), European cranberry, grosse moosebeere, isokarpalo, Kranbeere, Kronsbeere, large cranberry, low cranberry, marsh apple, moosebeere, mossberry, mountain cranberry, *Oxycoccus hagerupii, Oxycoccus macrocarpus, Oxycoccus microcarpus, Oxycoccus palustris, Oxycoccus quadripetalus,* pikkukarpalo, preisselbeere, ronce d'Amerique, trailing swamp cranberry, Tsuru-kokemomo, *Vaccinium edule, Vaccinium erythrocarpum, Vaccinium hageruppi, Vaccinium microcarpum, Vaccinium occycoccus, Vaccinium plaustre, Vaccinium vitis.*

BACKGROUND

- There is some clinical evidence supporting the use of cranberry juice and cranberry supplements to *prevent* urinary tract infection (UTI), although most available studies are of limited strength. There are no clear dosing guidelines, but given the safety of cranberry, it may be reasonable to recommend the use of moderate amounts of cranberry juice cocktail to prevent UTI in otherwise healthy individuals.
- Cranberry has not been shown effective as a *treatment* for documented UTI. Although cranberry may be used as an adjunct therapy in some cases, given the proven efficacy of antibiotics, cranberry should not be considered a first-line treatment.
- Cranberry has been investigated for numerous other medicinal uses, and promising areas of investigation include prevention of *Helicobacter pylori* infection, which causes gastrointestinal ulcers and dental plaque.

EVIDENCE

Uses Based on Scientific Evidence	Grade
Helicobacter pylori Infection Based on early research, cranberry may reduce the ability of *Helicobacter pylori* bacteria to live in the stomach and cause ulcers. Further research is needed to confirm these results.	B
Urinary Tract Infection (Prevention) There are multiple studies of cranberry (juice or capsules) for the prevention of urinary tract infections in healthy women and nursing home residents. While no single study convincingly demonstrates the ability of cranberry to prevent UTIs, the cumulative favorable evidence combined with laboratory research tends to support this use. It is not clear what dose is best. Cranberry seems to work by preventing bacteria from sticking to cells that line the bladder. Contrary to prior belief, urine acidification does not appear to play a role. Notably, many studies have been sponsored by the cranberry product manufacturer Ocean Spray. Additional research is needed in this area before a strong recommendation can be made.	B

	Grade
Achlorhydria and B_{12} Absorption Preliminary research suggests that cranberry juice may increase vitamin B_{12} absorption in patients taking drugs that reduce stomach acid (antacids), such as proton pump inhibitors like lansoprazole (Prevacid). However, this effect may be due to the acidity of the juice rather than an active component of cranberry itself. Further studies are needed before a recommendation can be made.	C
Antibacterial Studies using cranberry as an antibacterial have produced conflicting results.	C
Antioxidant Based on laboratory study, cranberry may have antioxidant properties. However, clinical evidence is lacking.	C
Antiviral and Antifungal Limited laboratory research has examined the antiviral and antifungal activity of cranberry. There is a lack of clinical evidence to support this use.	C
Cancer Prevention Based on a small amount of laboratory research, cranberry has been proposed for cancer prevention. However, cranberry should be used cautiously to treat cancer, as some evidence suggests that cranberry pills have a strong positive association with bladder cancer.	C
Dental Plaque Because of its activity against some bacteria, cranberry juice has been proposed as helpful for mouth care. However, many commercial cranberry juice products are high in sugar and may not be suitable for this purpose. There is not enough research in this area to make a clear recommendation.	C
Kidney Stones Based on preliminary research, it is not clear if drinking cranberry juice increases or decreases the risk of kidney stone formation. Cranberry juice is reported to decrease urine levels of calcium, increase urine levels of magnesium and potassium, and increase urine levels of oxalate.	C
Memory Improvement Preliminary study results show that cranberry juice may increase overall ability to remember.	C
Radiation Therapy Side Effects (Prostate Cancer) There is preliminary evidence that cranberry is not effective in preventing urinary symptoms related to pelvic radiation therapy in patients with prostate cancer.	C

Uses Based on Scientific Evidence	Grade
Reduction of Odor from Incontinence/Bladder Catheterization There is preliminary evidence that cranberry juice may reduce urine odor from incontinence or bladder catheterization.	C
Urinary Tract Infection (Treatment) There is a lack of well-designed human studies of cranberry for the treatment of urinary tract infections. Laboratory research suggests that cranberry may not be an effective treatment when used alone, although it may be helpful as an adjunct to other therapies such as antibiotics.	C
Urine Acidification In large quantities, cranberry juice may lower urine pH, making it more acidic. Contrary to prior opinion, urine acidification does not appear to be the way that cranberry prevents urinary tract infections. More research is needed in this area.	C
Urostomy Care It is proposed that skin irritation at urostomy sites may be related to urine pH. Cranberry juice can lower urine pH and has been tested for this purpose.	C
Chronic Urinary Tract Infection Prevention: Children with Neurogenic Bladder The available evidence indicates that cranberry is not effective in preventing urinary tract infections in children with neurogenic bladder.	D

Uses Based on Tradition or Theory
Alzheimer's disease, anorexia, anticoagulant (blood thinner), anti-inflammatory, antiparasitic, atherosclerosis (hardening of the arteries), blood disorders, cancer treatment, cardiovascular disorders, cholecystitis (inflamed gall bladder), cystitis, decontamination (of meats), diuresis (increasing urine flow), gall bladder stones, high cholesterol, influenza, ischemic stroke, liver disorders, neurodegenerative diseases, periodontitis/gingivitis (gum diseases), rheumatoid arthritis, scurvy, stomach ailments, vomiting, wound care.

DOSING
Adults (18 Years and Older)

- For urinary tract infection *prevention*, the recommended doses range from 90 to 480 mL (3-16 oz) of cranberry juice cocktail twice daily, or 15-30 mL of unsweetened 100% cranberry juice daily. In well-designed research, 300 mL/day (10 oz) of commercially available cranberry juice cocktail (Ocean Spray) has been used.
- Other forms of cranberry used include capsules, concentrate, and tinctures. One to six 300- to 400-mg capsules of hard gelatin concentrated cranberry juice extract, twice daily by mouth, given with water 1 hour before or 2 hours after meals has been used. 1½ oz frozen juice concentrate twice daily by mouth has been used, as well as 4-5 mL of

cranberry tincture three times daily by mouth. One study suggests that 500 mL of cranberry juice with 1,500 mL of water was sufficient in helping prevent the formation of oxalate kidney stones.

Children (Younger than 18 Years)
- There is insufficient evidence to recommend cranberry supplementation in children (beyond amounts found in a normal balanced diet).

SAFETY
Allergies
- Cranberry should be avoided by people with an allergy/hypersensitivity to *Vaccinium* species (cranberries and blueberries).

Side Effects and Warnings
- Patients with diabetes or glucose intolerance may want to drink sugar-free cranberry juice to avoid a high sugar intake. High doses of cranberry may cause stomach distress and diarrhea, or may increase the risk of kidney stones in people with a history of oxalate stones. Some commercially available products are high in calories. On average, six ounces of cranberry juice contains approximately 100 calories. One study showed the possibility for occurrence of vaginal yeast infections in those women who often consume cranberry juice, although this has not been proven. Use cautiously if taking anticoagulants (blood thinners) such as warfarin, medications that affect the liver, or aspirin. Cranberry should be used cautiously in cancer patients, as some evidence suggests that cranberry pills have a strong positive association with bladder cancer.

Pregnancy and Breastfeeding
- Safety has not been determined in pregnancy and breastfeeding, although cranberry juice is believed to be safe in amounts commonly found in foods. Many tinctures contain high levels of alcohol and should be avoided during pregnancy.

INTERACTIONS
Interactions with Drugs
- In theory, due to its acidic pH, cranberry juice may counteract antacids. Cranberry juice theoretically may increase the effects of antibiotics in the urinary tract and increase the excretion of some drugs in the urine. Cranberry juice may increase absorption of vitamin B_{12} in patients using proton pump inhibitors such as esomeprazole (Nexium).
- Some cranberry tinctures may have high alcohol content and may lead to vomiting if used with the drug disulfiram (Antabuse) or metronidazole (Flagyl).
- Although controversial, some studies have shown that taking the prescription blood thinner warfarin (Coumadin) and cranberry products at the same time can elevate the international normalized ratio (INR), which could increase the risk of bleeding.
- Alzheimer's drugs, anthelmintics (expel worms), antifungals, cholesterol-lowering drugs, antineoplastics (anticancer agents), antiprotozoals, antiviral agents, clarithromycin, drugs broken down by the liver, diuretics, salicylates such as aspirin, and drugs eliminated by the kidneys may interact with cranberry.

Interactions with Herbs and Dietary Supplements

- In theory, cranberry juice may increase the excretion of some herbs or supplements in the urine.
- Theoretically, cranberry products may increase the risk of bleeding in people taking other herbs or supplements such as garlic or danshen.
- Inhibition of *Helicobacter pylori* bacteria, which may lead to gastrointestinal ulcers, may be increased when oregano and cranberry are taken together.
- Alzheimer's herbs and supplements, antacids, anthelminthics (expel worms), antibacterials, antifungals, cholesterol-lowering herbs and supplements, antineoplastics, antioxidants, antiparasitics, antivirals, herbs and supplements broken down by the liver, diuretics, lingonberry, salicylate-containing herbs such as willow bark, urine-acidifying herbs and supplements, and vitamin B_{12} may interact with cranberry.

For a complete list of references, please visit www.naturalstandard.com.

Creatine

RELATED TERMS

- Athletic series creatine, beta-GPA, Challenge Creatine Monohydrate, Cr, Creapure Creatine Monohydrate Powder, Creatine Booster, creatine citrate, creatine ethyl ester, Creatine Monohydrate Powder, creatine phosphate, Creatine Powder Drink Mix, Creatine Xtreme Punch, Creatine Xtreme Lemonade, creatinine, Creavescent, cyclocreatine, Hardcore Formula Creatine Powder, HPCE Pure Creatine Monohydrate, methyl guanidine-acetic acid, methylguanidine-acetic acid, N-amidinosarcosine, N-(aminoiminomethyl)-N methyl glycine, Neoton, Performance Enhancer Creatine Fuel, Phosphagen, Phosphagen Pure Creatine Monohydrate Power Creatine, Runners Advantage creatine serum, Total Creatine Transport.

BACKGROUND

- Creatine is naturally synthesized in the human body from amino acids primarily in the kidney and liver and transported in the blood for use by muscles. Approximately 95% of the body's total creatine content is located in skeletal muscle.
- Creatine was discovered in the 1800s as an organic constituent of meat. In the 1970s, Soviet scientists reported that oral creatine supplements may improve athletic performance during brief, intense activities such as sprints. Creatine gained popularity in the 1990s as a "natural" way to enhance athletic performance and build lean body mass. It was reported that skeletal muscle total creatine content increases with oral creatine supplementation, although response is variable. Factors that may account for this variation are carbohydrate intake, physical activity, training status, and muscle fiber type. The finding that carbohydrates enhance muscle creatine uptake increased the market for creatine multi-ingredient sports drinks.
- Use of creatine is particularly popular among adolescent athletes, who reportedly take doses that are not consistent with scientific evidence and to frequently exceed recommended loading and maintenance doses.
- Published reports suggest that approximately 25% of professional baseball players and up to 50% of professional football players consume creatine supplements. According to a survey of high school athletes, creatine use is common among football players, wrestlers, hockey players, gymnasts, and lacrosse players. In 1998, the creatine market in the United States was estimated at $200 million. In 2000, the National Collegiate Athletic Association (NCAA) banned colleges from distributing creatine to their players.
- Creatinine excreted in urine is derived from creatine stored in muscle.

EVIDENCE

Uses Based on Scientific Evidence	Grade
Enhanced Muscle Mass/Strength Several high-quality studies have shown an increase in muscle mass with the use of creatine. However, some weaker studies have reported mixed results. Overall, the available evidence suggests that creatine does increase lean body mass, strength, and total work. Future studies should consider the effects of individual fitness levels on treatment response.	A
Congestive Heart Failure (Chronic) Patients with chronic heart failure have low levels of creatine in their hearts. Several studies report that creatine supplements may improve heart muscle strength, body weight, and endurance in patients with heart failure. Studies comparing creatine with drugs used to treat heart failure are needed before a firm recommendation can be made. Heart failure should be treated by a qualified health care professional.	B
Adjunct to Surgery (Coronary Heart Disease) Preliminary studies suggest a potential benefit of creatine supplements in patients undergoing coronary artery surgery. Some evidence suggests that heart muscle may recover better and more rapidly after open heart surgery if intravenous creatinine is used during the operation. Larger, well-designed studies are warranted.	C
Apnea of Prematurity Preliminary studies have produced mixed results in infants with a breathing disorder called apnea of prematurity.	C
Bone Density Preliminary studies examining the effect of creatine in aging suggest that creatine may increase bone density when combined with resistance training. However, the efficacy remains unclear.	C
Chronic Obstructive Pulmonary Disease It is unclear if creatine can help treat chronic obstructive pulmonary disease. Study results are mixed.	C
Depression Preliminary research suggests a potential benefit of creatine supplements in depression. Creatine may have brought on a manic switch in patients with bipolar depression. However, effectiveness remains unclear.	C
Dialysis Preliminary studies suggest that creatine does not lower homocysteine levels in chronic hemodialysis patients. However, these patients were also using vitamin B_{12} and folate. Muscle cramps are also common complications of hemodialysis. Creatine may offer some benefit for this side effect.	C

(Continued)

Uses Based on Scientific Evidence	Grade
Enhanced Athletic Performance and Endurance It has been suggested that creatine may help improve athletic performance or endurance by increasing time to fatigue (possibly by shortening muscle recovery periods). It has been studied in cyclists, women, high-intensity endurance athletes, rowers, runners, sprinters (general), swimmers, and older adults. However, the results of research evaluating this claim are mixed.	C
GAMT Deficiency Some individuals are born with a genetic disorder in which there is a deficiency of the enzyme guanidinoacetate methyltransferase (GAMT). A lack of this enzyme causes severe developmental delays and abnormal movement disorders. The condition is diagnosed by a lack of creatine in the brain. However, there is limited evidence for the effect of creatine supplementation in this disorder. High-quality studies are needed.	C
High Cholesterol Preliminary studies did not find a benefit of creatine in the treatment of high cholesterol.	C
Huntington's Disease There is not enough scientific information to make a firm recommendation about the use of creatine in Huntington's disease. High-quality studies are needed to clarify this relationship.	C
Hyperornithinemia (High Levels of Ornithine in the Blood) Ornithine is normally formed in the liver. Some people are born with a genetic disorder that prevents them from appropriately breaking down ornithine, which causes blood levels to become too high. High amounts of ornithine may lead to blindness, muscle weakness, and reduced storage of creatine in muscles and the brain. Although there is limited research in this area, early evidence suggests that long-term daily creatine supplements may help replace missing creatine and slow vision loss.	C
Ischemic Heart Disease Preliminary studies suggest a potential benefit of creatine in people with ischemic heart disease.	C
McArdle's Disease In McArdle's disease, there is a deficiency of energy compounds stored in the muscles. This leads to muscle fatigue, exercise intolerance, and pain when exercising. Creatine has been proposed as a possible therapy for this condition. However, research is limited, and the results of existing studies are mixed. Therefore, it remains unclear if creatine offers any benefits to patients with McArdle's disease.	C
Memory Early studies show that creatine may improve cognition in certain populations, such as vegetarians and	C

older adults. Further research is required before a recommendation can be made.

	Grade
Multiple Sclerosis Preliminary studies suggest that creatine supplementation does not improve work production in people with multiple sclerosis.	C
Muscular Dystrophy Creatine loss is suspected to cause muscle weakness and breakdown in patients with Duchenne muscular dystrophy. Studies with creatine have found mixed results for this condition.	C
Myocardial Infarction (Heart Attack) There is some evidence that intravenous creatine after a heart attack may be beneficial to heart muscle function and may prevent irregular heart rhythms. It has been reported that the use of creatine phosphate may have a favorable effect on mental deterioration in "cardio-cerebral syndrome" following heart attacks in older adults.	C
Neuromuscular Disorders (General, Mitochondrial Disorders) Numerous studies suggest that creatine may help treat various neuromuscular diseases and may delay the onset of symptoms when used with standard treatment. However, creatine ingestion does not appear to have a significant effect on muscle creatine stores or high-intensity exercise capacity in people with multiple sclerosis, and supplementation does not seem to help people with tetraplegia. Although initial studies were encouraging, recent research reports no beneficial effects on survival or disease progression.	C
Spinal Cord Injury It is unclear if creatine is helpful in patients with spinal cord injuries. Results from early studies have been mixed.	C
Amyotrophic Lateral Sclerosis (ALS) Overall, the evidence suggests that creatine supplementation does not offer benefit to individuals with amyotrophic lateral sclerosis (ALS).	D
Surgical Recovery Early studies suggest that creatine has no effect on strength or body composition in people undergoing soft tissue surgery. Creatine supplements are likely ineffective in this condition and cannot be recommended without positive evidence.	D

Uses Based on Tradition or Theory

Arginine:glycine amidinotransferase (AGAT) deficiency, Alzheimer's disease, antiarrhythmic, anticonvulsant, anti-inflammatory, antioxidant, attention deficit hyperactivity disorder, bipolar disorder, brain

Uses Based on Tradition or Theory—Cont'd

damage, breast cancer, cervical cancer, circadian clock acceleration, colon cancer, diabetes, diabetic complications, disuse muscle atrophy, fibromyalgia, growth, herpes, hyperhomocysteinemia (an abnormally large level of homocysteine in the blood), mitochondrial diseases, mood disorder, neuroprotection, nutritional supplement, ophthalmological disorders (gyrate atrophy), osteoarthritis, Parkinson's disease, rheumatoid arthritis, seizures (caused by lack of oxygen to the brain), sexual dysfunction, wasting of brain regions.

DOSING

Adults (18 Years and Older)

- A wide range of dosing by mouth has been used or studied. A general dose of 400 mg/kg of body weight or up to 25 g/day has been studied for multiple conditions. Experts often recommend maintaining good hydration during creatine use.
- To increase anaerobic work capacity, studies have used a dose of 5 g four times daily for 5 days. For enhanced athletic strength and performance, studies have used a dose of 20 g/day for 4-7 days. Daily maintenance doses of 2-5 g or 0.3 mg/kg of body weight have been used.
- Numerous dosing regimens for intravenous or intramuscular administration have been used in studies in humans. Intravenous dosing should only be done under strict medical supervision.

Children (Younger than 18 Years)

- Dosing in children should be under medical supervision because of potential side effects. A daily dose of 5 g has been used in children with muscular dystrophy, and a range of doses (400 mg to 2 g/kg of body weight) have been used in children with guanidinoacetate methyltransferase (GAMT) deficiency. A dose of 100 mg/kg of body weight has been used for one week to treat motor sensory neuropathy in children.

SAFETY

Allergies

- Creatine has been associated with asthmatic symptoms. People should avoid creatine if they have known allergies to this supplement. Signs of allergy may include rash, itching, or shortness of breath.

Side Effects and Warnings

- There is limited systematic study of the safety, pharmacology, or toxicology of creatine. People using creatine, including athletes, should be monitored by a health care professional. Users are advised to inform their physicians or other qualified health care professionals.
- Some people may experience gastrointestinal symptoms, including loss of appetite, stomach discomfort, diarrhea, or nausea.
- Creatine may cause muscle cramps or muscle breakdown, leading to muscle tears or discomfort. Strains and sprains have been reported due to enthusiastic increases in workout regimens once starting creatine. Weight gain and increased body mass may occur. Heat intolerance, fever, dehydration, reduced blood volume, or electrolyte imbalances (and resulting seizures) may occur.

- There is less concern today than there used to be about possible kidney damage from creatine, although there are reports of kidney damage, such as interstitial nephritis. Patients with kidney disease should avoid use of this supplement. Similarly, liver function may be altered, and caution is advised in those with underlying liver disease.
- In theory, creatine may alter the activities of insulin. Caution is advised in patients with diabetes or hypoglycemia and those taking drugs, herbs, or supplements that affect blood sugar. Serum glucose levels may need to be monitored by a health care professional, and medication adjustments may be necessary.
- Long-term administration of large quantities of creatine is reported to increase the production of formaldehyde, which may potentially cause serious unwanted side effects.
- Creatine may increase the risk of compartment syndrome of the lower leg, a condition characterized by pain in the lower leg associated with inflammation and ischemia (diminished blood flow), which is a potential surgical emergency.
- Reports of other side effects include thirst, mild headache, anxiety, irritability, aggression, nervousness, sleepiness, depression, abnormal heart rhythm, fainting or dizziness, blood clots in the legs (called deep-vein thrombosis), seizure, or swollen limbs.

Pregnancy and Breastfeeding

- Creatine cannot be recommended during pregnancy or breastfeeding due to a lack of scientific information.
- Pasteurized cow's milk appears to contain higher levels of creatine than human milk. The clinical significance of this is not clear.

INTERACTIONS

Interactions with Drugs

- In theory, creatine may alter the activities of insulin, particularly when taken with carbohydrates. Caution is advised when using medications that may also alter blood sugar levels. Patients taking drugs for diabetes by mouth or insulin should be monitored closely by a qualified health care professional. Medication adjustments may be necessary.
- In theory, creatine may interact when taken in combination with acetaminophen/caffeine/central nervous system (CNS) depressants, aspirin/caffeine/CNS depressants, or caffeine/ergotamine. It may interact with stimulants such as caffeine.
- Use of creatine with probenecid may increase the levels of creatine in the body, leading to increased side effects.
- Use of creatine with diuretics such as hydrochlorothiazide or furosemide (Lasix) should be avoided because of the risks of dehydration and electrolyte disturbances. The likelihood of kidney damage may be greater when creatine is used with drugs that may damage the kidneys, such as trimethoprim, cimetidine (Tagamet), anti-inflammatory drugs such as ibuprofen (Advil, Motrin), cyclosporine (Neoral, Sandimmune), amikacin, gentamicin, or tobramycin.
- It is possible that creatine may increase the cholesterol-lowering effects of other drugs commonly used to lower cholesterol levels, such as lovastatin (Mevacor).
- The combination of creatine and nonsteroidal anti-inflammatory drugs is more effective at reducing inflammation than either agent used alone.
- Creatine and nifedipine, when used together, may enhance heart function, although research in this area is early.

- In theory, creatine may also interact with aminoglycoside antibiotics, gallium nitrate, lansoprazole, sodium bicarbonate, tacrolimus, and valacyclovir.
- Creatine supplements may enhance the activities and side effects of some cancer drugs.

Interactions with Herbs and Dietary Supplements

- Creatine may increase the risk of adverse effects, including stroke, when used with caffeine and ephedra. In addition, caffeine may reduce the beneficial effects of creatine during intense intermittent exercise.
- In theory, creatine may alter the activities of insulin. Caution is advised when using herbs or supplements that may also alter blood sugar. Blood glucose levels may require monitoring, and doses may need adjustment.
- Creatine may reduce the effectiveness of vitamins A, D, E, and K.

- Creatine may affect liver function and should be used cautiously with potentially hepatotoxic (liver-damaging) or nephrotoxic (kidney damaging) herbs and supplements.
- Use of creatine with diuretics should be avoided because of the risks of dehydration and electrolyte disturbances.
- It is possible that creatine may increase the cholesterol-lowering effects of herbs and supplements that lower cholesterol levels, such as red yeast (*Monascus purpureus*).
- In theory, creatine may interact with stimulants such as caffeine, which is found in green tea, black tea, and ephedra.
- Creatine may interact with alpha-lipoic acid, arginine, hydroxymethylbutyrate, magnesium, pyruvate, and herbs and supplements broken down by the liver or kidneys. Creatine may also interact with anti-inflammatory and antineoplastic supplements.

For a complete list of references, please visit www.naturalstandard.com.

Daisy
(*Bellis perennis*)

RELATED TERMS

- Apigenin glycosides, *Arnica montana*, Asteraceae (family), asterogenic acid glycosides, bairnwort, bayogenin, Bellidis flos, *Bellis sylvestris*, bellissaponin, Bellorita, besysaponin, bisdesmosidic glycosides, bruisewort, *Chrysanthemum leucanthemum* L., common daisy, Compositae (family), consolida, daisy, day's eye, dog daisy, English daisy, European daisy, flavonoids, flavonol glycosides, Gänseblümchen (German), glycosides, hen and chickens, Herb Margaret, La Paquerette (French), lawn daisy, little daisy, Madeliefje (Netherlands), Marguerite, Maslieben (German), Maya, meadow daisy, monodesmosidic glycosides, oxeye daisy, polyacetylenes, polygalacic acid, red daisy, saponins, Sedmikráska chudobka (Czech), triterpenoid glycosides, triterpenoid saponins, virgaureasaponin, wild daisy.

- **Note:** Daisy is also the common name for oxeye daisy, *Chrysanthemum leucanthemum* L., another weedy species found in fields and along roadsides throughout the United States. This species is native to Europe and Asia, and has also been naturalized as a weed in North America.

BACKGROUND

- *Bellis perennis* is a common European species of daisy. Although many other related plants are also called daisy, *Bellis perennis* is often considered the archetypal species. It is sometimes called common daisy or English daisy. It is native to western, central, and northern Europe, but is commonly found as an invasive plant in North America.

- The medicinal properties of *Bellis perennis* have been recorded in herbals as far back as the sixteenth century. John Gerard, the sixteenth century herbalist, recommended English daisy as a catarrh (inflammation of mucous membrane) cure, as a remedy for heavy menstruation, migraine, and to promote healing of bruises and swellings.

- Infusions of the flowers and leaves have been used to treat a wide range of other disorders, including rhinitis, rheumatoid arthritis, and liver and kidney disorders. An insect repellent spray has also been made from an infusion of the leaves. A strong decoction of the roots has been recommended for the long-term treatment of both scurvy and eczema, and a mild decoction may ease complaints of the respiratory tract.

- *Bellis perennis* has also been used traditionally for treating wounds. Chewing the fresh leaves is said to be a cure for mouth ulcers. In homeopathy, *Bellis perennis* is often used in combination with *Arnica montana* to treat bruising and trauma.

- Currently, common daisy is widely used in homeopathy, but is only rarely used in herbal medicine. Although homeopathic dosing has "generally recognized as safe" (GRAS) status by the U.S. Food and Drug Administration (FDA), there is a lack of available scientific evidence to support claims for effectiveness related to the use of *Bellis perennis*. More research is needed in this area. Recent research has explored the possibility of using the plant in HIV therapy.

EVIDENCE

Uses Based on Scientific Evidence	Grade
Bleeding (Postpartum, Mild) Homeopathic *Bellis perennis* has been used for bruising, bleeding, and recovery from surgery. There is insufficient evidence to recommend daisy for these indications.	C

Uses Based on Tradition or Theory

Analgesic (pain reliever), antifungal, anti-inflammatory, antimicrobial, antispasmodic, antitussive (suppresses coughs), arthritis, astringent, blood purifier, breast cancer, bronchitis, bruises, burns, bursitis (inflammation of bursa), childbirth (cesarean sections, episiotomy), cancer, catarrh (inflammation of mucous membrane), circadian clock acceleration, concussions, demulcent (soothes inflammation), digestion enhancement, diuretic, dysmenorrheal (painful menstruation), eczema, edema (post-operative and post-traumatic), emollient (soothes skin), expectorant (expels phlegm), fractures, HIV support, inflammation (tenosynovitis, styloiditis), insect repellent, jet lag, joint disorders (blood in joint), joint inflammation (epicondyle), joint problems (dislocations), kidney disorders, laxative, liver disorders, menorrhagia (heavy menstrual bleeding), migraines, mouth ulcers, ophthalmological (eye) uses, osteoarthritis, periarthritis humeroscapularis, periodontitis/gingivitis, pneumonia, post-surgical recovery (plastic surgery), purgative, rheumatism, scurvy, skin diseases, soft-tissue injury (acute), sports injuries, sprains, tissue healing after surgery (abdominal), tonic, trauma (pelvic organ), wounds.

DOSING

Adults (18 Years and Older)

- There is insufficient evidence to recommend a dose for *Bellis perennis*. A traditional dose is one cup of tea (made from 2 tsp of dried *Bellis perennis* herb steeped in 300 mL of boiling water for 20 minutes and then strained) taken two to four times daily.

- Typical homeopathic doses used are 1 or 2 tablets (6-c or 30-c potency) dissolved on the tongue. For general acute conditions, one dose every 2 hours, repeated for a maximum of six doses. For less acute conditions (e.g., seasonal or chronic), one dose three times daily between meals for no more than 1 month.

Children (Younger than 18 Years)

- There is insufficient evidence to recommend a dose for *Bellis perennis*. A general dose consists of 1 or 2 homeopathic 6-c or 30-c potency tablets dissolved on the tongue. For general acute conditions, one dose has been administered every 2 hours for up to six doses. For seasonal or chronic conditions, one dose three times a day between meals for no more than 1 month.

SAFETY
Allergies

- Avoid in individuals sensitive or allergic to *Bellis perennis* products or any of their ingredients. Respiratory allergies have occurred in sensitive individuals.

Side Effects and Warnings

- In general, *Bellis perennis* appears to be well tolerated when used at homeopathic doses.
- As an herb, however, *Bellis perennis* may affect the clotting cascade, resulting in blood clotting. Common daisy may also result in stunted growth, although there is a lack of scientific evidence supporting this.
- Patients at risk for coagulation disorders such as strokes or blood clots, or patients with anemia should use cautiously.

Pregnancy and Breastfeeding

- *Bellis perennis* is not recommended in pregnant or breastfeeding women due to a lack of available scientific evidence. Avoid use at traditional herbal doses during pregnancy and breastfeeding because of the possibility of growth retardation in the fetus and infant.

INTERACTIONS
Interactions with Drugs

- *Bellis perennis* may affect coagulation, and it is unclear how it may interact with medications that may increase the risk of bleeding. Examples include aspirin, anticoagulants (blood thinners) such as warfarin (Coumadin) or heparin, anti-platelet drugs such as clopidogrel (Plavix), and nonsteroidal anti-inflammatory drugs (NSAIDs) such as ibuprofen (Motrin, Advil) or naproxen (Naprosyn, Aleve). Caution is advised.

Interactions with Herbs and Dietary Supplements

- *Bellis perennis* may affect coagulation, and it is unclear how it may interact with herbs and supplements that may increase the risk of bleeding. Caution is advised when taking with herbs and supplements that may increase the risk of bleeding, such as garlic or *Ginkgo biloba*.

For a complete list of references, please visit www.naturalstandard.com.

Damiana
(Turnera diffusa, Turnera aphrodisiaca)

RELATED TERMS

- Bignoniaceae (family), bourrique, caryophyllene, caryophyllene oxide, *Damiana aphrodisiaca*, damiana de Guerrero, damiana herb, damiana leaf, delta-cadinene, elemene, flavone glycoside, herba de la pastora, flavonoids, Mexican damiana, Mexican holly, mizibcoc, old woman's broom, oreganillo, p-arbutin, ram goat dash along, rosemary, Turneraceae (family), *Turnera aphrodisiaca, Turnera diffusa, Turnera diffusa* Willd. ex Schult., *Turnera diffusa* Willd. var. *afrodisiaca* (Ward) Urb., *Turnerae diffusae* folium, *Turnerae diffusae* herba, *Turnera microphylla, Turnera ulmifolia*.

BACKGROUND

- Damiana includes the species *Turnera diffusa* and *Turnera aphrodisiaca*. These closely-related plants belong to the family of Turneraceae and grow wild in the subtropical regions of the Americas and Africa. Damiana is widely used in traditional medicine as an anti-cough, diuretic (increasing urine flow), and aphrodisiac agent. Recent studies in rats seem to support the folk reputation of *Turnera diffusa* as a sexual stimulant.
- In the Mexican culture, damiana is used for gastrointestinal disorders. Damiana extract has shown antibacterial activity against gram-positive and gram-negative bacteria, which may have gastrointestinal effects.
- Damiana appears on the U.S. Food and Drug Administration's (FDA) GRAS (generally recognized as safe) list and is widely used as a food flavoring. However, because damiana contains low levels of cyanide-like compounds, excessive doses may be dangerous.

EVIDENCE

Uses Based on Scientific Evidence	Grade
Female Sexual Dysfunction Traditionally, damiana has been used as a sexual stimulant. ArginMax for women contains damiana, but also L-arginine, ginseng, ginkgo, multivitamins, and minerals. There is a lack of clinical evidence to support this use.	C
Weight Loss (Obese Patients) YGD is an herbal preparation frequently used for weight loss that contains yerbe mate (leaves of *Ilex paraguayenis*), guarana (seeds of *Paullinia cupana*), and damiana (leaves of *Turnera diffusa* var. *aphrodisiaca*). The isolated affects of damiana are not clear.	C

Uses Based on Tradition or Theory

Antibacterial, anti-inflammatory, antioxidant, aphrodisiac, asthma, bedwetting, constipation, cough, depression, diabetes mellitus, diuretic, energy, gastrointestinal disorders, gastrointestinal motility, hallucinogenic, headache, impotence, laxative, respiratory problems, sexual dysfunction (female), sexual performance, muscle relaxant (smooth muscle), stimulant, ulcers, weight reduction.

DOSING

Adults (18 Years and Over)

- Traditional doses of damiana include 2-4 g of dried leaf (as tablets, capsules, or tea) has been taken three times daily by mouth. Also, 2-4 mL of liquid damiana extract or 0.5-1 mL of tincture has been taken three times daily. Dried extract (325 to 650 mg per dose) may also be used.

Children (Younger than 18 Years)

- There is insufficient evidence to recommend a dose of damiana in children.

SAFETY

Allergies

- Avoid in individuals with a known allergy or hypersensitivity to *Turnera diffusa* or *Turnera aphrodisiaca*, their constituents, or related plants in the Turneraceae family.

Side Effects and Warnings

- In general, few adverse effects have been reported for damiana, including diarrhea, headaches, mood changes, erotic dreams, insomnia, and hallucinations. Damiana appears on the U.S. Food and Drug Administration's (FDA's) GRAS (generally recognized as safe) list and is widely used as a food flavoring agent. However, because damiana contains low levels of cyanide-like compounds, excessive doses may be dangerous. Patients with psychiatric disorders, those taking medications for diabetes or to control blood sugar levels, or those with a history of breast cancer should use caution. Avoid use of damiana in patients with Alzheimer's disease, or Parkinson's disease, as ethanol (alcohol) extracts of the leaves and stem have shown central nervous system depressant activity.

Pregnancy and Breastfeeding

- Use of damiana is not recommended during pregnancy and breastfeeding due to a lack of reliable scientific study in this area. Traditionally, damiana has been used as an abortifacient (induces abortion) and is contraindicated during pregnancy.

INTERACTIONS
Interactions with Drugs
- Damiana may affect blood sugar levels. Caution is advised when using medications that may also lower blood sugar levels. Patients taking drugs for diabetes by mouth or insulin should be monitored closely by a qualified health care provider. Medication adjustments may be necessary.
- Damiana may interact with progestin drugs. Caution is advised.

Interactions with Herbs and Dietary Supplements
- Damiana may alter blood sugar levels. Caution is advised when using herbs or supplements that may also lower blood sugar levels. Blood glucose levels may require monitoring, and doses may need adjustment.
- Damiana may interact with herbs and supplements that alter progestin. Caution is advised.

For a complete list of references, please visit www.naturalstandard.com.

Dandelion
(Taraxacum officinale)

RELATED TERMS

- Artemetin, Asteraceae (family), beta-carotene, blowball, caffeic acid, cankerwort, Cichoroideae (sub-family), clock flower, common dandelion, Compositae (family), dandelion herb, dandelion T-1 extract, dent de lion, diente de lion, dudhal, dumble-dor, epoxide, esculetin, fairy clock, fortune teller, hokouei-kon, huang hua di ding, Irish daisy, Lactuceae (tribe), *Leontodon taraxacum*, lion's teeth, lion's tooth, lowenzahn (German), lowenzahnwurzel (German), maelkebotte, milk gowan, min-deul-rre, mok's head, mongoloid dandelion, pee in the bed, pissenlit, piss-in-bed, potassium, pries' crown, priest's crown, puffball, pu gong ying, pu kung ying, *Radix taraxaci*, swine snout, taraxaci herba, taraxacum, *Taraxacum mongolicum*, *Taraxacum palustre*, *Taraxacum vulgare*, taraxasteryl acetate, telltime, vitamin A, white endive, wild endive, witch gowan, witches' milk, yellow flower earth nail.

BACKGROUND

- Dandelion is a member of the Asteraceae/Compositae family closely related to chicory. It is a perennial herb native to the Northern hemisphere and found growing wild in meadows, pastures, and waste grounds of temperate zones. Most commercial dandelion is cultivated in Bulgaria, Hungary, Poland, Romania, and the United Kingdom.
- Dandelion was commonly used in Native American medicine. The Iroquois, Ojibwe, and Rappahannock prepared the root and herb to treat kidney disease, upset stomach, and heartburn. In traditional Arabian medicine, dandelion has been used to treat liver and spleen ailments. In traditional Chinese medicine (TCM), dandelion is combined with other herbs to treat liver disease; to enhance immune response to upper respiratory tract infections, bronchitis, or pneumonia; and as a compress for mastitis (breast inflammation).
- Dandelion root and leaf are used widely in Europe for gastrointestinal ailments. The European Scientific Cooperative on Phytotherapy (ESCOP) recommends dandelion root for the restoration of liver function, to treat upset stomach, and to treat loss of appetite. The German Commission E authorizes the use of combination products containing dandelion root and herb for similar illnesses. Some modern naturopathic physicians assert that dandelion can detoxify the liver and gallbladder, reduce side effects of medications metabolized (processed) by the liver, and relieve symptoms associated with liver disease.
- Dandelion is generally regarded as safe with rare side effects including contact dermatitis, diarrhea, and gastrointestinal upset.
- Dandelion is used as a salad ingredient, and the roasted root and its extracts are sometimes used as a coffee substitute.

EVIDENCE

Uses Based on Scientific Evidence	Grade
Anti-inflammatory Research in laboratory animals suggests that dandelion root may possess anti-inflammatory properties. There is a lack of clinical evidence supporting this use.	C
Antioxidant Several laboratory studies report antioxidant properties of dandelion flower extract, although this research is preliminary, and effects in humans are unclear.	C
Cancer Limited animal research does not provide a clear assessment of the effects of dandelion on tumor growth. There is a lack of clinical evidence supporting this use.	C
Colitis There is a report with several patients that suggests that a combination herbal preparation containing dandelion improved chronic pain associated with colitis. The Isolated effects of dandelion are not clear.	C
Diabetes There is limited research on the effects of dandelion on blood sugar levels in animals. Effects in humans are unclear.	C
Diuretic (Increased Urine Flow) Dandelion leaves have traditionally been used to increase urine production and excretion. Animal studies report mixed results, and there is a lack of clinical evidence supporting this use.	C
Hepatitis B One human study reports improved liver function in people with hepatitis B after taking a combination herbal preparation containing dandelion root, called Jiedu Yanggan Gao (also including *Artemisia capillaris*, *Taraxacum mongolicum*, *Plantago* seed, *Cephalanoplos segetum*, *Hedyotis diffusa*, *Flos chrysanthemi* indici, *Smilax glabra*, *Astragalus membranaceus*, *Salviae miltiorrhizae*, *Fructus polygonii* orientalis, *Radix paeoniae* alba, and *Polygonatum sibiricum*). The isolated the effects of dandelion are not clear.	C

Uses Based on Tradition or Theory

Abscess, acne, age spots, AIDS, alcohol withdrawal, allergies, analgesia, anemia, anorexia, antibacterial, antifungal, antioxidant, antiviral, aphthous ulcers, arthritis, benign prostate hypertrophy (enlarged prostate), bile flow stimulation, bladder irritation, blood purifier, boils, breast augmentation, breast cancer, breast infection, breast inflammation, breast milk stimulation, bronchitis, bruises, cardiovascular disorders, chronic fatigue syndrome, circulation, clogged arteries, coffee substitute, congestive heart failure, dandruff, diarrhea, dropsy (swelling), dyspepsia (upset stomach), eye problems, fertility, fever reduction, food uses, frequent urination, gallbladder disease, gallstones, gas, gastrointestinal inflammation (appendicitis), gout (painful inflammation), headache, heartburn, high blood pressure, high cholesterol, human immunodeficiency virus, hormonal abnormalities, immune stimulation, increased sweating, jaundice, kidney disease, kidney stones, laxative, leukemia, liver cleansing, liver disease, menopause, menstrual period stimulation, muscle aches, nutrition, obesity, osteoarthritis, pneumonia, pregnancy (including postpartum support), premenstrual syndrome (PMS), psoriasis, rheumatoid arthritis, skin conditions, skin toner, smoking cessation, spleen problems, stiff joints, stimulant, stomachache, urinary stimulant, urinary tract inflammation, warts, weight loss.

DOSING

Adults (18 Years and Older)

- There is insufficient evidence to recommend a dose for dandelion in adults. However, doses of 2-8 g of dried root taken by mouth in an infusion or decoction have been used.
- Doses of 4-8 mL of a 1:1 leaf fluid extract in 25% alcohol have been used.
- Doses of 1-2 tsp of a 1:5 root tincture in 45% alcohol have been used.

Children (Younger than 18 Years)

- There is insufficient evidence to recommend dandelion for use in children in amounts greater than those found in food.

SAFETY

Allergies

- Dandelion should be avoided by people with known allergy to honey, chamomile, chrysanthemums, yarrow, feverfew, or any members of the Asteraceae/Compositae plant families (ragweed, sunflower, daisies).
- The most common type of allergy is dermatitis (skin inflammation) after direct skin contact with dandelion, which may include itching, rash, or red/swollen or eczematous areas on the skin. Skin reactions have also been reported in dogs.
- Rhinoconjunctivitis and asthma have been reported after handling products, such as birdfeed, containing dandelion and other herbs with reported positive skin tests for dandelion hypersensitivity.

Side Effects and Warnings

- Dandelion has been well tolerated in a small number of available human studies. Safety of use beyond 4 months has not been evaluated.
- The most common reported adverse effects are skin allergy, eczema, and increased sun sensitivity following direct contact.

- According to traditional accounts, gastrointestinal symptoms may occur, including stomach discomfort, diarrhea, and heartburn.
- Parasitic infection due to ingestion of contaminated dandelion has been reported, affecting the liver and bile ducts, and characterized by fever, stomach upset, vomiting, loss of appetite, coughing, and liver damage.
- Dandelion may lower blood sugar levels based on one animal study, although another study noted no changes. Effects in humans are not known. Caution is advised in patients with diabetes or low blood sugar, and those taking drugs, herbs, or supplements that affect blood sugar. Serum glucose levels may need to be monitored by a health care professional, and medication adjustments may be necessary.
- In theory, due to chemicals called *coumarins* found in dandelion leaf extracts, dandelion may increase the risk of bleeding when taken with drugs that increase the risk of bleeding. Some examples include aspirin, anticoagulants (blood thinners) such as warfarin (Coumadin) or heparin, antiplatelet drugs such as clopidogrel (Plavix), and nonsteroidal anti-inflammatory drugs such as ibuprofen (Motrin, Advil) or naproxen (Naprosyn, Aleve).
- Historically, dandelion is believed to possess diuretic (increased urination) properties and to lower blood potassium levels. Use cautiously in patients with kidney failure.
- Dandelion may be prepared as a tincture containing high levels of alcohol. Tinctures should therefore be avoided during pregnancy or when driving or operating heavy machinery.

Pregnancy and Breastfeeding

- Dandelion cannot be recommended during pregnancy and breastfeeding in amounts greater than found in foods, due to a lack of scientific information. Many tinctures contain high levels of alcohol and should be avoided during pregnancy.

INTERACTIONS

Interactions with Drugs

- Drug interactions with dandelion have rarely been identified, although there is limited study in this area.
- Dandelion may reduce the effects of the antibiotic ciprofloxacin (Cipro) due to reduced absorption of the drug. In theory, dandelion may reduce the absorption of other drugs taken at the same time.
- Dandelion may lower blood sugar levels, although another study notes no changes. Although effects in humans are not known, caution is advised in patients taking prescription drugs that may also lower blood sugar levels. Those using oral drugs for diabetes or insulin should be monitored closely by a health care professional while using dandelion. Dosing adjustments may be necessary.
- Historically, dandelion is believed to possess diuretic (increased urination) properties and to lower blood potassium levels. In theory, the effects or side effects of other drugs may be increased, including other diuretics, lithium, digoxin (Lanoxin), or corticosteroids such as prednisone. However, dandelion also contains potassium, and human supportive evidence is lacking.
- The effects or side effects of niacin or nicotinic acid may be increased (such as flushing and gastrointestinal upset), due to small amounts of nicotinic acid present in dandelion.

- In theory, due to chemicals called *coumarins* found in dandelion leaf extracts, dandelion may increase the risk of bleeding when used with blood thinners. Examples include warfarin (Coumadin), heparin, and clopidogrel (Plavix). Some pain relievers may also increase the risk of bleeding if used with dandelion. Examples include aspirin, ibuprofen (Motrin, Advil), and naproxen (Naprosyn, Aleve, Anaprox). It is possible that dandelion may reduce the effectiveness of antacids or drugs commonly used to treat peptic ulcer disease. Examples include famotidine (Pepcid) and esomeprazole (Nexium).
- Dandelion may interfere with the way the liver breaks down certain drugs (using the P450 1A2 and 2E enzyme systems). As a result, levels of these drugs may be raised in the blood, and the intended effects or side effects may be increased. Patients using medications should check the package insert and speak with a health care professional, including a pharmacist, about possible interactions.
- Be aware that many tinctures contain high levels of alcohol and may cause nausea or vomiting when taken with metronidazole (Flagyl) or disulfiram (Antabuse).
- Although not well studied in humans, caution is advised in patients taking analgesics (pain relievers), anesthetics, anti-inflammatories, or certain types of antacids or peptic ulcer agents (Pepcid or Nexium). Dandelion may increase the effects and toxicity of blood pressure–lowering agents or niacin if taken together.
- Dandelion may also interact with cholesterol-lowering agents, such as bile acid sequestrants. Consult with a qualified health care professional, including a pharmacist, to check for interactions.
- Other potential interactions with dandelion that are lacking human scientific evidence include anticancer agents, appetite suppressants, hormonal agents (such as estrogens), laxatives, and agents used to treat gout.

Interactions with Herbs and Dietary Supplements

- Interactions of dietary supplements with dandelion have rarely been published, although there is limited study in this area.
- Based on an animal study, dandelion may lower blood sugar levels, although another study notes no changes. Although effects in humans are not known, caution is advised when using herbs or supplements that may also lower blood sugar. Blood glucose levels may require monitoring, and doses may need adjustment.
- Historically, dandelion is believed to possess diuretic (increased urination) properties and may increase the effects of other herbs with potential diuretic effects, such as artichoke, elder flower, or horsetail.
- In theory, due to chemicals called *coumarins* found in dandelion leaf extracts, dandelion may increase the risk of bleeding when taken with herbs and supplements that are believed to increase the risk of bleeding. Multiple cases of bleeding have been reported with the use of *Ginkgo biloba*, and fewer cases with garlic and saw palmetto. Numerous other agents may theoretically increase the risk of bleeding, although this has not been proven in most cases.
- Dandelion may interfere with the way the liver breaks down certain drugs (using the P450 1A2 and 2E enzyme systems). As a result, levels of other herbs or supplements may become too high in the blood. In theory, dandelion may also alter the effects that other herbs or supplements possibly have on the P450 system, such as bloodroot, grapefruit juice, or St. John's wort.
- Dandelion leaves contain vitamin A, niacin, lutein, and beta-carotene and thus, supplemental doses of these agents may have additive effects or side effects.
- Dandelion may reduce the effectiveness of the antibiotic ciprofloxacin (Cipro) and thus may have interactions with other antibacterial herbs or supplements.
- Although not well studied in humans, dandelion may interact with anti-inflammatory agents, antacids, analgesics, hormone replacement therapy (HRT), laxatives, nondigestible oligosaccharides (such as inulin), urine alkalinizing herbs or supplements, anticancer herbs or supplements, or other antioxidants. Dandelion may also decrease dehydroepiandrosterone, dehydroepiandrosterone-sulfate, androstenedione, and estrone-sulfate levels.
- Dandelion may increase the toxic effects when taken with supplements that lower blood pressure such as hawthorn (*Crataegus laevigata*). Toxic effects associated with herbs such as foxglove may increase when used in combination with dandelion.

For a complete list of references, please visit www.naturalstandard.com.

Danshen
(Salvia miltiorrhiza)

RELATED TERMS

- 3,4-dihydroxyphenyl-lactic acid, caffeic acid, Ch'ih Shen (scarlet sage), Chinese *Salvia*, cryptotanshisone, dangshem, Dan-Shen, Dan Shen, danshen root, danshensu, dihydrotanshinone, ethyl acetate, fufangdenshen, horse-racing grass, Huang Ken, Hung Ken (red roots), Labiatae (family), Lamiaceae (family), lithospermic acid B, miltirone, neo-tanshinlactone, phenolic acids, Pin-Ma Ts'ao (horse-racing grass), protocatechualdehyde, protocatechuic acid, protocatechuic aldehyde, *Radixsalvia miltiorrhiza*, rat-tail grass, red-rooted sage, red roots, red sage, red sage root, red saye root, roots of purple sage, *Salvia bowelyana, Salvia miltiozzhiza, Salvia miltiozzhiza bunge, Salvia przewalskii, Salvia przewalskii mandarinorum*, salvia root, *Salvia yunnanensis*, salvianolic acid B, scarlet sage, Sh'ih Shen, Shu-Wei Ts'ao (rat-tail grass), Tan Seng, Tan-Shen, tanshisone I, tanshisone IIA, tanshisone IIB, Tzu Tan-Ken (roots of purple sage), yunzhi danshen.
- **Note:** Danshen should not be confused with sage. Danshen is often used in combination with other products; combination products are not specifically discussed in this monograph.

BACKGROUND

- Danshen *(Salvia miltiorrhiza)* is widely used in traditional Chinese medicine (TCM), often in combination with other herbs. Remedies containing danshen are used traditionally to treat a diversity of ailments, particularly cardiac (heart) and vascular (blood vessel) disorders such as atherosclerosis (hardening of the arteries with cholesterol plaques) or blood clotting abnormalities.
- The ability of danshen to "thin" the blood and reduce blood clotting is well documented, although the herb's purported ability to "invigorate" the blood or improve circulation has not been demonstrated in high-quality human trials. Because danshen can inhibit platelet aggregation and has been reported to potentiate (increase) the blood-thinning effects of warfarin, it should be avoided in patients with bleeding disorders; prior to some surgical procedures; or when taking anticoagulant (blood-thinning) drugs, herbs, or supplements.
- In the mid-1980s, scientific interest was raised in danshen's possible cardiovascular benefits, particularly in patients with ischemic stroke or coronary artery disease/angina. More recent studies have focused on possible roles in liver disease (hepatitis and cirrhosis) and as an antioxidant. However, the available research in these areas largely consists of animal studies and small human trials of poor quality. Therefore, firm evidence-based conclusions are not possible at this time about the effects of danshen for any medical condition.

EVIDENCE

Uses Based on Scientific Evidence	Grade
Asthmatic Bronchitis Better studies are needed in which danshen is compared with more proven treatments before a clear conclusion can be drawn.	C
Burn Healing Although animal studies suggest that danshen may help speed healing of burns and wounds, there are limited human data supporting this claim.	C
Cardiovascular Disease/Angina A small number of poor-quality studies report that danshen may provide benefits for treating disorders of the heart and blood vessels, including heart attacks, cardiac chest pain (angina), or myocarditis. Danshen may have effects on blood clotting and therefore may be unsafe when combined with other drugs used in patients with cardiovascular disease. Patients should check with a physician and pharmacist before combining danshen with prescription drugs.	C
Chronic Prostatitis Early studies have found that danshen in combination with routine western medicine was not as effective as warming needle moxibustion. More studies are warranted in this area to draw a firm conclusion.	C
Diabetic Complications (Diabetic Foot) Early clinical trials suggest danshen may help treat diabetic foot. Well-designed clinical trials are needed before a strong recommendation can be made.	C
Dialysis (Peritoneal) Early studies suggest that danshen may speed peritoneal dialysis and ultrafiltration rates when added to dialysate solution. Although this evidence seems promising, it is not known whether danshen is safe for this use. Further research is necessary.	C
Glaucoma Danshen may be beneficial in glaucoma therapy, but further studies are needed in humans before a clear conclusion can be drawn. Danshen should not be used in place of more proven therapies, and patients with glaucoma should be evaluated by a qualified eye care specialist.	C
High Cholesterol Early studies suggest that danshen may improve blood levels of cholesterol (lowers low-density lipoprotein or "bad" cholesterol and triglycerides and raises high-density lipoprotein or "good" cholesterol). Large high-quality studies are needed before a strong recommendation may be made.	C
Kidney Disease Although early evidence is promising, it is not known whether danshen is safe for this use. Danshen injection may be helpful for recovery of kidney function after kidney transplant. Further research is needed to confirm these results.	C

Uses Based on Scientific Evidence	Grade
Liver Disease (Cirrhosis, Chronic Hepatitis B, Fibrosis) Some studies suggest that danshen may provide benefits for treating liver diseases such as cirrhosis, fibrosis, and chronic hepatitis B. However, it is unclear whether there are any clinically significant effects of danshen in patients with liver disease.	C
Pancreatitis (Acute) For many years, danshen has been used as a traditional Chinese medicine (TCM) remedy to treat acute pancreatitis. However, little research is currently available regarding the use of danshen in humans.	C
Stroke (Ischemic) Due to poor quality of evidence, unclear safety, and the existence of more proven treatments for ischemic stroke, this use of danshen cannot be recommended.	C
Syncope (Vasovagal) There is not enough evidence to recommend the use of danshen for vasovagal syncope.	C
Tinnitus (Ringing in the Ears) Limited evidence suggests that danshen in combination with other herbs and supplements may be a less effective treatment for tinnitus than acupuncture.	C
Weight Loss One study using a combination product that included danshen found that there was no effect on food intake or weight loss.	C

Uses Based on Tradition or Theory

Abdominal pain, acne, acute myocardial infarction (heart attack), alcohol dependence, Alzheimer's disease, anoxic brain injury, antibacterial, anti-inflammatory, antimicrobial, antioxidant, antiphospholipid syndrome, antiseptic, antithrombosis, antitumor, antiviral, anxiety, bleomycin–induced lung fibrosis, blood clotting disorders, breast cancer, bruising, cancer, cataracts, chemotherapy drug resistance, chronic obstructive pulmonary disease, circulation, clogged arteries, connective tissue disorders (external humeral epicondylitis), diabetes, diabetic nerve pain, ectopic pregnancy, eczema, gastric ulcers, gentamicin toxicity, hearing loss, heart palpitations, high blood pressure, human immuno virus, hypercoagulability, immunomodulator, insomnia, intrauterine growth retardation, kidney failure, kidney protection, left ventricular hypertrophy, leukemia, liver cancer, liver protection, lung fibrosis, menstrual problems, myocardial ischemia/reperfusion injury, nasopharyngeal carcinoma, neurasthenia, neuroprotection, organ transplantation, pre-eclampsia/pregnancy-induced hypertension (high blood pressure), psoriasis, pulmonary embolism, pulmonary hypertension, radiation-induced lung damage, restlessness, sedative, skin conditions, sleep difficulties, stimulation of GABA (gamma-aminobutyric acid) release, stomach ulcers, tennis elbow, vitiligo, wound healing.

DOSING
Adults (18 Years and Older)

- There is insufficient evidence to recommend a dose of danshen in adults.
- In research from the 1970s, an 8-mL injection of danshen (16 g of the herb) was given intravenously (diluted in 500 mL of a 10% glucose solution) for up to 4 weeks for ischemic stroke. Safety and effectiveness have not been established for this route of administration, and it cannot be recommended at this time.

Children (Younger than 18 Years)

- There is insufficient evidence to recommend a dose of danshen in children, and it should be avoided because of potential adverse effects.

SAFETY
Allergies

- People with known allergy to danshen (*Salvia miltiorrhiza*), its constituents (such as protocatechualdehyde, 3,4-dihydroxyphenyl-lactic acid, tanshinone I, dihydrotanshinone, cryptotanshione, miltirone, or salvianolic acid B), or other plants of the genus *Salvia* should avoid this herb. Danshen is often found in combination with other herbs in various formulations, and patients should read product labels carefully. Signs of allergy may include rash, itching, or shortness of breath.

Side Effects and Warnings

- Danshen may increase the risk of bleeding. This herb is reported to inhibit platelet aggregation and to increase the blood-thinning effects of warfarin in humans. Caution is advised in patients with bleeding disorders, in patients taking drugs that may increase the risk of bleeding, and prior to some surgical procedures. Dosing adjustments may be necessary.
- Some people may experience stomach discomfort, reduced appetite, or itching.
- In theory, danshen may lower blood pressure and should be used cautiously by patients with blood pressure abnormalities or those taking drugs that alter blood pressure.
- In theory, a chemical found in danshen called *miltirone* may increase drowsiness. Caution is advised while driving or operating machinery.
- Convulsions, mental changes, and dystonia syndrome may occur.

Pregnancy and Breastfeeding

- Danshen should be avoided during pregnancy and breastfeeding. In theory, the blood-thinning properties of danshen may increase the risk of miscarriage or bleeding, and effects on the fetus or nursing infants are not known.

INTERACTIONS
Interactions with Drugs

- Danshen may increase the risk of bleeding when taken with drugs that also increase the risk of bleeding. This herb is reported to inhibit platelet aggregation and to cause over-anticoagulation (excessive blood-thinning effects) in patients taking the blood thinner warfarin (Coumadin). Examples of drugs that increase the risk of bleeding include aspirin, anticoagulants such as warfarin (Coumadin) or heparin, antiplatelet drugs such as clopidogrel (Plavix), and

D

nonsteroidal anti-inflammatory drugs such as ibuprofen (Motrin, Advil) or naproxen (Naprosyn, Aleve).

- In theory, the risk of side effects or toxicity from digoxin (Lanoxin) may be increased if taken with danshen. In addition, danshen may cause laboratory measurements of digoxin blood levels to be inaccurate (too high or too low).
- Danshen may result in hypotension (dangerously low blood pressure) if taken with drugs that also lower blood pressure, such as angiotensin-converting enzyme inhibitors such as captopril (Capoten) or lisinopril (Prinivil) and beta-blockers like atenolol (Tenormin) or propranolol (Inderal). In addition, the use of danshen with beta-blockers may cause bradycardia (dangerously slow heart rate).
- In theory, a chemical found in danshen called *miltirone* may increase sleepiness or other side effects associated with some drugs taken for anxiety or insomnia, such as lorazepam (Ativan), alprazolam (Xanax), and diazepam (Valium), or alcohol. In addition, based on animal studies, danshen may affect the absorption of alcohol into the blood.
- Antibiotics, antilipemic agents, antineoplastic agents, antioxidants, antivirals, drugs broken down by the liver, immunosuppressants, nitrates, and steroids may interact with danshen.

Interactions with Herbs and Dietary Supplements

- Danshen may increase the risk of bleeding when taken with herbs and supplements that are believed to increase the risk of bleeding. Multiple cases of bleeding have been reported with the use of *Ginkgo biloba*, and fewer cases with garlic and saw palmetto.
- In theory, danshen may add to the effects of other herbs, such as hawthorn, with potential cardiac glycoside properties, potentially resulting in slow heart rate or toxicity.
- Danshen should be used cautiously with herbs/supplements that may also lower blood pressure.
- In theory, a chemical found in danshen called *miltirone* can increase the amount of drowsiness that may be caused by other herbs or supplements.
- Antibacterials, anti-inflammatory herbs, antilipemics, antineoplastics, antioxidants, antivirals, steroids, astragalus, chronotropic herbs, herbs and supplements broken down by the liver, immunosuppressants, Gexia zhuyu decoction, licorice, *Ligusticum chuanxiong, Ligustrum lucidum, Polyporus, Serissa, Sophora subprostrata,* and Yun zhi (*Coriolus* mushroom) may interact with danshen.

For a complete list of references, please visit www.naturalstandard.com.

Dehydroepiandrosterone (DHEA)

RELATED TERMS

- 5-androsten-3-ol-17-one, C19 steroid, dehydroepiandrosterone, dehydroepiandrosterone sulfate, DHA, DHAS, DHEA-enanthate, DHEA-FA, DHEA-S, DHEAS, DS, 7-KETO DHE, 7-oxo-DHEA, dehydroepiandrosterone (DHEA), the mother steroid, prasterone.
- **Note:** DHEA can be synthesized in a laboratory using wild yam extract. However, it is believed that wild yam cannot be converted into DHEA by the body. Therefore, information that markets wild yam as a "natural DHEA" may be inaccurate.

BACKGROUND

- DHEA (dehydroepiandrosterone) is an endogenous hormone that is made in the human body and secreted by the adrenal gland. DHEA serves as a precursor to male and female sex hormones (androgens and estrogens). DHEA levels in the body begin to decrease after age 30 and are reported to be low in some people with anorexia, end-stage kidney disease, type 2 diabetes (non-insulin–dependent diabetes), acquired immunodeficiency syndrome, adrenal insufficiency, and in the critically ill. DHEA levels may also be depleted by a number of drugs, including insulin, corticosteroids, opiates, and danazol.
- There is sufficient evidence supporting the use of DHEA for treating adrenal insufficiency, depression, induction of labor, and systemic lupus erythematosus.
- No studies on the long-term effects of DHEA have been conducted. DHEA can cause higher than normal levels of androgens and estrogens in the body and theoretically may increase the risk of prostate, breast, ovarian, and other hormone-sensitive cancers. Therefore, it is not recommended for regular use without supervision by a licensed health professional.

EVIDENCE

Uses Based on Scientific Evidence	Grade
Adrenal Insufficiency Several studies suggest that DHEA may improve well-being, quality of life, exercise capacity, sex drive, and hormone levels in people with insufficient adrenal function (Addison's disease). Though promising, additional studies are needed to make a strong recommendation. Adrenal insufficiency is a serious medical condition and should be treated under the supervision of a qualified health care professional, including a pharmacist.	B
Depression The majority of clinical trials investigating the effect of DHEA on depression support its use for this purpose under the guidance of a specialist.	B
Obesity The majority of clinical trials investigating the effect of DHEA on weight or fat loss support its use for this purpose.	B
Systemic Lupus Erythematosus The majority of clinical trials investigating the effect of DHEA for systemic lupus erythematosus support its use as an adjunct treatment.	B
Alzheimer's Disease Initial research reports that DHEA does not significantly improve cognitive performance or change symptom severity in patients with Alzheimer's disease, but some experts disagree.	C
Bone Density The ability of DHEA to increase bone density is under investigation. Effects are not clear at this time.	C
Cardiovascular Disease Initial studies report possible benefits of DHEA supplementation in patients with cholesterol plaques (hardening) in their arteries. There is conflicting scientific evidence regarding the use of DHEA supplements in patients with heart failure or diminished ejection fraction. Other therapies are more proven in this area, and patients with heart failure or other types of heart disease should discuss treatment options with a cardiologist.	C
Cervical Cancer Initial research reports that the use of intravaginal DHEA may be safe and may promote regression of low-grade cervical lesions. However, further studies are necessary in this area before a firm conclusion can be drawn. Patients should not substitute the use of DHEA for more established therapies and should discuss management options and follow-up with a primary health care professional or gynecologist.	C
Chronic Fatigue Syndrome The scientific evidence remains unclear regarding the effects of DHEA supplementation in patients with chronic fatigue syndrome.	C
Cocaine Withdrawal Preliminary studies show that DHEA is not beneficial in treating cocaine dependence.	C
Critical Illness Unclear scientific evidence exists surrounding the safety or effectiveness of DHEA supplementation in	C

(Continued)

Uses Based on Scientific Evidence	Grade
critically ill patients. At this time, it is recommended that severe illness in the intensive care unit be treated with more proven therapies.	
Crohn's Disease Initial research reports that DHEA supplements are safe for short-term use in patients with Crohn's disease. Preliminary research suggests possible beneficial effects, although the overall evidence is insufficient.	C
HIV/AIDS Although some studies suggest that DHEA supplementation may be beneficial in patients with HIV, results from different studies do not agree with each other. There is currently not enough scientific evidence to recommend DHEA for this condition.	C
Induction of Labor Preliminary evidence suggests that DHEA may help to induce labor. Further research is needed, and people who are pregnant should not self-treat.	C
Infertility DHEA supplementation may be beneficial in women with ovulation disorders. There is currently insufficient evidence to support this indication.	C
Menopausal Disorders Many different aspects of menopause have been studied using DHEA as a treatment, such as vaginal pain; osteoporosis; hot flashes; and emotional disturbances such as fatigue, irritability, anxiety, depression, insomnia, difficulties with concentration or memory; and decreased sex drive (which may occur near the time of menopause). Studies have produced conflicting results.	C
Myotonic Dystrophy There is conflicting scientific evidence regarding the use of DHEA supplements for myotonic dystrophy.	C
Psoriasis Overall study results suggest that DHEA likely offers no benefit to people with psoriasis, but some disagree.	C
Rheumatoid Arthritis Preliminary evidence from a case series suggests that DHEA likely offers no benefit to people with rheumatoid arthritis.	C
Schizophrenia Initial research reports benefits of DHEA supplementation in the management of negative, depressive, and anxiety symptoms of schizophrenia. Some of the side effects from prescription drugs used for schizophrenia may also be relieved.	C
Septicemia (Serious Bacterial Infections in the Blood) Unclear scientific evidence exists surrounding the safety or effectiveness of DHEA supplementation in septic patients. At this time, more proven therapies are recommended.	C
Sexual Function/Libido/Erectile Dysfunction The results of studies vary on the use of DHEA in erectile dysfunction and sexual function in both men and women.	C
Sjögren's Syndrome DHEA showed no evidence of efficacy in Sjögren's syndrome in preliminary studies. Without evidence for efficacy, patients with Sjögren's syndrome should avoid using unregulated DHEA supplements because long-term adverse consequences of exposure to this hormone are unknown.	C
Skin Aging Preliminary studies suggest the possibility of using DHEA topically as an anti–skin aging agent. Further research is needed to confirm these results.	C
Fibromyalgia (Postmenopause) DHEA does not seem to improve quality of life, pain, fatigue, cognitive function, mood, or functional impairment in fibromyalgia.	D
Immune System Stimulant It is suggested by some textbooks and review articles that DHEA can stimulate the immune system. However, the available scientific evidence does not support this claim.	D
Memory Studies of the effects of DHEA on cognition have produced complex and inconsistent results. Overall, the evidence does not support this indication.	D
Muscle Strength Many study results in this area conflict, but overall evidence in this area is negative.	D

Uses Based on Tradition or Theory

Aging, allergic disorders, amenorrhea associated with anorexia, andropause/andrenopause, angioedema, anxiety, asthma, bone diseases, bone loss associated with anorexia, bladder cancer, breast cancer, burns, colon cancer, dementia, diabetes, fatigue, heart attack, high cholesterol, Huntington's disease, influenza, joint diseases, lipodystrophy in HIV, liver protection, malaria, malnutrition, movement disorders, multiple sclerosis, osteoporosis, pancreatic cancer, Parkinson's disease, performance enhancement, polycystic ovarian syndrome, post-traumatic stress disorder (PTSD), premenstrual syndrome, prostate cancer, Raynaud's disease, skin graft healing, sleep disorders, stress, tetanus, ulcerative colitis, viral encephalitis.

DOSING

Adults (18 Years and Older)

- DHEA is available as capsules, tablets, and injections. Commonly used doses range from 25-200 mg/day. Higher doses of 200-500 mg/day have been studied for depression in human immunodeficiency virus/acquired immunodeficiency syndrome. Daily use of DHEA has been studied up to one year in the available scientific studies.

- Topical (on the skin) application and intravenous (into the veins) injections have also been studied, but safety and effectiveness has not been proven. A 5%-10% cream containing DHEA has been used up to 4 weeks.

Children (Younger than 18 Years)

- The dosing and safety of DHEA are not well studied in children. In theory, DHEA could interfere with normal hormone balance and growth in children.

SAFETY

Allergies

- Patients should avoid if allergic to DHEA products.

Side Effects and Warnings

- Few side effects are reported when DHEA supplements are taken by mouth in recommended doses. Side effects may include fatigue, nasal congestion, headache, acne, or rapid/irregular heartbeats. In women, the most common side effects are abnormal menses, emotional changes, headache, and insomnia. People with a history of abnormal heart rhythms, blood clots or hypercoagulability, or a history of liver disease should avoid DHEA supplements.

- Because DHEA is a hormone related to other male and female hormones, there may be side effects related to its hormonal activities. For example, masculinization may occur in women, including acne, greasy skin, facial hair, hair loss, increased sweating, weight gain around the waist, or a deeper voice. Likewise, men may develop more prominent breasts (gynecomastia), breast tenderness, increased blood pressure, testicular wasting, or increased aggressiveness. Other hormonal-related side effects may include increased blood sugar levels, insulin resistance, altered cholesterol levels, altered thyroid hormone levels, and altered adrenal function. Caution is advised in patients with diabetes or hyperglycemia, high cholesterol, thyroid disorders, or other endocrine (hormonal) abnormalities. Serum glucose, cholesterol, and thyroid levels may need to be monitored by a health care professional, and medication adjustments may be necessary.

- In theory, DHEA may increase the risk of developing prostate, breast, or ovarian cancer. DHEA may contribute to tamoxifen resistance in breast cancer. Other side effects may include insomnia, agitation, delusions, mania, nervousness, irritability, or psychosis.

- High DHEA levels have been correlated with Cushing's syndrome, which may be caused by excessive supplementation.

Pregnancy and Breastfeeding

- DHEA is not recommended during pregnancy or breastfeeding. Because DHEA is a hormone, it may be unsafe to the fetus or nursing infants.

INTERACTIONS

Interactions with Drugs

- DHEA may interfere with the way the body processes certain drugs using the liver's cytochrome P450 enzyme system. As a result, levels of these drugs may be increased in the blood and may cause increased effects or potentially serious adverse reactions. Central nervous system agents, including carbamazepine and phenytoin, induce the P450 enzymes that metabolize DHEA and DHEA-S and therefore can decrease circulating concentrations of these hormones. Patients using any medications should check the package insert and speak with a qualified health care professional, including a pharmacist, about possible interactions.

- DHEA may increase blood sugar levels. Caution is advised when using medications that may also lower blood sugar levels such as metformin (Glucophage). A qualified health care professional should closely monitor patients taking drugs for diabetes by mouth or insulin. Medication adjustments may be necessary.

- DHEA may increase the risk of blood clotting. Patients who take anticoagulants (blood thinners) or antiplatelet drugs (such as aspirin) to prevent blood clots should discuss the use of DHEA with a health care professional. Examples of blood-thinning drugs include warfarin (Coumadin), heparin, and clopidogrel (Plavix). The risk of blood clots is also increased by smoking or by taking other hormones (such as oral contraceptives or hormone replacement therapy), and these should not be combined with DHEA unless under medical supervision.

- DHEA may alter heart rates or rhythm and should be used cautiously with heart medications or drugs that may also affect heart rhythm. Alcohol may increase the effects of DHEA.

- Although it is not widely studied, there are some reports that drugs such as canrenoate, anastrozole (Arimidex), growth hormones, methylphenidale, amlodipine, and nicardipine and other calcium channel blockers such as diltiazem (Cardizem) and alprazolam (Xanax) may increase DHEA levels in the body, which could lead to increased side effects when taken with DHEA supplements. In theory, increased hormone levels may occur if DHEA is used with estrogen or androgen hormonal therapies. DHEA may interact with psychiatric drugs such as clozapine (Clozaril).

- DHEA may interact with GABA-receptor drugs used for seizures or pain. DHEA may decrease the effectiveness of methadone. DHEA may add to the effects of clofibrate or contribute to tamoxifen resistance in breast cancer.

- DHEA use has been suggested to result in a decreased rate of developing protective antibody titer after influenza vaccination.

- Drugs that reduce the normal levels of DHEA produced by the body include dopamine, insulin, corticosteroids such as dexamethasone, drugs used to treat endometriosis such as danazol, opiate painkillers, antipsychotics, and estrogen-containing drugs. Metopirone, alprazolam, and benfluorex may increase blood DHEA levels. Many other interactions are possible; check with a qualified health care professional including a pharmacist, for a thorough list.

Interactions with Herbs and Dietary Supplements

- Based on laboratory and animal studies, DHEA may interfere with the way the body processes certain herbs or supplements using the liver's cytochrome P450 enzyme system. As a result, levels of other herbs or supplements may become too high in the blood. It may also alter the effects that other herbs or supplements possibly have on the P450 system.

- DHEA may raise blood sugar levels or cause insulin resistance and may add to the effects of herbs/supplements that may also increase blood sugar levels, such as arginine, cocoa, ephedra (when combined with caffeine), or melatonin. DHEA may work against the effects of herbs/supplements that may decrease blood sugar levels, such as *Aloe vera*, American ginseng, and bilberry. Serum glucose levels should be monitored closely by a qualified health care professional while using DHEA. Dosing adjustments may be necessary.

- In theory, DHEA may increase the risk of blood clotting and may add to the effects of herbs/supplements that may also increase the risk of clotting, such as coenzyme Q10 or *Panax ginseng*. DHEA may work against the effects of herbs/supplements that may "thin" the blood and reduce the risk of clotting, such as *Ginkgo biloba*, garlic, and saw palmetto.

- It is not known what effects occur when DHEA is used with herbs that are believed to have hormonal effects in the body. Examples of agents with possible estrogen-like (phytoestrogenic) effects in the body include alfalfa, black cohosh, and bloodroot.

- DHEA may alter heart rates or rhythms. Caution is advised in patients taking herbs/supplements that may alter heart function or that include cardiac glycosides. Examples include adonis, balloon cotton, and foxglove/digitalis.

- Chromium picolinate may increase blood DHEA levels. Carnitine and DHEA may have additive effects. Based on animal research, DHEA may increase melatonin secretion and prevent breakdown of vitamin E in the body.

- Although it is not widely studied, there are some reports that DHEA may also interact with fiber, flavanoids, polyunsaturated fatty acids, probiotics, soy protein, and yam. Caution is advised.

For a complete list of references, please visit www.naturalstandard.com.

Devil's Claw
(*Harpagophytum procumbens*)

RELATED TERMS

- Acteoside, Afrikanische Teufelskralle (German), Algophytum, ao ao, aromatic acids, arpagofito (Italian), Arthrosetten H, Arthrotabsm, Artigel, artiglio del diavolo, arpagofito (Italian), Artosan, beta-sitosterol, burdock, caffeic acid, cinnamic acid, Defencid, Devil's Claw Capsule, Devil's Claw Secondary Root, Devil's Claw Vegicaps, Doloteffin, duiwelsklou (Afrikaans), ekatata (Ndonga, Kwangali), elyata (Kwanyama), Fitokey Harpagophytum, grapple plant, griffe du diable (French), gum resins, Hariosen, Harpadol, HarpagoMega, Harpagon, Harpagophyti radix (Latin), *Harpagophytum procumbens, Harpagophytum zeyheri*, harpagoquinone, harpagoside, iridoid glycosides, isoacteoside, Jucurba N, khams, khuripe, kloudoring (Afrikaans), likakata (Gciriku, Shambyu), otjihangatene (Herero), Pedaliaceae (family), procumbide, procumboside, Rheuma-Sern, Rheuma-Tee, Salus, sengaparile (Senegalese), stigmasterol, Südafrikanische Teufelskralle, Trampelklette (German), triterpenes, Venustorn (Danish), Windhoek's root, wood spider, *xemta'eisa* (Kung bushman), xsamsa-oro6-acetylacteoside.

BACKGROUND

- Devil's claw *(Harpagophytum procumbens)* originates from the Kalahari and Savannah desert regions of South and Southeast Africa. In these parts of the world, devil's claw has historically been used to treat a wide range of conditions, including fever, malaria, and indigestion. The medicinal ingredient of the devil's claw plant is extracted from the dried out roots.
- Currently, the major uses of devil's claw are as an anti-inflammatory and pain reliever for joint diseases, back pain, and headache. There is currently widespread use of standardized devil's claw for mild joint pain in Europe.
- Potential side effects include gastrointestinal upset, low blood pressure, or abnormal heart rhythms (increased heart rate or increased heart squeezing effects).
- Traditionally, it has been recommended to avoid using devil's claw in patients with stomach ulcers or in people using blood thinners (anticoagulants such as warfarin [Coumadin]).

EVIDENCE

Uses Based on Scientific Evidence	Grade
Degenerative Joint Disease/Osteoarthritis There is increasing scientific evidence suggesting that devil's claw is safe and beneficial for the short-term treatment of pain related to degenerative joint disease or osteoarthritis (8-12 weeks); may be equally effective as drug therapies such as nonsteroidal anti-inflammatory drugs like ibuprofen (Advil, Motrin); and may allow for dose reductions or stopping of these drugs in some patients. However, most studies have been small with flaws in designs.	B
Low Back Pain There are several human studies that support the use of devil's claw for the treatment of low back pain. However, most studies have been small with design flaws, and many have been done by the same authors. It is unclear how devil's claw compares to other therapies for back pain.	B
Appetite Stimulant Traditionally, devil's claw was commonly used as an appetite stimulant, and this remains a popular use. However, there is no reliable scientific evidence in this area, and it remains unclear if devil's claw is beneficial as an appetite stimulant.	C
Cancer (Bone Metastases) Devil's claw is used to treat several types of pain, including osteoarthritis and low back pain. One case report indicates it may also be helpful for pain due to bone metastases. Clinical studies are warranted.	C
Digestive Tonic Devil's claw is popular as a digestive tonic for the relief of constipation, diarrhea, and flatulence. However, there is no reliable scientific evidence in this area, and it remains unclear if devil's claw is beneficial for these uses.	C

Uses Based on Tradition or Theory

Allergies, antiarrhythmic, anticoagulant, anti-inflammatory, antioxidant, arteriosclerosis (clogged arteries), arthritis, bitter tonic, blood diseases, boils (topical), choleretic, constipation, coronary artery disease, diabetes, diuretic, dysmenorrhea, edema, fever, fibromyalgia, flatulence, gall bladder tonic, gastrointestinal disorders, gout, headache, heartburn, high blood sugar, high cholesterol, hip pain, kidney disorders, knee pain, labor aid, liver tonic, malaria, menopausal hot flashes, menstrual pain, migraine, myalgia, nerve pain, nicotine poisoning, pain reliever, rheumatoid arthritis, sedative, skin cancer (topical), skin ulcers (topical), sores (topical), spasmolytic, tendonitis, urinary tract infection, vulnerary for skin injuries (topical), wound healing.

DOSING
Adults (18 Years and Older)

- In general, a liquid extract (1:1 in 25% ethanol) of 0.10-0.25 mL has been taken three times daily. For appetite loss or stomach discomfort, 1.5 g has been taken daily in decoction or preparations with adequate bitterness. For low back pain or osteoarthritis, 2-9 g daily of crude extract or equivalent amounts of extract has been used. As tablets, 600-1,200 mg (standardized to contain 50-100 mg of harpagoside) has been taken by mouth three times daily. For painful osteoarthritis, treatment for 2-3 months is often recommended. A doctor should be consulted if symptoms continue for longer.

Children (Younger than 18 Years)

- There is insufficient evidence to recommend a dose of devil's claw for children. The dosing and safety of devil's claw have not been studied thoroughly in children, and safety is not established.

SAFETY
Allergies

- People with allergies to *Harpagophytum procumbens* or related plants should avoid devil's claw products.

Side Effects and Warnings

- At recommended doses, devil's claw is traditionally believed to be well tolerated. Whether use of devil's claw for longer than 3-4 months is safe or effective is unknown.
- There are reports of headache, ringing in the ears, loss of taste and appetite, gastrointestinal upset, and diarrhea in those taking this herb. Devil's claw may affect levels of acid in the gastrointestinal tract and should be avoided by people with gastric (stomach) or duodenal (intestinal) ulcers. Devil's claw should be used cautiously in patients with gallstones.
- Devil's claw may change the rate and force of heartbeats (chronotropic and inotropic effects). Individuals with heart disease or arrhythmias (abnormal heart rhythms) should consult their cardiologist or primary care physician before taking devil's claw.
- In theory, devil's claw may lower blood sugar levels. Caution is advised in patients with diabetes or hypoglycemia, and in those taking drugs, herbs, or supplements that affect blood sugar. Serum glucose levels may need to be monitored by a health care provider, and medication adjustments may be necessary.
- In theory, devil's claw may increase the risk of bleeding. Caution is advised in patients with bleeding disorders or those taking drugs that may increase the risk of bleeding. Dosing adjustments may be necessary. Patients may need to stop taking devil's claw before some surgeries and should discuss this with their primary health care provider.
- Devil's claw products may be contaminated with other herbs, pesticides, herbicides, heavy metals, or drugs.

Pregnancy and Breastfeeding

- Devil's claw may stimulate contractions of the uterus and cannot be recommended during pregnancy and breastfeeding. Patients should be aware that many tinctures contain high levels of alcohol and should be avoided during pregnancy.

INTERACTIONS
Interactions with Drugs

- Devil's claw may lower blood sugar levels. Caution is advised when using medications that may also lower blood sugar levels. A qualified health care provider should closely monitor patients taking drugs for diabetes by mouth or insulin. Medication adjustments may be necessary.
- In theory, devil's claw may have an additive effect if taken with drugs used for pain, inflammation, high cholesterol, and gout. Drugs used for malaria may also interact.
- Devil's claw may increase stomach acidity and therefore may affect drugs used to decrease the amount of acid in the stomach, such as antacids, sucralfate, ranitidine (Zantac), and esomeprazole (Nexium). People taking any of these drugs should consult a qualified health care professional, including a pharmacist, before taking devil's claw.
- Because devil's claw may affect heart rhythm, heart rate, and the force of heartbeats, individuals taking prescription drugs such as antiarrhythmics or digoxin (Lanoxin) should consult a health care provider before taking devil's claw.
- In theory, devil's claw may increase the risk of bleeding when taken with drugs that increase the risk of bleeding. Some examples include aspirin, anticoagulants (blood thinners) such as warfarin (Coumadin) or heparin, antiplatelet drugs such as clopidogrel (Plavix), and nonsteroidal anti-inflammatory drugs such as ibuprofen (Motrin, Advil) or naproxen (Naprosyn, Aleve).

Interactions with Herbs and Dietary Supplements

- In theory, devil's claw may lower blood sugar levels. Caution is advised when using herbs or supplements that may also lower blood sugar. Blood glucose levels may require monitoring, and doses may need adjustment.
- In theory, devil's claw may interfere with other herbs and dietary supplements that affect heart rhythm, heart rate, and the force of heartbeats. Notably, bufalin (Chan Suis) is a Chinese herbal formula that has been reported as toxic or fatal when taken with cardiac glycosides.
- Devil's claw may add to the effects of herbs and dietary supplements that are used for pain or inflammation. Devil's claw may also interact with herbs or supplements used to treat malaria.
- Devil's claw may reduce cholesterol concentrations and may add to the lipid-lowering effects of fish oil or garlic.
- In theory, devil's claw may increase the risk of bleeding when taken with herbs and supplements that are believed to increase the risk of bleeding. Multiple cases of bleeding have been reported with the use of *Ginkgo biloba*, and fewer cases with garlic and saw palmetto. Numerous other agents may theoretically increase the risk of bleeding, although this has not been proven in most cases.

For a complete list of references, please visit www.naturalstandard.com.

Devil's Club
(Oplopanax horridus)

RELATED TERMS

- Alaska ginseng, American ginseng, Araliaceae, cukilanarpak, devil's club, devil's root, *Echinopanax horridum* (Sm.) Decne. & Planch, Fatsia, *Fatsia horrida* (Sm.) Benth. & Hook., *Oplopanax horrideum, Oplopanax horridum, Oplopanax horridus* ssp. *horridus, Oplopanax horridus* (Sm.) Miq., Pacific ginseng, *Panax horridum* Sm., prickly porcupine ginseng, *Riconophyllum horridum* Pall., suxt, wild armored Alaskan ginseng.

BACKGROUND

- Devil's club, a member of the ginseng family (Araliaceae), has long been used for many medical conditions by indigenous peoples of Alaska and the Pacific Northwest. Among the traditional medical uses of devil's club, the most widespread is for the treatment of external and internal infections.
- Traditionally, the inner bark of aerial stems was used. The most modern commercial preparations, however, use the root. Western herbalists use devil's club as a respiratory stimulant and expectorant, and for autoimmune conditions, eczema, external infections, internal infections, rheumatoid arthritis, sores, and type 2 diabetes. They also use it to lower blood sugar and increase general well-being, and as a pancreatic tonic. At this time, there are no high-quality human trials supporting the use of devil's club for any indication.
- As with many medicinal plants, there is concern about the commercialization of devil's club. This concern stems from the need to respect the intellectual property rights of the people from which the knowledge originated, compensate the original users of the plant, and align current uses ethically and culturally within the ethnobotanical context, all in the midst of the failures of the current legal mechanisms to accomplish these goals.

EVIDENCE

Uses Based on Scientific Evidence	Grade
Diabetes The hypoglycemic (blood sugar–lowering) effect is one of many reported uses for devil's club, which had a traditional use in diabetes, and continues to be used for this condition. Although the preliminary evidence is promising, there is a lack of conclusive evidence.	C

Uses Based on Tradition or Theory
Acne, antibacterial, antifungal, antiviral, appetite stimulant, arthritis, blood disorders, birth control, blood purifier, body balancing, boils, burns, cancer prevention, colds, constipation, cough, diphtheria, emetic (induces vomiting), fertility, fever, gall stones, heart disease, influenza, laxative, measles, menstruation, pain, pneumonia, psychiatric disorders, purgative (laxative), skin infections, sexually transmitted diseases (STDs), sores, stomach trouble, stomach ulcers, swollen glands, tuberculosis, vision, weight loss, wound healing.

DOSING

Adults (18 Years and Older)

- There is insufficient evidence to recommend a dose for devil's club. Decoctions, tinctures, and infusions have all been used. Traditionally, 15-30 drops of tincture (fresh 1:2, dry 1:5, both 60% alcohol) or 1-3 fluid ounces of cold infusion has been used three times daily.
- For blood sugar–lowering effects, 1.4-1.6 mL of an aqueous extract per pound of body weight has been used. For weight gain, colds, and other illnesses, 125 mL before meals has been used.
- Devil's club raw inner bark has also been chewed and spit on wounds for analgesia (pain relief), or laid in strips over a fracture to help with pain and swelling. The inner bark may also be dried, rubbed to a pulp, and put on wounds to reduce infection. An ointment has also been made by burning the stems and mixing the ashes with grease to alleviate swellings.

Children (Younger than 18 Years)

- There is insufficient evidence to recommend a dose for devil's club in children.

SAFETY

Allergies

- Avoid in people with a known allergy or hypersensitivity to devil's club. The spines on the stems and leaves are known to cause a topical allergic reaction.

Side Effects and Warnings

- The American Herbal Products Association lists devil's club as Class 1, or "Herbs which can be safely consumed when used appropriately," though a duration of safe use is not specified. Devil's club is not listed by the U.S. Food and Drug Administration (FDA) as "generally recognized as safe" (GRAS).
- Chronic ingestion of a devil's club infusion may cause too much weight gain. The spines on the stems and leaves have been known to cause a topical allergic reaction. Diarrhea has occurred in one patient taking an aqueous extract of inner root bark.
- Devil's club may also lower blood sugar levels. Caution is advised in patients with diabetes (high blood sugar) or hypoglycemia (low blood sugar), and in those taking drugs, herbs, or supplements that affect blood sugar. Serum glucose levels may need to be monitored by a qualified health care professional, including a pharmacist, and medication adjustments may be necessary.

Pregnancy and Breastfeeding

- Devil's club is not recommended in pregnant or breastfeeding women due to a lack of available scientific evidence. Devil's club may expel afterbirth and start postpartum menstrual flow.

INTERACTIONS

Interactions with Drugs

- Devil's club may lower blood sugar levels. Caution is advised when using medications that may also lower blood sugar levels. Patients taking drugs for diabetes by mouth or insulin should be monitored closely by a qualified health care professional, including a pharmacist. Medication adjustments may be necessary.

Interactions with Herbs and Dietary Supplements

- Devil's club may lower blood sugar levels. Caution is advised when using herbs or supplements that may also lower blood sugar levels. Blood glucose levels may require monitoring, and doses may need adjustment.

For a complete list of references, please visit www.naturalstandard.com.

Dimethyl sulfoxide (DMSO)

RELATED TERMS

- C_2H_6OS, dimethyl sulfoxide, dimethyl sulphoxide, dimethylis sulfoxidum, methyl sulphoxide, NSC-763, SQ-9453, Rimso-50, sulphinybismethane.

BACKGROUND

- Dimethyl sulfoxide (C_2H_6OS), or DMSO, is a sulfur-containing organic compound. DMSO occurs naturally in vegetables, fruits, grains, and animal products. DMSO was first synthesized in 1866 as a byproduct of paper manufacturing. Therapeutic interest began in 1963. DMSO was reported to penetrate through the skin and produce analgesia, decrease pain, and promote tissue healing. DMSO is available for both non-medicinal and medicinal uses. The major clinical use of DMSO is to relieve symptoms of interstitial cystitis.
- Potential toxic effects to the lens of the eye have been reported in animals, but similar effects have not been noted in humans. Topical application has been associated with redness and inflammation of skin, and a garlic-like taste and odor on the breath have been reported.
- DMSO has been used to treat amyloidosis, diabetic ulcers, extravasation, erosive gastritis, and ischemia prevention in surgical flaps, but well-designed clinical trials are lacking. Because of the limited scientific evidence, whether DMSO provides effective treatment of patients with closed head trauma, herpes zoster, tendopathies, and complex regional pain syndrome will require more research.

EVIDENCE

Uses Based on Scientific Evidence	Grade
Interstitial Cystitis (Chronic Bladder Infection) Intravesical (administered in the bladder) DMSO is approved by the U.S. Food and Drug Administration (FDA) for interstitial cystitis when given by a qualified health care professional. DMSO may work when other treatments have failed.	B
Amyloidosis DMSO may change the course of amyloidosis if treatment is started early. However, there is not much scientific support for this claim.	C
Anesthesia (for Kidney and Gallbladder Stone Removal) Extracorporeal shock wave lithotripsy (ESWL) is sometimes used to break down kidney or gallbladder stones so that they can be passed in the urine. Treatment with DMSO may help reduce the pain of ESWL. Also, the diuretic, anti-inflammatory, muscle relaxant, and hydroxyl radical scavenger effects may also be beneficial for patients undergoing ESWL. However, more research is needed in this area.	C
Diabetic Ulcers Currently, there is not enough scientific evidence available to recommend the use of topical DMSO for diabetic ulcers.	C
Extravasation (Drug Accidentally Going Outside of a Vein) DMSO applied to the skin may prevent tissue death after extravasation of anticancer agents. It can be applied alone or with steroids. However, there is insufficient evidence supporting this use.	C
Gastritis When used with acid-blocking drugs (like ranitidine), DMSO may help treat gastritis. However, there is insufficient evidence supporting this use.	C
Herpes Zoster (Shingles) DMSO may help treat herpes zoster. This treatment may work even better when used with the drug idoxuridine. However, there is insufficient evidence supporting this use.	C
Inflammatory Bladder Disease DMSO may relieve the symptoms of inflammatory bladder disease. However, there is insufficient evidence supporting this use.	C
Intracranial Pressure DMSO may help treat increased intracranial pressure (high pressure in the skull), but most research is vague and results are conflicting. The risks may be greater than the potential benefits.	C
Pressure Ulcers (Prevention) Based on early research, massage therapy with a DMSO cream does not appear to effectively prevent pressure ulcers (also called *bedsores*). However, there is insufficient evidence supporting this use.	C
Reflex Sympathetic Dystrophy Little research has been done to see if DMSO helps reflex sympathetic dystrophy.	C
Rheumatoid Arthritis Applying DMSO to the skin may help rheumatoid arthritis.	C
Surgical Skin Flap Ischemia One trial suggests that DSMO improves lack of blood flow (ischemia) in surgical flaps. More research is needed to confirm these results.	C

(Continued)

Uses Based on Scientific Evidence	Grade
Tendopathies A randomized, controlled, double-blind trial evaluating DMSO for acute tendopathies found a positive effect. Overall, there is insufficient evidence supporting this use.	C
Scleroderma DMSO does not seem to help treat scleroderma and is therefore not recommended.	D

Uses Based on Tradition or Theory
Acute herpes infection, Alzheimer's disease, burns, cancer, closed head trauma, colitis, complex regional pain syndrome, fibromyalgia, gallstones, high cholesterol, muscle pain, pancreatitis, schizophrenia, systemic lupus erythematosus (SLE), tuberculosis.

DOSING

Adults (18 Years and Older)

- Administering DMSO in the bladder (intravesically) is approved by the U.S. Food and Drug Administration (FDA) for interstitial cystitis when given by a qualified health care professional.
- There is insufficient evidence to recommend a dose for DMSO for other conditions. DMSO has been taken by mouth in doses between 7 and 15 g/day. Various solutions ranging from 10% to 100% DMSO have been applied on the skin. DMSO creams and gels have also been used.

Children (Younger than 18 Years)

- There is insufficient evidence to recommend the safe use of DMSO in children.

SAFETY

Allergies

- People with a known allergy or hypersensitivity to DMSO should avoid use.

Side Effects and Warnings

- Skin reactions are the most common side effects with topical (applied to the skin) administration and are usually reversible after discontinuing the drug. Erythema (reddening of the skin), pruritus (itching), burning, drying, scaling, blistering, dermatitis, and wheals have been reported. Cases of headache, dizziness, sedation, and agitation have also been reported. Encephalopathy, stroke, and heart attack have been reported after DMSO was used in stem cell transplantations.
- Cautious use is advised in patients with urinary tract malignancies and with hepatic (liver) and renal (kidney) dysfunction. One clinical trial reported increased urgency, dysuria (difficult or painful urination), hematuria (blood in the urine), and red urine discoloration.
- Cases of nausea, vomiting, constipation, halitosis (bad breath), garlic taste, and diarrhea have been reported. Other adverse effects that have been reported include anorexia, influenza-like symptoms, facial flushing from intravenous administration, and low blood pressure resulting from topical use. Negative effects on blood cell counts such as eosinophilia and hemolysis have been reported to result from intravenous (into the vein) administration. Based on one case report, seizure occurred following a dimethylsulfoxide-preserved stem cell infusion.

Pregnancy and Breastfeeding

- DMSO is not recommended due to lack of sufficient available evidence.

INTERACTIONS

Interactions with Drugs

- Using DMSO with sulindac (Clinoril) may cause peripheral neuropathy. Animal studies have reported that the action of sulindac may be decreased by DMSO. Although human data is lacking, this drug combination should be avoided.

Interactions with Herbs and Supplements

- There is insufficient available information.

For a complete list of references, please visit www.naturalstandard.com.

Dogwood
(*Cornus* spp.)

RELATED TERMS

- *Cornus controversa, Cornus kousa, Cornus macrophylla, Cornus nuttallii, Cornus officinalis, Cornus officinalis* Sieb et Zucc, *Cornus officinalis* Sieb. et Zuce, *Cornus stolonifera, Cornus stolonifera* Michx, dandi tablet, dogwood fruit, red-osier dogwood, zuo-gui-wan.

BACKGROUND

- Dogwood (*Cornus* spp.) is a deciduous tree that has showy, four-petaled flowers in early spring. The indigenous peoples of the boreal forest in Canada traditionally used *Cornus stolonifera* for diabetes or its complications. Elders of the Saanich and Cowichan Coast Salish people of the southern Vancouver Island used *Cornus nuttallii* bark to treat respiratory ailments.
- There is limited human evidence about the use of dogwood for use in cancer and as an antioxidant. However, future studies may investigate these areas further. Dogwood has been studied with other herbs to see its effects on hormone levels in postmenopausal and infertile women, although currently there is a lack of strong evidence for these conditions.

EVIDENCE

Uses Based on Scientific Evidence	Grade
Fertility A traditional Chinese combination of herbs reportedly helped a woman with postmenopausal levels of follicle stimulating hormone and luteinizing hormone to become pregnant. Although this result is interesting, further research is needed in this area.	C
Postmenopausal Symptoms There is currently insufficient available evidence to recommend dogwood for the treatment of postmenopausal symptoms.	C

Uses Based on Tradition or Theory
Antioxidant, cancer, cataracts, coronary heart disease, diabetes, diabetic complications, diabetic eye disease, diabetic microangiopathy (disease of very fine blood vessels), diabetic neuropathy (nerve damage), HIV/AIDS, hyperlipidemia (high cholesterol), respiratory ailments, sperm motility.

DOSING
Adults (18 Years and Older)

- There is insufficient evidence to recommend a dose for dogwood in adults.

Children (Younger than 18 Years)

- There is insufficient evidence to recommend a dose for dogwood in children.

SAFETY
Allergies

- Avoid in people with a known allergy or hypersensitivity to dogwood (*Cornus* spp.) or its constituents.

Side Effects and Warnings

- Use cautiously in patients taking aldose reductase inhibitors, as dogwood may inhibit these enzymes.
- Use cautiously in patients taking antineoplastic (anticancer) agents, as dogwood may have antineoplastic activity.
- Use cautiously in patients with HIV, as dogwood may inhibit virus replication.
- Use cautiously in patients attempting to become pregnant or who are postmenopausal, as dogwood may alter hormone levels.
- Avoid in patients who are using birth control pills, as dogwood may alter hormone levels.

Pregnancy and Breastfeeding

- Dogwood is not recommended in pregnant or breastfeeding women due to a lack of available scientific evidence.
- Dogwood should be used cautiously with estrogens, fertility agents, and birth control pills.
- Dogwood fruits may increase sperm motility.

INTERACTIONS
Interactions with Drugs

- Dogwood may protect against diabetic complications. Patients taking drugs for diabetes by mouth or insulin should be monitored closely by a qualified health care professional, including a pharmacist. Medication adjustments may be necessary.
- Dogwood fruit may alter cholesterol levels in the body. Use with caution.
- Dogwood may have anticancer activity. Use cautiously with anticancer agents due to possible additive effects.
- Dogwood may have antioxidant activity. Use cautiously with antioxidants due to possible additive effects.
- Use dogwood extracts (stem and leaf) cautiously with antiretroviral agents due to possible additive effects.
- Dogwood fruit may alter hormone levels and may increase fertility in infertile women. Use cautiously with estrogen, fertility agents, and birth control pills.

Interactions with Herbs and Dietary Supplements

- Dogwood fruit may alter cholesterol levels in the body. Use with caution.
- Dogwood may have antineoplastic activity; use cautiously with anticancer herbs and supplements due to possible additive effects.

- Dogwood may have antioxidant activity. Use cautiously with antioxidants due to possible additive effects.
- Use dogwood extracts (stem and leaf) cautiously with herbs and supplements with antiviral activity due to possible additive effects.
- Dogwood fruit may alter hormone levels and may increase fertility in infertile women. Use cautiously with fertility herbs and supplements and phytoestrogens.

- Dogwood may protect against diabetic complications. Patients taking herbs or supplements for diabetes by mouth or insulin should be monitored closely by a qualified health care professional, including a pharmacist. Dose adjustments may be necessary.

For a complete list of references, please visit www.naturalstandard.com.

dong quai
(*Angelica sinensis* [Oliv.] Diels)

RELATED TERMS

- American angelica, *Angelica acutiloba, Angelica archangelica, Angelica atropurpurea, Angelica dahurica, Angelica edulis, Angelica gigas, Angelica keiskei, Angelica koreana, Angelica-polymorpha* var. sinensis Oliv., *Angelica pubescens, Angelica radix, Angelica root, Angelica silvestris,* Angelique, *Archangelica officinalis* Moench or Hoffm, beta-sitosterol, Chinese Angelica, Chinese Danggui, Danggui, Dang Gui, Danggui-Nian-Tong-Tang (DGNTT), Dang quai, Dong Kwai, Dong qua, dong quai extract, dong quai root, Dong qui, dry-kuei, engelwurzel, European angelica, European dong quai, Female ginseng, FP3340010, FP334015, FT334010, garden angelica, Heiligenwurzel, Japanese angelica, Kinesisk Kvan (Danish), Kinesisk Kvanurt (Danish), *Ligusticum glaucescens* Franch. *Ligusticum officinale* Koch, Ligustilides, phytoestrogen, Qingui, radix Angelica sinensis, root of the Holy Ghost, Tan Kue Bai Zhi, Tang Kuei, Tang Kuei Root, Tang kwei, Tang quai, Tanggui (Korean), Tanggwi (Korean), Toki (Japanese), wild angelica, wild Chin quai, women's ginseng, Yuan Nan wild dong quai, Yungui.

BACKGROUND

- dong quai (*Angelica sinensis*), also known as Chinese Angelica, has been used for thousands of years in traditional Chinese, Korean, and Japanese medicine. It remains one of the most popular plants in Chinese medicine and is used primarily for health conditions in women. dong quai has been called "female ginseng," based on its use for gynecological disorders (such as painful menstruation or pelvic pain), recovery from childbirth or illness, and fatigue/low vitality. It is also given for strengthening *xue* (loosely translated as "the blood"), for cardiovascular conditions/high blood pressure, inflammation, headache, infections, and nerve pain.
- In the late 1800s, an extract of dong quai called *Eumenol* became popular in Europe as a treatment for gynecological complaints. Recently, interest in dong quai has resurged due to its proposed weak estrogen-like properties. However, it remains unclear if dong quai has the same effects on the body as estrogens, blocks the activity of estrogens, or has no significant hormonal effects. Additional research is necessary in this area before a firm conclusion can be drawn.
- In Chinese medicine, dong quai is most often used in combination with other herbs and is used as a component of formulas for liver *qi* stasis and spleen deficiency. It is believed to work best in patients with a *yin* profile, and is considered to be a mildly warming herb. dong quai is thought to return the body to proper order by nourishing the blood and harmonizing vital energy. The name dong quai translates as "return to order" based on its alleged restorative properties.
- Although dong quai has many historical and theoretical uses based on animal studies, there is little human evidence supporting the effects of dong quai for any condition. Most of the available clinical studies have either been poorly designed or reported insignificant results. Also, most have examined combination formulas containing multiple ingredients in addition to dong quai, making it difficult to determine which ingredient may cause certain effects.

EVIDENCE

Uses Based on Scientific Evidence	Grade
Amenorrhea (Lack of Menstrual Period) There is limited poor-quality research on dong quai as a part of herbal combinations given for amenorrhea.	C
Angina Pectoris/Coronary Artery Disease There is insufficient evidence to support the use of dong quai for the treatment of heart disease.	C
Arthritis dong quai is traditionally used in the treatment of arthritis. However, there is insufficient clinical evidence to recommend the use of dong quai alone or in combination with other herbs for osteoarthritis or rheumatoid arthritis.	C
Dysmenorrhea (Painful Menstruation) There are unclear results of preliminary, poor-quality human research on dong quai in combination with other herbs for dysmenorrhea. Reliable scientific evidence for dong quai alone in humans with dysmenorrhea is currently not available.	C
Glomerulonephritis There is insufficient evidence to support the use of dong quai as a treatment for kidney diseases such as glomerulonephritis. Preliminary poor-quality research of dong quai in combination with other herbs reports unclear results.	C
Idiopathic Thrombocytopenic Purpura (ITP) A poor-quality study reports benefits of dong quai in patients diagnosed with idiopathic thrombocytopenic purpura (ITP). However, these patients were not compared to those who were not receiving dong quai, and therefore the results can only be considered preliminary.	C
Menstrual Migraine Headache The effects of dong quai alone for this condition are not clear; supportive research is lacking.	C
Nerve Pain There is insufficient evidence to support the use of dong quai as a treatment for nerve pain. High-quality human research is lacking.	C

(Continued)

Uses Based on Scientific Evidence	Grade
Pulmonary Hypertension It remains unclear if dong quai is beneficial for other causes of pulmonary hypertension.	C
Menopausal Symptoms dong quai is used in traditional Chinese formulas for menopausal symptoms. It has been proposed that dong quai may contain phytoestrogens (chemicals with estrogen-like effects in the body). However, it remains unclear from laboratory studies if dong quai has the same effects on the body as estrogens, blocks the activity of estrogens, or has no significant effect on estrogens.	D

Uses Based on Tradition or Theory

Abdominal pain, abnormal fetal movement, abnormal heart rhythms, abscesses, age-related nerve damage, acquired immunodeficiency syndrome, allergy, anemia, anorexia nervosa, anti-aging, antibacterial, antifungal, antioxidant, antiseptic, antispasmodic, anti-tumor (brain tumors), antiviral, anxiety, asthma, back pain, bleomycin-induced lung damage, blood flow disorders, blood purifier, blurred vision, body pain, boils, bone growth, breast enlargement, bronchitis, Buerger's disease, cancer, central nervous system disorders, cervicitis (inflammation of the cervix), chilblains, chronic hepatitis, chronic obstructive pulmonary disease (COPD), chronic rhinitis, cholagogue (promotes the flow of bile), cirrhosis, colchicine-induced learning impairment, congestive heart failure (CHF), constipation, cough, cramps, dermatitis, diabetes, digestion disorders, dysentery, eczema, emotional instability, endometritis, expectorant, fatigue, fibrocystic breast disease, flatulence (gas), fluid retention, gastric ulcer, glaucoma, headache, heartburn, hematopoiesis (stimulation of blood cell production), hemorrhoids (bleeding), hemolytic disease of the newborn, hernia, high cholesterol, hormonal abnormalities, immune cytopenias, immune suppressant, infections, infertility, irritable bowel syndrome, joint pain, labor aid, laxative, leukorrhea (vaginal discharge), liver protection, lung disease, malaria, menorrhagia (heavy menstrual bleeding), menstrual cramping, miscarriage prevention, morning sickness, muscle relaxant, osteoporosis, ovulation abnormalities, pain, pain from bruises, palpitations, pelvic congestion syndrome, pelvic inflammatory disease, peritoneal dialysis, pleurisy, postpartum weakness, pregnancy support, premenstrual syndrome (PMS), psoriasis, prolapsed uterus, pulmonary fibrosis, Raynaud's disease, reperfusion injury, respiratory tract infection, rheumatic diseases, sciatica, sedative, sepsis, shingles (herpes zoster), skin pigmentation disorders, skin ulcers, stiffness, stomach cancer, stress, stroke, tinnitus (ringing in the ear), toothache, uterine fibroids, vaginal atrophy, vitamin E deficiency, wound healing.

DOSING
Adults (18 Years and Older)

- dong quai is used in numerous herbal combinations, and various doses have been used both traditionally and in research in China. Because of this variation and lack of high-quality studies, no specific recommendations can be made. Safety and effectiveness are not established for most

herbal combinations, and the amounts of dong quai present from batch to batch may vary.
- Powdered or dried root/root slices, fluid extracts, tinctures, decoctions, and dried leaf preparations of dong quai are available to be taken orally. Topical preparations are available to be applied to the skin. Safety of intravenous use is not established, although it has been reported in research.

Children (Younger than 18 Years)

- There is insufficient evidence to recommend a dose of dong quai for use in children, and it is not recommended due to potential side effects.

SAFETY
Allergies

- People with known allergy/hypersensitivity to *Angelica radix* or members of the Apiaceae/Umbelliferae family (anise, caraway, carrot, celery, dill, parsley) should avoid dong quai. Skin rash has been reported with the use of dong quai, although it is not clear if this was an allergic response. An asthma response has occurred after breathing in dong quai powder.

Side Effects and Warnings

- Although dong quai is accepted as being safe as a food additive in the United States and Europe, its safety in medicinal doses is not known. There are no reliable long-term studies of side effects. Most precautions are based on theory, laboratory research, tradition, or isolated case reports.
- Components of dong quai may increase the risk of bleeding due to anticoagulant and antiplatelet effects. Caution is advised in patients with bleeding disorders or those taking drugs that may increase the risk of bleeding. Dosing adjustments may be necessary. Discontinue use prior to surgical or major dental procedures.
- It remains unclear if dong quai has the same effects on the body as estrogens, if it blocks the activity of estrogens, or if it has no significant hormonal effects. It remains unclear if dong quai is safe in individuals with hormone-sensitive conditions such as breast cancer, uterine cancer, ovarian cancer, or endometriosis. It is not known if dong quai possesses the beneficial effects that estrogen is believed to have on bone mass or potential harmful effects such as increased risk of stroke or hormone-sensitive cancers.
- Increased sun sensitivity with a risk of severe skin reactions (photosensitivity) may occur due to chemicals in dong quai. Prolonged exposure to sunlight or ultraviolet light should be avoided while taking dong quai.
- Safrole, a volatile oil in dong quai, may be carcinogenic (cancer-causing). Long-term use should therefore be avoided, and suntan lotions that contain dong quai often limit the amount of dong quai to less than 1%.
- dong quai has traditionally been associated with gastrointestinal symptoms (particularly with prolonged use), including laxative effects/diarrhea, upset stomach, nausea, vomiting, loss of appetite, burping, or bloating. Published literature is limited in this area.
- dong quai preparations may contain high levels of sucrose and should be used cautiously by patients with diabetes or glucose intolerance.
- Various other side effects have rarely been reported with dong quai taken alone or in combination with other herbs. However, side effects have not been evaluated in

well-designed studies. These include headache, lightheadedness/dizziness, sedation/drowsiness, insomnia, irritability, fever, sweating, weakness, abnormal heart rhythms, blood pressure abnormalities, wheezing/asthma, hot flashes, worsening premenstrual symptoms, reduced menstrual flow, increased male breast size (gynecomastia), kidney problems (nephrosis), or skin rash.

- The safety of dong quai injected into the skin, muscles, or veins is not known and should be avoided.

Pregnancy and Breastfeeding

- dong quai is not recommended during pregnancy due to possible hormonal and anticoagulant/antiplatelet properties. Animal research has noted conflicting effects on the uterus, with reports of both stimulation and relaxation. There is a published report of miscarriage in a woman taking dong quai, although it is not clear that dong quai was the cause. dong quai is traditionally viewed as increasing the risk of abortion. There is insufficient evidence regarding the safety of dong quai during breastfeeding.

INTERACTIONS
Interactions with Drugs

- dong quai may increase the risk of bleeding due to anticoagulant and antiplatelet effects and may increase the risk of bleeding when taken with drugs that increase the risk of bleeding. Some examples include aspirin, anticoagulants (blood thinners) such as warfarin (Coumadin) or heparin, antiplatelet drugs such as clopidogrel (Plavix), and nonsteroidal anti-inflammatory drugs such as ibuprofen (Motrin, Advil) or naproxen (Naprosyn, Aleve).
- It remains unclear if dong quai has the same effects on the body as estrogens, if it blocks the activity of estrogens, or has no significant hormonal effects. It is not known if taking dong quai increases or decreases the effects of birth control pills or hormone replacement therapy such as Premarin, which contains estrogen, or the anti-tumor effects of selective estrogen receptor modulators (SERMs) such as tamoxifen.
- Chemicals in dong quai may cause increased sun sensitivity with a risk of severe skin reactions (photosensitivity), and dong quai should be avoided with other drugs that cause

photosensitivity, such as tretinoin (Retin-A, Renova) and with some types of antidepressants, cancer drugs, antibiotics, and antipsychotic medications. Patients taking medications should check with their doctor or pharmacist before starting dong quai.
- Based on laboratory research, dong quai may increase the effects of drugs that affect heart rhythms, such as digoxin, beta-blockers such as metoprolol (Lopressor, Toprol), calcium channel blockers such as nifedipine (Procardia), or other antiarrhythmic drugs.
- Based on laboratory research, some compounds in dong quai may increase the effects of anticancer drugs and antidepressant drugs called selective serotonin reuptake inhibitors (SSRIs).

Interactions with Herbs and Dietary Supplements

- In theory, due to anticoagulant and antiplatelet effects, components of dong quai may increase the risk of bleeding when taken with herbs and supplements that are believed to increase the risk of bleeding. Multiple cases of bleeding have been reported with the use of *Ginkgo biloba,* and fewer cases with garlic and saw palmetto. Numerous other agents may theoretically increase the risk of bleeding, although this has not been proven in most cases.
- It remains unclear if dong quai has the same effects on the body as estrogens, blocks the activity of estrogens, or has no significant hormonal effects. The effects of agents believed to have estrogen-like properties may be altered.
- Chemicals in dong quai may cause increased sun sensitivity with a risk of severe skin reactions (photosensitivity), and dong quai should not be taken with products containing *Hypericum perforatum* (St. John's wort) or capsaicin, which are also reported to cause photosensitivity.
- Based on laboratory research, some compounds in dong quai may increase the effects of anticancer herbs or supplements and antidepressants.
- dong quai may increase the effects of antioxidants.

For a complete list of references, please visit www.naturalstandard.com.

Echinacea
(*Echinacea* spp.)

RELATED TERMS

- Alkamides, American coneflower, Asteraceae (family), black Sampson, black Susan, cichoric acid, cock-up-hat, combflower, coneflower, *Echinacea angustifolia, Echinacea pallida,* Echinacea Plus, *Echinacea purpurea,* Echinacin, Echinacin EC31, Echinaforce, Echinaforce Forte, Echinaguard, Echinilin (Factors R & D Technologies, Burnaby, British Columbia, Canada), hedgehog, igelkopf, Indian head, Kansas snake root, kegelblume, narrow-leaved purple coneflower, Pascotox, polysaccharides, purple coneflower, red sunflower, rudbeckia, SB-TOX, scurvy root, snakeroot, solhat, sun hat.

BACKGROUND

- *Echinacea* is a genus of nine perennial species that belong to the Aster family and originate in eastern North America. Traditionally used for a range of infections and malignancies, the roots and herb (above ground parts) of echinacea species have attracted recent scientific interest due to purported immune stimulant properties. Oral preparations are popular in Europe and the United States for prevention and treatment of upper respiratory tract infections (URIs), and *Echinacea purpurea* herb is believed to be the most potent echinacea species for this indication. In the United States, sales of echinacea are believed to represent approximately 10% of the dietary supplement market.
- For URI treatment, numerous human trials have found echinacea to reduce duration and severity, particularly when initiated at the earliest onset of symptoms. However, the majority of trials, largely conducted in Europe, have been small or of weak design. Negative results exist of a U.S. trial in adults, which used a whole-plant echinacea preparation containing both *Echinacea purpurea* and *Echinacea angustifolia.* Another clinical trial reported in July 2005 also did not demonstrate any clinical benefit. However, a 2006 meta-analysis investigating the efficacy of echinacea found that the likelihood of experiencing a clinical cold was 55% higher with a placebo than with Echinacea (based on three trials). The sum of the current evidence is conflicting, and further well-designed studies are needed before a definitive conclusion can be drawn. Lack of benefit in children ages 2-11 has also been reported.
- For URI prevention (prophylaxis), daily echinacea has not been shown effective in human trials.
- Preliminary studies of echinacea taken by mouth for genital herpes and radiation-associated toxicity remain inconclusive. Topical *Echinacea purpurea* juice has been suggested for skin and oral wound healing, and oral/injectable echinacea for vaginal *Candida albicans* infections, but evidence is lacking in these areas.
- The German Commission E discourages the use of echinacea in patients with autoimmune diseases, but this warning is based on theoretical considerations rather than human data.
- In children, echinacea cannot be recommended due to reports of rash and apparent lack of benefits in the available literature.

EVIDENCE

Uses Based on Scientific Evidence	Grade
Prevention of Upper Respiratory Tract Infections (Adults and Children) Preliminary studies suggest that echinacea is not helpful for preventing the common cold in adults. A recent meta-analysis suggested that standardized extracts of echinacea were effective in the prevention of symptoms of the common cold after clinical inoculation, compared with placebo. In children, a combination of echinacea, propolis, and vitamin C has been reported to reduce the number and duration of cold episodes. However, prevention research overall has not been well designed, and strong evidence is still lacking.	B
Treatment of Upper Respiratory Tract Infections (Adults) Although multiple low-quality studies have previously suggested that taking echinacea by mouth by adults when cold symptoms begin may reduce the length and severity of symptoms, a clinical trial reported in July 2005 did not demonstrate any clinical benefit. Recent meta-analyses are conflicting; one suggested that standardized extracts of echinacea were effective in the prevention of symptoms of the common cold after clinical inoculation, compared with placebo, whereas the other reported no such benefit. Strong supportive evidence is still lacking.	B
Cancer There is a lack of conclusive clinical evidence that echinacea affects any type of cancer.	C
Immune System Stimulation Echinacea has been studied alone and in combination preparations for immune system stimulation (including in patients receiving cancer chemotherapy). It remains unclear if there are clinically significant benefits.	C
Low White Blood Cell Counts after X-Ray Treatment (Leukopenia) Studies have reported mixed results, and it is not clear whether echinacea has benefits for this use.	C
Uveitis (Eye Inflammation) Oral *Echinacea purpurea* may offer some benefits in people with low-grade uveitis. However, the available evidence is insufficient to support clinical efficacy.	C

Uses Based on Scientific Evidence	Grade
Vaginal Yeast Infections When echinacea is used at the same time as the prescription cream econazole nitrate (Spectazole), vaginal yeast infections *(Candida)* may occur less frequently. However, the available evidence is insufficient to support clinical efficacy.	C
Genital Herpes Initial human studies suggest that echinacea is not helpful in the treatment of genital herpes.	D
Treatment of Upper Respiratory Tract Infections (Children) Initial research suggests that echinacea may not be helpful in children for alleviation of cold symptoms, possibly because parents are not able to recognize the onset of common cold symptoms soon enough to begin treatment, or because the dose of echinacea for use in children is not clear. There are fundamental differences in causes of upper respiratory tract infection symptoms in children versus adults (e.g., bacterial versus viral causes, different viruses, different sites of infection). Until additional research is available, echinacea cannot be considered effective in children for this use. Furthermore, development of rash has been associated with echinacea use, and therefore the risks may outweigh the potential benefits in this population.	D

Uses Based on Tradition or Theory
Abscesses, acne, attention deficit hyperactivity disorder (ADHD), bacterial infections, bee stings, boils, burn wounds, diphtheria, dizziness, eczema, gingivitis, gum inflammation (pyorrhea), hemorrhoids, herpes labialis, human immunodeficiency virus/acquired immunodeficiency syndrome, influenza, malaria, menopause, migraine headache, mouth sores, nasal congestion/runny nose, pain, psoriasis, rheumatism, skin ulcers, snake bites, stomach upset, syphilis, tonsillitis, typhoid, urinary disorders, urinary tract infections, whooping cough (pertussis).

DOSING

Adults (18 Years and Older)

- There is insufficient evidence to recommend a dose for echinacea. Echinacea is commercially available as capsules, expressed juice, extract, tincture, and tea. A common dosing range studied in trials is 500-1,000 mg of echinacea in capsule form taken by mouth three times daily for 5 to 7 days. As an extract, 300-800 mg of echinacea has been taken by mouth two to three times daily for up to 6 months.
- When applied on the skin, echinacea 15% pressed herb (non-root) juice semisolid preparation has been used daily for wounds and skin ulcers. Injected echinacea is not available commercially. Severe reactions to injected echinacea have been reported, and echinacea injections are not recommended.

Children (Younger than 18 Years)

- There is insufficient evidence to recommend a dose for echinacea in children. Parents considering echinacea for their children should discuss this decision with the child's health care provider before starting therapy. Some natural medicine practitioners recommend basing children's doses based on weight. The safety of echinacea injections is not established, and injections are not advised.

SAFETY
Allergies

- People with allergies to plants in the Asteraceae or Compositae family (ragweed, chrysanthemums, marigolds, daisies) are theoretically more likely to have allergic reactions to echinacea. Multiple cases of anaphylactic shock (severe allergic reactions) and allergic rash have been reported with echinacea taken by mouth. Allergic reactions including itching, rash, wheezing, and facial swelling, and anaphylaxis may occur more commonly in people with asthma or other allergies. Echinacea injections have caused severe reactions and are not recommended.
- Echinacea has been associated with an increased incidence of rash in children. Therefore, the risks may outweigh potential benefits, and use in children is not recommended.

Side Effects and Warnings

- Few side effects from echinacea are reported when it is used at the recommended doses. Reported complaints include stomach discomfort, nausea, sore throat, rash (allergic, hives, or painful lumps called *erythema nodosum*), drowsiness, headache, dizziness, and muscle aches. Rare cases of hepatitis (liver inflammation), kidney failure, or irregular heart rate (atrial fibrillation) have been reported in people taking echinacea, although it is not clear that these were due to echinacea itself. Injected echinacea may alter blood sugar levels and cause severe reactions and should be avoided. Echinacea has been associated with an increased incidence of rash in children, and therefore the risks of use may outweigh potential benefits. Thrombotic thrombocytopenic purpura (TTP) has also been reported.
- Some natural medicine experts discourage the use of echinacea by people with conditions affecting the immune system, such as human immunodeficiency virus/acquired immunodeficiency syndrome, some types of cancer, multiple sclerosis, tuberculosis, and rheumatological diseases (such as rheumatoid arthritis or lupus). However, there is a lack of specific studies or reports in this area, and the risks of echinacea use with these conditions are not clear. Long-term use of this herb may cause low white blood cell counts (leukopenia).
- Liver transplant patients who consume large amounts of echinacea may have increased liver enzyme activity, which often indicates liver damage. Although the relevance of this is not clear, liver transplant patients should use echinacea cautiously due to its potential hazards.

Pregnancy and Breastfeeding

- At this time, echinacea cannot be recommended during pregnancy or breastfeeding. Although early studies show no effect of echinacea on pregnancy, there is not enough research in this area. Pregnant women should avoid tinctures because of the potentially high alcohol content.

INTERACTIONS
Interactions with Drugs

- Natural medicine practitioners sometimes caution that echinacea may lead to liver inflammation. There is no clear information from laboratory or human studies in this area. Nonetheless, caution should be used when combining echinacea by mouth with other medications that can harm the liver. Examples of such agents include anabolic steroids, amiodarone, methotrexate, acetaminophen (Tylenol), and antifungal medications taken by mouth (such as ketoconazole). Echinacea may affect the way certain drugs are broken down by the liver.
- In theory, echinacea's ability to stimulate the immune system may interfere with drugs that suppress the immune system (including azathioprine, cyclosporine, and steroids such as prednisone). Because clear human studies are lacking, people taking these drugs should consult a health care professional or pharmacist before using echinacea.
- Based on one vague case report, taking echinacea along with amoxicillin may cause life-threatening reactions. However, the details of this case are not very clear.
- Early information suggests that the use of echinacea with econazole nitrate cream (Spectazole) on the skin may lower the frequency of vaginal yeast infections after treatment.
- Many tinctures contain high levels of alcohol and may cause nausea or vomiting when taken with metronidazole (Flagyl) or disulfiram (Antabuse).
- Echinacea may also interact with anesthetics, antineoplastics, and caffeine. However, these potential interactions are not fully understood.

Interactions with Herbs and Dietary Supplements

- Natural medicine practitioners sometimes caution that echinacea may lead to liver inflammation. Although there is no clear information from laboratory or human studies, in theory echinacea may add to liver toxicity caused by other agents, such as kava. Echinacea may affect the way certain herbs and supplements are broken down by the liver.
- Echinacea is sometimes used in combination products that are thought to stimulate the immune system. For example, Esberitox (PhytoPharmica, Germany) contains *Echinacea purpurea*, *Echinacea pallida*, wild indigo root *(Baptisia tinctoria)*, and thuja (white cedar). Echinacea may be combined with goldenseal or other herbs in some cold relief preparations. There is a lack of high-quality human studies that have shown added benefits or interactions of these combinations.
- Echinacea is sometimes sold in combination with goldenseal *(Hydrastis canadensis)*, an herb that may reduce the body's ability to absorb vitamin B.
- Anesthetics, antineoplastics, antioxidants, and caffeine may interact with echinacea. However, these potential interactions are not fully understood.

For a complete list of references, please visit www.naturalstandard.com.

Elder
(*Sambucus* spp.)

RELATED TERMS

- Almindelig hyld, baccae, baises de sureau, battree, black berried alder, black elder, black elderberry, boor tree, bountry, boure tree, Busine (Russian), Caprifoliaceae (family), cyanidin-3-glucoside, cyanidin-3-sambubioside, devil's eye, elderberry, elderberry anthocyanins, elderberry bark agglutinin, elderberry juice, ellanwood, ellhorn, European alder, European elder, European elderberry, European elderflower, European elder fruit, frau holloe, German elder, Holunderbeeren, Holunderblüten, lady elder, nigrin b, old gal, old lady, peonidin 3-glucoside, peonidin 3-sambubioside, peonidin monoglucuronide, pipe tree, Rubini (elderberry extract), sambreo (Italian), sambuco (Italian), *Sambucus sieboldiana* (Japanese), Sambuci flos, Sauco (Spanish), Schwarzer holunder (German), sieboldin-b, stinking elder, Sureau noir (French), sweet elder, tree of doom, yakori bengestro.

BACKGROUND

- Several species of the genus *Sambucus* produce elderberries. Most research and publications refer to black elder (*Sambucus nigra*). Other species with similar chemical components include the American elder or common elder (*Sambucus canadensis*), antelope brush (*Sambucus tridentata*), blue elderberry (*Sambucus caerulea*), danewort or dwarf elder (*Sambucus ebulus*), red-fruited elder (*Sambucus pubens* or *Sambucus racemosa*), and *Sambucus formosana*. American elder (*Sambucus canadensis*) and European elder (*Sambucus nigra*) are often discussed simultaneously in the literature because they have many of the same uses and contain common constituents.

- European elder grows up to 30 feet tall, is native to Europe, but has been naturalized to the Americas. Historically, the flowers and leaves have been used for pain relief, swelling/inflammation, diuresis (urine production), and as a diaphoretic or expectorant. The leaves have been used externally for sitz baths. The bark, when aged, has been used as a diuretic, laxative, or emetic (induces vomiting). The berries have been used traditionally in food as flavoring and in the preparation of elderberry wine and pies.

- The flowers and berries (blue/black only) are used most often medicinally. They contain flavonoids, which are found to possess a variety of actions, including antioxidant and immunological properties. Although hypothesized to be beneficial, there is no definitive evidence from well-conducted human clinical trials currently available regarding the use of elder.

- The bark, leaves, seeds, and raw/unripe fruit contain the cyanogenic glycoside sambunigrin, which is potentially toxic.

EVIDENCE

Uses Based on Scientific Evidence	Grade
Influenza Elderberry juice may improve flu-like symptoms, such as fever, fatigue, headache, sore throat, cough, and aches, in less time than it normally takes to get over the flu.	B
Bacterial Sinusitis Elder has been observed to reduce excessive sinus mucus secretion in laboratory studies. There is only limited research specifically using elder to treat sinusitis in humans. Combination products containing elder and other herbs (such as Sinupret) have been reported to have beneficial effects when used with antibiotics to treat sinus infections, although the majority of this evidence is not high quality.	C
Bronchitis There is a small amount of research on the combination herbal product Sinupret in patients with bronchitis. This formula contains elder flowers (*Sambucus nigra*) as well as gentian root, verbena, cowslip flower, and sorrel. Although benefits have been suggested, because of design problems with this research, no clear conclusion can be drawn either for Sinupret or elder in the management of bronchitis.	C
High Cholesterol There is a lack of reliable research evaluating elder alone as a treatment for high cholesterol levels. Preliminary evidence suggests that elderberry juice may decrease serum cholesterol concentrations and increase low-density lipoprotein (LDL or "bad" cholesterol) stability. Additional research is needed in this area before a firm conclusion can be reached. Elder should not be used in the place of other more proven therapies, and patients are advised to speak with primary health care providers before using elderberry for treatment of high cholesterol levels.	C

Uses Based on Tradition or Theory

Alzheimer's disease, angioprotectant, antiinflammatory, antioxidant, antispasmodic, asthma, astringent, blood vessel disorders, burns, cancer, chafing, circulatory stimulant, cold sores, colds, colic, cough suppressant, dental plaque and gingivitis, diabetes, diuresis (urine production), edema, epilepsy, fever, flavoring, fragrance (perfume), gout, gut disorders, hair dye, hay fever, headache, herpes, human immunodeficiency virus (HIV), immune stimulant, increased sweating, insomnia, joint swelling, kidney disease, laryngitis, laxative, liver disease, measles, migraines, mosquito repellant, nerve pain, osteoporosis, psoriasis, respiratory distress, sedative, skin infections, stomach ulcers, stress reduction, syphilis, toothache, ulcerative colitis, vomiting, weight loss.

DOSING
Adults (18 Years and Older)

- Patients were given 400 mg spray-dried powder capsules containing 10% anthocyanins three times a day equivalent to 5 mL of elderberry juice for 2 weeks in one study for high cholesterol levels.

- For treating influenza or flu-like symptoms, a dose of 4 tbsp of elderberry extract taken daily by mouth for 3 days has been used.
- Cream has been prepared by taking several handfuls of fresh elder flowers, mixing in liquefied petroleum jelly, simmering for 40 minutes, heating, filtering, and allowing the formula to solidify. This has been applied to the hands at bedtime.
- For bacterial sinusitis, a dose of 2 tablets of Sinupret taken by mouth three times daily with antibiotics has been used. Sinupret contains elder and several other herbs.
- A dose of 15 mL of elderberry syrup has been taken four times a day for 5 days for influenza symptoms.
- A dose of 3-5 g of dried elder flowers steeped in 1 cup of boiling water for 10-15 minutes taken three times daily by mouth has been used. Be aware of possible toxicity.

Children (Younger than 18 Years)

- There is insufficient evidence to recommend the safe use of elder in children. Toxicity has been reported, and caution is recommended.

SAFETY
Allergies

- Avoid elder in patients with known allergy to plants in the Caprifoliaceae family (honeysuckle family). There are some reports of allergies in children playing with toys made from fresh elder stems.

Side Effects and Warnings

- Elderberry products should be used under the direction of a qualified health care provider because of the possible risk of cyanide toxicity, especially from elder bark, root, or leaves.
- There are reports of gastrointestinal distress, diarrhea, vomiting, abdominal cramps, and weakness after drinking elderberry juice made from crushed leaves, stems, and uncooked elderberries. Notably, the berries must be cooked to prevent nausea or cyanide toxicity.
- Allergies are possible from fresh elder stems and may include rash, skin irritation, or difficulty breathing.
- In theory, high doses or long-term use of elder flowers may have diuretic (urine-producing) effects. People taking diuretics or drugs that interact with diuretics should use caution when taking products containing elder.
- Elder may also lower blood sugar levels. Additional blood tests may be necessary. Dizziness, headache, convulsions, and rapid heart rate have also been reported.

Pregnancy and Breastfeeding

- Elder cannot be recommended during pregnancy or breastfeeding based on a theoretical risk of birth defects or spontaneous abortion. Gastrointestinal discomfort in pregnant women taking elderberry has been reported.

INTERACTIONS
Interactions with Drugs

- Elder may possess diuretic (urine-producing) effects and should be used cautiously with drugs that increase urination. Elder may possess laxative effects and should be used cautiously with other laxatives.
- Elder may lower blood sugar levels. Caution is advised when medications that may also lower blood sugar are used. A qualified health care provider should closely monitor patients taking drugs for diabetes by mouth or using insulin. Medication adjustments may be necessary.
- The flavonoid quercetin, which is found in elder, has been reported to inhibit xanthine oxidase and may affect caffeine and theophylline levels. Patients using theophylline should speak with their health care provider before using elder.
- Elder may increase the effects and possible adverse effects of some cancer chemotherapies.
- Based on preliminary research, increased benefits may be seen when elder is used in combination with antibiotics and decongestants, such as oxymetazoline (Afrin). Elder flowers may possess antiinflammatory properties and may add to the effects of some drugs that also decrease inflammation.

Interactions with Herbs and Dietary Supplements

- Elder may possess diuretic (urine-producing) effects and should be used cautiously with herbs that may increase urination, such as artichoke, dandelion, or horsetail.
- Elder may possess laxative effects and should be used cautiously with herbs that may also have laxative effects, such as alder buckthorn, Dong quai, or psyllium.
- Elder may lower blood sugar levels. Caution is advised when herbs or supplements are used that may also lower blood sugar, such as aloe, burdock, fenugreek, maitake mushroom, or milk thistle. Blood glucose levels may require monitoring, and doses may need adjustment.
- Increased effects may be seen when elder is used in combination with other antioxidants, such as vitamin C or flavonoids like quercetin.
- Taking sucrose (table sugar) and elder together may decrease elimination of the anthocyanin component of elder.
- Elder may also interact with herbs and supplements with anticancer, antibacterial, decongestant, and antiinflammatory activities.

For a complete list of references, please visit www.naturalstandard.com.

Elecampane
(*Inula helenium*)

RELATED TERMS

- Alant, alant camphor, alantolactone, alantopicrin, Asteraceae (family), *Aster helenium* (L.) Scop., *Aster officinalis* All., Compositae (family), dammaradienol, dammaradienyl acetate, elecampane, elecampane camphor, elfwort, eudesmanes, eudesmanolides, friedelin, germacrane, helenin, helenin camphor, *Helenium grandiflorum* Gilib., horseheal, inula, *Inula campana*, inula camphor, *Inula helenium*, *Inula racemosa*, inulin, isoalantolactone, isocostunolide, mucilage, scabwort, sesquiterpenes, sitosterols, stigmasterol, thymol derivatives, yellow starwort.

BACKGROUND

- Elecampane is a tall wildflower with oversized pointed leaves and yellow to orange daisy-like flowers. Elecampane is a natural source of food flavoring in Europe and is approved for use in alcoholic beverages in the United States.
- Traditionally, elecampane is used as an antifungal, antiparasitic, and general antimicrobial agent, as well as an expectorant for coughs, colds, and bronchial ailments. At this time, there is a lack of evidence from randomized, controlled trials to support these uses.

EVIDENCE

Uses Based on Scientific Evidence

No available studies qualify for inclusion in the evidence table.

Uses Based on Tradition or Theory

Angina pectoris (chest pain), antibiotic, antifungal, antimicrobial, antioxidant, antiparasitic (roundworm, threadworm, hookworm, whipworm), antiseptic, antispasmodic, antiviral, boils, bronchial congestion, bronchitis, cancer, cardiovascular disease, colds, cough, decongestant/expectorant, diabetes, digestive tonic, headaches, hypertension (high blood pressure), hypnotic/sleep (aromatherapy), hypoxia (low oxygen levels), immunostimulant, irritable bowel syndrome, laxative, muscle tension, myocardial infarction (heart attack), pain (various causes), pruritus (itchy skin), sedative, skin conditions, stress, tuberculosis.

DOSING

Adults (18 Years and Older)

- Secondary sources suggest 1.5-4 g rhizome/root in capsule form or as a decoction, three times daily, or 300 mg alantolactone daily for two courses of 5 days with an interval of 10 days.
- Secondary sources suggest 15-25 drops of tinctured elecampane root daily.

Children (Younger than 18 Years)

- Secondary sources suggest 50-200 mg alantolactone daily for two courses of 5 days with an interval of 10 days.

- Secondary sources suggest 7-12 drops of tinctured elecampane root daily.

SAFETY
Allergies

- Avoid in individuals with a known allergy or hypersensitivity to elecampane or members of the Compositae/Asteraceae family such as dandelion, goldenrod, ragweed, sunflower, and daisies.
- Five cases of occupational allergic contact dermatitis caused by the Compositae family were diagnosed in a 14-year period. Elecampane was one of four plants indicated in the five cases.

Side Effects and Warnings

- There is inadequate available information regarding adverse effects associated with elecampane. Contact allergic dermatitis is the most commonly reported adverse event.
- Use cautiously in patients using glucose-modifying agents because of the potential for additive or opposite effects.
- Use cautiously in patients using blood pressure–altering agents, anticancer agents, heart agents, laxatives, muscle relaxants, or sedatives because of the potential for additive effects.
- Avoid in patients with allergies to the Compositae/Asteraceae family such as dandelion, goldenrod, ragweed, sunflower, and daisies.

Pregnancy and Breastfeeding

- Elecampane is not recommended in pregnant or breastfeeding women because of a lack of available scientific evidence.

INTERACTIONS
Interactions with Drugs

- Traditionally, elecampane has been added to white wine for the treatment of bronchitis. Use cautiously with alcohol.
- Elecampane may have moderate antibacterial activity. Use cautiously with antibiotics because of possible additive effects.
- Elecampane may alter blood sugar levels. Caution is advised when medication that may also alter blood sugar are used. Patients taking drugs for diabetes by mouth or using insulin should be monitored closely by a qualified health care provider. Medication adjustments may be necessary.
- Elecampane may have moderate antifungal and antiparasitic activity; use cautiously.
- Elecampane may have additive effects with other blood pressure–altering agents, anticancer agents, and laxative agents in humans; use cautiously.
- Elecampane may have antioxidant properties.
- Elecampane may have additive effects with agents that induce muscle relaxation. Use cautiously with antispasmodic medications.
- Elecampane may have additive effects with cardiac agents in humans. Use cautiously with heart medications.
- Elecampane may increase the amount of drowsiness caused by some drugs. Examples include benzodiazepines such as

lorazepam (Ativan) or diazepam (Valium), barbiturates such as phenobarbital, narcotics such as caffeine, some antidepressants, and alcohol. Use caution while driving or operating machinery.

Interactions with Herbs and Dietary Supplements

- Elecampane may have moderate antibacterial activity, antifungal activity, anticancer activity, antioxidant properties, and antiparasitic activity. Use cautiously with herbs and supplements with similar effects.
- Elecampane may have additive effects with agents that induce muscle relaxation; use cautiously with herbs with such activity.
- Elecampane may have additive effects with cardiac agents in humans. Use cautiously with herbs and supplements taken for the heart.
- *Echinacea* and osha (*Ligusticum porteri*) root have been used in combination with elecampane for respiratory ailments. Use cautiously.

- There is a potential for additive effects between elecampane and ginger as laxative agents in humans. There is also a potential for additive effects between elecampane and ginger as anticancer agents in humans.
- Elecampane may alter blood sugar levels. Caution is advised when herbs or supplements that may also alter blood sugar are used. Blood glucose levels may require monitoring, and doses may need adjustment.
- Elecampane may have additive effects with other blood pressure–altering herbs and supplements in humans; use cautiously.
- Use cautiously with herbs and supplements with laxative effects and those taken for respiratory ailments.
- Elecampane may increase the amount of drowsiness caused by some herbs and supplements. Use caution while driving or operating machinery.

For a complete list of references, please visit www.naturalstandard.com.

Emu Oil

(Dromaius novaehollandiae)

RELATED TERMS

- Australian emu, Casuariidae (family), *Dromaius novaehollandiae*, emu oil cream, emu oil lotion, oleic acid, omega-3 fatty acids, omega-6 fatty acids, omega-9 fatty acids, ratite, Thunder Ridge Emu Oil.

BACKGROUND

- Emu oil is the refined and deodorized oil made from the back fat of the emu. Emu oil was used by the aboriginal tribes of Australia to protect against sun damage and was then introduced to European settlers.
- Emu oil is now recommended by manufacturers for improving arthritis, burns, cuts, eczema, hair loss, high cholesterol levels, nosebleeds, psoriasis, skin softness, and stretch marks. However, currently there is not enough evidence available in humans to support the use of emu oil for any indication.

EVIDENCE

Uses Based on Scientific Evidence	Grade
Cosmetic Uses Limited research has examined emu oil for cosmetic uses, such as in moisturizers.	C

Uses Based on Tradition or Theory
Alopecia (hair loss), antibacterial, antiinflammatory, arthritis, atherosclerosis (hardening of the arteries), bruising, burns, cirrhosis (liver disease), cramps, dermatitis, dysmenorrhea (painful menstrual period), eczema, gastrointestinal conditions, high blood pressure, high cholesterol levels, hot flashes, joint pain, leg ulcers, muscle pain, nosebleeds, pain, psoriasis, reproductive disorders (female), skin conditions, stretch marks, sun protection, tumors, wound healing.

DOSING

Adults (18 Years and Older)

- There is insufficient evidence to recommend a dose for emu oil in adults.

Children (Younger than 18 Years)

- There is insufficient evidence to recommend a dose for emu oil in children.

SAFETY

Allergies

- Avoid in individuals with a known allergy or hypersensitivity to emus (*Dromaius novaehollandiae*), emu oil, or its constituents.

Side Effects and Warnings

- Emu oil is likely safe when applied to the skin in healthy people short-term.
- Restless leg syndrome has been associated with emu oil, although it is not well proven.
- Use cautiously if taking antiinflammatory agents.
- Avoid in individuals with a known allergy or hypersensitivity to emus (*Dromaius novaehollandiae*), emu oil, or its constituents.

Pregnancy and Breastfeeding

- Emu oil is not recommended in pregnant or breastfeeding women because of a lack of available scientific evidence.

INTERACTIONS

Interactions with Drugs

- Emu oil applied to the skin may reduce local, short-term inflammation and therefore have additive effects with antiinflammatory drugs.

Interactions with Herbs and Dietary Supplements

- Emu oil applied to the skin may reduce local, short-term inflammation and therefore have additive effects with antiinflammatory herbs and supplements.

For a complete list of references, please visit www.naturalstandard.com.

Ephedra/Ma Huang
(*Ephedra sinica*)

RELATED TERMS

- Amp II, amsania, brigham tea, budshur, cao Ma huang (Chinese), cathine, chewa, Chinese ephedra, Chinese joint fir, D-pseudoephedrine, desert herb, desert tea, dextro-rotatory, EPH 833, *Ephedra altissima*, *Ephedra americana*, *Ephedra antisyphilitica*, *Ephedra distacha*, *Ephedra distachya*, *Ephedra equisetina* (Mongolian Ephedra), *Ephedra fasciculata*, *Ephedra gerardiana*, *Ephedra helvetica*, *Ephedra intermedia* (intermediate ephedra), *Ephedra likiangensis*, *Ephedra major*, *Ephedra minuta*, *Ephedra monosperma*, *Ephedra nebrodensis*, *Ephedra nevadensis*, *Ephedra przewalskii*, *Ephedra regeliana*, *Ephedra sinica*, *Ephedra shennungiana*, *Ephedra trifurca*, *Ephedra viridis*, *Ephedra vulgaris*, Ephedraceae (family), ephedra alkaloids, Ephedra soup medicines, ephedrae herba, ephedrine, ephedrine alkaloids, ephedrine hydrochloride, ephedrine sulphate, ephedroid, epicatechin, epitonin, European ephedra, Gnetales, herba ephedrae, horsetail, hum, huma, Indian joint fir, intermediate ephedra, isoephedrine, joint fir, khama, L-ephedrine, levorotatory ephedrine, mahoàng, máhuáng, "Mao" (Chinese), maokon, mahuuanggen, methylephedrine, methylpseudoephedrine, Mexican tea, môc tac ma hoàng, Mongolian ephedra, Mormon tea, mu-tsei-ma-huang, muzei mu huang, natural ecstasy, neuropeptide Y, norephedrine, norpseudoephedrine, O-coumaric acid beta-D-glucopyranoside (nebrodenside B), O-coumaric acid glucoside, phok, popotillo, pseudoephedrine, quinoline, san-ma-huang, sea grape, shrubby, soma, song tuê ma hoàng, squaw tea, synephrine, tannins, teamster's tea, trun aa hoàng, tsao-ma-huang, tutgantha, yellow astringent, yellow horse, zhong Ma huang.
- **Note:** There are approximately 40 species of ephedra.

BACKGROUND

- On February 6, 2004, the U.S. Food and Drug Administration (FDA) issued a final rule prohibiting the sale of dietary supplements containing ephedrine alkaloids (ephedra) because such supplements present an unreasonable risk of illness or injury. The rule became effective 60 days from the date of publication.
- In 2005 this rule was struck down in Utah but reversed again 4 months later, so ephedra is currently banned throughout the United States. It remains unclear whether ephedra will reappear on the market, despite widespread acknowledgment of significant safety risks, including serious potential cardiovascular events or death.
- *Ephedra sinica*, a species of ephedra (ma huang), contains the alkaloids ephedrine and pseudoephedrine, which have been found to induce central nervous system (CNS) stimulation, bronchodilation, and vasoconstriction. In combination with caffeine, ephedrine appears to elicit weight loss (in trials of 1-12 months' duration). However, studies of ephedra or ephedrine monotherapy have been equivocal. Numerous trials have documented the efficacy of ephedrine in the management of asthmatic bronchoconstriction and hypotension. However, commercial preparations of nonprescription supplements containing ephedra have not been systematically studied for these indications.

- Major safety concerns have been associated with ephedra or ephedrine use, including hypertension (high blood pressure), tachycardia, CNS excitation, arrhythmia, myocardial infarction (heart attack), and stroke.
- Despite widely publicized safety concerns and the highly publicized 2003 death of a U.S. major league baseball pitcher thought to be related to ephedra, before the ban on ephedra, 14% of individuals using nonprescription weight-loss products in the United States continued to take ephedra or ephedrine-containing products.

EVIDENCE

Uses Based on Scientific Evidence	Grade
Weight Loss Ephedra contains the chemical ephedrine, which appears to cause weight loss when used in combination with caffeine, based on the available scientific evidence. The results of research on ephedrine alone without caffeine are unclear. The amounts of ephedrine in commercially available products have varied widely. Other weight loss treatments have been more commonly recommended because of significant safety concerns with combination products containing ephedra and caffeine.	A
Bronchodilator (Asthma) Ephedra contains the chemicals ephedrine and pseudoephedrine, which are bronchodilators (expand the airways to assist in easier breathing). It has been used and studied to treat asthma and chronic obstructive pulmonary disease in both children and adults. Other treatments, such as beta-agonist inhalers (e.g., albuterol), are more commonly recommended because of safety concerns with ephedra or ephedrine.	B
Allergic Nasal Symptoms (Used as a Nose Wash) Early studies suggest that ephedrine nasal spray, a chemical in ephedra, may help treat symptoms of nasal allergies. Additional research is needed before a firm recommendation can be made.	C
Low Blood Pressure Chemicals in ephedra can stimulate the heart, increase heart rate, and raise blood pressure. Ephedrine, a component of ephedra, is sometimes used in hospitals to help control blood pressure. However, the effects of over-the-counter ephedra supplements taken by mouth are not well described in this area.	C
Sexual Arousal There is limited evidence that ephedra may increase sexual arousal in women.	C

DOSING
Adults (18 Years and Older)

- **Note:** The U.S. Federal Government has banned the sale of ephedra since 2004. Consumers are urged to stop using the herbal weight control supplement immediately as it has been linked to numerous adverse health effects, including death.

- Ephedra may cause serious adverse effects in any dose, particularly when used with other drugs such as caffeine. Because of serious safety concerns, ephedra cannot be recommended in any dose.

Children (Younger than 18 Years)

- Ephedrine is not recommended in children because of the risk of toxicity and death.

SAFETY
Allergies

- Persons with a known allergy to ephedra, ephedrine, or pseudoephedrine (Sudafed) should avoid ephedra. Signs of allergy may include rash, itching, or red, flaking skin.

Side Effects and Warnings

- The U.S. FDA has collected thousands of reports of serious adverse effects (including more than 100 deaths) from the use of various products containing ephedra or ephedrine. The U.S. federal government has banned the sale of ephedra since 2004. Consumers are urged to stop using the herbal weight control supplement immediately as it has been linked to numerous adverse health effects, including death.

- Some people may experience abdominal discomfort (nausea, vomiting, diarrhea, loss of appetite, constipation), anxiety, dizziness, headache, tremor, insomnia, dry mouth, delirium, or fainting. Ephedra may also cause irritability, euphoria, hallucinations, seizures, or stroke, as well as low potassium levels in the blood, exaggerated reflexes, weakness, muscle aches, muscle damage, depression, mania, agitation, suicidal ideas, or Parkinson's disease–like symptoms. Persons with prior strokes or transient ischemic attacks (TIAs/"mini-strokes"), tremor, or insomnia should avoid ephedra. Individuals with a history of a psychiatric illness, especially if treated with monoamine oxidase inhibitors (MAOIs), must first discuss ephedra with a qualified health care provider before taking supplements. Examples of MAOIs include isocarboxazid (Marplan), phenelzine (Nardil), and tranylcypromine (Parnate).

- Ephedra can cause chest tightness, irregular heart rhythms, damage to the heart muscle, high blood pressure, heart attack, inflammation of the heart, fluid retention in the lungs, breathing difficulties, dilated cardiomyopathy, left ventricular systolic dysfunction, coronary dissection, thrombosis, or cardiac arrest. Ephedra should be used with extreme caution in persons with a history of heart disease, heart rate disorders, or high blood pressure. Other side effects may include liver damage, kidney stones, difficulty passing urine or pain when urinating, increased urine production, or contractions of the uterus. These potential effects may limit the use of ephedra by people with kidney disease or enlarged prostate. Individuals with thyroid gland disorders or glaucoma should use ephedra cautiously. In theory, ephedra may lower blood sugar levels. Caution is advised in patients with diabetes or hypoglycemia, and in those taking drugs, herbs, or supplements that affect blood sugar. Serum glucose levels may need to be monitored by a qualified health care provider, and medication adjustments may be necessary.

- It has been recommended that ephedra (ma huang) use be stopped at least 1 week before major surgical or diagnostic procedures.

Pregnancy and Breastfeeding

- Ephedra should not be used during pregnancy because of risks to the mother and fetus. Ephedrine crosses the placenta and has been found to increase fetal heart rate. Ephedra may induce uterine contractions.

- Ephedra should not be used during breastfeeding because of risks to the mother and child. Ephedrine crosses into breast milk and has been associated with irritability, crying, and insomnia in infants.

INTERACTIONS
Interactions with Drugs

- Many drugs can cause increased stimulation when used with ephedra or ephedrine. Examples include caffeine and theophylline. When combined with ephedra, these drugs may lead to difficulty sleeping, nervousness, or stomach upset. The combination of ephedrine and caffeine may be fatal. Many products contain both ephedrine and caffeine and should be used with caution, if at all.

- Combined ingestion of caffeine and ephedrine has been observed to increase blood glucose and lactate concentrations. Ephedrine and dopamine concentrations are significantly increased. A case report exists of ephedra use associated with the onset of psychosis and autonomic hyperactivity after administration of risperidone.

- Bronchodilators used for asthma or the decongestant pseudoephedrine (Sudafed) may have increased bronchodilating effects when used with ephedra.

- If ephedra is taken with MAOI antidepressants, such as isocarboxazid (Marplan), phenelzine (Nardil), and tranylcypromine (Parnate), severe side effects may develop, including dangerously high blood pressure, muscle damage, fever, and irregular heart rate. Other antidepressants and medications for psychiatric disorders (e.g., phenothiazines, tricyclics, and selective serotonin reuptake inhibitors [SSRIs]) may reduce the effects of ephedra and cause low blood pressure and rapid heartbeat.

- Because ephedra affects blood pressure and heart rate, it may alter the effectiveness of medications given to control blood pressure or heart rhythm, including digoxin, alpha-blockers, beta-blockers, diuretics, calcium-channel blockers, or angiotensin-converting enzyme (ACE) inhibitors. The side effects of ephedra may be worsened by guanethidine, ergot alkaloids (bromocriptine, dihydroergotamine, ergotamine), oxytocin (Pitocin), diuretics, morphine, and anesthetic drugs (halothane, cyclopropane, propofol).

- Ephedra may lower blood sugar levels, although ephedra-caffeine combinations may increase blood sugar. Caution is advised when medications that may also alter blood sugar are used. Patients taking drugs for diabetes by mouth or using insulin should be monitored closely by a qualified health care provider. Medication adjustments may be necessary.
- Ephedra may reduce the effects of steroids such as dexamethasone. Ephedra may increase serum levels of thyroid hormones and may alter thyroid hormone treatments. Medications that alter the acidity of urine may reduce the effectiveness of ephedra.
- Effects of cholesterol-lowering medications may be altered by ephedra, although this has not been proven.
- Phenylpropanolamine, previously removed from the U.S. market, may lead to additive effects if taken with ephedra. Caution is advised when other agents taken for weight loss are used.
- Ephedra may also interact with alcohol, general anesthetics, and drugs taken for gout. Ephedra products should be stopped 24 hours before surgery.

Interactions with Herbs and Dietary Supplements

- The stimulant effects of ephedra may be increased when combined with herbs and supplements that have stimulant properties or with supplements that contain caffeine, such as guarana, cola nut, bitter orange, and yerba mate.

Commercially available products may contain combinations of ephedrine and caffeine or guarana. Ephedra may alter thyroid hormones and should be used cautiously with other herbs or supplements that affect thyroid hormones, such as bladderwrack (seaweed, kelp).

- Ephedra may decrease the effectiveness of cardiac glycosides (supplements taken for heart failure and irregular heart beat).
- Ephedra may raise blood pressure and may increase the blood pressure–raising effects of herbs such as American ginseng.
- Ephedra may lower blood sugar levels. Caution is advised when herbs or supplements that may also lower blood sugar are used. Blood glucose levels may require monitoring, and doses may need adjustment.
- Ephedra may increase the diuretic effects of herbs such as artichoke. Ephedra may also interact with urine acidifiers/alkalinizers.
- Combining ephedra with herbs that have possible MAOI antidepressant activity such as St. John's wort may cause severe side effects, including dangerously high blood pressure, muscle breakdown, fever, and irregular heartbeats. Ephedra may also interact with other antidepressant herbs such as those that have SSRI activity.
- Effects of cholesterol-lowering herbs and supplements may be altered by ephedra, although this has not been proven.
- Ephedra may also interact with herbs taken for gout or herbs with hormonal activity.

For a complete list of references, please visit www.naturalstandard.com.

Essiac

RELATED TERMS

- Burdock root *(Arctium lappa)* synonyms/related terms: Aku-jitsu, anthraxivore, arctii, *Arctium minus*, *Arctium tomentosa*, bardana, *Bardanae radix*, bardane, bardane grande (French), beggar's buttons, burr, burr seed, chin, clot-burr, clotbur, cocklebur, cockle button, cocklebuttons, cuckold, daiki kishi, edible burdock, fox's clote, grass burdock, great bur, great burdock, great burdocks, gobo (Japan), Grosse klette (German), happy major, hardock, hare burr, hurrburr, Kletterwurzel (German), lampazo (Spanish), lappola, love leaves, niu bang zi, oil of lappa, personata, Philanthropium, thorny burr, turkey burrseed, woo-bang-ja, wild gobo.
- Sheep sorrel *(Rumex acetosella)* synonyms/related terms: Acedera, acid sorrel, azeda-brava, buckler leaf, cigreto, common sorrel, cuckoo sorrow, cuckoo's meate, dock, dog-eared sorrel, field sorrel, French sorrel, garden sorrel, gowke-meat, greensauce, green sorrel, herba acetosa, kemekulagi, Polygonaceae (family), red sorrel, red top sorrel, round leaf sorrel, *Rumex scutatus*, *Rumex acetosa* L., sheephead sorrel, sheep's sorrel, sorrel, sorrel dock, sour dock, sour grass, sour sabs, sour suds, sour sauce, Wiesensauerampfer, wild sorrel.
- Slippery elm inner bark *(Ulmus fulva)* synonyms/related terms: Indian elm, moose elm, red elm, rock elm, slippery elm, sweet elm, Ulmaceae, Ulmi rubrae cortex, *Ulmus fulva* Michaux, *Ulmus rubra*, winged elm.
- Turkish rhubarb *(Rheum palmatum)* synonyms/related terms: Baoshen pill, Canton rhubarb, Chinesischer Rhabarber (German), Chinese rhubarb, chong-gi-huang, common rhubarb, da-huang, Da Huang, daio, Da huang Liujingao, English rhubarb, Extractum Rhei Liquidum, Himalayan rhubarb, Indian rhubarb, Japanese rhubarb, Jiang-Zhi Jian-Fei Yao (JZJFY), Jinghuang tablet, medicinal rhubarb, pie rhubarb, Polygonaceae (family), Pyralvex, Pyralvex Berna, racine de rhubarbee (French), RET (rhubarb extract tablet), rhabarber, rhei radix, rhei rhizoma, rheum, *Rheum australe*, *Rheum emodi* Wall., *Rheum officinale* Baill., *Rheum rhabarbarum*, *Rheum rhaponticum* L., *Rheum tanguticum* Maxim., *Rheum tanguticum* Maxim. ex. Balf., *Rheum tanguticum* Maxim. L., *Rheum undulatum*, *Rheum x cultorum*, *Rheum webbianum* (Indian or Himalayan rhubarb), rhizoma, rheirhubarbe de chine (French), rhubarb, rubarbo, ruibarbo (Spanish), shenshi rhubarb, tai huang, Turkey rhubarb.

BACKGROUND

- Essiac contains a combination of herbs, including burdock root *(Arctium lappa)*, sheep sorrel *(Rumex acetosella)*, slippery elm inner bark *(Ulmus fulva)*, and Turkish rhubarb *(Rheum palmatum)*. The original formula was developed in the 1920s by the Canadian nurse Reneé Caisse *(Essiac* is Caisse spelled backwards). The recipe is said to be based on a traditional Ojibwa (Native American) remedy, and Caisse administered the formula by mouth and injection to numerous cancer patients during the 1920s and 1930s. The exact ingredients and amounts in the original formulation remain a secret.
- During investigations by the Canadian government and public hearings in the late 1930s, it remained unclear if Essiac was an effective cancer treatment. Amidst controversy, Caisse

closed her clinic in 1942. In the 1950s, Caisse provided samples of Essiac to Dr. Charles Brusch, founder of the Brusch Medical Center in Cambridge, Massachusetts, who administered Essiac to patients. It is unclear if Brusch was given access to the secret formula). According to some accounts, additional herbs were added to these later formulations, including blessed thistle *(Cnicus benedictus)*, red clover *(Trifolium pratense)*, kelp *(Laminaria digitata)*, and watercress *(Nasturtium officinale)*.
- A laboratory at Memorial Sloan-Kettering Cancer Center tested Essiac samples (provided by Caisse) on mice during the 1970s. This research was not formally published, and there is controversy regarding the results; some accounts note no benefits and others report significant effects (including an account by Dr. Brusch). Questions were later raised of improper preparation of the formula. Caisse subsequently refused requests by researchers at Memorial Sloan-Kettering and the U.S. National Cancer Institute for access to the recipe.
- In the 1970s, Caisse provided the formula to Resperin Corporation Ltd., with the understanding that Resperin would coordinate a scientific trial in humans. Although a study was initiated, it was stopped early amidst questions of improper preparation of the formula and inadequate study design. This research was never completed. Resperin Corporation Ltd., which owned the Essiac name, formally went out of business after transferring rights to the Essiac name and selling the secret formula to Essiac Products Ltd., which currently distributes products through Essiac International.
- Despite the lack of available scientific evidence, Essiac and Essiac-like products (with similar ingredients) remain popular among patients, particularly among those with cancer. Essiac is most commonly taken as a tea. A survey conducted in the year 2000 found almost 15% of Canadian women with breast cancer to be using Essiac. It has also become popular in patients with human immunodeficiency virus (HIV) and diabetes and in healthy individuals for its purported immune-enhancing properties, although there is a lack of reliable scientific research in these areas.
- There are more than 40 Essiac-like products available in North America, Europe, and Australia. Flor-Essence includes the original four herbs (burdock root, sheep sorrel, slippery elm bark, and Turkish rhubarb) as well as herbs that were later added as "potentiators" (blessed thistle, red clover, kelp, watercress). Virginias Herbal E-Tonic contains the four original herbs along with echinacea and black walnut. Other commercial formulations may include additional ingredients, such as cat's claw *(Uncaria tomentosa)*.

EVIDENCE

Uses Based on Scientific Evidence	Grade
Cancer There is a lack of properly conducted published human studies using Essiac for cancer. Currently, there is not enough evidence to recommend for or against the use of this herbal mixture as a therapy for any type of cancer.	C

DOSING

Adults (18 Years and Older)

- Historically, Essiac was administered by mouth or injection. The most common current use is as a tea. There is a lack of reliable published human studies of Essiac or Essiac-like products, and safety or effectiveness has not been established scientifically for any dose. Instructions for tea preparation and dosing vary from product to product. Patients are advised to read product labels and speak with their cancer health care professional before starting any new therapy, such as Essiac or Essiac-like products.
- Women with breast cancer have taken low doses (total daily dose, 43.6 ± 30.8 mL) of Essiac that matched the label instructions on most Essiac products.

Children (Younger than 18 Years)

- There is insufficient evidence to recommend the safe use of Essiac or Essiac-like products in children.

SAFETY

Allergies

- Reports of Essiac allergies are lacking in the published scientific literature, although reactions in individuals with allergy to members of the Asteraceae/Compositae family, such as ragweed, potentially can occur because of any of the included herbs. Anaphylaxis has been reported after rhubarb leaf ingestion, and there are reports of allergic reactions to sorrel products taken by mouth. Contact dermatitis (skin rash after direct contact) has been reported with exposure to burdock, slippery elm bark, and rhubarb leaves. Cross-sensitivity to burdock may occur in individuals allergic to chrysanthemums, marigolds, and daisies.

Side Effects and Warnings

- The safety of Essiac is not well studied scientifically. Safety concerns are based on theoretical and known reactions associated with herbal components of Essiac: burdock root (*Arctium lappa*), sheep sorrel (*Rumex acetosella*), slippery elm bark (*Ulmus fulva*), and Turkish rhubarb (*Rheum palmatum*). However, the safety and toxic effects of these individual herbs are also not well studied. Various Essiac-like products may contain different or additional ingredients, and patients are advised to carefully review product labels.
- Potentially toxic compounds present in Essiac include tannins, oxalic acid, and anthraquinones. Tannins, present in burdock, sorrel, rhubarb, and slippery elm, may cause stomach upset and in high concentrations may lead to kidney or liver damage. In theory, long-term use of tannins may increase the risk of head and neck cancers, although there are no documented human cases.

- Oxalic acid, contained in rhubarb, slippery elm, and sorrel, can cause serious adverse effects when taken in high doses (particularly in children). Oxalic acid toxicity/poisoning may be associated with nausea, vomiting, mouth/throat burning, dangerously low blood pressure, blood electrolyte imbalances, seizure, throat swelling that interferes with breathing, and liver or kidney damage. Deaths from oxalic acid poisoning have been reported in an adult man eating soup containing sorrel and in a 4-year-old child eating rhubarb leaves. The amount of oxalic acid in Essiac preparations is not known. In cases of suspected oxalic acid poisoning, medical attention should be sought immediately. Regular intake of oxalic acid may increase the risk of kidney stones.
- Anthraquinones in rhubarb root or sheep sorrel may lead to diarrhea, intestinal cramping, and loss of fluid and electrolytes (such as potassium). Use of rhubarb may lead to discoloration of the urine (bright yellow or red) or of the inner mucosal surface of the intestine (a condition called melanosis coli). Fluoride poisoning has been reported with the use of rhubarb fruit juice. Rhubarb products manufactured in China have been contaminated with heavy metals. Chronic use of rhubarb products may lead to dependence.
- Based on animal research and limited human study, burdock may cause either increases or reductions in blood sugar levels. Caution is advised in patients with diabetes or hypoglycemia and in those taking drugs, herbs, or supplements that affect blood sugar. Serum glucose levels may need to be monitored by a health care professional, and medication adjustments may be necessary. Diuretic effects (increased urine flow) and estrogen-like effects have been reported with oral burdock use in patients with HIV.
- Reports of anticholinergic reactions (such as slow heart rate and dry mouth) with the use of burdock products in the 1970s are believed to be due to contamination with belladonna alkaloids, which resemble burdock and can be introduced during harvesting. Burdock itself has not been found to contain constituents that would be responsible for these reactions.

Pregnancy and Breastfeeding

- There is not enough scientific evidence to recommend the safe use of Essiac or Essiac-like products during pregnancy and breastfeeding, and there are potential risks from the included herbs. Oxalic acid and anthraquinone glycosides in the included herbs may be unsafe during pregnancy. Rhubarb and burdock may lead to contraction of the uterus; some publications note that whole slippery elm bark can lead to abortion, although there is limited supporting scientific evidence.

INTERACTIONS

Interactions with Drugs

- Essiac interactions are not well studied scientifically. Most potential interactions are based on theoretical and known reactions associated with herbal components of Essiac: burdock root (*Arctium lappa*), sheep sorrel (*Rumex acetosella*), slippery elm bark (*Ulmus fulva*), and Turkish rhubarb (*Rheum palmatum*). However, the interactions of these individual herbs are also not well studied. Various Essiac-like products may contain different or additional ingredients, and patients are advised to carefully review product labels.
- Essiac may interfere with the way the body processes certain drugs using the liver's "cytochrome P450" enzyme system.

As a result, the levels of these drugs may be increased in the blood and may cause increased effects or potentially serious adverse reactions. Patients using any medications should check the package insert and speak with a health care professional or pharmacist about possible interactions. This is based on a report of one patient in a research study taking the experimental drug DX-8951f (metabolized by CYP3A4 and CYP1A2), who experienced toxic side effects and drug clearance that was four to five times slower than in other patients. This patient was also taking "Essiac tea," although further details are not available and it is not clear whether the patient was taking Essiac or an Essiac-like product.

- Anthraquinones in rhubarb root or sheep sorrel may lead to diarrhea, dehydration, or loss of electrolytes (such as potassium) and may increase the effects of other laxative agents. Burdock has been associated with diuretic effects (increased urine flow) in one human report and in theory may cause excess fluid loss (dehydration) or electrolyte imbalances (such as changes in blood potassium or sodium levels). These effects may be increased when burdock is taken at the same time as diuretic drugs such as chlorothiazide (Diuril), furosemide (Lasix), hydrochlorothiazide (HCTZ), or spironolactone (Aldactone). The laxative and diuretic properties of herbs in Essiac may lead to low potassium blood levels that are potentially dangerous in people taking digoxin or digitoxin.
- Based on animal research and limited human study, burdock may either lower or raise blood sugar levels. Caution is advised when medications that may also affect blood sugar are used. Patients taking drugs for diabetes by mouth or using insulin should be monitored closely by a qualified health care professional. Medication adjustments may be necessary.
- Based on limited human evidence that is not entirely clear, burdock may have estrogen-like properties and may act to increase the effects of estrogenic agents, including hormone replacement therapies such as Premarin or birth control pills.
- Essiac may also interact with antibiotics, angiotensin-converting enzyme (ACE) inhibitors, antacids, corticosteroids, heart-regulating agents, or agents used for cancer, including radiotherapy or chemotherapy. Essiac may increase the risk of kidney or liver damage when taken with other agents that also affect the kidney or liver.
- There is early evidence suggesting that Essiac may have a positive interaction when used with nifedipine, an agent used for high blood pressure during pregnancy, although more studies are needed to confirm this finding. Based on human evidence, the combination of rhubarb with antipsychotic agents used in the management of schizophrenia may show promise.

Interactions with Herbs and Dietary Supplements

- Based on one human report, Essiac may interfere with the way the body processes certain herbs or supplements using the liver's cytochrome P450 enzyme system. As a result, the levels of other herbs or supplements may become too high in the blood. It may also alter the effects that other herbs or supplements possibly have on the P450 system.
- Anthraquinones in rhubarb root or sheep sorrel may lead to diarrhea, dehydration, or loss of electrolytes (such as potassium) and may increase the effects of agents with possible laxative properties.
- Burdock has been associated with diuretic effects (increased urine flow) in one human report and in theory may cause excess fluid loss (dehydration) or electrolyte imbalances (such as changes in blood potassium or sodium levels) when used with other diuretic herbs or supplements.
- The laxative and diuretic properties of herbs in Essiac may lead to low potassium blood levels that are potentially dangerous in people taking cardiac glycoside–containing herbs.
- Based on animal research and limited human study, burdock may either lower or raise blood sugar levels. Caution is advised when herbs or supplements that can also alter blood sugar are used. Blood glucose levels may require monitoring, and doses may need adjustment.
- Because burdock may contain estrogen-like chemicals, the effects of other agents believed to have estrogen-like properties may be altered.
- In theory, use of rhubarb and sheep sorrel may decrease the absorption of minerals such as calcium, iron, and zinc.
- Essiac may also interact with herbs or supplements with certain effects, such as antibacterial, antacid, steroid, or heart-regulating effects. There is unclear evidence as to whether Essiac interacts with agents used for cancer, and caution is advised when combining treatments. Essiac may increase the risk of kidney or liver damage when taken with other agents that also affect the kidney or liver. Some preparations contain added ingredients, such as blessed thistle, red clover, or cat's claw, that are thought to increase the effectiveness of the original formula, but supportive evidence is lacking.

For a complete list of reference, please visit www.naturalstandard.com.

Eucalyptus
(Eucalyptus spp.)

RELATED TERMS

- 1,8-Cineole, aerial eucalyptus, Australian fever tree leaf, blauer gommibaum, blue gum, $C_{10}H_{18}O$, cajuputol, camphor oil, catheter oil, cider gum, cineole, Citriodiol, crown gall, essence of eucalyptus rectifiee, essencia de eucalipto, eucalypti aetheroleum, eucalypti folium, eucalyptol, *Eucalyptus camaldulensis* (Red gum), *Eucalyptus citriodora* (Lemon-scented gum), *Eucalyptus coccifera* (Tasmanian snow gum), *Eucalyptus dalrympleana* (Mountain gum), eucalyptus dried leaves, eucalyptus essential oil, *Eucalyptus ficifolia* (red flowering gum), eucalyptus flower, *Eucalyptus fructicetorum* F. Von Mueller, eucalyptus globules tree, *Eucalyptus globulus* Labillardiere, *Eucalyptus gunnii* (cider gum), *Eucalyptus johnstonii* (yellow gum), eucalyptus leaf extract, *Eucalyptus leucoxylon* (white ironbark), *Eucalyptus maculata, Eucalyptus occidentalis, Eucalyptus parvifolia, Eucalyptus pauciflora* subsp. niphophila (snow gum), *Eucalyptus perriniana* (spinning gum), eucalyptus pollen, *Eucalyptus polybractea, Eucalyptus sideroxylon* (red ironbark), *Eucalyptus smithii* R.T. Baker, *Eucalyptus* spp., *Eucalyptus urnigera* (urn gum), *Eucalyptus viminalis* Labill. (euvimals), eucalypto setma ag, fevertree, gommier bleu, gum tree, kafur ag, lemon eucalyptus extract, lemon-scented gum, malee, Meijer (eucalyptus oil, camphor, menthol), mountain gum, Myrtaceae, oil of eucalyptus citriodora, oleum eucalypti, red flowering gum, red gum, red ironbark, schonmutz, snow gum, southern blue gum, spinning gum, stringy bark tree, Tasmanian blue gum, Tasmanian snow gum, urn gum, verbenone, white ironbark, yellow gum.

BACKGROUND

- Eucalyptus oil is used commonly as a decongestant and expectorant for upper respiratory tract infections or inflammations, as well as for various musculoskeletal conditions. The oil is found in numerous over-the-counter cough and cold lozenges as well as in inhalation vapors or topical ointments. Veterinarians use the oil topically for its reported antimicrobial activity. Other applications include as an aromatic in soaps or perfumes, as flavoring in foodstuffs or beverages, and as a dental or industrial solvent. High-quality scientific evidence is currently lacking.
- Eucalyptus oil contains 70%-85% 1,8-cineole (eucalyptol), which is also present in other plant oils. Eucalyptol is used as an ingredient in some mouthwash and dental preparations, as an endodontic solvent, and may possess antimicrobial properties. Listerine mouthrinse is a combination of essential oils (eucalyptol, menthol, thymol, methyl salicylate) that has been shown to be efficacious for the reduction of dental plaque and gingivitis.
- Topical use or inhalation of eucalyptus oil at low concentrations may be safe, although significant and potentially lethal toxicity has been consistently reported with oral use and may also occur with inhalation use. All routes of administration should be avoided in children.

EVIDENCE

Uses Based on Scientific Evidence	Grade
Arthritis Aromatherapy using eucalyptus has been studied for its effects on pain, depression, and feelings of satisfaction in life in arthritis patients. Aromatherapy may help reduce pain and depression but does not appear to alter the feeling of satisfaction in life. Overall, the benefits remain unclear.	C
Asthma There is insufficient clinical evidence of antiinflammatory and mucolytic activity. Further research is needed before eucalyptus can be recommended in upper and lower airway diseases.	C
Decongestant/Expectorant Although commonly used in nonprescription products, there is inconclusive scientific research of eucalyptus oil or eucalyptol.	C
Dental Plaque/Gingivitis (Mouthwash) Although studies on combination mouthwashes show effectiveness (such as Listerine), it is not clear that eucalyptus oil by itself is effective or safe for this purpose.	C
Headache (Applied to the Skin) Effectiveness of eucalyptus oil applied to the skin for headache relief has not been supported with reliable human research.	C
Skin Ulcers Limited evidence suggests that eucalyptus essential oil may be beneficial for patients with skin ulcers when combined with antibiotics.	C
Smoking Cessation Nicobrevin is a proprietary product marketed as an aid for smoking cessation that contains quinine, menthyl valerate, camphor, and eucalyptus oil. Despite use of this product, there is a lack of evidence suggesting benefit of this product or eucalyptus oil for smoking cessation.	C
Tick Repellent (Topical) Preliminary research shows that Citriodiol spray, containing eucalyptus, may reduce the number of tick bites and thus tick-borne infections, although additional studies are warranted.	C

Uses Based on Tradition or Theory

Acquired immunodeficiency syndrome (AIDS), alertness, antibacterial, antifungal, antimicrobial, antioxidant, antiviral, aromatherapy, astringent, athlete's foot, back pain, bronchitis, burns, cancer prevention, cancer treatment, chronic obstructive pulmonary disease (COPD), cleaning solvent, croup, deodorant, diabetes, diarrhea, dysentery, ear infections, emphysema, fever, flavoring, fragrance, herpes, hookworm, inflammation, inflammatory bowel disease, influenza, insect repellent, leukemia, liver protection, muscle/joint pain (applied to the skin), muscle spasm, nerve pain, onychomycosis (fungal infection), pain, parasitic infection, ringworm, runny nose, scabies, shingles, sinusitis, skin infections in children, snoring, stimulant, strains/sprains (applied to the skin), tuberculosis, urinary difficulties, urinary tract infection, whooping cough, wound healing.

DOSING
Adults (18 Years and Older)

- Eucalyptus has been used at concentrations 5%-20% in an oil-based formulation or 5%-10% in an alcohol-based formulation. Topical lemon eucalyptus extract spray (Citriodiol) was applied daily for 2 weeks to the lower extremities to reduce tick attachment.
- Eucalyptus oil should be taken with caution because small amounts of oil taken by mouth have resulted in severe and deadly reactions. Doses of 0.05-0.2 mL or 0.3-0.6 g daily have been used traditionally but may cause toxic side effects. For infusions prepared with eucalyptus leaf, a quantity of 2-3 g of eucalyptus leaf in 150 mL of water has been taken three times a daily but may result in toxic side effects.
- Tinctures with 5%-10% eucalyptus oil (or a few drops placed into a vaporizer) have been used as an inhalant.
- Eucalyptol (1,8-cineole) is a major chemical in eucalyptus oil, and it is used in some commercially sold mouthwashes.

Children (Younger than 18 Years)

- Severe side effects have been reported in children after small doses of eucalyptus have been taken by mouth or applied to the skin. Eucalyptus is not recommended for use by infants and young children, especially near the face and nose.

SAFETY
Allergies

- Case reports describe allergic rash after exposure to eucalyptus oil, either alone or as an ingredient in creams. One child developed a rash after taking eucalyptus oil by mouth. Reports also describe hives after exposure to eucalyptus pollen.
- An herbal survey in asthmatic patients found 12% of asthmatic patients using eucalyptus. Ironically, eucalyptus may cause allergic reactions and the exacerbation of asthma. Worsening of rhinoconjunctivitis and vocal cord dysfunction within minutes of exposure to eucalyptus has been reported.

Side Effects and Warnings

- Severe and potentially deadly side effects have been reported with the use of eucalyptus oil by mouth in children and adults. These include slowing of the brain and central nervous system, drowsiness, seizures, and coma. Use caution if driving or operating heavy machinery. Anecdotal reports suggest that serious side effects can develop with as little as 1 tsp taken by mouth. Reports also suggest that inhaled eucalyptus products or bathtub exposure can cause symptoms. Avoid eucalyptus products in infants and young children, as reports describe severe reactions after exposure by mouth or by application to the skin. Ingestion by children of vaporizer formulas containing eucalyptus has been reported.
- Symptoms reported with eucalyptus oil taken by mouth include abdominal pain, nausea, vomiting, diarrhea, dizziness, muscle weakness, constricted pupils, a feeling of suffocation or difficulty breathing, wheezing, cough, blue discoloration of the lips or skin, delirium, or convulsions. Drowsiness, hyperactivity, difficulty walking, muscle weakness, slurred speech, fever, pneumonia, and headache have also been reported. Case reports describe several abnormalities in heart function after eucalyptus oil has been taken by mouth, including abnormal rhythms, loss of heartbeat, low blood pressure, and complete disruption of the heart and circulation. Individuals with seizure disorders, heart disease, disorders of the stomach or intestines, or lung disease should use caution.
- Published reports describe "attacks" in patients with acute intermittent porphyria (AIP), an inherited disorder affecting the liver and blood. Individuals with AIP should avoid eucalyptus products. Other case reports mention symptoms in individuals who have kidney or liver disease or who are taking other medications that are processed by the liver. Eucalyptus is reported to lower blood sugar in diabetic animals, although reliable human studies are not available in this area. Nonetheless, caution is advised in patients with diabetes or hypoglycemia and in those taking drugs, herbs, or supplements that affect blood sugar. Serum glucose levels may need to be monitored by a health care provider, and medication adjustments may be necessary.
- A strain of bacteria found on eucalyptus may cause infection. Worsening of asthma and rhinoconjunctivitis has been reported.
- Cardiovascular collapse and multiorgan failure have been reported following a massive ingestion of mouthwash containing phenolic compounds (eucalyptol, menthol, thymol).

Pregnancy and Breastfeeding

- Because of the known side effects of eucalyptus and the unknown effects during pregnancy or breastfeeding, eucalyptus should be avoided by pregnant and breastfeeding women.

INTERACTIONS
Interactions with Drugs

- Multiple case reports associate eucalyptus oil taken by mouth with slowing of the mind and nervous system. These symptoms may be worsened when eucalyptus is taken with sedating medications. Examples include benzodiazepines such as lorazepam (Ativan) or diazepam (Valium), barbiturates such as phenobarbital or pentobarbital, narcotics such as codeine, some antidepressants, and alcohol. Use caution while driving or operating machinery. Eucalyptus may also interact with amphetamine.
- Eucalyptus should be taken with caution if combined with medications that lower blood sugar. Patients taking drugs for diabetes by mouth or using insulin should be monitored

closely by a qualified health care provider. Medication adjustments may be necessary.

- Several components of eucalyptus interfere with the way the body processes certain drugs using the liver's cytochrome P450 enzyme system. As a result, the levels of these drugs may be decreased in the blood with reduced intended effects. Patients using any medications should check the package insert and speak with a health care provider or pharmacist about possible interactions.
- When applied to the skin with 5-fluorouracil lotion (5-FU, Efudex, Carac), eucalyptus may increase the absorption of 5-FU.
- Many tinctures contain high levels of alcohol and may cause nausea or vomiting when taken with metronidazole (Flagyl) or disulfiram (Antabuse).

Interactions with Herbs and Dietary Supplements

- Eucalyptus may increase the drowsiness caused by some herbs or supplements, such as German chamomile or lemon balm. Use caution while driving or operating machinery.
- Eucalyptus may lower blood sugar levels. Caution is advised when herbs or supplements that may also lower blood sugar are used. Blood glucose levels may require monitoring, and doses may need adjustment.
- Eucalyptus may interfere with the way the body processes certain herbs or supplements using the liver's cytochrome P450 enzyme system. As a result, the levels of other herbs or supplements may become too low in the blood. In addition, levels of eucalyptus in the body may be affected by herbs or supplements that affect the P450 system, such as bloodroot, cat's claw, or chamomile.
- Eucalyptus has been said to worsen the side effects of borage, coltsfoot, comfrey, hound's tooth, or *Senecio* species, although there is no reliable research in this area.

For a complete list of references, please visit www.naturalstandard.com.

Evening Primrose
(*Oenothera biennis*)

RELATED TERMS

- Bronchipret TP FCT, Echte Nachtkerze, EPO, fever plant, gamma-linolenic acid, herbe aux anes, Huile D'Onagre, kaempe natlys, king's cureall, la belle de nuit, linoleic acid, nachtkerzenol, night willow-herb, *Oenothera communis* Leveill, *Oenothera graveolens* Gilib., omega-6 essential fatty acid, *Onagra biennis* Scop., *Onogra vulgaris*, onagre bisannuelle, primrose, primrose oil, scabish, Spach, stella di sera, sun drop, Teunisbloem.

BACKGROUND

- Evening primrose oil (EPO) contains an omega-6 essential fatty acid, gamma-linolenic acid (GLA), which is believed to be the active ingredient. EPO has been studied in a wide variety of disorders, particularly those affected by metabolic products of essential fatty acids. However, high-quality evidence for its use in most conditions is still lacking.

EVIDENCE

Uses Based on Scientific Evidence	Grade
Atopic Dermatitis (Eczema) There are several studies of evening primrose oil taken by mouth for eczema. Large well-designed studies are needed before a strong recommendation can be made. Evening primrose oil is approved for skin disorders in several countries outside of the United States.	B
Breast Cancer Not enough information is available to advise the use of evening primrose oil for breast cancer. People with known or suspected breast cancer should consult with a qualified health care professional about possible treatments.	C
Breast Cysts The limited available research does not demonstrate that evening primrose oil has a significant effect on treating breast cysts.	C
Breast Pain (Mastalgia) Although primrose oil is used for breast pain in several European countries, high-quality human studies using this treatment are lacking. Therefore, the available information does not allow recommendation for or against the use of primrose oil in this condition.	C
Bronchitis There is evidence that primrose oil, in combination with thyme, may have some benefits in the treatment of acute bronchitis. However, it is unclear whether primrose alone is useful in treating bronchitis. More studies are needed to examine the effectiveness of primrose oil alone as a therapy for bronchitis.	C
Chronic Fatigue Syndrome/Postviral Infection Symptoms Not enough information is available to advise the use of evening primrose oil for symptoms of chronic fatigue syndrome or fatigue following a viral infection.	C
Diabetes A small number of laboratory studies and theory suggests that evening primrose oil may be helpful in diabetes, but more information is needed before a firm recommendation can be made.	C
Diabetic Neuropathy (Nerve Damage) Gamma-linolenic acid (GLA), one of the components of evening primrose oil, may be helpful in people with diabetic neuropathy. Additional studies are needed before a strong recommendation can be made.	C
Multiple Sclerosis (MS) It is theorized that primrose oil may be helpful in patients with MS based on laboratory studies. Limited evidence is available in humans.	C
Obesity/Weight Loss Initial human study is unclear about the effects that evening primrose oil may have on weight loss.	C
Osteoporosis Primrose oil has been suggested as a possible treatment for bone loss/osteoporosis. However, osteoporosis studies using primrose oil as a treatment are lacking. Well-designed human trials are needed before primrose oil can be recommended for osteoporosis therapy.	C
Preeclampsia/High Blood Pressure of Pregnancy Evening primrose oil is proposed to have effects on chemicals in the blood called prostaglandins, which may play a role in preeclampsia. However, more studies are needed before a firm conclusion can be drawn.	C
Raynaud's Phenomenon Not enough scientific information is available to advise the use of evening primrose oil for Raynaud's phenomenon.	C
Rheumatoid Arthritis Benefits of evening primrose oil in the treatment of arthritis have not clearly been shown. More information is needed before a firm recommendation can be made.	C

(Continued)

Uses Based on Scientific Evidence	Grade
Scalelike Dry Skin (Ichthyosis Vulgaris) Not enough scientific information is available to advise the use of evening primrose oil for dry skin.	C
Asthma Available evidence does not support the use of evening primrose oil as a treatment for asthma. Further research is needed to confirm this conclusion.	D
Attention Deficit Hyperactivity Disorder (ADHD) Small human studies show a lack of benefit from evening primrose oil in ADHD. Further research is needed to confirm this conclusion.	D
Cardiovascular Health Early study of evening primrose oil shows a lack of beneficial effects on cardiovascular function and health.	D
Menopause (Flushing/Bone Metabolism) Available studies do not show evening primrose oil to be helpful with these potential complications of menopause. More evidence of effectiveness is needed before primrose oil can be recommended as a treatment for menopausal symptoms.	D
Premenstrual Syndrome (PMS) Small human studies do not report that evening primrose oil is helpful for the symptoms of PMS.	D
Psoriasis Initial research does not show a benefit from evening primrose oil in the treatment of psoriasis.	D
Schizophrenia Results from studies of mixed quality do not support the use of evening primrose oil for schizophrenia. In contrast, fish oils have shown some promise in this disease, and further study is merited.	D

Uses Based on Tradition or Theory

Alcoholism, antioxidant, atherosclerosis, bruises (primrose oil applied to the skin), cancer, cancer prevention, chemotherapy-induced neuropathy (nerve damage), Crohn's disease, cystic fibrosis, disorders of the stomach and intestines, hangover remedy, heart disease, hemorrhoids, hepatitis B, high cholesterol levels, inflammation, irritable bowel syndrome, kidney stones, labor and delivery (preventing preterm delivery and promoting easier birth), melanoma, multiple sclerosis, pain, postnatal depression, scleroderma, Sjögren's syndrome, skin conditions due to kidney failure in dialysis patients, stomach pain, systemic lupus erythematosus (SLE), tumors (fibroadenomas), ulcerative colitis, whooping cough, wound healing (primrose oil poultice applied to the skin).

DOSING
Adults (18 Years and Older)

- Studies of the treatment of eczema have used doses of 4-8 g of evening primrose oil (EPO) daily, taken by mouth, divided into several smaller doses throughout the day. Studies treating breast pain have used doses of 3 g EPO daily, taken by mouth, divided into several smaller doses throughout the day.

Children (Younger than 18 Years)

- Studies in children treated for skin conditions have used 3 g of evening primrose oil daily, taken by mouth, divided into several smaller doses throughout the day. It is reported that the maximum dose should not be greater than 0.5 g/kg of body weight daily. Medical supervision is required.

SAFETY
Allergies

- Allergy or hypersensitivity to evening primrose oil has not been widely reported. Individuals with allergy or adverse reactions to plants in the Onagraceae family, GLA, or other ingredients in evening primrose oil should avoid its use. Contact dermatitis (skin rash) is possible.

Side Effects and Warnings

- Several reports describe seizures in individuals taking EPO. Some of these seizures developed in people with a previous seizure disorder or in individuals taking EPO in combination with anesthetics. On the basis of these reports, people with seizure disorders should not take EPO. EPO should be used cautiously with drugs used to treat mental illness such as chlorpromazine (Thorazine), thioridazine (Mellaril), trifluoperazine (Stelazine), or fluphenazine (Prolixin) because of an increased risk of seizure. Patients who plan to undergo surgery requiring anesthesia should stop taking EPO 2 weeks ahead of time because of the possibility of seizure.
- Other reports describe occasional headache, abdominal pain, nausea, and loose stools in people taking EPO. In animal studies, GLA (an ingredient of EPO) is reported to decrease blood pressure. Early results in human studies do not show consistent changes in blood pressure.

Pregnancy and Breastfeeding

- There is not enough information to recommend the safe use of EPO during pregnancy or breastfeeding.

INTERACTIONS
Interactions with Drugs

- Because of reported seizures in people taking EPO alone or in combination with certain medications used to treat mental illness, patients should use caution when combining EPO with medications such as chlorpromazine (Thorazine), thioridazine (Mellaril), trifluoperazine (Stelazine), or fluphenazine (Prolixin). Individuals undergoing surgery requiring general anesthesia may be more sensitive to developing seizures and should stop taking EPO 2 weeks ahead of time. In people with a history of seizures, doses of antiseizure medications may require adjustment because EPO may increase the risk of seizures.

- An ingredient of EPO, GLA, is reported to lower blood pressure in animal studies. Although human studies do not show clear changes in blood pressure, people taking certain blood pressure medications should consult with a health care professional before starting EPO.
- Possible additive effects may occur when primrose oil is taken with anticoagulants (blood thinners) and drugs used to treat arthritis.
- Possible interactions may occur with antidepressants, including monoamine oxidase inhibitors (MAOIs) and selective serotonin reuptake inhibitors (SSRIs). Interactions may also occur with the following: antineoplastic agents, antiobesity agents, antiviral agents, central nervous system (CNS) stimulants, drugs metabolized by the liver, gastrointestinal treatments, and neurological agents.

Interactions with Herbs and Dietary Supplements

- In animal studies, GLA (an ingredient of EPO) is reported to lower blood pressure. Therefore, in theory, EPO may have effects on blood pressure and should be used cautiously when combined with other agents that may lower blood pressure.
- Theoretically, EPO may have additive effects when taken concomitantly with thyme because a fixed combination of thyme fluid extract and primrose root tincture (Bronchicum Tropfen) has been used in studies to treat bronchitis.
- Primrose oil may potentially interact with herbs and supplements used to treat arthritis, gastrointestinal disorders, obesity, seizures, viral infections, and psychosis. Primrose oil may interact with stimulants and herbs and supplements that are metabolized in the liver. Antineoplastics may also interact with primrose.

For a complete list of references, please visit www.naturalstandard.com.

Eyebright
(Euphrasia officinalis)

RELATED TERMS

- Adhib, ambrosia, augentrost, Augentrostkraut (German), Augstenzieger, briselunettes (French), casse-lunette (French), clary, clary wort, clear eye, eufragia, eufrasia (Italian), Euphraise, Euphraisiae herba, Euphraisiae herbal (eyebright herb), *Euphrasia, Euphrasia mollis, Euphrasia officinalis, Euphrasia rostkoviana, Euphrasia sibirica*, euphrasy, ewfras, frasia, herbed euphraise, herbe d'euphraise officinale, hirnkraut, laegeojentrost (Danish), luminella, meadow eyebright, muscatel sage, red eyebright, sage, *Salvia sclarea*, schabab, Scrophulariaceae (family), see bright, Weisses Ruhrkraut, Wiesenaugetrost, Zwang-kraut.

BACKGROUND

- Eyebright's genus name, *Euphrasia*, is derived from the Greek "euphrosyne," the name of one of the three Graces who was distinguished for joy and mirth. Eyebright was used as early as the time of Theophrastus (Greek philosopher and biologist, student of Plato and Aristotle) and Dioscorides (Greek philosopher [circa AD 64] who authored a pharmacological account of plants), who prescribed infusions for topical applications in the treatment of eye infections. During the middle ages, eyebright was widely prescribed by medical practitioners as an eye medication and as a cure for "all evils of the eye."

- In Europe, the herb eyebright (*Euphrasia officinalis*) has been used for centuries as a rinse, compress, or bath against eye infections and other eye-related irritations (a use reflected in many of its vernacular names). When taken by mouth, eyebright has been used to treat inflammation of nasal mucous membranes and sinusitis.

- Eyebright is high in iridoid glycosides such as aucubin. In several laboratory studies, this constituent has been found to possess hepatoprotective (liver-protecting) and antimicrobial activity. There is limited clinical research assessing the efficacy of eyebright in the treatment of conjunctivitis (pink eye), and the use of eyebright for other indications has not been studied in clinical trials.

- Few data exist regarding the safety and toxicity of eyebright. A concern regarding the ophthalmological (eye) use of eyebright is the potential for contamination. The U.S. Food and Drug Administration (FDA) has not evaluated eyebright for "generally recognized as safe" (GRAS) status.

EVIDENCE

Uses Based on Scientific Evidence	Grade
Antiinflammatory Several iridoid glycosides isolated from eyebright, particularly aucubin, possess antiinflammatory properties comparable to those of indomethacin (a nonsteroidal antiinflammatory drug). Although early evidence is promising, there is currently insufficient evidence to recommend for or against eyebright as an antiinflammatory agent.	C
Conjunctivitis (Pinkeye) Eyebright has been used in ophthalmic (eye) solutions for centuries in the management of multiple eye conditions. Currently, there is insufficient scientific evidence to recommend for or against the use of eyebright in the treatment of conjunctivitis.	C
Hepatoprotection Aucubin, a constituent of eyebright, may aid in liver protection. However, there is currently insufficient evidence to recommend for or against the use of eyebright as a hepatoprotective agent.	C

Uses Based on Tradition or Theory

Allergies, antibacterial, antihelmintic (expels worms), antiviral, appetite stimulant, asthma, astringent, blepharitis (inflammation of the eyelid), bronchitis (chronic), cancer, cataracts, catarrh (inflammation of the mucous membranes) of the eyes, common cold, congestion, cough, digestive aid, earaches, epilepsy, expectorant, flavoring agent, gastric acid secretion stimulation, hay fever, headache, hoarseness, jaundice, liver disease, measles, memory loss, middle ear problems, ocular (eye) compress, ocular (eye) fatigue, ocular inflammation (acute, subacute, blood vessels of eye, eyelids), ocular (eye) rinse, ophthalmia (eye infection), respiratory infections, rhinitis (inflammation of nasal mucosa), sinusitis, skin conditions, sneezing (chronic), sore throat, sties, visual disturbances.

DOSING

Adults (18 Years and Older)

- There is insufficient evidence to recommend a dose of eyebright. Traditionally, 2-4 g of dried herb three times daily has been suggested for multiple indications. For conjunctivitis (pinkeye), studies have used one drop of eyebright one to five times daily for 3-17 days.

Children (Younger than 18 Years)

- There is insufficient evidence to recommend a dose of eyebright in children. However, children have tolerated four to five homeopathic pills of Euphrasia 30C daily for 3 days for prevention of viral conjunctivitis.

SAFETY

Allergies

- Avoid in individuals with a known allergy or hypersensitivity to eyebright. Hypersensitivity to members of the Scrophulariaceae family may lead to a cross-sensitivity reaction.

Side Effects and Warnings

- Systematic study of clinical safety and tolerability has been limited. Both children and adults have tolerated short-term ophthalmological use of eyebright for conjunctivitis (pinkeye). However, the potential exists for contamination of ophthalmological preparations of eyebright, and eyebright tincture has been associated with pruritus (severe itching), redness and swelling of the eye, vision changes, and photophobia (intolerance or fear of light). Other adverse effects reported include toothache, confusion, headache, sneezing, yawning, insomnia, raised ocular pressure, lacrimation (tears), cough, dyspnea (difficulty breathing), nasal congestion, hoarseness, nausea, constipation, expectoration, polyuria (excessive urination), and diaphoresis (excessive sweating).

- Eyebright is possibly safe when used in amounts commonly found in foods or when used as a flavoring agent.
- Eyebright is likely unsafe when homemade preparations are used for ophthalmic indications because of the likelihood of microbial contamination; when used in greater than studied doses or duration because of lack of safety data; and when used during pregnancy and breastfeeding or in pediatric patients.
- Although not well-studied in humans, eyebright may lower blood sugar levels. Caution is advised in patients with diabetes or hypoglycemia and in those taking drugs, herbs, or supplements that affect blood sugar. Serum glucose levels may need to be monitored by a qualified health care professional, including a pharmacist, and medication adjustments may be necessary.

Pregnancy and Breastfeeding

- Eyebright is not recommended in pregnant or breastfeeding women because of a lack of available scientific evidence.

INTERACTIONS
Interactions with Drugs

- Eyebright may interfere with the way the body processes certain drugs using the liver's cytochrome P450 enzyme system. As a result, the levels of these drugs may be altered in the blood and may cause increased effects or potentially serious adverse reactions. Patients using any medications should check the package insert and speak with a qualified health care professional, including a pharmacist, about possible interactions.
- Eyebright may lower blood sugar levels. Caution is advised when medications that may also lower blood sugar are used. Patients taking drugs for diabetes by mouth or using insulin should be monitored closely by a qualified health care professional, including a pharmacist. Medication adjustments may be necessary.

Interactions with Herbs and Dietary Supplements

- Eyebright may interfere with the way the body processes certain herbs or supplements using the liver's cytochrome P450 enzyme system. As a result, the levels of other herbs or supplements may become too high in the blood. It may also alter the effects that other herbs or supplements possibly have on the P450 system.
- Theoretically, eyebright may lower blood sugar levels. Caution is advised when herbs or supplements that may also lower blood sugar are used. Blood glucose levels may require monitoring, and doses may need adjustment.

For a complete list of references, please visit www.naturalstandard.com.

Fennel
(*Foeniculum vulgare*)

RELATED TERMS

- Adas, adas pedas, anason dulce, aneth doux, anis, *Anethum foeniculum, Anthemis cotula* (dog fennel), Apiaceae (parsley family), aptechnyj ukrop, apteegitilliseemne, badesopu, badishep, bitter fennel, carosella, cay thi la, common fennel, edeskomeny, fenchel, fenheli parastie, fenhelis, fenicol, fenikel, fenkel, fenkhel, fenkoli, fenkolo, fennel honey syrup, fennel oil, fenneru, fennika, fennikel, fenouil, fenoun, fenykl, *Ferula communis* (giant fennel), finocchio, finokio, florence fennel, *Foeniculi aetheroleum, Foeniculum capillaceum, Foeniculum officinale, Foeniculum vulgare,* Fructus foeniculi, funcho, garden fennel, guamoori, haras, harilik apteegitill, hinojo, hoehyang, hoehyang-pul, hoi huong, hui xiang, jinten manis, kama, koper wloski, komorac, koper, koromac, large cummin, large fennel, lus an t'saiodh, madhurika, maduru, marac, maratho, mehul, mellet karee, merula obisnuita, mieloi, miur belar, molura, morach, moti saunf, mouri, paciolis, pak chi duanha, pan mohuri, paprastasis pankolis, pedda jilakarra, pennel, perunjiragam, phak si, phong karee, phytoestrogen, razianaj, razianeh, razyana, rezene, samit, samong-saba, saunf, shamaar, shamar, shamari, shamraa, shatpushpa, shoap, shoumar, shumar, siu wuih heung, sladki komarcek, sladkij ukrop, so-hoehyang, sohikirai, sombu, sonf, sopu, spice of the angels, sulpha, sweet cumin, sweet fennel, thian-klaep, tian hi xiang, tieu hoi huong, tihm wuih heung, uikyo, ukrop sladki, Umbelliferae (parsley family), venkel, wariari, wild fennel, wuih heung, xiao hui xiang, yira.
- **Note:** Some languages do not differentiate between anise and fennel. Not to be confused with giant fennel (*Ferula communis*).

BACKGROUND

- Fennel is native to the Mediterranean region. For centuries, fennel fruits have been used as traditional herbal medicine in Europe and China. For the treatment of infants suffering from dyspeptic (indigestion) disorders, fennel tea is the remedy of first choice. Its administration as a carminative (digestive aid) is practiced in infant care in private homes and in maternity clinics, where it is highly appreciated for its mild flavor and good tolerance.
- There is evidence suggesting that fennel is effective in reducing infantile colic. Fennel has also been studied in human clinical trials for angiotensin-converting enzyme (ACE) inhibitor–induced cough, dysmenorrhea (painful menstruation), and ultraviolet protection, but additional research is merited in these areas.

EVIDENCE

Uses Based on Scientific Evidence	Grade
Infantile Colic An emulsion of fennel seed oil and an herbal tea containing fennel have reduced infantile colic. Additional studies are warranted to confirm these findings.	B

Cough (ACE Inhibitor–Induced) Fennel fruit may be helpful in relieving cough (a side effect of angiotensin converting enzyme inhibitor [ACEI]). However, there is insufficient evidence to recommend for or against its use for ACEI-induced cough.	C
Dysmenorrhea (Painful Menstruation) Fennel has been used to treat dysmenorrhea. Although preliminary study is promising, there is currently insufficient evidence to recommend for or against this use of fennel.	C
Ultraviolet Light Skin Damage Protection Topical fennel extract improved sun protection factor (SPF) and decreased ultraviolet (UV)-induced erythema (reddening of the skin) and demonstrated consistent inhibition of lipid peroxidation. However, results were not conclusive.	C

Uses Based on Tradition or Theory

Abdominal cramps, abortion (when used in combination), attention deficit hyperactivity disorder (ADHD), antibacterial, antifungal, antioxidant, bad breath, bone loss (inhibition of bone resorption), bronchitis, bust enhancer, cancer preventative (in combination with antioxidants), common cold/upper respiratory tract infection, cough, digestion, dyspepsia (upset stomach), eye disorders (improve eyesight), feeling of fullness, flatulence (gas), flavoring, flu, fragrance, galactagogue (stimulates milk production), gastrointestinal discomfort, intestinal cramps, labor and delivery (facilitates birth), libido, loss of appetite, promotes menstruation, prostate cancer, sedative, spastic colon (disorders of the gastrointestinal [GI] tract), visual disturbances.

DOSING
Adults (18 Years and Older)

- There is insufficient evidence to recommend a dose of fennel. For ACE inhibitor–induced cough, 1-1.5 g of fennel fruit has been used up to three times daily. Up to 4600 micrograms has been studied for its antioxidant effects. For dysmenorrhea (painful menstruation), 25 drops of a 2% concentration of fennel fruit has been taken every 4 hours for 5 days.
- Traditionally, numerous other doses and preparations have been used, in the form of tea, seed, tincture, oil, or dry extract.

Children (Younger than 18 Years)

- There is insufficient evidence to recommend a dose of fennel in children. For infantile colic (ages 2 to 12 weeks), 0.1% fennel seed oil in a water emulsion and 0.4% polysorbate-80 have been studied for 1 week. Traditional dosing for upper respiratory tract catarrh (inflammation of mucous membranes) in children is 0.5 g of the oil per kilogram.

For ages 1 to 4 years, 3-6 g has been used daily; for ages 4 to 10 years, 6-10 g has been used daily.

SAFETY
Allergies

- Avoid in individuals with a known allergy or hypersensitivity to fennel or other members of the Apiaceae family including carrot, celery, and mugwort because of the chance of cross-sensitization. Oral allergy syndrome has been reported with the use of fennel in a woman. Allergic reactions affecting the skin such as atopic dermatitis and photosensitivity may occur in patients who consume fennel.

Side Effects and Warnings

- Fennel is generally well tolerated. Allergic reactions, such as atopic dermatitis and photosensitivity, are the most common adverse effects but rarely occur. Fennel oil has "generally recognized as safe" (GRAS) status for food use in the United States. A maximum level of 0.119% is allowed in meat products.
- Epileptic seizures have been reported with the use of fennel oil. Respiratory problems including bronchial asthma, hay fever, occupational rhinoconjunctivitis (inflammation of the lining of the nose and the mucous membrane that covers the front of the eyes and lines the eyelids) and asthma have been reported in patients working with fennel seed.
- Inhalation of essential oils, including fennel oil, resulted in 1.2-2.5-fold increase in relative sympathetic activity, representing low frequency amplitude of systolic blood pressure.
- Use cautiously in diabetic patients. Fennel honey syrup is a source of carbohydrates.
- *Yersinia enterocolitica*, a bacterial pathogen, has been isolated in the Umbelliferae family, which could pose a potential threat of infection if fennel is consumed fresh. Fennel preparations, other than fennel seed infusions and fennel honey, should be avoided in infants and toddlers.
- The constituent estragoel is a procarcinogen (precursor of a cancer causing compound).

Pregnancy and Breastfeeding

- Fennel is not recommended in pregnant or breastfeeding women because of a lack of available scientific evidence. Based on expert opinion, fennel preparations, other than fennel seed infusions and fennel honey, are contraindicated during pregnancy.

INTERACTIONS
Interactions with Drugs

- Giant fennel (*Ferula communis*) may increase the risk of bleeding when taken with drugs that increase the risk of bleeding. Some examples include aspirin, anticoagulants ("blood thinners") such as warfarin (Coumadin) or heparin, antiplatelet drugs such as clopidogrel (Plavix), and nonsteroidal antiinflammatory drugs (NSAIDs) such as ibuprofen (Motrin, Advil) or naproxen (Naprosyn, Aleve).
- Concurrent use of fennel and ciprofloxacin (Cipro) may lead to decreased bioavailability of ciprofloxacin. Theoretically, fennel may also interfere similarly with other fluoroquinolone antibiotics.

Interactions with Herbs and Dietary Supplements

- Fennel may increase the risk of bleeding when taken with herbs and supplements that are believed to increase the risk of bleeding. Multiple cases of bleeding have been reported with the use of *Ginkgo biloba*, and fewer cases have been reported with garlic and saw palmetto. Numerous other agents may theoretically increase the risk of bleeding, although this has not been proven in most cases.

For a complete list of references, please visit www.naturalstandard.com.

Fenugreek
(Trigonella foenum-graecum)

RELATED TERMS

- Abish, alholva, bird's foot, bockhornsklover, bockshornklee, bockshornsamen, cemen, chilbe, diosgenin, fenegriek, fenogreco, fenogrego, fenigreko, fenugree, fenugreek seed, fenu-thyme, foenugraeci semen, gorogszena, graine de fenugrec, gray hay, Greek hay seed, griechische Heusamen, fieno greco, halba, hilbeh, hulba, hu lu ba, kasoori methi, kozieradka pospolita, kreeka lambalaats, mente, mentikura, mentula, methi, methika, methini, methri, methro, mithiguti, pazhitnik grecheskiy, penantazi, sag methi, sambala, sarviapila, shabaliidag, shambelile, trigonella, trigonelline, trogonella semen, uluhaal, uwatu, vendayam, venthiam.

BACKGROUND

- Fenugreek has a long history of medical uses in Indian and Chinese medicine and has been used for numerous indications, including labor induction, aiding digestion, and as a general tonic to improve metabolism and health.
- Preliminary evidence suggests possible hypoglycemic (blood sugar lowering) and antihyperlipidemic properties of fenugreek seed powder when taken by mouth. However, at this time, the evidence is not sufficient to recommend either for or against fenugreek for diabetes or hyperlipidemia. Nonetheless, caution is warranted in patients taking blood sugar–lowering agents, in whom blood glucose levels should be monitored. Hypokalemia (lowered potassium levels in the blood) has also been reported, and potassium levels should be followed in patients taking concomitant hypokalemic agents or with underlying cardiac disease.

EVIDENCE

Uses Based on Scientific Evidence	Grade
Diabetes Mellitus Type 1 Review of the literature suggests a possible efficacy of fenugreek in type 1 diabetes. Although promising, these data cannot be considered definitive. At this time there is insufficient evidence to recommend either for or against the use of fenugreek for type 1 diabetes.	C
Diabetes Mellitus Type 2 Fenugreek has been found to lower serum glucose levels both acutely and chronically. Although promising, these data cannot be considered definitive, and at this time there is insufficient evidence to recommend either for or against fenugreek for type 2 diabetes.	C
Galactagogue (Breast Milk Stimulant) Traditionally in India, fenugreek has been used to increase milk flow. However, supportive clinical evidence is lacking.	C
Hyperlipidemia There is insufficient evidence to support the use of fenugreek as a hyperlipidemic agent.	C

Uses Based on Tradition or Theory

Abortifacient (induces abortion), abscesses, antioxidant, aphthous ulcers, appetite stimulant, asthenia, atherosclerosis (hardening of the arteries), baldness, beriberi (vitamin B$_1$ deficiency), boils, breast enhancement, bronchitis, burns, cancer, cellulitis, chapped lips, colic, colon cancer, constipation, convalescence (gradual healing), cough (chronic), dermatitis, diarrhea, digestion, dropsy, dysentery, dyspepsia (upset stomach), eczema, energy enhancement, food uses, furunculosis (acute skin disease), gas, gastric ulcers, gastritis, gout (foot inflammation), heart conditions, *Helicobacter pylori* infection, hepatic disease, hepatomegaly, hernia, high blood pressure, immunomodulator, impotence, indigestion, infections, inflammation, inflammatory bowel disease, insecticide, labor induction (uterine stimulant), leg edema, leg ulcers, leukemia, lice, liver damage, low energy, lymphadenitis (inflammation of the lymph nodes), menopausal symptoms, myalgia (muscle pain), postmenopausal vaginal dryness, protection against alcohol toxicity, rickets, splenomegaly (enlarged spleen), stomach upset, thyroxine-induced hyperglycemia, tuberculosis, vitamin deficiencies, wound healing.

DOSING

Adults (18 Years and Older)

- Products rich in fenugreek fiber may interfere with the absorption of oral medications because of its mucilaginous fiber content and high viscosity in the gut. Medications should be taken separately from such products. However, it should be noted that fenugreek is rarely used for its fiber content.
- There is insufficient evidence to recommend a dose of fenugreek in adults. For type 1 diabetes, 100 g of debitterized powdered fenugreek seeds divided into two equal doses has been used. For type 2 diabetes, 2.5 g of fenugreek seed powder in capsule form, twice daily for 3 months, or 25 g seed powder, divided into two equal doses has been used. For hyperlipidemia, 2.5 g of fenugreek seed powder in capsule form, twice daily for 3 months, or 100 g debitterized powdered seeds divided into two equal doses has been used.

Children (Younger than 18 Years)

- There is insufficient evidence to recommend a dose of fenugreek in children.

SAFETY

Allergies

- Caution is warranted in patients with known fenugreek allergy or with allergy to chickpeas because of possible cross-reactivity. Inhaling fenugreek seed powder may cause allergic or asthmatic reactions, including bronchospasm.

Side Effects and Warnings

- Fenugreek has traditionally been considered safe and well tolerated. There are rare reports of dizziness, diarrhea, gas, facial swelling, numbness, difficulty breathing (after inhalation from occupational exposure), fainting, increased risk of bleeding, reduction of blood sugar levels, reduction of serum potassium levels, and alteration of thyroid hormone levels.

- Blood sugar levels should be followed in patients with diabetes. Patients should be monitored if taking anticoagulants or drugs that affect potassium levels.

Pregnancy and Breastfeeding

- Literature review reveals no reliable human data or systematic study of fenugreek during pregnancy or lactation. Caution is warranted during pregnancy because of potential hypoglycemic effects. In addition, both water and alcoholic extracts of fenugreek exert a stimulating effect on isolated guinea pig uterus, especially during late pregnancy. As a result, fenugreek may possess abortifacient effects and is usually not recommended for use during pregnancy in doses higher than found in foods.

INTERACTIONS
Interactions with Drugs

- Products rich in fenugreek fiber may interfere with the absorption of oral medications because of its mucilaginous fiber content and high viscosity in the gut. Medications should be taken separately from such products.
- Fenugreek is thought to possess both acute and chronic hypoglycemic properties. Concomitant use with other hypoglycemic agents may lower serum glucose more than expected, and levels should be monitored closely

- Fenugreek should be used cautiously with medications that decrease blood potassium levels, diuretics, laxatives, mineralocorticoids, hormone replacement therapy (HRT), birth control pills, thyroid medications, corticosteroids, anticoagulants, cardiac glycosides, and monoamine oxidase inhibitors. Use cautiously when taking with drugs used for cancer or high cholesterol or when taking with alcohol.

Interactions with Herbs and Dietary Supplements

- Fenugreek may lower blood sugar levels. Caution is advised when herbs or supplements that may also lower blood sugar are used. Blood glucose levels may require monitoring, and doses may need adjustment.
- Fenugreek may increase the risk of bleeding when taken with herbs and supplements that are believed to increase the risk of bleeding. Multiple cases of bleeding have been reported with the use of *Ginkgo biloba*, and fewer cases have been reported with garlic and saw palmetto. Numerous other agents may theoretically increase the risk of bleeding, although this has not been proven in most cases.
- Fenugreek should also be used cautiously with agents that decrease blood potassium levels, diuretic agents, laxatives, phytoestrogens, and herbs with monoamine oxidase inhibitor properties. Use cautiously when taking with drugs used for cancer, pain, heart conditions, thyroid conditions, or high cholesterol levels. Fenugreek may interact with antioxidants.

For a complete list of references, please visit www.naturalstandard.com.

Feverfew
(Tanacetum parthenium, syn. Chrysanthemum parthenium, Pyrethrum parthenium)

RELATED TERMS

- 6-Hydroxykaempferol, alpha-pinene, altamisa, apigenin, bachelor's button, camomille grande, camphene, camphor, *Chrysanthemum parthenium*, (E)-beta-ocimene, (E)-chrysanthenol, (E)-chrysanthenyl acetate, featherfew, featherfoil, febrifuge plant, federfoy, flirtwort, gamma-terpinene, golden feverfew, *Leucanthemum parthenium*, limonene, linalool, lipophilic flavonoids, luteolin 7-glucuronides, *Matricaria capensis*, matricaria eximia hort, *Matricaria parthenium* L., melatonin, midsummer daisy, MIG-99, Mig-RL, monoterpenes, mother herb, mutterkraut, nosebleed, p-cymene, *Parthenium hysterophorus*, parthenolide, *Pyrethrum parthenium* L., quercetagetin, Santa Maria, sesquiterpene lactones, sesquiterpenes, *Tanacetum parthenium*, *Tanacetum parthenium* (L.) Schultz-Bip., Tanetin, tannins, wild chamomile, wild quinine.

BACKGROUND

- Feverfew is an herb that has been used traditionally for fevers, as its name denotes, although this effect has not been well studied.
- Feverfew is most commonly taken by mouth for the prevention of migraine headache. Several human trials have been conducted with mixed results. Overall, these studies suggest that feverfew taken daily as dried leaf capsules may reduce the incidence of headache attacks in patients who experience chronic migraines. However, this research has been poorly designed and reported.
- There is currently inconclusive evidence regarding the use of feverfew for symptoms associated with rheumatoid arthritis.
- Feverfew appears to be well tolerated in clinical trials, with a mild and reversible side effects profile. The most common adverse effect appears to be mouth ulceration and inflammation with direct exposure to leaves. In theory, there may be an increased risk of bleeding.

EVIDENCE

Uses Based on Scientific Evidence	Grade
Migraine Headache Prevention Feverfew is often taken by mouth for the prevention of migraine headaches. Laboratory studies show that feverfew can reduce inflammation and prevent blood vessel constriction (squeezing) that may lead to headaches. Most of the available human studies are not high quality and report mixed results. However, overall they do suggest that feverfew may reduce the number of headaches that occur in people with frequent migraines. A large, well-designed study comparing feverfew with other migraine treatments is needed before a strong recommendation can be made.	A
Rheumatoid Arthritis It is not clear whether feverfew is helpful for treating rheumatoid arthritis symptoms such as joint stiffness or pain.	C

Uses Based on Tradition or Theory

Abdominal pain, anemia, antiinflammatory, asthma, blood vessel dilation (relaxation), blood vessel disorders (antiangiogenic), breast cancer, cancer, central nervous system diseases, colds, colorectal cancer, constipation, cystic fibrosis, diarrhea, digestion, dizziness, fever, gastrointestinal distress, heart muscle injury, induction of labor/abortion, insect bites, insect repellant, joint pain, leukemia, menstrual cramps, neurological complications of malaria, pancreatic cancer, parasitic infections (leishmaniasis), promotion of menstruation, rash, ringing in the ears, skin cancer, toothache, tranquilizer, uterine disorders.

DOSING
Adults (18 Years and Older)

- Dosing for feverfew includes two to three dried leaves (approximately 60 mg) or 50-250 mg of a dried leaf preparation has been taken daily, standardized to 0.2% parthenolide (a common dose is 125 mg daily). Human studies have used 50-114 mg of feverfew powdered leaves daily, packed into capsules, standardized to 0.2% parthenolide, or 0.50 mg of parthenolide daily. Another common dose is 70-86 mg of dried chopped feverfew leaves in capsules, taken once daily.

Children (Younger than 18 Years)

- There is insufficient evidence to safely recommend feverfew for use in children.

SAFETY
Allergies

- Feverfew may cause allergy in people allergic to chrysanthemums, daisies, marigolds, or other members of the Compositae family, including ragweed. There are multiple reports of allergic skin rashes after contact with feverfew.

Side Effects and Warnings

- Few side effects are reported in human studies of feverfew. The side effects that do occur are usually mild and reversible. Mouth inflammation or ulcers, including swelling of the lips, tongue irritation, bleeding of the gums, and loss of taste, have been reported and usually occur after direct contact of the mouth with the leaves, although some people report burning after swallowing a capsule containing dried leaf. Photosensitivity (sensitivity to sunlight or sunlamps) has been reported with other herbs in the Compositae plant family and may also be possible with feverfew. Indigestion, nausea, flatulence, constipation, diarrhea, abdominal bloating, and heartburn have been reported rarely in human studies. Gardeners may develop skin irritation at sites of contact with feverfew plants. Feverfew can also cause allergic rashes. One small study reported increased heart rate in some patients.
- Long-term feverfew users who stop treatment suddenly may experience feverfew withdrawal symptoms, including

rebound headaches, anxiety, difficulty sleeping, muscle stiffness, and joint pain.

- Laboratory tests suggest that feverfew affects blood platelets and in theory may increase the risk of bleeding. However, this has not been clearly shown in humans. Nonetheless, caution is advised in patients with bleeding disorders or in those taking drugs that may increase the risk of bleeding. Dosing adjustments may be necessary. Use caution before some surgeries or dental procedures because of a theoretical increase in bleeding risk.

Pregnancy and Breastfeeding

- There is not enough information about safety to recommend feverfew during pregnancy or breastfeeding. Traditional experience suggests that feverfew may stimulate menstrual flow and induce abortion and therefore should be avoided.

INTERACTIONS
Interactions with Drugs

- Based on laboratory research, feverfew theoretically may increase the risk of bleeding when taken with drugs that increase the risk of bleeding. However, this has not been clearly shown in humans. Some examples include aspirin, anticoagulants ("blood thinners") such as warfarin (Coumadin) or heparin, antiplatelet drugs such as clopidogrel (Plavix), and nonsteroidal antiinflammatory drugs such as ibuprofen (Motrin, Advil) or naproxen (Naprosyn, Aleve).
- Sun sensitivity caused by certain drugs like doxycycline or Retin A may be increased by feverfew. Feverfew may also alter the way that certain drugs are broken down by the liver.

- Feverfew may have an additive effect if taken along with drugs taken for cancer, histamine release, fungal or protozoal infections, and drugs that increase blood flow. Feverfew may also interact with anesthetics and antibiotics.
- In theory, feverfew may interact with antidepressants and should be used with caution in people with a history of depression and/or other mental illness.

Interactions with Herbs and Dietary Supplements

- In theory, feverfew may increase the risk of bleeding when taken with herbs and supplements that are believed to increase the risk of bleeding. This is based on laboratory research and has not been reported clearly in humans. Multiple cases of bleeding have been reported with the use of *Ginkgo biloba* and fewer cases have been reported with garlic and saw palmetto. Numerous other agents may theoretically increase the risk of bleeding, although this has not been proven in most cases.
- Sun sensitivity caused by certain herbs and supplements may be increased by feverfew. Feverfew may alter the way that certain herbs and supplements are broken down by the liver.
- Feverfew may theoretically interact with herbs that act as antidepressants, such as St. John's wort.
- Feverfew may also interact with herbs taken for cancer, parasitic infection, fungal infection, bacterial infection, protozoal infection, and drugs that increase blood flow.

For a complete list of references, please visit www.naturalstandard.com.

F

Fig
(Ficus carica)

RELATED TERMS

- Caricae fructus, feigen, *Ficus benjamina* (weeping fig), *Ficus carica*, *Ficus elastica* (rubber plant).

BACKGROUND

- Figs are thought to have been first cultivated in Egypt. They spread to ancient Crete and subsequently to ancient Greece, where they became a staple in the traditional diet. Figs were regarded with such esteem that laws were created forbidding the export of the best quality figs. Figs were respected in ancient Rome and thought of as a sacred fruit. According to Roman myth, the twin founders of Rome, Romulus and Remus, rested under a fig tree.
- Traditionally, figs have been used to treat constipation, bronchitis, hyperlipidemia (high cholesterol levels), eczema, psoriasis (chronic skin disease), vitiligo (white skin patches), and diabetes (high blood sugar). Topically, its latex has been used to remove warts and treat skin tumors.
- At this time, there are no high-quality human trials supporting the effectiveness of fig for any indication. However, the antioxidant activity and cytotoxicity against various cancer cell lines reported in fig are potentially promising in its future therapeutic uses.

EVIDENCE

Uses Based on Scientific Evidence	Grade
Diabetes (Type 1) Preliminary evidence suggests that fig has antioxidant properties and may be beneficial in type 1 diabetes.	C

Uses Based on Tradition or Theory
Antioxidant, cancer, hemostatic potency (stops bleeding), photosensitization (abnormal sensitivity to sunlight).

DOSING

Adults (18 Years and Older)

- There is insufficient evidence to recommend a dose for fig. However, as a tea decoction, 1 cup daily of 13 g of *Ficus carica* leaf has been used.

Children (Younger than 18 Years)

- There is insufficient evidence to recommend a dose for fig in children, and use is not recommended.

SAFETY

Allergies

- Avoid in individuals with a known allergy or hypersensitivity to fig or herbs in the Moraceae family. Some oral allergy syndromes in people have been attributed to cross-sensitivity to grass and birch pollens. Food allergy to fig has also been reported due to cross sensitization to weeping fig (*Ficus benjamina*) or mulberry. Sensitization to fig with cross-sensitization to weeping fig and natural rubber latex has also been reported.
- Allergic reactions to fresh or dried figs can occur as a consequence of primary sensitization to airborne *Ficus benjamina* allergens independent of sensitization to rubber latex allergens. Kiwi fruit, papaya, and avocado as well as pineapple and banana may be other fruits associated with sensitization to *Ficus* allergens.

Side Effects and Warnings

- There are few reports of adverse effects associated with fig. At least one report has indicated no adverse effects in subjects who were treated with an oral (by mouth) fig leaf decoction for 1 month. However, because fig leaf contains psoralens, it may cause photodermatitis when applied to the skin. Excessive sunlight or ultraviolet light exposure should be avoided while products that contain fig leaf are used.
- Many cases of occupational allergy to weeping fig in plant keepers have been reported, and side effects may include conjunctivitis, rhinitis, anaphylactic shock or asthma.
- Although rare, obstructive ileus (intestinal/bowel obstruction), hemolytic anemia (deficiency of red blood cells), and retinal hemorrhages (bleeding of the retina) have been reported. Use cautiously in patients with bleeding disorders.

Pregnancy and Breastfeeding

- Fig, taken as a medicinal agent, is not recommended in pregnant or breastfeeding women because of a lack of available scientific evidence. However, fresh or dried fruit is likely safe when taken by mouth in amounts commonly found in foods.

INTERACTIONS

Interactions with Drugs

- Theoretically, because fig leaf contains furocoumarins, it may increase the risk of bleeding when taken with drugs that increase the risk of bleeding. Some examples include aspirin, anticoagulants ("blood thinners") such as warfarin (Coumadin) or heparin, antiplatelet drugs such as clopidogrel (Plavix), and nonsteroidal antiinflammatory drugs (NSAIDs) such as ibuprofen (Motrin, Advil) or naproxen (Naprosyn, Aleve).
- Theoretically, fig leaf may lower blood sugar levels. Caution is advised when medications that may also lower blood sugar are used. Patients taking drugs for diabetes by mouth or using insulin should be monitored closely by a qualified health care professional, including a pharmacist. Medication adjustments may be necessary.

Interactions with Herbs and Dietary Supplements

- Theoretically, because fig leaf contains furocoumarins, it may increase the risk of bleeding when taken with herbs

Fig 331

and supplements that are believed to increase the risk of bleeding. Multiple cases of bleeding have been reported with the use of *Ginkgo biloba*, and fewer cases have been reported with garlic and saw palmetto. Numerous other agents may theoretically increase the risk of bleeding, although this has not been proven in most cases.

- Theoretically, fig leaf may lower blood sugar levels. Caution is advised when herbs or supplements that may also lower blood sugar are used. Blood glucose levels may require monitoring, and doses may need adjustment.

For a complete list of references, please visit www.naturalstandard.com.

F

Flax
(Linum usitatissimum)

RELATED TERMS

- Alashi, alpha-linolenic acid, Barlean's Flax Oil, Barlean's Vita-Flax, brazen, common flax, eicosapentaenoic acid, flachssamen, flax, gamma-linolenic acid, Graine de Lin, leinsamen, hu-ma-esze, Linaceae, linen flax, lini semen, lino, lino usuale, linseed, linseed oil, lint bells, linum, *Linum catharticum, Linum humile* seeds, keten, omega-3 fatty acid, phytoestrogen, prebiotic bread, sufulsi, tesimosina, Type I Flaxseed/Flaxseed (51-55% alpha-linolenic acid), Type II Flaxseed/CDC-flaxseed (2-3% alpha-linolenic acid), winterlien.

BACKGROUND

- Flaxseed and its derivative flaxseed oil/linseed oil are rich sources of the essential fatty acid alpha-linolenic acid, which is a biological precursor to omega-3 fatty acids such as eicosapentaenoic acid. Although omega-3 fatty acids have been associated with improved cardiovascular outcomes, evidence from human trials is mixed regarding the efficacy of flaxseed products for coronary artery disease or hyperlipidemia.
- The lignin constituents of flaxseed (not flaxseed oil) possess in vitro antioxidant and possible estrogen receptor agonist/antagonist properties, prompting theories of efficacy for the treatment of breast cancer. However, there is not sufficient human evidence to make a recommendation. As a source of fiber mucilage, oral flaxseed (not flaxseed oil) may possess laxative properties, although only one human trial has been conducted for this indication. In large doses or when taken with inadequate water, flaxseed may precipitate bowel obstruction via a mass effect. The effects of flaxseed on blood glucose levels are not clear, although hyperglycemic effects have been reported in one case series.
- Flaxseed oil contains only the alpha-linolenic acid component of flaxseed and not the fiber or lignin components. Therefore, flaxseed oil may share the purported lipid-lowering properties of flaxseed but not the proposed laxative or anticancer abilities.

EVIDENCE

Uses Based on Scientific Evidence	Grade
Attention Deficit Hyperactivity Disorder (ADHD) Preliminary evidence supports the idea that deficiencies or imbalances in certain highly unsaturated fatty acids may contribute to attention deficit hyperactivity disorder (ADHD). Based on one trial, alpha linolenic acid–rich nutritional supplementation in the form of flax oil may improve symptoms of ADHD. More research is needed to confirm these results.	C
Breast Cancer (Flaxseed, Not Flaxseed Oil) There is a lack of information from human studies that flaxseed is effective in preventing or treating breast cancer.	C
Diabetes (Flaxseed, Not Flaxseed Oil) Human studies on the effect of flaxseed on blood sugar levels report mixed results. Flaxseed cannot be recommended as a treatment for diabetes at this time.	C
Dry Eye Syndrome Taking flaxseed oil capsules by mouth may reduce dry eyes associated with Sjögren's syndrome patients.	C
Heart Disease (Flaxseed and Flaxseed Oil) People who have had a heart attack are reported to benefit from diets rich in alpha-linolenic acid, which is found in flaxseed. It is unclear whether flaxseed supplementation alters the course of heart disease.	C
High Blood Pressure (Flaxseed, Not Flaxseed Oil) In animals, diets high in flaxseed have mixed effects on blood pressure. Limited clinical evidence suggests that flaxseed might lower blood pressure.	C
High Cholesterol or Triglycerides (Flaxseed and Flaxseed Oil) In laboratory and animal studies, flaxseed and flaxseed oil are reported to lower blood cholesterol levels. Effects on blood triglyceride levels in animals are unclear, with increased levels in some research and decreased levels in other research. Clinical studies in this area report mixed results, with decreased blood levels of total cholesterol and low-density lipoprotein ("bad cholesterol") in some studies but no effect in other studies.	C
HIV/AIDS There is a lack of strong evidence to support this indication.	C
Kidney Disease/Lupus Nephritis (Flaxseed, Not Flaxseed Oil) There is a lack of strong evidence to support this indication.	C
Laxative (Flaxseed, Not Flaxseed Oil) Preliminary clinical evidence suggests that flaxseed can be used as a laxative. However, the comparative effectiveness remains unclear.	C
Menopausal Symptoms There is preliminary evidence that flaxseed oil may help decrease mild menopausal symptoms. This remains an area of controversy. Patients should consult a doctor and pharmacist about treatment options before starting a new therapy. Overall effects on bone mineral density and lipid profiles remain unclear.	C
Menstrual Breast Pain (Flaxseed, Not Flaxseed Oil) Limited clinical evidence suggests that flaxseed may reduce menstrual breast pain.	C

Uses Based on Scientific Evidence	Grade
Obesity There is limited research on the effects of flaxseed flour and its effects in obese patients.	C
Pregnancy (Spontaneous Delivery) It has been proposed that alpha-linolenic acid, provided as flax oil capsules, may delay the timing of spontaneous delivery, but the available evidence does not support this use.	C
Prostate Cancer (Flaxseed, Not Flaxseed Oil) There is limited high-quality research on the effects of flaxseed or alpha-linolenic acid (found in flaxseed) on the risk of developing prostate cancer. This area remains controversial as there are some data reporting possible increased risk of prostate cancer with alpha-linolenic acid. Prostate cancer should be treated by a medical oncologist.	C

Uses Based on Tradition or Theory

Abdominal pain, acute respiratory distress syndrome (ARDS), allergic reactions, antioxidant, benign prostatic hypertrophy (BPH), bipolar disorder, bladder inflammation, blood thinner, boils, bowel irritation, bronchial irritation, burns (poultice), catarrh (inflammation of mucous membrane), colon cancer, cough (suppression or loosening of mucus), cystitis, depression, diabetic nephropathy, diarrhea, diverticulitis, dry skin, dysentery, eczema, emollient, enlarged prostate, enteritis, eye cleansing (debris in the eye), gastritis, gonorrhea, headache, infections, inflammation, irritable bowel syndrome, liver protection, malaria, melanoma, menstrual disorders, ovarian disorders, pimples, psoriasis, rheumatoid arthritis, skin infections, skin inflammation, sore throat, stomach upset, stroke, ulcerative colitis, upper respiratory tract infection, urinary tract infection, vaginitis, vision improvement.

DOSING
Adults (18 Years and Older)

- Flaxseed oil is available in liquid and capsule form, flaxseed powder, flour, and soluble fiber, and 10-250 g have been taken by mouth.
- Whole or bruised (not ground) flaxseed can be mixed with liquid and taken by mouth. Generally, 1 tablespoon in this form is mixed with 6-12 oz of liquid and taken by mouth up to three times a day. Some studies use doses of soluble flaxseed mucilage/fiber as high as 60-80 g/kg (1 kg = 2.2 lb) of the person's weight. These liquid forms of flaxseed should not be confused with preparations of flaxseed oil.
- Anecdotally, 30-100 g of flaxseed flour can be mixed with warm or hot water to form a moist compress and can be applied to the skin up to three times a day. It is not clear how long a flaxseed poultice should be used.

Children (Younger than 18 Years)

- There is insufficient evidence to recommend a dose of flaxseed or flaxseed oil in children.

SAFETY
Allergies

- People with known allergy to flaxseed, flaxseed oil, or any other members of the Linaceae plant family or *Linum* genus should avoid flaxseed products. Severe allergic reactions have been reported.

Side Effects and Warnings

- There are few studies of flaxseed safety in humans. Flaxseed and flaxseed oil supplements do appear to be well tolerated in the available research, and there is long-standing historical use of flaxseed products without many reports of side effects. However, unripe flaxseed pods are believed to be poisonous and should not be eaten. Raw flaxseed or flaxseed plant may increase blood levels of cyanide, a toxic chemical (this effect has not been reported when flaxseed supplements are taken at recommended doses). Do not apply flaxseed or flaxseed oil to open wounds or broken skin.
- Based on animal studies, overdose of flaxseed may cause shortness of breath, rapid breathing, weakness, or difficulty walking and may cause seizures or paralysis. Theoretically, flaxseed (*not* flaxseed oil) may increase the risk of cell damage from a reaction called oxidative stress. Studies report conflicting results in this area. Based on one study, flaxseed or flaxseed oil taken by mouth may cause mania or hypomania in people with bipolar disorder. In theory, the laxative effects of flaxseed (*not* flaxseed oil) may cause diarrhea, increased number of bowel movements, and abdominal discomfort. Laxative effects are reported in several studies of people taking flaxseed or omega-3 acids. People with diarrhea, irritable bowel syndrome, diverticulitis, or inflammatory bowel disease (Crohn's disease or ulcerative colitis) should avoid flaxseed because of its possible laxative effects. Nausea, vomiting, and abdominal pain were reported in two individuals shortly after taking flaxseed products by mouth; these reactions may have been caused by allergy.
- Large amounts of flaxseed by mouth may cause the intestines to stop moving (ileus). People with narrowing of the esophagus or intestine, ileus, or bowel obstruction should avoid flaxseed (*not* flaxseed oil). Individuals with high blood triglyceride levels should avoid flaxseed and flaxseed oil because of unclear effects on triglyceride levels in animal research. People with diabetes should use caution if taking flaxseed products by mouth, as the omega-3 fatty acids in flaxseed and flaxseed oil may increase blood sugar levels.
- One study reports that the menstrual period may be altered in women who take flaxseed powder by mouth daily. Because of the possible estrogen-like effects of flaxseed (*not* flaxseed oil), it should be used cautiously in women with hormone-sensitive conditions such as endometriosis, polycystic ovary syndrome, uterine fibroids, or cancer of the breast, uterus, or ovary. Some natural medicine textbooks advise caution in patients with hypothyroidism, although little scientific information is available in this area. Flaxseed and flaxseed oil may increase the risk of bleeding, based on early studies that show decreased clotting of blood. Caution is advised in patients with bleeding disorders, in people taking drugs that increase the risk of bleeding, and in people planning to undergo medical, surgical, or dental procedures. Dosing of blood-thinning medications may need to be adjusted. In animal studies, flaxseed has increased the number of red blood cells.

F

- Several studies in humans report an increased risk of prostate cancer in men taking alpha-linolenic acid (which is present in flaxseed) by mouth. One small study of men with prostate cancer reports that flaxseed supplements do not increase prostate-specific antigen (PSA) levels. Until more information is available, men with prostate cancer or at risk of prostate cancer should avoid flaxseed and alpha-linolenic acid supplements.

Pregnancy and Breastfeeding

- The use of flaxseed or flaxseed oil during pregnancy and breastfeeding is not recommended. Animal studies show possible harmful effects, and there is little information in humans. Flaxseed may stimulate menstruation or have other hormonal effects and could be harmful to pregnancy.

INTERACTIONS

Interactions with Drugs

- Taking flaxseed (*not* flaxseed oil) by mouth may reduce the absorption of other medications. Drugs used by mouth should be taken 1 hour before or 2 hours after flaxseed to prevent decreased absorption. People taking mood stabilizers such as lithium should use caution. Flaxseed contains alpha-linolenic acid, which may theoretically lower blood pressure. Individuals taking medications to lower blood pressure should use caution when taking flaxseed. Laxatives and stool softeners may increase or enhance the laxative effects of flaxseed. Flaxseed and flaxseed oil can lower cholesterol levels in animals, but studies in humans show mixed results. In theory, flaxseed may increase the effect of other medications that lower lipid (cholesterol and triglyceride) levels in the blood. Hormonal drugs may be affected. Dietary flaxseed may increase the effects of tamoxifen, a medication used to treat cancer. Consult a qualified oncologist and pharmacist before making decisions about treatment or health conditions.

- Although studies report conflicting results, the omega-3 fatty acids in flaxseed and flaxseed oil may increase blood sugar, reducing the effects of diabetes treatments, including insulin and glucose-lowering medications taken by mouth. Flaxseed (*not* flaxseed oil) is a rich source of plant lignins. Lignins are sometimes referred to as phytoestrogens and may possess estrogen-like properties. It is not known if flaxseed can alter the effects of birth control pills or hormone replacement therapies. Flaxseed and flaxseed oil theoretically may increase the risk of bleeding, and caution should be used when flaxseed products are taken with drugs that increase the risk of bleeding. Some examples include aspirin, anticoagulants ("blood thinners") such as warfarin (Coumadin) or heparin, antiplatelet drugs such as clopidogrel (Plavix), and nonsteroidal antiinflammatory drugs such as ibuprofen (Motrin, Advil) or naproxen (Naprosyn, Aleve).

- Flaxseed may also interact with muscle relaxants (such as metaxalone), drugs used for acid reflex (proton pump inhibitors such as lansoprazole), or prostaglandins (such as iloprost or treprostinil).

Interactions with Herbs and Dietary Supplements

- Consumption of flaxseed (*not* flaxseed oil) may reduce the absorption of vitamins or supplements taken by mouth at the same time. Therefore, vitamins and supplements should be taken 1 hour before or 2 hours after a dose of flaxseed to prevent decreased absorption. Flaxseed may alter the effects of psyllium and vitamin E in particular.

- Use caution if combining flaxseed with other mood-altering herbs, including St. John's wort (*Hypericum perforatum*), kava (*Piper methysticum*), or valerian (*Valeriana officinalis*). Hormonal herbs and supplements may be affected. Flaxseed contains alpha-linolenic acid, which may theoretically lower blood pressure. Use caution when combining flaxseed with other herbs or supplements that can lower blood pressure.

- Because of the laxative effects of flaxseed, caution should be used when it is taken with other supplements that have laxative effects.

- Studies on the effects of flaxseed on blood sugar in people with type 2 diabetes report mixed results. Use caution when combining flaxseed products with supplements that may raise blood sugar levels. In theory, flaxseed may contain estrogen-like chemicals. Use caution when combining flaxseed (*not* flaxseed oil) with supplements believed to have estrogen-like properties.

- Early studies in humans show that flaxseed and flaxseed oil theoretically may increase the risk of bleeding. Caution should be used when flaxseed products are taken with herbs and supplements that are believed to increase the risk of bleeding.

- Flaxseed may lower blood cholesterol levels. Caution is advised when herbs or supplements that may also lower cholesterol levels are used. Cholesterol levels may require monitoring, and doses may need adjustment.

- Use cautiously when taking flaxseed with other herbs or supplements taken to treat or prevent cancer because of a possible interaction.

For a complete list of references, please visit www.naturalstandard.com.

Folate
(Folic Acid)

RELATED TERMS

- B complex vitamin, folacin, folate, folic acid, folinic acid, pteroylglutamic acid, pteroylmonoglutamic acid, pteroylpolyglutamate, vitamin B_9, vitamin M.

BACKGROUND

- Folate and folic acid are forms of a water-soluble B vitamin. Folate occurs naturally in food, and folic acid is the synthetic form of this vitamin. Folic acid is well-tolerated in amounts found in fortified foods and supplements. Sources include cereals, baked goods, leafy vegetables (spinach, broccoli, lettuce), okra, asparagus, fruits (bananas, melons, lemons), legumes, yeast, mushrooms, organ meat (beef liver, kidney), orange juice, and tomato juice. Folic acid is frequently used in combination with other B vitamins in vitamin B complex formulations.

EVIDENCE

Uses Based on Scientific Evidence	Grade
Folate Deficiency Folate deficiency will occur if the body does not get the adequate amount of folic acid from dietary intake. Folic acid has been shown to be effective in the treatment of megaloblastic and macrocytic anemias due to folate deficiency.	A
Megaloblastic Anemia (Due to Folate Deficiency) Folate deficiency can cause megaloblastic (or macrocytic) anemia. In this type of anemia, red blood cells are larger than normal, and the ratio of nucleus size to cell cytoplasm is increased. There are other potential causes of megaloblastic anemia, including vitamin B_{12} deficiency or various inborn metabolic disorders. If the cause is folate deficiency, then treatment with folate is the standard approach. Patients with anemia should be evaluated by a physician so that the underlying cause is diagnosed and addressed.	A
Prevention of Pregnancy Complications Studies have proven that folate consumption during pregnancy prevents deficiency and anemia in pregnant women. Low folate levels during pregnancy may contribute to birth defects and pregnancy loss. Consuming a high dietary intake of folate and taking folic acid supplements orally during pregnancy reduces the risk of neural tube birth defects or cleft palate in the infant.	A
Methotrexate Toxicity Folate supplementation is beneficial in patients being treated with long-term, low-dose methotrexate for rheumatoid arthritis (RA) or psoriasis. Development	B

of folate deficiency is associated with increased risk of certain side effects including gastrointestinal effects, stomatitis, alopecia, abnormal liver function tests, myelosuppression, megaloblastic anemia, and increased homocysteine levels, which are associated with cardiovascular disease. People who have experienced side effects may need to continue taking folic acid for the duration of methotrexate therapy. Patients receiving methotrexate for cancer should avoid folic acid supplements, unless recommended by their oncologist. There is some evidence that folic acid supplements reduce the efficacy of methotrexate in the treatment of acute lymphoblastic leukemia, and theoretically they could reduce its efficacy in the treatment of other cancers.

Alzheimer's Disease Preliminary evidence indicates that low folate concentrations might be related to Alzheimer's disease. Well-designed clinical trials of folate supplementation are needed before a conclusion can be drawn.	C
Arsenic Poisoning (Arsenic-Induced Illnesses) Folate may lower blood arsenic concentrations and thereby contribute to the prevention of arsenic-induced illnesses. Additional research is needed in this area.	C
Cancer Preliminary evidence surrounding the use of folate seems promising for decreasing the risk of breast, cervical, pancreatic, and gastrointestinal cancer. However, currently there is insufficient evidence available to recommend folate supplementation for any type of cancer prevention or treatment. Please follow the advice of a qualified health care provider in this area.	C
Chronic Fatigue Syndrome Some patients with chronic fatigue syndrome (CFS) also have decreased folic acid levels. Daily injections of a combination of folic acid, bovine liver extract, and vitamin B_{12} for 3 weeks were not beneficial for CFS in one study.	C
Depression Folic acid deficiency has been found among people with depression and has been linked to poor response to antidepressant treatment. Folate supplements have been used for enhancing treatment response to antidepressants. Limited clinical research suggests that folic acid is not effective as a replacement for conventional antidepressant therapy. Depression should be treated by a qualified health care provider.	C

(Continued)

Uses Based on Scientific Evidence	Grade
Folate Deficiency in Alcoholics Folate deficiency has been observed in alcoholics. Alcohol interferes with the absorption of folate and increases excretion of folate by the kidney. Many alcohol abusers have poor-quality diets that do not provide the recommended intake of folate. Increasing folate intake through diet or folic acid intake through fortified foods or supplements may be beneficial to the health of alcoholics.	C
Hearing Loss (Age-Associated Hearing Decline) Folic acid supplementation slowed the decline in hearing of speech frequencies associated with aging in a population from a country without folic acid fortification of food. The effect requires confirmation, especially in populations from countries with folic acid fortification programs.	C
Nitrate Tolerance Folic acid might prevent nitroglycerin-induced nitrate tolerance and cross-tolerance to endothelial nitric oxide, which plays a role in blood pressure control. These conditions need to be treated by a qualified health care provider.	C
Phenytoin-Induced Gingival Hyperplasia Early evidence shows that applying folic acid topically may inhibit gingival hyperplasia (overgrowth of gum tissue) secondary to phenytoin therapy. Oral folic acid supplementation has not been proven to be beneficial. More research is needed in this area.	C
Pregnancy-Related Gingivitis Based on preliminary data, applying folic acid topically may improve gingivitis in pregnant women. Well-designed clinical trials are needed to confirm these results.	C
Stroke Study results are mixed for the use of folate in stroke patients. Further research is needed in this area before a strong recommendation can be made.	C
Vascular Disease/Hyperhomocysteinemia Elevated homocysteine levels may be a marker of vascular disease. Preliminary data suggest that folic acid lowers homocysteine levels and might reduce the risk of vascular disease (cardiac, peripheral, or cerebral). Large randomized controlled trials are needed before a firm conclusion can be drawn.	C
Vitiligo Based on preliminary data, folic acid and vitamin B_{12} may improve the symptoms of vitiligo. Further research is needed to confirm these results.	C
Down's Syndrome One study does not show a protective effect of folic acid on heart anomalies among infants with Down's syndrome.	D
Lometrexol Toxicity Folic acid supplementation does not seem to reduce toxicity from the cancer drug lometrexol.	D
Fragile X Syndrome Folic acid supplementation has been shown not to improve symptoms of fragile X syndrome.	F

Uses Based on Tradition or Theory

Acquired immunodeficiency syndrome (AIDS), anti-aging (preventing signs of aging), aphthous ulcers, celiac disease, colorectal adenoma, Crohn's disease, diabetes (type 2), fracture (risk reduction), genetic damage (X-ray induced chromosomal damage), high blood pressure, infertility, insomnia, liver disease, macular degeneration, memory enhancement, osteoporosis, peripheral neuropathy, restless leg syndrome, sickle cell anemia, spinal cord injury (myelopathy), ulcerative colitis.

DOSING
Adults (18 Years and Older)

- U.S. recommended dietary allowance (RDA) for adults (oral): 400 mcg daily for males or females ages 14 years and older; 500 mcg daily for breastfeeding adult women; 600 mcg daily for pregnant adult women. All are given as dietary folate equivalents (DFE).
- Tolerable upper intake levels (UL) per day: The UL is the maximum daily level of intake that is likely not to pose a risk of adverse effects. The UL is 800 mcg daily for males or females ages 14-18 years old (including pregnant or breastfeeding women) and 1000 mcg daily for males or females ages 19 years and older (including pregnant or breastfeeding women).
- Adjunct treatment with conventional antidepressants: Doses of 200-500 mcg daily has been used for enhancing treatment response to antidepressants. Limited clinical research suggests that folic acid is not effective as a replacement for conventional antidepressant therapy.
- Anticonvulsant-induced folate deficiency: 15 mg (15,000 mcg) daily has been used under the supervision of a qualified health care provider.
- Cervical cancer: 0.8-10 mg (800-10,000 mcg) daily has been used, but further data are necessary before a strong recommendation can be made.
- Colon cancer: Doses of 400 mcg daily have been used to reduce the risk of colon cancer occurring, although supplementation has not been proven to be effective.
- Drug-induced toxicity: For reduction of toxicity symptoms (nausea and vomiting) associated with methotrexate therapy for rheumatoid arthritis (RA) or psoriasis, 1 mg/day (1000 mcg daily) may be sufficient, but up to 5 mg/day (5000 mcg daily) may be used.
- End-stage renal disease (ESRD): Doses of 0.8-15 mg (800-15,000 mcg) folic acid daily are generally used, but the degree of homocysteine reduction is variable (between 12%-50%), and normal homocysteine levels (<12 micromoles/L) cannot always be achieved. Folic acid 2.5-5 mg (2500-5000 mcg) three times weekly also reduces homocysteine levels in ESRD patients receiving dialysis.

Doses greater than 15 mg (15,000 mcg)/day do not provide additional benefit. Doses of 30-60 mg (30,000-60,000 mcg) seem to cause a rebound in homocysteine levels when treatment is stopped.

- Folate deficiency: The typical dose is 250-1000 mcg daily. For severe folate deficiency, such as in cases of megaloblastic anemia and malabsorption disorders, 1-5 mg (1000-5000 mcg)/day is often used until corrected blood tests are documented by a qualified health care professional.
- Hyperhomocysteinemia: Doses of 0.5-5 mg/day (500-15,000 mcg) have been used, although 0.8-1 mg/day (800-1000 mcg) appears to provide maximal reduction of homocysteine levels. Doses greater than 1 mg daily (1000 mcg) do not seem to produce any greater benefit except in some people with certain gene mutations that cause homocysteine levels of 20 micromoles/L or higher. However, initial data suggest that the U.S. government–mandated fortification of cereals and flour with 140 mcg folic acid per 100 g is reducing the mean homocysteine level in the general population by about 7%. Consumption of at least 300 mcg daily of dietary folate seems to be associated with a 20% lower risk of stroke and a 13% lower risk of cardiovascular disease when compared with consumption of less than 136 mcg of folate per day. Doses of 10 mg (10,000 mcg) daily of folic acid have been used to improve coagulation status, oxidative stress, and endothelial dysfunction.
- Megaloblastic anemia: In cases of megaloblastic anemia resulting from folate deficiency or malabsorption disorders such as sprue, oral doses of 1-5 mg (1000-5000 mcg) daily may be used until hematological recovery is documented by a qualified health care provider.
- Neural tube defects (prevention): Doses of at least 400 mcg of folic acid per day from supplements or fortified food should be taken by women capable of becoming pregnant and continued through the first month of pregnancy. Women with a history of previous pregnancy complicated by such neural tube defects usually take 4 mg (4000 mcg) daily beginning 1 month before and continuing for 3 months after conception under the guidance of a qualified health care professional.
- Pancreatic cancer: Consuming greater than 280 mcg daily of dietary folate is associated with a decreased risk of exocrine pancreatic cancer. Further research is needed to confirm these results.
- Phenytoin-induced gingival hyperplasia: Applying folic acid topically may inhibit gingival hyperplasia secondary to phenytoin therapy. However, taking folic acid by mouth does not seem to be beneficial for this indication.
- Pregnancy-related gingivitis: Applying folic acid topically may improve gingivitis in pregnancy.
- Preventing increases in homocysteine levels after nitrous oxide anesthesia: Folate 2.5 mg (2500 mcg) in combination with pyridoxine 25 mg (25,000 mcg) and vitamin B_{12} 500 mcg has been used daily for 1 week before surgery under the supervision of a qualified health care provider.
- Vitiligo: Doses of 5 mg (5000 mcg) have been taken twice daily to improve the symptoms of vitiligo.

Children (Younger than 18 Years)

- U.S. Recommended Dietary Allowance (RDA) or Adequate Intake (AI) for children (oral): For infants 0-6 months old, the AI is 65 mcg daily; for infants 7-12 months old, the AI is 80 mcg daily; for children 1-3 years old, the RDA is 150 mcg daily; for children 4-8 years old, the RDA is 200 mcg daily; for children 9-13 years old, the RDA is 300 mcg daily. All are given as dietary folate equivalents (DFE).
- Tolerable upper intake levels (UL) daily: The UL is the maximum daily level of intake that is likely not to pose a risk of adverse effects. For children 1-3 years old, the UL is 300 mcg; for children 4-8 years old, the UL is 400 mcg; for children 9-13 years old, the UL is 600 mcg; for adolescents 14-18 years old, the UL is 800 mcg.
- Caution: Folic acid injection contains benzyl alcohol (1.5%) as a preservative, and extreme care should be used in administration to neonates. Folic acid injections should be administered by a qualified health care provider.

SAFETY
Allergies

- Avoid folic acid supplements if hypersensitive or allergic to any of the product ingredients.

Side Effects and Warnings

- Folate appears to be well tolerated in recommended doses. Stomatitis, alopecia, myelosupression, and zinc depletion have been reported.
- An intravenous loading dose of folic acid, vitamin B_6, and vitamin B_{12} followed by oral administration of folic acid plus vitamin B_6 and vitamin B_{12}, taken daily after coronary stenting, might actually increase restenosis rates. Because of the potential for harm, this combination of vitamins should not be recommended for patients receiving coronary stents.
- Erythema, pruritus, urticaria, skin flushing, rash, and itching have been reported.
- Nausea, bloating, flatulence, cramps, bitter taste, and diarrhea have been reported.
- Color of urine may become more intense.
- Folic acid may mask the symptoms of pernicious, aplastic, or normocytic anemias caused by vitamin B_{12} deficiency and may lead to neurological damage.
- Irritability, excitability, general malaise, altered sleep patterns, vivid dreaming, overactivity, confusion, impaired judgment, increased seizure frequency, and psychotic behavior have been reported. Very high doses can cause significant central nervous system (CNS) side effects. Supplemental folic acid might increase seizures in people with seizure disorders, particularly in very high doses.
- Anaphylaxis and bronchospasm have also been reported.

Pregnancy and Breastfeeding

- Pregnancy: It is recommended that all women capable of becoming pregnant consume folate to reduce the risk of the fetus developing a neural tube defect. Folic acid supplementation in higher than recommended doses is categorized as U.S. Food and Drug Administration (FDA) Pregnancy Category C.
- Breastfeeding: Folic acid is present in the breast milk and is likely safe to use during breastfeeding under the supervision of a qualified health care provider.

INTERACTIONS
Interactions with Drugs

- Excessive use of alcohol increases the requirement for folic acid.

F

- Aminosalicylic acid can reduce dietary folate absorption, worsening the folate deficiency often seen with active tuberculosis or preventing its reversal during treatment. Megaloblastic anemia occurs rarely and usually when there are other contributing factors, such as concurrent vitamin B_{12} malabsorption. Patients being treated for tuberculosis may be advised to take folic acid supplements if their dietary folate intake is low.
- Chronic use of large doses of antacids can reduce folic acid absorption, but this is likely significant only if dietary folate intake is very low. Maintenance of the recommended daily intake of folic acid in the diet is recommended.
- Antibiotic therapy can disrupt the normal gastrointestinal (GI) flora, interfering with the absorption of folic acid. Folate supplements are not considered necessary.
- Aspirin may decrease serum folate levels, especially with chronic large doses. It is suggested that folate is just being redistributed in the body rather than there being an actual folate deficiency; therefore, folate supplementation is not considered necessary.
- Oral contraceptives (birth control pills) may impair folate metabolism, which may cause depletion, but the effect is unlikely to cause anemia or megaloblastic changes.
- Carbamazepine (Tegretol) can reduce serum folate levels, but megaloblastic anemia has not been reported. Pregnant women taking carbamazepine may be especially at risk from reduced folate levels.
- Chloramphenicol may antagonize some effects of folic acid on the blood (hematopoietic system).
- Cholestyramine reduces folic acid absorption. It can lower serum and red blood cell folate levels in children taking large doses for several months. Maintenance of dietary folate intake is recommended.
- Colestipol (Colestid) can interfere with absorption of folic acid, and reduced serum folate levels may occur. Maintenance of dietary folate intake is recommended.
- Cycloserine can reduce serum folate levels, and rare cases of megaloblastic anemia have occurred. Maintenance of dietary folate intake is recommended.
- Limited data suggest that diuretics ("water pills") may increase excretion of folic acid. Reduced red blood cell folate levels, possibly contributing to increased homocysteine levels, a risk factor for cardiovascular disease, were found in one group of people taking diuretics for 6 months or longer. The need for folic acid supplementation during diuretic therapy requires further study before a firm recommendation can be made. Currently, maintenance of dietary folate intake is recommended.
- Reduced serum and red blood cell folate levels can occur in some women taking conjugated estrogens (Premarin), but this is unlikely in women with adequate dietary folate intake. Supplements are recommended only for those women with inadequate dietary intake or other conditions that contribute to folate deficiency and for those diagnosed with or at increased risk of cervical dysplasia (e.g., because of family history).
- Folic acid absorption from the small intestine is optimal at pH of 5.5-6. The increased pH associated with the use of H_2 blockers (such as cimetidine [Tagamet], famotidine [Pepcid], nizatidine [Axid], and ranitidine [Zantac]) may therefore reduce folic acid absorption, but this is probably significant only if dietary folate intake is very low. Another class of prescription drugs that may affect folic acid absorption is proton pump inhibitors (PPIs). These are used for reflux disease and ulcers and include esomeprazole (Nexium), lansoprazole (Prevacid), omeprazole (Prilosec), pantoprazole (Protonix), and rabeprazole (AcipHex). Maintenance of dietary folate intake is recommended.
- Reduced vitamin B_{12} and, to a lesser extent, folate levels occur in some people with diabetes and can contribute to hyperhomocysteinemia, which adds to their already increased risk of cardiovascular disease. The reduced folate levels seen in diabetic patients have been linked to metformin use in some cases, possibly as a result of reduced folic acid absorption. Symptomatic folate deficiency is unlikely to occur with metformin, but people with diabetes may need folic acid supplements to reduce hyperhomocysteinemia. Diabetes should be treated by a qualified health care provider.
- Methotrexate is a folate antagonist that prevents the conversion of folic acid to its active form and lowers plasma and red blood cell folate levels. Folic acid supplements reduce side effects without reducing the efficacy of methotrexate in treating rheumatoid arthritis or psoriasis. Patients being treated with methotrexate for cancer should avoid folic acid supplements, unless recommended by their oncologist. Folic acid could interfere with the anticancer effects of methotrexate.
- Reduced serum folate levels have been noted in people with multiple sclerosis (MS) after treatment with methylprednisolone sodium succinate (Solu-Medrol). Clinical significance is unknown.
- Chronic cigarette smoking is associated with diminished folate status.
- Folate-dependent enzymes have been inhibited in laboratory experiments by certain nonsteroidal antiinflammatory drugs (NSAIDs) (ibuprofen [Advil, Motrin, Nuprin], naproxen [Anaprox, Aleve], indomethacin [Indocin], and sulindac [Clinoril]). Clinical significance is unknown.
- Reduced folate levels can occur in some people taking pancreatic extracts (such as Pancrease, Cotazym, Viokase, Creon, Ultrase) possibly because of reduced absorption. Folate levels should be checked in patients taking pancreatic enzymes for prolonged periods.
- Pentamidine is a prescription drug used to treat *Pneumocystis carinii* pneumonia (PCP). Decreased serum folate levels and megaloblastic bone marrow changes can occur rarely with prolonged intravenous pentamidine (Pentacarinat, Pentam 300) therapy. Most patients are unlikely to need folic acid supplements.
- Phenobarbital (Luminal) and primidone (Mysoline) can reduce serum folate levels, occasionally leading to megaloblastic anemia (usually in people with low dietary folate intake), and possibly contributing to neurological side effects, mental changes, and cerebral atrophy. Pregnant women taking phenobarbital or primidone may be especially at risk from reduced folate levels. Folic acid can have direct convulsant activity in some people, reversing the effects of phenobarbital or primidone and worsening seizure control. Folic acid may increase metabolism of phenobarbital. Seizure activity should be monitored closely.
- Pyrimethamine (Daraprim) is a folate antagonist that prevents conversion of folic acid to its active form. Patients taking pyrimethamine should avoid folic acid supplements because they can antagonize the therapeutic effects against *Toxoplasmosis* and *Pneumocystis carinii* pneumonia. Patients

taking lower doses of pyrimethamine for prolonged periods should maintain the recommended dietary folate intake and be monitored for folate deficiency. Folic acid does not antagonize the effects of pyrimethamine in the treatment of malaria. Folinic acid may be used as an alternative to folic acid when indicated. Pyrimethamine also reduces serum folate levels.

- One study found that administration of folic acid to pregnant women might not interfere with the protective effect of sulfadoxine/pyrimethamine combination when used for intermittent preventative treatment of malaria.
- Sulfasalazine inhibits absorption and metabolism of folic acid. Patients on chronic sulfasalazine therapy may be advised to increase their dietary folate intake and to take a supplement if they have any other condition, that could also contribute to deficiency.
- Triamterene (Dyrenium) is a folate antagonist that prevents conversion of folic acid to its active form and also reduces folate absorption. Reduced serum and red blood cell folate levels have occurred, as well as occasional cases of megaloblastic anemia, usually in people with other conditions contributing to folate deficiency. Patients on chronic triamterene therapy should maintain the recommended dietary folate intake or take a supplement if advised by their physician.
- There is a general belief that folic/folinic acid supplements do not interfere with the therapeutic effects of trimethoprim. However, this view has been challenged, and failure of trimethoprim therapy has occurred rarely when folinic acid is given concurrently.

Interactions with Herbs and Dietary Supplements

- Reduced serum and red blood cell folate levels can occur in some women taking conjugated estrogens (Premarin) or birth control pills, but this is unlikely in women with adequate dietary folate intake. Theoretically this interaction may also occur with estrogenic herbs and supplements.
- Taking folic acid along with vitamin B_{12} may increase the risk of vitamin B_{12} deficiency. Caution is advised when both of these vitamins are taken together.
- Normal supplemental doses of folic acid are unlikely to have an adverse effect on zinc balance in people with adequate dietary zinc intake. The data on the effects of supplemental folic acid on dietary zinc absorption are conflicting.

For a complete list of references, please visit www.naturalstandard.com.

Fo-ti
(*Polygonum multiflorum*)

RELATED TERMS

- Chinese climbing knotweed, Chinese cornbind, Chinese flowery knotweed, Chinese knotweed, fo ti, fo-ti-tient, fo-ti root, foti, he shou wu (Chinese), heshouwu (Chinese), ho shou wu (Chinese), Hoshouwu (Chinese), multiflori preparata, multiflori, *Polygonum*, *Polygonum multiflorum*, radix polygoni, radix polygoni multiflori, radix Polygoni Shen Min, "red" fo-ti, Shen Min, Shou Wu, Shou-Wu, Shouwu, shou-wu-pian, shou xing bu zhi, "white" fo-ti, zhihe shou wu, Zhihe Shou Wu, Zhihe-Shou-Wu, zhihe-shouwu, zi shou wu, Zi-Shou-Wu, zishouwu.
- **Note**: No fo-ti is contained in the product Fo-ti-Tieng.

BACKGROUND

- Fo-ti (Chinese name: he-shou-wu) is a plant native to China, where it continues to be widely grown. It also grows extensively in Japan and Taiwan. Fo-ti has a history of reversing and preventing the effects of aging.
- Fo-ti is available in both unprocessed and processed forms. Unprocessed fo-ti (also known as "white" fo-ti because its color is usually much lighter than the processed form) is taken by mouth for its laxative effect. Topically (applied on the skin), unprocessed fo-ti is used to treat skin conditions such as acne, athlete's foot, dermatitis, razor burn, and scrapes. Processed fo-ti, also known as "red" fo-ti because it is much darker in color than the unprocessed variety, is used to prevent or delay heart disease by blocking the formation of plaque in blood vessels.
- Currently, there are no high-quality human trials available supporting the use of fo-ti for any indication.

EVIDENCE

Uses Based on Scientific Evidence

No available studies qualify for inclusion in the evidence table.

Uses Based on Tradition or Theory

Acne, anemia (low red blood cell count resulting in weakness, fatigue, and paleness), angina pectoris (chest pain), antioxidant, atherosclerosis (hardening of the arteries), athlete's foot, autoimmune diseases, blood purification, cancer, carbuncles (clusters of boils on the skin), cerebral ischemia (inadequate blood flow to the brain), constipation, dermatitis, diabetes, dizziness (vertigo), energy, enhanced immune function, erectile dysfunction, hormone replacement therapy (HRT), hypercholesterolemia (high cholesterol levels), hypertension (high blood pressure), impotence (inability to develop or maintain an erection of the penis), infections, infertility, insomnia, itchiness, laxative, liver enlargement or disease, longevity/anti-aging, low back pain, memory (learning), muscle soreness, muscle strength, scrapes, skin eruptions, stomach disorders, tonic (liver, kidney), tuberculosis, vaginal discharge, weakness.

DOSING

Adults (18 Years and Older)

- There is insufficient evidence to recommend a dose for fo-ti. Capsules, dried herb preparations, teas, and topical creams or ointments are all commercially available. Doses of 560 mg (capsules) two to three times a day and 9-15 g of the dried herb daily have been taken.

Children (Younger than 18 Years)

- There is insufficient evidence to recommend a dose for fo-ti in children.

SAFETY

Allergies

- Avoid in individuals with a known allergy or hypersensitivity to unprocessed or processed forms of fo-ti.

Side Effects and Warnings

- Although not well studied in humans, fo-ti has been taken daily as a tonic by millions of individuals with no known severe adverse effects. Although rare, skin rash may be a sign of hypersensitivity to both forms of fo-ti.
- In some individuals, fo-ti may cause hepatitis. Avoid in patients with liver disease because it has been associated with hepatitis.
- High doses of unprocessed fo-ti may also lead to hypokalemia (potassium deficiency), muscle weakness, numbness in the arms or legs, and hallucinations.
- Use cautiously in patients with low iron levels. Theoretically, chronic use of anthraquinone laxatives may increase the risk for hypokalemia (potassium deficiency) and digoxin cardiotoxicity.
- Unprocessed fo-ti may cause diarrhea, abdominal pain, nausea, and vomiting. Avoid unprocessed fo-ti in patients with diarrhea, intestinal obstruction, acute intestinal inflammation (Crohn's disease, ulcerative colitis, appendicitis), ulcer, abdominal pain of unknown origin, nausea, and vomiting because of the probable mechanism of it irritating the lining of the gastrointestinal tract. Although the irritation is minor for most individuals, it can worsen inflammatory bowel conditions.
- Use cautiously in patients with constipation because anthraquinone compounds may lead to laxative dependency.

Pregnancy and Breastfeeding

- Fo-ti is not recommended in pregnancy because of a lack of sufficient data. Breastfeeding women should also avoid fo-ti because it is known to enter breast milk. Taking it while breastfeeding may cause diarrhea in the infant(s).

INTERACTIONS

Interactions with Drugs

- Fo-ti may lower blood sugar levels. Caution is advised when medications that may also lower blood sugar are used. Patients taking drugs for diabetes by mouth or using insulin should be monitored closely by a qualified health care professional, including a pharmacist. Medication adjustments may be necessary.

- Because fo-ti contains compounds that were found to inhibit the calcium channel, theoretically it may produce a synergistic effect when taken with these drugs. The effect may be beneficial in some cases, but studies need to be done to further investigate this effect.
- The possible effect of fo-ti in causing hypokalemia (potassium deficiency) may increase the risk of side effects from the use of digoxin. There are no documented cases of this interaction in the available literature.
- The effects of potassium loss may be enhanced if diuretics are used with fo-ti. This may lead to worsening of the symptoms of hypokalemia (potassium deficiency). However, there are no reports available in the literature.
- Theoretically, fo-ti may interact with estrogen-containing drugs because of its estrogen content. Caution is advised in patients taking hormone replacement therapy or birth control pills.
- Theoretically, concomitant use of fo-ti with other laxatives can increase the risk of fluid and electrolyte depletion.
- Fo-ti may interfere with the way the body processes certain drugs using the liver's cytochrome P450 enzyme system. As a result, the levels of these drugs may be increased in the blood and may cause increased effects or potentially serious adverse reactions. Patients using any medications should check the package insert and speak with a qualified health care professional, including a pharmacist, about possible interactions.

Interactions with Herbs and Dietary Supplements

- Theoretically, fo-ti may cause hypokalemia (potassium deficiency) and increase the risk of side effects from the use of herbs such as foxglove and oleander that contain cardiac glycosides that behave similarly to digoxin.
- Fo-ti may act as a weak diuretic and may reduce potassium levels. Use of fo-ti with other diuretic herbs and supplements may lead to hypokalemia (potassium deficiency). However, there are no reports available in the literature.
- Theoretically, fo-ti may interact with estrogen-containing herbs and supplements because of its estrogen content.
- Fo-ti may lower blood sugar levels. Caution is advised when herbs or supplements that may also lower blood sugar are used. Blood glucose levels may require monitoring, and doses may need adjustment.
- Taking fo-ti with other laxative herbs such as alder buckthorn, aloe, cascara, rhubarb, senna, and yellow dock, may contribute additively to the laxative effects of fo-ti.
- Licorice and fo-ti both have potassium-depleting properties and theoretically may increase the risk of hypokalemia (potassium deficiency).
- Fo-ti may interfere with the way the body processes certain herbs or supplements using the liver's cytochrome P450 enzyme system. As a result, the levels of other herbs or supplements may become too high in the blood. It may also alter the effects that other herbs or supplements possibly have on the P450 system.

For a complete list of references, please visit www.naturalstandard.com.

Gamma-Linolenic Acid (GLA)

RELATED TERMS

- Black currant berry, black currant dried leaf, black currant oil, black currant seed oil, borage oil (*Borago officinalis*), borage seed oil, BSO, bugloss, burage, burrage, casis, cassis, cureall, Efamol, European black currant, evening primrose (*Oenothera biennis*), European blackcurrant, evening primrose oil (EPO), fever plant, fungal oil, king's grosellero negro, hempseed oil, huile de hourrache, huile d'onagre, n-6 essential fatty acids, night willow-herb, omega-6, omega-6 fatty acids, omega 6 oil, omega-6 oil, polyunsaturated fatty acid, primrose, PUFA, quinsy berries, ribes nero, ribes nigri folium (*Ribes nigrum*), scabish, siyah frenkuzumu (Turkish), squinancy berries, starflower, starflower oil, sun drop, zwarte bes.

BACKGROUND

- Gamma-linolenic acid (GLA) is a dietary omega-6 fatty acid found in many plant oil extracts. Commercial products are typically made from seed extracts from evening primrose (average oil content, 7-14%), black currant (15-20%), borage oil (20-27%) and fungal oil (25%). GLA is not found in high levels in the diet. It has been suggested that some individuals may not convert the omega-6 fatty acid linoleic acid to longer chain derivatives, such as GLA, efficiently. Thus, supplementation with GLA-containing oils, such as borage oil and evening primrose oil, is occasionally recommended to increase GLA levels in the body.
- GLA is available commonly as a dietary supplement and is sold over the counter in capsules or oil to treat a variety of conditions such as eczema, oral mucoceles (mucus polyps), hyperlipidemia (high cholesterol levels), depression, postpartum depression, chronic fatigue syndrome (CFS), psoriasis (chronic skin disease), muscle aches, and menopausal flushing.
- There is currently good evidence for GLA treatment in rheumatoid arthritis, acute respiratory distress syndrome, and diabetic neuropathy (nerve damage). Little or no effect has been found in treatment of atopic dermatitis, attention deficit hyperactivity disorder (ADHD), cancer prevention, menopausal flushing, systemic sclerosis, and hypertension (high blood pressure). GLA has also been used to help with the body's response to tamoxifen in breast cancer patients.
- Today, production and extraction of oil from evening primrose and borage is done by companies primarily in China, New Zealand, and England. Pharmaceutical licensing for GLA oil products has had only limited success worldwide.

EVIDENCE

Uses Based on Scientific Evidence	Grade
Diabetic Neuropathy Diabetic neuropathy is a degenerative state of the nervous system that causes pain, tingling, burning, numbness, and resultant loss of balance. The most common type, which is said to affect nearly half of diabetic patients, is distal polyneuropathy, which	B
affects the peripheral nervous system in the legs, feet, arms, and hands. GLA may be a viable treatment, although additional study is needed in this area to confirm these findings.	
Acute Respiratory Distress Syndrome (ARDS) Acute respiratory distress syndrome is respiratory failure in adults or children resulting in diffuse injury to the alveoli (tiny air sacs) and lung capillary endothelium. GLA may promote the production of prostaglandin-E_1, an eicosanoid with known antiinflammatory and immunoregulatory properties, which in turn may aid in treating ARDS. Additional study is warranted in this area.	C
Atopic Dermatitis Atopic dermatitis (AD) is one of the most common chronic inflammatory skin diseases, associated with at least 10% of children and 0.5-1% of adults. Studies in the past 20 years reveal minimal therapeutic improvements with GLA as therapy for atopic dermatitis, noted by only marginal to no improvement in inflammation and itching.	C
Attention Deficit Hyperactivity Disorder (ADHD) Clinical trials investigating the effect of GLA on symptoms associated with attention-deficit disorder are limited. There is no evidence of effectiveness of treatment with GLA, but more study is needed to confirm these results.	C
Blood Pressure Control Preliminary study has investigated GLA on blood pressure changes. The evidence suggests that GLA may offer benefits in terms of blood pressure reduction; however, better designed trials are required before definite conclusions can be made.	C
Cancer Treatment (Adjunct) Preliminary study has indicated that GLA may act as a cytotoxic agent or at least as an adjunct agent to a chemotherapy regimen. However, human studies are conflicting, and more study is needed before a strong conclusion can be made.	C
Immune Enhancement Few clinical trials have investigated the effect of GLA on immune responses in healthy human subjects. GLA, as black currant seed oil, may offer some benefits. Further study is required before a definite conclusion can be made.	C
Mastalgia Cyclical mastalgia is breast pain experienced by women and typically associated with the menstrual cycle. The pain can vary in severity and usually occurs between ovulation and menstruation.	C

Uses Based on Scientific Evidence	Grade
Evidence for efficacy of GLA treatment is very limited, although since the 1990s, GLA has been recommended historically as a therapy.	
Menopausal Hot Flashes Some research has examined the effect of GLA (evening primrose oil) on menopausal flushing; however, the effectiveness remains unclear. No improvement in the number of flushes was noted as compared with placebo.	C
Migraine Preliminary research has examined the effect of fatty acids, including GLA, on severity, frequency, and duration of migraine attacks. The effectiveness remains unclear.	C
Osteoporosis Some evidence suggests that GLA and eicosapentaenoic acid (EPA) enhance the effects of calcium supplementation in elderly patients with senile osteoporosis. The contribution of GLA to any observed effect remains unclear.	C
Preeclampsia A study of GLA plus fish oil suggests there is a potential for benefit in terms of reducing edema (swelling) in pregnancy. However, clinical evidence of GLA monotherapy is lacking.	C
Premenstrual syndrome (PMS) There is limited evidence that Efamol (containing GLA) may be beneficial in terms of PMS symptoms.	C
Pruritus Abnormalities of plasma fatty acids may be associated with pruritus (severe itching) in patients undergoing hemodialysis. GLA as evening primrose oil may improve skin conditions in these patients; however, clinical evidence is lacking.	C
Rheumatoid Arthritis Several clinical studies indicate significant therapeutic improvements in rheumatoid arthritis symptoms through reductions in scores on joint tenderness, joint swelling, physician global assessment, and pain. Some studies also suggest that GLA may be a more tolerable alternative to the standard pain-reduction therapies, such as COX/COX-2 inhibitors, and NSAIDs and their adverse events. However, there is some concern about dosage control, and strong clinical evidence is lacking.	C
Sjögren's Syndrome Currently, there is limited evidence showing that GLA is effective in treating Sjögren's syndrome.	C

Ulcerative Colitis Currently, there is insufficient available evidence supporting the use of GLA for ulcerative colitis.	C

Uses Based on Tradition or Theory

Cancer, cystic fibrosis, red blood cell aplasia, systemic sclerosis (rare chronic disease), venous (vein) disorders.

DOSING
Adults (18 Years and Older)

- There is insufficient evidence to recommend a dose for GLA in adults. GLA is likely safe when taken by mouth short-term (up to 18 months) in recommended doses. GLA is possibly safe when used long-term (up to 36 months). Doses as high as 6 g daily have been taken for treatment of hyperlipidemia (high cholesterol levels), and doses as high as 2.8 g have been taken for rheumatoid arthritis and as an adjuvant treatment with tamoxifen, however, there is some concern that these high levels may have adverse effects. However, studies following up patients taking large doses, for example, 1.4 g-2.8 g daily for up to 1 year, have found GLA to be nontoxic.
- Common doses of GLA range between 500-1000 mg daily. For atopic eczema, up to 920 mg has been taken daily. For diabetic neuropathy, up to 480 mg has been taken daily. Intravenous preparations (injections) have also been studied, although injections should be given only under the supervision of a qualified health care professional, including a pharmacist.

Children (Younger than 18 Years)

- There is insufficient evidence to recommend a dose for GLA in children. However, 360-460 mg daily has been used for atopic eczema.

SAFETY
Allergies

- Avoid in individuals with allergy or sensitivity to GLA. However, there are no reports of allergy or hypersensitivity in the available literature.

Side Effects and Warnings

- GLA is generally considered nontoxic and well tolerated for up to 18 months. Possible side effects may include upset and bloated stomach, soft stool, nausea and vomiting, flatulence (gas), and belching.
- Supplementation with GLA at high levels and for a long duration has been suggested to produce excess levels of arachidonic acid. Chronic use may result in changes in the blood and increased bleeding time. However, studies of diets rich in GLA did not reveal any significant change in blood parameters. Until more research resolves this controversy, caution is advised in those using anticoagulant or antiplatelet (blood-thinning) agents.

Pregnancy and Breastfeeding

- GLA is not recommended in pregnant or breastfeeding women because of a lack of available scientific evidence.

G

INTERACTIONS
Interactions with Drugs

- GLA may increase the risk of bleeding when taken with drugs that increase the risk of bleeding. Some examples include aspirin, anticoagulants ("blood thinners") such as warfarin (Coumadin) or heparin, antiplatelet drugs such as clopidogrel (Plavix), and nonsteroidal antiinflammatory drugs (NSAIDs) such as ibuprofen (Motrin, Advil) or naproxen (Naprosyn, Aleve).
- Theoretically, GLA may increase the effectiveness of ceftazidime, an antibiotic in a class known as cephalosporins, against a variety of bacterial infections. It is unknown whether effectiveness of other cephalosporin antibiotics are likewise affected.
- GLA may alter the effects of certain anticancer treatments. Caution is advised.
- Theoretically, taking omega-6 fatty acids, such as GLA, during therapy with cyclosporine, a medication used to suppress the immune system after an organ transplant, for example, may increase the immunosuppressive effects of cyclosporine and may protect against kidney damage associated with cyclosporine.

- Individuals taking phenothiazines (such as chlorpromazine, fluphenazine, perphenazine, promazine, and thioridazine) to treat schizophrenia should not take evening primrose oil, a source of GLA, because it may interact with these medications and increase the risk of seizures. Theoretically, the same may be true for other GLA-containing supplements.

Interactions with Herbs and Dietary Supplements

- GLA may increase the risk of bleeding when taken with herbs and supplements that are believed to increase the risk of bleeding. Multiple cases of bleeding have been reported with the use of *Ginkgo biloba*, and fewer cases have been reported with garlic and saw palmetto. Numerous other agents may theoretically increase the risk of bleeding, although this has not been proven in most cases.
- Although not well studied in humans, coenzyme Q10 and vitamin E reversed the inhibition of cell growth associated with GLA. Thus, nutritional antioxidants may inhibit certain effects associated with GLA.

For a complete list of references, please visit www.naturalstandard.com.

Gamma Oryzanol

RELATED TERMS

- Beta-sitosterol, beta-sitosteryl ferulate calclate, campesterol, campesteryl ferulate, compestanyl ferulate, crude rice bran oil, cycloartenol, cycloartenyl ferulate, cyclobranol, ferulic acid, ferulic acid derivatives, ferulic acid esters, gamma-orizanol, gamma-oryzanol, gamma oryzanol Fine Particle, gamma-oz, gammariza, gammatsul, guntrin, Hi-Z, maspiron, oliver, oryvita, oryzaal, oryzanol, oz, rice bran oil, sitostanyl ferulate, sitosteryl ferulate, sterols, stigmasterol, stigmasteryl ferulate, thiaminogen, triterpene alcohol, triterpenyl alcohol.

BACKGROUND

- Gamma oryzanol is a mixture of ferulic acid esters of sterol and triterpene alcohols, and it occurs in rice bran oil at a level of 1-2%, although it has also been extracted from corn and barley oils. It is theorized that some of the health benefits from rice bran oil, namely, its cholesterol-lowering effects, may be due to its gamma oryzanol content.
- Gamma oryzanol was first isolated and purified in the 1950s. In the 1960s, it was used medically in Japan for anxiety. Each year Japan manufactures 7500 tons of gamma oryzanol from 150,000 tons of rice bran. Not surprisingly, most of the research on oryzanol has been performed in Japan.
- Gamma oryzanol is frequently sold as a bodybuilding aid, specifically to increase testosterone levels, stimulate the release of endorphins (pain-relieving substances made in the body), and promote the growth of lean muscle tissue. However, most currently available studies do not support these claims.

EVIDENCE

Uses Based on Scientific Evidence	Grade
Hyperlipidemia (High Cholesterol Levels) Preliminary evidence indicates that gamma oryzanol may reduce hyperlipidemia. Gamma oryzanol seems to reduce total cholesterol, low-density lipoprotein (LDL), high-density lipoprotein (HDL), and triglycerides. Additional study is needed to establish gamma oryzanol's effect on hyperlipidemia.	B
Gastritis Little research has examined the effects of gamma oryzanol on gastritis.	C
Hypothyroidism Preliminary evidence has indicated that gamma oryzanol affects several parts of the endocrine system and may reduce thyroid-stimulating hormone (TSH) in patients with hypothyroidism. Effectiveness has not been conclusively shown.	C
Menopausal Symptoms Gamma oryzanol may reduce menopausal symptoms. However, these results must be viewed cautiously as treatment of menopausal symptoms has a high placebo effect.	C
Prevention of Restenosis after Percutaneous Transluminal Coronary Angioplasty (PTCA) Gamma oryzanol has been used to reduce restenosis (return of blood vessel blockages after treatment) after coronary dilation, in combination with ticlopidine and probucol. Although restenosis was not affected by any of the treatments, the potential effects of gamma oryzanol alone remain unclear.	C
Skin Conditions A few studies have used gamma oryzanol by mouth or applied on the skin to treat skin conditions. Although these studies seem to indicate that gamma oryzanol may be useful, its effectiveness has not been established.	C
Bodybuilding Gamma oryzanol has been touted as a bodybuilding aid, specifically to increase testosterone levels, stimulate the release of endorphins (pain-relieving substances made in the body), and promote the growth of lean muscle tissue. However, there is little or no conclusive evidence to support these claims.	D

Uses Based on Tradition or Theory

Anemia, anticoagulant, antiinflammatory, antioxidant, anxiety, atherosclerosis (hardening of the arteries), atopic dermatitis, body fat reducer, cancer, central nervous system disorders (autonomic imbalance), cosmetics, diabetes, digestive complaints, exercise recovery, fatty liver, food uses, gynecological disorders (hypoovarianism), heartburn, heart disease, hypercalciuria (excessive amounts of calcium in the urine), immunostimulant, kidney stones, muscle soreness, nausea, nervous system function (suppressant), pain, sports or other physical injuries, ulcers, vomiting, whiplash.

DOSING

Adults (18 Years and Older)

- There is insufficient evidence to recommend a dose for gamma oryzanol. A common dose of gamma oryzanol is 300 mg, which has been taken up to 6 months for hyperlipidemia (high cholesterol levels). This dose has also been used for hypothyroidism as a single dose. Another common dose is 100 mg of Hi-Z (Otsuka Pharmaceutical Co, Tokyo, Japan), which has been taken for skin conditions (up to 4 weeks) or hyperlipidemia (up to 16 weeks). For bodybuilding, 500 mg daily has been used according to manufacturer's instructions for up to 9 weeks. For menopausal symptoms or hyperlipidemia, 1.5 g of gamma oryzanol Fine Particle (300 mg gamma oryzanol included) for up to 8 weeks has been used.

Children (Younger than 18 Years)

- There is insufficient evidence to recommend a dose for gamma oryzanol in children. However, 20 mL of 0.5% gamma oryzanol solution has been dissolved in the bathtub to form a medicinal bath for up to 6 months in children.

SAFETY
Allergies

- Avoid in individuals with a known allergy or hypersensitivity to gamma oryzanol, its components, or rice bran oil.

Side Effects and Warnings

- Many clinical trials have been conducted and have reported no adverse effects with gamma oryzanol. It is likely safe when taken at normal doses, and it is not considered toxic or carcinogenic (cancer causing).

Pregnancy and Breastfeeding

- Gamma oryzanol is not recommended in pregnant or breastfeeding women because of a lack of available scientific evidence. Although not well studied in humans, gamma oryzanol may alter hormone production.

INTERACTIONS
Interactions with Drugs

- Although not well studied in humans, oryzanol combined with a high cholesterol diet may increase the risk of bleeding. Gamma oryzanol has also shown significant cholesterol-lowering effects. Caution is advised when gamma oryzanol is taken with other cholesterol-lowering agents because of additive effects.
- In pharmacological tests, cycloartenol ferulic acid ester, a component of gamma oryzanol, may have a suppressant effect on the central nervous system; its properties seemed different from those of existing major and minor tranquilizers.
- Although not well studied in humans, gamma oryzanol may suppress growth hormone synthesis, prolactin release, and luteinizing hormone release.
- Gamma oryzanol may increase insulin sensitivity in diabetic patients. Patients taking insulin or agents that alter blood sugar levels should use gamma oryzanol with caution. Dosing adjustments may be necessary.
- Gamma oryzanol may moderately stimulate the immune system, and caution is advised in patients taking immunomodulating agents.
- Gamma oryzanol may reduce thyroid-stimulating hormone (TSH) in patients with hypothyroidism.

Interactions with Herbs and Dietary Supplements

- Although not well studied in humans, oryzanol combined with a high cholesterol diet may increase the risk of bleeding. Caution is advised.
- In pharmacological tests, cycloartenol ferulic acid ester, a component of gamma oryzanol, may have a suppressant effect on the central nervous system; its properties seemed different from those of existing major and minor tranquilizers.
- Although not well studied in humans, gamma oryzanol may increase insulin sensitivity in diabetic patients. Patients using herbs that alter blood sugar levels should use gamma oryzanol with caution. Dosing adjustments may be necessary.
- Gamma oryzanol may moderately stimulate the immune system. Caution is advised in patients taking immunomodulating herbs because of possible additive effects.
- Gamma oryzanol may reduce TSH in patients with hypothyroidism.

For a complete list of references, please visit www.naturalstandard.com.

Garcinia, Hydroxycitric Acid

(*Garcinia cambogia*, HCA)

RELATED TERMS

- Bitter kola, brindal berry, brindall berry, brindleberry, Cambodia, Camboge, *Cambogia gummi-guta* L., *Cambogia gutta* L., *Cambogia gutta* Lindl., CitriLean, CitriMax, citrin, Citrinate, Criton K, desoxygambogenin, gambodge, gamboge (French), gambogellic acid, gambogenic acid, gambogin, gambogenin, gambogenin dimethyl acetal, Gambogium, gambooge, ganburin, *Garcinia atroviridis*, *Garcinia bracteata*, Garcinia Cambogi, *Garcinia Cambogia*, *Garcinia hanburyi*, *Garcinia indica*, *Garcinia kola*, *Garcinia mangostana*, *Garcinia multiflora*, *Garcinia neglecta*, *Garcinia puat*, *Garcinia pyrifera*, garushinia kanbogia (Japanese), geelhars (Dutch), Gomaguta, Gomma guta, Gomme Gutte, gomme-gutte (French), gorikapuli, Gumme gutte, Gummigut, Gummigutt (German), Gummiguttbaum (German), gummi-gutti (Italian), gummiguttræ (Danish), gummiharpiks (Danish), Gummiresina gutti, Gutta gamba, guttegom (Dutch), Gutti, Guttiferae (family), hydroxycitrate, (-)-hydroxycitric acid (HCA), isogambogenin, isomoreollin B, korakkaipuli (Sinhalese), Malabar tamarind, *Mangostana cambogia* (Gaertn.), mangosteen, Mangoustanier du Cambodge (French), morellin dimethyl acetal, moreollic acid, rubber resin, Tamarinier de Malabar (French), uppagi.

BACKGROUND

- Garcinia (*Garcinia cambogia*) is a diminutive purple fruit native to India and Southeast Asia. It is used as a weight loss aid, but the evidence is inconclusive. The rind is rich in hydroxycitric acid (HCA) and has been used for centuries throughout Southeast Asia as a food preservative, flavoring agent, and carminative (induces expulsion of gas from the stomach or intestines). According to Indian folk tradition, *Garcinia cambogia* is used for rheumatism and bowel complaints.

- Neither acute nor chronic toxicity is reported with regular consumption of garcinia products as either food or tonics. These products have been used routinely in the coastal areas of Southeast Asia for centuries, and they continue to be consumed in large amounts. There is preliminary evidence for the use of garcinia in exercise performance and weight loss; although current, available evidence is mixed.

EVIDENCE

Uses Based on Scientific Evidence	Grade
Exercise Performance Hydroxycitric acid, a constituent in garcinia, may increase fat metabolism and enhance exercise performance. However, long-term safety and efficacy have not been conclusively demonstrated.	C
Weight Loss Evidence supporting hydroxycitric acid, the active ingredient in *Garcinia cambogia*, for weight loss is mixed.	C

Uses Based on Tradition or Theory

Anthelmintic (expels worms), antibacterial, antifungal, anti-inflammatory, antimicrobial, antioxidant, antitumor, antiviral, appetite suppressant, bowel disorders, bronchodilator (relaxes the muscles of the airways), cancer, carminative (reduces gas), catarrh (inflammation of mucous membrane), cathartic (produces bowel movements), constipation, diabetes, diuretic, dropsy (edema), dysmenorrhea (painful menstruation), edema (swelling), Ebola virus (*Garcinia kola*), flavoring agent, food uses, gastric ulcer prophylaxis, hepatoprotection (liver protection), human immunodeficiency virus (HIV), influenza (*Garcinia kola*), intestinal motility disorders, menstrual disorders, rheumatism, sore throat, tumors, urinary tract disorders, uterus disorders.

DOSING

Adults (18 Years and Older)

- Dosing evidence is conflicting, and there is insufficient evidence to recommend a dose for garcinia. There is sufficient available scientific evidence suggesting that intake of HCA at levels up to 2800 mg/day is safe for human consumption. Garcinia has been well tolerated for up to 12 weeks in available human trials.

- For exercise performance, 250 mg of HCA capsules administered for 5 days may be beneficial. However, a dose of 3000 mg was not effective in three daily doses for 3 days in adult untrained males. For weight loss, 1500 mg of HCA per day (three times daily as 500-mg caplets) given in combination with a high-fiber, low-energy diet has been studied with no effect on weight loss. However, HCA given three times daily 30-60 minutes before meals for a total of 4667 mg/day reduced body weight index and body mass index in 60 moderately obese subjects.

Children (Younger than 18 Years)

- There is insufficient evidence to recommend a dose for garcinia in children, and use is not recommended.

SAFETY

Allergies

- Avoid in individuals with a known allergy or hypersensitivity to *Garcinia cambogia*.

Side Effects and Warnings

- Garcinia has been well tolerated for up to 12 weeks in available human trials. HCA from the rind given by mouth is likely safe in recommended doses.

- Garcinia may lower blood sugar levels. Caution is advised in patients with diabetes (high blood sugar) or hypoglycemia (low blood sugar) and in those taking drugs, herbs, or supplements that affect blood sugar. Serum glucose levels may need to be monitored by a qualified health care professional, including a pharmacist, and medication adjustments may be necessary.

G

- Rhabdomyolysis (serious and potentially fatal disease involving degeneration of skeletal muscle) has been reported 3 hours after ingestion of a weight-loss herbal medicine containing ma huang (ephedrine), guarana (active alkaloid caffeine), chitosan, *Gymnema sylvestre*, *Garcinia cambogia* (50% HCA), and chromium. Because there were multiple substances, it cannot exclusively be attributed to *Garcinia cambogia*. Nevertheless, use cautiously in patients with a history of rhabdomyolysis or in patients taking 3-hydroxy-3-methylglutaryl coenzyme A (HMG-CoA) reductase inhibitors ("statins"), as they may increase the risk for rhabdomyolysis.
- Avoid in patients with Alzheimer's disease and other dementia syndromes because of the theoretical possibility of forming acetylcholine in the brain.

Pregnancy and Breastfeeding

- Garcinia is not recommended in pregnant or breastfeeding women because of a lack of available scientific evidence.

INTERACTIONS

Interactions with Drugs

- Garcinia may lower blood sugar levels. Caution is advised when medications that may also lower blood sugar are used. Patients taking drugs for diabetes by mouth or using insulin should be monitored closely by a qualified health care professional, including a pharmacist. Medication adjustments may be necessary.
- Taking HCA with statin medications, such as atorvastatin calcium (Lipitor), may increase the risk of rhabdomyolysis (disease involving the degeneration of skeletal muscle). An incidence of rhabdomyolysis was reported in a case report of a patient taking a weight-loss herbal medicine that contained 50% HCA.

Interactions with Herbs and Dietary Supplements

- Garcinia may lower blood sugar levels. Caution is advised when herbs or supplements that may also lower blood sugar are used. Blood glucose levels may require monitoring, and doses may need adjustment.
- The combination of HCA-SX (calcium/potassium-bound hydroxycitric acid complex) with niacin-bound chromium or *Gymnema sylvestre* may increase the effects on weight loss. Consult with a qualified health care professional, including a pharmacist, before combining therapies.

For a complete list of references, please visit www.naturalstandard.com.

Garlic
(Allium sativum)

RELATED TERMS

- Aged garlic extract (AGE), ajoene, alisat, alk(en)yl thiosulfates, allicin, Allicor, Allii sativi bulbus, alliinase, *Allium*, allitridium, allyl mercaptan, alubosa elewe, Amaryllidaceae (family), ayo-ishi, ayu, banlasun, camphor of the poor, clove garlic, da-suan, dai toan, dasuan, dawang, diallyl, diallyl disulphide (DADS), diallyl sulfide (DAS), diallyl sulphide, diethyl disulfide, diethyl hexasulfide, diethyl monosulfide, diethyl pentasulfide, diethyl tetrasulfide, diethyl trisulfide, dipropyl disulphide, dipropyl sulphide, dra thiam, (E)-ajoene, foom, garlic clove, garlic corns, garlic extract, garlic oil, garlic powder extract, Gartenlauch, hom khaao, hom kia, hom thiam, hua thiam, Karinat (beta-carotene 2.5 mg, alpha-tocopherol 5 mg, ascorbic acid 30 mg, and garlic powder 150 mg per tablet), kesumphin, kitunguu-sumu, knoblauch, kra thiam, Krathiam, krathiam cheen, krathiam khaao, Kwai, Kyolic, l'ail, lahsun, lai, la-juan, lasan, lashun, la-suan, lasun, lasuna, lauch, lay, layi, lehsun, lesun, Liliaceae (family), lobha, majo, methyl allyl, naharu, nectar of the gods, Ninniku, pa-se-waa, poor man's treacle, rason, rasonam, rasun, rust treacle, rustic treacles, S-alk(en)yl cysteine sulfoxide, S-allylcysteine (SAC), seer, skordo, sluon, stinking rose, sudulunu, tafanuwa, ta-suam, ta-suan, tellagada, Tellagaddalu, thiam, thioallyl derivative, thiosulfinates, toi thum, tum, umbi bawang putih, vallaippundu, Velluli, vellulli, verum, vinyl dithiin, vinyldithiin, (Z)-ajoene.

BACKGROUND

- Numerous controlled trials have examined the effects of oral garlic on serum lipids. Long-term effects on lipids or cardiovascular morbidity and mortality remain unknown. Other preparations (such as enteric-coated or raw garlic) have not been well studied.
- Small reductions in blood pressure (<10 mm Hg), inhibition of platelet aggregation, and enhancement of fibrinolytic activity have been reported and may exert effects on cardiovascular outcomes, although evidence is preliminary in these areas.
- Numerous case-control/population-based studies suggest that regular consumption of garlic (particularly unprocessed garlic) may reduce the risk of developing several types of cancer, including gastric and colorectal malignancies. However, prospective controlled trials are lacking.
- Multiple cases of bleeding have been associated with garlic use, and caution is warranted in patients at risk of bleeding or before some surgical/dental procedures. Garlic does not appear to significantly affect blood glucose levels.

EVIDENCE

Uses Based on Scientific Evidence	Grade
High Cholesterol Level Multiple studies in humans have reported small reductions in total blood cholesterol and low-density lipoprotein levels ("bad cholesterol") over short periods	B

of time (4-12 weeks). It is not clear whether there are benefits after this amount of time. Effects on high-density lipoprotein levels ("good cholesterol") are not clear. This remains an area of controversy.

Antifungal (Applied to the Skin) Several studies describe the application of garlic to the skin to treat fungal infections, including yeast infections. Use caution as garlic can cause severe burns and rash when applied to the skin of sensitive individuals.	C
Antiplatelet Effects (Blood Thinning) The effects of garlic on platelet aggregation have been assessed in several human trials. Because garlic has been associated with several cases of bleeding, therapy should be applied with caution (particularly in patients using other agents that may precipitate bleeding).	C
Atherosclerosis ("Hardening" of the Arteries) Preliminary research in humans suggests that deposits of cholesterol in blood vessels may not grow as quickly in people who take garlic. It is not clear if this is due to the ability of garlic to lower cholesterol levels or to other effects of garlic.	C
Cancer Preliminary human studies suggest that regular consumption of garlic (particularly unprocessed garlic) may reduce the risk of developing several types of cancer, including gastric and colorectal malignancies. Some studies use multiingredient products, so it is difficult to determine whether garlic alone may play a beneficial role.	C
Cryptococcal Meningitis Preliminary evidence suggests potential benefits of oral plus intravenous garlic in the management of cryptococcal meningitis. The lack of definitive evidence precludes garlic in the treatment of this potentially serious condition, for which other treatments are available.	C
Familial Hypercholesterolemia Familial hypercholesterolemia is a genetic disorder in which very high cholesterol levels run in families. Research in children with an inherited form of high cholesterol suggests that garlic does not have a large effect in lowering cholesterol levels in these patients.	C
Heart Attack Prevention in Patients with Known Heart Disease It is not clear whether garlic prevents future heart attacks in people who have already had a heart attack. The effects of garlic on cholesterol levels may be beneficial in such patients.	C

(Continued)

G

Uses Based on Scientific Evidence	Grade
High Blood Pressure Numerous human studies report that garlic can lower blood pressure by a small amount, but larger, well-designed studies are needed to confirm this possible effect.	C
Peripheral Vascular Disease (Blocked Arteries in the Legs) Some human studies suggest that garlic may improve circulation in the legs by a small amount, but this issue remains unclear. Better-designed studies are needed.	C
Tick Repellant Self-reports of tick bites were significantly less in people receiving garlic over a placebo "sugar" pill. However, strong clinical evidence is lacking.	C
Upper Respiratory Tract Infection Preliminary reports suggest that garlic may reduce the severity of upper respiratory tract infections. However, this has not been demonstrated in well-designed human studies.	C
Diabetes Animal studies suggest that garlic may lower blood sugar and increase the release of insulin, but studies in humans do not confirm this effect.	D
Stomach Ulcers Caused by *Helicobacter pylori* Bacteria Overall, studies in humans show no effect of garlic on gastric or duodenal ulcers.	D

Uses Based on Tradition or Theory

Abortion, age-related memory problems, AIDS, allergies, amoeba infections, antibacterial, antioxidant, antitoxin, antiviral, aphrodisiac, atrophic gastritis, arthritis, ascariasis (worms in the gut or liver), asthma, athlete's foot, benign breast disease, bile secretion problems, bladder cancer, bloody urine, breast fibromatosis, bronchitis, cholera, claudication (leg pain due to poor blood flow), colds, cough, cytomegalovirus infection, dental pain, digestive aid, diphtheria, diuretic (water pill), dysentery, dysmenorrhea (painful menstruation), earache, fatigue, fever, gallstones, hair growth, headache, heart rhythm disorders, hemorrhoids, hepatopulmonary syndrome, HIV, hormonal effects, immune system stimulation, improved digestion, induction of vomiting, inflammation, inflammatory bowel disease, influenza, kidney damage from antibiotics, kidney problems, leukemia, liver health, liver tumors, malaria, mucous thinning, muscle spasms, nephrotic syndrome, obesity, parasites and worms, perspiration, pneumonia, premenstrual syndrome (PMS), psoriasis, Raynaud's disease, ringworm (tinea corporis, tinea cruris), sedative, sinus decongestant, snake venom protection, spermicide, stomachache, stomach acid reduction, stomach lining protection, stress (anxiety), stroke, thrush, toothache, traveler's diarrhea, tuberculosis, typhus, urinary tract infections, vaginal irritation, vaginal trichomoniasis, warts, well-being, whooping cough.

DOSING
Adults (18 Years and Older)
- Human studies report the use of 4-12.3 mg of garlic oil by mouth daily. Some sources report that steam-distilled oils, oil from crushed garlic, and aged-garlic in alcohol may be less effective for some uses, particularly as a blood thinner.
- A range of 600-900 mg daily of noncoated, dehydrated garlic powder in three divided doses, standardized to 1.3% allicin content, has been used in human studies. The European Scientific Cooperative on Phytotherapy (ESCOP) recommends 3-5 mg allicin daily (1 clove or 0.5-1.0 g dried powder) for prevention of atherosclerosis. The World Health Organization (WHO) recommends 2-5 g fresh garlic, 0.4-1.2 g of dried powder, 2-5 mg oil, 300-1000 mg of extract, or other formulations that are equal to 2-5 mg of allicin daily.
- The ESCOP recommends 2-4 g of dried bulb or 2-4 mL of tincture (1:5 dilution in 45% ethanol) by mouth three times a day for upper respiratory tract infections.

Children (Younger than 18 Years)
- Safety or effectiveness of garlic supplements has not been proven in children. Garlic in amounts found in food is likely safe in most children.

SAFETY
Allergies
- People with a known allergy to garlic, any of its ingredients, or to other members of the Liliaceae (lily) family, including hyacinth, tulip, onion, leek, and chives, should avoid garlic. Allergic reactions have been reported with garlic taken by mouth, inhaled, or applied to the skin. Some of these reactions are severe, including throat swelling and difficulty breathing (anaphylaxis). It has been suggested that some cases of asthma from inhaling garlic may be due to mites on the garlic. Fresh garlic applied to the skin may be more likely to cause rashes than garlic extract.

Side Effects and Warnings
- Bad breath, body odor, and allergic reactions are the most common reported side effects of garlic. Fresh garlic has caused rash or skin burns, both in people taking garlic therapy and in food preparers handling garlic. Most reactions improve after stopping garlic therapy. Garlic products should not be applied to the skin of infants or children because of multiple reports of skin burns and should be used cautiously in adults. Other reported side effects include dizziness, increased sweating, headache, itching, fever, chills, asthma flares, and runny nose.
- Bleeding is a potentially serious side effect of garlic use, including bleeding after surgery and spontaneous bleeding. Several cases of bleeding are reported, which may be due to effects of garlic on blood platelets or to increased breakdown of blood clots (fibrinolysis). There is debate about the effects of garlic in people treated with warfarin

(Coumadin), but studies suggest that garlic does not alter the international normalized ratio (INR) values that are used to measure the effect of warfarin on blood thinning. Garlic should be stopped before some surgical or dental procedures because of an increased risk of bleeding. Caution is urged in people who have bleeding disorders or who take blood thinning medications (anticoagulants, aspirin/antiplatelet agents, nonsteroidal antiinflammatory drugs such as ibuprofen or naproxen) or herbs/supplements that may increase the risk of bleeding. Dosing adjustments may be necessary.

- Garlic or its ingredients may lower blood sugar levels and increase the release of insulin. However, studies in humans do not show changes in blood sugar control in people with or without diabetes. Nonetheless, caution is advised in people with diabetes or hypoglycemia and in those taking drugs, herbs, or supplements that affect blood sugar. Blood sugar levels may need to be monitored by a health care professional, and medication adjustments may be necessary. Informal reports describe low iodine absorption in the thyroid and low levels of thyroid hormone (hypothyroidism) with garlic supplementation. A few reports suggest that garlic and garlic-like plants may be linked to nodules or tumors of the thyroid. Reduced sperm counts have been reported in rats.

- Dehydrated garlic preparations or raw garlic taken by mouth may cause burning of the mouth, bad breath, abdominal pain or fullness, poor appetite, gas, belching, nausea, vomiting, irritation of the stomach lining, changes in the bacteria in the gut, heartburn, diarrhea, or constipation. One report describes bowel obstruction in a man who ate a whole garlic bulb. Garlic should be used cautiously by people with stomach ulcers or who are prone to stomach irritation.

- Multiple studies show a small reduction in blood cholesterol levels after garlic supplements are taken by mouth. Small reductions in blood pressure are also commonly reported. One case of heart attack is noted in a healthy man after taking a large amount of garlic by mouth.

- Contamination of garlic products has been reported.

- In Vancouver, British Columbia, Canada, a commercial preparation of chopped garlic was linked to botulism. One report describes overdose of colchicine and even death after meadow saffron (*Colchicum autumnale*) was mistaken for wild garlic (*Allium ursinum*).

- Garlic and Pycnogenol have been shown to increase human growth hormone secretion in laboratory experiments.

Pregnancy and Breastfeeding

- Garlic is likely safe during pregnancy in amounts usually eaten in food, based on historical use. However, garlic supplements or large amounts of garlic should be avoided during pregnancy because of a possible increased risk of bleeding. In addition, early animal studies suggest that garlic may cause contraction of the uterus. Many tinctures contain high levels of alcohol and should be avoided during pregnancy.

- Garlic is likely safe during breastfeeding in amounts usually eaten in food, based on historical use. However, some mothers who take garlic supplements report increased nursing time, milk odor, and reduced feeding by the infant.

The safety of garlic supplements during breastfeeding is not known.

INTERACTIONS
Interactions with Drugs

- Human reports suggest that garlic may increase the risk of bleeding when taken with drugs that also increase the risk of bleeding. Examples include aspirin, anticoagulants ("blood thinners") such as warfarin (Coumadin) or heparin, antiplatelet drugs such as clopidogrel (Plavix), and nonsteroidal antiinflammatory drugs such as ibuprofen (Motrin, Advil) or naproxen (Naprosyn, Aleve). Animal and human studies show that garlic can lower blood pressure. Use caution when combining with other medications that lower blood pressure. Several human studies report lower cholesterol levels in people taking garlic. These effects may be increased if garlic is taken with medications that lower blood cholesterol like lovastatin (Mevacor) or other "statins" (HMG-CoA reductase inhibitors).

- Levels of the drug saquinavir, used in human immunodeficiency virus (HIV) treatment, may be reduced if garlic is taken, and its effectiveness may therefore be reduced. Other antiviral drugs like ritonavir may also be affected.

- Garlic may lower blood sugar levels. Although this is theoretical in humans, caution is advised when medications that may also lower blood sugar are used. Patients taking drugs for diabetes by mouth or using insulin should be monitored closely by a qualified health care professional. Medication adjustments may be necessary. Individuals with thyroid disorders or who take thyroid medications should use caution in taking garlic supplements as they may affect the thyroid.

- Garlic may alter levels of certain drugs metabolized by the liver's cytochrome P450 enzyme system.

- Many tinctures contain high levels of alcohol and may cause nausea or vomiting when taken with metronidazole (Flagyl) or disulfiram (Antabuse).

- Garlic may alter levels of various anticancer drugs. Check with your oncologist and pharmacist before starting to take garlic supplements.

Interactions with Herbs and Dietary Supplements

- Garlic may increase the risk of bleeding. In theory, this risk may be further increased when garlic is taken with other herbs or supplements that also increase the risk of bleeding. Multiple cases of bleeding have been reported with the use of *Ginkgo biloba*, and two cases have been reported with saw palmetto. Numerous other agents may theoretically increase the risk of bleeding, although this has not been proven in most cases.

- Garlic may have a small effect in lowering blood pressure. Caution should be used if garlic is taken with other supplements that can lower blood pressure.

- Garlic may lower blood sugar levels. Caution is advised when herbs or supplements that may also lower blood sugar are used. Blood glucose levels may require monitoring, and doses may need adjustment.

- Garlic may lower cholesterol levels by a small amount. These effects may be larger than expected if taken with other cholesterol-lowering supplements such as fish oil.

- Garlic may interact with herbals and dietary supplements that are metabolized by the liver's cytochrome P450 enzyme system.
- Garlic and Pycnogenol have been shown to increase human growth hormone secretion in laboratory experiments.

Effects of herbs and supplements that act on the thyroid may be affected by garlic.

For a complete list of references, please visit www.naturalstandard.com.

Germanium (Ge)

RELATED TERMS

- Azaspirane compounds, carboxyethyl germanium sesquioxide, Ge-132, germanium citrate lactate, germanium dioxide (GeO_2), germanium elixir, germanium lactate citrate, germanium salts, inorganic germanium, lactate-citrate-germanate, Mu-trioxo-bis [betacarboxyethyl] germanic anhydride, organogermanium compound, poly-*trans*-(2-carboxyethyl) germansesquioxane, propagermanium (3-oxygermylpropionic acid polymer), proxigermanium, proxygermanium, repagermanium, S 99 A, sanumgerman, Serocion, SG, Spiro 32, spirogermanio (Spanish), Spirogermanium 32, Spirogermanium dihydrochloride, spirogermanium hydrochloride, vitamin O.
- **Note:** This monograph reviews the therapeutic benefit of organic germanium compounds, specifically spirogermanium and carboxyethyl germanium sesquioxide. Inorganic germanium compounds (germanium dioxide, germanium citrate lactate, and elemental germanium) are potentially toxic and should not be confused with organic germanium.

BACKGROUND

- There are two general forms of germanium: organogermanium compounds, which are carbon-containing compounds (carboxyethyl germanium sesquioxide, spirogermanium, propagermanium, Ge-132); and inorganic (non–carbon containing) germanium compounds (Ge, germanium citrate lactate, germanium dioxide). In this monograph, elemental germanium is classified as inorganic. Inorganic germanium is present in all living plant and animal matter in microtrace quantities.
- In recent years, inorganic germanium salts and novel organogermanium compounds have been sold as nutritional supplements in some countries for their purported immunomodulatory effects or as health-producing elixirs. Bis (2-carboxyethyl germanium sesquioxide), simply called germanium sesquioxide, has been shown in animal studies to have antiviral and immunological properties including the induction of gamma-interferon, macrophages, and T-suppressor cells and augmentation of natural killer cell activity. Another organic germanium, spirogermanium (3-(8,8-diethyl-3-aza-8-germaspiro [4.5]dec-3-yl)-N,N-dimethyl-propan-1-amine), is a heavy metal compound in which germanium has been substituted in an azaspirane ring structure. The supposed therapeutic attributes of organogermaniums include immunoenhancement, oxygen enrichment, free radical scavenging, analgesia, and heavy metal detoxification. However, because of the possibility of contaminated organic germanium products on the market and several unclear and poor quality scientific reviews, all types of germanium are currently thought of as unsafe.
- The National Nutritional Foods Association continues to support a voluntary ban on the sale of germanium. Based on information accessed on February 2, 2007, the import alert against germanium products (see related terms) remains in effect. This import alert was created in 1988 and amended in 1995 to prevent the importation of germanium-containing products that are deemed as "poisonous and deleterious substances (PSNC)" or "unapproved new drugs" (DRND) by the U.S. Food and Drug Administration (FDA).

EVIDENCE

Uses Based on Scientific Evidence	Grade
Hepatitis B There is some evidence supporting the use of propagermanium (an organogermanium) for treating hepatitis B. However, the comparative effectiveness with established therapies remains uncertain.	C
Multiple myeloma There is some evidence supporting the use of propagermanium (an organogermanium) in the treatment of multiple myeloma. However, its efficacy remains uncertain.	C

Uses Based on Tradition or Theory
Amyloidosis (disease), analgesia, angina, antioxidant, antiviral, arteriosclerosis (hardening of the arteries), arthritis, asthma, Behçet's disease, breast cancer, burns, cancer, cancer (intestinal), carcinoma (renal cell), cardiac abnormalities, cataracts, cerebral sclerosis, cervical cancer, chemotherapy (adjuvant), chronic fatigue syndrome, circulatory disorders, corns, depressive symptoms, detoxification, diabetes, digestion disorders, eczema, epilepsy, Epstein-Barr virus, eye diseases, gastritis, glaucoma, heart attack (acute myocardial infarction), heart disease, herpes, HIV/AIDS, hypertension (high blood pressure), immune stimulant, inflammation (retina and optic nerves), influenza, leukemia, lung cancer, lupus erythematosus, lymphoma, malaria, mental disorders, neuropathy, non-Hodgkin's lymphoma, osteoporosis, ovarian cancer, Parkinson's disease, prostate cancer, radiation toxicity, Raynaud's disease, rheumatoid arthritis, schizophrenia, skin eruptions, stress, tumors, ulcers, warts.

DOSING

Adults (18 Years and Older)

- There is insufficient evidence to recommend a dose for germanium. For cancer, intermittent administration of germanium sesquioxide (trade name: Ge-132) 1000 mg has been shown to augment natural killer cell activity for up to 10 days. For Epstein-Barr virus syndrome, 150-500 mg daily of Ge-132 (germanium sesquioxide) has caused marked symptom relief. For advanced malignant neoplasms, spirogermanium, one type of organogermanium, had limited and acceptable toxicity in utilizing a dose of $120 \, mg/m^2$ infused over 2 hours, three times weekly; however, the benefits of this dosing remain unclear.

Children (Younger than 18 Years)

- There is insufficient evidence to recommend a dose for germanium, and use in children is not recommended.

SAFETY
Allergies

- Avoid in individuals with a known allergy or hypersensitivity to germanium. Skin rash occurred in a patient taking a germanium preparation (main component was germanium dioxide with some organic compound present). There have been no available reports of allergy to germanium sesquioxide, spirogermanium, or other pure organogermanium compounds.

Side Effects and Warnings

- Pure organic germanium (germanium sesquioxide, Ge-132) is possibly safe when used at recommended doses and monitored by a qualified health care professional, including a pharmacist. However, more study is needed to make a firm recommendation. To date, there have been no clinical trials studying germanium sesquioxide, but one available case report indicated no side effects.
- Most trials have been conducted on spirogermanium and have reported neurotoxicity and neurological adverse effects, although there is at least one trial that has reported no adverse effects. Lethargy, dizziness, ataxia, lightheadedness, visual blurring, partial loss of taste, extreme weakness, ataxia, paresthesia, nausea, and grand mal seizure have occurred. Rash and diarrhea have also been reported in patients taking spirogermanium, although it is unclear whether spirogermanium was the cause. There are relatively few reports of hepatic (liver) or renal (kidney) adverse effects with spirogermanium. However, hematological (blood) toxicity and pulmonary (lung) toxicity have been observed in patients taking spirogermanium and 5-fluorouracil. Spirogermanium is likely unsafe when taken long-term or at high doses.
- Depression was observed in two patients receiving propagermanium.

- Peripheral neuropathy, anemia, kidney dysfunction, kidney tubular degeneration, myopathy (muscle disease), and germanium accumulation have occurred in those who ingested marketed organic germanium contaminated with germanium dioxide, carboxyethyl germanium sesquioxide, germanium lactate citrate, and/or unspecified forms. Avoid inorganic germanium products because of potential toxic effects. Also avoid ingesting organic germanium from unregulated sellers as it may be contaminated with toxic inorganic germanium.

Pregnancy and Breastfeeding

- High doses of germanium may result in an increased embryonic resorption, but possible malformations have been reported only after administration of dimethyl germanium oxide (GeO_2; inorganic germanium) to pregnant animals. Inorganic germanium should be avoided during pregnancy, and organic germanium is not recommended because of insufficient scientific evidence. It is not recommended during breastfeeding because of insufficient available scientific evidence.

INTERACTIONS
Interactions with Drugs

- Two toxic deaths, both attributable to neutropenia and sepsis, were reported in a phase II trial studying spirogermanium in combination with 5-fluorouracil. Significant toxicity has occurred, and caution is advised.
- Ge-132 (germanium sesquioxide) may enhance morphine analgesia in humans following both oral and intraperitoneal injection. Caution is advised.

Interactions with Herbs and Dietary Supplements

- Insufficient evidence is available.

For a complete list of references, please visit www.naturalstandard.com.

Ginger
(Zingiber officinale)

RELATED TERMS

- African ginger, *Amomum zingiber* L., black ginger, bordia, chayenne ginger, cochin ginger, curcumin gan jiang, gegibre, gingembre, gingerall, ginger BP, ginger oil, ginger power BP, ginger root, ginger trips, ingwer, Jamaica ginger, kankyo, oleoresins, race ginger, rhizoma zinziberis, sheng jiang, vanillyl ketones, verma, zenzero, *Zingiber capitatum*, *Zingiber officinale* Roscoe, *Zingiber zerumbet* Smith, *Zingiber blancoi* Massk, *Zingiber majus* Rumph, zingerone, zingibain, Zingiberis rhizoma, Zinopin (Pycnogenol and standardized ginger root extract), Zintona EC.

BACKGROUND

- The rhizomes and stems of ginger have assumed significant roles in Chinese, Japanese, and Indian medicine since the 1500s. The oleoresin of ginger is often contained in digestive, antitussive, antiflatulent, laxative, and antacid compounds.
- There is supportive evidence from one randomized controlled trial and an open-label study that ginger reduces the severity and duration of chemotherapy-induced nausea/emesis. Effects appear to be additive to prochlorperazine (Compazine). The optimal dose remains unclear. Ginger's effects on other types of nausea/emesis, such as postoperative nausea or motion sickness, remain indeterminate.
- Ginger is used orally, topically, and intramuscularly for a wide array of other conditions, without scientific evidence of benefit.
- Ginger may inhibit platelet aggregation/decrease platelet thromboxane production, thus theoretically increasing bleeding risk.

EVIDENCE

Uses Based on Scientific Evidence	Grade
Nausea and Vomiting of Pregnancy (Hyperemesis Gravidarum) Early studies suggest that ginger may be safe and effective for nausea and vomiting of pregnancy when used at recommended doses for short periods of time. Some publications discourage large doses of ginger during pregnancy because of concerns about mutagenicity or abortions. Long-term safety remains unclear.	B
Antiplatelet Agent There is limited evidence that ginger may have a synergistic effect on antiplatelet aggregation in patients with high blood pressure when used in combination with nifedipine.	C
Migraine There is not enough available scientific evidence in this area.	C
Motion Sickness/Seasickness There is mixed evidence in this area, with some studies reporting that ginger has no effect on motion sickness and other research noting that ginger may reduce vomiting (but not nausea).	C
Nausea (Due to Chemotherapy) Initial human research reports that ginger may reduce the severity and length of time that cancer patients feel nauseous after chemotherapy. Other studies show no effects. Additional studies are needed to confirm these results and to determine safety and dosing. Numerous prescription drugs are highly effective at controlling nausea in cancer patients undergoing chemotherapy, and the available options should be discussed with the patient's medical oncologist.	C
Nausea and Vomiting (after Surgery) Some human studies report improvement in nausea or vomiting after surgery if patients take ginger before surgery. However, other research shows no difference.	C
Osteoarthritis Ginger has been studied as a possible treatment for osteoarthritis. However, results of these studies are mixed.	C
Rheumatoid Arthritis There is limited scientific evidence in this area, and it is not clear whether ginger is beneficial.	C
Urinary Disorders (Poststroke) It is unclear whether ginger can help treat urinary disorders in patients recovering from strokes.	C
Shortening Labor There is not enough available scientific evidence in this area.	C
Weight Loss Ginger has been suggested as a possible weight loss aid, but effectiveness has not been clearly demonstrated.	C

Uses Based on Tradition or Theory

Alcohol withdrawal, antacid, antibacterial, antiinflammatory, antioxidant, antiseptic, antispasm, antiviral, aphrodisiac, asthma, atherosclerosis, athlete's foot, baldness, bile secretion problems, bleeding, blood circulation, blood thinner, bronchitis, burns (applied to the skin), cancer, cholera, colds, colic, coronary artery

(Continued)

Uses Based on Tradition or Theory—Cont'd

disease, cough suppressant, depression, diarrhea, digestive aid, diminished appetite, diuresis, dysmenorrhea (painful menstruation), dysentery, dyspepsia, elevated cholesterol levels, energy metabolism, flatulence (gas), flu, fungal infections, gallbladder disease, gonarthritis, headache, heart disease, *Helicobacter pylori* infection, hepatitis, high blood pressure, immune stimulation, immune system disorders (Kawasaki disease), impotence, increased drug absorption, insecticide, intestinal parasites, kidney disease, kidney toxicity, laxative, leukemia, liver disease, liver toxicity, low blood pressure, low blood sugar, malaria, neuroblastoma, orchitis (painful or swollen testes), pain relief, poisonous snake bites, promotion of menstruation, psoriasis (applied to the skin), respiratory infections, selective serotonin reuptake inhibitor discontinuation or tapering, serotonin-induced hypothermia, stimulant, stomachache, sweating, thrombosis (traveler's thrombosis), tonic, toothache, ulcers.

DOSING
Adults (18 Years and Older)

- Common forms of ginger include fresh root, dried root, tablets, capsules, liquid extract, tincture, and tea. Many publications note that the maximum recommended daily dose of ginger is 4 g. It is believed that the mild stomach upset sometimes caused by ginger may be reduced by taking ginger capsules rather than powder.
- Many experts and publications suggest that ginger powder, tablets, or capsules or freshly cut ginger can be used in doses of 1-5 g daily, by mouth, divided into smaller doses.

Children (Younger than 18 Years)

- There is insufficient scientific evidence to recommend the use of ginger in children.

SAFETY
Allergies

- Ginger supplements should be avoided by individuals with a known allergy to ginger, its components, or other members of the Zingiberaceae family, including *Alpinia formosana*, *Alpinia purpurata* (red ginger), *Alpinia zerumbet* (shell ginger), *Costus barbatus*, *Costus malortieanus*, *Costus pictus*, *Costus productus*, *Dimerocostus strobilaceus*, or *Elettaria cardamomum* (green cardamom). Allergic contact rashes have been reported, and these rashes may be more likely in people who work with ginger, who apply ginger to the skin, or who have a positive allergy test for Balsam of Peru. An allergic eye reaction has also been reported.

Side Effects and Warnings

- Few side effects have been associated with ginger at low doses. There is a lack of available studies that confirm the long-term, safe use of ginger supplements. The most commonly reported side effects of ginger involve the stomach and intestines. Irritation or bad taste in the mouth, heartburn, belching, bloating, gas, and nausea have been reported, especially with powdered forms of ginger. There are several reports that fresh ginger that is swallowed without enough chewing can result in blockage of the intestines. Individuals who have had ulcers, inflammatory bowel disease, or blocked intestines should use ginger supplements cautiously and should avoid large amounts of freshly cut ginger. People with gallstones should use ginger with caution.

- In theory, ginger can cause abnormal heart rhythms, although reports in humans are lacking. Some publications suggest that ginger may raise or lower blood pressure, although limited scientific information is available.

- In addition, ginger may theoretically prevent blood clotting by preventing the clumping of platelets. In one study, gingerol compounds and their derivatives were shown to be more potent antiplatelet agents than aspirin. This raises a concern that individuals who are treated with medications that slow blood clotting or who undergo surgery may have a high risk of excessive bleeding if they take ginger supplements. Ginger is traditionally said to reduce blood sugar levels at high doses, but there is a lack of scientific evidence available. In one study, two of eight participants reported an intense urge to urinate 30 minutes after ingesting ginger. Ginger has also been associated with pinkeye (conjunctivitis), but this was considered a rare occurrence.

Pregnancy and Breastfeeding

- Some authors suggest that pregnant women should not take ginger in amounts greater than found in food (or more than 1 g dry weight per day). There are reports that ginger can increase discharge from the uterus in menstruating women and possibly lead to abortion, mutations of the fetus, or increased risk of bleeding. However, other reports state that there is a lack of scientific evidence that ginger endangers pregnancy. Little scientific study is available in this area to support either perspective, although ginger has been studied in a small number of pregnant women (to assess effects on nausea), without reports of adverse pregnancy outcomes. There is controversy in this area. The use of ginger in pregnancy is cautioned against in traditional Chinese medicine (TCM). However, higher doses of ginger are generally used in Chinese medicine.

INTERACTIONS
Interactions with Drugs

- There is evidence that ginger may increase stomach acid production. As a result, it theoretically may work against the effects of antacids, sucralfate (Carafate), or antireflux medications such as H_2 blockers like ranitidine (Zantac) or proton pump inhibitors like lansoprazole (Prevacid). In contrast, other laboratory and animal studies report that ginger may act to protect the stomach.
- In theory, ginger may increase the risk of bleeding when taken with blood thinners (although clear human evidence is lacking). Some examples include aspirin, anticoagulants such as warfarin (Coumadin) or heparin, antiplatelet drugs such as clopidogrel (Plavix), and nonsteroidal antiinflammatory drugs such as ibuprofen (Motrin, Advil) or naproxen (Naprosyn, Aleve).
- In theory, large doses of ginger may increase the effects of medications that slow thinking or cause drowsiness.
- Ginger may also interfere with medications that change the contraction of the heart, including beta-blockers, digoxin, and other heart medications.

- Because ginger can theoretically lower blood sugar levels, it may interfere with the effects of insulin or diabetes medications that are taken by mouth.
- Ginger may interact with drugs broken down by the liver or with xanthine oxidase drugs.
- Ginger may also interact with drugs taken for nausea/vomiting, arthritis, blood disorders, high cholesterol levels, high/low blood pressure, allergies (antihistamines), cancer, inflammation, vasodilators, or weight loss. Caution is advised when ginger is taken with drugs that weaken the immune system because of a possible interaction.

Interactions with Herbs and Dietary Supplements

- Ginger may increase stomach acid production. As a result, it theoretically may work against the effects of antacids.
- In theory, ginger may increase the risk of bleeding when taken with herbs and supplements that are believed to increase the risk of bleeding (although clear human evidence is lacking). Multiple cases of bleeding have been reported with the use of *Ginkgo biloba*, and fewer cases have been reported with garlic and saw palmetto. Numerous other agents may theoretically increase the risk of bleeding, although this has not been proven in most cases.

- In theory, ginger with large amounts of calcium may increase the risk of abnormal heart rhythms. Study results suggest that dietary phytochemicals, such as capsaicin, curcumin, and resveratrol, have inhibitory effects on P-glycoprotein and potencies to result in interactions with food, drugs, herbs, or supplements.
- Ginger may also theoretically lower blood sugar levels. Caution is advised when herbs or supplements that may also affect blood sugar are used.
- Ginger may interact with herbs broken down by the liver or with xanthine oxidase herbs.
- Ginger may also interact with herbs or supplements taken for nausea/vomiting, pain, arthritis, blood disorders, high cholesterol levels, high/low blood pressure, allergies (antihistamines), cancer, inflammation, vasodilators, or weight loss. Caution is advised when ginger is taken with herbs or supplements that affect the immune system because of possible interactions. Ginger may have antioxidant properties, and use with other antioxidants may result in additive effects.

For a complete list of references, please visit www.naturalstandard.com.

Ginkgo
(*Ginkgo biloba*)

RELATED TERMS

- Adiantifolia, AKL1, arbre aux quarante écus, ArginMax, bai guo ye, baiguo, BioGinkgo, Blackmores Ginkgo Brahmi (*Bacopa monniera*), BN-52063, duck foot tree, EGb, EGb 761, Elefantenohr, Eun-haeng, facherblattbaum, Fossil tree, GBE, GBE 24, GBX, gin-nan, ginan, Gincosan, Ginexin Remind, Gingopret, Ginkai, ginkgo balm, *Ginkgo biloba* blätter, Ginkgo biloba exocarp polysaccharides (GBEP), Ginkgo folium, Ginkgo Go, Ginkgo Phytosome, Ginkgo Powder, Ginkgoaceae (family), ginkgoblätter, ginkgogink, ginkgold, Ginkgold, ginkgopower, Ginkopur, ginkyo, Herbal vX, icho, ityo, Japanbaum, Japanese silver apricot, kew tree, kung sun shu, LI 1370, maidenhair tree, noyer du Japon, oriental plum tree, pei kuo, pei-wen, *Pterophyllus*, *Pterophyllus salisburiensis*, Rokan, Rö Kan, salisburia, *Salisburia adiantifolia*, *Salisburia macrophylla*, Seredyn, silver apricot, sophium, tanakan, tanakene, Tebofortan, Tebonin, tempeltrae, temple balm, tramisal, Valverde, vasan, Vital, ya chio, yin-guo, yin-hsing.

BACKGROUND

- *Ginkgo biloba* has been used medicinally for thousands of years. Today, it is one of the top selling herbs in the United States.
- Ginkgo is used for the treatment of numerous conditions, many of which are under scientific investigation. Available evidence demonstrates ginkgo's efficacy in the management of intermittent claudication, Alzheimer's/multiinfarct dementia, and "cerebral insufficiency" (a syndrome thought to be secondary to atherosclerotic disease, characterized by impaired concentration, confusion, decreased physical performance, fatigue, headache, dizziness, depression, and anxiety).
- Although not definitive, there is promising early evidence favoring the use of ginkgo for memory enhancement in healthy subjects, altitude (mountain) sickness, symptoms of premenstrual syndrome (PMS), and reduction of chemotherapy-induced end-organ vascular damage.
- Although still controversial, a recent large trial has shifted the evidence against the use of ginkgo for tinnitus.
- The herb is generally well tolerated, but because of multiple case reports of bleeding, it should be used cautiously in patients receiving anticoagulant therapy, with known coagulopathy, or before some surgical or dental procedures.

EVIDENCE

Uses Based on Scientific Evidence	Grade
Claudication (Painful Legs from Clogged Arteries) Numerous studies suggest that *Ginkgo biloba* taken by mouth causes small improvements in claudication symptoms (leg pain with exercise or at rest due to clogged arteries). However, ginkgo may not be as helpful for this condition as exercise therapy or prescription drugs. Additional evidence is needed.	A
Dementia (Multiinfarct and Alzheimer's Type) The scientific literature overall does suggest that ginkgo benefits people with early stage Alzheimer's disease and multiinfarct dementia and may be as helpful as acetylcholinesterase inhibitor drugs such as donepezil (Aricept). Well-designed research comparing ginkgo with prescription drug therapies is needed.	A
Cerebral Insufficiency Multiple clinical trials have evaluated ginkgo for a syndrome called "cerebral insufficiency." This condition, more commonly diagnosed in Europe than the United States, may include poor concentration, confusion, absent-mindedness, decreased physical performance, fatigue, headache, dizziness, depression, and anxiety. It is believed that cerebral insufficiency is caused by decreased blood flow to the brain due to clogged blood vessels. Some research reports benefits of ginkgo in patients with these symptoms, but most have been poorly designed without reliable results. Better studies are needed before a strong recommendation can be made.	B
Acute Hemorrhoidal Attacks In early study ginkgo was shown to be effective in the treatment of patients with acute hemorrhoidal attacks. Further research is needed to confirm these results.	C
Age-Associated Memory Impairment (AAMI) AAMI is a nonspecific syndrome that may be caused by early Alzheimer's disease or multiinfarct dementia (conditions for which ginkgo has been shown to have benefit). There is preliminary research showing small improvements in memory and other brain functions in patients with AAMI, although some studies disagree. Overall, there is currently not enough clear evidence to recommend for or against ginkgo for this condition.	C
Altitude (Mountain) Sickness A small amount of poorly designed research reports benefits of ginkgo for the treatment of altitude (mountain) sickness. Additional study is needed before a recommendation can be made.	C
Asthma Ginkgo may reduce symptoms in patients with asthma. More study is needed to make a firm recommendation.	C
Cardiovascular Disease Animal and limited human data suggest a role in heart blood flow. More research is needed in this area.	C

Uses Based on Scientific Evidence	Grade
Chemotherapy Side Effects (Reduction) In limited human study, ginkgo has been examined in addition to 5-fluorouracil (5-FU) in the treatment of pancreatic and colorectal cancer to measure possible benefits on side effects. At this time, there is a lack of conclusive evidence in this area.	C
Chronic Venous Insufficiency Research is unclear in this area. However, a multiingredient product called Ginkor Fort may aid in treatment of patients with lower limb chronic venous insufficiency. Further study is needed, and recommendations cannot be made at this point.	C
Cocaine Dependence It is not clear whether ginkgo is helpful in treating cocaine dependence. More study is needed.	C
Deafness (Cochlear) Preliminary clinical study has been conducted on the effect of ginkgo in chronic cochleovestibular disorders. Further research is needed before a recommendation can be made.	C
Depression and Seasonal Affective Disorder (SAD) Preliminary study of SAD suggests that ginkgo is not effective in preventing the development of winter depression. Other research in elderly patients with depression shows possible minor benefits. Overall, there is not enough evidence to form a clear conclusion.	C
Diabetic Neuropathy Research is unclear in this area. Ginkgo may help improve some laboratory parameters associated with diabetic neuropathy, but more study is needed to make a firm recommendation.	C
Dyslexia Ginkgo is traditionally used for improved memory or cognition, and research supports a possible use for patients with dyslexia. More study is needed in this area.	C
Gastric Cancer *Ginkgo biloba* exocarp polysaccharides (GBEP) capsule preparation has been studied for upper digestive tract malignant tumors of middle and late stage with positive results. However, further research is needed before a recommendation can be made.	C
Glaucoma It is not clear whether ginkgo may improve intraocular pressure and blood flow in patients with glaucoma. Some study results conflict or have not been significant. Further research is needed before a recommendation can be made.	C

Graves' Disease Ginkgo may decrease damage to cells caused by radioiodine therapy in patients with Graves' disease. Further study is needed.	C
Macular Degeneration Preliminary research suggests that ginkgo may improve eye blood flow, although it remains unclear whether macular degeneration is significantly affected by ginkgo. More research is needed in this area before a conclusion can be drawn.	C
Memory Enhancement (in Healthy People) It remains unclear whether ginkgo is effective. Further well-designed research is needed, as existing study results conflict.	C
Mood and Cognition in Postmenopausal Women It remains unclear whether ginkgo is effective for mood and cognition improvement. Further well-designed research is needed, as existing study reports conflicting evidence.	C
Multiple Sclerosis Based on laboratory study, it has been suggested that ginkgo may provide benefit in multiple sclerosis (MS). Human research is limited to several small studies, which have not found consistent benefit. Additional research is needed before a recommendation can be made.	C
Premenstrual Syndrome (PMS) Initial study in women with premenstrual syndrome or breast discomfort suggests that ginkgo may relieve symptoms including emotional upset. Further well-designed research is needed before a recommendation can be made.	C
Pulmonary Interstitial Fibrosis Based on early study, ginkgo may be effective in treating pulmonary interstitial fibrosis. Further research is needed to confirm these results.	C
Quality of Life Early studies suggest that ginkgo may aid in quality of life. More randomized controlled trials are needed before a conclusion can be made.	C
Raynaud's Disease Results from one clinical trial suggest that *Ginkgo biloba* may be effective in reducing the number of Raynaud's attacks in patients suffering from Raynaud's disease. To confirm these results, further clinical trials are required.	C
Retinopathy (Diabetes Mellitus Type 2) Early study suggests *Ginkgo biloba* extract may offer benefit to individuals with retinopathy. Further clinical trials are required to determine efficacy.	C

G

(Continued)

Uses Based on Scientific Evidence	Grade
Ringing in the Ears (Tinnitus) There is conflicting research regarding the use of ginkgo for tinnitus. Additional well-designed research is needed to resolve this controversy.	C
Schizophrenia Based on ginkgo's proposed antioxidant effects, ginkgo has been studied in the treatment of schizophrenia. Although early study is promising, there is currently not enough scientific evidence to make a strong recommendation.	C
Sexual Dysfunction Ginkgo has been used and studied for the treatment of sexual dysfunction in men and women. In general, studies are small and not well designed. Additional research is needed before a recommendation can be made.	C
Stroke Laboratory studies suggest that ginkgo may be helpful immediately after strokes because of possible antioxidant or blood vessel effects. However, initial study of ginkgo in people having strokes found a lack of benefit. Further research is needed in this area.	C
Vertigo A small amount of poorly designed research reports benefits of ginkgo for the treatment of vertigo. Additional study is needed before a recommendation can be made.	C
Vitiligo Early study using oral *Ginkgo biloba* extract reports that ginkgo appears to arrest the progression of this disease. Better designed studies are needed to confirm these results.	C
Mental Performance (after Eating) The results of one study investigating the effect of *Ginkgo biloba* on postprandial mental alertness are unclear. Ginkgo may benefit some but not all end points. Further clinical trials are required before recommendations can be made.	D

Uses Based on Tradition or Theory

Acidosis, aging, alcoholism, allergies, angina, antibacterial, antifungal, antiinflammatory, antioxidant, antiparasitic, antirheumatic, antitumor, anxiety, attention deficit hyperactivity disorder, autoimmune disorders, bladder disorders, blood clots, blood vessel disorders, body fat reducer (cellulite), brain damage, breast disease, breast tenderness, bronchitis, cancer, cataracts, chest pain, chilblains (inflammation of toes, fingers, ears, or face with exposure to cold), chronic rhinitis, colorectal cancer, congestive heart failure, cough, cyanosis, degenerative diseases (prevention), dermatitis, diabetes, digestion, dizziness, dysentery (bloody diarrhea), eczema, edema, encephalopathy (circulatory), fatigue, fibromyalgia, freckle-removing, genitourinary disorders, headache, heart attack, hepatitis B, high blood pressure, high cholesterol levels, hypoxia (lack of oxygen), immunomodulator, insomnia, labor induction, menstrual pain, migraine, mouth cancer, respiratory tract illnesses, scabies (ginkgo cream), seizures, sepsis, skin sores (ginkgo cream), spermicide, swelling, traumatic brain injury, ulcer (trophic lesions), ulcerative colitis, vaginal dryness, varicose veins, vision (color).

DOSING
Adults (18 Years and Older)

- From 80-240 mg of a 50:1 standardized leaf extract has been taken daily by mouth in two to three divided doses. Extracts are typically standardized to 24%-25% ginkgo flavone glycosides and 6% terpine lactones. Other forms used include tea (bags usually contain 30 mg of extract), 3-6 mL of 40 mg/mL extract daily in three divided doses, and "fortified" foods. Ginkgo seeds are potentially toxic and should be avoided. The German ginkgo product Tebonin, given intravenously (IV; through the veins), was removed from the German market because of significant side effects.

Children (Younger than 18 Years)

- There is insufficient evidence to recommend use of ginkgo in children.

SAFETY
Allergies

- Allergy/hypersensitivity to *Ginkgo biloba* or members of the Ginkgoaceae family may occur. A severe reaction called Stevens-Johnson syndrome, which includes skin blistering and sloughing-off, has been reported with use of a combination product. There may be cross-sensitivity to ginkgo in people allergic to the plant toxin urushiols (found in mango rind, sumac, poison ivy, poison oak, cashews), and an allergic cross-reaction has been reported with poison ivy.

Side Effects and Warnings

- Overall, ginkgo leaf extract (used in most commercial products) appears to be well tolerated in most healthy adults at recommended doses for up to 6 months. Minor symptoms including headache, nausea, and intestinal complaints have been reported.
- Bleeding has been associated with the use of ginkgo taken by mouth, and caution is advised in patients with bleeding disorders or taking drugs/herbs/supplements that may increase the risk of bleeding. Dosing adjustments may be necessary. Ginkgo should be stopped before some surgical or dental procedures. Reports of bleeding range from nose bleeds to life-threatening bleeding in several case reports. In some of these reports, ginkgo has been used with other agents that may also cause bleeding.
- Eating the seeds is potentially deadly because of risk of tonic–clonic seizures and loss of consciousness.
- Based on human study, ginkgo may theoretically affect insulin and blood sugar levels. Caution is advised in patients with diabetes or hypoglycemia, and in those taking drugs, herbs, or supplements that affect blood sugar. Serum glucose levels may need to be monitored by a health care professional, and medication adjustments may be necessary.

- There have been uncommon reports of dizziness, stomach upset, diarrhea, vomiting, muscle weakness, loss of muscle tone, restlessness, racing heart, rash, and irritation around the mouth with the use of ginkgo. There is a case report of "coma" in an elderly Alzheimer's patient taking trazodone and ginkgo, although it is not clear that ginkgo was the cause. Based on laboratory and human research, ginkgo may decrease blood pressure, although there is one report of ginkgo possibly raising blood pressure in a person taking a thiazide diuretic ("water pill"). Based on theory, high concentrations of ginkgo may reduce male and female fertility. Contamination with the drug colchicine has been found in commercial preparations of *Ginkgo biloba*.
- Ginkgo may affect the outcome of electroconvulsive therapy (ECT). Adverse effects on the eyes have also been reported.

Pregnancy and Breastfeeding

- Use of ginkgo is not recommended during pregnancy and breastfeeding because of lack of reliable scientific study in this area. The risk of bleeding associated with ginkgo may be dangerous during pregnancy.

INTERACTIONS
Interactions with Drugs

- Overall, controlled trials of ginkgo report few adverse effects and good tolerance, with rates of complications similar to placebo. However, use of ginkgo with drugs that may cause bleeding may further increase the risk of bleeding, based on multiple case reports of spontaneous bleeding in patients using ginkgo alone, with warfarin (Coumadin), or with aspirin. One case report documents a possible increase in bleeding risk with ticlodipine (Ticlid) and ginkgo. Examples of drugs that may increase the risk of bleeding include aspirin, anticoagulants ("blood thinners") such as warfarin (Coumadin) or heparin, antiplatelet drugs such as clopidogrel (Plavix), and nonsteroidal antiinflammatory drugs such as ibuprofen (Motrin, Advil) or naproxen (Naprosyn, Aleve). However, not all studies agree with the existence of this risk, and it is not clear whether particular types of patients may be at greater risk.
- Based on preliminary research, ginkgo may affect insulin and blood sugar levels. Caution is advised when medications that may also lower blood sugar are used. Patients taking drugs for diabetes by mouth or using insulin should be monitored closely by a qualified health care professional. Medication adjustments may be necessary.
- Ginkgo has been found to decrease blood pressure in healthy volunteers, although some studies disagree. Theoretically, ginkgo may add to the effects of medications that also lower blood pressure, although raised blood pressure has been reported in a patient taking a thiazide diuretic (water pill) with ginkgo. It has been suggested that *Ginkgo biloba* leaf extract (GBE) and nifedipine should not be ingested at the same time.
- Monoamine oxidase (MAO) inhibition by ginkgo was reported in one animal study but has not been confirmed in humans. In theory, if taken with MAOI drugs, such as isocarboxazid (Marplan), phenelzine (Nardil), or tranylcypromine (Parnate), additive effects and side effects may occur. Based on laboratory research, ginkgo may also add to the effects of selective serotonin reuptake inhibitor (SSRI) antidepressants such as sertraline (Zoloft), with an increased risk of causing serotonin syndrome, a condition characterized by stiff muscles, fast heart rate, hyperthermia, restlessness, and sweating.

- Based on human use, ginkgo may decrease side effects of antipsychotic drugs, although scientific information in this area is limited. There is a case report of "coma" in an elderly Alzheimer's patient taking trazodone and ginkgo, although it is not clear that this reaction was due to ginkgo. In theory, ginkgo may increase the actions of drugs used for erectile dysfunction such as sildenafil (Viagra).
- There may be a risk of seizure when ginkgo is taken, particularly in people with a history of seizure disorder. Although most reports of seizures have been due to eating ginkgo seeds (not leaf extract, which is found in most products), an animal study found that the antiseizure properties of sodium valproate or carbamazepine were reduced if ginkgo was given. In theory, drugs such as donepezil (Aricept) and tacrine (Cognex) may have an additive effect when used at the same time as ginkgo, potentially increasing cholinergic effects (such as salivation and urination).
- 5-Fluorouracil-induced side effects and cyclosporine kidney toxicity may in theory be improved by ginkgo, although evidence is not conclusive in these areas. Colchicine has been found in commercial preparations of ginkgo and may increase blood concentrations in patients using colchicine.
- Ginkgo may alter the way the liver breaks down certain drugs.

Interactions with Herbs and Dietary Supplements

- Use of ginkgo with herbs or supplements that may cause bleeding may increase the risk of bleeding, although some studies disagree. Several cases of bleeding have been reported with the use of garlic, and two cases have been reported with saw palmetto. Numerous other agents may theoretically increase the risk of bleeding, although this has not been proven in most cases.
- Ginkgo has been found to decrease blood pressure in healthy volunteers, although some studies disagree. Theoretically, ginkgo may have additive effects when used with herbs or supplements that also decrease blood pressure. However, high blood pressure was reported in a patient taking a thiazide diuretic (water pill) plus ginkgo. Although it remains unclear whether ginkgo has clinically significant effects on blood pressure, caution may be warranted when ginkgo is used with other agents that affect blood pressure.
- Based on human study, ginkgo may theoretically affect insulin and lower blood sugar levels. Caution is advised when herbs or supplements that may also affect blood sugar are used. Blood glucose levels may require monitoring, and doses may need adjustment.
- Effects on monoamine oxidase (inhibition) by ginkgo are reported in animals but not confirmed in humans. In theory, ginkgo may add to the side effects of herbs or supplements that also inhibit monoamine oxidase, such as 5-HTP (5-hydroxytryptophan).
- Based on laboratory research, ginkgo may add to the effects of herbs or supplements that affect levels of serotonin in the blood or brain and could increase the risk of serotonin syndrome (a condition characterized by muscle stiffness, increased heart rate, hyperthermia, restlessness, and sweating).
- Ginkgo may increase the actions of agents used for erectile dysfunction, including yohimbine.
- Ginkgo may alter the way the liver breaks down herbs and supplements.

For a complete list of references, please visit.www.naturalstandard.com.

Ginseng
(*Panax* spp.)

RELATED TERMS

- General: Acetylenic alcohol, acidic polysaccharides, acupuncture-moxibustion, aglycones, Allheilkraut, American ginseng (AG), American wild ginseng, Araliaceae (family), Asian ginseng, Asiatic ginseng, chikusetsaponin-L8, chikusetsu ginseng, chosen ninjin, CPPQ (coarse polysaccharide from Panax quinquefolium), CVT-E002, dae-jo-hwan (DJW), dwarf ginseng, *Eleutherococcus senticosus*, five-fingers, five-leaf ginseng, G115, ginsan, ginsenan PA (phagocytosis-activating polysaccharide), ginseng acidic polysaccharide, ginseng radix, ginseng saponins, ginseng tetrapeptide, Ginsengwurzel (German), ginsenoside, ginsenosides (Rb1, Rb2, Rc, Rd, Re, Rf and Rg1), ginsenosides compound (shen-fu), GTTC (Ginseng and Tang-kuei Ten Combination), hakusan, hakushan, higeninjin, hongshen, hua qi shen, hungseng, hungsheng, hunseng, insam, jenseng, jenshen, jinpi, kao-li-seng, Korean ginseng, Korea red ginseng (KRG), Kraftwurzel (German), man root, memory enhancer, minjin, nhan sam, ninjin, ninzin, niuhan, North American ginseng, notoginsenoside, oleanolic acid, Oriental ginseng, otane ninjin, panax de chine, *Panax ginseng*, *Panax ginseng* C.A. Meyer, *Panax notoginseng*, *Panax pseudoginseng* Wall. var. notoginseng, *Panax pseudoginseng* var. major, *Panax pseudoginseng*, *Panax quinquefolium*, *Panax* spp., *Panax trifolius* L., *Panax vietnamensis* (Vietnamese ginseng), panaxadiol, panaxans, panaxatriol, panaxydol, panaxynol, panaxytriol, pannag, polyacetylenic compounds, poly-furanosyl-pyranosyl-saccharides, proprietary ginseng root extract (Cold-FX, CV Technologies Inc., Edmonton, AB, Canada), protopanaxadiol ginsenosides, quinqueginsin, racine de ginseng, red ginseng, renshen, sam, sanchi ginseng, san-qi, sang, schinsent, sei yang seng, shanshen, shen-fu, shen-sai-seng, shenghaishen, shenlu, shenshaishanshen, siyojin, stressbuster, sun ginseng, t'ang-sne, tartar root, tienchi ginseng, to-kai-san, triterpenoids, true ginseng, tyosenninzin, vanillic acid, Vietnamese ginseng, Western ginseng, Western sea ginseng, white ginseng, wild ginseng, woods-grown (wild-simulated) ginseng root, xi shen, xi yang shen, yakuyo ninjin, yakuyo ninzin, yang shen, yeh-shan-seng, yuan-seng, yuansheng, zhuzishen.
- *Panax ginseng* synonyms: *Aralia* (botanical synonym), Aralia ginseng Mey, Araliaceae (family), Asian ginseng, Asiatic ginseng, Chinese ginseng, G115, Gincosan (a combination of 120 mg *Ginkgo biloba* and 200 mg *Panax ginseng*), Ginsai, ginseng asiatique, ginsengjuuri, ginseng radix, ginseng root, Japanese ginseng, jintsam, Korean ginseng, Korean Panax ginseng, Korean red, Korean red ginseng, kuhuang shenmai injection (KHSM), ninjin, Oriental ginseng, Panax, *Panax ginseng*, *Panax ginseng* C. Meyer, *Panax schinseng*, *Panax schinseng* Nees, *Panax* spp., radix ginseng rubra, red ginseng, ren shen (traditional Chinese medicine [TCM]), renshen (TCM), Renxian, sang, schinsent, seng, shen, shenmai, shenmai huoxue decoction (SMHXD), shenmai injection (SMI), shengmai, shengmai chenggu capsule, shengmai injection (SI), shengmai san (SMS), shengmai-san, shengmaisan, shengmaiyin, white ginseng.

- American ginseng synonyms: American ginseng, amerikan ginseng, amerikanischer Ginseng, amerikkalainen ginseng, Sanchi ginseng, *Aralia quinquefolia* Decne. & Planch (botanical synonym), Araliaceae (family), Canadian ginseng, CVT-E002, five fingers, five leafed ginseng, garantoquen, ginseng, ginseng d'Amerique, ginsenosides poly-furanosyl-pyranosyl-saccharides, man-root, man's health, North American ginseng, Occidental ginseng, Ontario ginseng, Panax quincefolium, Panax quinquefolium, *Panax quinquefolius*, redberry, red berry, sang, shang, tartar root, tienchi ginseng, traditional Chinese medicine (TCM), wild American ginseng, Wisconsin ginseng, xi yang shen.
- Siberian ginseng synonyms: *Acanthopanax senticosus*, ci wu jia, ciwujia, devil's bush, devil's shrub, eleuthera, eleuthero, eleuthero ginseng, eleutherococ, eleutherococci radix, *Eleutherococcus*, *Eleutherococcus senticosus*, phytoestrogen, shigoka, touch-me-not, wild pepper, wu-jia, wu-jia-pi, ussuri, ussurian thorny pepperbush.
- **Note:** Siberian ginseng (*Eleutherococcus senticosus*) is distinct from true ginseng (*Panax* spp.) and not covered in this review. Other distinct plants may be referred to as ginseng as well, including *Pseudostellaria heterophylla* (prince ginseng), *Angelica sinensis* (female ginseng, or dong quai), *Withania somnifera* (Indian ginseng or ashwagandha), *Pfaffia paniculata* (Brazilian ginseng), *Lepidium meyenii* (Peruvian ginseng or maca), *Gynostemma pentaphyllum* (southern ginseng or jiaogulan).

BACKGROUND

- The term *ginseng* refers to several species of the genus *Panax*. For more than 2000 years, the roots of this slow-growing plant have been valued in Chinese medicine. The two most commonly used species are Asian ginseng (*Panax ginseng* C. A. Meyer), which is almost extinct in its natural habitat but is still cultivated, and American ginseng (*P. quinquefolius* L.), which is both harvested from the wild and cultivated. *Panax ginseng* should not be confused with Siberian ginseng (*Eleutherococcus senticosus*). In Russia, Siberian ginseng was promoted as a cheaper alternative to ginseng and was believed to have identical benefits. However, Siberian ginseng does not contain the ginsenosides found in the *Panax* species, which are believed to be active ingredients and have been studied.

EVIDENCE

Uses Based on Scientific Evidence	Grade
Heart Conditions Ginseng appears to have antioxidant effects that may benefit patients with heart disorders. Some studies suggest that ginseng also reduces oxidation of low-density lipoprotein (LDL or "bad") cholesterol and brain tissue. Better studies are needed to make a firm recommendation.	B

Uses Based on Scientific Evidence	Grade
High Blood Sugar/Glucose Intolerance Several studies suggest ginseng may lower blood sugar levels in patients with type 2 diabetes before and after meals. These results are promising, especially because ginseng does not seem to lower blood sugar to dangerous levels. Future research should focus on the long-term effects of ginseng in managing blood sugar levels.	B
Immune System Enhancement Several studies report that ginseng may boost the immune system, improve the effectiveness of antibiotics in people with acute bronchitis, and enhance the body's response to flu vaccines. Additional studies are needed before a clear conclusion can be reached.	B
Type 2 Diabetes (Adult-Onset) Several human studies report that ginseng may lower blood sugar levels in patients with type 2 diabetes. Long-term effects are not clear, and it is not known what doses are safe or effective. People with diabetes should seek the care of a qualified health care practitioner and should not use ginseng instead of more proven therapies. Effects of ginseng in type 1 diabetes (insulin dependent) are not well studied.	B
Aplastic Anemia Weak studies suggest that ginseng in combination with other herbs may improve cell activity, immune function, and red and white blood cell counts in patients with aplastic anemia. Other studies have found decreases in blood cell counts. High-quality studies of ginseng alone are needed.	C
Attention Deficit Hyperactivity Disorder (ADHD) Preliminary small studies suggest that American ginseng may help treat attention deficit hyperactivity disorder in children. However, there is currently not enough evidence to support this use of ginseng.	C
Birth Outcomes (Anoxemic Encephalopathy) There is currently not enough evidence to support the use of ginseng for this condition. High-quality studies are needed to understand this relationship.	C
Bronchodilator Limited research suggests that ginseng has positive effects on breathing. Further studies are needed in this area.	C
Cancer Chemotherapy Preliminary studies suggest that ginseng injections may help patients undergoing chemotherapy for various types of cancer. Ginseng may improve body weight, quality of life, and the immune response. Although this evidence is promising, the effect of ginseng alone is not clear. More research using ginseng alone is needed.	C
Cancer Prevention A few studies report that ginseng taken by mouth may lower the risk of developing some cancers, especially if ginseng powder or extract is used. Study results are controversial, and more research is needed before a clear conclusion can be reached.	C
Cardiovascular Risk Reduction Current evidence does not support the use of ginseng to reduce the risk of heart disease. Some evidence suggests that ginseng may improve blood pressure, blood sugar, and cholesterol levels. High-quality studies are needed.	C
Chronic Hepatitis B Preliminary studies show that ginseng may improve some aspects of liver function but not others. More research is needed in this area.	C
Chronic Obstructive Pulmonary Disease (COPD) Ginseng was reported to improve lung function and exercise capacity in patients with COPD. Further research is needed to confirm these results.	C
Congestive Heart Failure Based on limited research, it is unclear whether ginseng improves congestive heart failure. High-quality studies looking at the effect of ginseng alone are needed.	C
Coronary Artery Disease Several studies from China report that ginseng in combination with various other herbs may reduce symptoms of coronary artery disease. Without further evidence on the effects of ginseng specifically, a firm conclusion cannot be reached.	C
Dementia Preliminary small studies report that Fuyuan mixture, an herbal combination that contains ginseng, may improve symptoms of multiinfarct dementia. The effects of ginseng alone are not clear, and no firm conclusion can be drawn.	C
Diabetic Complications (Kidney Damage) Preliminary evidence suggests that a form of ginseng not commonly available in the United States may improve kidney damage in patients with diabetes. Some research suggests that *Panax notoginseng* may be as effective as ticlopidine (Ticlid). However, more research is needed.	C
Erectile Dysfunction Preliminary studies suggest that ginseng may help treat erectile dysfunction. Additional high-quality studies are needed.	C
Exercise Performance Athletes commonly use ginseng as a potential way to improve stamina. However, it remains unclear	C

(Continued)

Uses Based on Scientific Evidence	Grade
whether ginseng taken by mouth significantly affects exercise performance. Many studies have been published in this area, with mixed results. Better studies are necessary before a clear conclusion can be reached.	
Fatigue A few studies using ginseng extract G115 (with or without multivitamins) report improvements in patients with fatigue of various causes. However, these results are preliminary, and studies have not been a high quality.	C
Fistula (Anal) Preliminary evidence in infants with perianal abscesses or anal fistulas suggests that GTTC (Ginseng and Tang-kuei Ten Combination) may speed up recovery. Further research is needed to confirm these results.	C
Heart Damage (Cardiac Bypass Complications) Preliminary studies suggest that ginseng may have a positive effect on complications of cardiac bypass surgery, including decreasing damage to the lining of the digestive tract. Well-designed studies are needed before a strong recommendation can be made.	C
High Blood Pressure Early research suggests that ginseng may lower blood pressure (systolic and diastolic). It is not clear what doses may be safe or effective. Well-conducted studies are needed to confirm these preliminary results.	C
High Cholesterol Several low-quality studies have examined the effects of *Panax ginseng* on cholesterol levels. Results are mixed. More studies are needed to understand the effects of ginseng on cholesterol levels.	C
Idiopathic Thrombocytopenic Purpura (Refractory) Combination herbal products containing ginseng may help treat refractory idiopathic thrombocytopenic purpura, a blood disorder that does not respond well to treatment. Studies that use ginseng alone are needed.	C
Intracranial Pressure (ICP) Preliminary research reports that Xuesaitong injection (XSTI), a preparation of *Panax notoginseng*, may help decrease pressure inside the skull and benefit coma patients. Further study is needed to confirm these results.	C
Kidney Dysfunction (Hemorrhagic Fever with Renal Syndrome) A combination of herbs that included ginseng was not better than treatment with a conventional medicine plus traditional Chinese medicine. More research is needed in this area because the effects of ginseng alone are unknown.	C
Liver Protection Preliminary studies suggest that ginseng may have protective effects on the liver. Additional human study is warranted in this area.	C
Lung Conditions Several studies have looked at the effects of ginseng in a variety of lung conditions. Preliminary results are promising, but many studies have used combination products, which makes it difficult to evaluate the effect of ginseng. More research using ginseng alone is needed in this area.	C
Male Infertility Preliminary evidence suggests that ginseng may improve male fertility by increasing the number and movement of sperm. Further studies are needed to determine what dose may be safe and effective.	C
Menopausal Symptoms Based on limited research, it is unclear whether ginseng may help treat menopausal symptoms. Some studies report improvements in depression and sense of well-being, without changes in hormone levels.	C
Mental Performance Several studies report that ginseng may modestly improve thinking or learning. Benefits have been seen both in healthy young people and in older ill patients. Effects have also been reported with a combination of ginseng and *Ginkgo biloba*. However, some mixed results have also been reported. Therefore, even though most available evidence supports this use of ginseng, better research is needed before a strong recommendation can be made.	C
Methicillin-Resistant *Staphylococcus aureus* (MRSA) In patients treated with Hochu-ekki-to, which contains ginseng and several other herbs, urinary MRSA has been reported to decrease after 10 weeks. Further study of ginseng alone is necessary to draw firm conclusions.	C
Mood and Cognition in Postmenopausal Women A review of several studies suggested that ginseng may improve mood and anxiety in postmenopausal women. Additional studies are needed before a firm conclusion may be drawn.	C
Neurological Disorders Preliminary studies suggest that ginseng may have beneficial effects on neurological disorders. High-quality studies are needed in this area.	C
Postoperative Recovery (Breast Cancer) Preliminary studies have tested the effect of a combination product containing ginseng on recovery after surgery among breast cancer patients. Results suggest no benefits in cell counts but a slightly faster	C

Uses Based on Scientific Evidence	Grade
recovery of the iron-carrying component of red blood cells (called hemoglobin). Studies using ginseng alone are needed.	
Pregnancy Problems (Intrauterine Growth Retardation) Early studies have found that components of *Panax ginseng* might be useful in treating intrauterine growth retardation. Larger, well-designed studies are needed in this area.	C
Premature Ejaculation Preliminary studies suggest that applying an herbal combination containing *Panax ginseng* on the penis may help treat premature ejaculation. However, because ginseng was tested with other herbs, its individual effects are unclear.	C
Quality of Life There is preliminary evidence that *Panax ginseng* or American ginseng may help improve quality of life in both healthy and ill patients, although effects may not be long-lasting unless ginseng is taken continually. More research is needed in this area before a firm conclusion can be reached.	C
Radiation Therapy Side Effects Preliminary studies suggest that ginseng may improve fatigue and measures of well-being among patients receiving radiation therapy. However, there is not enough evidence to recommend the use of *Panax ginseng* or American ginseng for this use.	C
Respiratory Infections Ginseng (CVT-E002) may be safe, well tolerated, and potentially effective for preventing acute respiratory illnesses caused by the flu or the respiratory syncytial virus. More study is needed in this area.	C
Sexual Arousal (in Women) Preliminary studies suggest that a product containing *Panax ginseng*, L-arginine, *Ginkgo biloba*, damiana, and multivitamin/minerals may improve sexual function in menopausal women and women with decreased sex drives. Studies with *Panax ginseng* alone are needed before strong recommendations can be made.	C
Viral Myocarditis Research in patients injected with the ginseng preparation Shenmai suggests that it may improve heart function. However, evidence is insufficient to support efficacy.	C
Well-being Several studies have examined the effects of ginseng (with or without multivitamins) on overall well-being in healthy and ill patients, for up to 12 weeks. Most studies have produced weak evidence, and results are mixed. It remains unclear whether ginseng is beneficial for well-being in any patient.	C

Uses Based on Tradition or Theory

Acrocyanosis (circulatory insufficiency of the extremities), adaptogen, adrenal tonic, aerobic fitness, aggression, aging, AIDS/HIV, air pollution protection, alcoholism, allergy, altitude (mountain) sickness, Alzheimer's disease, amnesia, antibacterial, antidepressant, antifungal, antiinfective, antiinflammatory, antioxidant, antipsychotic, antitumor, anxiety, appetite stimulant, asthma, atherosclerosis, autoimmune disorders, bile flow stimulant, bleeding disorders, breast enlargement, breathing difficulty, burns, central nervous system diseases, chronic cough, chronic fatigue syndrome, colitis, convulsions, demulcent, diabetic nerve pain, dialysis, digestive complaints, diuretic (water pill), dizziness, dysentery, dyspnea (shortness of breath), earache, female infertility, fetal development, fever, fibromyalgia, frequent urination, gastritis, gastrointestinal motility, gynecological disorders, hair tonic, hangovers, head injury (severe intractable), headaches, hemolytic anemia, herpes, hoarse voice, improved memory and thinking after menopause, improvement of blood supply, improving resistance to disease, inflammation (systemic inflammatory reaction syndrome), influenza, insomnia, irritability, ischemia-reperfusion injury prevention, ischemic injury (brain), ischemic stroke, jaundice, Kaposi's sarcoma, kidney disease, learning, leukemia, liver diseases, long-term debility, longevity, low back pain, lumbar disk herniation, lymphoma (Burkitt's and Hodgkin's lymphoma), malaise, malignant tumors, migraine, mood enhancement, morphine tolerance, multiple myeloma, muscle weakness, nausea, neuralgia (pain due to nerve damage or inflammation), neurasthenia, neuroblastoma, neurodegenerative diseases, neuroprotective, organ dysfunction (multiple organ failure), organ prolapse, ovulation disorders, oxygen absorption, pain relief, palpitations, Parkinson's disease, physical work capacity, pneumonia, postherpetic neuralgia, *Pseudomonas* infection in cystic fibrosis, psychoasthenia, pulmonary edema, qi-deficiency and blood-stasis syndrome in heart disease (Eastern medicine), rehabilitation, rheumatism, salivary stimulant, scar healing (acne), sciatica, sedative, sexual symptoms, skin care, skin irritation (mucus membranes), spleen disorders, stimulant, stomach ulcers, stomach upset, stress, strokes, sweating, tonic, toxicity, tuberculosis, upper respiratory tract infection, vein clots, vitality, vomiting, weight loss, wound healing, wrinkle prevention.

DOSING

Adults (18 Years and Older)

- Many different doses are used traditionally. Practitioners sometimes recommended that after using ginseng continuously for 2-3 weeks, people should take a break for 1-2 weeks. Long-term dosing should not exceed 1 g of dry root daily.
- Capsules containing 100-200 mg of a standardized ginseng extract (4% ginsenosides) have been taken by mouth once or twice daily for up to 12 weeks. A range of 0.5-2 g of dry ginseng root, taken daily by mouth in divided doses, has also been used. *E. senticosus* dry extract at a dose of 300 mg daily was used for 8 weeks to improve quality of life in elderly patients. A ginseng root extract has been studied in athletes for 28 days at a dose of 400 mg daily. Higher doses are sometimes given in studies or under the supervision of a qualified health care provider. A decoction of 1-2 g added to 150 mL of water has been taken by mouth daily. A 1:1 (grams per milliliter) fluid extract has been taken as 1-2 mL by mouth daily.

Approximately 5-10 mL (about 1-2 teaspoons) of a 1:5 (grams per milliliter) tincture has been taken by mouth daily.

- *Panax ginseng* tea may be made by soaking about 3000 mg (3 g) of chopped fresh root or 1500 mg (1.5 g) of dried root powder in about 5 oz of boiling water for 5-15 minutes and then straining the tea. Some sources suggest consuming ginseng tea via the above method three to four times daily for 3-4 weeks.
- When applied on the skin, 0.20 g of SS-cream containing ginseng has been used to treat premature ejaculation.

Children (Younger than 18 Years)

- There is not enough scientific information available to recommend the safe use of ginseng in children.

SAFETY
Allergies

- People with known allergies to *Panax* species and/or plants in the Araliaceae family should avoid ginseng. Signs of allergy may include rash, itching, or shortness of breath. Inhalation of ginseng root dust has been associated with immediate and late-onset asthma.

Side Effects and Warnings

- Ginseng has been well tolerated by most people in scientific studies when used at recommended doses, and serious side effects appear to be rare.
- Based on limited evidence, long-term use may be associated with skin rash or spots, itching, diarrhea, sore throat, loss of appetite, excitability, anxiety, depression, or insomnia. Less common reported side effects include headache, fever, dizziness, chest pain, difficult menstruation, heartburn, heart palpitations, rapid heart rate, leg swelling, nausea/vomiting, or manic episodes in people with bipolar disorder.
- Consumption of ginseng may increase or decrease blood pressure. Caution should be used in those with high or low blood pressure or in those taking drugs for either of these conditions.
- Seizures have been reported after excessive consumption of energy drinks containing caffeine, guarana, and herbal supplements, including ginseng.
- Based on human research, ginseng may lower blood sugar levels. This effect may be greater in patients with diabetes than in those without diabetes. Use cautiously in patients with diabetes or hypoglycemia and in those taking drugs, herbs, or supplements that affect blood sugar. Blood glucose levels may need to be monitored by a health care provider, and medication adjustments may be necessary.
- There are reports of nosebleeds and vaginal bleeding with ginseng use, although scientific study is limited in this area. There is also evidence in humans of ginseng reducing the effectiveness of the "blood thinning" medication warfarin (Coumadin). Caution is advised in patients with bleeding disorders or taking drugs that may affect the risk of bleeding or blood clotting. Dosing adjustments may be necessary.
- Several cases of severe drops in white blood cell counts were reported in people using a combination product containing ginseng in the 1970s; this may have been due to contamination.
- Ginseng may have estrogen-like effects and has been associated with reports of breast tenderness, loss of menstrual periods, vaginal bleeding after menopause, breast enlargement (reported in men), difficulty developing or maintaining an erection, or increased "sexual responsiveness." Avoid use of ginseng in patients with hormone sensitive conditions, such as breast cancer, uterine cancer, or endometriosis.
- A severe life-threatening rash known as Stevens-Johnson syndrome occurred in one patient and may have been due to contaminants in a ginseng product. A case report describes liver damage (cholestatic hepatitis) after taking a combination product containing ginseng.
- High doses of ginseng have been associated with rare cases of temporary swelling of blood vessels in the brain (cerebral arteritis), abnormal dilation of the pupils of the eye, or confusion.

Pregnancy and Breastfeeding

- Ginseng has been used traditionally in pregnant and breastfeeding women. Animal studies and preliminary human research suggests that ginseng may be safe, although safety has not been clearly established in humans. Therefore, ginseng use cannot be recommended during pregnancy or breastfeeding. Neonatal death and the development of male characteristics in a developing baby girl after her mother was exposed to ginseng during pregnancy has been reported.
- Many tinctures contain high levels of alcohol and should be avoided during pregnancy.

INTERACTIONS
Interactions with Drugs

- Research in humans suggests that American ginseng may reduce the anticoagulant (blood thinning) effects of warfarin (Coumadin). In addition, based on limited animal research and individual reports of nosebleeds and vaginal bleeding in humans, ginseng may increase the risk of bleeding when taken with other drugs that increase the risk of bleeding. Examples include aspirin, anticoagulants ("blood thinners") such as heparin, antiplatelet drugs such as clopidogrel (Plavix), and nonsteroidal antiinflammatory drugs such as ibuprofen (Motrin, Advil) or naproxen (Naprosyn, Aleve). In contrast, there is a case of the effectiveness of the blood thinner warfarin (Coumadin) being reduced when taken at the same time as ginseng.
- Based on human research, ginseng may lower blood sugar levels. This effect may be greater in patients with diabetes than in nondiabetic individuals. Caution is advised when medications that may also lower blood sugar are used. Patients taking drugs for diabetes by mouth or injection should be monitored closely by a qualified health care provider. Medication adjustments may be needed.
- Headache, tremors, mania, or insomnia may occur if ginseng is combined with prescription antidepressant drugs called monoamine oxidase inhibitors (MAOIs), such as isocarboxazid (Marplan), phenelzine (Nardil), and tranylcypromine (Parnate).
- Ginseng may alter the effects of blood pressure or heart medications, including calcium channel blockers such as nifedipine (Procardia). There is a reported case of decreased effects of the diuretic drug furosemide (Lasix) when used with ginseng. A Chinese study reports that the effects of the cardiac glycoside drug digoxin (Lanoxin) may be increased when used with ginseng in patients with heart failure. Do not combine ginseng with heart or blood pressure medications without first talking to a qualified health care provider.

- There is limited laboratory evidence that ginseng may contain estrogen-like chemicals and may affect medications with estrogen-like or estrogen-blocking properties. This has not been well demonstrated in humans.
- In theory, ginseng may interfere with the way the body processes certain drugs using the liver's cytochrome P450 enzyme system. As a result, the levels of these drugs may be increased in the blood and may cause increased effects or potentially serious side effects. A pharmacist should be consulted before taking any herbs or supplements concomitantly with drugs.
- The analgesic effect of opioids may be inhibited by ginseng. Ginseng may interact with sedatives.
- Many tinctures contain high levels of alcohol and may cause nausea or vomiting when taken with metronidazole (Flagyl) or disulfiram (Antabuse). In preliminary research, ginseng has been reported to increase removal of alcohol from the blood, although this has not been well substantiated.
- Ginseng may also interact with cholesterol-lowering, anticancer, antiviral, antipsychotic, erectile dysfunction, immunomodulator, and glucocorticoid drugs, as well as caffeine.

Interactions with Herbs and Dietary Supplements

- Based on human research, ginseng may lower blood sugar levels. This effect may be greater in patients with diabetes than in non-diabetic individuals. Caution is advised when herbs or supplements that may also lower blood sugar are used. Blood glucose levels may require monitoring, and doses may need adjustment.
- Headache, tremors, mania, and insomnia may occur if ginseng is combined with supplements that have MAOI activity or that interact with MAOI drugs.
- Based on case reports, ginseng may raise or lower blood pressure. Use cautiously if combining ginseng with other products that affect blood pressure.
- There is preliminary evidence that ginseng may increase the QTc interval (thus increasing the risk of abnormal heart rhythms) and decrease diastolic blood pressure 2 hours after ingestion in healthy adults. Therefore, caution is advised when other agents that may cause abnormal heart rhythms are taken.
- Based on limited animal research and anecdotal reports of nosebleeds and vaginal bleeding in humans, ginseng may increase the risk of bleeding when taken with herbs and supplements that are believed to increase the risk of bleeding. Multiple cases of bleeding have been reported with the use of *Ginkgo biloba*, some cases have been reported with garlic, and fewer cases have been reported with saw palmetto. Numerous other agents may theoretically increase the risk of bleeding, although this has not been proven in most cases.
- In theory, ginseng may decrease the effects of diuretic herbs, such as horsetail or licorice. Ginseng may interact with sedatives or other supplements that affect the central nervous system.
- In theory, ginseng may interfere with the way the body processes certain herbs or supplements using the liver's cytochrome P450 enzyme system. As a result, the levels of other herbs or supplements may be too high in the blood. It may also alter the effects that other herbs or supplements possibly have on the P450 system, such as cat's claw or echinacea.
- There is limited laboratory evidence that ginseng may contain estrogen-like chemicals and may affect agents with estrogen-like or estrogen-blocking properties. This has not been proven in humans.
- Ginseng may also interact with cholesterol-lowering, antiinflammatory, anticancer, antiviral, antipsychotic, steroid, glucocorticoid, immunomodulator, and erectile dysfunction herbs and supplements as well as dehydroepiandrosterone (DHEA), caffeine, mate, and guarana.

For a complete list of references, please visit www.naturalstandard.com.

G

Globe Artichoke
(Cynara scolymus)

RELATED TERMS

- Alcachofa, alcaucil, artichaut (French), artichiocco, artichoke, artichoke inulin, artichoke juice, Artischocke (German), artiskok, carciofo, cardo, cardo de comer, cardon d'Espagne, cardoon, chlorogenic acid, Cynara, *Cynara cardunculus, Cynara scolymus* L., *Cynarae folium,* cynarin, cynaroside, French artichoke, garden artichoke, Gemuseartischocke (German), golden artichoke, Hekbilin A, Hepar SL forte, inulin, kardone, LI220, Listrocol, luteolin, Raftiline, scolymoside, tyosen-azami, Valverde Artischoke bei Verdauungsbeschwerden.
- **Note:** Globe artichoke should not be mistaken for Jerusalem artichoke, which is the tuber of *Helianthus tuberosa* (a species of sunflower).

BACKGROUND

- Globe artichoke *(Cynara scolymus)* is a species of thistle. The edible part of the plant is the base of the artichoke head flower bud, which is harvested well before any fruit develops. In traditional European medicine, the leaves of the artichoke (not the flower buds, which are the parts commonly cooked and eaten as a vegetable) were used as a diuretic to stimulate the kidneys and as a choleretic to stimulate the flow of bile from the liver and gallbladder.
- Cynarin, luteolin, cynardoside (luteolin-7-O-glycoside), scolymoside, and chlorogenic acid are believed to be artichoke's active constituents. The most studied component, cynarin, is concentrated in the leaves.
- Artichoke has been used in the treatment of hypercholesterolemia (high cholesterol) and alcohol-induced hangover, and for its choleretic (stimulates bile release) and antioxidant properties.
- Artichoke extracts are becoming increasingly available in the United States, with public interest and the availability of standardized extracts resulting in more rigorous clinical research on the beneficial effects of artichoke.

EVIDENCE

Uses Based on Scientific Evidence	Grade
Choleretic (Stimulates the Release of Bile) Globe artichoke leaf extract has been found to increase bile secretion in animal and human and laboratory studies. Additional human studies are needed to show the effectiveness of artichoke as a choleretic.	B
Lipid-Lowering Agent Preliminary human studies suggest that cynarin and (and perhaps other constituents in artichoke extracts) may reduce serum cholesterol and triglyceride levels.	B

Alcohol-Induced Hangover Artichoke extract has been used and marketed as a hangover remedy. However, the effectiveness remains uncertain.	C
Antioxidant Antioxidant properties of artichoke have been noted, although long-term effects in humans are unclear.	C
Dyspepsia (Upset Stomach) One proposed etiology of non-ulcer dyspepsia is bile duct dyskinesia. Because globe artichoke extract has been studied as a choleretic, it has been hypothesized that it may also function as an antidyspeptic agent. Preliminary evidence supports this hypothesis.	C
Irritable Bowel Syndrome (IBS) There is insufficient available evidence to recommend the use of artichoke in relieving the symptoms of irritable bowel syndrome.	C

Uses Based on Tradition or Theory

Allergies, anemia, antifungal, arthritis, atherosclerosis (hardening of the arteries), bitter tonic, cholelithiasis (stops bile flow), constipation, cystitis (bladder inflammation), diuretic, eczema, emesis (vomiting), gout (foot inflammation), hepatoprotection (liver protection), jaundice, nausea, nephrolithiasis/urolithiasis (kidney stones), nephrosclerosis (kidney disease), probiotic, peripheral edema, pruritis (severe itching), rheumatic diseases, snakebite.

DOSING

Adults (18 Years and Older)

- There is insufficient evidence to recommend a dose for artichoke. A typical dosage of standardized artichoke extract is 320-1,800 mg daily for 6 weeks. The expert panel German Commission E recommends 6 g of the dried herb or its equivalent daily (usually divided into three doses).
- Also, 3-8 mL of 1:2 liquid extract daily is often recommended in clinical practice. Up to 10 mL of pressed juice from fresh leaves and flower buds of the artichoke has been used in clinical trials. The German Commission E has recommended 6 mL of tincture (1:5 g per mL) given three times daily.
- Daily doses of up to 1,900 mg have been used in clinical trials. However, optimal dosing is not clear.
- Daily doses of 4-9 g of dried leaves are often recommended in clinical practice. The German Commission E has recommended 0.5 g of a 12:1 (w/w) dried extract given as a single daily dose.

Children (Younger than 18 Years)

- There is no proven safe or effective dose for artichoke in children, and use is not recommended.

SAFETY
Allergies

- Avoid in individuals with a known allergy or hypersensitivity to globe artichoke (*Cynara scolymus*), its constituents, or members of the Asteraceae or Compositae family (including chrysanthemums, daisies, marigolds, ragweed, and arnica) due to possible cross-reactivity. Symptoms of allergy may include worsening of asthma, skin rash, anaphylactic shock, dyspnea (difficulty breathing), cough, and chest tightness. While rare, individuals with a known inulin allergy should avoid artichokes and artichoke extracts.

Side Effects and Warnings

- Artichoke is likely safe when taken by mouth for short periods of time. The adverse effects associated with artichoke are generally mild and include gastrointestinal symptoms. However, there have been reports of kidney failure and/or toxicity from the use of artichoke leaves. Use cautiously in patients with kidney disease.
- Contact dermatitis (rash) and contact urticaria have been noted after application to the skin, with symptoms spontaneously subsiding hours or days after exposure.
- Mild flatulence (gas), diarrhea, hunger, redness in the face, increased bile secretion, and nausea have been reported. Use cautiously in patients with cholelithiasis (gallstones) or biliary/bile duct obstruction.
- Artichoke extract may increase the risk of bleeding, although causality is unclear. Caution is advised in patients with bleeding disorders or those taking drugs that may increase the risk of bleeding. Dosing adjustments may be necessary.
- Dyspnea (difficulty breathing), cough, chest tightness, and severe asthma exacerbation may occur. Severe anaphylactic shock in response to artichoke inulin as an ingredient in commercially available products has also been reported. People with a noted sensitivity to artichokes should consume inulin with caution. While rare, individuals with a known inulin allergy should avoid artichokes and artichoke extracts.

Pregnancy and Breastfeeding

- There is currently a lack of available scientific evidence to recommend the use of artichoke in pregnant or breastfeeding women.

INTERACTIONS
Interactions with Drugs

- Artichoke may increase the risk of bleeding when taken with drugs that increase the risk of bleeding. Some examples include aspirin, anticoagulants such as warfarin (Coumadin) or heparin, antiplatelet drugs such as clopidogrel (Plavix), and nonsteroidal anti-inflammatory drugs (NSAIDs) such as ibuprofen (Motrin, Advil) or naproxen (Naprosyn, Aleve).
- There are multiple published reports of cholesterol-lowering effects of artichoke, although the quality of most studies is not sufficient to make a recommendation. Artichoke may add to the cholesterol-lowering effects of other agents.

Interactions with Herbs and Dietary Supplements

- Artichoke may increase the risk of bleeding when taken with herbs and supplements that also increase the risk of bleeding. Multiple cases of bleeding have been reported with the use of *Ginkgo biloba*, and fewer cases with garlic and saw palmetto. Numerous other agents may theoretically increase the risk of bleeding, although this has not been shown conclusively in most cases.
- There are multiple published reports on the cholesterol-lowering effects of artichoke, although the quality of most studies is not sufficient to make a recommendation. Artichoke may add to the lipid-lowering effects of other agents, such as fish oil, garlic, or niacin.

For a complete list of references, please visit www.naturalstandard.com.

G

Glucosamine

($C_6H_{13}NO_5$)

RELATED TERMS

- 2-Acetamido-2-deoxyglucose, acetylglucosamine, Arth-X Plus, chitosamine, ChitoSeal, Clo-Sur PAD, D-glucosamine, disease modifying drugs for osteoarthritis (DMOAD), enhanced glucosamine sulfate, Flexi-Factors, glucosamine chlorohydrate, Glucosamine Complex, glucosamine hydrochloride, glucosamine hydroiodide, Glucosamine Mega, glucosamine N-Acetyl, glucosamine sulfate, glucosamine sulphate, Joint Factors, N-acetyl D-glucosamine (NAG, N-A-G), Nutri-Joint, poly-N-acetyl glucosamine (pGlcNAc), Poly-NAG, Syvek Patch, Ultra Maximum Strength Glucosamine Sulfate.

BACKGROUND

- Glucosamine is a natural compound that is found in healthy cartilage. Glucosamine sulfate is a normal constituent of glycosaminoglycans in cartilage matrix and synovial fluid.
- Overall, the evidence from randomized controlled trials supports the use of glucosamine sulfate in the treatment of osteoarthritis, particularly of the knee. It is believed that the sulfate moiety provides clinical benefit in the synovial fluid by strengthening cartilage and aiding glycosaminoglycan synthesis. If this hypothesis is confirmed, it would mean that only the glucosamine sulfate form is effective and non-sulfated glucosamine forms are not effective.
- Glucosamine is commonly taken in combination with chondroitin, a glycosaminoglycan derived from articular cartilage. Use of complementary therapies, including glucosamine, is common in patients with osteoarthritis and may allow for reduced doses of nonsteroidal antiinflammatory agents.

EVIDENCE

Uses Based on Scientific Evidence	Grade
Knee Osteoarthritis (Mild-to-Moderate) Based on human research, there is good evidence to support the use of glucosamine sulfate in the treatment of mild-to-moderate knee osteoarthritis. Most studies have used glucosamine sulfate supplied by one European manufacturer (Rotta Research Laboratorium), and it is not known whether glucosamine preparations made by other manufacturers are equally effective. Although some studies of glucosamine have not found benefits, these have either included patients with severe osteoarthritis or used products other than glucosamine *sulfate*. The evidence for the effect of glycosaminoglycan polysulfate is conflicting and merits further investigation. More well-designed clinical trials are needed to confirm safety and effectiveness and to test different formulations of glucosamine.	A
Osteoarthritis (General) Several human studies and animal experiments report benefits of glucosamine in treating osteoarthritis of various joints of the body, although the evidence is	B
less plentiful than that for knee osteoarthritis. Some of these benefits include pain relief, possibly due to an antiinflammatory effect of glucosamine, and improved joint function. Overall, these studies have not been well designed; thus stronger evidence is needed.	
Chronic Venous Insufficiency *Chronic venous insufficiency* is a syndrome that includes leg swelling, varicose veins, pain, itching, skin changes, and skin ulcers. The term is more commonly used in Europe than in the United States. Currently, there is not enough reliable scientific evidence to recommend glucosamine in the treatment of this condition.	C
Diabetes (and Related Conditions) Early research suggests that glucosamine does not improve blood sugar control, lipid levels, or apolipoprotein levels in diabetic patients. However, the effectiveness remains unlcear.	C
Inflammatory Bowel Disease (Crohn's Disease, Ulcerative Colitis) Preliminary research reports improvements with N-acetyl glucosamine as an added therapy in inflammatory bowel disease. However, the effectiveness remains unlcear.	C
Pain (Leg Pain) Preliminary human research reports benefits of injected glucosamine plus chondroitin in the treatment of leg pain arising from advanced lumbar degenerative disk disease. However, the evidence thus far has not been definitive.	C
Rehabilitation (after Knee Injury) Glucosamine has been given to athletes with acute knee injuries. Although glucosamine did not improve pain, it did help improve flexibility. However, the evidence thus far has not been definitive.	C
Rheumatoid Arthritis Early human research reports benefits of glucosamine in the treatment of joint pain and swelling in rheumatoid arthritis. In other research, glucosamine did not exert antirheumatic effects, but it did improve symptoms of the disease. However, the evidence thus far has not been definitive. The treatment of rheumatoid arthritis can be complicated, and a qualified health care provider should follow up patients with this disease.	C
Temporomandibular Joint (TMJ) Disorders There is a lack of sufficient evidence to recommend for or against the use of glucosamine (or the combination of glucosamine and chondroitin) in the treatment of TMJ disorders.	C

Uses Based on Scientific Evidence	Grade
High Cholesterol Glucosamine does not appear to alter low-density lipoprotein (LDL) or high-density lipoprotein (HDL) levels in patients with chronic joint pain or diabetes.	D

Uses Based on Tradition or Theory
Acquired immunodeficiency syndrome (AIDS), athletic injuries, back pain, bleeding esophageal varices (blood vessels in the esophagus), cancer, congestive heart failure, depression, fibromyalgia, immunosuppression, kidney stones, migraine headache, osteoporosis, pain, psoriasis, skin rejuvenation, spondylosis deformans (growth of bony spurs on the spine), topical hypopigmenting agent (combination product containing multiple ingredients), wound healing.

DOSING
Adults (18 Years and Older)

- In most available studies, 500 mg of glucosamine sulfate has been taken by mouth as tablets or capsules three times daily for 30-90 days. Once-daily dosing as 1.5 g (1500 mg) has also been used. Limited research has used 1500 mg daily as a crystalline powder for oral solution or 500 mg of glucosamine *hydrochloride* three times daily. Dosing of 20 mg/kg of body weight daily has also been recommended in some publications. One study used a dose of 2000 mg/day for 12 weeks.
- Another kind of glucosamine that has been used is a topical form in combination with chondroitin for a 4-week period. Safety and effectiveness of these formulations are not clearly proven.
- Glucosamine hydrochloride provides more glucosamine than glucosamine sulfate, although this difference likely does not matter when products are prepared to provide a total of 500 mg of glucosamine per tablet.

Children (Younger than 18 Years)

- There is insufficient evidence to recommend the use of glucosamine in children.
- Research in children has shown that there could be a relationship between the ingestion of MSM (methylsulfonylmethane) and autism; whether it is beneficial or harmful is unclear. MSM is often marketed with glucosamine as a dietary supplement and at this time should be avoided in children.

SAFETY
Allergies

- Because glucosamine can be made from the shells of shrimp, crab, and other shellfish, people with shellfish allergy or iodine hypersensitivity may have an allergic reaction to glucosamine products. However, some research suggests that there is not enough shrimp allergen in glucosamine supplements to trigger reactions in patients who are allergic to shrimp. Nevertheless, caution is warranted. A serious hypersensitivity reaction including throat swelling has been reported with glucosamine sulfate. There are reported cases suggesting a link between glucosamine/chondroitin products and asthma exacerbations.

Side Effects and Warnings

- In most human studies, glucosamine sulfate has been well tolerated for 30-90 days.
- Side effects may include upset stomach, drowsiness, insomnia, headache, skin reactions, sun sensitivity, and nail toughening. There are rare reports of abdominal pain, loss of appetite, vomiting, nausea, flatulence (gas), constipation, heartburn, and diarrhea. Based on several human cases, temporary increases in blood pressure and heart rate, as well as palpitations, may occur with glucosamine/chondroitin products. Based on animal research, glucosamine theoretically may increase the risk of eye cataract formation.
- It remains unclear whether glucosamine alters blood sugar levels. Several human studies suggest that glucosamine taken by mouth has no effects on blood sugar, while other research reports mixed effects on insulin. When glucosamine is injected, it appears to cause insulin resistance and endothelial dysfunction. Preliminary studies show no effect on mean hemoglobin A1c concentrations in patients with type 2 diabetes mellitus. Caution is advised in patients with diabetes or hypoglycemia and in those taking drugs, herbs, or supplements that affect blood sugar. Serum glucose levels may need to be monitored by a health care provider, and medication adjustments may be necessary.
- In theory glucosamine may increase the risk of bleeding. Caution is advised in patients with bleeding disorders or taking drugs that may increase the risk of bleeding. Dosing adjustments may be necessary.
- In several human cases, abnormally high amounts of protein were found in the urine of patients receiving glucosamine/chondroitin products. The clinical meaning of this is unclear. Glucosamine is removed from the body mainly in the urine, and elimination of glucosamine from the body is delayed in people with reduced kidney function. Acute interstitial nephritis, a condition that causes the kidneys to become swollen and possibly dysfunctional, has been reported in a patient taking glucosamine. Increased blood levels of creatine phosphokinase may occur with glucosamine/chondroitin, which may be due to impurities in some products. This may alter certain laboratory tests measured by health care providers.
- Preliminary evidence suggests that glucosamine may modulate the immune system, although the clinical relevance of this is not clear.
- One patient developed liver inflammation (acute cholestatic hepatitis) after taking glucosamine forte.

Pregnancy and Breastfeeding

- Glucosamine is not recommended during pregnancy or breastfeeding because of lack of scientific evidence.

INTERACTIONS
Interactions with Drugs

- In theory, glucosamine may decrease the effectiveness of insulin or other drugs used to control blood sugar levels. However, there is limited human research to suggest that glucosamine may not have significant effects on blood sugar. Nonetheless, caution is advised when insulin is used or drugs for diabetes are taken by mouth. Patients with diabetes or hypoglycemia should be monitored closely by a qualified health care provider, and medication adjustments may be necessary. Based on limited evidence, the combination of glucosamine with diuretics (water pills), such as furosemide (Lasix), may cause an increased risk of glucosamine side effects.

- In theory, glucosamine may increase the risk of bleeding when taken with drugs that increase the risk of bleeding. Some examples include aspirin, anticoagulants ("blood thinners") such as warfarin (Coumadin) or heparin, antiplatelet drugs such as clopidogrel (Plavix), and nonsteroidal antiinflammatory drugs such as ibuprofen (Motrin, Advil) or naproxen (Naprosyn, Aleve).

Interactions with Herbs and Dietary Supplements

- In theory, glucosamine may decrease the effectiveness of herbs or supplements that lower blood sugar levels. Caution is advised when herbs or supplements that may alter blood sugar are used.
- Based on limited human study, side effects of glucosamine may be increased when it is used at the same time as diuretic herbs or supplements.
- In theory, glucosamine may increase the risk of bleeding when taken with herbs and supplements that are believed to increase the risk of bleeding
- There are preliminary reports that use of glucosamine with vitamin C, bromelain, chondroitin sulfate, or manganese may lead to increased beneficial glucosamine effects on osteoarthritis. Simultaneous use with fish oil may have additive beneficial effects in the treatment of psoriasis, based on preliminary research.

For a complete list of references, please visit www.naturalstandard.com.

Glyconutrients

RELATED TERMS

- Ambrotose, Ambrotose complex, dietary saccharide, fucose, galactose, glucose, Glycentials, glycoconjugates, glycobiology, glycoform, glyconutritional, glycoprotein, Manapol, mannose, N-acetylgalactosamine, N-acetylglucosamine, N-acetylneuraminic acid, saccharide, sialic acid, sugars, xylose.

BACKGROUND

- Glyconutrients are dietary supplements that supply sugars such as glucose, galactose, mannose, fucose, xylose, N-acetylglucosamine, N-acetylgalactosamine, and N-acetylneuraminic acid. These sugars are thought to be necessary for cells to communicate with each other in the body.
- Glyconutrient research (glycobiology) has increased in the last few years. A company called Mannatech is the leading manufacturer of glyconutrient supplements. They market glyconutrients under the product line Ambrotose.
- There is currently a lack of available scientific evidence showing effectiveness for any condition. Advocates of this therapy claim that only glucose and galactose are readily found in a normal diet, and that glyconutrient supplementation is needed to prevent disease states. Critics of glyconutrient therapy argue that the body can synthesize any sugar it requires from protein intake, so unless a person has a genetic mutation, most glyconutrients are not cost-effective.

EVIDENCE

Uses Based on Scientific Evidence	Grade
Attention Deficit Hyperactivity Disorder (ADHD) Glyconutrients may cause a decrease in the number and severity of symptoms in children with attention deficit hyperactivity disorder. However, the available evidence is not definitive.	C
Failure-to-Thrive Glyconutrients may cause an increase in weight and height in toddlers with failure-to-thrive. However, the available evidence is not definitive.	C

Uses Based on Tradition or Theory
Acquired immunodeficiency syndrome (AIDS), alcoholism, allergy, Alzheimer's disease, antibacterial, anxiety, asthma, athletic performance, bladder cancer, bone density, brain wave frequency alteration, burns, cancer, canker sores, cataracts, cerebral palsy, chronic fatigue, cognitive function, colitis, cystic fibrosis, depression, diabetes, Down's syndrome, dyslexia, eczema, fever blisters, fibromyalgia, heart disease, hepatitis, herpes, high cholesterol levels, hormonal imbalances, immune disorders, infections, infections (streptococcal toxic shock syndrome), infertility, inflammation, inflammation (muscle tissue), insomnia, lupus, Lyme disease, memory, menopause, metabolic disorders, multiple

sclerosis, muscle mass, muscular dystrophy (adjuvant), myasthenia gravis, myofascial pain, organ transplantation (heart), osteoporosis (prevention), Parkinson's disease, pemphigus vulgaris, periodontal disease, premenstrual syndrome, psoriasis, rash, retinal protection (from detaching), rheumatoid arthritis, sleep, stomatitis, stress, stroke, Sturge Weber syndrome, Tay-Sachs disease, Tourette's syndrome, tumor (eye), wound healing.

DOSING

Adults (18 Years and Older)

- There is insufficient evidence to recommend a dose for glyconutrients in adults.

Children (Younger than 18 Years)

- There is insufficient evidence to recommend a dose for glyconutrients in children.

SAFETY

Allergies

- Plant sources containing glyconutrients may cause allergy or adverse effects in some people; it is recommended to be knowledgeable before herbal extracts or supplements are used.

Side Effects and Warnings

- Glyconutrients are likely safe when derived from food or supplements in recommended doses. However, use cautiously in patients taking iron supplements and in patients with a history of copper deficiency or vitamin B_{12} deficiency.

Pregnancy and Breastfeeding

- Glyconutrients are essential in cellular communication and are important for pregnant and lactating women. However, scientific evidence investigating the therapeutic use of these nutrients is currently lacking.

INTERACTIONS

Interactions with Drugs

- Glyconutrient commercial products that contain vitamin K may interact with blood thinners and thus should be avoided. Similarly, glyconutrients containing ubidecarenone may diminish the response to warfarin (Coumadin), and patients should be monitored.

Interactions with Herbs and Dietary Supplements

- Glyconutritional supplements may decrease copper levels, increase iron levels, or increase folic acid levels in the body. Dosing of supplements may need adjustment when glyconutrients are taken.
- Glyconutrient commercial products that contain vitamin K may interact with blood thinners and thus should be avoided.

For a complete list of references, please visit www.naturalstandard.com.

Goldenseal
(Hydrastis canadensis)

RELATED TERMS

- BBR, berberine bisulfate, curcuma, eye balm, eye root, golden root, goldensiegel, goldsiegel, ground raspberry, guldsegl, hydrastis rhizoma, *Hydrophyllum*, Indian dye, Indian paint, Indian plant, Indian turmeric, jaundice root, kanadische gelbwurzel, kurkuma, Ohio curcuma, orange root, turmeric root, warnera, wild curcuma, wild turmeric, yellow eye, yellow Indian plant, yellow paint, yellow paint root, yellow puccoon, yellow root, yellow seal, yellow wort.
- **Note:** Goldenseal is sometimes referred to as "Indian turmeric" or "curcuma" but should not be confused with turmeric (*Curcuma longa* Linn.).

BACKGROUND

- Goldenseal is one of the five top-selling herbal products in the United States. However, there is little scientific evidence about its safety or effectiveness. Goldenseal can be found in dietary supplements, eardrops, feminine cleansing products, cold/flu remedies, allergy remedies, laxatives, and digestive aids.
- Goldenseal is often found in combination with echinacea in treatments for upper respiratory infections and is suggested to enhance the effects of echinacea. However, the effects when these agents are combined are not scientifically proven.
- Goldenseal has been used by some people because of the popular notion that detection of illegal drugs in urine may be hidden by use of the herb, although scientific information is limited in this area.
- The popularity of goldenseal has led to a higher demand for the herb than growers can supply. This high demand has led to the substitution of other herbs such as Chinese goldthread (*Coptis chinensis* Franch.) and Oregon grape (*Mahonia aquifolium* [Pursh] Nutt.), that do not contain exactly the same isoquinoline alkaloids and may not affect the body in the same way as goldenseal.
- Studies of the effectiveness of goldenseal are limited to one of its main chemical ingredients, berberine salts (there are few published human studies of goldenseal itself). Because of the small amount of berberine actually present in most goldenseal preparations (0.5-6%), it is difficult to extend the research of berberine salts to the use of goldenseal. Therefore, there is not enough scientific evidence to support the use of goldenseal in humans for any medical condition.

EVIDENCE

Uses Based on Scientific Evidence	Grade
Chloroquine-Resistant Malaria A small amount of research reports that berberine, a chemical found in goldenseal, may be beneficial in the treatment of chloroquine-resistant malaria when used in combination with pyrimethamine. Because of the very small amount of berberine found in most goldenseal preparations, it is unclear whether goldenseal contains enough berberine to have these effects.	C
Common Cold/Upper Respiratory Tract Infection Goldenseal has become a popular treatment for the common cold and upper respiratory tract infections and is often added to echinacea in commercial herbal cold remedies. Animal and laboratory research suggests that the goldenseal component berberine has effects against bacteria and inflammation. However, because of the very small amount of berberine in most goldenseal preparations, it is unclear whether goldenseal contains enough berberine to have the same effects.	C
Heart Failure Limited evidence suggests that berberine in addition to a standard prescription drug regimen for chronic congestive heart failure (CHF) may improve quality of life and decrease ventricular premature complexes (VPCs) and mortality. However, the evidence is insufficient to support the effectiveness.	C
High Cholesterol Berberine, a compound isolated from a Chinese herb, may lower cholesterol and triglyceride levels with a mechanism of action different from that of statin drugs.	C
Immune System Stimulation Goldenseal is sometimes suggested to be an immune system stimulant. However, there is little clinical or laboratory evidence in this area.	C
Infectious Diarrhea Berberine has been used as a treatment for diarrhea caused by bacterial infections (including diarrhea from cholera). Because of the very small amount of berberine in most goldenseal products, it is unclear whether goldenseal contains enough berberine to have the same effects.	C
Narcotic Concealment (Urinalysis) It has been suggested that taking goldenseal can hide the presence of illegal drugs from urine tests. However, there is limited research to support this idea. The National Institute on Drug Abuse, National Institutes of Health, examined marijuana and cocaine use and suggested that goldenseal probably does not have this effect.	C

Uses Based on Scientific Evidence	Grade
Trachoma (*Chlamydia trachomatis* Eye Infection) The goldenseal component berberine has effects against bacteria and inflammation. There is some weak clinical evidence that berberine used in the eye may help treat trachoma.	C

Uses Based on Tradition or Theory

Abnormal heart rhythms, acne, acquired immunodeficiency syndrome (AIDS), alcoholic liver disease, anal fissures, anesthetic, antibacterial, anticoagulant ("blood thinning"), antifungal, antihistamine, antiinflammatory, anxiety, appetite stimulant, arthritis, asthma, astrocytoma (brain tumor), atherosclerosis ("hardening" of the arteries), athlete's foot, bile flow stimulant, blood circulation stimulant, boils, bronchitis, cancer, canker sores, cervicitis (inflammation of the cervix), chemotherapy adjuvant, chickenpox, chronic fatigue syndrome, colitis (intestinal inflammation), conjunctivitis, constipation, Crohn's disease, croup, cystic fibrosis, cystitis, dandruff, deafness, diabetes mellitus, diarrhea, diphtheria, diuretic (increases urine flow), eczema, eyewash, fever, fistula problems, flatulence (gas), gallstones, gangrene, gastroenteritis, genital disorders, gingivitis, glioblastoma, headache, *Helicobacter pylori* infection, hemorrhage (bleeding), hemorrhoids, hepatitis, hernia, herpes, high blood pressure, high tyramine levels, hypoglycemia (low blood sugar levels), impetigo, indigestion, inducing (causing) abortion, infections, influenza, insulin potentiation, itching, jaundice, keratitis (inflammation of the cornea of the eye), leishmaniasis, liver disorders, lupus, menstruation problems, morning sickness, mouthwash, muscle pain, muscle spasm, night sweats, obesity, osteoporosis, otorrhea (fluid from the ear), pain, pneumonia, premenstrual syndrome, prostatitis, psoriasis, sciatica, seborrhea, sedative, sinusitis, stimulant, stomach ulcers, strep throat, syphilis, tetanus, thrombocytopenia (low blood platelets), tinnitus (ringing in the ears), tonsillitis, tooth disease, trichomoniasis (vaginal infection), tuberculosis, urinary tract disorders, uterine inflammation, uterine stimulant, vaginal irritation, varicose veins, yeast infection.

DOSING
Adults (18 Years and Older)

- For general use, various types of goldenseal dosing have been used, each taken by mouth three times daily, including 0.5-1 g tablets or capsules, 0.3-1 mL of liquid/fluid extract (1:1 in 60% ethanol), 0.5-1 g as a decoction, or 2-4 mL as a tincture (1:10 in 60% ethanol).
- For infectious diarrhea, 100-200 mg of berberine hydrochloride taken by mouth four times daily or a single dose of 400 mg taken by mouth has been studied. Berberine sulfate is also often used, and the hydrochloride and sulfate forms are generally thought to be equivalent.

Children (Younger than 18 Years)

- There is insufficient evidence to safely recommend the use of goldenseal in children.

SAFETY
Allergies

- Goldenseal should be avoided by people with known allergy/hypersensitivity to goldenseal or any of its constituents, including berberine and hydrastine.

Side Effects and Warnings

- Goldenseal is rarely reported to cause nausea, vomiting, breathing failure, or a feeling of numbness in the arms or legs. Large doses of goldenseal may cause mucus membrane irritation and worsening of stomach ulcers. Goldenseal used on the skin may cause irritation or ulcers.
- Goldenseal may cause low sodium levels in the blood.
- Possible effects of berberine, a chemical found in small amounts in goldenseal, include headache, slow heart rate, nausea, vomiting, abdominal bloating, and low white blood cell count. It is not clear whether the amount of berberine in goldenseal products is enough to cause these reactions. Toxic doses of berberine may cause seizures or irritation of the esophagus and stomach when taken by mouth. Berberine used intravenously (through the veins) may cause abnormal heart rhythms. Berberine may increase blood concentrations of bilirubin. Berberine theoretically may cause low blood pressure, although a different chemical in goldenseal, hydrastine, may actually cause increased blood pressure.
- Goldenseal or berberine could increase the risk of bleeding. Caution is advised in patients with bleeding disorders or taking drugs that may increase the risk of bleeding. Dosing adjustments may be necessary.
- Goldenseal or berberine may cause increased sun sensitivity, although this is not a commonly reported symptom.
- Berberine may lower blood sugar levels. Caution is advised in patients with diabetes or hypoglycemia and in those taking drugs, herbs, or supplements that affect blood sugar. Serum glucose levels may need to be monitored by a health care provider, and medication adjustments may be necessary.
- The popularity of goldenseal has led to the substitution of other alkaloid-containing herbs, including Chinese goldthread (*Coptis chinensis*) and Oregon grape, which do not contain the same active components and may increase the risk of serious toxicity or adverse events.

Pregnancy and Breastfeeding

- Use of goldenseal or berberine is not recommended during pregnancy or breastfeeding. The chemical hydrastine (found in goldenseal) may induce labor when taken by mouth during pregnancy and could have dangerous effects.

INTERACTIONS
Interactions with Drugs

- Goldenseal or its component berberine could increase the risk of bleeding when taken with drugs that increase the risk of bleeding. Some examples include aspirin, anticoagulants ("blood thinners") such as warfarin (Coumadin) or heparin, antiplatelet drugs such as clopidogrel (Plavix), and nonsteroidal antiinflammatory drugs such as ibuprofen (Motrin, Advil) or naproxen (Naprosyn, Aleve).
- Goldenseal may interfere with the way the body processes certain drugs using the liver's cytochrome P450 enzyme system. As a result, the levels of these drugs may be increased in the blood, and this may cause increased effects or potentially serious adverse reactions. Chemicals in goldenseal may increase the effects of L-phenylephrine and decrease the effects of tetracycline, neostigmine, or yohimbine.
- Berberine may reduce the gastrointestinal absorption of P-glycoprotein–mediated substrates including chemotherapeutic agents such as daunomycin.

G

- Berberine may lower blood sugar levels. Caution is advised when medications that may also lower blood sugar are used. Patients taking drugs for diabetes by mouth or using insulin should be monitored closely by a qualified health care provider. Medication adjustments may be necessary.
- Berberine may lower cholesterol and triglyceride levels, increasing the effects of some drugs like lovastatin (Mevacor).
- Interactions with beta-blockers or 1,3,-bis-(2-chloroethyl)-1-nitrosourea (BCNU) may occur.

Interactions with Herbs and Dietary Supplements

- Goldenseal or its component berberine could increase the risk of bleeding when taken with herbs or supplements that are believed to increase the risk of bleeding. Multiple cases of bleeding have been reported with the use of *Ginkgo biloba*, and fewer cases have been reported with garlic and saw palmetto. Numerous other agents may theoretically increase the risk of bleeding, although this has not been proven in most cases.

- Goldenseal may interfere with the way the body processes certain herbs and supplements using a liver enzyme called cytochrome P450. As a result, the levels of other herbs or supplements may become too high in the blood. It may also alter the effects that other herbs or supplements possibly have on the P450 system, such as bloodroot, cat's claw, or chamomile. The goldenseal component berberine may reduce the effectiveness of yohimbine, which is found in small amounts in yohimbe bark extract.
- Berberine may lower blood sugar levels. Caution is advised when herbs or supplements that may also lower blood sugar are used. Blood glucose levels may require monitoring, and doses may need adjustment.
- Berberine may lower cholesterol and triglyceride levels, increasing the effects of some herbs and supplements like red yeast rice and guggul.

For a complete list of references, please visit www.naturalstandard.com.

Gotu Kola
(Centella asiatica)

RELATED TERMS

- Antanan gede, asiaticoside, Asiatic pennywort, asiatischer wassernabel, bevilacqua, Blastoestimulina, brahmi, brahmi-buti, brahmi manduc(a) parni, calingan rambat, Centasium, Centalase, Centellase, *Centella coriacea, Centella asiatica* triterpenic fraction (CATTF), coda-gam, Emdecassol, Fo-Ti-Teng, gagan-gagan, gang-gagan, HU300, hydrocotyle, *Hydrocotyle asiatica*, hydrocotyle asiatique, idrocotyle, Indian pennywort, Indian water navelwort, indischer wassernabel, kaki kuda, kaki kuta, kerok batok, kos tekosan, lui gong gen, Madecassol, marsh penny, pagaga, panegowan, papaiduh, pegagan, pepiduh, piduh, puhe beta, rending, sheep rot, talepetrako, tete kadho, tete karo, thankuni, thick-leaved pennywort, titrated extract from *Centella asiatica* (TECA), total triterpenic fraction of *Centella asiatica* (TTFCA), Trofolastin, tsubo-kusa, tungchian, tungke-tunfke, water pennyrot, white rot.

BACKGROUND

- Gotu kola is from the perennial creeping plant, *Centella asiatica* (formerly known as *Hydrocotyle asiatica*), which is a member of the parsley family. It is native to India, Madagascar, Sri Lanka, Africa, Australia, China, and Indonesia.
- Gotu kola has a long history of use, dating back to ancient Chinese and Ayurvedic medicine. Gotu kola is mentioned in the *Shennong Herbal*, compiled in China roughly 2000 years ago, and has been widely used medicinally since 1700 AD. It has been used to treat leprosy in Mauritius since 1852; to treat wounds and gonorrhea in the Philippines; and to treat fever and respiratory infections in China.
- The most popular use of gotu kola in the United States is the treatment for varicose veins or cellulitis. Preliminary evidence suggests short-term efficacy (6-12 months) of the total triterpenic fraction of *Centella asiatica* (TTFCA) in the treatment of "chronic venous insufficiency" (a syndrome characterized by lower extremity swelling, varicosities, pain, itching, atrophic skin changes, and ulcerations, possibly due to venous valvular incompetence or a post-thrombotic syndrome).
- Although quality human evidence on the efficacy of gotu kola is still lacking, gotu kola can now be found worldwide as a component of skin creams, lotions, hair conditioners, shampoos, tablets, drops, ointments, powders, and injections. Gotu kola is not related to the kola nut (*Cola nitida, Cola acuminata*). Gotu kola is not a stimulant and does not contain caffeine.

EVIDENCE

Uses Based on Scientific Evidence	Grade
Chronic Venous Insufficiency/Varicose Veins *Chronic venous insufficiency* (CVI) is a term more commonly used in Europe than in the United States. It describes a syndrome characterized by lower extremity swelling, varicosities, pain, itching, atrophic skin changes, and ulcerations. Multiple small trials	B

suggest that the total triterpenoid fraction of *Centella asiatica* (TTFCA) (from gotu kola) may have small to moderate benefits on objective and subjective parameters associated with chronic venous insufficiency. However, the available evidence is not definitive.

Anxiety In Ayurvedic (traditional Indian) medicine, gotu kola is said to develop the crown chakra, the energy center at the top of the head, and to balance the right and left hemispheres of the brain. Preliminary evidence has demonstrated anxiolytic properties of gotu kola, although this activity may or may not apply to humans. Although preliminary findings are promising, the available evidence is not definitive.	C
Cognitive Function Study results on gotu kola and liver disease are mixed.	C
Diabetic Microangiopathy Preliminary studies have suggested beneficial effects of the total triterpenoid fraction of *Centella asiatica* (TTFCA) on subjective and objective parameters of venous insufficiency of the lower extremities. However, the available evidence is not definitive.	C
Liver Cirrhosis Study results on gotu kola and liver disease are mixed.	C
Wound Healing Preliminary study has demonstrated the ability of *Centella asiatica* extracts to promote wound healing, possibly through the stimulation of collagen synthesis. However, the available evidence is not definitive.	C

Uses Based on Tradition or Theory

Abscesses, airline flight–induced lower extremity edema, Alzheimer's disease, amenorrhea, anemia, antidepressant, antifertility agent, antiinfective, antioxidant, antivenom, aphrodisiac, asthma, bladder lesions, blood purifier, bronchitis, bruises, burns, cancer, cellulitis, cerebrovascular disease, cholera, colds, corneal abrasion, dehydration, diarrhea, diuretic, dysentery, eczema, elephantiasis, energy, epilepsy, eye diseases, fatigue, fever, fungal infections, gastric ulcers, gastric ulcer prophylaxis, gastritis, gonorrhea, hair growth promoter, hemorrhoids, hepatic disorders, hepatitis, herpes simplex virus-2, high blood pressure, hot flashes, immunomodulator, inflammation, influenza, jaundice, keloid formation prevention, leprosy, leukoderma, libido, longevity, malaria, memory enhancement, menstrual disorders, mental disorders, mood disorders, neuroprotection, pain, periodontal disease, peripheral vasodilator, physical exhaustion, psoriasis, radiation-induced

(Continued)

Uses Based on Tradition or Theory—Cont'd

behavioral changes, respiratory infections, restless leg syndrome, rheumatism, scabies, scar healing, scleroderma, shigellosis, shingles (postherpetic neuralgia), skin diseases, skin graft donor wounds, snakebites, striae gravidarum (stretch marks), sunstroke, syphilis, systemic lupus erythematosus, tonsillitis, tuberculosis, urinary retention, urinary tract infection, vaginal discharge, vascular fragility, venous disorders.

DOSING

Adults (18 Years and Older)

- There is no proven effective dose for gotu kola in adults. For chronic venous insufficiency, varicose veins, or venous hypertension, various dosing regimens have been studied, including 60-120 mg daily Centellase (TTFCA); 30 mg twice daily Centellase; 30 mg three times daily TTFCA; 60 mg twice daily TTFCA; 60 mg TTFCA three times daily. Preliminary studies suggest a dose-dependent response, and results were better with 60 mg three times daily TTFCA. TECA has also been studied at a dose of 60-120 mg daily. For diabetic microangiopathy, 60 mg twice daily of TTFCA has been studied. Combination products such as Cogno-Blend have been studied for liver cirrhosis and cognitive enhancement.

Children (Younger than 18 Years)

- There is insufficient evidence to recommend a dose for gotu kola in children.

SAFETY

Allergies

- Avoid in individuals with a known allergy or hypersensitivity to gotu kola or any of its constituents, including asiaticoside, asiatic acid, or madecassic acid. There are numerous reports of allergic contact dermatitis after topical gotu kola use. Allergic contact dermatitis has been reported after the use of topical Blastoestimulina cream, containing *Centella asiatica* extract and after the application of topical Madecassol ointment.

Side Effects and Warnings

- Studies suggest that gotu kola has few side effects when taken by mouth. Reported symptoms include stomach upset and nausea. In animal research, large doses of gotu kola cause drowsiness, increase cholesterol levels, and raise blood sugar levels. Individuals with diabetes or high cholesterol levels should avoid gotu kola. Use caution if driving or operating heavy machinery while taking gotu kola as it may cause drowsiness. Asiaticoside, an ingredient of gotu kola, may have weak cancer-causing effects when applied to the skin. There is also a report of night eating syndrome associated with gotu kola.
- Gotu kola is not related to the kola nut (*Cola nitida, Cola acuminata*). Gotu kola is not a stimulant and does not contain caffeine.

Pregnancy and Breastfeeding

- In animal studies, gotu kola reduces the ability of a female to become pregnant, but it is not known whether this effect occurs in humans. Gotu kola is not recommended during pregnancy or breastfeeding because there is little safety and efficacy information available.

INTERACTIONS

Interactions with Drugs

- In theory, gotu kola may increase the amount of drowsiness caused by sedating drugs. Examples include benzodiazepines such as lorazepam (Ativan), barbiturates such as phenobarbital, narcotics such as codeine, and alcohol. Use caution while driving or operating heavy machinery.
- In animals, gotu kola can raise blood sugar levels. Patients taking medications for diabetes or using insulin should be monitored closely by a qualified health care professional while using gotu kola. Dosing adjustments may be necessary.
- In theory, gotu kola may increase cholesterol levels and may work against the activity of cholesterol-lowering drugs.
- Although not well studied in humans, gotu kola may also interact with drugs taken for Alzheimer's disease, anxiety, or cancer. Gotu kola may have antiinflammatory, antibacterial, or antiviral effects. Use caution when taking gotu kola with other medications that have similar effects. Gotu kola may also interact with drugs that relax and dilate the blood vessels, which allows increased blood flow (vasodilators).
- Gotu kola may also interact with the way other drugs are broken down by the liver. It may also cause liver damage. Consult a qualified health care professional, including a pharmacist, to check for interactions.
- Gotu kola may have a positive interaction when taken with diuretics (water pills) or hormones.

Interactions with Herbs and Dietary Supplements

- In theory, gotu kola may increase the amount of drowsiness caused by some herbs or supplements. Use caution while driving or operating heavy machinery.
- Although not well studied in humans, gotu kola may raise blood sugar levels and may therefore counteract the effects of products that lower blood sugar levels. Use caution when taking herbs or supplements that may also lower blood sugar levels. Blood glucose levels may require monitoring, and doses may need adjustment.
- Studies in animals suggest that gotu kola may increase cholesterol levels. It may therefore interfere with the effectiveness of lipid-lowering agents such as fish oil, garlic, or niacin.
- Although not well studied in humans, gotu kola may also interact with drugs taken for Alzheimer's disease, anxiety, or cancer. Gotu kola may have antiinflammatory, antibacterial, antioxidant, or antiviral effects. Use caution when taking gotu kola with other herbs or supplements that have similar effects. Gotu kola may also interact with herbs or supplements that relax and dilate the blood vessels, which allows increased blood flow (vasodilators).
- Gotu kola may also interact with the way other herbs or supplements are broken down by the liver. It may also increase the risk of liver damage when used with other liver-damaging herbs or supplements. Consult a qualified health care professional, including a pharmacist, to check for interactions.
- Although not well studied in humans, gotu kola may have a positive interaction when taken with diuretics (water pills). It may also have a positive interaction with herbs and supplements with hormonal effects.

- Gotu kola may have additive affects when taken concomitantly with herbs that stimulate the immune system, such as astragalus, ginger, goldenseal, or propolis. Gotu kola may have additive effects when taken with herbs and supplements that increase blood flow, such as aconite, black cohosh, fenugreek, or garlic.

For a complete list of references, please visit www.naturalstandard.com.

Grape

(*Vitis* spp.)

RELATED TERMS

- ActiVin, bioflavinols, catechin, condensed tannins, drue kerne, Endotelon, enocianina, epicatechin, extrait de pepins de raisin, gallic acid, grape complex, grape seed oil, grape skin extract, grapeseed, grapeseed extract (GSE), grapeseed oil, IH636 grape seed proanthocyanidin, Indena's Grape Seed Standardized Extract, leucoanthocyanidins, Leucoselect-phytosome, Masquelier's Original OPCs, muscat, nonhydrolyzable tannins, oligomeres procyanidoliques, pine bark extract, procyanidolic oligomers (PCOs), polyphenolic oligomers, pycnogenol, Pycnogenol, tannins, Vitaceae (family), *Vitis coignetiae, Vitis vinifera* L.
- **Note:** Pycnogenol is a patented nutrient supplement extracted from the bark of European coastal pine *Pinus maritima*. Pycnogenol consists of flavonoids, catechins, procyanidins, and phenolic acids, which are the same things found in grape seed, but not the same supplement. See the monograph on Pycnogenol for more information.

BACKGROUND

- Grape leaves, sap, and fruit have been used medicinally since the time of the Greek empire. Preparations from different parts of the plant have been used historically to treat a variety of conditions, including skin and eye irritation, bleeding, varicose veins, diarrhea, cancer, and smallpox.
- Interest in grape products for heart disease prevention increased with reporting of possible protective effects from wine consumption in French men who also consume a high fat diet (the so-called French paradox). However, well-designed controlled trials of the proposed active component of grape seed extract (GSE), the oligomeric proanthocyanidins (OPCs), are lacking. It is important to note that GSE and Pycnogenol are not the same even though they both contain oligomeric proanthocyanidins. Pycnogenol is a patented nutrient supplement extracted from the bark of European coastal pine *Pinus maritima*.
- The antioxidant properties of OPCs have made products containing these extracts candidate therapies for a wide range of human disease. Randomized controlled trials have documented the effectiveness of OPCs from grape seed in relieving symptoms of chronic venous insufficiency, injury-related extremity edema, diabetic retinopathy, arteriosclerosis, and high blood pressure. Grape seed extract has been used by natural practitioners in Europe to treat venous insufficiency, promote wound healing, alleviate inflammatory conditions, and as a "cardioprotective" therapy.
- OPCs appear to be well tolerated with few side effects noted in the available literature. However, long-term studies assessing safety are lacking.

EVIDENCE

Uses Based on Scientific Evidence	Grade
Chronic Venous Insufficiency Human studies report that extract from grape seed can reduce the symptoms of poor circulation in leg veins.	A
Symptoms that showed significant improvements include itching, swelling, heaviness, nighttime cramps, tingling, burning, numbness, and nerve pain.	
Edema (Swelling) Several small human studies show that grape seed ingredients may speed the reduction of swelling after many types of injury, including surgery.	A
Diabetic Retinopathy Diabetic retinopathy is a disease of the small blood vessels in the retina of the eye. Preliminary study using OPCs and the brand name product Endotelon has shown beneficial effects in stopping the disease progression.	B
Vascular Fragility Small human studies suggest that ingredients from grape seed may make small blood vessels less fragile and less likely to leak.	B
Agitation in Dementia Grape seed oil is a popular (nonscented) carrier oil used in aromatherapy. Although grape seed has been compared with lavender oil and thyme oil to reduce agitation in patients with dementia, there is not enough scientific evidence of effectiveness.	C
Antioxidant Studies have found grape seed to be an antioxidant, which may help prevent or relieve symptoms of certain conditions, such as vision problems associated with diabetes and wound healing. The safety of long-term use of grape seed is unknown.	C
Cancer There is little information available on the use of grape seed extract in the treatment of human cancer (prostate, skin, breast, and others).	C
High cholesterol Historical statistics suggest that wine may reduce the risk of heart disease. Animal studies suggest that grape seed may decrease cholesterol deposits in blood vessels and may reduce the amount of injury to heart muscle during a "heart attack."	C
Inhibition of Platelet Aggregation Preliminary human and animal studies show that extracts of grape seed can block the ability of platelets to form a clot (resulting in "thinner" blood). This effect seems to be more prominent in smokers.	C
Melasma (Chloasma) Chloasma (melasma) is a skin discoloration that may occur due to hormonal imbalances. Antioxidants are thought to improve chloasma, and grape seed extract	C

Uses Based on Scientific Evidence	Grade
is thought to have antioxidant activity. However, clinical evidence is insufficient.	
Pancreatitis A small human study suggests that grape seed may reduce abdominal pain in chronic pancreatitis. Animal studies suggest that some grape seed ingredients may protect the liver from injury. Definitive clinical evidence is lacking.	C
Premenstrual Syndrome Little information is available for the use of grape seed extract in the treatment of premenstrual symptoms. Preliminary study shows positive results, but further research is necessary before a recommendation can be made.	C
Radiation (UV) Protection (Skin) Some grape seed ingredients may protect the skin from the harmful effects of UV radiation by acting as antioxidants. One human study reports a small benefit from grape seed in reducing redness after exposure to UV light. Grape seed may also promote hair growth. Strong clinical evidence is lacking.	C
Skin Aging (Postmenopausal Women) Epicatechin is an antioxidant component of grape seed extract that has become increasingly popular in skin products. Combination products that include grape seed extract have shown promising effects. The isolated effects of grape seed are unclear.	C
Vision Problems Several small studies suggest that grape seed may slow the progression of retinopathy (damage to the retina caused by diabetes or high blood pressure). Visual performance may also be improved in healthy patients. Stronger evidence is needed.	C
Allergic Rhinitis Grape seed has been used to treat immune system disorders because of its antioxidant effects. However, a well-designed human study of allergic rhinitis sufferers showed no improvement in allergy symptoms with administration of grape seed extract ingredients.	D
Radioprotection Grape seed extract has been studied for its radioprotective effects in breast cancer patients with tissue hardening after radiotherapy. Overall, the results show a lack of benefit.	D

Uses Based on Tradition or Theory

Alzheimer's disease, antiaging, antimicrobial, antiviral, arteriosclerosis, arthritis, ascites (Ehrlich ascites carcinoma), asthma, astringent, atherosclerosis, attention deficit hyperactivity disorder (ADHD), bleeding, blood vessel dilation (telangiectasia), body fat reducer (cellulite), bruising, cachexia, chemoprotectant, cholera, chronic fatigue syndrome, circulatory disorders, connective tissue disorders, constipation, corneal abrasion, cough, cramps (menstrual), dental caries, detoxification, diabetes, diabetic neuropathy, diarrhea, diuresis, dysmenorrhea (painful menstrual bleeding), gastrointestinal disorders, glaucoma, hemorrhoids, human immunodeficiency virus/acquired immunodeficiency syndrome (HIV/AIDS), immunostimulant, inflammation, liver cirrhosis, liver protection, lymphedema (acrocyanosis), macular degeneration, nausea, nephrotoxicity, pain (acroparesthesia), Parkinson's disease, photoprotection, psoriasis, respiratory tract infections, retinopathy, scurvy, shock, skin care, skin diseases, skin irritation, smallpox, sore throat, tonic, ulcers (gastroduodenal), urinary disorders (increased urination), varicose veins, vascular disorders (prevention in diabetic patients), weight loss (maintenance), wound healing.

DOSING

Adults (18 Years and Older)

- Grape seed is commercially available as grape seed extract, which is typically standardized to its proanthocyanidin content. OPCs found in grape seed (as well as pine bark extract) are also available. Two popularly studied products are Acti-Vin and Endotelon. Grape seed extract is also sold as tinctures, capsules, and as an ingredient in topical creams.
- There is strong scientific evidence that Endotelon (procyanidolic oligomers, which are found in grape seed) taken in a dose of 150-300 mg/day for 28-30 days is an effective dosing range for poor circulation in leg veins. Other doses have been studied but show unclear effectiveness. For instance, 150-400 mg Endotelon for up to 2 months for conditions such as postoperative swelling, diabetic retinopathy, vascular fragility, and other vision problems has been studied. For diabetic retinopathy, 100-200 mg of OPCs has been taken for up to 1 year. Grape seed extract, standardized to its proanthocyanidin content, in a dose of 100-400 mg has also been taken three times a day for up to 6 months for radioprotection. ActiVin 200-300 mg/day has also been studied for chronic pancreatitis.

Children (Younger than 18 Years)

- There is insufficient evidence to recommend a dose of grape seed or OPCs in children.

SAFETY

Allergies

- There are reports of people with allergy to grapes or other grape compounds, including anaphylaxis. Individuals allergic to grapes should not take grape seed and related products.

Side Effects and Warnings

- Natural medicine practitioners generally regard OPCs as safe. Reported side effects include scalp dryness or itching, hives, headache, high blood pressure, nausea, indigestion, or dizziness. There are mixed reports as to whether compounds found in grape seed can damage the liver, but grape seed extract as a whole is thought to protect the liver.
- Use cautiously in patients taking anticoagulants such as warfarin, aspirin, nonsteroidal antiinflammatory drugs (NSAIDs), or antiplatelet agents, as OPCs may alter platelet function and the ability to form clots. Based on animal studies, grape seed may increase the risk of bleeding. Caution is advised in patients with bleeding disorders or taking

G

drugs that may increase the risk of bleeding. Dosing adjustments may be necessary. Avoid in people with disorders that increase their risk of bleeding or who have active bleeding disorders (e.g., stomach ulcers or bleeding into the brain). Stop all use of grape seed extract at least 2 weeks before surgery or dental procedures.

- Grape seed may interfere with the way the body processes certain drugs using the liver's cytochrome P450 enzyme system. Therefore, the levels of these drugs may be altered in the blood and may cause potentially serious effects. If using any medications, check the package insert and speak with a qualified health care provider and pharmacist about possible interactions.
- Caution is also advised in patients with blood pressure disorders or those taking angiotensin-converting enzyme (ACE) inhibitors.

Pregnancy and Breastfeeding

- The use of grape seed during pregnancy or breastfeeding is not recommended because of lack of safety information.

INTERACTIONS
Interactions with Drugs

- In theory, grape seed extract or OPCs may increase the risk of bleeding when taken with drugs that increase the risk of bleeding. Some examples include aspirin, anticoagulants ("blood thinners") such as warfarin (Coumadin) or heparin, antiplatelet drugs such as clopidogrel (Plavix), and nonsteroidal antiinflammatory drugs such as ibuprofen (Motrin, Advil) or naproxen (Naprosyn, Aleve). However, reports of human cases are lacking. OPCs may theoretically alter the effectiveness of prescribed blood pressure medications that are ACE inhibitors like captopril (Capoten).
- OPCs may interact with medications such as methotrexate and allopurinol leading to severe side effects in people taking these medications. OPCs may interfere with the way the body processes certain drugs using the liver's cytochrome P450 enzyme system. As a result, the levels of these drugs may be increased or decreased in the blood and may change the intended effects.
- Grape seed may lower cholesterol levels and may have additive effects with other cholesterol-lowering medications such as 3-hydroxy-3-methylglutaryl coenzyme A (HMG-CoA) reductase inhibitors (statins) like lovastatin (Mevacor).
- OPCs may also interact with agents used to control nausea and vomiting (antiemetics), agents used for cancer, and folate analogs. A qualified health care professional, including a pharmacist, should be consulted to check for interactions.

Interactions with Herbs and Dietary Supplements

- In theory, grape seed or OPCs may increase the risk of bleeding when taken with herbs and supplements that are believed to increase the risk of bleeding. Multiple cases of bleeding have been reported with the use of *Ginkgo biloba*, fewer cases have been reported with garlic, and some have been reported with saw palmetto. Numerous other agents may theoretically increase the risk of bleeding, although this has not been proven in most cases.
- OPCs may interfere with the way the body processes certain herbs or supplements using the liver's cytochrome P450 enzyme system. As a result, the levels of other herbs or supplements in the blood may be too high or too low. OPCs may also alter the effects that other herbs or supplements possibly have on the P450 system.
- One study reports that Leucoselect-phytosome (an OPC preparation) has no effect on vitamin C levels, although unofficial reports suggest that some ingredients from grape seed may enhance the absorption and effectiveness of vitamins C and E.
- Grape seed may lower cholesterol levels and may have additive effects with other cholesterol-lowering herbs or supplements such as niacin and red yeast rice.
- OPCs may also interact with herbs or supplements used to control nausea and vomiting (antiemetics) or for cancer. OPCs may also have additive effects with antioxidants or alter folate metabolism. Taking grape seed and the probiotic *Lactobacillus acidophilus* may prevent colonization of the gastrointestinal tract. Also use caution when taking grape seed or OPCs with herbs that affect the heart or blood pressure; interactions are possible. A qualified health care professional, including a pharmacist, should be consulted to check for interactions.

For a complete list of references, please visit www.naturalstandard.com.

Grapefruit
(*Citrus x paradisi*)

RELATED TERMS

- Antioxidizers, bergamottin, bergapten, bergaptol, blond grapefruits, citricidal, *Citrus decumana*, *Citrus maxima*, *Citrus paradisi*, *Citrus paradisi* Macf., *Citrus x paradisi* Macfad., *Citrus x paradisi*, citrus seed, citrus seed extract, flavonoids, Fresca, furanocoumarins, geranylcoumarin, grapefruit juice, grapefruit pectin, grapefruit seed, grapefruit seed extract, naringenin, naringin, nootkatone, organic grapefruit juice, paradiesapfel, ParaMicrocidin, pomelo, pummelo grapefruit, red grapefruit, Red Mexican grapefruit, Rio Red Grapefruit, Rutaceae (family), sesquiterpen, shaddock oil, Sun Drop, toronja, vitamin C, white grapefruit.

BACKGROUND

- The grapefruit was first described in the 1750s as the "forbidden fruit" of Barbados. It was introduced to Florida in the 1820s. Most grapefruit in the United States is still grown in Florida. Grapefruit juice has been used in folk medicine for the treatment of diabetes as well as to strengthen the immune system. Grapefruit is also added to cosmetics and hair care products as a fragrance.
- Grapefruit has been suggested as a treatment for several conditions, but there is currently insufficient scientific evidence to support the use of grapefruit for any medical disorder. The use of supplemental grapefruit pectin in the prevention of cardiovascular disease and the use of grapefruit seed extract in atopic eczema warrants further scientific investigation before a strong recommendation can be made. There is conflicting research regarding the use of grapefruit for kidney stones.
- Grapefruit juice alters the way some drugs are broken down in the liver. Grapefruit may increase the effects of calcium channel blockers, benzodiazepines, immunosuppressants, and 3-hydroxy-3-methylglutaryl coenzyme A (HMG-CoA) reductase inhibitors.

EVIDENCE

Uses Based on Scientific Evidence	Grade
Atopic Eczema There is preliminary but inconclusive evidence to support the use of grapefruit seed extract for treating atopic eczema.	C
Endocrine Disorders (Metabolic Syndrome) Preliminary studies suggest grapefruit may have some benefit in the management of metabolic syndrome.	C
Heart Disease Grapefruit pectin supplementation may inhibit high cholesterol levels. There is promising but inconclusive human evidence to support the use of grapefruit pectin in the prevention of heart disease.	C
Kidney Stones There is limited and mixed research regarding the use of grapefruit for kidney stones.	C

Uses Based on Tradition or Theory

Alzheimer's disease, antibacterial, antifungal, antioxidant, antiparasitic, antiseptic, antiviral, cancer, common cold, cosmetic uses, Crohn's disease, diabetes, diarrhea, eye diseases, immune function, insecticidal, liver disease, Parkinson's disease, preservative, stomach ulcers, tonic, weight loss.

DOSING

Adults (18 Years and Older)

- There is insufficient evidence to recommend a dose for grapefruit. Grapefruit is typically taken as a fruit, seed extract, or pectin by mouth. It has also been applied on the skin as a disinfectant for skin wounds. For atopic eczema, 150 mg of grapefruit seed extract has been taken by mouth three times daily for 1 month. For heart disease, 15 g of grapefruit pectin in divided doses with meals for 16 weeks has been taken. For metabolic syndrome, studies have used grapefruit capsules, fresh grapefruit, or 8 oz of grapefruit juice three times daily before each meal for 12 weeks.

Children (Younger than 18 Years)

- There is insufficient evidence to recommend a dose for grapefruit in children. Grapefruit is likely safe when used in amounts commonly found in foods by individuals not receiving concurrent drug therapy.

SAFETY

Allergies

- Avoid in individuals with a known allergy or hypersensitivity to grapefruit.

Side Effects and Warnings

- Grapefruit appears to be well-tolerated. Grapefruit is likely safe when used in amounts commonly found in foods by individuals not receiving concurrent drug therapy. Grapefruit has "generally recognized as safe" (GRAS) status in the United States. Adverse effects from grapefruit juice have been reported only rarely and have been limited to those in combination with drug therapy. The severity of the interaction may depend on how much and how often the grapefruit juice is consumed, the timing of the grapefruit juice, the specific brand of juice, and the medication dose.
- Experts report that topically applied grapefruit seed extract can be irritating to the skin.
- High doses may cause pseudohyperaldosteronism (Liddle's syndrome), increases in potassium clearance, mineralocorticoid excess, lowered or elevated hematocrit values, the

development of kidney stones, or increases in enamel loss and tooth surface loss.

- Use cautiously in patients who drink red wine. Red wine in combination with grapefruit juice appears to have an additive inhibitory effect on the way liver breaks down some agents, theoretically increasing the risk for interactions with other drugs.
- Use cautiously in patients who drink tonic water or smoke.
- Use cautiously in patients with liver cirrhosis, at risk of kidney stones, or who have undergone gastric bypass surgery.

Pregnancy and Breastfeeding

- Grapefruit is not recommended in pregnant or breastfeeding women because of a lack of available scientific evidence.

INTERACTIONS

Interactions with Drugs

- Grapefruit juice may interfere with the way the body breaks down certain drugs in the liver. As a result, the levels of some drugs may be increased in the blood and may cause increased effects or potentially serious adverse reactions. Patients using medications such as amitriptyline, clomipramine, clozapine, cyclobenzaprine, haloperidol, naproxen, ondansetron, propranolol, theophylline, and verapamil should check the package insert and speak with a qualified health care professional, including a pharmacist, about possible interactions.
- Grapefruit juice may also interact with nonsteroidal antiinflammatory drugs (NSAIDs) (e.g., diclofenac, ibuprofen, meloxicam, piroxicam), oral antidiabetic agents (tolbutamide, glipizide), and angiotensin II blockers (e.g., losartan).
- Caution is advised when grapefruit juice is mixed with proton pump inhibitors (e.g., lansoprazole, omeprazole, pantoprazole), antiepileptics (e.g., diazepam, phenytoin), carisoprodol, citalopram, and nelfinavir.
- Grapefruit juice may increase drug levels and the risk of adverse effects when taken with macrolide antibiotics (e.g., erythromycin, clarithromycin), antiarrhythmics (e.g., quinidine), benzodiazepines (e.g., alprazolam, midazolam, diazepam, triazolam), immune modulators (e.g., cyclosporine, tacrolimus), protease inhibitors (e.g., ritonavir, saquinavir), prokinetic agents (e.g., cisapride), antihistamines (e.g., terfenadine), calcium channel blockers (e.g., amlodipine, felodipine, diltiazem), HMG-CoA reductase inhibitors (e.g., atorvastatin, lovastatin), alfuzosin, and others.
- Although not well studied in humans, numerous other potential interactions with grapefruit juice may occur with acebutolol, alfentanil, alprazolam, amlodipine, amprenavir, anthelmintics (e.g., praziquantel), antiarrhythmics (e.g., amiodarone, propafenone, quinidine), anticonvulsants (e.g., carbamazepine), antifungal agents (e.g., itraconazole), antimalarial agents (e.g., halofantrine, artemether, quinine), antineoplastic agents, aripiprazole, atorvastatin, beta-blocking agents, benzodiazepines, budesonide, buspirone, celiprolol, digoxin, eplerenone, etoposide, felodipine, fentanyl, hormone replacement, imatinib, indinavir, lovastatin, levothyroxine, oral contraceptives (e.g., estradiol, progesterone), methylprednisolone, mifepristone, nifedipine, nimodipine, nitrendipine, opioids, pranidipine, ranolazine, scopolamine, selective serotonin reuptake inhibitors (e.g., sertraline), simvastatin, sufentanil, sunitinib, talinolol, tolterodine, trazodone, triazolam, and zolpidem. Check with a qualified health care professional, including a pharmacist, for any interactions.

- Grapefruit may increase the risk of bleeding when taken with drugs that increase the risk of bleeding. Some examples include aspirin, anticoagulants ("blood thinners") such as warfarin (Coumadin) or heparin, antiplatelet drugs such as clopidogrel (Plavix), and nonsteroidal antiinflammatory drugs such as ibuprofen (Motrin, Advil) or naproxen (Naprosyn, Aleve).
- Grapefruit has been shown to modestly increase the absorption of sildenafil, an erectile dysfunction agent. Theoretically, grapefruit may have similar effects if used with other erectile dysfunction agents, such as tadalafil or vardenafil.
- Clinical studies show that the ingestion of grapefruit juice should not cause any pharmacokinetic or pharmacodynamic interactions when coadministered with caffeine.
- Grapefruit may reduce the effectiveness of antihistamines such as fexofenadine.
- Theoretically, grapefruit juice may inhibit the hepatic metabolism of oxybutynin, leading to increased drug levels and associated adverse events.
- Grapefruit juice was found to have no significant effect on the metabolism of prednisone or prednisolone in one study of kidney transplant patients.
- Based on laboratory study, grapefruit may inhibit the absorption of vinblastine or alter the permeation of vincristine across the blood–brain barrier.

Interactions with Herbs and Dietary Supplements

- Theoretically, grapefruit may increase the adverse effects associated with antiarrhythmic, anticonvulsant, antihistamine, immunosuppressant, anticancer, beta-blocking, or estrogen-containing herbs and supplements. Concomitant use of grapefruit and green tea may increase caffeine levels, which may lead to an increased risk of cardiovascular and central nervous system stimulatory effects, along with other caffeine-related adverse effects due to caffeine in green tea. However, currently, this effect has not been reported in humans.
- In theory, grapefruit juice may increase concentrations of digitalis (foxglove) and vitamin C levels, although clinical significance is unknown.
- Theoretically, grapefruit may increase the risk of bleeding when taken with herbs and supplements that are believed to increase the risk of bleeding. Multiple cases of bleeding have been reported with the use of *Ginkgo biloba*, and fewer cases have been reported with garlic and saw palmetto. Numerous other agents may theoretically increase the risk of bleeding, although this has not been proven in most cases.
- Preliminary evidence suggests that grapefruit juice may interfere with the way the body processes certain herbs or supplements using the liver's cytochrome P450 enzyme system. As a result, the levels of other herbs or supplements may become too high in the blood. It may also alter the effects that other herbs or supplements possibly have on the P450 system.
- Grapefruit may interfere with the body's conversion of cortisol to cortisone. If both licorice and grapefruit are taken together, the risk of high blood pressure and other side effects may be increased.
- Grapefruit juice has a weak interaction with theophylline-containing drugs. In theory, grapefruit may interact with xanthine-containing herbs, and caution is advised.

For a complete list of references, please visit www.naturalstandard.com.

Green-lipped mussel
(Perna canaliculus)

RELATED TERMS

- Betain, brevetoxin B analog B4, BTXB4, chondroitin sulfate, eicosatetraenoic acids, freeze-dried mussel powder, glycosaminoglycans, green lipped mussel, Green Lips, green shell mussel, Greenback, Greenshell, Greenshell Mussel, heparin, Lyprinol, marine oils, mollusk, Mytilidae (family), New Zealand green-lipped mussel, okadaic acid, pectenotoxins, *Perna canaliculus,* pernin, shellfish lipid extract, Seatone, sterol esters, yessotoxins.

BACKGROUND

- The green-lipped mussel is native to the New Zealand coast and is a staple in the diet of the indigenous Maori culture. The antiinflammatory effects of green-lipped mussel have been studied since the observation of a lower incidence of arthritis in coastal Maoris compared with European or inland Maori people.
- Products containing green-lipped mussel are used to treat inflammatory conditions such as asthma, osteoarthritis, and rheumatoid arthritis. Evidence of an effect in asthma and osteoarthritis is unclear, while evidence suggests green-lipped mussel is not effective in treating rheumatoid arthritis.

EVIDENCE

Uses Based on Scientific Evidence	Grade
Asthma Limited evidence suggests that green-lipped mussel supplementation may help allergic diseases, such as atopic asthma.	C
Osteoarthritis There is conflicting evidence of the effect of green-lipped mussel supplementation for treating osteoarthritis.	C
Rheumatoid Arthritis There is conflicting evidence of the effect of green-lipped mussel supplementation for treating rheumatoid arthritis. Overall, the evidence does not support this use.	D

Uses Based on Tradition or Theory
Abortion inducing, antihistamine, antiinflammatory, breast cancer, connective tissue disorders, eye disorders (retinal disorders), heart disease, inflammatory bowel disease, inflammatory joint disease (bursitis, ankylosing spondylitis), Lyme disease, menstrual pain, mucositis (inflammation of mucus membranes of the digestive tract), multiple sclerosis, nerve disorders, prostate cancer, psoriasis, skin inflammation (atopic dermatitis), sports injuries, systemic lupus erythematosus (prevention), ulcers (NSAID-induced).

DOSING
Adults (18 Years and Older)

- Two capsules of Lyprinol (containing 50 mg of omega-3 polyunsaturated fatty acids and 100 mg olive oil per capsule) have been used twice daily for 8 weeks for asthma.
- For the treatment of osteoarthritis, the following doses have been used: 1050 mg green-lipped mussel extract (three capsules) daily for 3-6 months; six capsules Seatone daily for 6 months; 210 mg Lyprinol (or 1150 mg green-lipped mussel powder) daily for 3-6 months; four capsules Lyprinol daily for 2 months followed by 4 months of two capsules daily.
- For the treatment of rheumatoid arthritis, the following doses have been used: 210 mg Lyprinol daily for 3-6 months; Sanhelios Mussel Lyprinol Lipid Complex (containing Lyprinol and omega-3 fatty acids) for 12 weeks.

Children (Younger than 18 Years)

- There is insufficient evidence to recommend a dose for green-lipped mussel in children.

SAFETY
Allergies

- Avoid in individuals with allergy or sensitivity to green-lipped mussel or other shellfish. Allergy symptoms may include rash (itching and hives), swelling of the face or hands, swelling or tingling in the mouth or throat, chest tightness, and difficulty breathing.

Side Effects and Warnings

- Green-lipped mussel is generally considered safe. Adverse effects that have been associated with green-lipped mussel include metallic taste, nausea, stomach upset, intestinal gas, skin rash, fluid retention, gout, lung dysfunction, respiratory symptoms, heart failure, abnormal liver function, toxic hepatitis, neurotoxic shellfish poisoning, and temporary worsening of rheumatoid arthritis symptoms.
- Use with caution in patients taking antiinflammatory drugs, herbs, or supplements, as green-lipped mussel may enhance both the effects and the side effects of these agents.
- Use with caution in patients with asthma because of the risk of lung dysfunction and other respiratory symptoms. Avoid in patients with liver disease because of potential toxic hepatitis associated with green-lipped mussel.

Pregnancy and Breastfeeding

- Green-lipped mussel is not recommended in pregnant or breastfeeding women because of a lack of available scientific evidence.

INTERACTIONS
Interactions with Drugs

- Green-lipped mussel may add to the effects of antiasthma agents, leukotriene receptor antagonists, agents that affect the immune system, uterotrophic agents, and antihistamines.

In addition, green-lipped mussel may interact with corticosteroids, particularly pentoxifylline (Pentoxil). Green-lipped mussel may add to the effects and side effects of antiinflammatory agents.

Interactions with Herbs and Dietary Supplements
- Green-lipped mussel may add to the effects of antiasthma herbs and supplements, leukotriene receptor antagonists, herbs and supplements that affect the immune system, antihistamines, and uterotrophic herbs and supplements. In addition, green-lipped mussel may interact with omega-3 fatty acids. Green-lipped mussel may add to the effects and side effects of antiinflammatory herbs and supplements.

For a complete list of references, please visit www.naturalstandard.com.

Green tea
(Camellia sinensis)

RELATED TERMS

- AR25, Camellia, *Camellia assamica*, *Camellia sinensis*, *Camellia sinensis* (L.) Kuntze, Camellia tea, catechins, Chinese tea, epigallocatechin gallate (EGCG), epigallocatechin-3-gallate, Exolise, flavonol, green tea extract (GTE), Matsu-cha Tea, polyphenols, Polyphenon E, *Thea bohea*, *Thea sinensis*, *Thea viridis*, Theanine, Theifers, Veregen T.

BACKGROUND

- Green tea is made from the dried leaves of *Camellia sinensis*, a perennial evergreen shrub. Green tea has a long history of use, dating back to China approximately 5000 years ago. Green tea, black tea, and oolong tea are all derived from the same plant.
- Tea varieties reflect the growing region (e.g., Ceylon or Assam), the district (e.g., Darjeeling), the form (e.g., pekoe is cut, gunpowder is rolled), and the processing method (e.g., black, green, or oolong). India and Sri Lanka are the major producers of green tea.
- Historically, tea has been served as a part of various ceremonies and has been used to stay alert during long meditations. A legend in India describes the story of Prince Siddhartha Gautama, the founder of Buddhism, who tore off his eyelids in frustration at his inability to stay awake during meditation while journeying through China. A tea plant is said to have sprouted from the spot where his eyelids fell, providing him with the ability to stay awake, meditate, and reach enlightenment. Turkish traders reportedly introduced tea to Western cultures in the sixth century.

EVIDENCE

Uses Based on Scientific Evidence	Grade
Genital Warts Polyphenon E, a proprietary extract of green tea, has been approved in the United States for external topical use as a prescription for genital warts caused by human papilloma virus.	B
Anxiety L-theanine is a predominant amino acid found in green tea. Preliminary research exists on the effects of this amino acid in comparison with the prescription drug alprazolam on experimentally induced anxiety. No benefit was found.	C
Arthritis Research indicates that green tea may benefit arthritis by reducing inflammation and slowing cartilage breakdown. Further studies are required before a recommendation can be made.	C
Asthma Research has shown caffeine to cause improvements in airflow to the lungs (bronchodilation). However, it is not clear whether caffeine or tea use has significant benefits	C

in people with asthma. Better research is needed in this area before a strong conclusion can be drawn.

	Grade
Cancer (General) Overall, the relationship of green tea consumption and human cancer remains inconclusive. One clinical trial showed minimal benefit using green tea extract capsules for the treatment of hormone refractory prostate cancer. Further research is needed before a recommendation can be made.	C
Cardiovascular Conditions There is early suggestive evidence that regular intake of green tea may reduce the risk of heart attack or atherosclerosis (clogged arteries). Further well-designed clinical trials are needed before a firm recommendation can be made in this area.	C
Common Cold Prevention In humans, preliminary data suggest that a specific formulation of green tea may help prevent cold and flu symptoms. Further well-designed clinical trials are needed to confirm these results.	C
Dental Cavity Prevention There is limited study of tea as a gargle (mouthwash) for the prevention of dental cavities (caries). It is not clear whether this is a beneficial therapy.	C
Diabetes More studies are required to determine whether green tea and polyphenols have any therapeutic benefit for diabetes prevention or treatment.	C
Fertility Early research using a combination product called FertilityBlend has been associated with some success in helping women to conceive. Further well-designed research on green tea alone for this use is needed before a strong conclusion can be drawn.	C
High cholesterol Laboratory studies, animal studies, and limited human research suggest possible effects of green tea on cholesterol levels. Better human evidence is necessary in this area.	C
Hypertension Green tea has been shown to increase or have no effect on blood pressure in several studies in humans.	C
Hypertriglyceridemia Laboratory, animal, and limited human research suggest possible effects of green tea on triglyceride levels. Better human evidence is necessary in this area.	C

(Continued)

Uses Based on Scientific Evidence	Grade
Menopausal Symptoms A study conducted in healthy postmenopausal women showed that a morning/evening menopausal formula containing green tea was effective in relieving menopausal symptoms including hot flashes and sleep disturbance. However, evidence thus far has not been definitive.	C
Mental Performance/Alertness Several preliminary studies have examined the effects of caffeine, tea, or coffee use on short and long-term memory and cognition. It remains unclear whether tea is beneficial for this use. Limited, low-quality research reports that the use of green tea may improve cognition and sense of alertness. Green tea contains caffeine, which is a stimulant.	C
Photoprotection There is limited animal and human study of green tea as a protective agent of skin from ultraviolet light injury. Some study results conflict. Comparisons have not been made with well-established forms of sun protection such as ultraviolet-protective sunscreen. The effects of green tea on skin damage caused by the sun remain unclear.	C
Viral Infection (Human T-Cell Lymphocytic Virus [HTLV]) Preliminary research suggests that green tea decreases viral load in carriers of the HTLV-1 virus. Additional well-designed controlled research is needed before a recommendation can be made for or against green tea in the treatment of HTLV-1 carriers.	C
Weight Loss (Maintenance) There are several small human studies addressing the use of green tea extract (GTE) capsules for weight loss or weight maintenance in overweight or average weight individuals. Study results are mixed.	C

Uses Based on Tradition or Theory

Adenocarcinoma, antioxidant, astringent, atherosclerosis, autoimmune disorders (encephalomyelitis), bleeding of gums or tooth sockets, bone density improvement, cancer treatment side effects, cataracts, cognitive performance enhancement, coronary heart disease, Crohn's disease, dementia, detoxification from alcohol or toxins, diarrhea, digestion, exercise performance, fibrosarcoma, flatulence, fungal infections, gastritis, gingivitis, gum swelling, hair growth, headache, heart disease, *Helicobacter pylori* infection, human immunodeficiency virus/acquired immunodeficiency syndrome (HIV/AIDS), improving blood flow, improving resistance to disease, improving urine flow, inhibition of platelet aggregation, ischemia-reperfusion injury protection, joint pain, kidney stone prevention, leukoplakia, longevity, lymphocytic leukemia, memory, neuroprotection, osteoporosis, Parkinson's disease (prevention), protection against asbestos lung injury, regulation of body temperature, stimulant, stomach disorders, stroke prevention, tired eyes, vascular tumors, vomiting.

DOSING
Adults (18 Years and Older)

- Benefits of specific doses of green tea are not established. Most studies have examined green tea in the form of a brewed beverage rather than in capsule form. One cup of tea contains approximately 50 mg of caffeine and 80-100 mg of polyphenol content, depending on the strength of the tea and the size of cup.
- Studies have examined the effects of habitually drinking anywhere from 1-10 cups/day (or greater).
- In capsule form, there is considerable variation in the amount of GTE; there may be anywhere from 100-750 mg per capsule. Currently, there is no established recommended dose for GTE capsules.
- In topical form, local treatment with Polyphenon E ointment for genital warts has been used three times daily for up to 16 weeks.

Children (Younger than 18 Years)

- Green tea is not recommended for infants or children because of the caffeine content.

SAFETY
Allergies

- People with a known allergy or hypersensitivity to caffeine or tannin should avoid green tea. Skin rash and hives have been reported with caffeine ingestion.

Side Effects and Warnings

- Studies of the side effects of green tea specifically are limited. However, green tea is a source of caffeine, for which multiple reactions are reported.
- Caffeine is a stimulant of the central nervous system and may cause insomnia in adults, children, and infants (including nursing infants of mothers taking caffeine). Caffeine acts on the kidneys as a diuretic (increases urine and urine sodium/potassium levels and potentially decreases blood sodium/potassium levels) and may worsen incontinence. Caffeine-containing beverages may increase the production of stomach acid and may worsen ulcer symptoms. Tannin in tea can cause constipation. Certain doses of caffeine can increase heart rate and blood pressure, although people who consume caffeine regularly do not seem to experience these effects in the long-term.
- An increase in blood sugar levels may occur. Caffeine-containing beverages such as green tea should be used cautiously in patients with diabetes. In contrast, lowering of blood sugar levels from drinking green tea has also been reported in preliminary research. Additional study is needed in this area.
- People with severe liver disease should use caffeine cautiously, as levels of caffeine in the blood may build up and last longer. Skin rashes have been associated with caffeine ingestion. In laboratory and animal studies, caffeine has been found to affect blood clotting, although effects in humans are not known.
- Caffeine toxicity is possible with high doses. Chronic use can result in tolerance and psychological dependence and may be habit forming. Abrupt discontinuation may result in withdrawal symptoms.

- Several population studies initially suggested a possible association between caffeine use and fibrocystic breast disease, although more recent research has not found this connection. Limited research reports a possible relationship between caffeine use and multiple sclerosis, although evidence is not definitive in this area. Animal study reports that tannin fractions from tea plants may increase the risk of cancer, although it is not clear that the tannin present in green tea has significant carcinogenic effects in humans.
- Drinking tannin-containing beverages such as tea may contribute to iron deficiency, and in infants tea has been associated with impaired iron metabolism and microcytic anemia.
- In preliminary research, green tea has been associated with decreased levels of estrogens in the body. It is not clear whether significant side effects such as hot flashes may occur.
- In human study, topical use of ointment containing Polyphenon E may result in local irritation.

Pregnancy and Breastfeeding

- Large amounts of green tea should be used cautiously in pregnant women, as caffeine crosses the placenta and has been associated with spontaneous abortion, intrauterine growth retardation, and low birth weight.
- Caffeine is readily transferred into breast milk. Caffeine ingestion by infants can lead to sleep disturbances/insomnia.

INTERACTIONS
Interactions with Drugs

- Studies of the interactions of green tea with drugs are limited. However, green tea is a source of caffeine, for which multiple interactions have been documented.
- The combination of caffeine with ephedrine, an ephedra alkaloid, has been implicated in numerous severe or life-threatening cardiovascular events such as very high blood pressure, stroke, or heart attack. Stroke has also been reported after the nasal ingestion of caffeine with amphetamine.
- Caffeine may add to the effects and side effects of other stimulants including nicotine, beta-agonists such as albuterol (Ventolin), or other methylxanthines such as theophylline. Conversely, caffeine can counteract drowsy effects and mental slowness caused by benzodiazepines like lorazepam (Ativan) or diazepam (Valium). Phenylpropanolamine and caffeine should not be used together because of reports of numerous potentially serious adverse effects; forms of phenylpropanolamine taken by mouth have been removed from the U.S. market because of reports of bleeding into the head.
- When taken with caffeine, a number of drugs may increase caffeine blood levels or the length of time caffeine acts on the body, including disulfiram (Antabuse), birth control pills or hormone replacement therapy (HRT), ciprofloxacin (Cipro), norfloxacin, fluvoxamine (Luvox), cimetidine (Tagamet), verapamil, and mexiletine. Caffeine levels may be lowered by taking dexamethasone (Decadron). The metabolism of caffeine by the liver may be affected by multiple drugs, although the effects in humans are not clear.
- Caffeine may lengthen the effects of carbamazepine or increase the effects of clozapine (Clozaril) and dipyridamole. Caffeine may affect serum lithium levels, and abrupt cessation of caffeine use by regular caffeine users taking lithium may result in high levels of lithium or lithium toxicity. Levels of aspirin or phenobarbital may be lowered in the body, although clinical effects in humans are not clear.
- Although caffeine by itself does not appear to have pain-relieving properties, it is used in combination with ergotamine tartrate in the treatment of migraine or cluster headaches (e.g., Cafergot). It has been shown to increase the headache-relieving effects of other pain relievers such as acetaminophen and aspirin (e.g., Excedrin). Caffeine may also increase the pain-relieving effects of codeine or ibuprofen (Advil, Motrin).
- As a diuretic, caffeine increases urine and sodium losses through the kidneys and may add to the effects of other diuretics such as furosemide (Lasix).
- Green tea may contain vitamin K, which, when used in large quantities, can reduce the blood thinning effects of warfarin (Coumadin), a phenomenon that has been reported in a human case.
- Based on preliminary data, theanine, a specific glutamate derivative in green tea, may reduce the adverse reactions caused to the heart and liver by the prescription cancer drug doxorubicin. Further research is needed to confirm these results.
- Based on preliminary data, ingestion of green tea may lower low-density lipoprotein (LDL) cholesterol levels and thus may theoretically interact with other cholesterol-lowering drugs.
- Other potential interactions may include drugs such as adenosine, alcohol, anticoagulants, antidiabetics, antipsychotics, fluconazole, hydrocortisone, levodopa, monoamine oxidase inhibitor (MAOI) antidepressants, methoxsalen, phenytoin, proton pump inhibitors (PPIs), riluzole, terbinafine, theophylline, and timolol.

Interactions with Herbs and Dietary Supplements

- Studies of green tea interactions with herbs and supplements are limited. However, green tea is a source of caffeine, for which multiple interactions have been documented.
- Caffeine may add to the effects and side effects of other stimulants. The combination of caffeine with ephedrine, which is present in ephedra (ma huang), has been implicated in numerous severe or life-threatening cardiovascular events such as very high blood pressure, stroke, or heart attack.
- Cola nut, guarana (*Paullinia cupana*), and yerba mate (*Ilex paraguariensis*) are also sources of caffeine and may add to the effects and side effects of caffeine in green tea. A combination product containing caffeine, yerba mate (*Ilex paraguariensis*), and damiana (*Turnera diffusa*) has been reported to cause weight loss, slowing of the gastrointestinal tract, and a feeling of stomach fullness.
- As a diuretic, caffeine increases urine and sodium losses through the kidneys and may add to the effects of other diuretic agents.
- Based on preliminary data, ingestion of green tea may lower LDL ("bad") cholesterol levels and thus may theoretically interact with other cholesterol-lowering herbs and supplements.
- Bitter orange, calcium, iron, MAOIs, and tannin-containing herbs and supplements may also interact with green tea.

For a complete list of references, please visit www.naturalstandard.com.

Guarana
(Paullinia cupana)

RELATED TERMS

- Brazilian cocoa, caffeine, caffeine–tannin complex, Dark Dog Lemon, elixir of youth, gift of the gods, Go Gum, guarana bread, guarana gum, guarana paste, Guarana Rush, guarana seed paste, guaranin, guaranine, Guts, Happy Motion, Josta, mysterious Puelverchen, pasta guarana, Paullinia, *Paullinia cupana, Paullinia sorbilis,* Sapindaceae (family), Superguarana, tetramethylxanthine, Uabano, Uaranzeiro, Zoom.

BACKGROUND

- Guarana is native to South America and has stimulating properties when taken by mouth. Guarana is also used to enhance athletic performance and reduce fatigue. It has been used as an aphrodisiac, diuretic, astringent, and to prevent malaria, dysentery, diarrhea, fever, headache, and rheumatism.

- The active ingredient in guarana was formerly called guaranine (tetramethylxanthine) but was later found to be caffeine. Guarana has one of the highest caffeine contents of all plants (up to 7%) and has been used by manufacturers for its caffeine content (e.g., Dark Dog Lemon, Guts, and Josta).

- Although there is no scientific evidence that guarana itself increases mental alertness, its relationship to caffeine makes it probable that it would possess the same effects. It is proposed that the stimulatory effect of guarana is more gradual and sustained than caffeine because of the caffeine–tannin complex. Guarana is generally regarded as safe when used in moderation and not combined with other stimulatory agents, such as ephedra.

EVIDENCE

Uses Based on Scientific Evidence	Grade
Cognitive Enhancement Guarana has not been shown to alter cognitive function or arousal in preliminary studies. Caffeine found in guarana may improve simple reaction time but may not improve immediate memory. Additional study is needed in this area.	C
Mood Enhancement Caffeine may have positive effects on mood and may increase alertness and feelings of well-being. Limited research has been conducted on guarana in this area, and more study is needed.	C
Weight Loss Caffeine has been used as a weight loss agent because of its thermogenic effects (the process of fat or calorie burning caused by increasing heat output). In available studies, guarana has been studied with other herbs, which makes it difficult to draw a conclusion based on the effects of guarana alone.	C

DOSING

Adults (18 Years and Older)

- There is insufficient evidence to recommend a dose for guarana. Teas, capsules, and energy drinks are all commercially available. For cognitive enhancement, a single dose of 150 mg guarana dry extract, standardized to 11-13% alkaloid concentration has been used. One gram of guarana up to four times a day has been taken to relieve diarrhea or dysentery. As a diuretic, 486 mg of guarana daily has been used. One to two tablets or capsules (200-800 mg guarana extract) before breakfast or lunch, not to exceed 3 g daily, has reportedly been used for energy enhancement.

Children (Younger than 18 Years)

- There is insufficient evidence to recommend a dose for guarana in children.

SAFETY

Allergies

- Avoid in individuals with a known allergy or hypersensitivity to guarana (*Paullinia cupana*), caffeine, tannins, or related species of the Sapindaceae family. Caffeine, a prominent constituent of guarana, may have an inhibitory effect on type I allergic reactions.

Side Effects and Warnings

- Guarana is generally well tolerated. A majority of information related to adverse effects of guarana is based in theory on the adverse effect profile of caffeine. The effects of caffeine are likely more pronounced at age extremes: in the elderly and in children. The chronic use of caffeine, especially in large amounts, may produce tolerance, habituation, and psychological dependence. Abrupt discontinuation of caffeine can result in physical withdrawal symptoms including headache, irritation, nervousness, anxiety, and dizziness.

- Caffeinism and caffeine withdrawal may be indistinguishable from anxiety neurosis (physical symptoms of anxiety), and caffeine intoxication may cause psychosis (mental disorder). In various cases, anxiety disorders and somatic dysfunctions could be linked to caffeine intake. However, in a study of schizophrenic inpatients, no correlation was found between levels of anxiety, depression, or other behavior and caffeine consumption. Caffeine has been reported to increase mental alertness and physical energy and enhance mood, physical performance, and endurance. Avoid use in patients with psychological or psychiatric disorders, as guarana may exacerbate symptoms.
- Seizures, muscle spasms, and convulsions have been reported from caffeine overdose. Lifetime caffeinated coffee intake equivalent to 2 cups a day without daily milk consumption (or calcium intake below recommended dietary allowance [RDA]) in women has been associated with significantly decreased bone density and bone loss in older women. Use cautiously in individuals at risk of osteoporosis, as caffeine may increase urinary excretion of calcium. Cases of rhabdomyolysis and myoglobinuria have been related to toxic effects of caffeine. Caffeine-induced insomnia has also been extensively studied.
- Consuming large amounts of caffeine per day may increase the risk of breast disease, tachycardia (increased heart rate), or high blood pressure, although there is controversy in this area. Nevertheless, use cautiously in patients with preexisting mitral valve prolapse, as intractable ventricular fibrillation has been reported in a case associated with high dosage caffeine consumption.
- Several studies have found no connection between coronary heart disease and habitual coffee drinking. The Framingham Study did not find an association between coffee-drinking and atherosclerotic (hardening of the blood vessels) cardiovascular disease in the general population. In another large study, there was no significant association between coffee consumption and angina (chest pain).
- An increase in blood glucose may occur after low caffeine ingestion. Caution is advised in patients with diabetes or hypoglycemia and in those taking drugs, herbs, or supplements that affect blood sugar. Serum glucose levels may need to be monitored by a qualified health care professional, including a pharmacist, and medication adjustments may be necessary.
- Theoretically, the caffeine in guarana may increase the bioavailability and absorption of tannins, thus decreasing the absorption of nutrients. Weight loss, delayed gastric emptying time, and perceived gastric fullness have been attributed to a combination guarana product also containing yerba mate and damiana. "Burning in the stomach," worsening of ulcer symptoms, and urticaria ("hives") have also been reported.
- Guarana may increase the risk of bleeding. Caution is advised in patients with bleeding disorders or taking drugs that may increase the risk of bleeding. Dosing adjustments may be necessary.

- Adverse effects reported secondary to ingestion of a combination of ma huang and guarana included insomnia, anxiety, headache, irritability, poor concentration, blurred vision, and dizziness. Other symptoms include hyperexcitation, tremor, nervousness, cerebral infarction (stroke), changes in voice quality, and palpitations (with and without chest pain). Avoid use in combination with other stimulatory agents, especially ephedra, because of reports of death and permanent disability associated with this combination.
- Ingestion of caffeine has increased intraocular pressure in two glaucoma patients. Use cautiously in individuals with glaucoma.
- Guarana may produce a diuretic effect. A reduction of caffeine may reduce the episodes of leakage per day in patients with symptoms of urinary frequency, and/or urge incontinence. Caffeine may cause dysuria (difficulty or pain urinating). High caffeine intake has been shown to worsen the condition of detrusor instability (unstable bladder) in older women. Use cautiously in patients with impaired kidney function.
- Use cautiously in individuals with an iron deficiency because of possible association with the development of anemia.
- Avoid in patients with liver impairment, as the clearance of caffeine may be impaired.

Pregnancy and Breastfeeding

- Studies on caffeine, the active constituent in guarana, indicate that consumption of caffeine may increase certain risks in pregnant women, although there is controversy in this area. For instance, high levels of caffeine consumption may result in delayed conception among women who are nonsmokers. Several studies found an association between caffeine and low birth weight. Heavy caffeine intake throughout pregnancy may increase the risk of sudden infant death syndrome (SIDS). Three cases of birth defects have been associated with excessive caffeine intake. Studies in pregnant women drinking moderate amounts of caffeine have shown inconsistent results, with more recent studies reporting no adverse effects on the fetus.
- Caffeine consumption may increase the risk of an early spontaneous abortion among nonsmoking women. Heavy caffeine consumers reporting nausea had a doubled risk of spontaneous abortion. Light caffeine use has been associated with risk of spontaneous abortion among women who aborted in their last pregnancy.
- Caffeine is readily transferred into breast milk. Infant caffeine ingestion can lead to infant sleeping disturbances. The effect of other substances contained in guarana is unknown. Breastfeeding may inhibit the caffeine metabolism in infants because of human milk components. Babies from mothers who consumed large amounts of caffeine daily have experienced tremors, and some experienced cardiac rhythm disturbances.

INTERACTIONS
Interactions with Drugs

- Although the interactions for guarana are quite limited, there are numerous theoretical interactions based on guarana's caffeine content.
- Caffeine combined with analgesics (pain relievers) has been reported to increase analgesic effects. For example, in treatment of migraine, a combination of N-acetyl-para-aminophenol acetaminophen (APAP), aspirin, and

caffeine was found to be highly effective. Caffeine may also be beneficial when taken with ibuprofen or propyphenazone. Caffeine increases the peak plasma concentration, rate of absorption, and bioavailability of aspirin. The addition of caffeine to aspirin has significant benefits on mood and performance. An aspirin-butalbital-caffeine-codeine combination is considered superior to acetaminophen/codeine in relieving oral surgery pain.

- Caffeine is an adenosine antagonist and inhibits A1-receptors. Therefore the actions of caffeine and adenosine are mutually antagonistic.
- Alcohol consumption may increase caffeine serum concentrations and the risk of caffeine adverse effects.
- There is one case report of ischemic stroke after the nasal ingestion of amphetamine and caffeine. Caution is advised with this combination.
- Caffeine has been reported to have antiplatelet activity and may increase the risk of bleeding when taken with drugs that increase the risk of bleeding. Some examples include aspirin, anticoagulants ("blood thinners") such as warfarin (Coumadin) or heparin, antiplatelet drugs such as clopidogrel (Plavix), and nonsteroidal antiinflammatory drugs (NSAIDS) such as ibuprofen (Motrin, Advil) or naproxen (Naprosyn, Aleve). Caffeine was also shown to attenuate the hemodynamic response to dipyridamole, a rheological agent that inhibits platelet aggregation.
- Caffeine may also alter blood sugar levels. Caution is advised when medications that may also alter blood sugar are used. Patients taking drugs for diabetes by mouth or using insulin should be monitored closely by a qualified health care professional, including a pharmacist. Medication adjustments may be necessary.
- Caffeine may interact with benzodiazepines. When lorazepam and caffeine were given and mental performance tests were administered and compared, the effect of caffeine counteracted both the effect of reducing anxiety and the reduction in mental performance caused by lorazepam alone. Caffeine with diazepam (Valium) may produce similar results by counteracting the drowsy effects and mental slowness of diazepam. The caffeine in guarana may also negate the hypnotic effects of pentobarbital. Sedative doses may need to be monitored.
- Concomitant use of guarana may increase the inotropic effects of beta-adrenergic agonists.
- Caffeine may alter the effects of carbamazepine (Tegretol) and reduce the bioavailability. Consult with a qualified health care professional, including a pharmacist, as dosing adjustments may be necessary.
- The antihistamine cimetidine (Tagamet) may decrease caffeine clearance by inhibiting the microsomal metabolism of caffeine. Caution is advised in patients taking cimetidine along with caffeine or guarana.
- The antibiotic ciprofloxacin (Cipro) significantly inhibits caffeine elimination. Caution is advised in patients taking certain antibiotics and caffeine.
- Caffeine taken with the antipsychotic clozapine (Clozaril, Leponex) may increase the risk of unwanted side effects, such as tardive dyskinesia, hallucinations, and akathisia. Caution is advised.
- Concomitant use of central nervous system stimulants and caffeine may increase the risk of stimulant adverse effects.
- Caffeine may interfere with the way the body processes certain drugs using the liver's cytochrome P450 enzyme system. As a result, the levels of these drugs may be decreased or increased in the blood and may alter the intended effects. Patients taking any medications should check the package insert and speak with a qualified health care professional, including a pharmacist, about possible interactions. Examples of agents that may interact include riluzole or fluvoxamine.

- Numerous agents alter the clearance, metabolism, and pharmacokinetics of caffeine when taken concurrently. For instance, when caffeine is taken with the steroid agent dexamethasone (Decadron), the clearance of caffeine may increase. Antibacterial agents such as enoxacin may significantly inhibit caffeine elimination. Impaired iron metabolism and microcytic anemia may occur in infants of breastfeeding women consuming caffeine. Methoxsalen and mexiletine have been shown to decrease the clearance of caffeine. Concomitant use of birth control pills and caffeine may increase serum caffeine concentrations and increase the risk of adverse effects, as birth control pills decrease the rate of caffeine clearance. Disulfiram decreased clearance of caffeine in healthy volunteers. Caffeine administration in patients pretreated with quinolones (norfloxacin or pipemidic acid) may result in decreased caffeine clearance. Caffeine degradation may be impaired by phenytoin (Dilantin), an anticonvulsant drug.
- Caffeine may increase diuresis and urinary sodium, potassium, and osmol excretion. Caution is advised in patients taking other diuretic agents because of additive effects.
- Ephedrine in combination with guarana may increase blood pressure and therefore the risk of stroke and other cardiovascular events. Thermogenic synergism between ephedrine and caffeine may enhance the activity of ephedrine. Theoretically, pseudoephedrine (Sudafed) would be expected to have the same effect on blood pressure when used in combination with guarana.
- Caffeine may enhance the effectiveness of ergotamine tartrate (Cafergot) in the treatment of migraine headaches. Caffeine may enhance topically applied (on the skin) hydrocortisone in the treatment of atopic dermatitis.
- In preterm infants, caffeine has been found to be equivalent to theophylline in altering erythropoietin production, a hormone made in the kidneys. Theophylline is also used as a bronchodilator agent and given to patients with asthma. Caffeine may decrease the total body clearance and elimination rate of theophylline. Caution is advised.
- In a case report, esmolol was an effective treatment for caffeine toxicity resulting from a suicide attempt of ingesting excessive amounts of caffeine.
- Caffeine may increase the renal (kidney) clearance of lithium and may reduce the plasma levels in stabilized patients. Abrupt discontinuation of a consistent caffeine intake may cause an increase in lithium tremors and an increase in serum lithium levels. Monitoring of doses may be necessary.
- Although not well studied in humans, caffeine and monoamine oxidase inhibitors (MAOIs) may cause encephalopathy (degenerative brain disease), neuromuscular irritability, hypotension (low blood pressure), sinus tachycardia (increased heartbeat), rhabdomyolysis (potentially fatal disease involving destruction or degeneration of skeletal muscle), and hyperthermia (abnormally high body temperature). Consult with a qualified health care professional, including a pharmacist, to check for any interactions.
- Caffeine may have additive effects on cardiovascular parameters when taken with nicotine. Concomitant consumption of caffeine and cigarettes during pregnancy

may place the developing fetus at higher risk of diminished growth.

- The combination of phenylpropanolamine and caffeine caused a manic psychosis in one woman with no previous history of mental disturbances. It is noted that phenylpropanolamine can increase the peak levels reached by caffeine by almost fourfold. An additive increase in blood pressure has occurred when the combination of phenylpropanolamine and caffeine was used. Caution is advised.
- Terbinafine (Lamisil) is an antifungal agent that may increase serum caffeine concentrations and increase the risk of adverse effects. Caution is advised when terbinafine is taken concurrently with caffeine.
- Verapamil is a calcium channel blocker agent. When taken with caffeine, verapamil may increase the risk of side effects.

Interactions with Herbs and Dietary Supplements

- Herb and supplement interactions associated with guarana are predominantly theoretical and generally based on the adverse effect profile of caffeine.
- Caffeine may increase the risk of bleeding when taken with herbs and supplements that are believed to increase the risk of bleeding. Multiple cases of bleeding have been reported with the use of *Ginkgo biloba*, and fewer cases have been reported with garlic and saw palmetto. Numerous other agents may theoretically increase the risk of bleeding, although this has not been proven in most cases.
- Caffeine might increase or decrease blood sugar levels. Caution is advised when herbs or supplements that may also lower blood sugar are used. Blood glucose levels may require monitoring, and doses may need adjustment.
- Bitter orange may add to the possible hypertensive (blood pressure–increasing) effects of caffeine. Caution is advised in patients with high blood pressure or those taking other herbs that have blood pressure–altering effects.

- Other caffeine-containing products (e.g., black tea, cocoa, coffee, cola nut, green tea, and yerba mate) used in combination with guarana may have additive effects.
- Caffeine may interfere with the way the body processes certain herbs or supplements using the liver's cytochrome P450 enzyme system. As a result, the levels of other herbs or supplements may become too low in the blood. It may also alter the effects that other herbs or supplements potentially may have on the P450 system.
- Caffeine may increase the flow of urine (diuresis) and may have additive effects with other herbs or supplements that have diuretic effects.
- Avoid use of combination products of ma huang (ephedra) and guarana because of the reports of death and permanent disability associated with this combination (such as Metabolife-356).
- Caffeine may interact with herbs with estrogenic effects; caffeine metabolism was inhibited in postmenopausal women using hormone replacement estrogen.
- Impaired iron metabolism and microcytic anemia may occur in infants of breastfeeding women consuming caffeine. Caution is advised.
- Caffeine and MAOIs may cause encephalopathy (degenerative brain disease), neuromuscular irritability, hypotension (low blood pressure), sinus tachycardia (increased heartbeat), rhabdomyolysis (potentially fatal disease involving destruction or degeneration of skeletal muscle), and hyperthermia (abnormally high body temperature).
- Additive effects on cardiovascular parameters may occur with nicotine or tobacco. Concomitant consumption of caffeine and cigarettes during pregnancy may place the developing fetus at higher risk of diminished growth.

For a complete list of references, please visit www.naturalstandard.com.

Guggul
(Commiphora mukul)

RELATED TERMS

- African myrrh, Arabian myrrh, *Commiphora mukul*, *Commiphora myrrha*, guggal, guggulsterone, guggulsterone (4,17 (20)-pregnadiene-3,16-dione), guggulu, gum guggul, gum guggulu, Gugulmax, guggulipid C+, Guglip, gum myrrh, fraction A, myrrha, Somali myrrh, yemen myrhh.

BACKGROUND

- Guggul (gum guggul) is a resin produced by the mukul myrrh tree. Guggulipid is extracted from guggul and contains plant sterols (guggulsterones E and Z), which are believed to be its bioactive compounds.
- Before 2003, the majority of scientific evidence suggested that guggulipid elicits significant reductions in serum total cholesterol, low-density lipoprotein (LDL), and triglyceride levels and elevations in high-density lipoprotein (HDL) levels. However, recent research provides preliminary evidence against the efficacy of guggul for hypercholesterolemia; thus, further study is necessary before a definitive conclusion can be reached.
- Guggulsterones are antagonists of the farsenoid X receptor (FXR) and the bile acid receptor (BAR), nuclear hormones that are involved with cholesterol metabolism and bile acid regulation.

EVIDENCE

Uses Based on Scientific Evidence	Grade
Hypercholesterolemia Before 2003, the majority of scientific evidence suggested that guggulipid elicits significant reductions in serum total cholesterol, low-density lipoprotein (LDL), and triglyceride levels and elevations in high-density lipoprotein (HDL) levels. However, recent research provides preliminary evidence against the efficacy of guggul for hypercholesterolemia. This contradicts prior research and historical use.	C
Acne Guggulipid has been found to possess antiinflammatory properties and has been suggested as an oral therapy for nodulocystic acne vulgaris. Preliminary data suggest possible short-term improvements in the number of acne lesions.	C
Obesity There is insufficient evidence to support the use of guggul or guggul derivatives for the management of obesity.	C
Rheumatoid Arthritis There is insufficient evidence to support the use of guggul or guggul derivatives for the management of rheumatoid arthritis.	C
Osteoarthritis There is insufficient evidence to support the use of guggul or guggul derivatives for the management of osteoarthritis.	C

Uses Based on Tradition or Theory

Asthma, bleeding, colitis, diabetes, gingivitis, hemorrhoids, leprosy, leukorrhea, menstrual disorders, mouth infections, neuralgia, obesity, pain, psoriasis, rhinitis, sore throat, sores, tumors, weight loss, wound healing.

DOSING
Adults (18 Years and Older)

- There is insufficient evidence for guggul in adults. For hyperlipidemia, 500-1000 mg of guggulipid (standardized to 2.5% guggulsterones) has been taken two to three times daily. An equivalent dose of commercially prepared guggulsterone is 25 mg three times daily or 50 mg taken twice daily by mouth. A higher dose has been studied (2000 mg three times daily, standardized to 2.5% guggulsterones), although this dose may be associated with a greater risk of hypersensitive skin reactions. For nodulocystic acne, a dose of guggulipid equivalent to 25 mg guggulsterone has been taken daily.

Children (Younger than 18 Years)

- There is insufficient evidence to recommend a dose for guggul in children.

SAFETY
Allergies

- Avoid in individuals with a known allergy or hypersensitivity to guggul or any of its constituents. Hypersensitive skin reactions have been noted, in most cases within 48 hours of starting therapy, and have resolved spontaneously within 1 week of therapy discontinuation.

Side Effects and Warnings

- Standardized guggulipid is generally regarded as safe in healthy adults at recommended doses for up to 6 months. Gastrointestinal upset is the most common adverse effect, as well as diarrhea, nausea, vomiting, burping, and hiccough. Headache, restlessness, and anxiety have been noted in studies. Allergic skin rash (especially at higher doses) has been reported.
- Guggulipid has been associated with inhibition of platelets and increased fibrinolysis (blood clot breakdown), and in theory the risk of bleeding may increase.
- Although not well studied in humans, weight loss and stimulation of thyroid function may occur.

Pregnancy and Breastfeeding

- Guggul is not recommended in pregnant or breastfeeding women because of a lack of available scientific evidence.

INTERACTIONS

Interactions with Drugs

- Coadministration of guggulipid to humans has been reported to decrease the bioavailability of the beta-blocker propranolol and the calcium channel blocker diltiazem.
- Guggulipid has been associated with inhibition of platelets and increased blood clot breakdown. In theory, guggul may increase the risk of bleeding when taken with drugs that increase the risk of bleeding. Some examples include aspirin, anticoagulants ("blood thinners") such as warfarin (Coumadin) or heparin, antiplatelet drugs such as clopidogrel (Plavix), and nonsteroidal antiinflammatory drugs such as ibuprofen (Motrin, Advil) or naproxen (Naprosyn, Aleve).
- The effect of guggul on serum lipids remains controversial. Guggul may affect serum lipid levels (decreasing cholesterol, triglyceride, and LDL levels and increasing HDL levels) and may thus increase the effects of lipid-lowering drugs such as statins.
- Animal studies suggest that the guggul constituent Z-guggulsterone may stimulate thyroid function. Therefore, additional effects may occur in patients taking thyroid drugs and guggul together.

Interactions with Herbs and Dietary Supplements

- The effect of guggul on serum lipids remains controversial. Guggul may affect serum lipid levels (decreasing cholesterol, triglyceride, and LDL levels and increasing HDL levels) and may thus increase the effects of lipid-lowering agents such as niacin, garlic, or fish oil (omega-3 fatty acids).
- Guggulipid has been associated with inhibition of platelets and increased blood clot breakdown. In theory, guggul may increase the risk of bleeding when taken with herbs and supplements that are believed to increase the risk of bleeding. Multiple cases of bleeding have been reported with the use of *Ginkgo biloba*, and fewer cases have been reported with garlic or saw palmetto. Numerous other agents may theoretically increase the risk of bleeding, although this has not been proven in most cases.

For a complete list of references, please visit www.naturalstandard.com.

Gymnema
(*Gymnema sylvestre*)

RELATED TERMS

- Asclepiadaceae (family), *Asclepias geminata* roxb., GS4 (water soluble extract of the leaves), gur-mar, gurmar, gur-marbooti, gurmari, *Gymnema inodum, Gemnema melicida, Gymnema montanum, Gymnema sylvestre,* kogilam, madhunashini, mangala gymnema, merasingi, meshashringi, meshavalli, miracle plant, periploca of the woods, *Periploca sylvestris,* podapatri, Proeta, ram's horn, small Indian ipecac, sarkaraikolli, shardunika, sirukurinjan, vishani.

BACKGROUND

- Preliminary human evidence suggests that gymnema may be effective in the management of blood sugar levels in type 1 and type 2 diabetes, as an adjunct to conventional drug therapy, for up to 20 months. Gymnema appears to lower serum glucose and glycosylated hemoglobin (HbA1c) levels following chronic use but may not have significant acute effects. High-quality human trials are lacking in this area. Some of the available research has been conducted by authors affiliated with manufacturers of gymnema products.

EVIDENCE

Uses Based on Scientific Evidence	Grade
Diabetes Preliminary human research reports that gymnema may be beneficial in patients with type 1 or type 2 diabetes when it is added to diabetes drugs being taken by mouth or to insulin. Further studies of dosing, safety, and effectiveness are needed.	B
High Cholesterol Preliminary research in people with type 2 diabetes reports decreased cholesterol and triglyceride levels. Better evidence is needed before a clear conclusion can be drawn.	C
Weight Loss *Gymnema sylvestre* extract (GSE) has been shown to be effective for weight loss when used in combination with other products. The effects of gymnema remain unclear.	C

Uses Based on Tradition or Theory
Allergy, antimicrobial, antioxidant, aphrodisiac, cancer, cardiovascular disease, constipation, cough, dental caries, digestive stimulant, diuresis, gout, high blood pressure, laxative, liver disease, liver protection, malaria, metabolic disorders, rheumatoid arthritis, snake venom antidote, stomach ailments, uterine stimulant, viral infection.

DOSING
Adults (18 Years and Older)

- A total of 200 mg of extract GS4 has been taken by mouth twice daily. Similarly, 2 mL of an aqueous decoction (10 g of shade-dried powdered leaves per 100 mL) has been taken three times daily.
- The manufacturer PharmaTerra recommends the dose for their product Proeta (GS4) to be two 250-mg capsules taken twice daily at mealtimes (for adults weighing more than 100 lbs) or one 250-mg capsule taken twice daily at mealtimes (for adults weighing less than 100 lbs).

Children (Younger than 18 Years)

- There is insufficient evidence to safely recommend gymnema for use in children.

SAFETY
Allergies

- Allergy to gymnema may occur. In theory, allergic cross-reactivity may exist with members of the Asclepiadaceae (milkweed) family.

Side Effects and Warnings

- Aside from lowered blood sugar levels and increased effects of antidiabetic drugs following chronic use of gymnema, no significant adverse effects were reported with the herb in multiple studies up to 20 months long. Caution is advised in patients with diabetes or low blood sugar levels and in those taking drugs, herbs, or supplements that affect blood sugar. Serum glucose levels may need to be monitored by a qualified health care professional, and medication adjustments may be necessary. Based on human and animal studies, gymnema may lower blood cholesterol levels.
- Gymnema is reported to suppress the ability to detect sweet tastes because of the component gurmarin. This phenomenon prompted the Hindi name *gurmar* or "sugar destroyer."

Pregnancy and Breastfeeding

- Gymnema should not be used during pregnancy or breastfeeding because of a lack of reliable safety information.

INTERACTIONS
Interactions with Drugs

- Gymnema may lower blood sugar levels. Caution is advised when medications that may also lower blood sugar are used. Patients taking drugs for diabetes by mouth or using insulin should be monitored closely by a qualified health care professional. Medication adjustments may be necessary.
- Gymnema may lower blood cholesterol levels. Therefore, increased effects may occur if gymnema is taken in combination with drugs that lower cholesterol levels such as "statins" (3-hydroxy-3-methylglutaryl coenzyme A [HMG-CoA] reductase inhibitors) like lovastatin (Mevacor) or atorvastatin (Lipitor).

- Gymnema may have additive effects with weight loss drugs.

Interactions with Herbs and Dietary Supplements

- Gymnema may lower blood sugar levels. Caution is advised when herbs or supplements that may also lower blood sugar are used. Blood glucose levels may require monitoring, and doses may need adjustment.
- Gymnema may lower blood cholesterol levels. Therefore, increased effects may occur if gymnema is taken in combination with herbs or supplements that lower cholesterol levels, such as fish oil, garlic, guggul, or niacin.
- Absorption of oleic acid (a fatty acid) may be decreased by gymnema.
- Gymnema may have additive effects with herbs and supplements that help with weight loss. It may interact with chromium, fat-soluble vitamins, and garcinia.

For a complete list of references, please visit www. naturalstandard.com.

G

Hawthorn
(*Crataegus* spp.)

RELATED TERMS

- Aubepine, bei shanzha, bianco spino, bread and cheese tree, Cardiplant, Chinese hawthorn, cockspur, cockspur thorn, Crataegi flos, Crataegi folium, Crataegi folium cum flore, Crataegi fructus, Crataegi herba, Crataegisan, *Crataegus azarolus*, *Crataegus cuneata*, Crataegus fructi, *Crataegus monogyna*, *Crataegus nigra*, *Crataegus oxyacanthoides*, *Crataegus pentagyna*, *Crataegus pinnatifida*, Crataegus sinaica boiss, Crataegus special extract WS 1442, Crataegutt, English hawthorn, epicatechin, epine blanche, epine de mai, Fructus oxyacanthae, Fructus spinae albae, gazels, haagdorn, hagedorn, hagthorn, halves, harthorne, haw, Hawthorne Berry, Hawthorne Formula, Hawthorne Heart, Hawthorne Phytosome, Hawthorne Power, hawthorn tops, hazels, hedgethorn, huath, hyperoside, isoquercitrin, ladies' meat, LI 132, may, mayblossoms, maybush, mayhaw, maythorn, mehlbeerbaum, nan shanzha, northern Chinese hawthorn, oneseed, oneseed hawthorn, quickset, red haw, RN 30/9, sanza, sanzashi, shanza, shan zha rou, southern Chinese hawthorn, thorn-apple tree, thorn plum, tree of chastity, Washington thorn, weissdorn, Weissdornblaetter mit Blueten, whitethorn, whitethorn herb, WS 1442.

BACKGROUND

- Hawthorn, a flowering shrub of the rose family, has an extensive history of use in cardiovascular disease, dating back to the first century. Flavonoids and other compounds found in hawthorn may synergistically improve performance of the damaged heart muscles and, further, may prevent or reduce symptoms of coronary artery disease.
- Hawthorn is widely used in Europe for treating New York Heart Association (NYHA) Class I-II heart failure, with standardization of its leaves and flowers. Overall, hawthorn appears to be effective, safe, and well tolerated and, in accordance with its indication, best used under the supervision of a medical professional.
- The therapeutic equivalence of hawthorn extracts to drugs considered standard-of-care for heart failure (such as angiotensin-converting enzyme [ACE] inhibitors, diuretics, or beta-adrenergic receptor blockers) remains to be established, as does the effect of concomitant use of hawthorn with these drugs. Nonetheless, hawthorn is a potentially beneficial therapy for patients who cannot or will not take prescription drugs and may offer additive benefits to prescription drug therapy.

EVIDENCE

Uses Based on Scientific Evidence	Grade
Congestive Heart Failure Extracts of the leaves and flowers of hawthorn have been reported as effective in the treatment of mild-to-moderate congestive heart failure (CHF), improving exercise capacity and reducing symptoms of cardiac insufficiency. However, whether hawthorn is as effective as drugs considered standard-of-care for heart failure (such as ACE inhibitors, diuretics, or beta-adrenergic receptor blockers) is unclear, as is the effect of the combined use of hawthorn with these drugs. Nonetheless, hawthorn is a potentially beneficial treatment for patients who cannot or will not take prescription drugs and may offer additive benefits to established therapies.	A
Anxiety Hawthorn in combination with other herbs may help to reduce anxiety and anxious mood. It is unknown whether hawthorn specifically had beneficial effects.	C
Coronary Artery Disease (Angina) Hawthorn has not been tested in the setting of concomitant drugs such as beta-blockers or ACE-inhibitors, which are often considered to be standard-of-care. At this time, there is not enough evidence to recommend for or against hawthorn for coronary artery disease or angina.	C
Functional Cardiovascular Disorders Herbal combinations containing hawthorn have been found effective in the treatment of functional cardiovascular symptoms. However, because of a lack of information on the use of hawthorn alone, there is not enough evidence to recommend for or against hawthorn for functional cardiovascular disorders.	C
High Blood Pressure Studies in patients with type 2 diabetes support the historic use of hawthorn to lower blood pressure.	C
Orthostatic Hypotension (Low Blood Pressure on Standing Up) Fresh hawthorn berries may improve orthostatic hypotension (a lowering of blood pressure that occurs when a person goes from a lying down position to a standing position).	C

Uses Based on Tradition or Theory

Abdominal colic, abdominal pain, acne, amenorrhea (lack of menstrual period), antioxidant, appetite stimulant, arteriosclerosis, asthma, astringent, bacterial infections, bladder disorders, blood vessel disorders (Buerger's disease), cancer, cardiac murmurs, circulation, diabetes mellitus, diarrhea, dysentery, dyspnea (shortness of breath), edema, frostbite, heart rhythm disorders, hemorrhoids, human immunodeficiency virus (HIV), hyperlipidemia, hypoxia (lack of oxygen), indigestion, insomnia, kidney disease, kidney stones, migraine, nephrosis, nervous disorders, peripheral artery disease, skin sores, sore throat, spasmolytic, stomachaches, sweating, varicose veins.

DOSING
Adults (18 Years and Older)

- For congestive heart failure, high-quality trials have used doses of 60 mg three times daily or 80 mg twice daily for products containing standardized extract WS 1442 (18.75% oligomeric procyanidins). The U.S. brand HeartCare (Nature's Way) is standardized in this fashion.
- Other high-quality trials have used doses of 100 mg three times daily, 200 mg twice daily, and up to 300 mg three times daily for products containing standardized extract LI 132 (2.2% flavonoids).
- The dosage range recommended in review literature is 160-900 mg hawthorn extract per day in two to three divided doses (corresponding to 3.5-19.8 mg flavonoids or 30-168.8 mg oligomeric procyanidines). Some sources recommend a range of 240-480 mg/day for extracts standardized to 18.75% oligomeric procyanidines.

Children (Younger than 18 Years)

- There is insufficient evidence to recommend a dose for hawthorn in children.

SAFETY
Allergies

- Avoid if allergic to hawthorn or to members of the *Crataegus* genus. There is a case report of an immediate-type hypersensitivity reaction to hawthorn plants. It is not known whether this applies to formulations taken by mouth.

Side Effects and Warnings

- There are limited reports of adverse effects associated with hawthorn. Numerous human trials, observational studies including more than 4500 patients, and case reports have noted rare adverse effects, including abdominal discomfort, nausea, agitation, dizziness, headache, fatigue, shortness of breath, skin rash, insomnia, sweating, and rapid heart rate.

Pregnancy and Breastfeeding

- Hawthorn is not recommended because of lack of sufficient data.

INTERACTIONS
Interactions with Drugs

- Additive inotropic effects when used with cardiac glycoside drugs such as digoxin have been noted in animals without added toxicity. In humans, hawthorn has been used with the intention of decreasing digoxin doses, although data on safe and efficacious dosing in this setting is still limited.
- Hawthorn may have additive activity with medications that lower blood pressure. Hawthorn may add to the activity of drugs that dilate blood vessels and may decrease the effects of vasoconstrictors such as phenylephrine (Neo-Synephrine), ephedrine, or norepinephrine. Hawthorn may interact with cholesterol-lowering agents.

Interactions with Herbs and Dietary Supplements

- Hawthorn may add to the effects on the heart of agents containing cardiac glycosides, such as foxglove (*Digitalis purpurea*).
- Hawthorn may add to the effects of agents that lower blood pressure and may also interact with agents that increase blood pressure.
- Hawthorn may have additive activity with agents that reduce cholesterol levels such as garlic, niacin, or fish oil (omega-3 fatty acids).

For a complete list of references, please visit www.naturalstandard.com.

H

Heartsease
(Viola tricolor)

RELATED TERMS

- Ackerveilchen (German), banewort, banwort, banwurt, bird's eye, blue violet, bonewort, bouncing bet, bullweed, call-me-to-you, cuddle me, cull me, cull me to you, European field pansy, European wild pansy, field pansy, field violet, flower o'luce, godfathers and godmothers, heart-ease herb, Heart's ease, herb constancy, herb trinitatis, herba jaceae, herbe de pensee sauvage (French), Jack jump-up-and-kiss-me, Johnny jump up, Jupiter flower, kiss-her-in-the-buttery, kit-run-about, kit-run-in-the-fields, ladies' delight, live-in-idleness, love idol, love-in-idleness, love lies bleeding, love-lies-bleeding, loving idol, meet-me-in-the-entry, pancies, pansy, pawnce, pensée (French), pensee sauvage (French), pink-eyed-John, pink-o'-the-eye, pink of my John, stepmother, stepmother herb, Stiefmuetterchenkraut (German), three-faces-in-a-hood, three-faces-under-a-hood, viola, *Viola arvensis*, *Viola lutea*, *Viola ocellata*, *Viola tricolor* L., *Viola tricolor* (Linn.), *Viola tricolor* var. arvensis (Murr.) Boiss., Violaceae (family), Violae tricoloris herba, violette tricolore, violine, violutoside, wild pansy.

BACKGROUND

- Heartsease, also referred to as wild pansy, is the forerunner of cultivated pansies. The flowers and leaves are edible.
- Heartsease has been used by herbalists for centuries in the treatment of respiratory complaints (such as asthma, bronchitis, and whooping cough) and skin diseases (such as eczema and seborrhea). It has also been used for arthritis, rheumatism, and epilepsy and for its purported antiinflammatory, diuretic, mucus-thinning, laxative, soothing, and wound-healing properties.
- There is limited scientific evidence to confirm the many traditional uses of heartsease. Early research suggests that heartsease may have anticancer and antimicrobial properties.

EVIDENCE

Uses Based on Scientific Evidence

No available studies qualify for inclusion in the evidence table.

Uses Based on Tradition or Theory

Acne, antiinflammatory, antimicrobial, antispasmodic, arthritis, asthma, autoimmune diseases, bedwetting, bile flow stimulation, bladder inflammation, breast inflammation, bronchitis, bruises, childbirth (labor induction), colds, convulsions, cough, demulcent (soothes inflamed tissue), diarrhea, diuretic (increases urine flow), eczema, emetic (induces vomiting), epilepsy, eruptions, expectorant, eye inflammation, gonorrhea (suppressed), gout, heart disorders, hyperglycemia (high blood sugar levels), inflammatory conditions, itching, laxative, mucilage, pain relief, pleurisy, respiratory problems, rheumatism, ringworm, seborrhea, skin diseases (inflammation), skin infections (impetigo), sore throat, sweat stimulant, syphilis, testicular inflammation, tonic, ulcers (throat), urinary difficulties, urinary tract inflammation, uterine tonic, vaginal discharge, warts, whooping cough, wound healing.

DOSING
Adults (18 Years and Older)

- An infusion of heartsease made from 1-4 g dried heartsease has been used three times daily. One cup of heartsease tea (made with 1.5 g of the above-ground parts steeped in 150 mL boiling water for 5-10 minutes and then strained) has been taken three times daily. Two to four milliliters full-strength heartsease tincture has been taken three times daily.
- A tea or poultice prepared with heartsease has been applied to the skin three times daily.

Children (Younger than 18 Years)

- There is insufficient evidence to recommend a dose for heartsease, and use in children is not recommended.

SAFETY
Allergies

- Avoid in individuals with a known allergy or hypersensitivity to heartsease, violets, or pansies.

Side Effects and Warnings

- There is limited information regarding adverse effects of heartsease.
- In theory, heartsease may increase the risk of bleeding. Caution is advised in patients with bleeding disorders or in those taking drugs that may increase the risk of bleeding. Dosing adjustments may be necessary.

Pregnancy and Breastfeeding

- Heartsease is not recommended in pregnant or breastfeeding women because of a lack of available scientific evidence. Many tinctures contain high levels of alcohol and should be avoided during pregnancy.

INTERACTIONS
Interactions with Drugs

- Heartsease may increase the risk of bleeding when taken with drugs that increase the risk of bleeding. Some examples include aspirin, anticoagulants ("blood thinners") such as warfarin (Coumadin) or heparin, antiplatelet drugs such as clopidogrel (Plavix), and nonsteroidal antiinflammatory drugs such as ibuprofen (Motrin, Advil) or naproxen (Naprosyn, Aleve).
- Heartsease may have additive effects when taken with antibiotic, anticancer, and antiinflammatory drugs and drugs that clear mucus from the lungs.
- Many tinctures contain high levels of alcohol and may cause nausea or vomiting when taken with metronidazole (Flagyl) or disulfiram (Antabuse).

Interactions with Herbs and Dietary Supplements

- Heartsease may increase the risk of bleeding when taken with herbs and supplements that are believed to increase the risk of bleeding. Multiple cases of bleeding have been reported with the use of *Ginkgo biloba*, and fewer cases have been reported with the use of garlic and saw palmetto.

Numerous other agents may theoretically increase the risk of bleeding, although this has not been proven in most cases.

- Heartsease may have additive effects when taken with antibacterial, antifungal, antiinflammatory, and anticancer herbs and supplements and herbs and supplements that clear mucus from the lungs. In theory, because of its salicylic acid content, heartsease may have additive effects when taken with willow bark.

For a complete list of references, please visit www.naturalstandard.com.

H

Hibiscus
(*Hibiscus* spp.)

RELATED TERMS

- Ambary plant *(Hibiscus cannabinus)*, burao *(Hibiscus tiliaceus)*, chemparathampoo, erragogu, esculetin, gogu *(Hibiscus cannabinus)*, hibiscus protocatechuic acid (PCA), *Hibiscus mutabilis, Hibiscus rosa-sinensis, Hibiscus sabdariffa, Hibiscus syriacus, Hibiscus taiwanensis, Hibiscus tiliaceus,* Jamaican red sorrel, Karkadi, karkada, karkade (Arabic), kenaf *(Hibiscus cannabinus L.)*, Malvaceae (family), red sorrel (English), roselle (English), sour tea, tellagogu, Zobo drink.
- **Note:** This monograph does not include okra *(Abelmoschus esculentus,* formerly classified as *Hibiscus esculentus)* or Norfolk Island hibiscus *(Lagunaria patersonii).*

BACKGROUND

- The *Hibiscus* genus contains several species, many of which have been used medicinally. For instance, *Hibiscus rosa-sinensis* has been documented in the ancient Indian scriptures. *Hibiscus sabdariffa* has been used as a folk medicine in Canada and appears promising in treatment of hypertension (high blood pressure). *Hibiscus cannabinus* has been studied to treat head lice, although there is currently insufficient available evidence in this area.
- *Hibiscus sabdariffa* and compounds isolated from it (e.g., anthocyanins and hibiscus protocatechuic acid) are likely candidates for future studies. There are limited reported safety data about hibiscus, although it is popularly used as a tea.
- Based on ethnobotanical study, *Hibiscus tiliaceus* has been used throughout the Vanuatu archipelago to speed childbirth. *Hibiscus sabdariffa* L. has been used as a folk medicine in Canada. *Hibiscus rosa-sinensis* has been documented to have been used for several ailments in the ancient Indian scriptures.

EVIDENCE

Uses Based on Scientific Evidence	Grade
Hypertension (High Blood Pressure) Extracts of hibiscus may lower systolic and diastolic pressure. Additional studies are needed to confirm these results, although the use of hibiscus for lowering blood pressure looks promising.	B
Lice Currently, there is limited available evidence evaluating the effects of hibiscus for the treatment of lice.	C

Uses Based on Tradition or Theory
Antibacterial (melioidosis), antifungal, antioxidant, antipyretic (fever reducer), antiviral, atherosclerosis (hardening of the arteries), cancer, contraceptive, flavoring agent, hypercholesterolemia (high cholesterol levels), leukemia, liver diseases, liver protection, pain (antinociceptive), renal stone disease, weight loss.

DOSING

Adults (18 Years and Older)

- There is no proven effective dose for hibiscus, although an herbal infusion prepared with 10 g of dry calyx from *Hibiscus sabdariffa* with 0.5 L water (9.6 mg anthocyanins content) daily before breakfast showed similar results as captopril 25 mg twice a day for 4 weeks.

Children (Younger than 18 Years)

- There is insufficient evidence to recommend a dose for hibiscus in children.

SAFETY

Allergies

- Avoid in individuals with a known allergy or hypersensitivity to hibiscus, its constituents, or members of the Malvaceae family. Reported allergy symptoms include skin rash and hives.

Side Effects and Warnings

- There are limited reported safety data about hibiscus, although it is popularly used as a tea.
- Although not well studied in humans, excessive doses of hibiscus for relatively long periods may have antifertility effects. One study found that hibiscus tea contained polycyclic aromatic hydrocarbons (PAHs). PAHs have been associated with birth defects and cancer. The sources of PAHs in food are predominantly from environmental pollution and food processing. Use cautiously in patients with hypertension or hypotension (high or low blood pressure), as hibiscus may lower blood pressure.

Pregnancy and Breastfeeding

- Hibiscus is not recommended in pregnant or breastfeeding women because of a lack of available scientific evidence. However, *Hibiscus tiliaceus* has been used throughout the Vanuatu archipelago to speed childbirth. In theory, excessive doses of hibiscus for relatively long periods may have antifertility activity, and caution is advised.

INTERACTIONS

Interactions with Drugs

- Although not well studied in humans, hibiscus may have anticancer effects. Thus, caution is advised when taking hibiscus with other anticancer agents.
- Extracts of hibiscus may lower systolic and diastolic pressure. Patients taking blood pressure–lowering agents should use hibiscus cautiously because of additive effects. Consult with a qualified health care professional, including a pharmacist, to check for interactions.
- Zobo drink (made from hibiscus) may change the way certain antiinflammatory agents, such as acetaminophen, are processed in the body. Caution is advised when antiinflammatory agents and hibiscus are taken within a 2-hour period of one another.
- Karkadi beverage *(Hibiscus sabdariffa)* may reduce antimalarial (quinine, chloroquine) efficacy.

- Antiviral effects have been observed in preliminary laboratory study. In theory, hibiscus taken with other antiviral agents may have additive effects.
- *Hibiscus rosa-sinensis* may have estrogenic activity, although the clinical significance is unclear. Use hibiscus cautiously in patients taking hormone-altering agents, such as hormone replacement therapy or birth control pills.

Interactions with Herbs and Dietary Supplements

- Although not well studied in humans, hibiscus may have anticancer effects. Thus, caution is advised when hibiscus is taken with other anticancer agents.
- Extracts of hibiscus may lower systolic and diastolic pressure. Patients taking herbs that lower blood pressure should use hibiscus cautiously because of additive effects. Consult with a qualified health care professional, including a pharmacist, to check for interactions.
- In theory, Karkadi beverage (*Hibiscus sabdariffa*) may reduce the efficacy of antimalarial herbs and supplements.
- Antiviral effects have been observed in preliminary laboratory study. In theory, hibiscus taken with other herbs with antiviral activity may have additive effects.
- *Hibiscus rosa-sinensis* may have estrogenic activity, although the clinical significance is unclear. Use hibiscus cautiously in patients taking hormone altering herbs or supplements.

For a complete list of references, please visit www.naturalstandard.com.

Holy Basil
(*Ocimum sanctum*)

RELATED TERMS

- Ajaka, bai gka-prow, bai gkaprow, baranda, basilici herba, brinda, common basil, garden basil, green holy basil, hot basil, Indian basil, kala tulasi, kala tulsi, kemangen manjari, Krishna tulsi, krishnamul, Manjari tulsi, *Ocimum sanctum*, *Ocimum sanctum* seed oil, *Ocimum tenuiflorum*, orientin, parnasa, patra-puspha, Rama tulsi, red holy basil, sacred basil, sacred purple basil, shayama tulsi, St. Joseph's wort, suvasa tulasi, Thai basil, thulasi, thulsi, Trittavu, tulasi, tulshi, tulsi, tulsi cha-jadha, vicenin, Vishnu priya.
- **Note:** Not included in this review is sweet basil (*Ocimum basilicum*).

BACKGROUND

- The two primary types of basil are closely related: *Ocimum basilicum* (sweet basil), which is a staple of Italian and Asian cooking, and *Ocimum sanctum* (holy basil), which has a religious use or origin in different cultures. Both forms are native to India and Southeast Asia, although they are grown around the world.
- Holy basil has been used extensively for its medicinal values by a number of cultures. Chinese medicine uses holy basil for stomach spasms, kidney conditions, promotion of blood circulation, and treatment of snake and insect bites.
- In India, holy basil is known as *tulsi*, which translates as "incomparable one." The plant, which is considered sacred, is used extensively in religious ceremonies and is believed to protect any home where it is grown. According to Ayurvedic tradition, tulsi is one of the best herbs to prepare the heart and mind for spiritual practices, resolve colds and flu, treat various skin conditions, and reduce fever.
- Modern research on holy basil suggests that holy basil contains powerful antioxidants and it may be hepatoprotective (liver protecting). Also, preliminary clinical studies are investigating holy basil's effect on ulcers and blood sugar levels in patients with type 2 diabetes. Holy basil is generally recognized as having safe status in the United States (GRAS).

EVIDENCE

Uses Based on Scientific Evidence	Grade
Diabetes Mellitus Holy basil may have blood sugar–lowering effects and may be useful as an adjunct to dietary therapy and drug treatment in mild to moderate diabetes mellitus. It is unknown whether common culinary basil (*Ocimum basilicum*) would have similar effects.	C

Uses Based on Tradition or Theory
Adaptogen, allergies, analgesic (pain reliever), anthelmintic (expels worms), antibacterial, anticarcinogenic, antifertility, antifungal, antiinflammatory, antioxidant, antipyretic (fever reducer), antispasmodic, antitumor, appetite stimulant, arthritis, asthma, atherosclerosis (hardening of the arteries), bad breath, bronchitis, cancer, canker sores, cardiopathy, carminative (digestive aid), cataracts, catarrh (inflammation of the mucous membranes), cerebral reperfusion injury, cholera, common cold, conjunctival xerosis (dry eye), conjunctivitis (pink eye), constipation, cough, dacryocystitis (inflammation of the tear sac), demulcent (soothes inflamed tissue), diarrhea, dysentery (severe diarrhea), earache, eczema, enteritis (inflammation of the small intestine), exercise performance, expectorant (relieves cough/congestion), eye disorders, fever (chronic), galactagogue (promotes lactation), genitourinary disorders, gonorrhea (STD), gum disease, headaches, heart disease, hemopathy, hepatic disorders, hiccups, high cholesterol levels, immune system stimulant, improving circulation, indigestion, influenza, insect bites, kidney disorders, kidney stones, leukoderma (skin disorder), longevity, lumbar pain, malaria, mercury toxicity, metabolic disorders, mouth sores, ophthalmia (inflamed eye), phlegm removal, pinguecula (thickening of the white part of the eye), psoriasis (skin disease), pterygium (eye condition), quality of life, radioprotection, ringworm, skin diseases, snakebite, sore throat, stomach problems, stress, tonic, tuberculosis, ulcers, verminosis (parasitic worm disease), vomiting, whooping cough, wound healing.

DOSING

Adults (18 Years and Older)

- There is insufficient evidence to recommend a dose of holy basil. Traditionally, 300-2000 mg as a single dose of dried leaves has been used daily for preventive therapy, and 600-1800 mg in divided doses has been used daily for curative therapy. As a tea, 2 g holy basil has been infused in 1 cup of water. Also, 10-20 mL of fresh leaf juice or 1 oz of dried herb in 16 oz of water has been taken three times daily in 5-oz doses. For diabetes, 2.5 g of dried leaf powder by mouth every morning or 1 teaspoon dried herb brewed in 1 cup of water has been taken three times daily.

Children (Younger than 18 Years)

- There is insufficient evidence to recommend a dose for holy basil in children.

SAFETY

Allergies

- Avoid in individuals with a known allergy or hypersensitivity to holy basil (*Ocimum sanctum*).

Side Effects and Warnings

- Holy basil seems to be well tolerated in most people, and it has GRAS status in the United States.
- Holy basil may lower blood sugar levels. Caution is advised in patients with diabetes (high blood sugar) or hypoglycemia (low blood sugar) and in those taking drugs, herbs, or supplements that affect blood sugar. Serum glucose levels may need to be monitored by a qualified health care professional, including a pharmacist, and medication adjustments may be necessary.
- Although not well studied in humans, holy basil may have antispermatogenic (sperm-blocking) and antifertility effects.

- Holy basil may prolong bleeding time. Caution is advised in patients with bleeding disorders or taking drugs that may increase the risk of bleeding. Dosing adjustments may be necessary.

Pregnancy and Breastfeeding

- Holy basil is not recommended in pregnant or breastfeeding women. Based on traditional use, holy basil may stimulate uterine contractions.

INTERACTIONS
Interactions with Drugs

- Ursolic acid isolated from holy basil may somewhat protect against adriamycin-induced lipid peroxidation of liver and heart microsomes.
- Holy basil may increase the risk of bleeding when taken with drugs that increase the risk of bleeding. Some examples include aspirin, anticoagulants ("blood thinners") such as warfarin (Coumadin) or heparin, antiplatelet drugs such as clopidogrel (Plavix), and nonsteroidal antiinflammatory drugs (NSAIDS) such as ibuprofen (Motrin, Advil) or naproxen (Naprosyn, Aleve).
- Holy basil may interfere with the way the body processes certain drugs using the liver's cytochrome P450 enzyme system. As a result, the levels of these drugs may be increased in the blood and may cause increased effects or potentially serious adverse reactions. Patients using any medications should check the package insert and speak with a qualified health care professional, including a pharmacist, about possible interactions.
- Holy basil may reduce the amnesic (memory loss) effect of diazepam or scopolamine. Holy basil may increase the sedative effects of pentobarbital. Use caution if driving or operating heavy machinery.

- Holy basil may lower blood sugar levels. Caution is advised when medications that may also lower blood sugar are used. Patients taking drugs for diabetes by mouth or using insulin should be monitored closely by a qualified health care professional, including a pharmacist. Medication adjustments may be necessary.
- Caution is advised in patients taking statins or other cholesterol-lowering agents, as holy basil may reduce serum lipid levels.

Interactions with Herbs and Dietary Supplements

- Holy basil may increase the risk of bleeding when taken with herbs and supplements that are believed to increase the risk of bleeding. Multiple cases of bleeding have been reported with the use of *Ginkgo biloba*, and fewer cases have been reported with garlic and saw palmetto. Numerous other agents may theoretically increase the risk of bleeding, although this has not been proven in most cases.
- Holy basil may interfere with the way the body processes certain herbs or supplements using the liver's cytochrome P450 enzyme system. As a result, the levels of other herbs or supplements may become too high in the blood. It may also alter the effects that other herbs or supplements possibly have on the P450 system.
- Caution is advised in patients taking cholesterol-lowering agents, such as red yeast rice, as holy basil may reduce serum lipid levels.
- Holy basil may lower blood sugar levels. Caution is advised when herbs or supplements that may also lower blood sugar are used. Blood glucose levels may require monitoring, and doses may need adjustment.

For a complete list of references, please visit www.naturalstandard.com.

RELATED TERMS

- Acacia honey, adular, älskling, amour, andromedotoxin-containing honey, *Apis mellifera* (honey bee), apitherapy product, azalea honey, bee products, blackberry honey, blueberry honey, borage honey, buckwheat honey, chou, cielo, *Citrus sinensis* Osbeck, clarified honey, clover honey, coisa doce, comb honey, crystallized honey, deli bal, dried honey, endulzar, falar docemente, feng mi, flavonoids, grayanotoxin honey, hachimitsu, honeydew honey, honig, honing, honingkleur, honung, iets beeldigs, jelly bush honey, kamahi honey, kanuka honey, lastig portret, lavender honey, lief doen, liefje (aanspreekvorm), ling honey, ljuvhet, mad honey, madu, Manuka honey, mel, mel depuratum, melliferous products, miel, miel blanc, miele, mi vida, mooi praten, mountain laurel honey, namorado, nectar, Nigerian citrus honey, nodding thistle honey, orange blossom honey, pasture honey, purified honey, rata honey, raw honey, rewarewa honey, rhododendron honey, schatz, smöra, sourwood honey, strained honey, sunflower honey, tala smickrande, tansy ragwort honey, Tasmanian leatherwood honey, tawari honey, tesoro, toppensak, toxic honey, tupelo honey, tutan bal, versuikeren, vipers bugloss honey, vleien, whipped honey, wild thyme honey, zoet maken.

BACKGROUND

- Honey is a sweet, viscid fluid produced by honeybees (*Apis melliflera*) from the nectar of flowers. It is "generally recognized as safe" (GRAS), but there have been numerous reports of certain types of honey produced from the nectar of flowering plants from the genus *Rhododendron* and others that have toxic effects in humans and in animals.
- Honey is easily absorbed and utilized by the body. It contains about 70-80% sugar; the rest is water, minerals, and traces of protein, acids, and other substances. Honey has been used by ancient Egyptians, Assyrians, Chinese, Romans, and Greeks as a medicinal remedy for the management of wounds, skin ailments, and various gastrointestinal diseases.
- Honey's therapeutic importance as a known antibacterial agent has been recognized since 1892. Modern research has been conducted on the role of honey in chronic wound management and other indications. However, high-quality studies are lacking, and further research is warranted to establish the therapeutic effect of honey in any indication.

EVIDENCE

Uses Based on Scientific Evidence	Grade
Burns Preliminary evidence suggests that honey may reduce burn-healing time. Additional study is needed to make a firm recommendation.	C
Dermatitis (Dandruff) The evidence supporting the use of honey in the treatment of dermatitis and dandruff is limited.	C
Further investigation is needed to make a firm recommendation.	
Diabetes Mellitus Type 2 Preliminary evidence suggests that honey may help lower blood sugar levels in diabetic patients. However, the overall evidence is insufficient to support this use.	C
Fournier's Gangrene Currently, there is insufficient available evidence for the use of honey in the treatment of Fournier's gangrene.	C
Gastroenteritis (Infantile) Currently, there is insufficient human evidence to recommend honey for the treatment of infantile gastroenteritis.	C
Herpes Preliminary study found honey effective in treating labial but not genital herpes. More research is needed in this area to draw a firm conclusion.	C
Hypercholesterolemia (High Cholesterol) In general, the evidence supporting the use of honey to treat high cholesterol levels is weak.	C
Hypertension (High Blood Pressure) Currently, there is preliminary evidence that suggests benefit in the use of honey in the treatment of high blood pressure. However, the evidence is not sufficient to support this use.	C
Leg Ulcers Honey dressings have been used on leg ulcers with no apparent clinical benefit.	C
Plaque/Gingivitis Currently there is limited research showing a small benefit in the use of honey in the treatment of gingival plaque and gingivitis.	C
Radiation Mucositis Currently, there is insufficient available evidence to recommend for or against the use of honey for radiation mucositis.	C
Rhinoconjunctivitis Currently there is insufficient human evidence to recommend honey for the treatment of rhinoconjunctivitis. Preliminary study suggests no benefit.	C
Skin Graft Healing (Split Thickness) Currently there is insufficient human evidence to recommend honey for the treatment of split-thickness skin graft.	C

Uses Based on Scientific Evidence	Grade
Wound Healing The primary studied use of honey is for wound management, particularly in promoting rapid wound healing, deodorizing, and debriding necrotic tissue. The types of wounds studied are varied; most are nonhealing wounds such as chronic ulcers, postoperative wounds, and burns.	C

Uses Based on Tradition or Theory

Acidosis (excessive acidity), antacid, antiaging, antiinflammatory, antimicrobial, antimycotic (antifungal), antioxidant, antiparasitic, antitumor, asthma, atopic dermatitis, breast ulcers, cancer prevention, cataracts, conjunctivitis (pink eye), cough, dental caries, dental surgery adjunct, diarrhea, edema (swelling), expectorant, eye infections/inflammation, fever, *Helicobacter pylori* infection, hyperglycemia (high blood sugar), immunostimulant, infections, leprosy, oral rehydration, pain, postherpetic corneal opacities, pressure sores, psoriasis, respiratory infections, septicemia, skin care, skin disorders, tinea corporis, tinea cruris, tinea faciei.

DOSING
Adults (18 Years and Older)

- There is insufficient evidence to recommend a dose for honey in adults. Commercial preparations of honey are available, and honey is typically taken by mouth or applied on the skin. Doses for topical use are often nonspecific, but 15-30 mL is a common dose for Fournier's gangrene, burns, radiation-induced mucositis, skin ulcers, and other wounds. Various types of honey and honey products have been studied, including honey from wildflowers, *Camellia sinensis* honey, Medihoney dressings, Manuka honey, and Honey-Soft (honey-medicated dressing).
- For dermatitis and dandruff, a diluted solution of honey and warm water containing 90% water has been rubbed gently into the scalp for 2-3 minutes and then left on the scalp for 3 hours. For type 2 diabetes mellitus and hypertension (high blood pressure), honey solutions with 30-90 g of natural unprocessed honey with 250 mL of water have been studied.

Children (Younger than 18 Years)

- There is insufficient evidence to recommend a dose for honey in children, and use is not recommended. However, for neonatal postoperative infected wounds, 5-10 mL of commercial, unprocessed, nonpasteurized and nonirradiated honey applied locally to the wound and covered with a sterile gauze dressing has been used. Dressings were changed twice daily. Do not give honey to infants under 12 months of age because of potential toxicity of contaminated honey.

SAFETY
Allergies

- The components of honey responsible for allergic reactions, ranging from cough to anaphylaxis, are usually thought to be pollens, glandular secretions, and bee body material. There is some disagreement with the idea that honey allergies are primarily caused by the pollen particles found in the honey. Patients with polyvalent pollen or food allergies such as an allergy to celery, as well as patients with other bee-related allergens, should avoid honey consumption.
- Chronic pruritic cheilitis (dry, itchy lips), occupational asthma, urticaria on the hands, chronic bronchitis, bronchial asthma, angioedema (swelling under the skin) with dysphagia (difficulty swallowing), dysphonia (abnormal voice), and dyspnea (difficulty breathing) have all been reported.

Side Effects and Warnings

- In general, honey is well tolerated in the recommended doses and for daily consumption. Honey has GRAS status in the United States. However, there are reported cases of honey intoxication documented in the literature as an adverse effect of consuming toxic honey, also known as "mad honey," which is produced from the nectar of certain flowering plants such as those of the genus *Rhododendron*. The symptoms of honey intoxication vary from case to case and may include weakness, sweating, hypotension (low blood pressure), bradycardia (lowered heart rate), Wolff-Parkinson-White syndrome, gastritis (inflammation of the stomach), peptic ulcer, nausea, vomiting, faintness, leukocytosis (abnormally high white blood cell count), mild paralysis, dizziness, vertigo, blurred vision, convulsions, and respiratory rate depression. Avoid the use of honey that is produced from the nectar of flowering plants of the genus *Rhododendron*.
- There is a concern in some third world countries that the topical use of honey on deep leprotic (of leprosy) ulcers may increase the risk of maggot infestation in the wound by houseflies and bluebottle flies. Topically, honey may cause excessive dryness of wounds, which may delay healing. Applying saline packs as needed may treat this.
- Honey contains fructose in excess of glucose, which may lead to incomplete fructose absorption associated with abdominal symptoms and/or diarrhea.
- Many cases of infant botulism (bacterial illness) caused by consumption of honey containing *Clostridium botulinum* spore have been reported. *Clostridium botulinum* spores can proliferate in the intestines of infants and cause botulism poisoning. However, this potential risk does not pertain to older children or adults. Do not give honey to infants under 12 months of age. Because of honey's acidity, another concern is that the practice of keeping honey in the mouth for a prolonged period may erode dental enamel.

Pregnancy and Breastfeeding

- There are some concerns regarding the use of honey in pregnant and breastfeeding women. Potentially harmful contaminants such as *C. botulinum* and grayanotoxins can be found in some types of honey and may be harmful to pregnant or breastfeeding woman and to the growing fetus.

INTERACTIONS
Interactions with Drugs

- Theoretically, honey used in combination with other antibiotics may have an additive effect. Caution is advised.

- Although not well studied in humans, honey may interact with carbamazepine. Patients taking anticonvulsants should use honey with caution.
- Nigerian *Citrus sinensis* Osbeck honey reduces peak blood alcohol (ethanol) levels. Interactions with alcohol are possible, and patients should consult with a qualified health care professional, including a pharmacist.
- Although honey has been investigated in the treatment of diabetes and lowering plasma glucose, honey is composed of sugars (mainly fructose and glucose). Based on its composition, honey may increase blood sugar levels when taken orally, and caution is advised in patients taking antidiabetic agents.

Interactions with Herbs and Dietary Supplements

- Theoretically, honey used in combination with other antibiotics may have an additive effect. Caution is advised.
- Although honey has been investigated in the treatment of diabetes and lowering plasma glucose, honey is composed of sugars (mainly fructose and glucose). Based on its composition, honey may increase blood sugar levels when taken orally, and caution is advised in patients taking herbs or supplements that alter blood sugar.

For a complete list of references, please visit www.naturalstandard.com.

Honeysuckle

(*Lonicera* spp.)

RELATED TERMS

- Caprifoliaceae (family), Chinese honeysuckle, coral honey-suckle, eglantine, European honeysuckle, Hall's Japanese honeysuckle, Japanese honeysuckle, *Lonicera caerulea, Lonicera japonica, Lonicera japonica* halliana, *Lonicera periclymenum, Lonicera sempervirens, Lonicera* spp., trumpet honeysuckle, white honeysuckle, woodbine honeysuckle, woodbine.

BACKGROUND

- There are at least 180 species of honeysuckle, with most species found in Asia and a few in Europe and the Americas.
- In homeopathy, honeysuckle has been used for asthma, breathing difficulties, irritability with violent outbursts, and syphilis. However, currently there is a lack of clinical evidence supporting the use of honeysuckle for these conditions or any other indication.
- Honeysuckle poisoning from ingestion by children may cause severe gastrointestinal symptoms and cramping.

EVIDENCE

Uses Basedon Scientific Evidence

No available studies qualify for inclusion in the evidence table.

Uses Based on Tradition or Theory

Asthma, breathing difficulties, irritability (with violent outbursts), syphilis (STD).

DOSING

Adults (18 Years and Older)

- There is insufficient evidence to recommend a dose for honeysuckle in adults.

Children (Younger than 18 Years)

- There is insufficient evidence to recommend a dose for honeysuckle in children.

SAFETY

Allergies

- Avoid in individuals with a known allergy or hypersensitivity to honeysuckle (*Lonicera* spp.) or its constituents. Itchy raised blisters on the wrist have been reported after pulling Hall's Japanese honeysuckle (*Lonicera japonica* halliana).

Side Effects and Warnings

- There is insufficient evidence in humans to support the use of honeysuckle for any indication. Honeysuckle poisoning from ingestion may cause severe gastrointestinal symptoms and cramping. In addition, honeysuckle may cause contact dermatitis.

Pregnancy and Breastfeeding

- Honeysuckle is not recommended in pregnant or breastfeeding women because of a lack of available scientific evidence.

INTERACTIONS

Interactions with Drugs

- Insufficient evidence is available.

Interactions with Herbs and Dietary Supplements

- Insufficient evidence is available.

For a complete list of references, please visit www.naturalstandard.com.

Hoodia
(Hoodia gordonii)

RELATED TERMS

- Apocynaceae (family), cactus, Ghaap, hoodia cactus, *Hoodia gordonii*, hoodia P57, Hoodoba, Kalahari cactus, Kalahari diet, P57, South African desert cactus, South African hoodia, Xhoba, xhooba.

BACKGROUND

- *Hoodia* is a genus in the plant family Apocynaceae. Although hoodia was introduced to the West in early 2004, the Bushmen of the Kalahari have been eating it for a long time to help ward off hunger and thirst during long trips in the desert.
- Unlike ephedra, hoodia does not work as a stimulant; it acts as an appetite suppressant. The pharmaceutical company, Phytopharm, finds hoodia promising and is currently trying to isolate the appetite-suppressing molecule, P57, to create a patented diet drug in the future. P57 was at one time licensed to Pfizer for development but was discontinued in 2003.
- There are no available reliable human trials demonstrating efficacy and safety. BBC news reports from 2003 suggested that some samples of hoodia products sold on the Internet might show no evidence of containing actual hoodia.

EVIDENCE

Uses Based on Scientific Evidence

No available studies qualify for inclusion in the evidence table.

Uses Based on Tradition or Theory

Appetite suppressant, energy improvement, mood enhancement, nutritional deficiencies, thirst, weight reduction.

DOSING

Adults (18 Years and Older)

- There is insufficient evidence to recommend a dose for hoodia. However, hoodia is popularly used for weight loss, and dried extracts (20:1) with a dosage ranging from 400-800 mg daily have been used.

Children (Younger than 18 Years)

- There is insufficient evidence to recommend a dose for hoodia in children, and use is not recommended.

SAFETY

Allergies

- Avoid in individuals with a known allergy or hypersensitivity to hoodia.

Side Effects and Warnings

- Currently, there is a lack of available information about the safety of hoodia. Hoodia is popularly used as a weight loss agent, and use may suppress appetite. Safety in children is unknown.

Pregnancy and Breastfeeding

- The use of hoodia during pregnancy and breastfeeding should be avoided because of a lack of safety studies.

INTERACTIONS

Interactions with Drugs

- There is not enough available scientific evidence to report drug interactions. However, hoodia is popularly used for weight loss, and it may interact with other medications that are appetite suppressants.

Interactions with Herbs and Dietary Supplements

- There is not enough available scientific evidence to report herb and supplement interactions. However, hoodia is popularly used for weight loss, and it may interact with other appetite-suppressing herbs and supplements.

For a complete list of references, please visit www.naturalstandard.com.

Hop
(Humulus lupulus)

RELATED TERMS

- 2-Methyl-3-butene-2-ol, 8-prenylnaringenin (8-PN), beer, Cannabaceae (family), colupulone, common hop, European hops, hop, hop strobile, Hopfen (German), houblon (French), humulon, humulus, *Humulus lupulus*, iso-alpha-acids, lupulin, lupulus, Lupuli strobulus, prenylated 2'-hydroxychalcones, prenylflavonoids, spent hop, xanthohumol, Ze 91019.

BACKGROUND

- The hop is a member of the Cannabaceae family, traditionally used for relaxation, sedation, and to treat insomnia. A number of methodologically weak human trials have investigated hop in combination with valerian (*Valeriana officinalis*) for the treatment of sleep disturbances, and several animal studies have examined the sedative properties of hop alone. However, the results of these studies are equivocal, and there is currently insufficient evidence to recommend hop alone or in combination for any medical condition.

- Hop is also sometimes found in combination products with passionflower (*Passiflora incarnata*), skullcap (potentially damaging to the liver), or with a high percentage of alcohol (up to 70% grain alcohol), which confounds the association between the herb and possible sedative or hypnotic effects.

- Hop contains phytoestrogens that may possess estrogen receptor agonist or antagonist properties with unclear effects on hormone-sensitive conditions, such as breast, uterine, cervical, or prostate cancer or endometriosis.

EVIDENCE

Uses Based on Scientific Evidence	Grade
Insomnia/sleep quality Animal studies report that hop may have sedative and sleep-enhancing (hypnotic) effects. However, little human research has evaluated the effects of hop on sleep quality.	C
Menopausal symptoms When used in combination with other products, hop may help alleviate menopausal symptoms, such as hot flashes and difficulty sleeping, because it has estrogen-like activity. However, clinical evidence is not sufficient to establish effectiveness.	C
Rheumatic diseases Preliminary clinical research suggests that a combination formula containing hop may help reduce symptoms of rheumatic diseases, such as osteoarthritis, rheumatoid arthritis, and fibromyalgia. The isolated effects of hop alone are unclear to determine whether these positive effects are specifically the result of hop.	C
Sedation Hop has been used traditionally as a sedative, for relaxation and reduction of anxiety. Although some animal studies suggest possible sedative properties, there is limited human research in this area.	C

Uses Based on Tradition or Theory

Analgesic, antibacterial (antimycobacterial), antidepressant, antifungal, antiinflammatory, antispasmodic, antiviral (anti-hepatitis C virus [HCV], anti-rhino, anti-herpes virus), anxiety, aphrodisiac, appetite stimulant, asbestosis, atherosclerosis (hardening of the arteries), atopic dermatitis, breast enhancer, cancer (breast, uterine, cervical, prostate), Crohn's disease, depression, diabetes, digestion, dysentery, dyspepsia, Epstein-Barr virus, estrogen-like activity, heartburn, high cholesterol levels, irritable bowel syndrome (IBS), kidney disorders, leprosy, leukemia (HL-60), mood disturbances, muscle spasm, nervous disorders, obesity, osteoporosis, pain, parasites and worms, restlessness, skin ulcers (topical), spine problems (scoliosis), tuberculosis.

DOSING
Adults (18 Years and Older)

- For insomnia or sleep disturbances, studies have used 300-400 mg of hop extract combined with 240-300 mg of valerian extract, taken by mouth before bed. Traditionally, doses of 0.5-1.0 g of dried hop extract or 0.5-1.0 mL of liquid hop extract (1:1 in 45% alcohol) have been taken up to three times daily, although using hop alone has not been well studied.

- Intravenous/intramuscular dosing is not recommended.

Children (Younger than 18 Years)

- Hop extract is traditionally considered to be one of the milder sedative herbs and to be safe for children. However, there is limited research in this area, and safety has not been clearly established.

SAFETY
Allergies

- Rash (contact dermatitis) and difficulty breathing have been reported, mainly in hop harvesters. Allergy to hop pollen has also been reported. Hop allergy has been reported in a patient with previous severe allergic reactions to peanut, chestnut, and banana. Therefore people allergic to any of these agents should avoid hop.

Side Effects and Warnings

- Dry cough, difficulty breathing, chronic bronchitis, and other occupational respiratory diseases have been associated with hop. Dust from hop can contain harmful bacteria. Long-term breathing problems have been reported.

- Hop may cause mild central nervous system (CNS) depression (drowsiness and slowed breathing and thinking), especially when taken with drugs or herbs or supplements that also cause CNS depression. Use caution while driving or operating machinery.
- Eating hop in large quantities may cause seizure, hyperthermia, restlessness, vomiting, stomach pain, and increased stomach acid. It is unclear what effects may occur in hormone-sensitive conditions such as cancer (breast, uterine, cervical, prostate) or endometriosis.
- Hop may lower blood sugar levels in healthy individuals but may actually increase blood sugar in those with diabetes. Caution is advised in patients with diabetes or hypoglycemia and in those taking drugs, herbs, or supplements that affect blood sugar. Serum glucose levels may need to be monitored by a health care provider, and medication adjustments may be necessary.

Pregnancy and Breastfeeding

- Hop is not recommended during pregnancy or lactation because of possible hormonal and sedative effects. Limited research is available in these areas. Many tinctures contain high levels of alcohol and should be avoided during pregnancy.

INTERACTIONS
Interactions with Drugs

- Hop may cause mild CNS depression (drowsiness and slowed breathing and thinking) and may add to the effects of drugs that also cause CNS depression or sedation. Examples include benzodiazepines such as lorazepam (Ativan) or diazepam (Valium), barbiturates such as phenobarbital, narcotics such as codeine, some antidepressants, and alcohol. Use caution while driving or operating machinery.
- Based on preliminary animal studies, hop may lower blood sugar levels in healthy individuals but may actually increase blood sugar levels in those with diabetes. Caution is advised when medications that may also lower blood sugar are used. Patients taking drugs for diabetes by mouth or using insulin should be monitored closely by a qualified health care provider. Medication adjustments may be necessary.
- Laboratory research shows that estrogen-like substances in hop may have stimulatory or inhibitory effects on estrogen-sensitive parts of the body. It is not clear what interactions may occur when used with other hormonal therapies such as birth control pills, hormone replacement therapy, tamoxifen, or aromatase inhibitors like letrozole (Femara).
- Hop may interfere with the way the body processes certain drugs using the liver's cytochrome P450 enzyme system. As a result, the levels of these drugs may be decreased in the blood and the intended effects may be reduced. Patients using any medications should check the package insert and speak with a health care professional or pharmacist about possible interactions.
- Taking phenothiazine antipsychotic drugs with hop is said to possibly increase the risk of hyperthermia (increased body temperature), although there is a lack of reliable human studies in this area.
- Many tinctures contain high levels of alcohol and may cause nausea or vomiting when taken with metronidazole (Flagyl) or disulfiram (Antabuse).
- Hop compounds have also been shown to reduce triglyceride and free fatty acid blood levels and therefore may have additive effects with cholesterol-lowering drugs such as lovastatin (Mevacor).
- Hop may also interact with antibiotic, antidepressant, antifungal, antiinflammatory, and gastrointestinal drugs.

Interactions with Herbs and Dietary Supplements

- Hop may cause mild CNS depression (drowsiness and slowed breathing and thinking) and may add to the effects of herbs or supplements that also cause CNS depression or sedation. Use caution while driving or operating machinery.
- Based on preliminary animal studies, hop may lower blood sugar levels in healthy individuals but may actually increase blood sugar levels in those with diabetes. Caution is advised when herbs or supplements that may also affect blood sugar are used. Blood glucose levels may require monitoring, and doses may need adjustment.
- Hop may interfere with the way the body processes certain drugs using the liver's cytochrome P450 enzyme system. As a result, the levels of other herbs or supplements may become too low in the blood. It may also alter the effects that other herbs or supplements potentially may have on the P450 system. Patients using any medications should check the package insert and speak with a health care professional, including a pharmacist, about possible interactions.
- Because hop contain estrogen-like chemicals, the effects of other agents believed to have estrogen-like properties may be altered.
- Hop compounds have also been shown to reduce triglyceride and free fatty acid blood levels and therefore may have additive effects with cholesterol-lowering herbs and supplements such as guggul or red yeast rice.
- Hop may also interact with antibacterial, antidepressant, antifungal, antiinflammatory, antineoplastic, antioxidant, antipsychotic, and gastrointestinal supplements.

For a complete list of references, please visit www.naturalstandard.com.

Horny Goat Weed
(Epimedium grandiflorum)

RELATED TERMS

- Acetylicariin, apigenin, baohuoside I, baohuoside II, barren-wort, benzene, Berberidaceae (family), breviflavone B, bux-ueyangyan mixture, caohuoside B, chrysoeriol, desmethylanhydroicaritin, desmethylicaritin, diphylloside B, Epimedii, Epimedii Herba, epimedin A, epimedin B, epimedin C, *Epimedium acuminatum* Franch., *Epimedium brevicornum* Maxim., *Epimedium cremeum*, *Epimedium coactum*, *Epimedium davidii*, *Epimedium diphyllum*, *Epimedium flavone*, *Epimedium grandiflorum* Morr., *Epimedium grandiflorum* var. *flavescens*, *Epimedium hunanense*, *Epimedium koreanum* Nakai, *Epimedium leptorrhizum*, *Epimedium pubescens* Maxim., *Epimedium sagittatum* (Sieb. et Zucc.) Maxim., *Epimedium sempervirens*, *Epimedium truncatum*, *Epimedium wushanense* T.S. Ying, epimedokoreanoside-I, epimedoside A, epimedoside E, Herba Epimedii, huichun zhibao, hyperin, icariin, icarisid II, icaritin, ikarisoside A, ikarisoside C, ikarisoside F, Japanese epimedium, kaempferol, korepimedoside A, korepimedoside B linolenic acid, luteolin, magnoflorine, O-methylicariin, oleic acid, palmitic acid, prenylflavone, quercetin, sagittatoside A, sagittatoside B, sterols, syringaresinol, tannin, vitamin E, wanepimedoside A, xian ling pi, xin-qin granule (long-spur epimedium), yin yang huo, zuo-gui-wan.

BACKGROUND

- The leaves of as many as 15 species of *Epimedium* are used as the herb known as yin yang huo in traditional Chinese medicine. *Yin yang huo* is usually translated as horny goat weed because the Chinese characters literally mean "obscene goat leaves of pulse plants."

- In traditional Chinese medicine, *Epimedium* (yin yang huo) is used as a bodybuilding agent, a yang supporter, an agent to reinforce muscles and bones, and a supporter of the health of the liver and kidneys. This herb is also commonly used to treat angina pectoris (chest pain), chronic bronchitis, and neurasthenia (nervous exhaustion). As with many other herbs in Chinese medicine, horny goat weed is rarely used as a single ingredient. Horny goat weed is traditionally used as an ingredient in a yang tonic and for combating wind-damp-cold blocking qi circulation.

- Despite its traditional and popular use, there is little scientific evidence in support of horny goat weed. Currently, there exists a potential benefit for the treatment of atherosclerosis symptoms and quality of life associated with hemodialysis. Other promising areas include sexual function.

EVIDENCE

Uses Based on Scientific Evidence	Grade
Atherosclerosis Horny goat weed is traditionally used to treat cardiovascular disease. Preliminary evidence suggests that horny goat weed may improve symptoms associated with ischemic cardiocerebral vascular diseases. However, clinical evidence is insufficient to support this use.	C

Sexual Dysfunction (in Renal Failure Patients) Horny goat weed is traditionally used to increase fertility. One study suggests that horny goat weed may improve sexual performance and quality of life in patients with renal failure on chronic hemodialysis. However, evidence is insufficient to support this use.	C

Uses Based on Tradition or Theory

Abortion, adrenal cortex function (atrophy), aging, allergy/hay fever, Alzheimer's disease, amenorrhea (absence of menstruation), analgesia, angina, antibacterial, antiinflammatory, antimicrobial, antioxidant, antitussive (preventing or relieving cough), antiviral, aphrodisiac, asthma, cancer, chronic bronchitis, chronic hepatitis, cognitive improvement, cold prevention, coronary heart disease, erectile dysfunction, exercise performance enhancement, expectorant, fatigue, hepatoprotection, human immunodeficiency syndrome/acquired immunodeficiency syndrome (HIV/AIDS), hypercholesterolemia (high cholesterol levels), hyperhomocysteinemia, hypertension (high blood pressure), immunosuppression, impotence, infertility, kidney protection, leukopenia, memory, menopause, muscle ache, myocarditis/endocarditis, neurasthenia, osteoporosis, ovulation disorders, paralysis, platelet aggregation inhibition, prostate cancer, quality of life, renal failure (insufficiency), respiratory distress, thyroid disorders, tonic, viral infection (polio), yang insufficiency.

DOSING
Adults (18 Years and Older)

- There is insufficient evidence to recommend a dose for horny goat weed. In general, 6-15 g daily has been used. A decoction (5 g of horny goat weed simmered in 250 mL of water for 10-15 minutes) three times daily has been used. A similar amount of horny goat weed has been used in the form of granules (freeze-dried grains made from decocted herb) or powdered herb in capsules. Also, 5 mL of 20% tincture has been used three times daily before meals.

- For angina pectoris, chronic bronchitis, and neurasthenia, four to six 0.3-g tablets (equivalent to 2.7 g of raw material in each tablet) has been used twice daily for 1 month, stopping administration for 7-10 days and then resuming in a second series if required.

- Intramuscular injections have also been used in ampoules of 2 mL (equivalent to 1 g of raw material). Injections should be given only under the guidance of a qualified health care professional, including a pharmacist.

Children (Younger than 18 Years)

- There is insufficient evidence to recommend a dose for horny goat weed in children, and use is not recommended.

SAFETY
Allergies

- Avoid in individuals with a known allergy or hypersensitivity to horny goat weed (*Epimedium grandiflorum*).

Side Effects and Warnings

- In general, horny goat weed is well tolerated. Based on long-term traditional use in Chinese culture, horny goat weed is possibly safe when taken by mouth at recommended doses. However, avoid use of horny goat weed in patients with fire from yin deficiency (people with too much "yang" or heat, masculinity, and activity, based on Chinese philosophy).
- Gastrointestinal complaints, such as nausea, vomiting, and dryness of the mouth, are the most common side effects. Other side effects may include tachyarrhythmia (disturbance in the regular rhythm of the heartbeat), fever, or hypomania (a mild form of mania). Horny goat weed may also dilate coronary vessels and lower blood pressure. Long-term use may cause aggressiveness, irritability, or respiratory arrest. Extended use of Japanese Epimedium taken by mouth may result in nosebleed, exaggeration of tendon reflexes to the point of spasm, or dizziness. Certain compounds isolated from *Epimedium davidii* may affect immune responses in some individuals. Use cautiously in patients with immune function disorders because of the potential for worsening symptoms.
- Based on these side effects, horny goat weed is possibly unsafe when used in patients with tachyarrhythmia, decreased blood pressure, frequent nosebleeds, musculoskeletal disorders, bipolar disorder, immune function disorders, homocysteine disorders, thyroid disorders, respiratory distress, hormone-sensitive conditions, or cardiovascular disease.

Pregnancy and Breastfeeding

- Horny goat weed is not recommended in pregnant or breastfeeding women because of a lack of available scientific evidence. Horny goat weed may increase testosterone and estrogen levels in the body.

INTERACTIONS
Interactions with Drugs

- Horny goat weed may increase the risk of bleeding. Caution is advised in patients with bleeding disorders or taking drugs that may increase the risk of bleeding. Dosing adjustments may be necessary.
- Horny goat weed may lower cholesterol levels or blood pressure. Caution is advised in patients taking medications that also lower cholesterol levels or blood pressure. Consult with a qualified health care professional, including a pharmacist, before combining therapies.
- Horny goat weed has hormonal effects and may interact with certain medications, such as menopausal agents or birth control pills.
- Based on preliminary study, horny goat weed may also interact with immunostimulating, immunosuppressing, or thyroid medications. Caution is advised.
- One species, *Epimedium brevicornum*, may inhibit the activity of monoamine oxidase in the hypothalamus. Caution is advised when horny goat weed is taken with other monoamine oxidase inhibitors (MAOIs), such as MAOI antidepressants.

Interactions with Herbs and Dietary Supplements

- Horny goat weed may increase the risk of bleeding. Caution is advised in patients with bleeding disorders or taking herbs or supplements that may increase the risk of bleeding. Dose adjustments may be necessary.
- Horny goat weed may lower cholesterol levels or blood pressure. Caution is advised in patients taking herbs and supplements that also lower cholesterol levels or blood pressure. Consult with a qualified health care professional, including a pharmacist, before combining therapies.
- Horny goat weed may have hormonal effects and may interact with certain herbs and supplements that also have hormonal effects, such as black cohosh or St. John's wort.
- Based on preliminary study, horny goat weed may also interact with immunostimulating, immunosuppressing, or thyroid herbs and supplements. Caution is advised.
- One species, *Epimedium brevicornum*, may inhibit the activity of monoamine oxidase in the hypothalamus. Caution is advised when horny goat weed is taken with other herbs and supplements with MAOI activity.

For a complete list of references, please visit www.naturalstandard.com.

Horse Chestnut
(*Aesculus hippocastanum*)

RELATED TERMS

- Aescin, aescine, Aesculaforce, aescule, aesculetin, buckeye, bongay, chestnut, conkers, conquerors, coumarins, eschilo, escin, escina, escine, fatty acids, fish poison, flavonoids, graine de marronier d'Inde, fraxetin glucoside, fraxin, HCSC, *Hippocastani vulgare* Gaertnhestekastanje, *Hippocastani folium*, Hippocastanaceae (family), Hippocastani semen, horsechestnut, horse chestnut seed extract (HCSE), linolenic acid, Marron Europeen, Marronier, NV-101, palmitic acid, quinines, Rokastaniensamen, rosskastanie, scopoletin glucoside, scopolin, Spanish chestnut, steric acid, sterols, tannins, Venastat, Venoplant, Venostasin.

BACKGROUND

- HCSE is widely used in Europe for chronic venous insufficiency (CVI), a syndrome that may include leg swelling, varicose veins, leg pain, itching, and skin ulcers. Although HCSE is traditionally recommended for a variety of medical conditions, CVI is the only condition for which there is strong supportive scientific evidence.
- Side effects from HCSE have been similar to placebo in clinical trials. However, because of an increased risk of low blood sugar levels, caution is advised in children and people with diabetes.

EVIDENCE

Uses Based on Scientific Evidence	Grade
Chronic Venous Insufficiency Chronic venous insufficiency (CVI) is a condition that is more commonly diagnosed in Europe than in the United States and may include leg swelling, varicose veins, leg pain, itching, and skin ulcers. There is evidence from laboratory, animal, and human research that horse chestnut seed extract (HCSE) may be beneficial to patients with this condition. Studies report significant decreases in leg size, leg pain, itchiness, fatigue, and "tenseness." There is preliminary evidence that HCSE may be as effective as compression stockings.	A

Uses Based on Tradition or Theory
Angiogenesis, benign prostatic hypertrophy (BPH or enlarged prostate), bladder disorders (incontinence, cystitis), bruising, cough, diarrhea, dizziness, fever, fluid in the lungs (pulmonary edema), gall bladder disease, gall bladder infection (cholecystitis), gall bladder pain (colic), gall bladder stones (cholelithiasis), hemorrhoids, kidney diseases, leg cramps, liver congestion, lung blood clots (pulmonary embolism), menstrual pain, nerve pain, osteoarthritis, pancreatitis, postoperative/posttraumatic soft tissue swelling, rectal complaints, rheumatoid arthritis, ringing in the ears (tinnitus), skin conditions, ulcers, varicose leg ulcers, varicose veins, vein clots (deep venous thrombosis), whooping cough.

DOSING

Adults (18 Years and Older)

- A dose of 300 mg every 12 hours, for up to 12 weeks (containing 50-75 mg of escin per dose), has been taken by mouth. A dose of 600 mg of chestnut seed extract per day has also been studied.
- A gel preparation of horse chestnut containing 2% escin (applied to the skin three to four times daily) has been studied for bruising, without clear benefits.
- Severe allergic reaction (anaphylactic shock) has been reported with intravenous use. Horse chestnut leaf has been associated with liver inflammation (hepatitis) after injection into muscle.

Children (Younger than 18 Years)

- There is insufficient scientific evidence to recommend use of horse chestnut in children. Deaths have been reported in children who ate raw horse chestnut seeds or tea made from horse chestnut leaves and twigs.

SAFETY

Allergies

- HCSE may cause an allergic reaction in patients with known allergy to horse chestnuts, esculin, or any of its ingredients (flavonoids, biosides, trisides of quertins, and oligosaccharides including 1-ketose and 2-ketose). Anaphylactic shock (severe allergic reaction) has been reported with intravenous (through the vein) use.
- Allergic skin rashes (contact dermatitis) have been reported after use of a skin cream containing HCSE.

Side Effects and Warnings

- Unprocessed horse chestnut seeds have been associated with significant toxicity and death. Symptoms associated with horse chestnut poisoning may include vomiting, diarrhea, headache, confusion, weakness, muscle twitching, poor coordination, coma, or paralysis. HCSE standardized to escin content should not contain significant levels of esculin and should not have the same risks.
- Standardized HCSE is generally considered to be safe in adults at recommended doses for short periods of time. Stomach upset, muscular (calf) spasm, headache, dizziness, nausea, and itching have been reported. Contact skin irritation (dermatitis) has been reported following application of HCSE to the skin.
- Based on animal study, HCSE may cause lowered blood sugar levels. Caution is advised in patients with diabetes or hypoglycemia and in those taking drugs, herbs, or supplements that affect blood sugar. Serum glucose levels may need to be monitored by a qualified health care provider, and medication adjustments may be necessary.
- In theory, horse chestnut may increase the risk of bleeding. Caution is advised in patients with bleeding disorders or taking drugs that may increase the risk of bleeding. Monitoring is recommended, and dosing adjustments may be necessary. Liver and kidney toxicity

has been associated with horse chestnut. Aflatoxins, considered to be cancer-causing agents, have been identified in commercial skin products containing horse chestnut but not in HCSE.

- Several studies report the development of pseudolupus (a syndrome characterized by recurrent fever, muscle pain, and lung and heart muscle inflammation) in patients taking Venocuran or Venopyronum, which contains phenopyrazone, horse chestnut extract, and cardiac glycosides. Because these are combination products, these effects may not be accounted for by horse chestnut alone.

Pregnancy and Breastfeeding

- There is not enough scientific research to recommend the safe use of horse chestnut or HCSE during pregnancy and breastfeeding.

INTERACTIONS
Interactions with Drugs

- In theory, because of its esculin constituents, horse chestnut (but not HCSE, which when properly prepared does not contain esculin) may theoretically increase the risk of bleeding when taken with drugs that increase the risk of bleeding. Some examples include aspirin, anticoagulants ("blood thinners") such as warfarin (Coumadin) or heparin, antiplatelet drugs such as clopidogrel (Plavix), and nonsteroidal antiinflammatory drugs such as ibuprofen (Motrin, Advil) or naproxen (Naprosyn, Aleve).
- In theory and based on limited animal study, HCSE may have an additive effect when taken with drugs that cause hypoglycemia (low blood sugar levels). Caution is advised when medications that may also lower blood sugar are used. Patients taking drugs for diabetes by mouth or using insulin should be monitored closely by a qualified health care provider. Medication adjustments may be necessary.
- Escin in HCSE may theoretically interfere with protein-bound drugs such as phenytoin (Dilantin), warfarin (Coumadin), or amiodarone (Cordarone), although human evidence is lacking.
- HCSE has been demonstrated to have antiangiogenic activity and may thus interact with antiangiogenic drugs.

Interactions with Herbs and Dietary Supplements

- In theory, because of its esculin constituents, horse chestnut (but not HCSE, which when properly prepared does not contain esculin) may theoretically increase the risk of bleeding when taken with herbs or supplements that increase the risk of bleeding. Multiple cases of bleeding have been reported with the use of *Ginkgo biloba*, and fewer cases have been reported with garlic and saw palmetto. Numerous other agents may theoretically increase the risk of bleeding, although this has not been proven in most cases.
- In theory, and based on limited animal study, horse chestnut seed extract may have an additive effect when taken with other herbs or supplements that may lower blood sugar levels. Blood glucose levels may require monitoring, and doses may need adjustment.
- In theory, horse chestnut may interact with neurological herbs and supplements.

For a complete list of references, please visit www. naturalstandard.com.

Horseradish
(Armoracia rusticana, syn. Cochlearia armoracia)

RELATED TERMS

- Allyl isothiocyanate, allylisothiocyanate, *Armoracia lapathifolia* Gilib., *Armoracia rusticana*, *Armoracia rusticana* Gaertner, *Armoracia sativa* Heller, Amoraciae Rusticanae Radix, Bohemian horseradish, Brassicaceae (family), *Cochlearia armoracia*, *Cochlearia rusticana* Lamarck, common horseradish, glucobrassicin, gluconasturtiin, glucosinolates, great raifort, horseradish peroxidase, horseradish peroxidase/indole-3-acetic acid, isoenzymes, isothiocyanates, Meerrettich (German), mountain radish, myrosinase, neoglucobrassicin, pepperrot, phosphatidylcholines, red cole, seiyowasabi (Japanese), sinigrin, thioglucoside conjugates, Western wasabi.
- **Note:** This monograph does not include wasabi (*Wasabia japonica*), for which horseradish is a common substitute. The U.S. Food and Drug Administration (FDA) defines horseradish as the root of *Armoracia lapathifolia* Gilib. This monograph uses the more common scientific name *Armoracia rusticana*, which is used by the U.S. Department of Agriculture (USDA).

BACKGROUND

- Horseradish (*Armoracia rusticana*) is a hardy perennial plant of the Brassicaceae family, which includes mustard and cabbage. Large doses by mouth can cause gastrointestinal upset, bloody vomiting, diarrhea, and irritation of mucous membranes and the urinary tract. Horseradish may also provoke allergic reactions.
- Although horseradish may be irritating, it is frequently used as a condiment or spice, especially for beef, sausages, and fish. The U.S. FDA has given horseradish (*Armoracia lapathifolia* Gilib.) "generally recognized as safe" (GRAS) status as a seasoning, spice, and flavoring (the FDA currently accepts *Armoracia lapathifolia* as the binomial name for horseradish, although *Armoracia rusticana* is more commonly used and is the preferred name by the USDA).
- Traditionally, horseradish has been used for pain, rheumatism, and cancer. It has also been studied for bronchitis, sinusitis, and urinary tract infections, but additional study is needed before making firm recommendations.

EVIDENCE

Uses Based on Scientific Evidence	Grade
Bronchitis Horseradish may have antibiotic activity and has been used in combination with other herbs to treat bronchitis. However, the effectiveness of horseradish as a single therapy is unclear.	C
Sinusitis Horseradish may have antibiotic activity and has been used in combination with other herbs to treat sinusitis. However, the effectiveness of horseradish as a single therapy is unclear.	C

Urinary Tract Infection	C
Horseradish may have antibiotic activity and has been used in combination with other herbs to treat urinary tract infections. However, the effectiveness of horseradish as a single therapy is unclear.	

Uses Based on Tradition or Theory

Abortion, allergies, anodyne (pain reliever), antibiotic, anticoagulant (blood thinner), antihypertensive (blood pressure–lowering), antiinflammatory, antimutagenic, arthritis, blood cleanser, bruises, cancer, carminative (relieves gas), childbirth (expelling afterbirth), colic, cough, diaphoretic (promotes sweating), digestive, diuretic (increases urine flow), dropsy (swelling), edema (swelling), emetic (induces vomiting), expectorant (encourages coughing up of mucus), fever, food uses, gallbladder disorders, gout (foot inflammation), headaches, hoarseness, infections, inflammation, intestinal worms (in children), lower back pain, muscle aches, neuralgia (facial nerve pain), paralysis, pleurisy (lung inflammation), respiratory disorders, rheumatism (painful disorder of the joints, muscle, or connective tissue), saliva stimulant, sciatica (irritation of the sciatic nerve resulting in pain or tingling running down the inside of the leg), scurvy, skin conditions (rubefacient), skin fairness, stimulant, tuberculosis, urinary stones, wounds.

DOSING
Adults (18 Years and Older)

- There is insufficient evidence to recommend a dose of horseradish in adults.

Children (Younger than 18 Years)

- There is insufficient evidence to recommend a dose of horseradish in children.

SAFETY
Allergies

- Avoid in individuals with a known allergy or hypersensitivity to horseradish (*Armoracia rusticana*), its constituents, or members of the Brassicaceae family. Large doses taken by mouth may provoke allergic reactions.

Side Effects and Warnings

- Horseradish is likely safe when the root is used in food amounts. The U.S. FDA has given horseradish GRAS status as a seasoning, spice, and flavoring.
- There are few reported adverse effects associated with horseradish. Possible side effects include abortion, aggravated stomach ulcers, esophageal irritation or other stomach conditions, allergic reactions, blistering, bloody vomiting, burning pain at the epigastrium, depressed thyroid function, diarrhea, diuresis, gastrointestinal upset, irritation of the mouth, pharynx, esophagus, and stomach, irritation of

mucous membranes and the urinary tract, nausea, sinus and eye irritation, skin irritation, stimulated bladder, stimulation of the stomach and salivation, violent sneezing, vomiting, and worsened kidney conditions.

- Use cautiously in patients with low blood pressure or taking antihypertensives, as horseradish in medicinal amounts may lower blood pressure.
- Use cautiously in patients taking antiinflammatory agents, as horseradish may inhibit cyclooxygenase-1 (COX-1) enzymes.
- Use cautiously in patients undergoing treatment for cancer, as horseradish and horseradish combined with indole-3-acetic acid may have antineoplastic (anticancer) activity.
- Use cautiously in patients with thyroid disorders or taking thyroid hormones, as medicinal amounts of horseradish may interact with thyroid medications.
- Avoid medicinal amounts of horseradish in patients who are pregnant or breastfeeding, as glucosinolates from horseradish are considered a toxin that can be excreted through breast milk and may pose a toxicity hazard.
- Use cautiously in patients with kidney disorders, kidney inflammation, gastrointestinal conditions, or ulcers, as horseradish may have strong diuretic (increased urination) effects.
- Use cautiously in patients with stomach ulcers.

Pregnancy and Breastfeeding

- Avoid if pregnant or breastfeeding. Horseradish has been used to induce abortion. Certain chemicals, such as glucosinolates, from horseradish are considered toxins that can be excreted through breast milk and may pose a toxicity hazard.

INTERACTIONS
Interactions with Drugs

- Horseradish may have antibiotic activity. Use cautiously with antibiotics because of additive effects.
- Horseradish may increase the risk of bleeding when taken with drugs that increase the risk of bleeding. Some examples include aspirin, anticoagulants ("blood thinners") such as warfarin (Coumadin) or heparin, antiplatelet drugs such as clopidogrel (Plavix), and nonsteroidal antiinflammatory drugs (NSAIDS) such as ibuprofen (Motrin, Advil) or naproxen (Naprosyn, Aleve).
- Horseradish in medicinal amounts may have hypotensive (blood pressure–lowering) activity. Use cautiously with blood pressure medications.

- Horseradish may inhibit COX-1 enzymes. Use cautiously with antiinflammatory agents because of possible additive effects.
- Horseradish may have antineoplastic activity. Use cautiously with anticancer medications because of possible additive effects.
- Horseradish root may have oxidative activity; use cautiously with other antioxidants because of possible additive effects.
- Medicinal amounts of horseradish may interact with thyroid medications.
- Horseradish may have strong diuretic (increased urination) effects.
- Medicinal amounts of horseradish may interact with thyroid medications; use cautiously.

Interactions with Herbs and Dietary Supplements

- Horseradish may have antibiotic activity. Use cautiously with antibacterial herbs and supplements because of possible additive effects.
- Horseradish may increase the risk of bleeding when taken with herbs and supplements that are believed to increase the risk of bleeding. Multiple cases of bleeding have been reported with the use of *Ginkgo biloba*, and fewer cases have been reported with garlic and saw palmetto.
- Horseradish may inhibit COX-1 enzymes. Use cautiously with antiinflammatory herbs and supplements.
- Horseradish may have antineoplastic activity. Use cautiously with anticancer herbs or supplements.
- Horseradish root may have oxidative activity. Use cautiously with herbs or supplements with antioxidant activity.
- Horseradish may have strong diuretic effects. Horseradish may also have beneficial effects when taken with the phytohormone indole-3-acetic acid, although human evidence is lacking in this area.
- Horseradish in medicinal amounts may have hypotensive (blood pressure–lowering) activity; use cautiously with blood pressure medications.
- Horseradish contains tannins and vitamin C, which may have additive effects when taken with other tannin-containing herbs or vitamin C supplements.
- Medicinal amounts of horseradish may interact with thyroid herbs or supplements; use cautiously.

For a complete list of references, please visit www.naturalstandard.com.

Horsetail
(Equisetum arvense)

RELATED TERMS

- Bottle brush, cola de caballo (Spanish), common horsetail, common scouring rush, corn horsetail, corncob plant, Dutch rush, Equisetaceae (family), *Equisetum arvense*, *Equisetum myriochaetum*, *Equisetum ramosissimum*, *Equisetum telmateia*, field horsetail, Herba Equiseti Hiemalis, hippuric acid, homovanillic acid, horse willow, horsetail grass, horsetail rush, mokuzoku (Japanese), mokchok, mokjeok (Korean), muzei (*Equisetum hyemale*), paddock pipes, pewterwort, prele, pribes des champs, running clubmoss, Schachtelhalm (German), scouring rush, shave grass, shenjincao (Chinese), toadpipe, Wenjing, Zinnkraut (German).
- Crude drugs derived from *Equisetum arvense* include Wenjing, Jiejiecao, and Bitoucai.
- **Note:** *Equisetum arvense* should not be confused with members of the genus *Laminaria*, kelp, or brown alga, for which *horsetail* has been used as a synonym.

BACKGROUND

- Horsetail (*Equisetum arvense*) has traditionally been used in Europe as a diuretic for the treatment of edema (swelling/fluid retention). The German Commission E expert panel has approved horsetail for this indication. Horsetail is also occasionally used for osteoporosis, nephrolithiasis (kidney stones), urinary tract inflammation, and wound healing (topical). It is also used in cosmetics and shampoos. These uses have largely been based on anecdote and clinical tradition rather than scientific evidence.
- There is preliminary human evidence supporting the use of horsetail as a diuretic. One poorly designed human trial found horsetail to effectively raise bone density equally to calcium supplements.
- In theory (based on mechanism of action), horsetail ingestion in large amounts may cause thiamine deficiency, hypokalemia (low potassium levels), or nicotine toxicity. Reported adverse effects include dermatitis.

EVIDENCE

Uses Based on Scientific Evidence	Grade
Diuresis (Increased Urine) Use of horsetail dates to ancient Roman and Greek medicine. The name *Equisetum* is derived from equus, "horse," and seta, "bristle." Preliminary human and laboratory research suggests that horsetail may increase the amount of urine produced by the body. More studies are needed to determine whether horsetail is safe or useful for specific health conditions.	B
Osteoporosis (Weakening of the Bones) Silicon may be beneficial for bone strengthening. Because horsetail contains silicon, it has been suggested as a possible natural treatment for osteoporosis. Preliminary human study reports benefits, but more	C

detailed research is needed before a firm recommendation can be made. People with osteoporosis should speak with a qualified health care provider about possible treatment with more proven therapies.

Uses Based on Tradition or Theory

Antibacterial, antioxidant, astringent, bedwetting, benign prostate hyperplasia (enlarged prostate), bladder disturbances, bleeding, brittle fingernails, cancer, cosmetic uses, cystic ulcers, diabetes, dropsy, dyspepsia, edema, fever, fluid in the lungs, frostbite, gonorrhea, gout, hair loss, hematuria (blood in the urine), hepatitis, itch, itching (chronic), kidney disease, kidney stones, leg swelling, liver protection, malaria, menorrhagia (heavy menstrual bleeding), menstrual pain, nosebleeds, prostate inflammation, Reiter's syndrome, rheumatism, sedative, stomach upset, styptic (to stop bleeding cuts on the skin), thyroid disorders, tuberculosis, urinary incontinence, urinary tract infection (UTI), urinary tract inflammation, urolithiasis (urinary tract stones), vaginal discharge, wound healing.

DOSING
Adults (18 Years and Older)

- Most reported doses for horsetail are based on historical use or expert opinion. There is a lack of reliable studies available in humans that show horsetail to be effective or safe at any specific dose. Different doses of horsetail have been used, starting at 300-mg capsules taken three times per day, up to 6 g daily. A maximum of 6 cups of tea, containing 1.5 g of dried stem in 1 cup of hot water, is a dose that has been used. A common dose for a tincture (1:1 in 25% alcohol) is 1-4 mL three times daily. To treat osteoporosis, a supplement containing 270 mg of Osteosil calcium (a combination of horsetail and calcium) has been taken twice daily for 1 year. A wash prepared by mixing 10 teaspoons of horsetail in cold water and soaking for 10-12 hours has been applied on the skin.

Children (Younger than 18 Years)

- There is insufficient evidence to recommend the use of horsetail in children. Poisonings have been reported in children using horsetail stems as whistles.

SAFETY
Allergies

- People with allergies to *Equisetum arvense*, related substances, or to nicotine should avoid horsetail. Rash has been reported in a patient taking horsetail who was known to be sensitive to nicotine.

Side Effects and Warnings

- There are few scientific studies or reports of side effects with horsetail. It is more often used in Germany and Canada, where it is traditionally considered to be safe when taken in appropriate doses. *Equisetum palustre* (marsh horsetail) contains a poisonous ingredient and should be avoided. There are reports that some batches of *Equisetum arvense* (horsetail) have been contaminated with *Equisetum palustre*.

- Large doses of horsetail may cause symptoms of nicotine overdose, including fever, cold hands and feet, abnormal heart rate, difficulty walking, muscle weakness, and weight loss. People who smoke or who use nicotine patches or nicotine gum should avoid horsetail. Reports from animal studies and one report of a nicotine-allergic person describe a rash occurring after the use of white horsetail. Other reports from use in animals describe nausea, increased frequency of bowel movements, increased urination, loss of the body's potassium stores, and muscle weakness. People with kidney disorders should avoid horsetail.

- Studies in mice suggest that horsetail may change the activity of the kidneys, which may cause abnormal control of the amount of water and potassium released. Low potassium, which in theory may occur with horsetail, can have negative effects on the heart. Individuals who have heart rhythm disorders or who take digoxin should be cautious. Studies suggest that horsetail does not change blood pressure.

- Horsetail contains an ingredient that destroys thiamine (vitamin B_1), which could lead to deficiency with long-term use. This may cause permanent damage to the brain and nervous system, including confusion, difficulty walking, difficulties with vision and eye movement, and memory loss. People who have thiamine (vitamin B_1) deficiency or poor nutrition should avoid horsetail, as it may affect levels of thiamine even more. Alcoholic or malnourished individuals are often thiamine deficient, and their condition may be worsened by horsetail.

- Avoid use in children because of anecdotal reports of poisonings after use of horsetail stems as whistles.

- Avoid use in patients taking antidiabetic agents, as a different horsetail species (*Equisetum myriochaetum*) has reportedly caused low blood sugar levels in type 2 diabetic patients. However, the effects of *Equisetum arvense* are unclear.

- Avoid use in patients with gout or in those taking antigout agents, as horsetail has been shown to increase the formation of uric acid crystals in the urine.

Pregnancy and Breastfeeding

- Horsetail is not recommended during pregnancy or breastfeeding because little information is available about its safety. Its potential to cause thiamine (vitamin B_1) depletion, low potassium levels, and nicotine-like effects are of particular concern. Many tinctures contain high levels of alcohol and should be avoided during pregnancy.

INTERACTIONS
Interactions with Drugs

- Some diuretic drugs ("water pills") can cause the body to lose water and potassium, for example, loop diuretics such as furosemide (Lasix). The use of horsetail with certain diuretics may cause dehydration or further potassium deficiency. Some steroids and laxative drugs can also lower potassium levels and should not be combined with horsetail. Individuals with heart rhythm disorders who are treated with digoxin (Lanoxin) or digitoxin may be especially sensitive to low potassium levels, and potassium levels should be monitored in such individuals.

- Nicotine, a stimulant, may be found in horsetail. Because horsetail can stimulate the brain and nervous system, caution should be used when horsetail is combined with stimulant drugs and nicotine.

- Horsetail may interact with antigout agents because horsetail has been shown to increase the formation of uric acid crystals in the urine.

- Other horsetail species have caused low blood sugar levels; therefore horsetail may increase the effects of diabetes medications. However, clinical effects on diabetes therapies are unclear.

- Horsetail may have additive effects when taken with agents that treat osteoporosis because horsetail may increase bone density. However, horsetail's antiosteoporosis effects are not well established.

- Many tinctures contain high levels of alcohol and may cause nausea or vomiting when taken with metronidazole (Flagyl) or disulfiram (Antabuse).

Interactions with Herbs and Dietary Supplements

- Increased urine production, dehydration, or electrolyte imbalances may theoretically occur when horsetail is used with herbs that may increase urination. Dehydration or low potassium levels also may theoretically occur if horsetail is used with laxatives. Horsetail may also interact with herbs or supplements taken for gout or osteoporosis, although supportive evidence is currently lacking.

- In theory, low potassium levels caused by horsetail may be dangerous in people using herbs that have cardiac glycoside activity on the heart, such as foxglove and oleander. Other potassium-depleting herbs, such as licorice, should also be avoided when taking horsetail.

- Horsetail may interact with stimulants and herbs and supplements with similar properties such as ephedra and licorice.

- Other horsetail species have caused low blood sugar levels; therefore horsetail may increase effects of diabetes medications. However, clinical effects on diabetes therapies are unclear.

- Horsetail may break down thiamine and may cause thiamine deficiency. Horsetail may also have additive effects in patients taking antioxidants.

For a complete list of references, please visit www.naturalstandard.com.

Hoxsey Formula

RELATED TERMS

- Antimony trisulfide, Aromatic USP 14, arsenic sulfide, berberis root, bloodroot, buckthorn bark, burdock, cascara, licorice, pokeroot, prickly ash bark, red clover, stillingia root, sulfur, talc, trichloroacetic acid, zinc chloride.

BACKGROUND

- "Hoxsey formula" is a misleading name because it is not a single formula but rather is a therapeutic regimen consisting of an oral tonic, topical (on the skin) preparations, and supportive therapy. The tonic is individualized for cancer patients based on their general condition, the location of their cancer, and their previous history of treatment. An ingredient that usually remains constant for every patient is potassium iodide. Other ingredients are then added and may include licorice, red clover, burdock, stillingia root, berberis root, pokeroot, cascara, Aromatic USP 14, prickly ash bark, and buckthorn bark. A red paste may be used, which tends to be caustic (irritating), and contains antimony trisulfide, zinc chloride, and bloodroot. A topical yellow powder may be used and contains arsenic sulfide, talc, sulfur, and a "yellow precipitate." A clear solution may also be administered and contains trichloroacetic acid.

EVIDENCE

Uses Based on Scientific Evidence	Grade
Cancer The original "Hoxsey formula" was developed in the mid-1800s, when a horse belonging to John Hoxsey was observed to recover from cancer after feeding in a field of wild plants. These plants were collected and used to create a remedy that was initially given to ill animals. Different historical accounts state various herbs included in the original formula. The formula was passed down in the Hoxsey family, and John Hoxsey's great-grandson Harry Hoxsey, an Illinois coal miner, marketed an herbal mixture for cancer and promoted himself as an herbal healer. The first Hoxsey clinic opened in the 1920s in Illinois, and Hoxsey therapy became popular for cancer in the United States during the 1940s and 1950s, with clinics operating in multiple states. The Hoxsey clinic in Dallas was one of the largest privately owned cancer hospitals in the world. However, after legal conflicts with the American Medical Association and the U.S. Food and Drug Administration (FDA), the last U.S. clinic closed in the 1950s. The formula was passed to Mildred Nelson, a nurse in the clinic, who used the formula to open and operate a Hoxsey clinic in Tijuana, Mexico. There is a lack of strong evidence of the safety or effectiveness of Hoxsey formula.	C

Uses Based on Tradition or Theory
Elimination of toxins, improving/normalizing cell metabolism.

DOSING

Adults (18 Years and Older)

- There is insufficient evidence to recommend a dose of Hoxsey formula.

Children (Younger than 18 Years)

- There is insufficient evidence to support the safe or effective use of the Hoxsey formula in children.

SAFETY

Allergies

- Allergy or hypersensitivity to burdock root, potassium iodide, licorice, red clover, stillingia root, berberis root, pokeroot, cascara, prickly ash bark, and buckthorn bark (which all may be contained in the oral Hoxsey tonic) may cause an allergic reaction.

Side Effects and Warnings

- Well-designed safety studies of the Hoxsey formula are currently unavailable. It is not known whether concentrations of the various ingredients are great enough to cause side effects that may be associated with those ingredients when used alone in therapeutic amounts.

Pregnancy and Breastfeeding

- There is a lack of reliable scientific study of the Hoxsey formula in pregnant or breastfeeding women. Safety is unknown; therefore use cannot be recommended.

INTERACTIONS

Interactions with Drugs

- There is a lack of published scientific evidence available on drug interactions with the Hoxsey formula. It is not known whether concentrations of the various ingredients are great enough to cause interactions that may be associated with those ingredients when used alone in therapeutic amounts. The formula may include administration of antimony trisulfide, Aromatic USP 14, arsenic sulfide, berberis root, bloodroot, buckthorn bark, burdock, licorice, pokeroot, cascara, potassium iodide, prickly ash bark, red clover, stillingia root, sulfur, talc, trichloroacetic acid, and/or zinc chloride.

Interactions with Herbs and Dietary Supplements

- Scientific evidence of herb or supplement interactions with the Hoxsey formula is currently unavailable. It is not known whether concentrations of the various ingredients are great enough to cause interactions that may be associated with those ingredients when used alone in therapeutic amounts. The formula may include administration of antimony trisulfide, Aromatic USP 14, arsenic sulfide, berberis root, bloodroot, buckthorn bark, burdock, licorice, pokeroot, cascara, potassium iodide, prickly ash bark, red clover, stillingia root, sulfur, talc, trichloroacetic acid, and/or zinc chloride.

For a complete list of references, please visit www.naturalstandard.com.

Hydrazine Sulfate (HS)

($H_6N_2O_4S$)

RELATED TERMS

- 2,4-Dinitro-phenylhydrazine, alpha-methyldopa-hydrazine, beta-phenylisopropylhydrazine, carbidopa, diamide, diamine, dimethylhydrazine, hydrazine, hydrazine monosulphate, hydrazine sulphate, hydrazinium sulphate, idrazina solfato (Italian), Sehydrin.

BACKGROUND

- Cachexia is defined as physical wasting with loss of weight and muscle mass caused by disease. Patients with advanced cancer, acquired immunodeficiency syndrome (AIDS), and some other major chronic progressive diseases may appear cachectic. Anorexia (lack of appetite) and cachexia often occur together. Cachexia can occur in people who are eating enough but who cannot absorb the nutrients. Cachexia is not the same as starvation. A healthy person's body can adjust to starvation by slowing down its use of nutrients, but in cachectic patients, the body does not make this adjustment.

- Hydrazine is an industrial chemical marketed as having the potential to repress weight loss and cachexia associated with cancer and to improve general appetite status. However, in large randomized controlled trials, hydrazine has not been proven effective for improving appetite, reducing weight loss, or improving survival in adults with small cell lung cancer (when used as adjuvant therapy) or metastatic colorectal cancer (when used alone).

- Hydrazine sulfate causes liver damage in rodents. It is associated with nausea and vomiting, fatigue, sensory and motor neuropathies, and a significantly reduced quality of life in cancer patients. It is currently being investigated as a potential treatment for endotoxin-mediated shock. Hydrazine sulfate has demonstrated significant mutagenic and carcinogenic potential in animal studies.

- Hydrazine has not been well evaluated for safety or toxicity during pregnancy, lactation, or childhood.

- Other applications of hydrazine include corrosion inhibitor, herbicide and pesticide component, laboratory reagent, refining rare metals, soldering flux for light metals, silvering of mirrors, and rocket fuel.

EVIDENCE

Uses Based on Scientific Evidence	Grade
Cachexia (Cancer Related) The results of multiple clinical studies for the use of hydrazine sulfate in cancer-related cachexia are conflicting. The use of hydrazine sulfate cannot be fully recommended because of the lack of well-designed studies and potential risks.	C
Cancer Treatment The National Cancer Institute (NCI) sponsored studies of hydrazine sulfate that claimed efficacy in improving survival for some patients with advanced cancer.	C

Trial results found that hydrazine sulfate did not prolong survival for cancer patients. The U.S. Food and Drug Administration (FDA) has received requests from individual physicians for approval to use hydrazine sulfate on a case-by-case "compassionate use" basis on the chance that patients with no other available effective therapy might benefit. The overall controversy in the use of hydrazine sulfate is ongoing, and relevance to clinical practice is unknown. The use of hydrazine sulfate needs to be evaluated further before any recommendations can be made. Side effects have been reported.

Uses Based on Tradition or Theory

Analytical tests for blood, anorexia, antidepressant, antioxidant, biocide for molds and fungi (onychomycosis), chemotherapy, impaired glucose tolerance, multidrug resistance (tachyphylaxis), normalizing laboratory indices, nutritional support (improving caloric intake), pain, Parkinson's disease, sickle-cell anemia, tuberculosis, weight loss (prevention).

DOSING

Adults (18 Years and Older)

- Various clinical trials have used 60 mg of hydrazine sulfate taken by mouth one to three times daily for 30 days in patients with cancer and or cachexia. Injections have also been given by a health care provider.

Children (Younger than 18 Years)

- There is insufficient evidence to recommend hydrazine sulfate in children.

SAFETY

Allergies

- Avoid if known allergy or hypersensitivity exists to hydrazine sulfate or any of its constituents.
- Hydrazine sulfate is a sensitizer and can potentially cause allergic reactions. Rash has been reported.

Side Effects and Warnings

- Hydrazine sulfate is a severe skin and mucus membrane irritant; effects when used internally include weakness and excitability. Side effects include nausea, vomiting, pruritus, headache, dizziness, drowsiness, insomnia, weakness, irregular breathing, confusion, low blood sugar, lethargy, violent behavior, restlessness, seizures, coma, and peripheral neuropathies (a disease or abnormality of the nervous system). Sweating has been reported in two patients in a small clinical trial.
- Periarteritis nodosa and lupus have also been associated with hydrazine. Polyarteritis nodosa is a serious blood vessel disease in which small and medium-sized arteries become swollen and damaged when they are attacked by rogue immune cells. Lupus is a chronic inflammatory disease that

can affect various parts of the body, especially the skin, joints, blood, and kidneys.

- Hydrazine has been associated with low blood pressure, abnormal heart rhythms, septic shock, congestive heart failure, and facial swelling. A fatal case of liver and kidney failure has been reported.
- Anorexia, heartburn, diarrhea, constipation, and hunger have been reported. Elevation of liver enzymes and "bad" or low-density lipoprotein (LDL) cholesterol have been reported.
- In a clinical trial, there was a report of possible thrombophlebitis (vein inflammation), although it was unclear whether it was drug related. One report suggested hydrazine-induced platelet aggregation. Methemoglobinemia, a condition in which the iron in the hemoglobin molecule (the red blood pigment) is defective and is unable to carry oxygen effectively to the tissues, has been noted.
- Hydrazine sulfate has been reported to cause paresthesia (of the upper and lower extremities), arthralgia or pain, depression, distorted sense of taste, palpebral tic, slurred speech, and hiccup; it may also affect fine motor functions. Paresthesia is a sensation of burning, prickling, tingling, or creeping on the skin that is often seen in multiple sclerosis (MS). Hydrazine sulfate either inhaled or used topically may cause irritation, burns, and permanent damage to the eye. Mydriasis (dilation of the pupil) and nystagmus (rapid involuntary oscillation/movement back and forth of the eyes) have been reported.
- In a clinical trial, one patient had visual and auditory hallucinations.
- A chest x-ray of a person who handled hydrazine for 6 months showed fluid in the lungs. An autopsy revealed severe trachea inflammation, bronchitis, and death due to pneumonia. Oral hydrazine sulfate may cause irregular breathing. Inhaled or topical use of hydrazine sulfate may cause bronchial mucus destruction, pulmonary edema, cancer, and death. Dyspnea (shortness of breath), rhinitis (inflammation of nasal mucosa), and cough have also been reported.

Pregnancy and Breastfeeding

- Hydrazine sulfate is not recommended in pregnant or breastfeeding women because of a lack of sufficient data.

INTERACTIONS
Interactions with Drugs

- One clinical study reported that a patient with lung cancer experienced flushing after alcohol ingestion while receiving hydrazine sulfate therapy.
- Hydrazine is a monoamine oxidase inhibitor (MAOI). Therefore, use of hydrazine with selective serotonin reuptake inhibitors (SSRIs), tricyclic antidepressants (TCAs), tetracyclic, antidepressants (TeCAs), or MAOI antidepressants should be avoided as it may result in hypertensive crisis (dangerously high blood pressure) and/or serotonin syndrome.

A derivative of hydrazine has been used as an antidepressant in the MAOI family for the treatment of minor depressive states but failed to show any beneficial results.

- Dr. Joseph Gold, the pioneer in hydrazine use in cancer patients, has conducted several studies on the effects of hydrazine sulfate; he suggested that patients using hydrazine sulfate refrain from using benzodiazepines and barbiturates.
- Hydrazine sulfate used with bleomycin, a chemotherapy drug, may lead to an additive effect of both agents. Hydrazine sulfate used with cyclophosphamide, a chemotherapy drug, may lead to enhanced antitumor effects of cyclophosphamide.
- Hydrazine sulfate may induce hypoglycemia (low blood sugar levels) or hyperglycemia (high blood sugar levels). Use of hydrazine sulfate with diabetes medications/oral hypoglycemic agents may result in either additive or negative effects.
- Hydrazine sulfate used along with isoniazid may lead to enhanced effects of hydrazine.
- Hydrazine may increase the length of time that levodopa works.
- Hydrazine sulfate used with methotrexate may lead to an additive effect of both agents.
- Hydrazine sulfate used with mitomycin C may lead to enhanced antitumor effects of mitomycin C when these agents are administered 6 hours apart from each other. A study found that if hydrazine sulfate and mitomycin C are mixed in the same syringe, they inactivate each other.

Interactions with Herbs and Dietary Supplements

- Interactions may occur with herbs and supplements with the following properties: amphetamine-like, anesthetic-like, anti-depressant-like, anxiolytic-like, barbiturate-like, beta-blocker-like, central adrenergic-like, demerol-like, hypoglycemic-like, insulin-like, sympathomimetic-like, or theophylline-like.
- Hydrazine sulfate may alter blood sugar levels (induce hypoglycemia or hyperglycemia). Use with other herbs or supplements that alter blood sugar may result in either additive or negative effects when taken with hydrazine.
- Based on animal studies, hydrazine is an MAOI; therefore use of hydrazine with SSRIs, TCAs, tetracyclic, or other MAOI-acting herbs or supplements should be avoided as it may result in hypertensive crisis and/or serotonin syndrome. An example is St. John's wort. A derivative of hydrazine has been used as an antidepressant in the MAOI family for treatment of minor depressive states but failed to show any beneficial results.
- Hydrazine sulfate is typically suggested as a cancer treatment; thus hydrazine sulfate may interact with herbs or supplements also used for cancer. Caution is advised.

For a complete list of references, please visit www.naturalstandard.com.

Hyssop

(Hyssopus officinalis)

RELATED TERMS

- Azob, bitter aperitifs, borneol, bornylacetate, caffeic acid, camphene, chartreuse, decoction of qingre huoxue (QHR), diosmin, diterpenoid, European mint, ezob (Hebrew), flavonoids, geraniol, giant-hyssop herb, herb hyssop, hesperidin, holy herb, hyssop decoction, hyssop leaf extract, hyssop oil, hyssopin, hyssopos of Dioscorides, *Hyssopus ambiguus* (Trautv.) Iljin, *Hyssopus cretaceus* Dubjan., *Hyssopus cuspidatus* Boriss., *Hyssopus ferganensis* Boriss., *Hyssopus latilabiatus* C.Y.Wu & H.W.Li, *Hyssopus lophanthoides* Buch.-Ham.ex D. Don, *Hyssopus macranthus* Boriss., *Hyssopus ocymifolius* Lam., *Hyssopus officinalis*, *Hyssopus officinalis* L., *Hyssopus seravschanicus* (Dub.) Pazij, *Hyssopus tianschanicus* Boriss, isopinocamphone, Lamiaceae (family), limonene, linalool, marrubiin, oleanolic acid, *Origanum aegypticum*, *Origanum syriacum*, phellandrene, pinene, pinocamphone, polysaccharide MAR-10, QHR, resin, tannins, terpenoids, thujone, ursolic acid, volatile oil.

BACKGROUND

- The use of hyssop as an herbal remedy dates back to Biblical times. It is mentioned in both the Old and New Testaments of the Christian Bible as a cleansing agent (although these references may be to other species of hyssop, such as *Origanum aegypticum* or *Origanum syriacum*, rather than *Hyssopus officinalis*).
- Hyssop has been prescribed for a multitude of medical conditions, although there are few high-quality human trials researching these uses. It has been used traditionally as an antispasmodic, expectorant, emmenagogue (stimulates menstruation), stimulant, carminative (digestive aid), peripheral vasodilator, antiinflammatory, anticatarrhal, antispasmodic, tonic, and sweat-inducer. However, both the alcoholic extract and decoction have been used to inhibit sweating. Hyssop is used specifically for cough, bronchitis, and chronic catarrh and also for its tonic effects on the digestive, urinary, nervous, and bronchial systems. Hot hyssop decoction vapors have also been used to treat inflammation and tinnitus.

EVIDENCE

Uses Based on Scientific Evidence

No available studies qualify for inclusion in the evidence table.

Uses Based on Tradition or Theory

Abscess (peritonsillar), anemia, anthelmintic (expels worms), antifungal, antiinflammatory, antioxidant, antispasmodic, antitussive (preventing or relieving cough), antiviral, anxiety, asthma, bronchitis, bruises, burns, calming, cancer, cardiovascular conditions, carminative (digestive aid), catarrh (inflammation of mucous membranes), chronic venous insufficiency (CVI), circulatory disorders, common cold, cosmetic, cough, depression, diabetes mellitus type 1, diaphoretic (promotes sweating), digestive tonic, diuretic, dyspepsia (upset stomach), emmenagogue (stimulates menstruation), epilepsy, exhaustion, expectorant, fever, food flavoring, flu, gallbladder disorders, gout (foot inflammation), herpes simplex, HIV, hyperlipidemia (high cholesterol levels), hysteria, influenza, intestinal inflammation, intestinal worms, Kaposi's sarcoma, leukemia, liver conditions, melanoma, nephritis (inflamed liver), night sweats, ophthalmia (inflamed eye), perfume, peripheral vasodilator, pleurisy (inflamed membranes around the lungs), poor circulation, respiratory congestion, respiratory infections, rheumatism (painful disorder of the joints, muscles, or connective tissues), rhinitis (hay fever), sedative, seizure (petit mal), sore throat, stimulant, stress, tinnitus, tonic, tonsillitis, toothache, vulnerary (wound healing).

DOSING

Adults (18 Years and Older)

- There is insufficient evidence to recommend a dose for hyssop. In general, 2 g of dried herb infused in boiling water three times daily has been given. Avoid sustained use of hyssop oil (10-30 drops daily for adults) because of a slight risk of seizures.

Children (Younger than 18 Years)

- Avoid in children because of possible seizures, as hyssop is a known convulsant.

SAFETY

Allergies

- Avoid in individuals with a known allergy or hypersensitivity to hyssop, any of its constituents, or any related plants in the Lamiaceae family.

Side Effects and Warnings

- Hyssop has been reported to cause vomiting and seizures, especially at high doses. The essential oil contains the ketone pinocamphone, which is known to cause convulsions. Avoid in patients with epilepsy, fever, hypertension (high blood pressure), or pregnancy.

Pregnancy and Breastfeeding

- Hyssop is not recommended in pregnant or breastfeeding women because of a lack of available scientific evidence.

INTERACTIONS

Interactions with Drugs

- Hyssop may lower the seizure threshold and theoretically may interact with antiepileptic medications.
- Daflon 500 (a mixture of diosmin [90%] and hesperidin [10%]) may interact additively with antihyperglycemic (blood sugar–altering) drugs. Caution is advised in patients with diabetes (high blood sugar levels) or hypoglycemia (low blood sugar levels) and in those taking drugs, herbs, or supplements that affect blood sugar levels. Serum glucose levels may need to be monitored by a qualified health care professional, including a pharmacist, and medication adjustments may be necessary.

- Hyssop constituents oleanolic acid and ursolic acid have recognized antihyperlipidemic (cholesterol-lowering) properties and may interact additively with antihyperlipidemia drugs.
- Early studies showed that crude extracts of hyssop produced antiviral activity against herpes simplex and human immunodeficiency virus (HIV-1). Therefore, hyssop may theoretically interact with antiviral medications.
- A decoction of qingre huoxue, which includes hyssop, may interact additively with glucocorticoids.
- Hyssop is proposed to possess immunomodulatory activity and may theoretically interact with immunosuppressant medications.
- Hyssop is proposed to affect the seizure threshold and may therefore theoretically interact with medications that affect the seizure threshold.

Interactions with Herbs and Dietary Supplements

- Hyssop may lower the seizure threshold and theoretically may interact with antiepileptic herbs.
- Daflon 500 (a mixture of diosmin [90%] and hesperidin [10%]) may interact additively with antihyperglycemic herbs (blood sugar–lowering). Caution is advised when herbs or supplements that may also lower blood sugar are used. Blood glucose levels may require monitoring, and doses may need adjustment.
- Hyssop constituents oleanolic acid and ursolic acid have recognized antihyperlipidemic (cholesterol-lowering) properties and may interact additively with antihyperlipidemia herbs, such as red yeast rice.
- Early studies showed that crude extracts of hyssop produced antiviral activity against herpes simplex and HIV-1. Therefore hyssop may theoretically interact with antiviral herbs and supplements.
- QHR contains hyssop and therefore may theoretically cause additive effects when taken together.
- Hyssop is proposed to affect the seizure threshold and may therefore theoretically interact with herbs that affect the seizure threshold.
- Hyssop is proposed to possess immunomodulatory activity and may therefore theoretically interact with immunosuppressant medications.

For a complete list of references, please visit www.naturalstandard.com.

Ignatia
(Strychnos ignatii)

RELATED TERMS

- Ignatia, Ignatia amara, Ignatius bean, Lu Song Guo, Saint Ignatius bean, St. Ignatius bean, *Strychnos ignatii.*

BACKGROUND

- Ignatia amara is a homeopathic remedy derived from the seeds of the St. Ignatius bean, *Strychnos ignatii,* a tree found in the Philippines and other parts of Southeast Asia. It is used as a homeopathic remedy because of its effects on the nervous system.
- Commonly called "homeopathic Prozac," ignatia is often used in treating grief stages. Ignatia was commonly used in the 1800s but has not been studied in modern scientific trials. Although there is little scientific evidence regarding the medicinal use of ignatia, it was added to Materia Medica (book of written descriptions of homeopathic medicines) in the early 1800s.
- Chinese doctors have used ignatia for emotional disorders such as depression and anxiety. Folk healers also used ignatia to treat headaches, sore throats, coughs, and menstrual problems.
- Ignatia is not widely used because it contains strychnine, which can be fatal to humans.

EVIDENCE

Uses Based on Scientific Evidence	Grade
Emotional Disorders (Emergency Use) Currently, there is insufficient evidence to recommend homeopathic ignatia for emergency use of emotional disorders.	C

Uses Based on Tradition or Theory
Allergies, antiinflammatory, anxiety, apprehension, atonic dyspepsia (upset stomach), backaches, bedwetting, belching, bereavement, chills, choking, climacteric symptoms, constipation, coughs, cravings, delusions, depression, faintness, fever, follicular inflammation, gastralgia (stomach pain), grief, hallucinations, headaches, hemorrhoids, hiccups, hysteria, inability to work, indigestion, inflammation, irritability, itching, loss of appetite, menopausal symptoms, menstrual problems, mood swings, mouth dryness, nasal problems, nausea and vomiting, nervousness, oversensitivity to all stimuli, pain, perspiration, placebo alternative, postpartum depression, rectal prolapse (rectum drops down outside the anus), rectal spasms, refresh body function, restless legs syndrome, sensitivity to noise, sleeplessness, sore throat, spasm in vocal cords, spasmodic conditions, sweat, thrush (mouth infection), tonic, trembling, unconsciousness, uncontrollable grief, weakness, weepiness.

DOSING

Adults (18 Years and Older)

- There is insufficient evidence to recommend a dose for ignatia.

Children (Younger than 18 Years)

- There is insufficient evidence to recommend a dose for ignatia in children.

SAFETY

Allergies

- Avoid in individuals with a known allergy or hypersensitivity to ignatia or to a member of the Loganiaceae family.

Side Effects and Warnings

- Ignatia is possibly safe when used as a homeopathic remedy. However, because of the strychnine content, taking Ignatius bean by mouth may cause restlessness, anxiety, heightened sense perception, enhanced reflexes, equilibrium disorders, painful back and neck stiffness, twitching, spasms of jaw and neck muscles, convulsions triggered by visual or touch stimulation with possible opisthotonos (rigid muscle contraction), extreme muscle tension, hyperthermia (abnormally high body temperature), seizures, metabolic acidosis (blood is too acidic), fatal cardiac arrest, rhabdomyolysis (degeneration of skeletal muscle), agitation, and difficulty breathing after respiratory spasms. The U.S. Food and Drug Administration (FDA) banned strychnine from nonregulated products in 1989.
- Avoid ignatia in patients with liver disease because strychnine accumulates in individuals with liver damage and can cause further damage. Ignatia may also cause myoglobinuric renal failure, and caution is advised in patients with compromised kidney function.

Pregnancy and Breastfeeding

- Ignatia is not recommended in pregnant or breastfeeding women because of toxic effects.

INTERACTIONS

Interactions with Drugs

- Concomitant use of analeptics (agents that stimulate breathing, heart activity) or phenothiazines (antipsychotic drugs) with ignatia may cause symptoms of ignatia poisoning. Avoid combined use.

Interactions with Herbs and Dietary Supplements

- Insufficient evidence is available.

For a complete list of references, please visit www.naturalstandard.com.

Iodine (I)

RELATED TERMS

- Atomic number 53, Betadine, cadexomer iodine, I, Iodin, iodine-125, iodine-131, iodized poppy seed oil, iodized salt, iodothyronine, iodotyrosine, Licartin, Lipiodol, Lugol solution, Lugol's iodine, potassium iodide (KI), polyvinyl-pyrrolidone-iodine (PVP-I), povidone-iodine, radioiodine, SSKI, strong iodine, tincture of iodine.
- **Note:** This review does not discuss the medical uses of radio-active iodine or iodine contrast agents used for imaging studies such as computerized tomographic (CT) scanning.

BACKGROUND

- Iodine is an element (atomic number 53) that is required by humans for the synthesis of thyroid hormones (triiodothyronine [T_3] and thyroxine [T_4]).
- Chronic iodine deficiency can lead to numerous health problems in children and adults, including thyroid gland dysfunction (including goiter) and various neurological, gastrointestinal, and skin abnormalities. Iodine deficiency in pregnant or nursing mothers can lead to significant neurocognitive deficits in their infants. "Cretinism" or severe mental retardation is a rare outcome of severe iodine deficiency during early development. Growth stunting, apathy, impaired movement, or speech/hearing problems may occur. Many individuals living in developing countries may be at risk of iodine deficiency and its complications, and iodine deficiency is considered to be a preventable cause of mental retardation.
- Iodine deficiency is rare in industrialized countries such as the United States because of the enrichment of table salt and cattle feed with iodine. However, deficiency is common in developing countries, and supplementation should be considered.
- Humans obtain iodine from their diets. The amount of iodine in food or water depends on the amount of iodine in the local soil. Areas with mountainous (glacier) water or heavy rainfall tend to be low in iodine content, which increases the risk of iodine deficiency.
- This review does not discuss medical uses of radioactive iodine or iodine contrast agents used for imaging studies such as CT scanning.

EVIDENCE

Uses Based on Scientific Evidence	Grade
Goiter Prevention Iodine deficiency is one of the causes of goiter (hypertrophy of the thyroid gland as it tries to make more thyroid hormone in the absence of iodine). Physically, goiter appears as an abnormal enlargement of the thyroid gland in the neck. Other causes of goiter include autoimmune thyroiditis, excess iodine, other hormonal disorders, radiation exposure, infectious causes, or inborn errors of metabolism. Although goiter due to low iodine intake is rare in developed countries, it may occur in regions with endemic low iodine levels. To avoid iodine deficiency in the United States, table salt is enriched with iodine (iodized salt) and iodine is added to cattle feed and used as a dough conditioner. Iodine supplementation is generally not recommended in developed countries where sufficient iodine intake is common, and excess iodine can actually cause medical complications (including goiter). Iodine supplementation should be considered in cases of known iodine deficiency and should be administered with medical supervision if possible. Notably, the treatment of goiter usually involves the administration of thyroid hormone, most commonly levothyroxine sodium (Synthroid, Levoxyl, Levothroid). Iodine generally does not play a role in the acute management of this condition.	A
Iodine Deficiency In regions with low iodine intake or cases of known deficiency, iodine enrichment of foods or supplementation should be considered. To avoid iodine deficiency in the United States, table salt is enriched with iodine (iodized salt), and iodine is added to cattle feed and used as a dough conditioner. While iodine deficiency is not common in developed countries, it is common in other parts of the world. When considering iodine enrichment or supplementation, supervision by medical personnel or public health officials is recommended because of the potential complications involved with iodine replacement in the setting of previous deprivation, particularly if supplementation is being considered in pregnant women or children.	A
Radiation Emergency (Potassium Iodide Thyroid Protection) Potassium iodide (KI) can be taken in the setting of radiation exposure to reduce levels of radioactive iodine uptake by the thyroid, thus reducing the risk of later development of thyroid cancer. It is important to note that KI does not provide immediate protection from radiation damage and does not have protective effects against other complications of radiation exposure. KI can serve as a part of a general strategy in cases of radiation emergencies, in conjunction with shelter and control of foodstuffs. Many radiation emergency kits include KI.	A
Skin Disinfectant/Sterilization Iodine is commonly used in topical disinfectant preparations for cleaning wounds, sterilizing skin before surgical/invasive procedures, or sterilizing catheter entry sites. Betadine solution, for example, contains povidone-iodine. Other topical disinfectants include alcohol and antibiotics, and iodine is sometimes used in combination with these. Commercially prepared iodine products are recommended to ensure appropriate concentrations.	A

(Continued)

Uses Based on Scientific Evidence	Grade
Water Purification Iodine can be used as an antimicrobial agent for the emergency purification of water. Tablets and solutions are commercially available. Effects generally occur within 15 minutes.	A
Bacterial Conjunctivitis Povidone-iodine solutions have been used in the management of childhood bacterial conjunctivitis and may be as effective as other antibacterial solutions such as neomycin-polymyxin B-gramicidin. This is not an effective treatment for viral conjunctivitis. Medical supervision is recommended.	B
Graves Disease (Adjunct Iodine/Iodides) Graves disease is an immune-mediated disorder that causes hyperthyroidism. Thyroid-stimulating immunoglobulins bind to the thyroid stimulating hormone (TSH) receptor, mimic the action of TSH, and stimulate thyroid growth and thyroid hormone overproduction. Standard treatments for Graves disease target the thyroid gland (rather than the source of the disorder) and include antithyroid drugs such as propylthiouracil or methimazole, radioactive iodine to ablate (destroy) thyroid cells, or surgery to remove thyroid tissue. Beta-blocker drugs may be used to control symptoms. Iodide preparations can be used to suppress thyroid hormone release from the thyroid, such as strong iodine solution (Lugol solution), potassium iodide (SSKI), and iodinated radiographic contrast agents (sodium ipodate). Patients undergoing thyroid surgery are commonly treated preoperatively with antithyroid drugs to achieve a euthyroid state, then SSKI.	B
Hearing Loss (Iodine Deficiency) Auditory disturbances may be present in iodine deficient children, and continuous iodine supplementation may improve the auditory thresholds.	B
Ocular Surgery Infection Prevention/Cataract Surgery Antisepsis Topical iodine solutions, such as povidone-iodine, are used preoperatively to sterilize before ophthalmological procedures. For example, povidone-iodine solution has been studied and used preoperatively for cataract surgery antisepsis.	B
Ophthalmia Neonatorum Prevention "Ophthalmia neonatorum" is defined as conjunctivitis with eye discharge that occurs during the first month of life. Various bacteria can cause this condition, including gonococcus and *Chlamydia trachomatis*. Several agents have been used as drops in the eyes to prevent this condition in infants, including erythromycin, silver nitrate, gentamicin, and povidone-iodine. Tetracycline and penicillin drops have also been used. Although this condition is now uncommon in industrialized nations, it remains a problem in the developing world with an incidence as high as 20%-30% and cases of blindness reported in Africa each year.	B
Povidone-iodine ophthalmic solution appears to have broad-spectrum activity against bacteria and is less expensive than many antibiotics. It therefore may be a cost-effective option in some populations.	
Oral Mucositis There is limited research to suggest that iodine mouth rinses may decrease the severity of mucositis in the mouth related to cancer chemotherapy or radiation therapy. The management of mucositis should be discussed with the cancer care team.	B
Thyrotoxicosis/Thyroid Storm (Adjunct Iodides) Hyperthyroid crisis (thyroid storm) is a medical emergency caused by excessive release of thyroid hormones into the circulation. Initial management of this condition involves inhibition of thyroid function with thioamide drugs such as propylthiouracil or methimazole. Iodides (such as potassium iodide) can then be administered to block the release of thyroid hormone but should only be given an hour after thioamides to ensure that the iodide is not used by the thyroid to make more thyroid hormone and worsen symptoms. Caution is warranted because iodide preparations carry a risk of causing serum sickness. Iodides should not be used for long-term treatment of thyrotoxicosis.	B
Bladder Irrigation Povidone-iodine bladder irrigation has been suggested before catheter removal or before prostatectomy surgery to reduce the risk of infection. There is limited research in this area.	C
Bleeding Early research suggests that povidone-iodine may control bleeding better than saline. Additional research is needed before a strong recommendation can be made.	C
Bowel Irrigation Povidone-iodine irrigation before large bowel resection has been suggested as a sterilization technique.	C
Cancer The potential role of nonradioactive iodine in cancer care remains unknown. Antioxidant and antitumor effects have been proposed based on laboratory research. In contrast, some scientists have asserted that tumors may uptake more iodine than normal tissues. It has been suggested that high rates of gastric (stomach) cancer or low rates of breast cancer in coastal Japan may be due to high iodine intake, although this has not been demonstrated scientifically. Povidone-iodine solutions have been used as a part of alternative cancer regimens, such as the Hoxsey formula. Preliminary study has also indicated povidone-iodine solution as a potential rectal washout for rectal cancer. Overall, no clear conclusion can be drawn based on the currently available evidence.	C

Uses Based on Scientific Evidence	Grade
Cognitive Function Iodine is required for the production of thyroid hormones, which are necessary for normal brain development and cognition. There some evidence that oral iodized oil significantly improved performance on cognitive tests in 10-12 year-old school children. However, evidence is insufficient to support this use.	C
Corpus Vitreous Degeneration Topical administration of iodine eye drops may reduce corpus vitreous degeneration. However, evidence is insufficient to support this use.	C
Goiter Treatment Iodine deficiency can cause goiter (hypertrophy of the thyroid gland). Other causes of goiter should be considered in patients with this condition, such as autoimmune thyroiditis, excess iodine, other hormonal disorders, radiation exposure, infectious causes, or inborn errors of metabolism. Although goiter due to low iodine intake is rare in developed countries, it may occur in regions with endemic low iodine levels. Initial management of goiter should involve a medical evaluation to identify the underlying cause and assessment of levels of thyroid hormones in the body. Treatment usually involves the administration of thyroid hormone, most commonly levothyroxine sodium (Synthroid, Levoxyl, Levothroid). Iodine plays a role in goiter prevention but not in acute management of this condition. Iodine deficiency should be corrected with supplementation, if found.	C
Lymphedema (Filarial) Footcare with Betadine may help in the management of filarial lymphedema.	C
Molluscum Contagiosum Povidone-iodine has been suggested as a topical treatment for molluscum. However, evidence is insufficient to support this use.	C
Oral Intubation Gargling with povidone-iodine before oral intubation reduces the transport of bacteria into the trachea.	C
Pelvic Infection Vaginal douching with aqueous povidone-iodine followed by normal saline irrigation immediately before oocyte retrieval seems effective in preventing the pelvic infection without compromising the outcome of in vitro fertilization treatment.	C
Periodontitis/Gingivitis Povidone-iodine mouthwash has been suggested to reduce mouth flora in the setting of periodontitis or around oral surgery. Evidence in this area is not conclusive.	C

	Grade
Pneumonia Based on one prospective randomized study, regular oropharyngeal application of povidone-iodine may decrease the prevalence of ventilator-associated pneumonia in patients with severe head trauma. Evidence in this area is not conclusive.	C
Postcesarean Endometritis Preoperative vaginal scrub with povidone-iodine decreases the incidence of postcesarean endometritis. This intervention does not seem to decrease the overall risk of postoperative fever or wound infection.	C
Renal Pelvic Instillation Sclerotherapy (RPIS) Povidone-iodine 0.2% has been shown to be as effective for RPIS as 1% silver nitrate.	C
Septicemia (Serious Bacterial Infections in the Blood) Rinsing with povidone-iodine may help reduce the incidence and severity of bacterial infections of the blood.	C
Wound Healing It is not clear whether healing of wounds or skin ulcers is improved with the application of topical iodine solutions. Iodine solutions may assist with sterilization as a part of a larger approach to the healing process.	C
Kidney Problems (Kidney Cysts) Iodine has been suggested as a possible treatment for kidney cysts, or small, fluid-filled sacs in the kidneys. Early research suggests that povidone-iodine injections after kidney cysts are drained are not effective.	D
Visual Outcomes in Corneal Ulceration Povidone-iodine does not seem to improve visual outcomes in corneal ulceration.	D

Uses Based on Tradition or Theory

Anemia, blood circulation improvement, burn wound healing, chronic otitis media, diabetic foot ulcers, energy level enhancement, fibrocystic breast disease, fungal skin infections, hyperlipidemia, infant mortality improvement, Kashin-Beck osteoarthropathy, keratitis, keratoconjunctivitis, parasites, respiratory congestion, thyroid adenoma, vaginitis, venous leg ulcers, weight loss.

DOSING
Adults (18 Years and Older)
- The U.S. Recommended Dietary Allowance (RDA) is 150 mcg daily in adults ages 18 years and older (220 mcg daily for pregnant women, 290 mcg daily for breastfeeding women). The Tolerable Upper Intake Levels (UL) for adults ages 18 years and older is 1100 mcg daily.

- Cataract surgery antisepsis: 1% povidone-iodine solution used preoperatively. Eye drops containing 0.8% povidone-iodine solution have been used three times every 5 minutes before surgery.
- Chronic suppurative otitis media: 5% povidone-iodine ear drops, three drops taken three times daily for 10 days have been used, although other approaches such as antibiotics should be considered and discussed with a supervising health care professional.
- Hyperthyroidism, Graves disease, thyroid storm: As an adjunct to prescription drug inhibitors of thyroid function (such as propylthiouracil or methimazole), saturated solution of potassium iodide (SSKI, Pima) 1-5 drops by mouth every 8 hours, or Lugol solution (8 mg iodide per drop) 2-6 drops (1 mL) every 8 hours, have been used. For thyrotoxicosis, parenteral treatment may be used, and sodium iodide 1 g by slow intravenous drip every 8-12 hours has been given. Management should be under the supervision of a licensed health care professional. Lower doses may be used in pregnancy.
- Iodine deficiency and goiter: Iodine deficiency is rare in industrialized countries because of supplementation of table salt and cattle feed with iodine. In areas of endemic iodine deficiency, various doses of iodine have been used as prevention or treatment, including 200 mg or 2 mL of iodized oil daily by mouth. For prolonged supplementation, a single annual intramuscular injection with 1 mL Lipiodol UF (480 mg of iodine) or 570 mg of oral iodine has been used. In those with goiter induced by iodine deficiency, correction may not be practical and treatment should involve thyroid hormone replacement with levothyroxine sodium (Synthroid, Levoxyl, Levothroid).
- Mouthwash: As an antibacterial mouthwash, 10-20 mL of povidone-iodine mouthwash has been used as a rinse and gingival sulcus irrigant. For prevention of plaque and gingivitis, mouth rinses have been used up to twice daily. For chemotherapy mucositis prevention, povidone-iodine rinses have been used up to four times daily.
- Pneumonia: 20 mL of a 10% povidone-iodine aqueous solution, reconstituted in a 60-mL solution with sterile water, has been used as a nasopharynx and oropharynx rinse in patients with pneumonia and head trauma.
- Preoperative before thyroidectomy: Lugol solution 5-10 drops three times daily or 2-6 drops twice or three times daily, given 10-21 days before surgery, has been used. Use for longer than 14 days can lead to "iodide escape" with rebound thyrotoxicosis and should be avoided. In pregnant women, there is a risk of fetal goiter, although brief administration of lower doses (6-40 mg/day) can be considered. Potassium iodide (SSKI, Pima) 1-2 drops three times daily mixed in juice or water has also been given. Administration of these preparations should be under the direction of the operating surgeon.
- Radiation emergencies: Potassium iodide (KI) should be taken just before or as soon as possible after exposure. For adults exposed to 10 centigrays (cGy) of radiation or more, KI 130 mg is given (for pregnant or lactating women, 120 mg KI is administered for radiation exposure of 5cGy or more).
- Septicemia (serious bacterial infections in the blood): Patients with gingivitis have rinsed with 7.5% povidone-iodine for 2 minutes before ultrasonic scaling of the teeth.

- Skin/wound sterilization: Various concentrations of iodine have been used, for example, 2% tincture or 2% aqueous solution to affected areas, 10% povidone-iodine applied before insertion of catheters, 0.9% iodine ointment for diabetic foot ulcers, and 1% povidone-iodine for wound irrigation. Use as directed.
- Upper airway sterilization: 1% povidone-iodine solution inhaled via nebulizer twice daily has been used, with gargle twice daily.
- Water sterilization: Salt iodization of water supplies on a large-scale basis can be performed with the addition of iodide or iodate salt with an iodine content varying from 7-100 mg/kg of salt. For individual use, tincture of iodine 3-10 drops per quart of water has been used, with 15 minutes for antimicrobial effects to occur.

Children (Younger than 18 Years)

- The U.S. Recommended Dietary Allowance (RDA) is 50 mcg daily for infants 0-12 months; 90 mcg daily for children 1-8 years; 120 mcg daily for children 9-13 years; 150 mcg daily for children 14-18 years. The Adequate Intake (AI) for infants is 110 mcg daily for ages 0-6 months; 130 mcg daily for 7-12 months. The Tolerable Upper Intake Levels (UL) are 200 mcg daily for ages 1-3 years; 300 mcg daily for ages 4-8 years; 600 mcg daily for ages 9-13 years; 900 mcg daily for ages 14-18 years (including pregnancy and lactation).
- Iodine deficiency: Iodine deficiency is rare in industrialized countries because of supplementation of table salt and cattle feed with iodine. In areas of endemic iodine deficiency, various doses of iodine have been used as prevention or treatment in children, including 150 mcg daily.
- Ophthalmia neonatorum prevention: 1 drop of 2.5% povidone-iodine applied at birth has been used. No advantage of a second drop has been found.
- Radiation emergencies: Potassium iodide (KI) should be taken just before or as soon as possible after exposure. For infants, babies, and children, KI is administered for exposure of 5 centigrays (cGy) or more. For birth through 1 month, 16 mg can be administered; for ages 1 month through 3 years, 32 mg can be administered; for ages 3-12 years, 65 mg can be administered; for adolescents ages 12-18 years, 65 mg can be administered (or up to 120 mg if the adolescent is approaching adult size).
- Skin/wound sterilization: Various concentrations of iodine have been used, for example, 2% tincture or 2% aqueous solution to affected areas.
- Thyroid disorders: Children should be managed under medical supervision.

SAFETY
Allergies

- Some individuals are allergic or hypersensitive to iodide or to organic preparations containing iodine. Hypersensitivity reactions may involve rash, angioedema (throat swelling), cutaneous/mucosal hemorrhage (bleeding), fever, arthralgias (joint pains), eosinophilia (abnormal blood counts), urticaria (hives), thrombotic thrombocytopenic purpura, or severe periarteritis (inflammation around blood vessels). Reactions can be severe and deaths have occurred with exposure.

- Topical use of iodine preparations may irritate or burn tissues and cause sensitization in some individuals.
- This review does not comprehensively cover the use of iodine-based intravenous contrast media for CT scan imaging, although serious life-threatening allergic reactions have been associated with use. Individuals with known or suspected iodine hypersensitivity should inform their physician before receiving contrast media.

Side Effects and Warnings

- **Note:** This review does not cover adverse effects associated with intravenous iodine-based contrast agents used for CT scan imaging or radioactive iodine.
- Iodine preparations used orally (by mouth) or topically (on the skin) are generally considered to be safe in healthy non-allergic individuals when used in recommended amounts, not exceeding tolerated upper limits. Higher amounts taken acutely or chronically may result in adverse effects.
- Acute iodine poisoning is rare and generally occurs only with doses of many grams. Symptoms may include burning of the mouth, throat, and stomach, fever, nausea, vomiting, diarrhea, cardiovascular compromise, and loss of consciousness/coma.
- Chronic iodism, also known as iodide intoxication, may cause eye irritation, eyelid swelling, unpleasant/metallic taste, burning or swelling of the mouth/throat, soreness of the gums/teeth, increased salivation, gastrointestinal upset, diarrhea, anorexia, flu-like symptoms, sneezing, cough, pulmonary edema (fluid in the lungs), confusion, headache, fatigue, depression, numbness, tingling, pain, weakness, muscle aches, easy bruising, irregular heartbeat, or acne-like skin lesions. Prolonged excess intake of iodine can lead to thyroid gland dysfunction including hypothyroidism or hyperthyroidism, parotitis, thyroid gland hyperplasia (enlargement), thyroid adenoma, goiter, autoimmunity, and elevated thyroid stimulating hormone (TSH) levels.
- Individuals with autoimmune thyroid disease (AITD) may have increased sensitivity to adverse effects of iodine. Those with previous iodine deficiency or nodular goiter may be particularly susceptible. Patients should be aware that kelp supplements also contain iodine, as a kelp-containing tea has been reported to cause iodine-induced hypothyroidism.
- Topical cadexomer iodine has been associated with local burning sensation in clinical trials. Cutaneous (skin) intolerance may develop with the topical use of iodinated polyvidone. Other reported reactions to tinctures include rash, blistering, crusting, irritation, itching, or erythema (reddening) of skin. Topical use of iodine may stain the skin.
- Sodium iodide should be used cautiously in those with gastrointestinal obstruction.
- Povidone-iodine bladder irrigation has been associated with increased risk of urinary tract infection.
- It has been suggested that application of povidone-iodine to wounds (particularly surgical wounds) may locally suppress immune cells and wound healing and increase susceptibility to local infection.
- Internal administration of povidone may cause serious side effects that may even lead to kidney failure or death.
- Lugol solution and saturated solution of potassium iodide (SSKI, Pima) should be avoided in patients with pulmonary edema, bronchitis, or known tuberculosis.
- Sodium iodide should be used cautiously in those with renal failure. Lugol solution and SSKI (Pima) should be avoided in those with hyperkalemia.

Pregnancy and Breastfeeding

- Iodine requirements are increased during pregnancy. Iodine supplementation during pregnancy may be particularly relevant in areas of endemic iodine deficiency, such as nonindustrialized nations. Iodine deficiency during pregnancy has been associated with an increased incidence of miscarriage, stillbirth, birth defects, and mental retardation. Moreover, severe iodine deficiency during pregnancy may result in congenital hypothyroidism in the newborn. In contrast, excess iodine intake by pregnant women may lead to effects of excess iodine in the fetus/newborn, including thyroid dysfunction or skin irritation.
- It has been suggested to avoid topical use of povidone-iodine for perianal preparation during delivery or postpartum antisepsis because of possible iodine absorption by the newborn or absorption by the mother leading to increased breast milk iodine concentrations. Other reports suggest that this may not be a significant concern.
- Iodine supplementation during breastfeeding may be particularly relevant in areas of endemic iodine deficiency, such as nonindustrialized nations. Infants are particularly vulnerable to the effects of iodine deficiency, and iodine deficient women may not be able to provide sufficient iodine in their breast milk.

INTERACTIONS
Interactions with Drugs

- Amiodarone (Cordarone) contains significant amounts of iodine. Plasma iodine levels may be increased and additive with iodine supplements. Thyroid function should be monitored.
- Concomitant use of angiotensin-converting enzyme inhibitors (ACE-I) or angiotensin receptor blockers (ARB) with potassium iodide increases the risk of hyperkalemia (high blood potassium levels). Examples of ACE inhibitors include benazepril (Lotensin), captopril (Capoten), enalapril (Vasotec), fosinopril (Monopril), lisinopril (Prinivil, Zestril), moexipril (Univasc), perindopril (Aceon), quinapril (Accupril), ramipril (Altace), and trandolapril (Mavik). The ARBs include losartan (Cozaar), valsartan (Diovan), irbesartan (Avapro), candesartan (Atacand), telmisartan (Micardis), and eprosartan (Teveten).
- Additive hypothyroid effects may occur with the use of iodine products in combination with antithyroid drugs (methimazole, propylthiouracil).
- Additive hypothyroid effects may occur with the use of iodine products such as potassium iodide in combination with lithium salts. Lugol solution can increase lithium toxicity by inducing additive hypothyroid effects.
- Concomitant use of potassium iodide with potassium-sparing diuretics may increase the risk of hyperkalemia (high blood potassium levels). Examples of potassium-sparing diuretics include spironolactone (Aldactone), triamterene (Dyrenium), and amiloride (Midamor).

Interactions with Herbs and Dietary Supplements

- Bugleweed (*Lycopus virginicus*, *Lycopus europaeus*) may reduce iodine uptake.
- High iodine content can be found in kelp/seaweed/bladderwrack and may add to the effects of iodine supplementation.
- Ingestion of lithospermum may lower thyroid hormone blood levels and may interact with the effects of iodine on thyroid hormone levels.

- Selenium deficiency may exacerbate the effects of iodine deficiency.
- Iodine may interact with herbs and supplements with diuretic effects; use cautiously.

For a complete list of references, please visit www.naturalstandard.com.

Iron (Fe)

RELATED TERMS

- Atomic number 26, carbonyl iron, dextran-iron, elemental iron, Fe, Fer, ferrous carbonate anhydrous, ferrous fumarate, ferrous gluconate, ferrous pyrophosphate, ferrous sulfate, iron dextran, iron-polysaccharide, iron sorbitol, iron sucrose, sodium ferric gluconate.
- Selected U.S. brand names: DexFerrum, Femiron, Feosol Caplets, Feosol Tablets, Feostat, Feostat Drops, Feratab, Fer-gen-sol, Fergon, Fer-In-Sol Drops, Fer-In-Sol Syrup, Fer-Iron Drops, Fero-Gradumet, Ferospace, Ferralet, Ferralet Slow Release, Ferralyn Lanacaps, Ferra-TD, Ferretts, Ferrlecit, Fumasorb, Fumerin, Hemocyte, Hemofer, Hytinic, INFeD, Ircon, Mol-Iron, Nephro-Fer, Niferex, Niferex-150, Nu-Iron, Nu-Iron 150, Simron, Slow Fe, Span-FF, Venofer.

BACKGROUND

- Iron is an essential mineral and an important component of proteins involved in oxygen transport and metabolism. Iron is also an essential cofactor in the synthesis of neurotransmitters such as dopamine, norepinephrine, and serotonin. About 15% of the body's iron is stored for future needs and mobilized when dietary intake is inadequate. The body usually maintains normal iron status by controlling the amount of iron absorbed from food.
- There are two forms of dietary iron: heme and nonheme. Sources of heme iron include meat fish, and poultry. Sources of nonheme iron, which is not absorbed as well as heme iron, include beans, lentils, flours, cereals, and grain products. Other sources of iron include dried fruit, peas, asparagus, leafy greens, strawberries, and nuts.
- The World Health Organization considers iron deficiency to be the largest international nutritional disorder. Although much of the ethnic disparity in iron deficiency anemia remains unexplained, socioeconomic factors may be involved.
- Iron deficiency can be determined by measurement of iron levels within the body, mainly serum ferritin levels, which can also help distinguish between iron deficiency anemia and anemia associated with chronic disease.
- Herbal preparations such as yellow dock root may be used in iron deficiency, although scientific evidence may be lacking.

EVIDENCE

Uses Based on Scientific Evidence	Grade
Anemia of Chronic Disease Taking iron orally with epoetin alfa (erythropoietin, EPO, Epogen, Procrit) is effective for treating anemia associated with chronic renal failure and chemotherapy.	A
Iron Deficiency Anemia Ferrous sulfate (Feratab, Fer-Iron, Slow-FE) is the standard treatment for treating iron deficiency anemia. Dextran-iron (INFeD) is given intravenously by health care providers to restore adequate iron levels in bone marrow when oral iron therapy has failed.	A
ACE Inhibitor–Associated Cough Taking iron orally seems to inhibit coughs associated with angiotensin-converting enzyme (ACE) inhibitors, such as captopril (Capoten), enalapril (Vasotec), and lisinopril (Prinivil, Zestril).	B
Preventing Iron Deficiency in Menstruating Women Iron supplementation has been shown to improve iron status in menstruating women.	B
Prevention of Iron Deficiency Anemia in Pregnancy Iron supplements have been shown to help prevent iron deficiency anemia in pregnant women. Anemia in pregnant women is associated with adverse outcomes such as low birth weight, premature birth, and maternal mortality. Screening by a qualified health care provider is needed. Low doses are generally well tolerated and associated with better compliance.	B
Attention Deficit Hyperactivity Disorder (ADHD) Based on preliminary data, taking iron orally might improve symptoms of attention deficit hyperactivity disorder (ADHD). However, evidence is insufficient to support effectiveness.	C
Fatigue in Women with Low Ferritin Levels Ferrous sulfate may improve fatigue primarily in women with borderline or low serum ferritin concentrations. However, evidence is insufficient to support effectiveness.	C
Improving Cognitive Performance Related to Iron Deficiency Taking iron by mouth seems to improve cognitive function related to iron deficiency in iron-deficient children and adolescents. Further research is needed to confirm the potential benefit of iron in this indication. Iron supplements are not recommended for improving cognitive performance in non–iron-deficient people.	C
Lead Toxicity Iron deficiency may increase the risk of lead poisoning in children. However, the use of iron supplementation in lead poisoning should be reserved for those individuals who are truly iron deficient or for those individuals with continuing lead exposure, such as continued residence in lead-exposed housing.	C
Preventing Anemia Associated with Preterm/ Low Birth Weight Infants There is insufficient evidence to recommend iron for treating anemia on preterm/low birth weight infants.	C

(Continued)

Uses Based on Scientific Evidence	Grade
Preventing Iron Deficiency in Exercising Women Preliminary studies suggest that iron supplementation can reverse mild anemia after exercise, improve energy, and enhance performance. However, other studies disagree. However, evidence is insufficient to support effectiveness.	C
Prevention of Iron Deficiency after Blood Donation The results of early study indicate that elemental iron can adequately compensate for iron loss in men and women who donate whole blood up to 4 (women) or 6 times per year (men).	C
Prevention of Iron Deficiency Anemia Due to Gastrointestinal Bleeding Intravenous high-dose iron sucrose therapy in patients with iron deficiency anemia due to gastrointestinal blood loss appears to be safe and therefore is a therapeutic option that may save time and improve patient compliance. However, evidence is insufficient to support effectiveness.	C
Treatment of Predialysis Anemia Adequate iron supplementation may be beneficial as an adjunct therapy to erythropoietin in the treatment of predialysis anemia. Predialysis anemia should be treated by a qualified health care provider. However, evidence is insufficient to support effectiveness.	C
Therapy for Anemia after Orthopedic Surgery Early study reports that iron taken after elective hip or knee replacement surgery does not result in higher hemoglobin levels after surgery or a faster rate of increase in hemoglobin levels than placebo.	D

Uses Based on Tradition or Theory

Anemia in anorexia nervosa, arm tremor, athletic performance enhancement, canker sores, Crohn's disease, cystic fibrosis, depression, enhanced immune function, fatigue, female infertility, growth, menorrhagia (abnormally heavy menstrual bleeding), pagophagia (compulsive eating of ice), prevention of anemia in blood donors, restless leg syndrome.

DOSING
Adults (18 Years and Older)
- The Recommended Dietary Allowance (RDA) for males (19-50 years) is 8 mg daily; females (19-50 years), 18 mg daily; adults (51 years and older), 8 mg daily; pregnant women (all ages), 27 mg daily; breastfeeding women (19 years and older), 9 mg daily.
- The Tolerable Upper Intake Level (UL) for adults (19 years and older) is 45 mg daily.
- The RDA for iron in a completely vegetarian diet should be adjusted as follows: 14 mg daily for adult men and

postmenopausal women, 33 mg daily for premenopausal women, and 26 mg daily for adolescent girls.
- Doses ranging from 60-180 mg of elemental iron have been used for iron deficiency/anemia. Dextran-iron (INFeD) is given by health care providers to replenish depleted iron stores in the bone marrow, where it is incorporated into hemoglobin. The usual adult dose is 2 mL daily (100 mg iron).

Children (Younger than 18 Years)
- The Recommended Dietary Allowance (RDA) is 11 mg for ages 7-12 months; 7 mg for ages 1-3 years; 10 mg for ages 4-8 years; 8 mg for ages 9-13 years (male and female); 11 mg for males 14-18 years; 15 mg for females 14-18 years; 27 mg for pregnant females 14-18 years; 10 mg for breastfeeding females 14-18 years. For infants 0-6 months, 0.27 mg is recommended as the adequate intake level (AI), which is used when RDA cannot be determined.
- The Tolerable Upper Intake Level (UL) for infants (1-12 months) is not possible to establish; the UL for children (1-13 years) is 40 mg daily; the UL for adolescents (14-18 years) is 45 mg daily.
- Dextran-iron (INFeD) is an intravenous preparation given by qualified health care providers to replenish depleted iron stores in the bone marrow, where it is incorporated into hemoglobin. Doses of 50 mg iron (1 mL) (5-10 kg) and 100 mg iron (2 mL) (10-50 kg) have been used.

SAFETY
Allergies
- Iron is a trace mineral, and hypersensitivity is unlikely. Avoid in individuals with a known allergy or hypersensitivity to products containing iron.

Side Effects and Warnings
- In general, people with a history of kidney disease, intestinal disease, peptic ulcer disease, enteritis, colitis, pancreatitis, and hepatitis and people who consume excessive alcohol, plan to become pregnant, or are older than 55 years and have a family history of heart disease should consult a doctor and pharmacist before taking iron.
- Liquid oral iron preparations can possibly blacken teeth.
- Acute overdosage or iron accumulation symptoms may include arthritis, signs of gonadal failure (amenorrhea, early menopause, loss of libido, impotence), and shortness of breath/dyspnea. High doses may cause vomiting and diarrhea followed by cardiovascular or metabolic toxicity and death. It is unclear whether high levels are associated with cancer, coronary heart disease, or myocardial infarction (MI or heart attack).
- Gastrointestinal upset, including nausea, vomiting, constipation, diarrhea, and dark stools, has been reported. Gastrointestinal side effects are relatively common, and corrective bowel regimens such as increasing dietary fiber or over-the-counter medication might be recommended to balance these side effects. Supervision by a qualified health care provider is recommended.
- Individuals with blood disorders who require frequent blood transfusions are also at risk of iron overload and should not take iron supplements without direction by a qualified health care provider. Long-term use of high doses of iron can cause hemosiderosis that clinically resembles hemochromatosis. Iron overload is associated with several genetic diseases including hemochromatosis (a defect in

iron metabolism with build-up of iron in the body). The most commonly associated early hemochromatosis symptoms include fatigue, weakness, weight loss, abdominal pain, and arthralgia (joint pain). Iron overload is possible in very low birth weight infants after multiple blood transfusions because of an increased liver iron concentration. Prenatal iron overload might contribute to the pathogenesis of the disease, but further studies are needed to confirm the assumption. Accumulation of excess iron is being investigated as a potential contributor to neurodegenerative diseases such as Alzheimer's and Parkinson's disease.

- Hepatitis C virus (HCV) infection and iron loading may aggravate oxidative stress in dialysis patients.
- A case of hypersiderosis (uncontrollable sweating) has been reported with long-term iron supplementation in uremic patients treated with periodic dialysis.
- One study indicates that higher consumption of total red meat, especially various processed meats, may increase risk of developing type 2 diabetes in women.

Pregnancy and Breastfeeding

- Pregnant or breastfeeding women should seek guidance from a qualified health care provider before taking dietary supplements. Iron status of the pregnant woman should be measured early (before the fifteenth week of gestation), and iron supplements should be given as selective prophylaxis based on the serum ferritin level.
- U.S. Food and Drug Administration (FDA) Pregnancy Category B: Usually safe but benefits must outweigh the risks.
- FDA Pregnancy Category C: Safety for use during pregnancy has not been established for replenishing depleted iron stores in the bone marrow, where it is incorporated into hemoglobin.

INTERACTIONS
Interactions with Drugs

- Acetohydroxamic acid (AHA, Lithostat) is prescribed to decrease urinary ammonia and may help with antibiotics to work with other kidney stone treatment. Use with iron supplements may cause either medicine to be less effective.
- Allopurinol (Zyloprim), a medication used to treat gout, may increase iron storage in the liver and should not be used in combination with iron supplements.
- Aminosalicylic acid (paraaminosalicylic acid, PAS, Paser) may cause a malabsorption syndrome (weight loss, iron and vitamin depletion, excessive fat in the stools [steatorrhea]). A qualified health care provider should be contacted immediately if any of these symptoms is experienced.
- Antacids may reduce iron absorption, and reduced efficacy has occurred occasionally. Clinically significant effects are unlikely with adequate dietary iron intake. However, it is recommended to avoid antacids or separate the doses of antacids and iron.
- Aspirin and nonsteroidal antiinflammatory drugs (NSAIDs) can cause mucosal damage and bleeding throughout the gastrointestinal tract. Chronic blood loss associated with long-term use of these agents may contribute to iron deficiency anemia. Because iron supplements may also irritate the gastrointestinal tract, patients should not use them concurrently with NSAIDs unless recommended by a physician. Iron-rich food intake may be advised as an alternative.
- Iron can decrease absorption of prescription drug bisphosphonates by forming insoluble complexes. Bisphosphonates include alendronate (Fosamax), etidronate (Didronel), risedronate (Actonel), and tiludronate (Skelid). Doses of bisphosphonates should be separated by at least 2 hours from doses of all other medications, including supplements such as iron.
- Chloramphenicol (Chloromycetin) can reduce the response to iron therapy in iron deficiency anemia.
- Cholestyramine (Questran) and colestipol (Colestid) may bind iron in the gut, reducing its absorption. Clinically significant iron deficiency induced by these drugs has not been reported, and supplements are not likely to be needed. If iron supplements are taken for other causes of deficiency, it is recommended that the iron and cholestyramine or colestipol doses be separated by at least 4 hours.
- Desferrioxamine (DFO) is an iron-chelating drug that lowers iron levels.
- Iron supplements and dimercaprol may combine in the body to form a harmful chemical.
- Bone marrow iron deposits have been shown to decrease significantly in patients taking human recombinant erythropoietin (EPO-R).
- Iron decreases the absorption of fluoroquinolone antibiotics. Fluoroquinolones include ciprofloxacin (Cipro), levofloxacin (Levaquin), ofloxacin (Floxin), and others. It is recommended to take these antibiotics at least 2 hours before or 2 hours after iron-containing supplements.
- Gastric acid is important for the absorption of iron, particularly dietary nonheme (plant-derived) iron. Adequate dietary iron intake is recommended when H_2 blockers such as cimetidine (Tagamet), ranitidine (Zantac), famotidine (Pepcid), or nizatidine (Axid) are taken. Iron supplements are not usually required unless they are being used for another indication.
- There is some evidence in healthy people that iron forms chelates with levodopa (Sinemet), which reduces the amount of levodopa absorbed by around 50%. Until further research is available, doses of levodopa and iron should be separated as much as possible.
- Iron can decrease the absorption and efficacy of levothyroxine (Levoxyl, Synthroid) by forming insoluble complexes in the gastrointestinal tract. It is recommended that levothyroxine and iron doses be separated by at least 2 hours.
- Iron can decrease the absorption of methyldopa (Aldomet), which results in increases in blood pressure. It is recommended that methyldopa and iron doses be separated by at least 2 hours.
- Oral iron supplements markedly reduce absorption of mycophenolate mofetil (CellCept). It is recommended that iron be taken 4-6 hours before or 2 hours after mycophenolate mofetil.
- There is some evidence that pancreatic enzyme supplements (pancrelipases such as Cotazym, Creon, Pancrease, Ultrase, and Viokase) can reduce iron absorption by possibly binding iron or altering pH. Clinical significance is unlikely, except in people with cystic fibrosis who need pancreatic enzyme supplements for prolonged periods and who have other factors contributing to iron deficiency. Iron status should be monitored by a qualified health care provider.
- Oral iron supplements can reduce absorption of penicillamine (Cuprimine, Depen) by 30%-70%, probably because of chelate formation. Efficacy of penicillamine is reduced in Wilson's disease; the clinical significance in people with

rheumatoid arthritis (RA) has not been determined. Patients should be advised to take penicillamine at least 2 hours before or after iron-containing supplements.

- Gastric acid is important for the absorption of iron. However, long-term treatment, up to 12.5 years, with proton pump inhibitors, such as esomeprazole (Nexium), lansoprazole (Prevacid), omeprazole (Prilosec), rabeprazole (AcipHex), and pantoprazole (Protonix, Pantoloc) has not been associated with iron depletion or anemia in people with normal iron stores. Maintaining adequate dietary iron intake is recommended.
- Concomitant use can decrease the absorption of tetracycline antibiotics by 50%-90%. Patients should be advised to take tetracyclines at least 2 hours before or after iron-containing supplements. Some of these drugs include doxycycline (Vibramycin), minocycline (Minocin), tetracycline (Achromycin), and others.

Interactions with Herbs and Dietary Supplements

- Acacia forms an insoluble gel with ferric iron. Clinical significance is unknown.
- Calcium supplements have been shown to inhibit absorption of iron supplements when taken with food. However, in people with adequate iron stores, this does not appear to be clinically significant. The recommendation for people at risk of iron deficiency is to take calcium supplements at bedtime, instead of with meals, to avoid inhibiting dietary iron absorption.
- Copper metabolism may be altered by iron supplements, but the clinical importance of this observation is unknown.
- Citric, malic, tartaric, and lactic acids have some enhancing effects on nonheme iron absorption.
- Phytic acid is present in legumes, grains, and rice and is an inhibitor of nonheme iron absorption. Small amounts of phytic acid can reduce nonheme iron absorption by 50%. The absorption of iron from legumes, such as soybeans, black beans, lentils, mung beans, and split peas, has been shown to be as low as 2%.
- Polyphenols, found in some fruits, vegetables, coffees, teas, wines, and spices, can markedly inhibit the absorption of nonheme iron. This effect is reduced by the presence of vitamin C.
- Riboflavin (vitamin B_2) supplements may improve the hematological response to iron supplements in some people with anemia.
- Based on preliminary data, iron may decrease selenium levels. Further research is needed to confirm these results.
- Soy protein reduces the absorption of dietary nonheme (plant-derived) iron, probably because of binding of iron by phytate and calcium present in soy. Fermented soy products seem to inhibit iron absorption less.
- Vitamin A appears to be involved in mobilizing iron from tissue stores for delivery to developing red blood cells in the bone marrow. Vitamin A may also be involved in the differentiation and proliferation of blood stem cells in the bone marrow and in the synthesis of erythropoietin. Preliminary evidence also suggests that vitamin A and beta-carotene may enhance nonheme iron absorption from iron-fortified wheat and corn flour and rice. It is unlikely that vitamin A supplements would have significant effects on iron status in people without vitamin A deficiency.
- The amount of vitamin C in the diet is a factor in dietary iron absorption and iron status. Vitamin C can counteract the effects of substances that inhibit iron absorption. Supplemental or dietary vitamin C improves absorption of supplemental or dietary nonheme (plant-derived) iron ingested at the same time. Taking a vitamin C supplement to improve the absorption of dietary or supplemental iron probably is not necessary for most people, especially if their diet contains adequate amounts of vitamin C.
- Use of oral iron preparations in premature infants with low serum vitamin E levels may cause hemolysis and hemolytic anemia. Vitamin E deficiency should be corrected before administering supplemental iron.
- Iron may decrease zinc absorption, but there does not seem to be a clinically significant interaction between dietary iron and zinc or between supplemental iron and zinc dietary sources.

For a complete list of references, please visit www.naturalstandard.com.

Jackfruit
(*Artocarpus heterophyllus*)

RELATED TERMS

- Artocarpus, *Artocarpus asperulus, Artocarpus heterophyllus, Artocarpus incisa, Artocarpus integer, Artocarpus integrifolia, Artocarpus masticata, Artocarpus melinoxylus, Artocarpus parva, Artocarpus petelotii*, breadfruit, jacalin, jack fruit, jackfruit seed, Moraceae (family).

BACKGROUND

- Jackfruit (*Artocarpus heterophyllus*), which refers to both a species of tree and its fruit, is native to southwestern India and Sri Lanka. Jackfruit was reportedly cultivated for food as early as the sixth century BC in India. At approximately 25 cm in diameter, jackfruit is reportedly the largest tree-borne fruit in the world. The fruit juices are extremely sticky, so people often oil their hands before preparing the fruit.
- The fruit can be ingested, and the wood is used for furniture and musical instruments. Recent laboratory studies show that lectins found in jackfruit and its seeds may have antibacterial, antifungal, antiviral, and immunostimulative properties. However, clinical study is lacking. The currently available research examines the role of jackfruit leaves in increasing glucose tolerance. More studies in humans are needed to define jackfruit's potential role in diabetes.

EVIDENCE

Uses Based on Scientific Evidence	Grade
High Blood Sugar/Glucose Intolerance Jackfruit leaves may improve glucose tolerance. However, there is little available research in this area.	C

Uses Based on Tradition or Theory
Antibacterial, antifungal, antiviral, contraception, food uses, immunostimulation.

DOSING

Adults (18 Years and Older)

- There is insufficient evidence to recommend a dose of jackfruit in adults. A hot-water extract of *Artocarpus heterophyllus* leaves equivalent to 20 g/kg of starting material has been taken by mouth for high blood sugar/glucose intolerance.

Children (Younger than 18 Years)

- There is insufficient evidence to recommend a dose of jackfruit in children.

SAFETY

Allergies

- Avoid in individuals with a known allergy or hypersensitivity to jackfruit (*Artocarpus heterophyllus*). In some patients, jackfruit is a Bet v 1 (birch pollen allergen)–related food allergy.

Side Effects and Warnings

- Jackfruit has few reported side effects. Use cautiously in patients with birch pollen allergies.
- Although not well studied in humans, jackfruit may increase coagulation. Caution is advised in patients with blood disorders. Jackfruit may also alter glucose tolerance, and patients with diabetes should consult with a qualified health care professional, including a pharmacist, to check for interactions.
- Jackfruit seeds may have immunostimulative effects. Use cautiously in patients using immunosuppression therapy or with transplanted tissues.
- Use cautiously in patients attempting to become pregnant because jackfruit seeds may markedly inhibit libido, sexual arousal, sexual vigor, and sexual performance (induce mild erectile dysfunction) in males. However, jackfruit seeds do not appear to alter ejaculating competence or fertility.

Pregnancy and Breastfeeding

- Jackfruit is not recommended in pregnant or breastfeeding women because of a lack of available scientific evidence. Although not well studied in humans, jackfruit seeds may transiently inhibit libido, sexual arousal, sexual vigor, and sexual performance (induce mild erectile dysfunction). However, jackfruit seeds do not appear to alter ejaculating competence or fertility.

INTERACTIONS

Interactions with Drugs

- Various jackfruit plant parts, including the bark, wood, leaves, fruit, and seeds, may exhibit a broad spectrum of antibacterial activity. Caution is advised in patients taking antibiotics because of possible additive effects.
- Jackfruit seeds may increase the risk of bleeding when taken with drugs that increase the risk of bleeding. Some examples include aspirin, anticoagulants ("blood thinners") such as warfarin (Coumadin) or heparin, antiplatelet drugs such as clopidogrel (Plavix), and nonsteroidal antiinflammatory drugs (NSAIDS) such as ibuprofen (Motrin, Advil) or naproxen (Naprosyn, Aleve).
- Jackfruit leaves may improve glucose tolerance in normal and type 2 diabetes patients. Caution is advised when medications that may also alter blood sugar are used. Patients taking drugs for diabetes by mouth or using insulin should be monitored closely by a qualified health care professional, including a pharmacist. Medication adjustments may be necessary.
- Although not well studied in humans, jackfruit may inhibit the growth of *Fusarium moniliforme* and *Saccharomyces cerevisiae*. However, there are conflicting data regarding jackfruit's antifungal activity. Caution is advised in patients taking other antifungal agents because of possible additive effects.
- Jackfruit may exhibit inhibitory activity with a cytopathic effect toward herpes simplex virus type 2, varicella-zoster virus, and cytomegalovirus. Caution is advised in patients

taking other antiviral agents because of possible additive effects.

- Jackfruit seeds may markedly inhibit libido, sexual arousal, sexual vigor, and sexual performance (induce mild erectile dysfunction) in males. However, jackfruit seeds do not appear to alter ejaculating competence and fertility. Caution is advised in patients taking jackfruit with agents for sexual dysfunction or agents with sexual side effects.
- Jackfruit and jackfruit seeds may have immunostimulative effects. Use cautiously when taking immunomodulators or immunostimulants.

Interactions with Herbs and Dietary Supplements

- Various jackfruit plant parts, including the bark, wood, leaves, fruit, and seeds, may exhibit a broad spectrum of antibacterial activity. Caution is advised when other herbs or supplements with antibacterial activity are taken because of possible additive effects.
- Jackfruit seeds may increase the risk of bleeding when taken with herbs and supplements that are believed to increase the risk of bleeding. Multiple cases of bleeding have been reported with the use of *Ginkgo biloba*, and fewer cases have been reported with garlic and saw palmetto. Numerous other agents may theoretically increase the risk of bleeding, although this has not been proven in most cases.
- Although not well studied in humans, jackfruit may inhibit the growth of *Fusarium moniliforme* and *Saccharomyces cerevisiae*. However, results are conflicting. Nonetheless, caution is advised in patients taking other herbs or supplements with antifungal activity because of possible additive effects.
- Jackfruit may exhibit inhibitory activity with a cytopathic effect toward herpes simplex virus type 2, varicella-zoster virus, and cytomegalovirus. Caution is advised in patients taking other herbs or supplements with antiviral activity because of possible additive effects.
- Jackfruit seeds may markedly inhibit libido, sexual arousal, sexual vigor, and sexual performance (induce mild erectile dysfunction) in males. However, jackfruit seeds do not appear to alter ejaculating competence or fertility. Caution is advised in patients taking jackfruit with herbs or supplements for sexual dysfunction or herbs or supplements with sexual side effects.
- Jackfruit leaves may improve glucose tolerance in normal and type 2 diabetes patients. Caution is advised when herbs or supplement that may alter blood sugar are used. Blood glucose levels may require monitoring, and doses may need adjustment.
- Jackfruit and jackfruit seeds may have immunostimulative effects. Use cautiously when taking immunomodulators or immunostimulants.

For a complete list of references, please visit www.naturalstandard.com.

Jasmine
(*Jasminum* spp.)

RELATED TERMS

- Catalonian jasmine, common jasmine, common white jasmine, Italian jasmine, jasmin, jasmine flower, Jasmini Flos, *Jasminum, Jasminum grandiflorum, Jasminum officinale*, jati, jessamine, mo li hua, pikake (Hawaiian), poet's jasmine, poet's jessamine, royal jasmine, sambac (Pilipino), Spanish jasmine, yasmin (Persian), yeh-hsi-ming.

BACKGROUND

- Jasmine (*Jasminum* spp.) is a woody perennial climbing plant that is well known for its sweet, highly scented flowers. The flowers and oil are used in perfumes, essential oils, food flavorings, and tea.
- Jasmine flower has been used in aromatherapy for depression, nervousness, coughs, relaxation, and tension. Early studies have shown that jasmine may help with alertness and memory improvement.

EVIDENCE

Uses Based on Scientific Evidence	Grade
Alertness Jasmine is commonly used in aromatherapy as a relaxing, yet stimulating herb. However, preliminary study did not show an increase in alertness in subjects who used jasmine essential oil. The effectiveness remains unclear.	C
Lactation Suppression In the Ayurvedic tradition, jasmine has been used to reduce the secretion of breast milk. Preliminary human studies found that application of jasmine flowers to the breast decreased breast engorgement and milk production. However, the evidence is insufficient to support this use.	C
Memory Improvement Preliminary human studies have not shown a benefit of jasmine scent for memory recall. However, the evidence is not definitive.	C
Stroke Limited population study found that tea drinking may decrease the risk of stroke; however, use of jasmine tea had less of an effect than black or green teas. This indicates that the reduction of stroke risk may not be related to jasmine. The isolated effects of jasmine remain unclear.	C

Uses Based on Tradition or Theory
Acne, air purification, amenorrhea (lack of menstruation), anger, antibacterial, antifungal, antiseptic, antiviral, aphrodisiac (especially in women), aromatherapy, astringent, breast milk stimulant, burning eyes, calming, cancer, canker sores, childbirth, conjunctivitis, constipation, corns, cough, depression, ear discharge, earache, exhaustion, eye disorders, facial paralysis, fragrance, gas, hair growth, headaches, hearing loss, heart rate abnormalities, high blood pressure, hoarseness, impotence, infections, insect bites, insomnia, laryngitis, leprosy, liver disease, liver inflammation, loose teeth, menstrual flow stimulant, mood enhancement, muscle spasms, muscle tension, nervous system function, painful menstruation, palpitations, paralysis, parasitic worm infections, premenstrual syndrome, pruritus, respiratory tract mucous membrane inflammation, sedative, skin inflammation, sprains, sterility, stress, sunstroke, toothache, ulcers, urinary disorders, uterine disorders, wound healing.

DOSING

Adults (18 Years and Older)

- Jasmine has been taken by mouth as a tea or tincture. Jasmine essential oil is used in aromatherapy. Jasmine essential oil should not be taken by mouth.

Children (Younger than 18 Years)

- There is insufficient evidence to recommend a dose for jasmine, and use in children is not recommended.

SAFETY

Allergies

- Avoid with a known allergy or sensitivity to jasmine, its constituents, or members of the Oleaceae family, or with a known allergy or sensitivity to fragrances such as ylang-ylang, lemongrass, narcissus, and sandalwood.

Side Effects and Warnings

- When essential oils, including jasmine essential oil, are consumed orally, they are potentially unsafe as they are extremely potent and can be poisonous.

Pregnancy and Breastfeeding

- Jasmine is not recommended in pregnant or breastfeeding women. When jasmine flowers are applied to the breast, breast milk production may stop.

INTERACTIONS

Interactions with Drugs

- Jasmine may cause low blood pressure. Caution is advised in patients taking drugs that lower blood pressure.
- Jasmine may also have additive effects when taken with antifungals, antianxiety drugs, and diuretics.

Interactions with Herbs and Dietary Supplements

- Jasmine may cause low blood pressure. Caution is advised in patients taking herbs or supplements that lower blood pressure.
- Jasmine may also have additive effects when taken with antifungals, antianxiety herbs or supplements, and diuretics.

For a complete list of references, please visit www.naturalstandard.com.

J

Jequirity
(Abrus precatorius)

RELATED TERMS

- Abrin, abrin A, abrin B, abrin C, abrus a chapelet, *Abrusabrus* (L.) W. Wight, *Abrus cantoniensis, Abrus precatorius,* Linn., *Abrus pulchellus,* abrus seed, aivoeiro, arraccu-mitim, ayurvedic phytomedicine, bead vine, black-eyed Susan, blackeyed Susan, Buddhist rosary bead, cain ghe, Carolina muida, colorine, coral bean, crab's eye, crabs eye, deadly crab's eye, *Glycine abrus* L., graines reglisse, gunchi, gunja, hint meyankoku, hung tou, Indian bead, Indian licorice, Indian liquorice, jequerit, jequirity bean, jequirity seed, jumble beads, juquiriti, lady bug bean, lady bug seed, legume, Leguminosae (family), liane reglisse, love bean, lucky bean, ma liao tou, ojo de pajaro, paratella, paternoster, peonia de St. Tomas, peonia, peronilla, phytotoxin, Pois rouge, prayer beads, prayer head, precatory bean, rakat, reglisse, rosary beads, rosary pea, ruti, rutti, Seminole bead, tentos da America, temtos dos mundos, tento muido, to-azuki, tribal pulse, weather plant, weesboontje, wild licorice.

BACKGROUND

- Abrin, a constituent of jequirity *(Abrus precatorius),* is toxic, and ingestion of one bean by a child may be fatal. However, the boiled seeds of *Abrus precatorius* L. are eaten by the residents of the Andaman Islands in India; boiling the seeds reportedly deactivates the toxins. Abrin is being investigated for the treatment of experimental cancers and is used as a "molecular probe" to investigate cell function.
- In folk medicine, jequirity is used orally to quicken labor, as an abortifacient (induces abortion), as an oral contraceptive, to treat diabetes and chronic nephritis (kidney inflammation), and as an analgesic (pain reliever) in terminally ill patients. The whole plant has been used for ophthalmic (eye) inflammations.

EVIDENCE

Uses Based on Scientific Evidence

No available studies qualify for inclusion in the evidence table.

Uses Based on Tradition or Theory

Abdominal pain, abortifacient (induces abortion), abscesses, acne, allergies, animal bites, anodyne (pain reliever), anthelmintic (expels worms), anticonvulsant, anti-inflammatory, antimicrobial, antiplatelet agent, antisuppurative (drains pus), antitumor, aphrodisiac, asthma, blennorrhea (mucous discharge), boils, bronchitis, cancer, colds, colic, conjunctivitis (pink eye), contraceptive, convulsions, cough, diabetes, diarrhea, diuretic, emetic (induces vomiting), epilepsy, evil spirits, expectorant (promotes coughing up of mucus), emollient (softens and soothes skin), febrifuge (fever reducer), fever, fractures in animals, gastritis (inflamed stomach), gonorrhea (STD), graying hair, headache, hemostat, insecticide, jaundice, laxative, leukemia, leukoderma (loss of skin pigmentation), malaria, nephritis (kidney inflammation, chronic), nightblindness, purgative (strongly laxative), rabies (prevention), rheumatism, sedative, snakebite, sores, spermatorrhea (involuntary loss of semen without orgasm), tetanus, schistosomiasis (tropical parasitic disease, urinary), uterine tonic.

DOSING

Adults (18 Years and Older)

- There is insufficient evidence to recommend a dose for jequirity. Abrin, a constituent of *Abrus precatorius* seeds, is toxic, and its ingestion can be fatal. A common traditional dose is 5 g of ground jequirity root paste daily, which has been used for cramping, diarrhea, spermatorrhea (involuntary loss of semen without orgasm), and abdominal pain. To expel worms (anthelmintic), 1 tsp of ground, dried jequirity seeds once a day for 2 days has been taken by mouth. Ground *Abrus precatorius* and *Curcumalonga* roots have also been applied to wounds.

Children (Younger than 18 Years)

- There is insufficient evidence to recommend a dose for jequirity in children.

SAFETY

Allergies

- Avoid in people with a known allergy or hypersensitivity to jequirity and related plants in the Leguminosae family.

Side Effects and Warnings

- Ingestion of jequirity seeds has many toxic side effects, predominantly vomiting, diarrhea (possibly bloody), edema (swelling), vascular leak syndrome, coma, circulatory collapse, and death. Ingestion of seeds may cause hypertension (high blood pressure), tachycardia (fast heart rate), coma, or circulatory collapse.
- Seeds that are sucked, chewed, or ingested with cracked shells can cause stomach cramping and nausea. Eye contact with the seeds' contents may cause necrotizing conjunctivitis (pinkeye, eye infection). Jewelry made of the seeds may cause dermatitis.
- Although not well studied in humans, jequirity may cause kidney or liver damage, dyspnea (difficulty breathing), pulmonary hemorrhage, or emphysema.
- Jequirity may increase the risk of bleeding. Caution is advised in patients with bleeding disorders or those taking agents that may increase the risk of bleeding. Dosing adjustments may be necessary.

Pregnancy and Breastfeeding

- Jequirity is not recommended in pregnant or breastfeeding women due to a lack of available scientific evidence. Avoid taking the seeds by mouth in all patients, as the toxin abrin is present in potentially lethal amounts in the seeds.

INTERACTIONS
Interactions with Drugs

- Although not well studied in humans, jequirity seeds may increase the risk of bleeding when taken with drugs that increase the risk of bleeding. Some examples include aspirin, anticoagulants (blood thinners) such as warfarin (Coumadin) or heparin, antiplatelet drugs such as clopidogrel (Plavix), and nonsteroidal anti-inflammatory drugs (NSAIDs) such as ibuprofen (Motrin, Advil) or naproxen (Naprosyn, Aleve).
- Jequirity seeds may cause necrosis of hepatocytes (death of liver cells) and may have additive effects with hepatotoxic (liver-damaging) drugs. Caution is advised.
- Jequirity seeds may cause hypertension (high blood pressure) and may interact with agents that alter blood pressure, such as ACE inhibitors or beta-blockers.
- Jequirity seeds may cause necrosis (death) of renal (kidney) convoluted tubules and may have additive effects with nephrotoxic (kidney-damaging) drugs.

Interactions with Herbs and Dietary Supplements

- Although not well studied in humans, jequirity seeds may increase the risk of bleeding when taken with herbs and supplements that are believed to increase the risk of bleeding. Multiple cases of bleeding have been reported with the use of *Ginkgo biloba*, and fewer cases with garlic and saw palmetto. Numerous other agents may theoretically increase the risk of bleeding, although this has not been proven in most cases.
- Jequirity seeds may cause necrosis of hepatocytes (death of liver cells) and may have additive effects with hepatotoxic (liver-damaging) herbs. Caution is advised.
- Jequirity seeds may cause hypertension (high blood pressure) and may interact with herbs that alter blood pressure.
- Jequirity seeds may cause necrosis (death) of renal (kidney) convoluted tubules and may have additive effects with nephrotoxic (kidney-damaging) herbs.

For a complete list of references, please visit www.naturalstandard.com.

J

Jewelweed, Impatiens
(*Impatiens* spp.)

RELATED TERMS

- Balsaminaceae (family), calcium oxalate, common jewelweed, *Impatiens biflora*, *Impatiens pallida*, pale jewelweed, pale touch-me-not, touch-me-not.

BACKGROUND

- Jewelweed is a flowering plant from North America that can be found in roadside ditches and marshy areas.
- Jewelweed has been used for the treatment of poison ivy/oak. However, human studies do not support this use.
- There is currently not enough scientific evidence available in humans to support the use of jewelweed for any indication.

EVIDENCE

Uses Based on Scientific Evidence	Grade
Contact Dermatitis (Poison Ivy/Oak Skin Rash) Although jewelweed has been used for centuries as a treatment for poison ivy/oak rashes, human studies show that it is no better than a placebo.	C

Uses Based on Tradition or Theory
Bee stings, burns, constipation, diuretic (increases urine flow), fevers, fungal skin disorders, hair dye, hemorrhoids, jaundice, measles, nettle rash, rheumatism, stomach cramps, warts (removal).

DOSING

Adults (18 Years and Older)

- There is insufficient evidence to recommend a dose for jewelweed in adults.

Children (Younger than 18 Years)

- There is insufficient evidence to recommend a dose for jewelweed in children.

SAFETY

Allergies

- Avoid in people with a known allergy or hypersensitivity to jewelweed *(Impatiens* spp.) or its constituents.

Side Effects and Warnings

- Jewelweed has been used as a food source as well as medicinally to treat a variety of ailments. However, due to a potential high mineral content, it is considered dangerous when consumed in excess amounts.
- Use cautiously if taking calcium supplements or if prone to kidney stones, as jewelweed may have high calcium oxalate content.

Pregnancy and Breastfeeding

- Jewelweed is not recommended in pregnant or breastfeeding women due to a lack of available scientific evidence. Jewelweed should be avoided due to reports of high mineral content, such as calcium oxalate.

INTERACTIONS

Interactions with Drugs

- There is not enough available scientific evidence.

Interactions with Herbs and Dietary Supplements

- Jewelweed may have high calcium oxalate content.

For a complete list of references, please visit www.naturalstandard.com.

Jiaogulan
(*Gynostemma pentaphyllum*)

RELATED TERMS

- Amachazuru, Cucurbitaceae (family), dammarane-type saponins, *Gynostemma pentaphyllum*, gypenoside XLIX, gypenosides, miracle grass, southern ginseng, *Vitis pentaphyllum*, xianxao.

BACKGROUND

- Jiaogulan (*Gynostemma pentaphyllum*) is best known as a traditional Chinese medicine herb. In the Guizhou Province it is used as an anti-aging herb, and many people who drink jiaogulan tea reach very old age. However, no link between jiaogulan tea and living many years has been scientifically proven.
- Jioagulan has shown some promise for treating cancer. Jiaogulan may also reduce nonalcoholic fatty liver disease, although more studies are needed in both of these areas before a recommendation can be made.

EVIDENCE

Uses Based on Scientific Evidence	Grade
Cancer Preliminary evidence indicates that gypenosides extracted from *Gynostemma pentaphyllum* decrease cancer cell viability, arrest the cell cycle, and induce apoptosis (cell death) in human cancer cells. Immune function in cancer patients has also been studied. However, evidence thus far has not been conclusive.	C
Fatty Liver (Nonalcoholic) *Gynostemma pentaphyllum* extract may be helpful for those with nonalcoholic fatty liver disease when combined with other treatment. However, evidence thus far has not been conclusive.	C

Uses Based on Tradition or Theory
Aging, anticoagulant (blood thinner), anti-inflammatory, atherosclerosis (hardening of the arteries), bleeding (subarachnoid hemorrhage), diabetes, hepatoprotection (liver protection), hypercholesterolemia (high cholesterol).

DOSING

Adults (18 Years and Older)

- There is insufficient evidence to recommend a dose for jiaogulan, although 80 mL of *Gynostemma pentaphyllum* extraction has been taken for 4 months in conjunction with a controlled diet for fatty liver.

Children (Younger than 18 Years)

- There is insufficient evidence to recommend a dose for jiaogulan in children.

SAFETY

Allergies

- Avoid in people with a known allergy or hypersensitivity to jiaogulan (*Gynostemma pentaphyllum*) or its constituents.

Side Effects and Warnings

- Currently, there is not enough available evidence about the side effects of jiaogulan. Nonetheless, use cautiously in patients with hematological (blood) conditions or those taking anticoagulants or antiplatelet agents (blood thinners). Also, use cautiously in patients with diabetes as *Gynostemma pentaphyllum* may decrease insulin levels and insulin index scores.

Pregnancy and Breastfeeding

- Jiaogulan is not recommended in pregnant or breastfeeding women due to a lack of available scientific evidence.

INTERACTIONS

Interactions with Drugs

- Although not well studied in humans, gypenosides extracted from *Gynostemma pentaphyllum* may have anti-cancer effects. Caution is advised when taking jiaogulan with other anticancer agents.
- *Gynostemma pentaphyllum* may decrease serum triglyceride levels. Thus, caution is advised when combining jiaogulan with other cholesterol-lowering agents.
- *Gynostemma pentaphyllum* may inhibit nuclear factor-kappaB activation, an important inflammatory factor. Caution is advised in patients taking anti-inflammatory agents.
- *Gynostemma pentaphyllum* may increase the risk of bleeding when taken with drugs that increase the risk of bleeding. However, current evidence is mixed. Some examples include aspirin, anticoagulants (blood thinners) such as warfarin (Coumadin) or heparin, antiplatelet drugs such as clopidogrel (Plavix), and nonsteroidal anti-inflammatory drugs (NSAIDs) such as ibuprofen (Motrin, Advil) or naproxen (Naprosyn, Aleve).
- *Gynostemma pentaphyllum* may decrease alanine aminotransferase, alkaline phosphatase, or aspartate aminotransferase levels in patients with nonalcoholic fatty liver disease. Caution is advised when combining jiaogulan with any potentially liver-damaging (hepatotoxic) agents.
- *Gynostemma pentaphyllum* may decrease insulin levels and insulin index scores in patients with nonalcoholic fatty liver disease. Caution is advised when combining jiaogulan with diabetes agents.

Interactions with Herbs and Dietary Supplements

- Although not well studied in humans, gypenosides extracted from *Gynostemma pentaphyllum* may have anti-cancer effects. Caution is advised when taking jiaogulan with other herbs or supplements that have potential anti-cancer effects.
- *Gynostemma pentaphyllum* may decrease serum triglyceride levels. Thus, caution is advised when combining jiaogulan

with other cholesterol-lowering herbs or supplements, such as red yeast rice.

- *Gynostemma pentaphyllum* may inhibit nuclear factor-kappaB activation, an important inflammatory factor. Caution is advised in patients taking anti-inflammatory herbs or supplements.
- *Gynostemma pentaphyllum* may increase the risk of bleeding when taken with herbs and supplements that are believed to increase the risk of bleeding. However, current evidence is mixed. Multiple cases of bleeding have been reported with the use of *Ginkgo biloba,* and fewer cases with garlic and saw palmetto. Numerous other agents may theoretically increase the risk of bleeding, although this has not been proven in most cases.

- *Gynostemma pentaphyllum* may decrease alanine aminotransferase, alkaline phosphatase, or aspartate aminotransferase levels in patients with nonalcoholic fatty liver disease. Caution is advised when combining jiaogulan with any potentially liver-damaging (hepatotoxic) herbs or supplements.
- *Gynostemma pentaphyllum* may decrease insulin levels and insulin index scores in patients with nonalcoholic fatty liver disease. Caution is advised when combining jiaogulan with herbs or supplements taken to control blood sugar.

For a complete list of references, please visit www.naturalstandard.com.

Jimson Weed

(Datura spp.)

RELATED TERMS

- Alkaloids, angel's trumpet, apple of peru, atropine, belladonna alkaloids, complex-type oligosaccharide binding lectin, crazy tea, *Datura arborea, Datura aurea, Datura candida, Datura inoxia, Datura L., Datura metel, Datura sanguinea, Datura stramonium, Datura stramonium* agglutinin, *Datura stramonium* L. var. *tatula* (L.) Torr., *Datura suaveolens, Datura tatula* L., devil's seed, devil's snare, devil's trumpet, DSA, endemic nightshade, hyoscamine, Jamestown weed, jimsonweed, lectins, "loco" weed, mad hatter, malpitte, moonflower seed, nightshade, pods, scopolamine, sobi-lobi, Solanaceae (family), stinkweed, TAL, thorn apple, thornapple leaf, tolguacha, toxic alkaloids, tropane belladonna alkaloids, trumpet lily, zombie's cucumber.

BACKGROUND

- Jimson weed *(Datura stramonium)* grows throughout the world and has been known as a hallucinogenic plant for centuries. It has reportedly been used by Shamans and native peoples during sacred rituals. In India, the smoke of jimson weed has been used to treat asthma.
- Jimson weed may cause extreme toxicity, including death. Even very small amounts may cause death. Jimson weed is therefore not used medicinally today, although some alkaloids from jimson weed are approved drugs.
- In early research, jimson weed has been studied for asthma and chronic bronchitis; however, clinical evidence supporting any safe or effective use of jimson weed is lacking at this time.

EVIDENCE

Uses Based on Scientific Evidence

No available studies qualify for inclusion in the evidence table.

Uses Based on Tradition or Theory

Antibacterial, antimicrobial, antitumor, asthma, colorectal cancer, hallucinogenic, insecticide, muscle spasms, Parkinson's disease (saliva production control), sedative, whooping cough.

DOSING

Adults (18 Years and Older)

- There is insufficient evidence to recommend a dose for jimson weed. Jimson weed may cause extreme toxicity.

Children (Younger than 18 Years)

- There is insufficient evidence to recommend a dose for jimson weed, and use in children is not recommended. Jimson weed may cause extreme toxicity, and even small amounts may cause death in children.

SAFETY

Allergies

- Avoid with a known allergy or hypersensitivity to jimson weed, its constituents, other *Datura* species, or other plants in the nightshade family, such as tobacco, peppers, eggplant, potatoes, and tomatoes.

Side Effects and Warnings

- Jimson weed may cause extreme toxicity, including death. Even very small amounts may cause death.
- Jimson weed may cause rapid heart rate, life-threatening abnormal heart rhythm, high blood pressure, respiratory arrest, psychosis, delirium, disorientation, hallucinations, seizures, amnesia, and coma, and it may worsen neurological disorders.
- Jimson weed may increase the risk of bleeding. Caution is advised in patients with bleeding disorders or those taking drugs that may increase the risk of bleeding. Dosing adjustments may be necessary.
- Jimson weed may also cause liver damage, kidney damage, difficulty urinating or urinary retention, and blurred vision.

Pregnancy and Breastfeeding

- Jimson weed is not recommended in pregnant or breastfeeding women due to potential for extreme toxicity.

INTERACTIONS

Interactions with Drugs

- Jimson weed may increase the risk of bleeding when taken with drugs that increase the risk of bleeding. Some examples include aspirin, anticoagulants (blood thinners) such as warfarin (Coumadin) or heparin, antiplatelet drugs such as clopidogrel (Plavix), and nonsteroidal anti-inflammatory drugs such as ibuprofen (Motrin, Advil) or naproxen (Naprosyn, Aleve).
- Jimson weed may increase the amount of drowsiness caused by some drugs. Examples include benzodiazepines such as lorazepam (Ativan) or diazepam (Valium), barbiturates such as phenobarbital, narcotics such as codeine, some antidepressants, and alcohol. Caution is advised while driving or operating machinery.
- Jimson weed may alter blood pressure. Caution is advised in patients taking drugs that alter blood pressure.
- Jimson weed may have additive effects when taken with anticholinergics; beta-blockers; cardiac glycosides; antimicrobials; analgesics; antipsychotics; diuretics; stimulants; drugs used for the eye; drugs used to alter heart rate or heart rhythm; drugs toxic to the liver; or drugs with antiasthmatic, anticancer, antiseizure, or immune-altering properties.

Interactions with Herbs and Dietary Supplements

- Jimson weed may increase the risk of bleeding when taken with herbs and supplements that are believed to increase the risk of bleeding. Multiple cases of bleeding have been reported with the use of *Ginkgo biloba*, and fewer cases with garlic and saw palmetto. Numerous other agents may theoretically increase the risk of bleeding, although this has not been proven in most cases.

- Jimson weed may increase the amount of drowsiness caused by some herbs or supplements.
- Jimson weed may alter blood pressure. Caution is advised in patients taking herbs or supplements that alter blood pressure.
- Jimson weed may have additive effects when taken with anticholinergics; beta-blockers; alkaloids; cardiac glycosides; antimicrobials; analgesics; antipsychotics; diuretics; stimulants; herbs or supplements used for the eye; herbs or supplements used to alter heart rate or heart rhythm; herbs or supplements toxic to the liver; or herbs or supplements with antiasthmatic, anticancer, antiseizure, or immune-altering properties.

For a complete list of references, please visit www.naturalstandard.com.

Jojoba
(*Simmondsia chinensis*)

RELATED TERMS

- D-pinitol, jojoba beans, jojoba bean oil, jojoba cotyledons, jojoba esters, jojoba liquid wax (JLW), JLW, jojoba meal, jojoba meal phospholipids, jojoba oil (Joj), jojoba protein, jojoba seed, jojoba seedlings, jojoba seed meal, jojoba seed xyloglucan, jojoba wax, jojoba xyloglucan oligosaccharides, lysophosphatidylcholine (LPC), myo-inositol sucrose, phosphatidylcholine (PC), pinitol alpha-D-galactosides, rimethylsilyl derivatives, *Simmondsia* chinensis, Simmondsiaceae (family), simmondsin, simmondsin ferulates, simmondsins, simmondsin derivative.

BACKGROUND

- Jojoba (*Simmondsia chinensis*) is a shrub native to deserts in Arizona, California, and Mexico and is also found in some arid African countries. The oil (or liquid wax) in jojoba seeds contains extremely long (C36-C46) straight chain fatty acids in the form of wax esters, as opposed to triglycerides. It is this structure that allows it to be easily refined for use in cosmetics and as a carrier oil for fragrances. Jojoba meal, remaining after oil extraction, is rich in protein. In Japan, jojoba oil (wax) is used as a food additive.
- Jojoba oil is used most commonly as a carrier oil for topical application or aromatherapy. At this time, there are no high-quality human trials available supporting the efficacy of jojoba oil for any indication. Potential effects of jojoba oil include anti-inflammatory, cholesterol-reduction, and mosquito-repellent effects.

EVIDENCE

Uses Based on Scientific Evidence	Grade
Dementia Jojoba oil is traditionally used as a carrier or massage oil. There is currently insufficient evidence to recommend the use of jojoba oil for dementia.	C
Mosquito Repellent There is currently insufficient evidence to recommend the use of jojoba oil as a mosquito repellent.	C

Uses Based on Tradition or Theory
Antiaging, anti-inflammatory, appetite suppressant, cosmetic uses, food uses (additive), insecticidal, reflexology treatment, skin disorders (dry skin), topical (applied to the skin) drug delivery, weight loss, wound healing.

DOSING

Adults (18 Years and Older)

- There is insufficient evidence to recommend a dose for jojoba in adults. Avoid taking jojoba products by mouth.

Children (Younger than 18 Years)

- There is insufficient evidence to recommend a dose for jojoba in children. Avoid taking jojoba products by mouth.

SAFETY

Allergies

- Avoid in people with a known allergy or hypersensitivity to jojoba or its constituents. Contact dermatitis to jojoba oil has been described in case reports.

Side Effects and Warnings

- Side effects of jojoba are mainly limited to contact dermatitis and gastrointestinal concerns in animals fed large amounts of jojoba meal. Avoid oral consumption of jojoba products.

Pregnancy and Breastfeeding

- Jojoba is not recommended in pregnant or breastfeeding women due to a lack of available scientific evidence. Although not well studied in humans, ingesting jojoba meal may lower fetal and placental weights.

INTERACTIONS

Interactions with Drugs

- Jojoba liquid wax may have anti-inflammatory effects. Thus, caution is advised when taking jojoba with other anti-inflammatory agents.
- Consumption of jojoba meal in combination with appetite suppressants may have additive effects.
- Although not well studied in humans, jojoba oil may alter blood cholesterol levels. Caution is advised when combining it with other cholesterol-lowering agents.
- A South African commercial oil containing coconut, jojoba, and rapeseed oils has shown ability to act as a mosquito repellent for humans. Thus, use of jojoba oil in combination with other mosquito repellents may have additive effects.

Interactions with Herbs and Dietary Supplements

- Jojoba liquid wax may have anti-inflammatory effects. Thus, caution is advised when taking jojoba with other anti-inflammatory herbs or supplements.
- Although not well studied in humans, jojoba oil may alter blood cholesterol levels. Caution is advised when combining with other cholesterol-lowering herbs or supplements, such as red yeast rice.
- Consumption of jojoba meal in combination with appetite suppressant herbs or supplements may have additive effects.
- Jojoba oil is commonly used as a carrier oil in aromatherapy. Combinations with other carrier oils, such as almond and apricot, with the essential oils from lavender, marjoram, eucalyptus, rosemary, and peppermint, may offer clinical benefits.
- A South African commercial oil containing coconut, jojoba, and rapeseed oils has shown the ability to act as a mosquito repellent. Thus, use of jojoba oil in combination with other mosquito repellent herbs may have additive effects.

For a complete list of references, please visit www.naturalstandard.com.

Juniper
(*Juniperus* spp.)

RELATED TERMS

- Cade oil, cedar, cedarwood, cedron, common juniper berry, Cupressaceae (family), empyreumatic oil, enebro, Geniévre, ginepro, juniper bark, juniper berry, juniper bush, juniper oil, juniper tar, juniper wood, Juniperi Fructus, *Juniperus californica, Juniperus communis, Juniperus deppeana, Juniperus mexicana, Juniperus occidentalis, Juniperus oxycedrus, Juniperus phoenicea, Juniperus scopulorum, Juniperus therifera, Juniperus virginiana*, pencil cedar, Pinaceae, red cedar, Sabina, Wacholderbeeren, zimbro.

BACKGROUND

- The genus *Juniperus* contains over 50 species that have been used by many people around the world but have also been recognized as toxic plants. Juniper is a flavoring in gin and other drinks and is used as a spice in small amounts. The plant displays significant toxicity to the kidneys and skin, which limits its use in medicine, except in small amounts. Juniper is safely used as a fragrance in soaps, shampoos, cosmetics, sachets, and other products.
- Juniper has been used in dyspepsia (upset stomach) as a berry tea and in eczema and other skin diseases as cade oil or juniper oil. Juniper is thought to be more effective and less irritating when combined with uva ursi, manzanita, or pipsissewa. There is a long history of juniper use in Europe and China, but there are no published clinical trials.

EVIDENCE

Uses Based on Scientific Evidence

No available studies qualify for inclusion in the evidence table.

Uses Based on Tradition or Theory

Abortifacient, analgesic, antirheumatic, arthritis, astringent (leaves), bladder infections, bladder stones, bloating, blood purification, cancer, carminative, colds, constipation, cosmetics, cystitis (bladder infection), disinfectant (berries), diuretic, dyspepsia (upset stomach), eczema, flatulence (gas), fumigant (pesticide), gastrointestinal infections, heartburn, hypoglycemia (low blood sugar), inflammation (volatile oil), intestinal worms, kidney infections, kidney stones, loss of appetite, plague, regulate menstruation, snakebites, stimulate stomach secretions, soaps, urethritis (inflammation of the urethra), urinary tract infections (UTIs), wounds.

DOSING
Adults (18 Years and Older)

- There is insufficient evidence to recommend a dose for juniper. Tinctures, tablets, capsules, and other forms of berry extracts are commercially available. As an infusion, 2-3 g of dried berries in 150 mL of hot water has been taken by mouth 3-4 times daily. For dyspepsia, 20-50 mg of the berry essential oil has been taken twice daily (up to a maximum of 100 mg). This is usually taken as juniper berry tea.
- Cade oil (juniper tar) or juniper oil has been typically used pure or partially diluted. It should be noted that application to the skin may be irritating or toxic to the skin. Volatile oil has been applied on the skin three or more times per day.

Children (Younger than 18 Years)

- There is insufficient evidence to recommend a dose for juniper in children, and use is not recommended.

SAFETY
Allergies

- Avoid in people with a known allergy or hypersensitivity to juniper. Repeated exposure to juniper pollen may cause occupational allergies that can affect the skin and respiratory tract.

Side Effects and Warnings

- The juniper berry has "generally recognized as safe" (GRAS) status in the United States. The maximum level used in food is 0.006% for the oil and 0.01% for the extract.
- Overdose may lead to kidney and skin damage. Overdose symptoms include albuminuria (excessive protein), hematuria (blood in the urine), purplish urine, tachycardia (increased heart rate), hypertension (high blood pressure), convulsions, and metrorrhagia (non-menstrual bleeding from the uterus).
- Other possible adverse effects include hypotension (low blood pressure), irritation, blisters, burns, liver toxicity, kidney damage, or kidney failure.
- Juniper may also lower blood sugar levels. Caution is advised in patients with diabetes or hypoglycemia (low blood sugar), and in those taking drugs, herbs, or supplements that affect blood sugar. Serum glucose levels may need to be monitored by a qualified health care professional, including a pharmacist, and medication adjustments may be necessary.
- Although not well studied in humans, juniper may also increase the risk of bleeding. Caution is advised in patients with bleeding disorders or those taking drugs that may increase the risk of bleeding. Dosing adjustments may be necessary.

Pregnancy and Breastfeeding

- Juniper is not recommended in pregnant or breastfeeding women due to the potential for abortions and/or the induction of labor contractions.

INTERACTIONS
Interactions with Drugs

- Juniper may increase the risk of bleeding when taken with drugs that increase the risk of bleeding. Some examples include aspirin, anticoagulants (blood thinners) such as warfarin (Coumadin) or heparin, antiplatelet drugs such as clopidogrel (Plavix), and nonsteroidal anti-inflammatory drugs such as ibuprofen (Motrin, Advil) or naproxen (Naprosyn, Aleve).

- Juniper may lower blood sugar levels. Caution is advised when using medications that may also lower blood sugar levels. Patients taking drugs for diabetes by mouth or insulin should be monitored closely by a qualified health care professional, including a pharmacist. Medication adjustments may be necessary.

Interactions with Herbs and Dietary Supplements

- Juniper may increase the risk of bleeding when taken with herbs and supplements that are believed to increase the risk of bleeding. Multiple cases of bleeding have been reported with the use of *Ginkgo biloba*, and fewer cases with garlic and saw palmetto. Numerous other agents may theoretically increase the risk of bleeding, although this has not been proven in most cases.
- Juniper may lower blood sugar levels. Caution is advised when using herbs or supplements that may also lower blood sugar levels. Blood glucose levels may require monitoring, and doses may need adjustment.

For a complete list of references, please visit www. naturalstandard.com.

Kava
(Piper methysticum)

RELATED TERMS

- (+)-dihydrokawain-5-ol, 11-methoxy-5, 5-hydroxydihydrokawain, 6-dihydroyangonin, antares, ava, ava pepper, ava pepper shrub, ava root, awa, bornyl cinnamate, cavain, flavokavines A and B, Fijian kava, gea, gi, grog, intoxicating long pepper, intoxicating pepper, kao, kava kava extract LI 140, kava kava rhizome, kavakava, kavalactones, kavapiper, kavapyrones, kavarod, kava root, kavasporal forte, kavain, kave-kave, kawa, kawa kawa, kawa pepper, Kawa Pfeffer, kew, LI150, long pepper, *Macropiper latifolium,* malohu, maluk, maori kava, meruk, milik, pepe kava, olanzapine, *Piper methysticum,* pipermethystine, piperis methystici rhizoma, Rauschpfeffer, rhizoma piperis methystici, rhizome di kava-kava sakaua, risperidone, sakau, sakua, tonga, wurzelstock, WS 1490, yagona, yangona, yaqona, yongona.

BACKGROUND

- Kava beverages, made from dried roots of the shrub *Piper methysticum,* have been used ceremonially and socially in the South Pacific for hundreds of years and in Europe since the 1700s.
- Several well-conducted human studies have demonstrated kava's efficacy in the treatment of anxiety with effects observed after as few as one to two doses and progressive improvements over 1-4 weeks. Preliminary evidence suggests possible equivalence to benzodiazepines.
- Many experts believe that kava is neither sedating nor tolerance-forming in recommended doses. Some trials report occasional mild sedation, although preliminary data from small studies suggest lack of neurological-psychological impairment.
- There is growing concern regarding the potential for liver toxicity from kava. Multiple cases of liver damage have been reported in Europe, including hepatitis, cirrhosis, and liver failure. Kava has been removed from shelves in several countries due to these safety concerns. The U.S. Food and Drug Administration (FDA) has issued warnings to consumers and physicians. It is not clear what dose or duration of use is correlated with the risk of liver damage. The quality of these case reports has been variable; several are vague, describe use of products that do not actually list kava as an ingredient, or include patients who also ingest large quantities of alcohol. Nonetheless, caution is warranted.
- Chronic or heavy use of kava has also been associated with cases of neurotoxicity, pulmonary hypertension, and dermatological changes. Most human trials have been shorter than two months, with the longest study being six months in duration.

EVIDENCE

Uses Based on Scientific Evidence	Grade
Anxiety Clinical studies have found at least moderate benefit of kava for treating anxiety. Preliminary evidence suggests that kava may be as effective as benzodiazepine drugs	A
such as diazepam (Valium). Kava's effects were reported to be similar to the prescription drug buspirone (Buspar) used for Generalized Anxiety Disorder (GAD) in one study. However, there is concern regarding the potential danger from taking kava based on multiple reports from Europe and the United States that included hepatitis, cirrhosis, and liver failure. The U.S. Food and Drug Administration (FDA) has issued warnings to consumers and physicians. Many products have been pulled from the market. Natural Standard has collaborated with the World Health Organization (WHO) to prepare a detailed report of kava and associated adverse effects, which is now available.	
Insomnia Kava may cause sedation or lethargy. However, early research suggests that kava may not be effective for insomnia.	C
Parkinson's Disease There is unclear evidence for the use of kava for Parkinson's disease. Kava has been shown to increase "off" periods in Parkinson's patients taking levodopa and can cause a semicomatose state when given with alprazolam. Consult with a qualified health care professional before taking kava due to the risk of harmful side effects.	C
Stress Preliminary studies suggest that kava and valerian may be beneficial to health by reducing the body's reactions during stressful situations and stress-induced insomnia.	C

Uses Based on Tradition or Theory

Addiction, anesthesia, anorexia, antifungal, anti-inflammatory, antipsychotic, aphrodisiac, arthritis, asthma, birth control, bladder inflammation, brain damage, bust enhancement, cancer, colds, depression, diuretic, dizziness, gonorrhea, hemorrhoids, incontinence, indigestion, infections, inflammation (ear), jet lag, joint pain or stiffness, kidney stones, leprosy, menopausal symptoms (hot flashes, sleep disturbances), menstrual disorders, migraine headache, muscle spasms, neuroprotective, pain, parasite infection, premenstrual syndrome (PMS), premenstrual dysphoric disorder (PMDD), protection of brain tissue against ischemic damage, renal colic, respiratory tract infections, rheumatism, seizures, stroke, syphilis, toothache, tuberculosis, urinary tract disorders, uterus inflammation, vaginal prolapse, vaginitis, weight reduction, wound healing.

DOSING
Adults (18 Years and Older)

- Many doctors recommend starting with a low dose and gradually increasing intake over time. Typical doses range from 50-280 mg of kava lactones per day at bedtime.

From 60-120 mg of kavapyrones have been taken daily. A dose of 50-100 mg taken by mouth has been used for up to 2 months. A dose of 100 mg of kava extract (WS 1490) has been taken three times daily. Doses as high as 800 mg/day of kava extract have been taken for short periods but have not been studied over the long term and safety is not clear.

Children (Younger than 18 Years)

- There is insufficient evidence to recommend the use of kava in children.

SAFETY
Allergies

- People with allergies to kava or kavapyrones should not take kava. Skin rashes have been reported after taking kava.

Side Effects and Warnings

- Until recently, kava was generally thought to be safe: when used in otherwise healthy people not taking any other drugs, herbs, or supplements; over short periods of time (one to two months); and at recommended doses. However, there have been numerous reports of severe liver problems in people using kava. Multiple cases of liver toxicity, including liver failure, have been reported following the use of kava in Europe. The U.S. Food and Drug Administration (FDA) has issued warnings to consumers and physicians and has requested that physicians report cases of liver toxicity that may be related to kava use. Although many natural medicine experts still believe that kava is safe at recommended doses, there is not enough scientific information to make a clear conclusion. Therefore, kava should be used only under the supervision of a qualified health care professional, should never be used above recommended doses, and should be avoided by people with liver problems or those taking drugs that affect the liver.
- Other serious side effects that have been observed with chronic or heavy use of kava include skin disorders, blood abnormalities, apathy, kidney damage, seizures, psychotic syndromes, and increased blood pressure in the lungs (pulmonary hypertension). Blood in the urine has also been reported.
- Mild side effects may include gastrointestinal (stomach) upset, allergic rash, or mild headache.
- Several cases of abnormal muscle movements have been reported after short-term use of kava (one to four days), including tightening, twisting, or locking of the muscles of the mouth, neck (torticollis), and eyes (oculogyric crisis). Worsening of symptoms of Parkinson's disease and several cases of abnormal whole body movements (choreoathetosis) following high doses of kava have also been noted. Tremor, poor coordination, headache, drowsiness, and fatigue have uncommonly been reported, particularly with large doses. A case of muscle cell breakdown (rhabdomyolysis) was reported in a 29-year-old man after taking an herbal combination of ginkgo, guarana, and kava.
- Sedation (drowsiness) has occasionally been reported with kava use, although there is early evidence from several small human studies that kava may not significantly cause this effect. Because this issue remains unclear, driving and operating heavy machinery is not recommend while taking kava.
- Eye disturbances and eye irritation have rarely been associated with chronic or heavy kava use. Rapid heart rate, electrocardiogram (ECG) abnormalities, and shortness of breath have been reported in heavy kava users. Laboratory tests suggest that kava may increase the risk of bleeding through effects on blood platelets.
- Kava may affect electroconvulsive therapy (ECT) outcome. It has also been associated with meningismus (pain caused by irritation in the layers around the brain and spinal cord), urinary retention, skin lesions, enhanced or decreased cognitive performance, anorexia, sleeplessness, abnormal sensations called *paresthesias,* vomiting, and dangerously high blood pressure.

Pregnancy and Breastfeeding

- Use of kava cannot be recommended during pregnancy or breastfeeding. There may be decreases in the muscle strength of the uterus with the use of kava, which may have harmful effects on pregnancy. Chemicals in kava may pass into breast milk with unknown effects, and therefore this herb should be avoided during breastfeeding.

INTERACTIONS
Interactions with Drugs

- Based on multiple human reports of liver toxicity, including hepatitis, cirrhosis, and liver failure, a theoretical increased risk of liver damage may occur if kava is taken with drugs that may injure the liver such as alcohol or acetaminophen (Tylenol). Chronic use of kava may lead to kidney damage. Agents broken down by the kidneys should be used cautiously with kava due to increased risk of kidney damage.
- In theory, kava may increase the effects of alcohol or other drugs that cause sedation (drowsiness). In theory, kava may interfere with the effects of dopamine or drugs that are similar to dopamine and may worsen the neurological side effects of drugs that block dopamine such as haloperidol (Haldol).
- Kava may have chemical properties similar to monoamine oxidase inhibitors (MAOIs). In theory, kava may add to the effects of MAOI antidepressants, such as isocarboxazid (Marplan), phenelzine (Nardil), or tranylcypromine (Parnate). Due to this possible effect, kava may also cause the effects of anesthesia to last longer; some practitioners recommend stopping kava two to three weeks before surgery.
- Laboratory tests suggest that kava may increase the risk of bleeding through effects on blood platelets. However, human evidence is lacking in this area. People using aspirin, anticoagulants (blood thinners) such as warfarin (Coumadin) and heparin, or antiplatelet drugs such as clopidogrel (Plavix) should be aware of possible interactions.
- Since kava has diuretic properties, it may have additive effects when taken with diuretic drugs such as furosemide or with ACE inhibitors such as benazepril or captopril. Avoid in patients with Parkinson's disease or those with a history of medication-induced extrapyramidal effects, because kava may cause additive effects. Kava may cause excessive drowsiness when taken with SSRI antidepressant drugs such as fluoxetine or sertraline. Buspirone and opipramol may have additive effects when taken with kava.
- Early evidence shows that kava may interfere with the way the body processes certain drugs using the liver's cytochrome P450 enzyme system. As a result, levels of these drugs may be altered in the blood, which may cause different effects or potentially serious adverse reactions.
- Kava may have additive sedative effects when taken concomitantly with the opioid analgesics oxycodone and propoxyphene.

K

- Kava may also interact with anticancer drugs or hormonal drugs, such as birth control pills.

Interactions with Herbs and Dietary Supplements

- Based on multiple human reports of liver toxicity, including hepatitis, cirrhosis, and liver failure, a theoretical increased risk of liver damage may occur if kava is taken with herbs or supplements that may damage the liver.
- Kava may increase the amount of sedation (drowsiness) caused by some herbs or supplements, such as valerian. Caution is advised while driving or operating machinery.
- In theory, kava may add to the effects of herbs and supplements that act like monoamine oxidase inhibitors (MAOIs) such as evening primrose oil. It may also add to the effects of herbs that have activity similar to the class of antidepressants known as selective serotonin reuptake inhibitors (SSRIs).
- Based on laboratory tests, it is suggested that kava may increase the risk of bleeding through effects on blood plate-lets. However, human evidence is lacking in this area. People using other herbs or supplements that may increase the risk of bleeding should speak with a health care professional before starting kava.
- Since kava has diuretic properties, it may have additive effects when taken with diuretic herbs or supplements like horsetail or licorice.
- Use cautiously with herbs or supplements that are broken down by the kidneys because kidney damage may occur.
- Preliminary evidence shows that kava may interfere with the way the body processes certain herbs or supplements using the liver's cytochrome P450 enzyme system. As a result, the levels of other herbs or supplements may be too high in the blood.
- Kava may interact with herbs and supplements with anticancer or hormonal activity; use cautiously.

For a complete list of references, please visit www.naturalstandard.com.

Khat

(Catha edulis)

RELATED TERMS

- Abyssinian tea, African salad, Arabian-tea, bushman's tea, cat, cathine, cathinone, *Catha edulis*, Celastraceae (family), *Celastrus edulis*, chat, chaat (Arabic), gat (Arabic), herbal ecstasy, kat (Arabic), kus es Salahin (Arabic), miraa, oat, phenylpropanolamine, qat (Yemen), qut, somali tea, tchaad (Arabic), tohai (Arabic), tohat (Arabic), tshcut (Arabic).

BACKGROUND

- Khat is believed to have originated in Ethiopia. It is a flowering evergreen plant native to tropical East Africa. Khat has been grown for use as a stimulant for centuries and predates the use of coffee.
- Khat is an agent that has been used in social settings to induce feelings of euphoria and pleasure. Medicinally, it has been used to treat depression and to enhance work capacity. Khat has also been used as an aphrodisiac, to treat premature ejaculation, and to enhance sexual desire.
- Currently, there is a lack of well-designed clinical trials evaluating khat for any indication. Two poorly documented trials evaluated khat in cognitive function. One study revealed no difference in cognitive function in the elderly with khat use. In the other study, cognitive functioning was negatively affected by khat use.
- Fresh khat leaves contain cathinone, a Schedule I drug under the Controlled Substances Act; however, the leaves typically begin to deteriorate after 48 hours, causing the chemical composition of the plant to break down. Once this occurs, the leaves contain cathine, a Schedule IV drug. Khat is currently illegal in the United States.

EVIDENCE

Uses Based on Scientific Evidence	Grade
Cognitive Function Khat has been evaluated for its cognitive effects; however, the results are mixed with some studies showing benefit and others showing negative effects.	C

Uses Based on Tradition or Theory
Appetite suppressant, depression, gastric ulcers, fatigue, male infertility, obesity, physical work capacity, premature ejaculation, sexual activity enhancement, stimulant.

DOSING

Adults (18 Years and Older)

- There is insufficient evidence to recommend a dose for khat. However, approximately 100-200 g of fresh leaves have been chewed, one at a time for their stimulant effects. The juice can be swallowed while the residue is retained in the cheek and later expelled. A juice has also been made by blending khat with water and lemon and then filtering the mixture. A tincture can be made by alcohol extraction of the active ingredients.

Children (Younger than 18 Years)

- There is insufficient evidence to recommend a dose for khat in children, and use is not recommended.

SAFETY
Allergies

- Avoid in people with a known allergy or hypersensitivity to *Cathus edulis* or members of the Celastraceae family.

Side Effects and Warnings

- Fresh khat leaves contain cathinone, a Schedule I drug under the Controlled Substances Act; however, the leaves typically begin to deteriorate after 48 hours, causing the chemical composition of the plant to break down. Once this occurs, the leaves contain cathine, a Schedule IV drug, which is similar in structure to amphetamine.
- The stimulatory effect associated with khat has been documented with delusions, paranoia, hypomania, mood swings, depression, irritability, insomnia, and increased alertness. There have also been reports of persistent hypnagogic hallucinations caused by khat use.
- Khat may cause nervousness, nightmares, aggressiveness, excitement, talkativeness, manic behavior, and hyperactivity. Khat chewing has dependency potential and may lead to dependence and addiction. Avoid using in patients with psychotic personalities. Use cautiously in patients with motor tics and Tourette's syndrome. Theoretically, khat may exacerbate motor tics and Tourette's syndrome. Khat is currently illegal in the United States.
- Although not well studied in humans, khat may increase respiratory rates, increase systolic and diastolic blood pressure and heart rate, or cause acute myocardial infarction (heart attack). Other reported side effects include gastritis (stomach inflammation), malnutrition, hemorrhoidal disease, constipation, and oral carcinoma. Avoid holding khat in the cheek for extended periods of time to avoid oral infection.
- Use cautiously in patients with hypertension (high blood pressure), tachycardia (fast heart rates), or cardiovascular disease because khat may increase blood pressure and heart rate. Khat should also be used cautiously in patients taking antihypertensives (blood pressure–lowering agents). Theoretically, khat may antagonize the effects of these drugs.
- Fasciola hepatica infection, a parasite infection, has been reported after the chewing of khat leaves. Loss of appetite and anorexia has also been noted.
- Methcathinone, a methyl derivative of cathinone, has been reported to cause mydriasis (dilation of the pupil).
- Use cautiously in patients taking stimulant drugs or herbs. Increased stimulant effects may occur. Avoid driving after khat use; there are reports of impaired driving and psychophysical function. Avoid using in patients with glaucoma.

Pregnancy and Breastfeeding

- Khat is not recommended for use in pregnant or breast-feeding women due to possible reductions in birth weight, birth defects, and breastfeeding inhibition.

INTERACTIONS
Interactions with Drugs

- Use khat cautiously in patients taking amoxicillin or ampicillin. Khat may reduce the effectiveness of these drugs. These two antibiotics, particularly ampicillin, should be taken 2 hours after khat chewing.
- Sympathomimetic effects of khat such as mydriasis (dilation of the pupil) and hypertension (high blood pressure) may be antagonized by antiadrenergic drugs including clonidine, reserpine, or terazosin.
- Theoretically, khat may antagonize the effects of heart medications or blood pressure–lowering agents. Khat has been reported to cause an increase in systolic and diastolic blood pressure and heart rate.
- Use cautiously in patients taking beta blockers or tricyclic antidepressants. Theoretically, khat may increase the risk of cardiovascular side effects with these drugs.

- Khat may cause central nervous system (CNS) stimulation, and use with other CNS stimulants may lead to additive effects. Stimulant and amphetamine-like effects are likely due to the phenylalkylamine alkaloid cathinone.
- Theoretically, concurrent use of khat with monoamine oxidase inhibitors (MAOIs) may cause hypertensive (high blood pressure) crisis.

Interactions with Herbs and Dietary Supplements

- Khat may antagonize the effects of antihypertensive (blood pressure–lowering) herbs and supplements. Khat has been reported to cause an increase in systolic and diastolic blood pressure and heart rate. Caution is advised.
- Theoretically, concurrent use of khat with herbs with monoamine oxidase inhibitor–like activity may cause hypertensive (high blood pressure) crisis.
- Theoretically, khat may increase the stimulant effects if taken with stimulant herbs and supplements such as guarana or ephedra.

For a complete list of references, please visit www.naturalstandard.com.

Khella
(Ammi visnaga)

RELATED TERMS

- Ammi, *Ammi daucoides, Ammi visnaga*, Bischofskrautfruchte, bishop's weed, bishop's weed fruit, daucus visagna, false Queen Anne's lace, fruits de khella, germakellin, honeyplant, khellin, picktooth, Spanish toothpick, toothpick plant, visnaga, visnagae, Visnagafruchte, visnagin.

BACKGROUND

- Khella *(Ammi visnaga)* was originally cultivated by the ancient Egyptians who used it to treat many ailments, including urinary tract diseases. It was also used in the Middle Ages as a diuretic.
- The whole fruit has traditionally been used to treat respiratory system diseases such as asthma, bronchitis, emphysema, and whooping cough, as well as cardiovascular disorders, premenstrual syndrome (PMS), liver and gallbladder disorders, and to stimulate diuresis (increase in urine production). Its purported effect is related to its antispasmodic action on smaller bronchial muscles, coronary arteries, and urinary tract tubules. *Ammi visnaga* may vasodilate the coronary arteries, which increases the blood supply to the myocardium and, as a result, can be used to treat mild forms of angina (chest pain). It is also used to treat problems associated with spasms and constriction of the gallbladder and bile duct and facilitates the discharge of kidney stones and gallstones.
- The clinical and therapeutic effectiveness of khellin, a constituent of khella, with respect to coronary, respiratory, and urological indications, has been demonstrated in experiments. Current khella indications include mild angina (chest pain) complaints, postoperative treatment of urinary calculus (kidney stones), and supportive treatment of mild forms of obstructive pulmonary diseases.
- Few clinical trials have investigated khella (the whole herb vs. its constituent khellin). However, based on traditional use, more studies of khella for the treatment of psoriasis (chronic skin disease) or lipid panel may be warranted.

EVIDENCE

Uses Based on Scientific Evidence	Grade
Psoriasis Preliminary evidence suggests that khellin, taken by mouth, may be an effective therapy for psoriasis. However, the available evidence is not definitive.	C
Vitiligo (Loss of Skin Pigment) Several studies have investigated the use of khellin for the treatment of vitiligo. However, the evidence of the efficacy of khellin is conflicting.	C

Uses Based on Tradition or Theory
Abdominal cramps, angina (chest pain), antispasmotic, arteriosclerosis (hardening of the arteries), asthma, bronchitis, colic (urinary), cardiovascular disorders, coronary insufficiency, diuretic, emphysema, gallbladder disorders, gallstones, gastroduodenal ulcer, gingivitis, hyperlipidemia (high cholesterol), inflammation, insect and spider bites (poisonous), irregular heartbeat, kidney stones, liver disorders, myocardial infarction (heart attack, recovery), chronic obstructive pulmonary disease, premenstrual syndrome (PMS), poisonous snake bites, spasms (muscle), spastic coughs, spastic heart, toothache, whooping cough, wounds.

K

DOSING

Adults (18 Years and Older)

- There is insufficient evidence to recommend a dose for khella. For vitiligo (loss of skin pigment), weekly applications of a 2% solution of khellin in acetone and propylene glycol (90% and 10%, respectively) with exposure to 90 minutes of sunlight for a period of 4 months has been studied. Traditionally, 30-60 drops of khella have been taken 3-5 times daily. An infusion of 1 tsp of crushed seeds per cup of water, infused for 25 minutes; or 1:3 dry liquid extract 20-60 drops of this infusion has been taken 1-4 times daily in a little water.

Children (Younger than 18 Years)

- There is insufficient evidence to recommend a dose for khella in children.

SAFETY

Allergies

- Avoid in people with a known allergy or hypersensitivity to khella *(Ammi visnaga)*. Long-term use of the monosubstance khellin in large doses may occasionally result in allergic manifestations.

Side Effects and Warnings

- It has been proposed that the observed side effects are of no practical relevance in the therapeutic use of *Ammi visnaga* extracts, as khella is thought to be clinically effective at moderate doses. However, there is a lack of clinical trials to support this claim. Use khella cautiously in asthmatics or after myocardial infarction (heart attack) because khella may act unreliably.
- Reported adverse effects include chest pain, skin rashes, hives, itchy or swollen skin, breathing problems, and tightness of the throat. Elevated liver enzymes or permanent jaundice (yellow skin color) may occur with the use of khella. When taken in high doses, khella may cause liver damage. Khella may also increase photosensitivity or increase the risk of skin cancer; avoid prolonged exposure to sunlight.
- Long-term use of khellin in high doses may occasionally result in nausea, constipation, loss of appetite, dizziness, headaches, or sleep disturbances.

Pregnancy and Breastfeeding

- Avoid if pregnant or breastfeeding as the active constituent in khella has uterine stimulant activity.

INTERACTIONS
Interactions with Drugs

- Khella may decrease the toxicity of the cardiac glycoside digoxin because it has coronary vasodilator and antiarrhythmic effects.

Interactions with Herbs and Dietary Supplements

- Khella may have beneficial effects when combined with other respiratory antispasmodics, such as skunk cabbage, lobelia, and thyme.

- Khella may decrease the toxicity of the cardiac glycoside digoxin in some herbs because it has coronary vasodilator and antiarrhythmic effects.

For a complete list of references, please visit www.naturalstandard.com.

Kinetin

RELATED TERMS

- Cytokinins, furfural, furfuryladenine, hyaluronidase, iso-pentenyladenine (IPA), kinerase, kinesin-I, kinetin, kinetin riboside.

BACKGROUND

- Kinetin is a chemical analogue of cytokinins, which are plant hormones that promote cell division. Kinetin is found in both plants and animals.
- Scientific studies have investigated whether kinetin might help lower side effects associated with cataract surgery, aid in the treatment of Ménière's disease, or decrease eye blood pressure. Currently, there is insufficient evidence to support any of these uses.

EVIDENCE

Uses Based on Scientific Evidence	Grade
Cataracts (Surgery) Side effects of cataract surgery may include pain, infection, swelling, bleeding, or retinal detachment. The use of kinetin during cataract surgery may lower adverse effects associated with cataracts. The available evidence is insufficient for this indication.	C
Ménière's Disease Ménière's disease is a disorder of the inner ear that causes hearing loss, ringing in the ear, and the sensation that one's surroundings are spinning. Kinetin may be beneficial for patients with Ménière's disease. However, evidence is insufficient to support this use.	C
Ocular Disorders (Eye Blood Pressure) Kinetin may decrease blood pressure in the eye, although currently there is insufficient available evidence to support this use.	C

Uses Based on Tradition or Theory
Aging, antioxidant, cancer, leukemia, nervous system disorders (familial dysautonomia), photoprotection, skin aging, surgical uses (adhesion prevention), thrombosis (blood clots).

DOSING

Adults (18 Years and Older)

- There is insufficient evidence to recommend a dose for kinetin in adults.

Children (Younger than 18 Years)

- There is insufficient evidence to recommend a dose kinetin for in children.

SAFETY

Allergies

- Avoid in people with a known allergy or hypersensitivity to kinetin.

Side Effects and Warnings

- Kinetin may have the following adverse effects: blood-thinning effects, increased coagulation (blood clotting) time, inhibited platelet aggregation, and prolonged or increased bleeding.
- Use cautiously in patients with coagulation or hematological (blood) disorders or those taking anticoagulants or antiplatelets (blood thinners).

Pregnancy and Breastfeeding

- Kinetin is not recommended in pregnant or breastfeeding women due to a lack of available scientific evidence.

INTERACTIONS

Interactions with Drugs

- Kinetin may have antioxidant effects. Use cautiously in patients taking antioxidants due to possible additive effects.
- Kinetin may increase the risk of bleeding when taken with drugs that increase the risk of bleeding. Some examples include aspirin, blood thinners such as warfarin (Coumadin) or heparin, antiplatelet drugs such as clopidogrel (Plavix), and nonsteroidal anti-inflammatory drugs (NSAIDs) such as ibuprofen (Motrin, Advil) or naproxen (Naprosyn, Aleve).
- Kinetin may inhibit cell growth, induce apoptosis, and stimulate cell differentiation. Use cautiously in patients with cancer or those taking anticancer agents.

Interactions with Herbs and Dietary Supplements

- Kinetin may have antioxidant effects. Use cautiously in patients taking antioxidant herbs or supplements due to possible additive effects.
- Kinetin may increase the risk of bleeding when taken with herbs or supplements that are believed to increase the risk of bleeding. Multiple cases of bleeding have been reported with the use of *Ginkgo biloba*, and fewer cases with garlic and saw palmetto.
- Kinetin may inhibit cell growth, induce apoptosis, and stimulate cell differentiation. Use cautiously in patients with cancer or those taking anticancer herbs or supplements.

For a complete list of references, please visit www.naturalstandard.com.

Kiwi
(Actinidia deliciosa, Actinidia chinensis)

RELATED TERMS

- *Actinidia arguta, Actinidia chinensis L., Actinidia coriacea, Actinidia kolomikta, Actinidia melanandra, Actinidia polygama, Actinidia purpurea, Actinidia sinensis* planch (ASP), Actinidiaceae, actinidin, Chinese egg gooseberry, China gooseberry, Chinese gooseberry, diethyl succinate, goat peach, hairy pear, hardy kiwi, hexyl hexanoate, kivi, kiivi, kiwi fruit, macaque peach, nonanal, octane, profilin, purple kiwi, red kiwi, silver vine, thiol-proteases, yang-tao.

BACKGROUND

- The kiwi fruit initially comes from China but is now produced in New Zealand, the United States, Italy, South Africa, and Chile.
- Kiwi is rich in vitamins C and E, serotonin, and potassium and is purported to have antioxidant activity. Kiwi fruit is also known to have the highest density of vitamin C for any fruit, and it is low in fat with no cholesterol. Claimed benefits of kiwi fruit, however, may be overshadowed by the growing number of reports of allergy.
- Kiwi has been used preventatively to protect against respiratory illness, increase lung function, and increase cardiovascular (heart) health.
- Currently, there is a lack of well-designed clinical regarding the medicinal use of kiwi fruit; however, additional research may be warranted to investigate its use in prevention of respiratory conditions and in energy enhancement.

EVIDENCE

Uses Based on Scientific Evidence	Grade
Energy Enhancement One study suggests that a kiwi-containing drink has beneficial effects on athletic performance. However, methodological weaknesses in this study preclude making any firm conclusions regarding kiwi's effectiveness at this time.	C
Respiratory Problems (Prevention) Current data on the therapeutic benefit of kiwi as a preventative for lung conditions is lacking. One survey study suggests that kiwi and other fruits high in vitamin C may have a protective effect on lung conditions in children, especially wheezing. However, properly controlled studies are lacking at this time.	C

Uses Based on Tradition or Theory
Antibacterial, antifungal, antioxidant, asthma, ATP-synthesis increase, cancer prevention, cardiovascular health, cell proliferation, collagen synthesis of fibroblasts, cytotoxic activity, digestion, human immunodeficiency virus, increasing proliferation, lung function, mitochondrial diseases, skin conditions.

DOSING
Adults (18 Years and Older)

- There is insufficient evidence to recommend a dose for kiwi. As an antioxidant, doses of 150-500 mL of kiwi fruit juice have been used. For cardiovascular health, studies have used two or three kiwi fruits per day for 28 days. For energy enhancement, studies have used 500-1,200 mL of kiwi fruit juice (*Actinidia sinensis* planch, ASP).

Children (Younger than 18 Years)

- One study reported beneficial effects on wheezing and other respiratory conditions in children from consuming between one and seven kiwi fruits per week.

SAFETY
Allergies

- Kiwi allergy is one of the more common allergies among fruits, and caution is advised. There are numerous reports of allergy and cross-sensitization with kiwi and birch pollen, banana, avocado, chestnut, melon, fig, nuts, poppy seeds, sesame seeds, rye grain, hazelnuts, flour, latex-containing plants, and grasses. Asthma, rash, hives, swelling, and anaphylaxis have been reported.

Side Effects and Warnings

- The most common adverse effect is allergy to kiwi, which may or may not clinically manifest in symptoms ranging from local mouth irritation to anaphylaxis. Urticaria (hives) and angioedema (swelling) due to allergy and cases of allergic contact dermatitis have been reported. Oral allergy syndrome (OAS), which includes itching and tingling with or without edema (swelling) of the lips, mouth, and tongue has been observed after consuming kiwi. Acute pancreatitis has also been reported.
- Kiwi is known to have high levels of vitamin C, E, potassium, and serotonin and may be capable of altering triglyceride levels. Nausea, vomiting, diarrhea, dysphagia (difficulty swallowing), and collapse have also been reported.

Pregnancy and Breastfeeding

- Kiwi is not recommended in pregnant or breastfeeding women due to a lack of available scientific evidence.

INTERACTIONS
Interactions with Drugs

- Based on preliminary laboratory evidence, kiwi may have antifungal activity and therefore have an additive effect when taken with other antifungals.
- Kiwi may increase the risk of bleeding when taken with drugs that increase the risk of bleeding. Some examples include aspirin, anticoagulants (blood thinners) such as warfarin (Coumadin) or heparin, antiplatelet drugs such as clopidogrel (Plavix), and nonsteroidal anti-inflammatory drugs such as ibuprofen (Motrin, Advil) or naproxen (Naprosyn, Aleve).
- Kiwi has a high serotonin concentration. Selective serotonin reuptake inhibitors (SSRIs) alter the levels of serotonin in the body usually by increasing them. Therefore,

theoretically, kiwi and SSRIs may have a synergistic effect on serotonin levels.

- Consumption of kiwi fruit may lower blood triglycerides.

Interactions with Herbs and Dietary Supplements

- Based on preliminary data, kiwi may have antifungal activity and therefore have an additive effect when taken with other antifungals.
- Based on preliminary data, kiwi may have antioxidant activity and therefore have an additive effect when taken with other antioxidants.
- In theory, kiwi may increase the risk of bleeding when also taken with other products that are believed to increase the risk of bleeding. Multiple cases of bleeding have been reported with the use of *Ginkgo biloba,* and fewer cases with garlic and saw palmetto. Numerous other agents may theoretically increase the risk of bleeding, although this has not been proven in most cases.

- Substantial amounts of lutein and zeaxanthin are present in kiwi fruit. Caution is advised when taking lutein supplements.
- Theoretically, kiwi may have an effect on the amount of potassium in the body because it is rich in potassium.
- Theoretically, kiwi is associated with an increased amount of serotonin. Kiwi plus herbs/supplements that alter serotonin levels may have an effect on the levels of serotonin in the body.
- Consumption of kiwi fruit may lower blood triglycerides.
- Kiwi may increase the amount of vitamin C in the body because it is rich in vitamin C. Based on urinary measurements, vitamin C status improved in athletes supplemented with *Actinidia sinensis* planch drink in one study.
- Theoretically, kiwi may have an effect on the amount of vitamin E in the body because it is rich in vitamin E.

For a complete list of references, please visit www. naturalstandard.com.

Kudzu
(Pueraria lobata)

RELATED TERMS

- Arrowroot, biochanin A, daidzein, daidzin, Fabaceae (family), Flos puerariae, ge-gen, gegen-tanj (TJ-1), genistein, genistin, glycitin, kaikasaponin III (KS-III), kakkonto, kampo, kudzu root, Kwao Kruea Khao, Leguminosae (family), pedunsaponin B2, pedunsaponin C3, puer, *Pueraria lobata, Pueraria lobata* L., *Pueraria lobata* Ohwi, *Pueraria lobata* root decoction, *Pueraria lobata* (Willd), *Pueraria mirifica, Pueraria montana, Pueraria omeiensis, Pueraria peduncularis, Pueraria phaseoloides, Pueraria thomsonii, Pueraria thunbergiana*, Pueraria flos, Pueraria radix, puerariae surculus, puerariae-flos, puerarin, Radix puerariae, spinasterol, tectoridin, tectorigenin, Tianbaokang, Yufengningxin.

BACKGROUND

- Kudzu originated in China and was brought to the United States from Japan in the late 1800s. It is widespread throughout much of the eastern United States and is most common in the southern part of the continent.
- Kudzu has traditionally been used in China to treat alcoholism, diabetes (high blood sugar), gastroenteritis (inflamed stomach or intestine), and deafness.
- Evidence suggests kudzu may improve signs and symptoms of unstable angina (chest pain), improve insulin resistance, and have a positive effect on cognitive function in postmenopausal women. However, most studies have suffered from methodological weaknesses and small sample sizes.
- Chinese healers have used kudzu to treat high blood pressure and chest pain and to minimize alcohol cravings. Research indicates that puerarin (a constituent of kudzu) may increase blood flow to the heart and brain, which helps explain certain traditional uses.

EVIDENCE

Uses Based on Scientific Evidence	Grade
Alcoholism Although preliminary studies indicate that kudzu may be useful in alcoholism, additional human studies are needed to make a firm recommendation.	C
Cardiovascular Disease/Angina Kudzu has a long history of use in the treatment of cardiovascular (heart) disorders, including angina (chest pain), acute myocardial infarction (heart attack), and heart failure. Preliminary studies have suggested that kudzu may reduce the frequency of angina events in human subjects. More research is needed in this area.	C
Deafness Kudzu was used in one clinical trial to treat sudden nerve deafness. Additional evidence is needed to confirm these results.	C
Diabetes Preliminary evidence suggests puerarin, a constituent of kudzu, may improve insulin resistance. Insulin resistance is a condition in which the cells of the body become resistant to the effects of insulin, and the normal response to a given amount of insulin is reduced. As a result, higher levels of insulin are needed in order for insulin to have its effects. Insulin resistance precedes the development of type 2 diabetes. Therefore, reversing insulin resistance can lessen chances of developing type 2 diabetes and heart disease. Additional studies are needed before a firm conclusion can be made.	C
Diabetic Retinopathy Preliminary evidence suggests that puerarin (a constituent of kudzu) injections may reduce blood viscosity, improve microcirculation, and play a positive therapeutic role in diabetic retinopathy. Well-designed clinical trials are needed to confirm these results before a recommendation can be made.	C
Glaucoma In China, the main herb-derived eye drops from glaucoma are pueraria flavonoids. The addition of puerarin to conventional drugs for glaucoma yielded favorable results. Additional research is needed to confirm these results.	C
Menopausal Symptoms There is conflicting evidence regarding the effects of kudzu on menopausal symptoms. Additional studies are needed to clarify these results.	C

Uses Based on Tradition or Theory

Allergic rhinitis, anti-inflammatory, antioxidant, antithrombotic (blood clots), breast enlargement cancer, cerebral ischemia (lack of adequate blood flow to the brain), circulation, cirrhosis (liver disease), colds, diarrhea, dysentery (severe diarrhea), elimination of toxins, encephalitis (brain infection), estrogenic effects, fever, gastritis (inflammation of the stomach), gastroenteritis (inflammation of stomach, intestine), hangovers, headaches, hypertension (high blood pressure), influenza, leukemia, macular degeneration (chronic eye disease), measles, menstrual irregularities, migraine, myalgia (muscle pain), reperfusion injury (myocardial, restoration of blood flow), neck stiffness, osteoporosis, pain, Parkinson's disease, pruritus (severe itching), psoriasis (chronic skin disease), pulmonary embolism, sinusitis, sweat stimulation, tinnitus, trauma, urticaria (hives), vasorelaxant (reduces tension of the blood vessel walls).

DOSING

Adults (18 Years and Older)

- Several doses of kudzu have been studied. For alcoholism, 1.2 g kudzu root extract has been taken twice daily for 1 month. For menopausal symptoms, 50 mg or 100 mg of *Pueraria mirifica* has been taken once daily for 6 months. Kudzu powder (containing 100 mg isoflavones) dissolved in water has been used once daily for 3 months.
- Puerarin 400 mg daily for 10 days has been taken by mouth to improve heart function in patients with chronic cardiac failure. Puerarin 500 mg has also been given as an injection daily for 2 weeks to reduce the size of infarction in patients with acute myocardial infarction (heart attack). Doses of 400-500 mg are typically used to treat diabetes, diabetic retinopathy, and unstable angina pectoris (chest pain). Injections should only be given under the guidance of a qualified health care professional, including a pharmacist.

Children (Younger than 18 Years)

- There is insufficient evidence to recommend a dose for kudzu.

SAFETY

Allergies

- Avoid in people with a known allergy or hypersensitivity to *Pueraria lobata* or the Fabaceae/Leguminosae family. There is one case report of allergic reaction following the use of a combination herbal product containing kudzu involving a maculo-papular (elevated, spotted rash-like skin condition) eruption starting on the thighs and spreading over the entire body.

Side Effects and Warnings

- Currently, there are no side effects reported of kudzu treatment when taken by mouth. Intravenous puerarin has caused intravascular hemolysis (destruction of red blood cells). Intraperitoneal administration of puerarin or crude extracts of *Pueraria lobata* caused hypothermia (low body temperature).
- In theory, intraperitoneal administration of puerarin or crude extracts of *Pueraria lobata* may cause hypothermia. Kudzu root may also cause weight loss, although this has not been well studied in humans.

Pregnancy and Breastfeeding

- Kudzu is not recommended in pregnant or breastfeeding women due to a lack of available scientific evidence.

INTERACTIONS

Interactions with Drugs

- Kudzu isoflavones are reported to have antiestrogenic activity. Theoretically, kudzu might competitively inhibit the effects of estrogen therapy.
- Kudzu extracts or individual isoflavones suppress voluntary alcohol intake in animal models of alcoholism.
- The kudzu constituent, daidzin, may have antiarrhythmic properties and, theoretically, kudzu may interfere with antiarrhythmic agents (used to treat irregular heartbeat). Daidzin may also act by inhibiting serotonin and dopamine metabolism. Theoretically, concurrent use of kudzu with drugs that affect the metabolism of serotonin and dopamine (e.g., MAOIs) may lead to increased serotonin levels and increased risk of serotonin syndrome.
- Kudzu may increase the risk of bleeding when taken with drugs that increase the risk of bleeding. Some examples include aspirin, anticoagulants (blood thinners) such as warfarin (Coumadin) or heparin, antiplatelet drugs such as clopidogrel (Plavix), and nonsteroidal anti-inflammatory drugs (NSAIDs) such as ibuprofen (Motrin, Advil) or naproxen (Naprosyn, Aleve).
- Kudzu may lower blood sugar levels. Caution is advised when using medications that may also lower blood sugar levels. Patients taking drugs for diabetes by mouth or insulin should be monitored closely by a qualified health care professional, including a pharmacist. Medication adjustments may be necessary.
- Although not well studied in humans, puerarin may lessen the feelings of anxiety and, theoretically, it may have an antagonistic effect with benzodiazepines. Puerarin may also suppress bone resorption, promote bone formation, and interfere with bisphosphonates. Puerarin may have vasorelaxant properties, possibly by blocking beta-adrenergic receptors.
- Kudzu inhibits and induces cytochrome P450 isoenzymes. It is unclear which cytochrome P450 isoenzymes are affected and to what degree. Concurrent use of drugs metabolized by the cytochrome P450 liver enzyme system may result in altered therapeutic levels.
- Theoretically, kudzu may interfere with blood pressure–lowering agents. Kudzu has vasodilatory (blood vessel–dilating) and hypotensive (blood pressure–lowering) effects.
- Kudzu may weaken the effects of mecamylamine.

Interactions with Herbs and Dietary Supplements

- The kudzu constituent, daidzin, may have antiarrhythmic (treats irregular heartbeat) properties and, theoretically, kudzu may interfere with these antiarrhythmic herbs and supplements.
- Kudzu isoflavones may increase the risk of bleeding when taken with herbs and supplements that are believed to increase the risk of bleeding. Multiple cases of bleeding have been reported with the use of *Ginkgo biloba,* and fewer cases with garlic and saw palmetto. Numerous other agents may theoretically increase the risk of bleeding, although this has not been proven in most cases.
- Kudzu may lower blood sugar levels. Caution is advised when using herbs or supplements that may also lower blood sugar levels. Blood glucose levels may require monitoring, and doses may need adjustment.
- Kudzu inhibits and induces cytochrome P450 isoenzymes; however, it is unclear which cytochrome P450 isoenzymes are affected and to what degree. Concurrent use of herbs and supplements metabolized by the cytochrome P450 liver enzyme system may result in altered therapeutic levels.
- Kudzu isoflavones are reported to have antiestrogenic activity. Theoretically, kudzu might competitively inhibit the effects of herbs and supplements with estrogen activity.
- Theoretically, kudzu may interfere with blood pressure–lowering herbs and supplements. Kudzu has vasodilatory (blood vessel–dilating) and hypotensive (blood pressure–lowering) effects.
- The daidzin in kudzu may act by inhibiting serotonin and dopamine metabolism. Theoretically, concurrent use of kudzu with herbs that affect the metabolism of serotonin and dopamine (e.g., MAOIs) may lead to increased serotonin levels and increased risk of serotonin syndrome.
- Puerarin may have vasorelaxant properties, possibly by blocking beta-adrenergic receptors.

For a complete list of references, please visit www.naturalstandard.com.

K

Labrador Tea
(*Ledum groenlandicum*)

RELATED TERMS

- Bog tea, finnmarkspors, getpors, Hudson's Bay tea, James tea, marsh tea, mose-post, muskeegobug aniibi (Ojibwe), muskeko-pukwa (Cree), skvattram, St. James tea, sumpf-porst, suopursu, swamp growing tea, swamp tea, vildpors, wish-a-ca-pucca (Chpewyan).

BACKGROUND

- Labrador tea is a small, aromatic shrub with a narrow, leathery leaf. It is also known as Hudson Bay tea and is used as a spice for meat.
- Native American tribes used labrador tea to treat a variety of ailments, including headaches, asthma, colds, stomachaches, and kidney ailments. It was also used topically as a wash for burns, ulcers, pruritus (severe itching), dry skin, dandruff, and lice. The plant is also said to have mild narcotic properties and was used by Native women before childbirth.
- Theoretically, if too much tea is ingested it may be cathartic (produces bowel movements) and may cause intestinal problems. Currently, no scientific studies in humans or animals are available involving labrador tea.

EVIDENCE

Uses Based on Scientific Evidence

No available studies qualify for inclusion in the evidence table.

Uses Based on Tradition or Theory

Analgesic (pain reliever), arthritis, asthma, childbirth (aid), burns, colds, cough, dandruff, diaphoretic (promotes sweating), diuretic, dizziness, elimination of blood toxins (blood purifier), fever, hangovers, headache, heartburn, kidney problems, laxative, narcotic, pruritus (severe itching), skin problems, skin ulcers, stomachache, tuberculosis.

DOSING

Adults (18 Years and Older)

- There is insufficient evidence to recommend a dose of labrador tea. Traditionally, 2-4 fl oz of labrador tea infusion, three to four times a day, has been used.
- Also, an ointment made of labrador tea has been applied on the skin to treat ulcers, cracked nipples, burns, and scalds.

Children (Younger than 18 Years)

- There is insufficient evidence to recommend a dose of labrador tea in children.

SAFETY

Allergies

- Avoid in people with a known allergy or hypersensitivity to labrador tea.

Side Effects and Warnings

- There is a lack of scientific studies reporting adverse effects of labrador tea. However, ingesting large quantities of labrador tea may cause stomachache and act as a laxative. Labrador tea overdoses may also cause violent headache, drowsiness, and symptoms of intoxication.

Pregnancy and Breastfeeding

- Labrador tea is not recommended in pregnant or breastfeeding women due to a lack of available scientific evidence.

INTERACTIONS

Interactions with Drugs

- Labrador tea has narcotic properties and theoretically may have additive effects with other central nervous system (CNS) depressants.

Interactions with Herbs and Dietary Supplements

- Labrador tea has narcotic properties and theoretically may have additive effects with other herbs and supplements that are central nervous system (CNS) depressants.

For a complete list of references, please visit www.naturalstandard.com.

Lady's Mantle
(*Alchemilla* spp.)

RELATED TERMS

- *Alchemillae herba,* bear's foot, common lady's mantle, ellagic acid, flavonoids, Frauenmantle, Frauenmantelkraut, lady's cloak, leontopodium, lion's foot, nine hooks, pied-de-lion, quercetol, quercetin, stellaria, tannins.

BACKGROUND

- Lady's mantle was named in the sixteenth century by Jerome Bock, also known as Tragus, and it appears under his name in the book *History of Plants,* published in 1532. Lady's mantle is referred to as lady's cloak or mantle because of its association with the Virgin Mary. The lobes of the leaf are said to resemble the scalloped edges of a mantle. It has also been referred to as lion's foot and bear's foot, most likely because of the resemblance of its spreading root leaves to such feet.
- Lady's mantle has been used for many centuries in Europe including in Sweden and Germany. Some experts consider lady's mantle to be good for treating wounds due to its coagulation (blood clotting), astringent, and styptic (stops bleeding) properties. It has also been used as a mouth rinse after dental procedures to help stop bleeding. Lady's mantle has been used for a variety of female conditions such as menstrual disorders, including excessive menstruation and menopause, as an aid during conception, in the prevention of miscarriages, and to help the body heal after childbirth. However, clinical evidence is lacking.

EVIDENCE

Uses Based on Scientific Evidence

No available studies qualify for inclusion in the evidence table.

Uses Based on Tradition or Theory

Acne, anticonvulsant, anti-inflammatory, antihemorrhagic, appetite stimulant, astringent, coagulation (blood clotting), diabetes, diarrhea, diuretic, fertility (conception aid), fibroids (benign tumors in or around the uterus that sometimes can cause miscarriages), childbirth (healing aid), high blood pressure, hormone imbalances (estrogen or testosterone), menopause, menorrhagia (excessive menstruation), miscarriage (prevention), rheumatism, sleep aid, stomach problems, styptic (stops bleeding), wound healing.

DOSING
Adults (18 Years and Older)

- There is insufficient evidence to recommend a dose for lady's mantle. Traditionally, drinking a tea made by steeping the chopped leaves in hot water for 15 minutes, then straining and ingesting for 20 consecutive days, has been used as a conception aid. To treat excessive menstruation, 1 oz of dried herb has been infused in 1 pint of boiling water to make a tea. This tea is then consumed in amounts similar to a teacupful (size of teacup not stated). Lady's mantle has also been used as a vaginal douche to treat leukorrhea (vaginal discharge).

Children (Younger than 18 Years)

- There is insufficient evidence to recommend a dose for lady's mantle in children.

SAFETY
Allergies

- Avoid in individuals with a known allergy or hypersensitivity to lady's mantle.

Side Effects and Warnings

- The lack of formal clinical trials makes it difficult to draw any conclusions regarding the safety of lady's mantle. Nonetheless, lady's mantle is possibly unsafe in patients using medications to prevent coagulation of the blood (e.g., warfarin) due to its theoretical use as a coagulant. It is also possibly unsafe in patients with iron deficiency anemia because lady's mantle may contain tannins, which may reduce the absorption of iron supplements.

Pregnancy and Breastfeeding

- Lady's mantle is not recommended in pregnant or breastfeeding women due to a lack of available scientific evidence. Traditionally, lady's mantle has been used as a conception aid and for excessive menstruation.

INTERACTIONS
Interactions with Drugs

- Theoretically, lady's mantle should be avoided in patients using anticoagulation therapy, such as warfarin (Coumadin). Lady's mantle may decrease the efficacy of these medications due to its proposed coagulation (blood clotting) effects.

Interactions with Herbs and Dietary Supplements

- Theoretically, lady's mantle should be avoided in patients taking anticoagulation (blood thinning) herbs or supplements. Lady's mantle may decrease the efficacy of these agents due to its proposed coagulation (blood clotting) effects.
- Lady's mantle contains tannins, which may reduce the absorption of iron supplements.
- Lady's mantle has been shown to have a weak mutagenic effect (cause changes in the DNA of cells) on bacteria, and it is proposed that the constituent quercetin is the cause of the mutagenic activity. Taking both quercetin and lady's mantle may increase this effect.

For a complete list of references, please visit www.naturalstandard.com.

RELATED TERMS

- American false-hellebore *(Veratrum viride)*, American valerian, bleeding heart, Cyripedium, *Cypripedium acaule, Cypripedium calceolus, Cypripedium californicum, Cypripedium candidum, Cypripedium fasciculatum, Cypripedium flavum, Cypripedium guttatum, Cypripedium japonicum, Cypripedium montanum, Cypripedium pubescens, Cypripedium tibeticum,* English lady's slipper *(Cypripedium calceolus)*, Indian valerian, Japanese lady's slipper *(Cypripedium japonicum)*, ladies slipper, moccasin flower, monkey flower, Noah's ark, Orchidaceae (family), pink lady's slipper *(Cypripedium acaule)*, ram's-head lady's-slipper *(Cypripedium arietinum)*, queen's lady slipper, showy lady's slipper *(Cypripedium reginae)*, slipper root, spotted lady's slipper *(Cypripedium guttatum)*, stemless lady's slipper *(Cypripedium acaule)*, two lips, venus shoe, virgin's shoe, yellow lady's slipper *(Cypripedium calceolus)*, yellows, nerve root.

BACKGROUND

- Lady's slipper is a wildflower in the orchid family (Orchidaceae). Yellow lady's slipper *(Cypripedium calceolus),* which comes from India and was named American valerian after Indian valerian *(Valeriana wallichii)*, shares similar medical properties with pink lady's slipper. Once commonly used to treat various nervous disorders, it is a mild stimulant and is antispasmodic. Lady's slipper has been described in the folklore as a stimulant and a sedative, and no reports are currently available to confirm these opposite proposed actions. It is also often used to treat depression related to female problems. Having been almost wiped out by collectors for such medical use, it is now too rare to be used medically.
- Pink lady's slipper *(Cypripedium acaule)* was considered a substitute for the preferred yellow lady's slipper as a medicinal plant. Used as a sedative and antispasmodic, it was substituted for the European valerian. It has also been used for male and female disorders.
- Presently, there are no high-quality human clinical trials available evaluating the safety and efficacy of lady's slipper. However, traditional users and some herbal experts suggest that more research may be warranted to investigate the antispasmodic and sedative/stimulant actions of lady's slipper.

EVIDENCE

Uses Based on Scientific Evidence

No available studies qualify for inclusion in the evidence table.

Uses Based on Tradition or Theory

Antispasmodic, anxiety, astringent, cramps, delirium tremens ("the shakes," an acute episode of delirium that is usually caused by withdrawal), depression (mild), diaphoretic (promotes sweating), diarrhea, enhancing recovery from surgery or illness, hypnotic, hysteria, insomnia, menorrhagia (heavy menstrual bleeding), mood (elevate), muscle spasms, nervousness, pain, pruritus (severe itching), sedative, stimulant, stress, styptic (stops bleeding), tension (emotional), tooth pain.

DOSING

Adults (18 Years and Older)

- There is insufficient evidence to recommend a dose of lady's slipper. Traditionally, 2-4 g dried rhizome/root, or a tea (2-4 g dried rhizome/root steeped in 150 mL of boiling water for 5-10 minutes and then strained) has been used three times daily. A liquid extract (1:1 in 45% alcohol) of 2-4 mL has also been used three times daily. In capsule form, one or two 570-mg capsules of 100% lady's slipper have been taken up to three times daily with water at mealtimes.

Children (Younger than 18 Years)

- There is insufficient evidence to recommend a dose of lady's slipper in children, and use is not recommended.

SAFETY

Allergies

- Avoid in people with a known allergy or hypersensitivity to lady's slipper. Contact with the leaves of lady's slipper may cause contact dermatitis. The stem of the showy lady's slipper, *Cypripedium reginae,* is covered with hairs containing a fatty acid that may cause blistering similar to that caused by poison ivy.

Side Effects and Warnings

- Adverse effects of lady's slipper are not well documented in the available literature. Dermatitis (inflammation of the skin), hallucinations, and restlessness are possible side effects, although the frequency and duration of these effects are unknown. Large doses have been associated with giddiness, restlessness, headache, and mental excitement. The stem of a related species, the showy lady's slipper *(Cypripedium reginae),* is covered with hairs containing a fatty acid that may cause blistering similar to that caused by poison ivy, although it is unclear if other species would have the same effect.

Pregnancy and Breastfeeding

- Lady's slipper is not recommended in pregnant or breastfeeding women due to a lack of available scientific evidence.

INTERACTIONS

Interactions with Drugs

- Lady's slipper contains quinines, which may have an additive effect when taken concomitantly with other quinine-containing agents, which are often used to treat malaria.
- Lady's slipper may contain tannins, glycosides, resins, and quinines. Patients taking cardiac glycosides or digoxin should use with caution.

- Based on traditional use, lady's slipper may have additive effects when used with other sedatives.

Interactions with Herbs and Dietary Supplements

- Lady's slipper may contain tannins, glycosides, resins, and quinines. Patients taking herbs with cardiac glycoside-like effects, such as foxglove, should use with caution. People taking herbs with high tannin content should also use with caution.

- Lady's slipper contains quinines, which may have an additive effect with other quinine-containing herbs.
- Based on traditional use, lady's slipper may have additive effects when used with other sedatives. Caution is advised in patients taking herbs such as valerian or chamomile.

For a complete list of references, please visit www. naturalstandard.com.

L

Lavender

(*Lavandula* spp.)

RELATED TERMS

- Common lavender, English lavender, garden lavender, *Lavandula burnamii*, *Lavandula dentate*, *Lavandula dhofarensis*, *Lavandula latifolia*, *Lavandula officinalis* L., *Lavandula stoechas*, limonene, NHED (contains *Allium sativum*, *Verbascum thapsus*, *Calendula flores*, *Hypericum perfoliatum*, lavender, and vitamin E in olive oil), perillyl alcohol, pink lavender, POH, true lavender, white lavender.

BACKGROUND

- Lavender is native to the Mediterranean, the Arabian Peninsula, Russia, and Africa. It has been used cosmetically and medicinally throughout history. In modern times, lavender is cultivated around the world and the fragrant oils of its flowers are used in aromatherapy, baked goods, candles, cosmetics, detergents, jellies, massage oils, perfumes, powders, shampoo, soaps, and tea. English lavender (*Lavandula angustifolia*) is the most common species of lavender used, although other species are in use, including *Lavandula burnamii*, *Lavandula dentate*, *Lavandula dhofarensis*, *Lavandula latifolia*, and *Lavandula stoechas*.
- Many people find lavender aromatherapy to be relaxing, and it has been reported to have anxiolytic (anti-anxiety) effects. Overall, the evidence suggests a small positive effect, although additional data from well-designed studies are required before the evidence can be considered strong.
- Lavender aromatherapy is also used as a hypnotic, although there is insufficient evidence in support of this use.
- Small Phase I human trials of the lavender constituent perillyl alcohol (POH) for cancer have suggested safety and tolerability, although efficacy has not been demonstrated.

EVIDENCE

Uses Based on Scientific Evidence	Grade
Agitated Behavior (Lavender Aromatherapy) Small studies of patients with severe dementia in nursing homes have found that lavender aromatherapy or pinning a cloth to the patient with lavender oil on it may help to decrease agitated behavior. However, the clinical evidence is insufficient to support this use.	C
Alopecia/Hair Loss (Lavender Used on the Skin) Small trials have shown that patients who massage essential oils (thyme, rosemary, lavender, and cedarwood) into their scalps daily showed more improvement than the control group. However, the clinical evidence is insufficient to support this use.	C
Antibacterial (Lavender Used on the Skin) Preliminary laboratory studies suggest that lavender oils may have antibiotic activity. However, this has not been well tested in animal or human studies.	C
Anxiety (Lavender Aromatherapy) Lavender aromatherapy is traditionally used for relaxation. It is reported to help relieve anxiety in several small studies, although negative results have also been reported. However, the clinical evidence is insufficient to support this use.	C
Cancer (Perillyl Alcohol) Perillyl alcohol (POH), derived from lavender, might be beneficial in the treatment of some types of cancer. This research has focused on cancers of the pancreas, breast, and intestine. Preliminary small studies in humans suggest safety and tolerability of POH, but effectiveness has not been established.	C
Cognitive Performance Although lavender is a sedative-type aroma, use during recess periods in a work environment after accumulation of fatigue seemed to prevent deterioration of performance in subsequent work sessions. However, the clinical evidence is insufficient to support this use.	C
Dementia Small trials investigating the effects of lavender aromatherapy on agitation and behavior in patients with Alzheimer's dementia report conflicting results. However, the clinical evidence is insufficient to support this use.	C
Depression Preliminary research suggests that lavender may be helpful as an adjunct to prescription antidepressant medications. However, the clinical evidence is insufficient to support this use.	C
Ear Pain A small clinical trial used a naturopathic eardrop called NHED (containing *Allium sativum*, *Verbascum thapsus*, *Calendula flores*, *Hypericum perfoliatum*, lavender, and vitamin E in olive oil) with and without an antibiotic and topical anesthetic. It was found that the ear pain was self-limiting and resolved after a few days with or without antibiotics. However, the clinical evidence is insufficient to support this use.	C
Eczema In a small clinical trial, essential oils were used in combination with massage to treat childhood atopic eczema. It was found that there was deterioration in the patient's eczema, which may have been caused by possible allergic contact dermatitis provoked by the essential oils themselves. However, the clinical evidence is insufficient to support this use.	C

Uses Based on Scientific Evidence	Grade
Hypnotic/Sleep Aid (Lavender Aromatherapy) Lavender aromatherapy is often promoted as a sleep aid. Although preliminary evidence suggests possible benefits, the clinical evidence is insufficient to support this use.	C
Low Back Pain Preliminary research suggests that the impression of pain intensity and unpleasantness may be reduced after treatment with lavender therapy. Other research has shown that lavender aromatherapy may be effective when used with acupressure for short-term relief of lower back pain. However, the clinical evidence is insufficient to support this use.	C
Neck Pain Preliminary human studies indicate a potential role for lavender aromatherapy in combination with massage in the short-term treatment of neck pain. However, the clinical evidence is insufficient to support this use.	C
Overall Well-Being (Lavender Used in a Bath) Preliminary evidence has shown that lavender oil in combination with grape seed oil used in a bath may help to improve overall well-being, and decrease anger and frustration. Lavender oil used as aromatherapy has also been shown to increase overall mood. However, the clinical evidence is insufficient to support this use.	C
Pain (Lavender Aromatherapy) Preliminary research suggests that the impression of pain intensity and unpleasantness may be reduced after treatment with lavender therapy. Other research has shown that lavender aromatherapy may be effective when used with acupressure for short-term relief of lower back pain. However, the clinical evidence is insufficient to support this use.	C
Perineal Discomfort after Childbirth (Lavender Added to Bath) Lavender has been evaluated as an additive to bathwater to relieve pain in the perineal area (between the vagina and anus) in women following birth. Preliminary poor-quality research reports no benefits. However, the clinical evidence is insufficient to support this use.	C
Quality of Life (Postpartum) Preliminary evidence suggests a potential role for lavender aromatherapy, especially in combination with massage or acupressure, in the improvement of measures of quality of life among new mothers. However, the clinical evidence is insufficient to support this use.	C
Rheumatoid Arthritis Pain Preliminary human studies have found conflicting results on the use of massage with lavender aromatherapy in this condition. However, the clinical evidence is insufficient to support this use.	C

	Grade
Spasmolytic (Oral) Preliminary laboratory and animal studies indicate a potential spasmolytic effect of lavender oil inhalation. However, the clinical evidence is insufficient to support this use.	C

Uses Based on Tradition or Theory

Acne, angioprotectant, antifungal, anti-inflammatory, antioxidant, aphrodisiac, appetite stimulant, asthma, bronchitis, carpal tunnel syndrome, circulation problems, cleanser (douche), colic, common cold, decrease in heart rate, diabetes, diuretic, dizziness, exercise recovery, fatigue, fever, gas, hangover, heartburn, HIV, indigestion, infertility, insect repellent, lice, low blood pressure, menopause, menstrual problems, migraine headache, minor burns, motion sickness, muscle spasm, nausea, neuroprotection, non-tubercular mycobacteria (NTM), parasites/worms, psychosis, seizures/epilepsy, snake repellent, sores, sprains, tension headache, toothache, varicose veins, vomiting, warts, wound healing.

DOSING
Adults (18 Years and Older)

- Lavender has been taken by mouth as a tea prepared from 1 to 2 tsp (5 to 10 g) of leaves steeped in 1 cup (250 ml) of boiling water for 15 minutes. As a tincture, a dose of 60 drops (1:5 in 50% alcohol) has been used daily.
- Lavender oil has been used in aromatherapy (inhaled) and massage therapy (applied on the skin). A naturopathic eardrop called NHED, which includes lavender, has been used at a dose of 5 drops three times a day with or without an antibiotic and topical anesthetic.
- To reduce perineal discomfort after childbirth, 6 drops of lavender oil have been added to a bath. Another technique reported is to add ¼ to ½ cup of dried lavender flowers to hot bath water.
- Preliminary cancer studies report doses of 800 to 1,200 mg per square meter of body surface, taken by mouth, four times daily in a 50:50 perillyl alcohol (a derivative of lavender):soybean oil preparation.

Children (Younger than 18 Years)

- There is not enough scientific evidence to safely recommend lavender for children.

SAFETY
Allergies

- People with allergies to lavender may experience skin irritation after contact and should avoid lavender in all forms.

Side Effects and Warnings

- Mild rash can develop after applying lavender oil. Reports describe increased sun sensitivity and changes in skin pigmentation after applying products containing lavender oil. Nausea, vomiting, loss of appetite, constipation, headache, chills, confusion, and drowsiness are sometimes reported after inhaling lavender, absorbing it through the skin, or taking large doses of lavender or perillyl alcohol (derived from lavender) by mouth. The essential oil of lavender may be poisonous if taken by mouth.

L

- Drowsiness can occur after lavender aromatherapy. More severe drowsiness or sedation may occur when lavender is used with other sedating agents. Use caution if driving or operating heavy machinery.
- In theory, lavender used by mouth may increase the risk of bleeding. People with bleeding disorders or those taking drugs that may increase bleeding should use caution. Dosing adjustments may be necessary.
- Some cancer patients have experienced low blood cell counts (neutropenia) after taking high doses of perillyl alcohol by mouth.

Pregnancy and Breastfeeding

- Lavender is not recommended during pregnancy or breastfeeding because of a lack of scientific evidence proving its safety. However, lavender has historically been used in pregnancy and breastfeeding with a lack of reported side effects.

INTERACTIONS

Interactions with Drugs

- Animal studies suggest that lavender used as aromatherapy or by mouth may increase the amount of drowsiness caused by some drugs. Examples include benzodiazepines such as lorazepam (Ativan) or diazepam (Valium), barbiturates such as phenobarbital, narcotics such as codeine, some antidepressants, and alcohol. Drowsiness caused by some seizure medicines may also be increased. Caution is advised while driving or operating machinery.
- In theory, lavender may add to the effects of cholesterol-lowering drugs.

- Lavender may have additive effects when used with prescription antidepressant medications, such as the tricyclic antidepressant imipramine.
- Lavender may increase the risk of bleeding when taken with drugs that increase the risk of bleeding. Some examples include aspirin, anticoagulants (blood thinners) such as warfarin (Coumadin) or heparin, anti-platelet drugs such as clopidogrel (Plavix), and non-steroidal anti-inflammatory drugs such as ibuprofen (Motrin, Advil) or naproxen (Naprosyn, Aleve).

Interactions with Herbs and Dietary Supplements

- Lavender used as aromatherapy or by mouth may increase the amount of drowsiness caused by some herbs or supplements, such as valerian. Caution is advised while driving or operating machinery.
- In theory, lavender may add to the cholesterol-lowering effects of some herbs or supplements such as fish oil, garlic, guggul, and niacin.
- Lavender may interact with herbs and supplements taken for depression; use cautiously.
- Lavender may increase the risk of bleeding when taken with herbs and supplements that are believed to increase the risk of bleeding. Multiple cases of bleeding have been reported with the use of *Ginkgo biloba,* and fewer cases with garlic and saw palmetto. Numerous other agents may theoretically increase the risk of bleeding, although this has not been proven in most cases.

For a complete list of references, please visit www.naturalstandard.com.

Lemon Balm
(Melissa officinalis)

RELATED TERMS

- Balm, balm mint, bee balm, blue balm, Citra, citronellae, citronmelisse, common balm, cure-all, dropsy plant, English balm, folia citronellae, folia melissae citratae, garden balm, gastrovegetalin, hjertensfryd, honey plant, kneipp melisse pflanzensaft, Labiatae/Lamiaceae (family), lemon melissa, lomaherpan, melissa, *Melissa officinalis, Melissa officinalis* L., melissae, melissae folium, Melisse (German and French), melissenblatt, melissengeist, sweet balm, sweet mary, toronjil (Spanish), valverde boutons de fievre crème.

BACKGROUND

- Lemon balm *(Melissa officinalis)* is an herb with a lemon scent native to southern Europe. Historically, lemon balm has been said to possess sedative/tranquilizing, anti-gas, fever-reducing, antibacterial, spasmolytic, hypotensive (blood pressure–lowering), memory-enhancing, menstrual-inducing, and thyroid-related effects and has been proposed by some to be an herbal cure-all. Laboratory data suggest that lemon balm may contain high concentrations of antioxidants.
- The German Commission E recommends lemon balm for nervous sleep disorders and functional gastrointestinal complaints. The European Scientific Cooperative on Phytotherapy (ESCOP) recommends its use for tenseness, restlessness, and irritability. Lemon balm has been placed on the U.S. Food and Drug Administration's GRAS (generally regarded as safe) list. No serious side effects have been reported, although there is limited research of long-term effects.

EVIDENCE

Uses Based on Scientific Evidence	Grade
Herpes Simplex Virus Infections Rigorous clinical data are lacking. Preliminary clinical studies demonstrate promising effects.	B
Agitation in Dementia There is limited evidence supporting the use of lemon balm as a treatment for agitation in dementia patients.	C
Anxiety Preliminary human evidence has been published that supports the use of lemon balm for anxiety, commonly referred to in the literature as psycho-vegetative disturbances. The evidence thus far has not been conclusive.	C
Cognitive Performance Clinical data suggest that the use of standardized lemon balm extract has some effect on particular self-reported measures of mood and cognition through cholinergic activities. However, the evidence thus far has not been conclusive.	C
Colitis Limited clinical evidence is available supporting the use of lemon balm for the treatment of chronic colitis.	C
Dyspepsia (Upset Stomach) Clinical evidence of varying quality suggests that lemon balm may help reduce dyspepsia as a component of combination products. However, the evidence thus far has not been conclusive.	C
Sleep Quality High-quality clinical evidence supporting the use of lemon balm as a sedative/hypnotic is lacking. The available evidence is conflicting.	C

Uses Based on Tradition or Theory

Analgesic (pain reliever), anorexia, anticholinergic (drug that blocks the action of acetylcholine, a neurotransmitter in the brain, often effective in reducing the tremor of Parkinson's disease), anti-gas, antihistaminic, antisecretory, antispasmodic, antiulcerogenic, antiviral, aromatic, attention deficit and hyperactivity disorder (ADHD), cancer, chronic bronchitis, chronic fatigue syndrome, colic, coughs, depression, digestive aid, fever reduction, flatulence, flatulent colic, gastrointestinal disorders, Graves' disease, heart conditions, high blood pressure, human immunodeficiency virus, influenza, insect bites, insomnia, irregular menstrual periods, irritable bowel syndrome (IBS), intestinal relaxant, memory enhancer, migraine, nausea, nervous palpitations, nervous stomach, neuralgia (nerve pain), neurasthenia (nervous exhaustion), promoting menstrual flow, promoting sweating, restlessness, sedative, shingles, skin irritations, sleep disorders, tension headache, toothache, tranquilizer, vasodilation, vomiting, wound healing (topical).

DOSING

Adults (18 Years and Older)

- There is insufficient evidence to recommend a dose for lemon balm. A common dose of lemon balm is 1 cup of tea taken several times per day as needed. A dosage of 2-6 mL three times per day (1:5 in 45% alcohol) as a tincture has been used historically. Lemon balm extract in a dose of 60 drops/day has been cited in research on patients with Alzheimer's disease for improvement in cognition.
- Lemon balm is also commonly used in combination with other herbs and supplements. Examples of some products include Songha Night (valerian extract and lemon balm extract), Klosterfrau Melissengeist (essential oils of lemon balm, orange peel, cinnamon, and myristica), and Iberogast (*Matricata recutita, Iberis amara, Angelica archangelica, Carum carvi, Silybum marianum,* lemon balm, *Chelidonium majus, Glycyrrhiza glabra,* and *Mentha* x *piperita*).

L

- Creams and teas containing lemon balm have also been applied on the skin to treat herpes.

Children (Younger than 18 Years)

- There is insufficient evidence to recommend a dose for lemon balm in children.

SAFETY
Allergies

- Avoid in people with a known allergy or hypersensitivity to lemon balm. Hypersensitivity reactions have been reported, including contact dermatitis.

Side Effects and Warnings

- Lemon balm is likely safe when applied on the skin or taken by mouth in recommended doses (up to 30 days) in otherwise healthy adults and when consumed in amounts found in foods. Lemon balm has been given "generally regarded as safe" (GRAS) status in the United States with a maximum level of 0.5% in baked goods. However, lemon balm preparations may contain trace amounts of lead. A study evaluating metal dispersion in food crops suggested that the soil in which some plants are grown may be contaminated by lead from environmental pollution and therefore may cause the plant to contain trace amounts of the element.
- Contact dermatitis, local reddening, burning sensation, paresthesia, residual pigmentation, and dermal irritation on application of cream have been reported. One case of irritation and one case of exacerbation of herpes symptoms were reported when lemon balm was applied on the skin. Cases of nausea and diarrhea have been reported.
- Lemon balm may also cause headache or EEG changes. It may also reduce alertness, so caution should be used when driving or operating heavy machinery. Sleep disturbances and tiredness have been reported with a combination of lemon balm and valerian (although sedative properties of *Valeriana officinalis* alone are well described, and the additional effects of lemon balm are not clear in this combination).
- Although not well studied in humans, lemon balm may also increase intraocular (inside the eye) pressure and cause palpitations. Use cautiously in patients with glaucoma, as anecdotal reports have suggested that lemon balm may increase intraocular pressure.
- Preliminary study suggests that constituents of lemon balm may block the binding of thyroid-stimulating hormone (TSH) to its receptor by acting both on the hormone and the receptor itself. Studies have suggested that patients with thyroid problems such as Graves' disease use caution due to the potential for thyroid hormone inhibition. Lemon balm may interfere with thyroid hormone replacement therapy.

Pregnancy and Breastfeeding

- Lemon balm is not recommended in pregnant or breastfeeding women due to a lack of available scientific evidence.

INTERACTIONS
Interactions with Drugs

- In theory, alcohol use with lemon balm may increase the sedative effects of alcohol. Combination use of lemon balm with other sedatives may also result in additive effects. However, no additive effects of alcohol were shown when combined with a *Valeriana officinalis-Humulus lupulus–*lemon balm combination product.
- Although not well studied in humans, lemon balm has been reported to increase the hypnotic effects of barbiturates.
- Although not well studied in humans, lemon balm may increase intraocular pressure, thereby diminishing effects of glaucoma medications. Caution is advised.
- Lemon balm may reduce pituitary and serum thyroid-stimulating hormone (TSH) concentrations. Constituents of lemon balm may block the binding of TSH to its receptor by acting on both the hormone and the receptor itself. Thus, in theory, lemon balm may interfere with thyroid hormone replacement therapy.
- Lemon balm may displace drugs bound to nicotinic and muscarinic receptors, as demonstrated in clinical trials with the displacement of nicotine and scopolamine from these receptors. Consult with a qualified health care professional, including a pharmacist, to check for interactions.
- Lemon balm may inhibit concentrations of serotonin and therefore may interact with drugs that affect concentrations of serotonin. Caution is advised in patients taking selective serotonin reuptake inhibitors (SSRIs) such as citalopram (Celexa), escitalopram oxalate (Lexapro), fluoxetine (Prozac), or paroxetine (Paxil).

Interactions with Herbs and Dietary Supplements

- A study examining efficacy and safety of herbal sedatives suggested that combination use of sedative herbs with lemon balm may result in additive effects. Such herbs include German chamomile, hops *(Humulus lupulus)*, or kava.
- Although not well studied in humans, lemon balm may increase intraocular pressure, thereby diminishing effects of glaucoma treatments. Caution is advised.
- Lemon balm may reduce pituitary and serum thyroid-stimulating hormone (TSH) concentrations. One study suggested that constituents of lemon balm may block the binding of TSH to its receptor by acting both on the hormone and the receptor itself. Consult with a qualified health care professional, including a pharmacist, to check for interactions.
- Lemon balm may inhibit concentrations of serotonin and therefore may interact with herbs that affect concentrations of serotonin. Caution is advised.
- Lemon balm may displace herbs or supplements bound to nicotinic and muscarinic receptors, as demonstrated in clinical trials with the displacement of nicotine and scopolamine from these receptors. Consult with a qualified health care professional, including a pharmacist, to check for interactions.

For a complete list of references, please visit www.naturalstandard.com.

Lemongrass
(*Cymbopogon* spp.)

RELATED TERMS

- Abafado (Portuguese), alpha-citral, alpha-terpineole, *Andropogon citratus, Andropogon nardus,* bai mak nao (Lao), beta-citral (neral), beta-myrcene, bhustrina (Indian), British Indian lemongrass, capim-cidrao, Ceylon citronella grass, citral, Cochin lemongrass, *Cymbopogon ambiguus, Cymbopogon citrates, Cymbopogon citratus* DC, *Cymbopogon excavatus, Cymbopogon flexuosus, Cymbopogon goeringii, Cymbopogon martinii, Cymbopogon nardus, Cymbopogon proximus, Cymbopogon schoenanthus* L., *Cymbopogon winterianus,* East Indian lemongrass, erba di limone (Italian), essência de capim-limão (Portuguese), farnesol, fever grass, geraniol, geranium grass, geranyl acetate, Graminaeae (family), Guatemala lemongrass, Halfa barr, herbe de citron (French), hierba de limon (Spanish), java citronella, lemon grass, lemon grass extract (LGE), lemongrass oil, lemongrass stalk, lemon herbs, Madagascar lemongrass, Melissa grass, myrcene, palmarosa, pinene, piperitone, Poaceae (family), proximadiol, *Santalum acuminatum,* sera (Indian, Sinhalese), serai (Malay), sere (Indonesian), sereh (Indonesian), Sudanese flora, takrai (Thai), terpene beta-myrcene, West Indian lemongrass, Zitronengras (German).
- **Note:** This review does not include citronella oil or stone root.

BACKGROUND

- Lemongrass *(Cymbopogon citrates)* is used in Cuban folk medicine to lower high blood pressure and as an anti-inflammatory. In India, lemongrass is used as a medicinal herb and in perfumes. It is also used in Brazilian folk medicine in a tea called *abafado* as a sedative, for gastrointestinal problems, and for fever. Lemongrass oil is a yellow/brown oil with a tinge of red. It has a fresh, strong, lemon-like and pungent odor with herbal and leaf aspects. Lemongrass oil is an essential oil used in deodorants, herbal teas, skin care products, fragrances, insect repellents, and for aromatherapy.
- Currently, there is very little scientific evidence investigating the use of lemongrass in humans, and more evidence is needed to make strong recommendations for its use as a sedative or for lowering high cholesterol. Lemongrass is not approved by the German Commission E, but does have "generally recognized as safe" (GRAS) status in the United States.

EVIDENCE

Uses Based on Scientific Evidence	Grade
Hypercholesterolemia (High Cholesterol) Early research has not shown any effect of lemongrass on serum cholesterol. However, more research is warranted in this area.	C
Sedation Lemongrass is used in Brazilian folklore for nervous disturbances; however, preliminary research of lemongrass has not confirmed this use.	C

Uses Based on Tradition or Theory

Abdominal pain, acne, analgesic (pain relieving), antibacterial, anticoagulant, antifungal, anti-inflammatory, antimicrobial, antineoplastic (antitumor), antioxidant, antiseptic, antispasmodic, antitussive (relieving cough), appetite stimulant, aromatherapy, arthritis, astringent, athlete's foot, bee stings, body fat reducer (cellulite), body odor, bruises, cancer, cardiovascular health (cardiac rate), cholera, circulation, colitis, common cold, connective tissue disorder (strengthening and detoxifying), convulsions, cough, cramps, detoxification, diabetes, digestion, diuretic, emmenagogue (promotes menstruation), exhaustion, excessive perspiration, fatigue, fever, flavoring, food additive, fragrance, gastroenteritis (inflammation of the stomach), gastrointestinal disorders, genetic damage, halitosis (bad breath), headache, hypertension (high blood pressure), infections, intestinal parasites, insecticide, insect repellent, irritability, jet lag, lactation stimulation, laryngitis, lymph flow enhancement, musculoskeletal pain, nausea, nervous exhaustion, neuralgia (nerve pain), pain, parasites (skin), radiation protection, rheumatism, ringworm, SARS, scabies, skin conditions (enlarged pores), skin toner, sleep, sore throat, stimulant, stomach spasms, stress, immunomodulator (T-lymphocyte activator), tonic, vasodilator, vomiting.

DOSING

Adults (18 Years and Older)

- There is insufficient evidence to recommend a dose of lemongrass for adults. However, 1-2 tsp of lemongrass in 6 oz of boiling water as a tea has been used. Also, 2 g of lemongrass herb, cut and powdered into 1 cup of boiling water, have been used. For hypercholesterolemia (high cholesterol), 140 mg of lemongrass oil in a capsule once a day for 90 days has been used for hypercholesterolemia with no significant benefit.

Children (Younger than 18 Years)

- There is insufficient evidence to recommend a dose of lemongrass for children.

SAFETY

Allergies

- Avoid lemongrass in people with a known allergy or hypersensitivity to lemongrass. Lemongrass and other essential oils, both applied on the skin and taken as a tea, may cause allergic contact skin reactions.

Side Effects and Warnings

- Lemongrass has "generally regarded as safe" (GRAS) status in the United States. There is no proven safe or effective dose for children or adults, or during pregnancy and breastfeeding.
- In general, a common side effect of lemongrass oil is rash. Lemongrass may also cause irritation and burning if not properly diluted when used on the skin. There are very

few reported side effects; however, this may be due to the lack of scientific evidence.

- Lemongrass may lower blood sugar levels. Caution is advised in patients with diabetes or hypoglycemia, and in those taking drugs, herbs, or supplements that affect blood sugar. Serum glucose levels may need to be monitored by a health care provider, and medication adjustments may be necessary.
- Lemongrass may cause slight increases in liver function tests, particularly bilirubin, or an increase in pancreatic tests, particularly amylase. Patient with liver conditions should use lemongrass with caution.

Pregnancy and Breastfeeding

- Lemongrass is not recommended during pregnancy or breastfeeding due to lack of sufficient human data. Early scientific evidence is conflicting, and some chemical compounds found in lemongrass (beta-myrcene) may cause decreased birth weight, increased perinatal mortality, and delay in development when taken at high doses. However, an infusion of lemongrass leaves did not show any toxic or harmful effects. More research is needed before a recommendation can be made.

INTERACTIONS

Interactions with Drugs

- Lemongrass may lower blood pressure and should be used cautiously with other drugs that alter blood pressure. Also, caution is advised in patients taking drugs that affect the heart as this combination may alter the effects of the drug or cause unwanted side effects.
- Lemongrass may lower blood sugar levels. Caution is advised when using medications that may also lower blood sugar. Patients taking drugs for diabetes by mouth or insulin should be monitored closely by a qualified health care provider. Medication adjustments may be necessary.
- Lemongrass may interfere with the way the body processes certain drugs using the liver's cytochrome P450 enzyme system. As a result, levels of these drugs may be altered in the blood and may cause increased or decreased effects or potentially serious adverse reactions. People using any medications should check the package insert and speak with a health care professional, including a pharmacist, about possible interactions.

Interactions with Herbs and Dietary Supplements

- Lemongrass may lower blood sugar levels. Caution is advised when using herbs or supplements that may also lower blood sugar levels. Blood glucose levels may require monitoring, and doses may need adjustment.
- Lemongrass may lower blood pressure and should be used cautiously with other herbs and supplements that alter blood pressure. Also, caution is advised in patients taking herbs or supplements that affect the heart as this combination may alter the effects of the herb or cause unwanted side effects.
- Lemongrass may interfere with the way the body processes certain herbs or supplements using the liver's cytochrome P450 enzyme system. As a result, levels of other herbs or supplements may become too high in the blood. Lemongrass may also alter the effects that other herbs or supplements possibly have on the cytochrome P450 system.

For a complete list of references, please visit www.naturalstandard.com.

Licorice

(Glycyrrhiza glabra)

RELATED TERMS

- Alcacuz (Portuguese), alcazuz (Spanish), asam boi, bois doux (French), carbenoxolone, Chinese licorice, deglycyrrhizinised liquorice, deglycyrrhizinized succus Liquiritiae, duogastrone, Fabaceae (family), gan cao, gan zao, glabrene, glabridin, glucoliquiritin, glycyrrhetenic acid, *Glycyrrhiza, Glycyrrhiza glabra, Glycyrrhiza uralensis* Fisher, glycyrrhizin, isoflavan, isoliquiritigenin, kanzo (Japanese), LA, Lakrids (Danish), lakritze, Lakritzenwurzel (German), Leguminoseae (family), licochalcone-A, licorice root, Liquiritiae radix, *Liquiritia officinalis,* liquirizia (Italian), liquorice, orozuz, phytoestrogen, Persian licorice, prenyllicoflavone, radix glycyrrhizae, réglisse (French), regliz, Russian licorice, Shakuyanu-kanzo-tou, shao-yao-gan-cao-tang, STW 5-11 (extracts from bitter candy tuft, matricaria flower, peppermint leaves, caraway, licorice root, and lemon balm), Suholzwurzel, sweet root, sweet wood, yashimadhu (Sanskrit), Yo Jyo Hen Shi Ko (Japanese).

BACKGROUND

- The medicinally used part of licorice is the root and dried rhizome of the low-growing shrub *Glycyrrhiza glabra.* Currently, most licorice is produced in Greece, Turkey, and Asia.
- Licorice has been used in ancient Greece, China, and Egypt, primarily for gastritis (inflammation of the stomach) and ailments of the upper respiratory tract. Ancient Egyptians prepared a licorice drink for ritual use to honor spirits of the pharaohs. Its use became widespread in Europe and Asia for numerous indications.
- In addition to its medicinal uses, licorice has been used as a flavoring agent, valued for sweetness (glycyrrhizin, a component of licorice, is 50 times sweeter than table sugar). The generic name *glycyrrhiza* stems from ancient Greek, meaning "sweet root." It was originally used as flavoring for licorice candies, although most licorice candy is now flavored with anise oil. Licorice is still used in subtherapeutic doses as a sweetening agent in herbal medicines, lozenges, and tobacco products (doses low enough that significant adverse effects are unlikely).
- Licorice has a long history of medicinal use in Europe and Asia. At high doses, there are potentially severe side effects, including hypertension (high blood pressure), hypokalemia (low blood potassium levels), and fluid retention. Most adverse effects have been attributed to the chemical component glycyrrhiza (or glycyrrhizic acid). Licorice can be processed to remove the glycyrrhiza, resulting in DGL (deglycyrrhizinated licorice), which does not appear to share the metabolic disadvantages of licorice.

EVIDENCE

Uses Based on Scientific Evidence	Grade
Adrenal Insufficiency (Addison's Disease) Addison's disease is a relatively common disorder to endocrinologists, but it is rare and potentially fatal when presenting acutely. Treatment now involves replacement of glucocorticoids and mineralocorticoids with synthetic compounds, although historically patients took common salt and plant-based preparations, including licorice.	C
Aplastic Anemia Limited evidence suggests that licorice may be beneficial in aplastic anemia, but results are inconclusive.	C
Apthous Ulcers/Canker Sores Some research suggests that licorice extracts, DGL, and the drug carbenoxolone may provide benefits for treating cankers sores. However, studies have been small with flaws in their designs. The safety of DGL makes it an attractive therapy if it does speed healing of these sores, but it is not clear at this time whether there is truly any benefit.	C
Atopic Dermatitis Topical licorice extract gel has been shown to be effective in the treatment of atopic dermatitis in preliminary human studies. However, the evidence thus far has not been definitive.	C
Bleeding Stomach Ulcers Caused by Aspirin Although there has been some study of DGL in this area, it is not clear what effects DGL has on gastrointestinal bleeding.	C
Dental Hygiene Further studies are needed prior to recommending the use of glycyrrhizin in dental hygiene.	C
Familial Mediterranean Fever (FMF) Preliminary research using a multi-ingredient preparation containing licorice called Immunoguard suggests possible effects in managing FMF. Further evidence is warranted.	C
Functional Dyspepsia Early studies indicate that the herbal preparation STW 5, which contains licorice among many other herbal extracts, may help improve symptoms in patients with functional dyspepsia.	C
Herpes Simplex Virus Laboratory studies have found that DGL may hinder the spread and infection of herpes simplex virus. Studies in humans have been small, but they suggest that topical application of carbenoxolone cream may improve healing and prevent recurrence.	C
High Potassium Levels Resulting from Abnormally Low Aldosterone Levels In theory, because of the known effects of licorice, there may be some benefits of licorice for high	C

(Continued)

L

Uses Based on Scientific Evidence	Grade
potassium levels caused by a condition called hypoaldosteronism. There is early evidence in humans in support of this use. However, research is preliminary, and a qualified health care provider should supervise treatment.	
HIV Early studies suggest that glycyrrhizin may inhibit HIV replication in patients with AIDS. However, clinical evidence is lacking.	C
Hyperprolactinemia (Neuroleptic-Induced) Shakuyaku-kanzo-to, an herbal medicine containing licorice, has been used for neuroleptic-induced hyperprolactinemia. However, the evidence is insufficient to support this use.	C
Idiopathic Thrombocytopenic Purpura Early studies have suggested that recombinant roasted licorice decoction combined with low-dose glucocorticoids may be more effective than glucocorticoids alone in treating idiopathic thrombocytopenic purpura. This combination has also shown a lower adverse effect rate than glucocorticoids alone.	C
Inflammation Many medical conditions are marked by inflammation. Because licorice can affect the metabolism of steroids, it is sometimes used to help decrease inflammation. However, the evidence is insufficient to support this use.	C
Polycystic Ovarian Syndrome Spironolactone is a synthetic steroid that is commonly used as a diuretic in women with polycystic ovary syndrome. Licorice has been used in combination with spironolactone to reduce side effects related to the diuretic activity of spironolactone.	C
Reducing Body Fat Mass Preliminary data shows that licorice may reduce body fat mass. However, the evidence is insufficient to support this use.	C
Upper Respiratory Tract Infections (Common Cold) Historically, licorice has been used for its expectorant and antitussive effects. The herbal combination product, KanJang, has been studied for the treatment of uncomplicated upper respiratory tract infections. Results are mixed, and the evidence is insufficient to support this use.	C
Viral Hepatitis The licorice extracts DGL and carbenoxolone have been proposed as possible therapies for viral hepatitis. However, the evidence is insufficient to support this use.	C

Peptic Ulcer Disease	D
Licorice extracts DGL and carbenoxolone have been studied for treating peptic ulcers. DGL (but not carbenoxolone) may offer some benefits. However, most studies are poorly designed, and some results conflict. Therefore, it is unclear whether there is any benefit from licorice for this condition.	

Uses Based on Tradition or Theory

Allergies, antimicrobial, antioxidant, antiparasitic, antispasmodic, antitumor, asthma, bacterial infections, bad breath, blood disorders, breast cancer, bronchitis, burns, cancer, chronic fatigue syndrome, colitis, colorectal cancer, constipation, coronavirus, cough, cysts, depression, detoxification, diabetes, diuretic, diverticulitis, dysmenorrhea (painful menstruation), Epstein-Barr virus, fever, fibromyalgia, gastroesophageal reflux disease, gentamicin-induced kidney damage, graft healing, heartburn, *Helicobacter pylori* infection, hepatoma, high cholesterol, hormone regulation, hot flashes, hyperpigmentation disorders, immune system stimulation, indigestion, infertility, inflammatory skin disorders, laryngitis, liver cancer, liver protection, lung cancer, melanoma, melasma, menopausal symptoms, metabolic abnormalities, methicillin-resistant *Staphylococcus aureus* (MRSA), muscle cramps, non-ulcer dyspepsia, obesity, osteoarthritis, postherpetic neuralgia, postural hypotension, premenstrual syndrome, prostate cancer, pruritus (rash), rheumatoid arthritis, RSV, SARS, skin disorders, sore throat, systemic lupus erythematosus, urinary tract inflammation, weight loss.

DOSING
Adults (18 Years and Older)
- Carbenoxolone gel or cream: A 2% cream or gel has been applied five times a day for 7-14 days for herpes simplex virus skin lesions.
- Commercial preparation: 3.5 g of a commercial preparation of licorice has been used daily for body fat mass reduction.
- DGL extract tablets (380-1,140 mg) have been taken three times daily by mouth 20 minutes before meals.
- Licorice fluid extract (10%-20% glycyrrhizin): Doses of 2-4 mL have been taken daily by mouth.
- Licorice powdered root (4%-9% glycyrrhizin): Doses of 1-4 g taken by mouth daily, divided into three or four doses, have been used.

Children (Younger than 18 Years)
- There is insufficient evidence to recommend licorice for use in children, and licorice is not recommended due to potential side effects.

SAFETY
Allergies
- People should avoid licorice if they have a known allergy to licorice, any component of licorice, or any member of the Fabaceae (Leguminosae) plant family (pea family). There is a report of rash after applying a cosmetic product containing licorice to the skin.

Side Effects and Warnings

- Licorice contains a chemical called glycyrrhizic acid, which is responsible for many of the reported side effects. DGL (deglycyrrhizinated licorice) has had the glycyrrhizic acid removed and therefore is considered safer for use.
- Many of the adverse effects of licorice result from actions on hormone levels in the body. By altering the activities of certain hormones, licorice may cause electrolyte disturbances. Possible effects include sodium and fluid retention, low potassium levels, and metabolic alkalosis.
- Electrolyte abnormalities may also lead to irregular heartbeats, heart attack, kidney damage, muscle weakness, or muscle breakdown. Licorice should be used cautiously by people with congestive heart failure, coronary heart disease, kidney or liver disease, fluid retention (edema), high blood pressure, underlying electrolyte disturbances, hormonal abnormalities, or those taking diuretics.
- Hormonal imbalances have been reported with the use of licorice, such as abnormally low testosterone levels in men or high prolactin levels and estrogen levels in women. However, study results conflict. These adverse effects may reduce fertility or cause menstrual abnormalities.
- Reduced body fat mass has been observed with the use of licorice, but weight gain is also possible. Acute pseudo-aldosteronism syndrome has been associated with licorice. Paralysis has been reported in a patient taking licorice that contributed to low potassium levels. Thyrotoxic periodic paralysis (TPP) has been associated with licorice. Metabolic alkalosis and seizure has been reported from licorice in antacid.
- Licorice has been reported to cause high blood pressure, including dangerously high blood pressure with symptoms such as headache, nausea, vomiting, and hypertensive encephalopathy with strokelike effects (for example, one-sided weakness).
- High doses of licorice may cause temporary vision problems or loss. Ocular side effects have been reported. Central retinal vein occlusion has been associated with licorice. A case report exists of licorice-induced hypokalemia associated with dropped head syndrome (DHS).

Pregnancy and Breastfeeding

- Licorice cannot be recommended during pregnancy and breastfeeding due to possible alterations of hormone levels and the possibility of premature labor.
- Hormonal imbalances reported with the use of licorice include abnormally low testosterone levels in men and high prolactin levels/estrogen levels in women. However, study results conflict. 17-OHP and LH levels may also be affected.

INTERACTIONS
Interactions with Drugs

- In general, prescription drugs should be taken 1 hour before licorice or 2 hours after licorice because licorice may increase the absorption of many drugs. Increased absorption may increase the activities and side effects of some drugs (for example, nitrofurantoin). Phosphate salts have been shown to increase licorice absorption. Liver metabolism of certain drugs may be affected by licorice, but further studies are needed before a conclusion can be drawn.
- Because the toxicity of digoxin (Lanoxin) is increased when potassium levels are low, people who take digoxin and are interested in using licorice should discuss this with their health care provider. Increased monitoring may be necessary. Other drugs that may increase the tendency for irregular heart rhythms are also best avoided when using licorice.
- Licorice may reduce the effects of blood pressure or diuretic (urine-producing) drugs, including hydrochlorothiazide and spironolactone. Use of licorice with the diuretics hydrochlorothiazide or furosemide (Lasix) may cause potassium levels to fall very low and subsequently lead to dangerous complications. Other drugs that can also cause potassium levels to fall too low and are best avoided when using licorice include insulin, sodium polystyrene (Kayexalate), and laxatives. Chewing tobacco may increase the toxicity of licorice gums by causing electrolyte disturbances.
- Licorice may increase the adverse effects associated with corticosteroids such as prednisolone and monoamine oxidase inhibitors such as isocarboxazid (Marplan), phenelzine (Nardil), or tranylcypromine (Parnate). Agents acting on serotonin may also interact with licorice.
- Licorice may reduce the effects of birth control pills, hormone replacement therapies, or testosterone therapy.
- In theory, licorice may increase the risk of bleeding when used with anticoagulants (blood thinners) or antiplatelet drugs. Examples include warfarin (Coumadin), heparin, clopidogrel (Plavix), or aspirin.
- Licorice may also interact with glucocorticoids, ulcer medications, interferon, or lithium.

Interactions with Herbs and Dietary Supplements

- Herbs with potential laxative properties may add to the potassium-lowering effects of licorice.
- Herbs with potential diuretic properties may increase adverse effects associated with licorice.
- Herbs and supplements that lower blood pressure may add to the blood pressure–lowering effects of licorice.
- Herbs with monoamine oxidase inhibitor activity may worsen side effects when used at the same time as licorice. Agents acting on serotonin may also interact with licorice.
- In theory, herbs and supplements that increase the risk of bleeding may further increase the risk of bleeding when taken with licorice.
- Liver metabolism of certain herbs and supplements may be affected by licorice, but further studies are needed before a conclusion can be drawn.
- Licorice may interact with herbs or supplements used for heart disorders. It may also interact with other herbs or supplements with hormonal effects.

For a complete list of references, please visit www.naturalstandard.com.

Lime
(*Citrus aurantiifolia*)

RELATED TERMS

- AA, acid lime, Adam's apple, agua de limón (Spanish), ascorbic acid, beta-pinene, baladi (Egypt, Sudan), bara nimbu, bijapura, bisabolene, citral, *Citrus acida, Citrus aurantiifolia, Citrus lima, Citrus limetta, Citrus limetta var. aromatica, Citrus limmerttioides, Citrus medica var. acida,* common lime, dayap (Tagalog), dayalap (Tagalog), dehydrofelodipine (primary metabolite of felodipine), doc (Morocco), felodipine, fenchone, furocoumarins, jeruk neepis (Malay), jeruk nipis (Indonesia), jeruk pecel (Indonesia), key lime, Krôôch chhmaa muul (Khmer), lamoentsji (Netherlands), lamunchi (Netherlands), large lime, lebu (India), lemmetje (Dutch), lime water, lima ácida (Portuguese, Spanish), lima boba (Spanish), lima chica (Spanish), limah (Arabic), limão galego (Portuguese), limau asam (Malaysia), limau neepis (Malay), limau nipis (Malay), limbu (India), lime (Danish), limeade, lime essential oil, lime flower (*Tilia cordata* Mill.), lime juice, lime mexicaine (French), lime oil, limetta (Italian), *Limettae fructus,* Limette, limette acide (French), Limettenbaum (German), Limettenzitrone (German), limettier (French), limey, limoen (Flemish), limón agria (Spanish), limón agrio (Spanish), limón chiquito (Spanish), limón corriente (Spanish), limón criollo (Spanish), limón sutil (Spanish), limonene, *Limonia aurantiifolia,* limun (India), limûn baladi (Egypt, Sudan), manao (Thai), Mexican lime, naaw (Laotian), ndimu (East African), nebu (India), nimbu (India), *Opuntia vulgaris* pads, oxypeucedanin, polyphenolic, *Rutaceae* (family), saure Limette (German), som manao (Thai), sour lime, suwa (Visayan), sweet limes, terpineol, turanj, West Indian lime.

BACKGROUND

- "Lime" refers to a number of citrus plants, typically with round, green to yellow fruits. Lime fruit, particularly its juice and zest, is used in food and beverages for its flavor and floral aroma. Due to its acidity, it is also used for pickling. Dried limes are typically used as flavoring in Persian cuisine. According to the U.S. Food and Drug Administration (FDA), lime has "generally recognized as safe" (GRAS) status for use in food in the United States when it is taken by mouth in amounts commonly found in foods.
- Lime is believed to be native to the tropical regions of Asia and the Malay Archipelago. It may have been brought to Persia, Palestine, Egypt, and Europe by Arabs from India at about the same time as sour orange and lemon. It is thought that lime was introduced to Florida in the United States during the establishment of St. Augustine in 1565. Today, south Florida is the source of more than 85% of North American limes.
- In the 1700s, British sailors consumed limes and other citrus fruits on board ships to prevent rickets, which occurs from a lack of vitamin C. Hence, the sailors derived the nickname "limey."
- Evidence of limeade's use in iron-deficient women is conflicting. Preliminary studies have observed a protective

effect of lime against cholera, but there are no well-designed clinical trials at this time evaluating the use of lime in the treatment of other conditions.

EVIDENCE

Uses Based on Scientific Evidence	Grade
Cholera (Prevention) There is some evidence that lime juice used in sauces might aid in the prevention of cholera. Other preliminary evidence suggests that using limes in the main meal may also have a protective effect. However, the available evidence is not sufficient to support this use.	C
Iron Deficiency There is conflicting evidence regarding the effectiveness of lime's ability to increase iron absorption.	C

Uses Based on Tradition or Theory
Acne, antimicrobial, antioxidant, antiseptic, arthritis, asthma, astringent, bad breath, cancer, chilblains (inflammation caused by the cold), colds, contraceptive (birth control), cough, detoxification, diarrhea (oral rehydration), diuretic (increases urine), dysentery (severe diarrhea), dyspepsia (upset stomach), fever, flu, genitourinary tract disorders, hair loss, headache, heart palpitations, hemorrhage (intestinal bleeding), hemorrhoids, human immunodeficiency virus, immunomodulator, indigestion, insect bites, jaundice, liver disorders, nausea, neuralgia (nerve pain), rheumatism, sexually transmitted disease (prevention), scurvy (vitamin C deficiency), stimulant, stomach ailments, tonic, ulcers, varicose veins.

DOSING
Adults (18 Years and Older)

- There is insufficient evidence to recommend a dose for lime. A limeade drink containing 25 mg ascorbic acid (vitamin C) has been studied but showed no clear benefit.

Children (Younger than 18 Years)

- There is insufficient evidence to recommend a dose for lime in children.

SAFETY
Allergies

- Avoid in individuals with a known allergy or hypersensitivity to lime. When applied on the skin, lime oil may cause hypersensitivity. Distilled lime oil may be nonirritating, nonsensitizing, and nonphototoxic to human skin, but expressed lime oil and lime peel may cause phototoxic skin reactions.

Side Effects and Warnings

- Lime juice, peel, and oil are generally considered safe to consume in food amounts, and few reported side effects, including photosensitivity, headaches, diarrhea, and dental effects, have been noted in case reports and clinical studies. Lime has GRAS (generally recognized as safe) status for use in foods in the United States.
- Lime is possibly safe for use when used orally in medicinal amounts or when lime oil is applied on the skin in cosmetics.
- Lime is possibly unsafe when applied on the skin in large amounts. Lime oil contains oxypeucedanin, which may cause photosensitization.
- Lemon and lime juice are widely used for douches among women at high risk of HIV transmission. However, there is no evidence that lime douche is effective for this use and caution is advised.
- Theoretically, distilled lime oils may promote tumors in the presence of carcinogenic chemicals.

Pregnancy and Breastfeeding

- Lime is not recommended for pregnant or breastfeeding women if using in amounts greater than those typically found in foods because of insufficient available evidence.

INTERACTIONS

Interactions with Drugs

- Based on laboratory studies, lime may interfere with the way the body processes certain drugs using the liver's cytochrome P450 (CYP450) enzyme system. As a result, levels of drugs metabolized via CYP450 may be affected in the blood and may cause potentially serious adverse reactions. Some drugs that may be affected are benzodiazepines, calcium channel blockers, some HIV antivirals, some HMG CoA reductase inhibitors, and some macrolide antibiotics.

- Based on laboratory studies, fresh lime juice in concentrations above 5% may increase the transport of digoxin across cell membranes. As a result, levels of digoxin may be affected in the blood and may cause altered effects or potentially serious adverse reactions, including overdose.
- Concentrations of lime juice may enhance the absorption of [(14)C]-mannitol. This could result in excessive diuresis and lead to electrolyte abnormalities or kidney failure. Caution is advised.
- Theoretically, use of lime oil with photosensitizing agents may increase the risk of phototoxicity.

Interactions with Herbs and Dietary Supplements

- Based on laboratory study, lime may interfere with the way the body processes certain herbs or supplements using the liver's cytochrome P450 (CYP450) enzyme system. As a result, use may cause the levels of other herbs or supplements to be too high or too low in the blood. It may also alter the effects that other herbs or supplements possibly have on the P450 system.
- Based on laboratory and human studies, there is conflicting evidence as to whether ascorbic acid (vitamin C) in limeade affects iron absorption. Preliminary study shows that limeade may increase iron absorption, but human studies did not show any therapeutic effect in iron-deficient women.
- Based on laboratory studies, a 30% concentration of lime juice may enhance the absorption of [(14)C]-mannitol. This could result in excessive diuresis and lead to electrolyte abnormalities or renal failure.
- Theoretically, use of lime oil with photosensitizing agents may increase the risk of phototoxicity.
- Theoretically, concomitant use of herbs and supplements containing psoralens might potentiate effects and adverse reactions. Caution is advised.

For a complete list of references, please visit www.naturalstandard.com.

Lingonberry
(*Vaccinium vitis-idaea*)

RELATED TERMS

- Alpine cranberry, anthocyanin, cowberry, cranberry, Ericaceae (family), evergreen, mountain cranberry, periwinkle leaf extracts, red berries, red bilberry, red whortleberry, *Vaccinium vitis-idaea*, *Vaccinium vitis-idaea* L, *Vaccinium vitis-idaea* cv. Amberland, *Vaccinium vitis-idea*.

BACKGROUND

- Lingonberry is a food native to Scandinavia. Lingonberry has shown antioxidant and anti-inflammatory effects in laboratory studies.
- Lingonberry has been used as a food and as a traditional medicine to treat inflammatory diseases and wounds in Sweden.

EVIDENCE

Uses Based on Scientific Evidence	Grade
Urinary Tract Infection (UTI) Prevention Cranberry juice is commonly used to prevent and treat urinary tract infections. There is limited clinical evidence that a combination of cranberry and lingonberry juice is more effective. The isolated effects of lingonberry remains unclear.	C

Uses Based on Tradition or Theory
Antihelminthic (expels worms), antibacterial, anti-inflammatory, antioxidant, antitussive (cough suppressant), antiviral, cancer, expectorant (encourages coughing-up of mucus), food uses, male contraception, periodontal (gum) disease, viral encephalitis (tick-borne), wound healing.

DOSING

Adults (18 Years and Older)

- There is insufficient evidence to recommend a dose for lingonberry supplements in adults.

Children (Younger than 18 Years)

- There is insufficient evidence to recommend a dose for lingonberry supplements in children.

SAFETY

Allergies

- Avoid in people with a known allergy or hypersensitivity to lingonberry *(Vaccinium vitis-idaea)* or its constituents.

Side Effects and Warnings

- Lingonberry is likely safe when used in food amounts.
- Lingonberry may not be safe in male patients in couples who are trying to become pregnant.

- There are few adverse effects associated with lingonberry reported in the available literature. However, one animal study indicates that *Vaccinium vitis* leaf extract may have adverse effects on the male reproductive system.

Pregnancy and Breastfeeding

- *Vaccinium vitis* leaf extract may have negative effects on fertility. Lingonberry should not be used by pregnant or breastfeeding women due to a lack of available scientific evidence.

INTERACTIONS

Interactions with Drugs

- Extracts from dry red bilberry fruit (*Vaccinium vitisidaea* L.) may expel or destroy intestinal worms. Use cautiously with medications that expel worms (anthelminthics), due to possible additive effects.
- Lingonberry may have antibacterial effects. Use cautiously with antibiotic medications, due to possible additive effects.
- Lingonberry may have anti-inflammatory effects.
- Lingonberry may have anticancer (antineoplastic) effects. Use cautiously in patients taking medications for the prevention or treatment of cancer, due to possible additive effects.
- Lingonberry may have antioxidant activity.
- Lingonberry may interact with cough suppressant medications; use cautiously.
- Aqueous (water) extracts of *Vaccinium vitis-idaea* berries may have antiviral activity. Use cautiously with antiviral medications, due to possible additive effects.
- *Vaccinium vitis* leaf extract may have negative effects on the reproductive system. Caution is advised in males who are part of couples trying to become pregnant.

Interactions with Herbs and Dietary Supplements

- Extracts from dry red bilberry fruit (*Vaccinium vitisidaea* L.) may expel or destroy intestinal worms. Use cautiously with herbs and supplements that expel worms (anthelminthics), due to possible additive effects.
- Lingonberry may have antibacterial effects. Use cautiously with herbs and supplements with antibacterial activity, due to possible additive effects.
- Lingonberry may have anti-inflammatory effects.
- Lingonberry may have anticancer (antineoplastic) activity; use cautiously with herbs and supplements used to prevent or treat cancer, due to possible additive effects.
- Lingonberry may have antioxidant activity.
- Lingonberry may interact with herbs and supplements taken as cough suppressants.
- Aqueous (water) extracts of *Vaccinium vitis-idaea* berries may have antiviral activity. Use cautiously with herbs and supplements with antiviral activity, due to possible additive effects.
- *Vaccinium vitis* leaf extract may have negative effects on the reproductive system. Caution is advised in males who are part of couples trying to become pregnant.

For a complete list of references, please visit www.naturalstandard.com.

Liver Extract

RELATED TERMS

- Alkaline phosphatase isoenzymes, aqueous liver, bovine liver extract, crude liver extract, cyanocobalamin, hydrolyzed liver extract, hydroxocobalamin, iron, LEx, liquid liver extract, liver, liver concentrate, liver extract lysate, liver factors, liver fractions, liver glandular products, liver hydrolysate, liver substance, purified liver extract, raw liver, Solcohepsyl, Solcohepsyl extralysate, subcellular liver fractions, vitamin B_{12}.
- **Note:** Although liver extract contains many constituents, such as vitamin B_{12}, this monograph focuses on liver extract research.

BACKGROUND

- Liver extract and desiccated (dried) liver have been marketed as iron supplements for over a century. The extract is processed cow or pig liver that may either be a freeze-dried brownish powder or a concentrated liquid that has had most of the fat and cholesterol removed.
- Preliminary clinical studies indicate that liver extract may be helpful in treating hepatic (liver) dysfunction. In addition, liver extract seems to work synergistically with interferon in treating hepatitis C and other viral infections. More research is needed in these areas.
- Laboratory studies indicate that liver extract may have some effects that could be useful for treating certain forms of cancer, such as the ability to direct migration of metastasizing cells and the inhibition of DNA, RNA, and protein formation.
- Some concern has been raised about the safety of liver extract, as it is made of animal liver, which may be infected with parasites, bacteria, or prion diseases. Although there are currently no available reports of diseases such as bovine spongiform encephalitis (BSE, or "mad cow disease") being transmitted by liver extract, the U.S. Food and Drug Administration (FDA) still cautions against the use of any animal organ extract. It is not clear how the processing of liver extract affects the transmission of these organisms.

EVIDENCE

Uses Based on Scientific Evidence	Grade
Pernicious Anemia Ingestion of liver increases red blood cell counts, and liver extract (by mouth or by injection) has the same effect. Both liver and liver extract have high vitamin B_{12} content. Today, pernicious anemia is typically treated with vitamin B_{12} injections.	A
Chronic Fatigue Syndrome An injectable solution of bovine liver extract containing folic acid and cyanocobalamin has been an advocated treatment of chronic fatigue syndrome. Preliminary evidence indicates that patients with chronic fatigue syndrome positively reacted to intramuscular bovine liver extract. Additional research is needed to make a firm recommendation.	C
Chronic Hepatitis (Hepatitis C) Hepatitis impairs liver function; liver extract has shown liver stimulatory and protective effects. The combination of liver extract and interferon may increase patients' response to interferon therapy alone. However, additional research is needed.	C
Hepatic Disorders Liver extract seems to stimulate liver function. Some studies demonstrated liver extract increased the liver function of patients with impaired liver function. However, the evidence thus far is insufficient to support this use.	C
Surgical Uses (Urological Operation Adjunct) Liver extract may help maintain liver function during urological surgery. However, the evidence thus far is insufficient to support this use.	C

Uses Based on Tradition or Theory

Allergies, anemia, antioxidant, antiviral, blood clots, cardiovascular disease, celiac disease, corneal abrasions/ulcers, deficiency (vitamin B_{12}), detoxification, drug addiction, enhanced muscle mass/strength, gastric acid secretion stimulation, hematopoiesis (stimulation of blood cell production), hepatoprotection, herpes simplex virus type 1, influenza virus infection, malabsorption (familial selective B_{12}), methylmalonic aciduria, multiple sclerosis, obstetrical and gynecological disorders, physical endurance, poisoning, renal failure (uremia), rheumatoid arthritis, stamina enhancer, tonic, tuberculosis, wound healing.

DOSING

Adults (18 Years and Older)

- There is insufficient evidence to recommend a dose for liver extract. A dose that has been used is 500 mg of liver extract one to three times per day. As an injection, 2 mL of liver extract has been administered daily for up to 5 days, although injections should only be given under the supervision of a qualified health care professional, including a pharmacist.

Children (Younger than 18 Years)

- There is insufficient evidence to recommend a dose for liver extract in children, and use is not recommended.

SAFETY

Allergies

- Avoid in people with a known allergy or hypersensitivity to liver extract or its constituents. Liver extract therapy has caused severe anaphylactic shock. Symptoms of sensitivity may include itching, slight flushing, tachycardia, cough, nasal and ocular discharges, and localized to generalized urticaria (hives), weakness, faintness, nausea, vomiting, bronchospasm, asthmatic reaction, substernal pain, collapse, rigor, profound shock, and, rarely, death.

Side Effects and Warnings

- Few adverse effects have been reported for liver extract, including anaphylactic shock and blood clotting changes. However, raw liver may contain liver flukes or the bacterium *Vibrio fetus*. The U.S. Food and Drug Administration (FDA) cautions against the consumption of any dietary supplement made from animal glands or organs, especially from cows and sheep from countries with known cases of bovine spongiform encephalitis (BSE, or "mad cow disease") or scrapie. It is thought that these extracts may contain viable prions that could infect humans. It is not clear how the processing of liver extract affects the transmission of these organisms. Currently, there are no available reports of transmission of BSE through liver extract.

- Other possible adverse effects of liver extract may include itching, slight flushing, tachycardia (fast heart rate), cough, nasal and ocular (eye) discharges, urticaria (hives), weakness, faintness, nausea, vomiting, bronchospasm, asthmatic reaction, substernal pain, collapse, rigor, profound shock, and, rarely, death.

- Use cautiously in patients taking antacids or those with acid reflux, as liver extract may increase gastric acid or pepsin output. Also use cautiously in patients with compromised immune function, as liver extract may inhibit lymphocyte proliferation. Use cautiously in hepatopathic patients with reduced human growth hormone metabolic clearance rate, as liver extract may tend to normalize its metabolism.

- Use cautiously in patients with clotting disorders, as liver extract may stimulate production of red blood cells, affect blood clotting, or improve hemoglobin concentration in patients with impaired hepatic function.

- Avoid liver extract in patients with iron metabolism disorders or iron shortage disorders, such as hemochromatosis (a metabolic disorder that causes increased absorption of iron).

Pregnancy and Breastfeeding

- Liver extract is not recommended in pregnant or breastfeeding women due to a lack of available scientific evidence. Raw liver may be a possible source of *Vibrio fetus* septicemia in humans, although there are no available reports of liver extract causing *Vibrio fetus* septicemia.

INTERACTIONS

Interactions with Drugs

- Liver extract may increase gastric acid and pepsin outputs. Study results are unclear, and caution is advised.

- Liver extract may affect blood clotting and may increase the risk of bleeding when taken with drugs that increase the risk of bleeding. Some examples include aspirin, anticoagulants (blood thinners) such as warfarin (Coumadin) or heparin, antiplatelet drugs such as clopidogrel (Plavix), and non-steroidal anti-inflammatory drugs (NSAIDs) such as ibuprofen (Motrin, Advil) or naproxen (Naprosyn, Aleve).

- Liver extract may improve plasma cholesterol levels in patients with impaired hepatic function. Patients taking any cholesterol-lowering medications should use cautiously, as dosing adjustments may be necessary.

- Liver extract may reversibly inhibit thymidine and uridine incorporation into DNA and RNA during cell growth and dose-dependently catalyze the removal of O6-methylguanine.

- Liver extract may tend to normalize the metabolic clearance rate of human growth hormone in hepatopathic patients. Caution is advised in patients taking human growth hormones. Monitoring may be necessary.

- Liver extract inhibits lymphocyte proliferation. Caution is advised when combining liver extract with immunomodulating drugs.

- Liver extract may increase the antiviral activity of interferon. It may also inhibit herpes simplex virus type 1 and influenza virus type A when used in combination with other antiviral agents.

- Liver extract may have a high content of heme iron and antioxidant superoxide dismutase.

Interactions with Herbs and Dietary Supplements

- Liver extract may increase gastric acid and pepsin outputs. Study results are unclear, and caution is advised.

- Liver extract may affect blood clotting, which may increase the risk of bleeding when taken with herbs and supplements that are believed to increase the risk of bleeding. Multiple cases of bleeding have been reported with the use of *Ginkgo biloba*, and fewer cases with garlic and saw palmetto. Numerous other agents may theoretically increase the risk of bleeding, although this has not been proven in most cases.

- Liver extract may improve plasma cholesterol levels in patients with impaired hepatic (liver) function. Patients taking any cholesterol-lowering herbs, such as red yeast rice, should use cautiously, as dosing adjustments may be necessary.

- Liver extract may interact with herbs used as cancer therapies. Although not well studied in humans, caution is advised.

- Liver extract may tend to normalize the metabolic clearance rate of human growth hormone in hepatopathic patients. Caution is advised in patients taking herbs or supplements similar to human growth hormones. Monitoring may be necessary.

- Liver extract inhibits lymphocyte proliferation. Caution is advised when combining liver extract with immunomodulating herbs.

- Liver extract may increase the antiviral activity of interferon. It may also inhibit herpes simplex virus type 1 and influenza virus type A when used in combination with other antiviral herbs.

- Liver extract may have a high content of heme iron and antioxidant superoxide dismutase. Liver extract and vitamin B_{12} may have a therapeutic effect in patients with liver diseases and rheumatoid arthritis.

For a complete list of references, please visit www.naturalstandard.com.

Lotus
(Nelumbo nucifera)

RELATED TERMS

- Alkaloids, aporphine, asimilobine, bean of India, benzylisoquinoline, beta-sitosterol glucopyranoside, bisbenzylisoquinoline alkaloids, carbohydrates, coclaurine, flavonoids, gallic acid, Indian lotus, isoliensinine, kaempferol, lian fang, lian xu, lian zi, liensinine, lirinidine, lotusine, methyl gallate, neferine, negferine, *Nelumbium speciosum* Willd., *Nelumbo nucifera*, *Nelumbo nucifera* Gaertn., Nelumbonaceae (family), norcoclaurine, nuciferine, phenolics, procyanidins, pronuciferine, quercetin, red lotus, sacred lotus, sacred water-lily, saponins.
- **Note:** This monograph does not include plants from the Lotus or Nymphaea genera, as these are distantly related plants from other botanical families.

BACKGROUND

- Lotus *(Nelumbo nucifera)* has been used throughout Egypt, the Middle East, India, and China since ancient times, primarily as a food, but also for gastrointestinal and bleeding-related disorders. The flowers, seeds, leaves, and rhizomes of the lotus are all edible. The petals of the flower are used as a wrap for foods in Asia, and the rhizome is a common ingredient in soups and stir-fry.
- The lotus flower has been used as a medicinal herb for generations in Asia. Lotus leaf juices alone are used for diarrhea and sunstroke when mixed with licorice. The flower is used for abdominal cramps, bloody discharges, bleeding gastric ulcers, excessive menstruation, and postpartum hemorrhage. The flower stamens of the lotus are used in urinary frequency, premature ejaculation, hemolysis (the breakdown of red blood cells), epistasis (gene interaction), and uterine bleeding.
- The fruit is used for agitation and fever. Lotus seed has been shown to lower cholesterol levels and to relax the smooth muscle of the uterus. It has been used for poor digestion, enteritis (inflammation of the small intestine), chronic diarrhea, insomnia, and palpitations. Currently, there is not enough scientific evidence to recommend the use of lotus for any indication.

EVIDENCE

Uses Based on Scientific Evidence

No available studies qualify for inclusion in the evidence table.

Uses Based on Tradition or Theory

Abdominal cramps, agitated behavior, antipyretic (fever reducer), astringent, vaginal discharge (bloody), cardiotonic (increases strength and tone of the heart), chronic diarrhea, contraception, diarrhea, enteritis (inflammation of small intestine), epistasis (gene interaction), gastric ulcers (bleeding), hemolysis (breakdown of red blood cells), hyperlipidemia (high cholesterol), hypertension (high blood pressure), indigestion, inflammation (tissue), insomnia, menorrhagia (heavy menstrual bleeding), muscle relaxant (smooth muscle), palpitations, postpartum hemorrhage, premature ejaculation, resolvent (reduces swelling), styptic (stops bleeding), sunstroke, tonic (stomach), urinary difficulties, uterine bleeding, vasodilator (dilates blood vessels).

DOSING

Adults (18 Years and Older)

- There is insufficient evidence to recommend a dose for lotus in adults, and use is not recommended.

Children (Younger than 18 Years)

- There is insufficient evidence to recommend a dose for lotus in children, and use is not recommended.

SAFETY

Allergies

- Avoid in people with a known allergy or hypersensitivity to lotus *(Nelumbo nucifera)*.

Side Effects and Warnings

- Few adverse effects in humans have been reported for lotus. Lotus may cause flatulence (gas), constipation, and other gastrointestinal irritation. Avoid in patients with constipation and stomach distension (swelling).
- Theoretically, lotus may lower blood pressure and have antiarrhythmic (treats abnormal heartbeat) and contraceptive activity. Lotus may also increase the risk of bleeding. Caution is advised in patients with bleeding disorders or those taking agents that may increase the risk of bleeding. Dosing adjustments may be necessary.

Pregnancy and Breastfeeding

- Lotus is not recommended in pregnant or breastfeeding women due to a lack of available scientific evidence. Although not well studied in humans, *Nelumbo nucifera* seed may have antifertility activity.

INTERACTIONS

Interactions with Drugs

- Alkaloids isolated from lotus have been noted to have antiarrhythmic activity and may interact with antiarrhythmic drugs. Patients taking medications aimed at maintaining sinus rhythm and suppressing atrial fibrillation should use lotus cautiously, as the effects may be additive.
- Neferine from *Nelumbo nucifera* may increase the risk of bleeding when taken with drugs that increase the risk of bleeding. Some examples include aspirin, anticoagulants (blood thinners) such as warfarin (Coumadin) or heparin, antiplatelet drugs such as clopidogrel (Plavix), and non-steroidal anti-inflammatory drugs (NSAIDs) such as ibuprofen (Motrin, Advil) or naproxen (Naprosyn, Aleve).

- Theoretically, lotus may lower blood sugar levels. Caution is advised when using medications that may also lower blood sugar levels. Patients taking drugs for diabetes by mouth or insulin should be monitored closely by a qualified health care professional, including a pharmacist. Medication adjustments may be necessary.
- Although not well studied in humans, lotus may cause low blood pressure. Caution is advised in patients taking herbs or supplements that lower blood pressure.

Interactions with Herbs and Dietary Supplements

- Theoretically, lotus may increase the risk of bleeding when taken with herbs and supplements that are believed to increase the risk of bleeding. Multiple cases of bleeding have been reported with the use of *Ginkgo biloba*, and fewer cases with garlic and saw palmetto. Numerous other agents may theoretically increase the risk of bleeding, although this has not been proven in most cases.

- Lotus may lower blood sugar levels. Caution is advised in patients with diabetes (high blood sugar) or hypoglycemia (low blood sugar) and in those taking drugs, herbs, or supplements that affect blood sugar levels. Serum glucose levels may need to be monitored by a qualified health care professional, including a pharmacist, and medication adjustments may be necessary.
- Alkaloids isolated from *Nelumbo nucifera*, including liensinine, daurisoline, and neferine, have been noted to have antiarrhythmic activity (treats irregular heartbeat). Patients taking herbs and supplements aimed at maintaining sinus rhythm and suppressing atrial fibrillation should use lotus cautiously, as the effects may be additive.
- Lotus may cause low blood pressure. Caution is advised in patients taking herbs or supplements that may lower blood pressure.

For a complete list of references, please visit www.naturalstandard.com.

Lutein

RELATED TERMS

- Anhydroluteins, C40H56O2, *Calendula officinalis*, carotenoids, Compositae, crystalline lutein, helenien, *Helenium autumnale* L., hydroxy-carotenoids, lutein dipalmitate, lutein ester, luteine, macular pigment, marigold extract, oxygenated carotenoids, *trans*-lutein, xantophyll, zeaxanthin.

BACKGROUND

- Lutein and zeaxanthin are found in high levels in foods such as green vegetables, egg yolk, kiwi fruit, grapes, orange juice, zucchini, squash, and corn. For some commercially available supplements, lutein is extracted from marigold petals.
- Lutein and zeaxanthin are carotenoids in the macular region of the retina of the eye (macular pigment), and thus lutein has been studied for its use in treating cataracts and preventing macular and retinal degeneration. Lutein and zeaxanthin also have antioxidant capabilities, as well as the ability to trap short-wavelength light. The potential for carotenoids, including lutein, to play a preventing role in cardiovascular disease and cancer was recognized in the 1990s.
- Most of the information surrounding lutein is based on blood and/or dietary intakes of lutein compared with disease states (e.g., cancer, eye disorders, lung function, muscle soreness, obesity, and preeclampsia). Clinical evidence is insufficient to support the use of lutein to treat any medical condition.

EVIDENCE

Uses Based on Scientific Evidence	Grade
Antioxidant Many laboratory studies have shown the antioxidant effect of lutein. However, these effects have not been confirmed with sufficient clinical evidence.	C
Atherosclerosis Currently, there is insufficient available evidence to recommend the use of lutein for atherosclerosis (hardening of the arteries).	C
Cancer Currently, there is insufficient available evidence to recommend the use of lutein for cancer. Available clinical evidence is conflicting.	C
Cataracts Human studies have not found a clear benefit of lutein supplementation on visual performance in people with cataracts.	C
Diabetes Mellitus Currently, there is insufficient available evidence to recommend the use of lutein for diabetes. Preliminary evidence is conflicting.	C
Eye Disorders (Lens Opacities) Spinach and collard greens, both rich in lutein, are associated with a reduced risk for age-related macular degeneration. However, preliminary evidence does not support a link between levels of lutein in the body and reduced risk for lens opacities.	C
Eye Disorders (Macular Degeneration) Macular degeneration is a chronic disease of the eyes caused by the deterioration of the central portion of the retina, known as the macula, which is responsible for focusing central vision in the eye. Preliminary evidence suggests that consumption of spinach and collard greens, both rich in lutein, may reduce the risk for age-related macular degeneration, and other preliminary studies support this. Nonetheless, additional studies are needed before a firm recommendation can be made.	C
Eye Disorders (Retinal Degeneration) Lutein supplementation may increase macular pigment optical density in patients with retinal degeneration. However, visual effects are still unknown. Clinical evidence is not sufficient to support this use.	C
Lung Function There is preliminary evidence of a role of carotenoids in lung function and severity of respiratory infections. However, there is no association between levels of lutein in the blood and illness severity in the elderly or in lung function in adults. However, clinical evidence is not sufficient to support this use.	C
Muscle Soreness Numerous laboratory studies have shown the antioxidant effect of lutein. Despite this, in one study a lutein-containing supplement had no effect on muscle soreness or measurements of muscle activity.	C
Obesity Currently, there is insufficient available evidence to recommend for or against the use of lutein for obesity.	C
Preeclampsia Preeclampsia is high blood pressure related to pregnancy. Preliminary evidence suggests that preeclampsia risk may decrease with increasing concentrations	C

(Continued)

L

Uses Based on Scientific Evidence	Grade
of lutein. However, clinical evidence is not sufficient to support this use.	
Sunburn Numerous laboratory studies have shown the antioxidant effect of lutein. However, clinical evidence is not sufficient to support this use.	C

Uses Based on Tradition or Theory
Burns, breast cancer, cardiovascular disease, colon cancer, cystic fibrosis, dementia, dry skin, eye disorders (glare sensitivity), hyperlipidemia (high cholesterol), immunostimulant, rheumatoid arthritis, skin conditions, sun protection, visual field loss.

DOSING

Adults (18 Years and Older)

- Lutein is likely safe when used at doses of up to 20 mg daily for up to 9 weeks, or 15 mg three times weekly for up to 2 years. Purified crystalline lutein is generally recognized as safe (GRAS) based on animal toxicity studies.
- Although there is no proven effective dose for lutein, lutein is commercially available in various doses. For instance, the manufacturer Twinlab (Ronkonkoma, NY) makes a 6-mg or 20-mg lutein preparation. Lutein 12-15 mg has been taken by mouth for up to 2 years as an antioxidant and to treat cataracts. Lutein 10-40 mg daily has been used for 6-12 months in the treatment of eye disorders.

Children (Younger than 18 Years)

- There is insufficient evidence to recommend a dose for lutein in children.

SAFETY

Allergies

- Avoid in people with a known allergy or hypersensitivity to lutein.

Side Effects and Warnings

- In general, lutein seems fairly safe. Purified crystalline lutein is "generally recognized as safe" (GRAS) based on animal toxicity studies.
- Nevertheless, use cautiously in people at risk for cardiovascular disease due to the possibility of increasing cardiovascular disease risk in those with higher plasma lutein levels. Also, use cautiously in patients at risk for cancer due to the possibility of an increased cancer risk in those with higher plasma lutein levels.
- Avoid in patients who are hypersensitive to lutein or zeaxanthin.

Pregnancy and Breastfeeding

- Due to the lack of available human studies, supplementation with lutein is not recommended in pregnant or breastfeeding women.

INTERACTIONS

Interactions with Drugs

- In humans, moderate consumption of various types of alcoholic beverages (red wine, beer, and spirits) may decrease plasma lutein/zeaxanthin.
- Although not well studied in humans, lutein may alter blood sugar levels. Caution is advised in patients taking drugs for diabetes by mouth or insulin. Blood sugar levels should be monitored closely by a qualified health care professional, including a pharmacist. Medication adjustments may be necessary.
- Although not well studied in humans, lutein may interfere with the way the body processes certain drugs using the liver's cytochrome P450 enzyme system. As a result, levels of these drugs and their intended effects may be altered. Patients taking any medications should check the package insert and speak with a qualified health care professional, including a pharmacist, about possible interactions.
- Cholesterol-altering medications, antioxidants, anticancer agents, cholestyramine, colestipol, mineral oil, nicotine, orlistat, and retinol all may alter lutein levels in the body. However, the effects of supplementation with lutein and these agents are unknown.

Interactions with Herbs and Dietary Supplements

- Alpha-tocopherol (vitamin E), antioxidants, anticancer agents, beta-carotene, cholesterol-altering herbs, carotenoids, mineral oil, retinol, and zeaxanthin all may alter lutein levels in the body. However, the effects of supplementation with lutein combined with these agents are unknown.
- Lutein may interfere with the way the body processes certain herbs or supplements using the liver's cytochrome P450 enzyme system. As a result, levels of other herbs or supplements may become too high in the blood.
- Dietary fiber may decrease the theoretical antioxidative effects of lutein supplements. Furthermore, the proposed antioxidant activity of lutein has the potential to inhibit fatty acid oxidation and increase levels of polyunsaturated fatty acids from supplements. Caution is advised due to possible additive effects.
- Although not well studied in humans, lutein may alter blood glucose levels. Caution is advised when using herbs or supplements that may also alter blood sugar levels. Blood glucose levels may require monitoring, and doses may need adjustment.

For a complete list of references, please visit www.naturalstandard.com.

Lycopene

RELATED TERMS

- Ψ-carotene, all-trans lycopene, Lyc-o-Mato, *Lycopersicon*, *Lycopersicon esculentum*, LycoRed, prolycopene, psi, psi-carotene, solanorubin, tangerine tomatoes, tomato, tomato paste.

BACKGROUND

- Lycopene is a carotenoid present in human serum and skin as well as the liver, adrenal glands, lungs, prostate, and colon. Lycopene has been found to possess antioxidant and antiproliferative properties in animal and laboratory studies, although activity in humans remains controversial.
- Numerous studies correlate high intake of lycopene-containing foods or high lycopene serum levels with reduced incidence of cancer, cardiovascular disease, and macular degeneration. However, estimates of lycopene consumption have been based on reported tomato intake, not on the use of lycopene supplements. Since tomatoes are sources of other nutrients, including vitamin C, folate, and potassium, it is not clear that lycopene itself is beneficial.
- There is no well-established definition of "lycopene deficiency," and direct evidence that repletion of low lycopene levels has any benefit is lacking.

EVIDENCE

Uses Based on Scientific Evidence	Grade
Antioxidant Laboratory research suggests that lycopene, like other carotenoids, may have antioxidant properties. However, it is not clear if lycopene has these effects in the human body. Results of different studies do not agree with each other.	C
Asthma Caused by Exercise Laboratory research suggests that lycopene, like other carotenoids, may have antioxidant properties. It has been suggested that antioxidants may be helpful in the prevention of asthma that is caused by exercise. There is limited research in this area, and further evidence is needed.	C
Atherosclerosis (Coronary Artery Disease) It has been suggested that lycopene may be helpful in people with atherosclerosis or high cholesterol, possibly due to antioxidant properties. Several studies have been published in this area, with most using tomato juice as a treatment. Results do not agree, and this issue remains unclear.	C
Benign Prostate Hyperplasia (BPH) Patients diagnosed with BPH or enlarged prostate are at increased risk of developing prostate cancer and may benefit from taking lycopene supplements. Initial evidence suggests that lycopene may help prevent disease progression in BPH. The available evidence is not sufficient to support this use.	C
Breast Cancer Prevention Research in animals and observations of large human populations have examined the relationship between developing breast cancer and tomato intake or lycopene levels in the body. The evidence in this area is not clear.	C
Cancer Prevention (General) Studies have examined large populations to identify the lifestyle factors that affect health. Many of these studies suggest a link between diets high in fruits and vegetables and a decreased risk of developing cancer. However, it is not entirely clear which foods are most beneficial, or if reduced cancer is due to other (non-dietary) aspects of a "healthy lifestyle."	C
Cervical Cancer Prevention Observations of large human populations suggest possible benefits of tomato product intake in preventing cervical cancer. However, other studies report no benefits. Research that specifically studies lycopene supplements is lacking.	C
Eye Disorders (Age-Related Macular Degeneration Prevention, Cataracts) Based on antioxidant properties observed in laboratory studies, lycopene has been suggested as a preventive therapy for age-related macular degeneration (AMD) and cataracts. However, recent studies have not found a clear benefit.	C
Gastrointestinal Tract and Colorectal Cancer Prevention Multiple studies have investigated whether intake of tomatoes or tomato-based products helps prevent digestive tract cancers, including oral, pharyngeal, esophageal, gastric, colon, and rectal. Results have been inconsistent with some studies reporting significant benefits and others finding no effects. Research that specifically studies lycopene supplements is limited.	C
Gingivitis There is some evidence that lycopene, administered systemically, may be an effective treatment for gingivitis. Further studies are needed to support these early findings and to examine lycopene in combination with other gingivitis treatments.	C
High Blood Pressure There is some evidence that short-term treatments of lycopene may reduce blood pressure. More research is needed, especially to examine the long-term effects of lycopene on blood pressure.	C

L

(Continued)

Uses Based on Scientific Evidence	Grade
High Blood Pressure Associated with Pregnancy (Preeclampsia) Based on preliminary studies, lycopene may reduce the development of preeclampsia and intrauterine growth retardation in women having their first child. However, the clinical evidence is not sufficient to support this use.	C
Infertility Based on preliminary evidence, taking lycopene seems to have a role in the management of idiopathic male infertility. However, the clinical evidence is not sufficient to support this use.	C
Kidney Disease There is very limited evidence that lycopene supplements may not reduce the risks of renal cell cancer, which affects the kidneys.	C
Lung Cancer Prevention Several studies observing large populations report a lower risk of developing lung cancer in people who regularly eat tomatoes. However, other studies report no benefits of tomato consumption. Research that specifically studies lycopene supplements is lacking.	C
Oral Mucositis Limited evidence suggests that lycopene, and lycopene and steroids, may help patients with oral submucous fibrosis.	C
Ovarian Cancer (Prevention) Based on population studies, lycopene intake in food seems to decrease the risk for ovarian cancer. However, research that specifically examines lycopene supplementation and ovarian cancer risk is lacking.	C
Prostate Cancer Studies of large populations report mixed results as to whether eating tomatoes/tomato-based products reduces the risk of developing prostate cancer. There is some evidence that lycopene may slow the progression of prostate cancer. Research that specifically studies lycopene supplements is limited.	C
Sun Protection Lycopene in combination with other carotenoids, such as beta-carotene, vitamins C and E, selenium, and proanthocyanidins, may help in reducing sunburn. Selected protective effects from UV rays have been observed in small, short-term studies. Further evidence is needed.	C
Immune Stimulation It has been proposed that lycopene and other carotenoids, such as beta-carotene, may stimulate the immune system. However, several studies of lycopene supplements and tomato juice intake in humans report no effects on the immune system.	D

	Grade
Lung Function after Exercise A daily dose of lycopene for 1 week does not seem to affect lung function after exercise and does not provide any protective effect against clinical difficulty in breathing in young athletes.	D

Uses Based on Tradition or Theory

Acquired immunodeficiency syndrome, breast cancer recurrence/secondary prevention, cognitive function, coronary death prevention, diabetes mellitus, inflammatory conditions, mesothelioma (tumor affecting the lining of the chest or abdomen), melanoma, myocardial infarction prevention, oral leukoplakia (formation of white patches on the tongue or cheek), pancreatitis, Parkinson's disease, periodontal disease, respiratory infections, rheumatoid arthritis, stroke prevention, stomach cancer, urinary tract cancer.

DOSING
Adults (18 Years and Older)
- There is insufficient evidence to recommend a dose of lycopene or lycopene-rich vegetables. A common dosing range is 2-30 mg of lycopene taken daily by mouth for up to 6 months. Commercially available products such as Lyc-O-Mato and Lyco-O-Pen have been studied for various conditions, as have lycopene oleoresin capsules.

Children (Younger than 18 Years)
- There is insufficient evidence to recommend the use of lycopene supplements in children.

SAFETY
Allergies
- Avoid lycopene in people with a known allergy/hypersensitivity to lycopene or tomatoes.

Side Effects and Warnings
- The safety of lycopene supplements has not been thoroughly studied. Review of available scientific literature finds tomatoes, tomato-based products, and lycopene supplements generally well tolerated. However, rare reports of diarrhea, nausea, stomach pain or cramps, gas, vomiting, and loss of appetite have been reported. Tomatoes and tomato-based products may be acidic and irritate stomach ulcers. Lycopene has been associated with death from a cancer-related hemorrhage, although causality is unclear.

Pregnancy and Breastfeeding
- There is not enough scientific research to recommend the use of lycopene supplements during pregnancy and breastfeeding. Amounts of lycopene found in foods are usually assumed to be safe. Tomato consumption has been shown to increase lycopene concentrations in breast milk and plasma of breastfeeding women.

INTERACTIONS
Interactions with Drugs
- Some drugs that lower cholesterol levels in the blood may also reduce the levels of carotenoids such as lycopene.

Examples of cholesterol-lowering drugs include "statin" drugs such as lovastatin (Mevacor) or atorvastatin (Lipitor), cholestyramine (Questran, Prevalite, LoCHOLEST), or colestipol (Cholestid). It is unknown if replacing lycopene levels with supplements has any benefit in people using these drugs. Some research suggests that lycopene may add to the cholesterol-lowering effects of statin drugs.

- It is proposed that nicotine (cigarette smoking) and alcohol may lower lycopene levels in the body, although this has not been proven.
- Based on human study, tomato-based foods may prevent platelet aggregation and thrombosis. Theoretically, lycopene may increase the risk of bleeding when taken with drugs that increase the risk of bleeding. Some examples include aspirin, anticoagulants (blood thinners) such as warfarin (Coumadin) or heparin, antiplatelet drugs such as clopidogrel (Plavix), and nonsteroidal anti-inflammatory drugs such as ibuprofen (Motrin, Advil) or naproxen (Naprosyn, Aleve).
- Lycopene may interact with drugs taken for cancer or high blood pressure. Lycopene may also interact with drugs that alter the body's immune response.
- In theory, lycopene may interact with fertility treatments, photosensitizing agents, or agents that affect the immune system, but these potential interactions have not been thoroughly studied.

Interactions with Herbs and Dietary Supplements

- Studies report mixed effects of taking lycopene with beta-carotene. Some studies report higher levels of lycopene, while others note no change or decreased levels.

Canthaxanthin has been shown to reduce lycopene uptake from dietary sources, and use may result in decreased lycopene levels in the blood.

- Laboratory studies suggest possible interactions between lycopene and other vitamins or supplements, although the significance of these interactions in the human body is not known. Examples include increased antioxidant effects when lycopene is combined with lutein or decreased growth of cancer-like cells when used with vitamin D or vitamin E.
- Red palm oil may increase blood levels of lycopene.
- Based on human study, tomato-based foods may prevent platelet aggregation and thrombosis. Theoretically, lycopene may increase the risk of bleeding when taken with herbs and supplements that are believed to increase the risk of bleeding. Multiple cases of bleeding have been reported with the use of *Ginkgo biloba*, and fewer cases with garlic and saw palmetto. Numerous other agents may theoretically increase the risk of bleeding, although this has not been proven in most cases.
- Lycopene may also interact with herbs or supplements taken for cancer, high blood pressure, or high cholesterol and those that alter the body's immune response.
- It has been suggested that when lycopene and soy isoflavones are taken together, the potential benefits of both supplements may be negated.
- In theory, lycopene may interact with herbs that affect fertility, photosensitizing agents, or agents that affect the immune system, but these potential interactions have not been thoroughly studied.

For a complete list of references, please visit www.naturalstandard.com.

L

Maca
(*Lepidium meyenii*)

RELATED TERMS

- Acyclic keto acid, alkaloids, amino, Andean Viagra, anthocyanines, aromatic glucosinolates, ayak chichira (Quechua/Spanish), ayuk willku (Quechua/Spanish), benzaldehyde, benzyl glucosinolate (glucotropaeolin), beta-ecdysone, Brassicaceae (family), calcium, carboline, cardiotonic glycosides, campesterol, chicha de maca (Spanish), Cruciferae (former family name), fatty acids, flavonoids, glucosinolate degradation products, glucotropaeolin, imidazole alkaloids, iron, isopteropodin, Lepidieae (tribe), lepidiline A, lepidiline B, *Lepidium apetalum, Lepidium meyenii, Lepidium peruvianum* Chacón, *Lepidium sativum* L., maca chicha, maca maca, macaenes, macamides, macaridine, mace, magnesium, maino, maka, malic acid, matia, methoxybenzyl isothiocyanate, natural Viagra, pepperweed, Peruvian ginseng, Peruvian maca, phenyl acetonitrile, phosphorus, potassium, prostaglandins, protein, quercitin, saponins, sitosterols, steroids, stigmasterol, tannins, uridine, vitamin B$_1$, vitamin B$_{12}$, vitamin C, vitamin E, vitamin K, zinc.

BACKGROUND

- Maca is a vegetable that has been cultivated as a root crop for at least 2,000 years. It can be found wild in Peru, Bolivia, Paraguay, and Argentina, but has primarily been cultivated in the highlands of the Peruvian Andes. Because of its ability to grow in harsh climates at high altitude, maca is an important staple food for native populations in the Peruvian highlands. It is highly nutritious with about 11% protein content and can be baked, roasted, prepared as a porridge, or used for making a fermented drink.
- Traditionally, maca has also been used to relieve stress, as an aphrodisiac, and for fertility enhancement in both males and females. Recently, commercial maca products have gained popularity in areas outside of South America as dietary supplements, with claims of boosting energy, enhancing fertility, balancing hormones, acting as an aphrodisiac, and enhancing sexual performance. However, evidence to support these claims is weak.
- Natives of the central Andes do not use fresh maca. It is considered harmful. When maca is harvested, the roots are dried by exposing them to sunlight for 4-6 days. After they have been dried, they can be stored in cool, dark places for several years. For consumption, the dried roots are rehydrated by boiling them in water until they are soft. Maca is also referred to as Peruvian ginseng, although it is not closely related to ginseng.

EVIDENCE

Uses Based on Scientific Evidence	Grade
Aphrodisiac (Male) In Peru, maca has been used traditionally as an aphrodisiac. Maca could improve sexual desire in healthy men independent of changes in mood, or serum testosterone, and estradiol levels. However, there is a lack of strong evidence to support this use.	C
Hormone Regulation (Male) Traditionally, maca has been used in Peru to enhance fertility. One study did not demonstrate that maca ingestion could change levels of luteinizing hormone, follicle-stimulating hormone, prolactin, hydroxyprogesterone, testosterone, or estradiol. The effectiveness of maca remains unclear for this use.	C
Spermatogenesis Maca has been traditionally used in Peru to enhance fertility of both people and animals. Maca may improve semen quality; however, the scientific evidence is insufficient to support this use.	C

Uses Based on Tradition or Theory

Adaptogen, acquired immunodeficiency syndrome, anabolic, anemia, anxiety, aphrodisiac (female), athletic performance, cancer, chronic fatigue syndrome, cognitive function, depression, fertility, food uses, hepatoprotection, hormonal imbalances (female), immunostimulant, joint diseases, leukemia, menstrual irregularities, metabolic enhancement, nutritional supplement, osteoporosis (postmenopausal), prostate enlargement, sexual function, sexual performance, stimulant, tonic, tuberculosis.

DOSING

Adults (18 Years and Older)

- Maca is likely safe when consumed by healthy adults in doses of 1,500-3,000 mg/day for up to 4 months as an aphrodisiac or to improve spermatogenisis; however, there is no proven effective dose for maca. Traditionally, up to 6,000 mg or more per day in divided doses has been used. Root powder containing 2,800 mg of maca root placed in 8 oz of water has also been used up to three times daily. Commercially prepared concentrated extracts containing 450 mg taken twice daily has been used as well.
- Common dietary consumption in native populations is greater than 100 g, or equivalent to greater than 1.4 g per kilogram, daily.

Children (Younger than 18 Years)

- There is insufficient evidence to recommend a dose of maca, and use in children is not recommended.

SAFETY

Allergies

- Avoid in people with a known allergy or hypersensitivity to maca (*Lepidium meyenii*).

Side Effects and Warnings

- Available studies in humans have only been performed on male subjects. In these trials, no side effects were noted and maca was generally considered safe. Maca has not been studied in women.

- Maca may cause changes in some sex hormones, although animal studies have demonstrated conflicting results. Preliminary evidence from studies in humans has failed to show that maca induces changes in luteinizing hormone, follicle-stimulating hormone, prolactin, testosterone, and estradiol. However, use cautiously in patients with hormone-responsive cancers such as breast cancer, or prostate cancer, and patients who are using birth control pills due to the potential effects of maca on sex hormone regulation.
- Consumption of large amounts of maca may cause bloating and flatulence. Consumption of fresh maca may cause stomach pain.
- The use of maca may increase leukocytes. The use of maca may decrease PT/INR values in patients being monitored for anticoagulation therapy.
- Maca may also lead to stimulation of the central nervous system. Use cautiously in patients with hypertension (high blood pressure), due to the possibility of central nervous system stimulation.

Pregnancy and Breastfeeding

- Maca is not recommended in pregnant or breastfeeding women due to a lack of available scientific evidence.

INTERACTIONS
Interactions with Drugs

- Plants in the Brassicaceae family, such as maca, are often rich in vitamin K. Thus, maca may increase the risk of bleeding when taken with drugs that increase the risk of bleeding. Some examples include aspirin, anticoagulants (blood thinners) such as warfarin (Coumadin) or heparin, antiplatelet drugs such as clopidogrel (Plavix), and non-steroidal anti-inflammatory drugs such as ibuprofen (Motrin, Advil) or naproxen (Naprosyn, Aleve).
- Maca may act as a stimulant and cause hypertension (high blood pressure). Patients taking medication for high blood pressure, or those taking other stimulant medications, should consult with a qualified health care professional, including a pharmacist, before combining therapies.
- Maca may alter the levels of sex hormones and may interfere with the effects of hormone replacement therapy or birth control pills. Caution is advised.

Interactions with Herbs and Dietary Supplements

- Plants in the Brassicaceae family, such as maca, are often rich in vitamin K. Maca may increase the risk of bleeding when taken with herbs and supplements that are believed to increase the risk of bleeding. Multiple cases of bleeding have been reported with the use of *Ginkgo biloba*, and fewer cases with garlic and saw palmetto. Numerous other agents may theoretically increase the risk of bleeding, although this has not been proven in most cases.
- Maca may act as a stimulant and cause hypertension (high blood pressure). Patients taking herbs or supplements for high blood pressure or those taking other stimulants should consult with a qualified health care professional, including a pharmacist, before combining therapies.
- Maca may alter the levels of sex hormones and may interfere with the effects of herbs or supplements with hormone effects, such as St. John's wort or chasteberry.

For a complete list of references, please visit www.naturalstandard.com.

M

Maitake Mushroom

(Grifola frondosa)

RELATED TERMS

- Beta-glucan, cloud mushroom, dancing mushroom, grifolan, Grifron Pro Maitake D-Fraction Extract, king of mushroom, Maitake Gold 404, MDF, MD-fraction, My-take.

BACKGROUND

- Maitake is the Japanese name for the edible fungus *Grifola frondosa*, which is characterized by a large fruiting body and overlapping caps. Maitake has been used traditionally both as a food and for medicinal purposes. Polysaccharide constituents of maitake have been associated with multiple bioactive properties in animal studies. Extracts of maitake mushroom, and particularly the beta-glucan polysaccharide constituent, have been associated with immune modulation in preclinical studies and are hypothesized to exert antitumor effects as a result of their immune properties. Human data are limited, and at this time there is insufficient evidence to recommend the use of oral maitake for any indication.

EVIDENCE

Uses Based on Scientific Evidence	Grade
Cancer Preliminary evidence suggests that beta-glucan extracts from maitake may increase the body's ability to fight cancer. However, these studies have not been well designed, and the evidence remains unclear.	C
Diabetes In animal studies, maitake extracts are reported to lower blood sugar levels. However, little is known about the effect of maitake on blood sugar in humans.	C
Immune Enhancement Animal and laboratory studies suggest that beta-glucan extracts from maitake may alter the immune system. However, clinical evidence is not sufficient to support this use.	C

Uses Based on Tradition or Theory
Antifungal, anti-infective, antitumor, antiviral, arthritis, bacterial infection, diagnostic agent, high blood pressure, high cholesterol, human immunodeficiency virus, liver inflammation (hepatitis), weight loss.

DOSING

Adults (18 Years and Older)

- As capsules, tablets, or liquid extract, doses of beta-glucan from maitake range from 0.5 to 1 mg/kg daily, taken in divided doses. Few studies in humans are available, and it is not known what doses may be safe or effective.
- It is not known what doses of raw mushroom are safe or effective.

Children (Younger than 18 Years)

- There is insufficient evidence to recommend a dose of maitake in children. Therefore, its use cannot be recommended.

SAFETY

Allergies

- A case report exists of hypersensitivity pneumonitis associated with maitake mushroom.

Side Effects and Warnings

- Maitake has not been studied thoroughly in humans, and its effects are not well known. Because it has been used historically as a food, it is thought that low doses may be safe. Studies in animals suggest that it may lower blood pressure. However, no information about these effects is reported for humans. Individuals who take blood pressure medications should use caution. Animal studies report that maitake may lower blood sugar levels. Caution is advised in patients with diabetes or hypoglycemia and in those taking drugs, herbs, or supplements that affect blood sugar. Blood glucose levels may need to be monitored by a health care professional, and medication adjustments may be necessary.

Pregnancy and Breastfeeding

- Little is known about the safety of maitake in pregnancy and breastfeeding, and therefore its use as a supplement cannot be recommended.

INTERACTIONS

Interactions with Drugs

- Based on animal studies, maitake may lower blood sugar levels. Caution is advised when using medications that may also lower blood sugar levels. Patients taking drugs for diabetes by mouth or insulin should be monitored closely by a qualified health care professional. Medication adjustments may be necessary. Animal studies suggest that maitake may lower blood pressure. People taking medications for blood pressure should use caution and should first discuss the use of maitake with a qualified health care professional.
- Use cautiously if taking drugs that affect the immune system, including interferons, because maitake may boost the immune response. Maitake may also increase the effects of antiviral or anticancer drugs.

Interactions with Herbs and Dietary Supplements

- Based on animal studies, maitake may lower blood sugar levels. Caution is advised when using herbs or supplements that may also lower blood sugar levels. Blood glucose levels may require monitoring, and doses may need adjustment. Animal studies suggest that maitake may lower blood pressure. Use cautiously when combining maitake with herbs that can lower blood pressure.
- Use cautiously if taking herbs or supplements that affect the immune system because maitake may boost the immune response. Maitake may increase the effects of antiviral or anticancer herbs or supplements.

For a complete list of references, please visit www.naturalstandard.com.

Malic Acid
($HO_2CCH_2CHOHCO_2H$)

RELATED TERMS

- Acidum malicum, lactic acid, malolactic fermentation, sodium malate, sour apples.
- **Note:** Maleic acid and malonic acid should not be confused with malic acid.

BACKGROUND

- Malic acid is an organic dicarboxylic acid found in wines, sour apples, and other fruits. Phosphoric acid is an acidulant added to cola drinks. An acidulant is a substance added to food or beverages to lower pH and to impart a tart taste. Malic acid is also used a flavoring agent in the processing of some foods. In addition to food uses, malic acid is sometimes used in cosmetics to adjust the pH.
- Preliminary studies indicate that malic acid may reduce injury from ischemic reperfusion injury and reduce blood pressure. However, there is insufficient available evidence in humans to support the use of malic acid for any medical indication.

EVIDENCE

Uses Based on Scientific Evidence

No available studies qualify for inclusion in the evidence table.

Uses Based on Tradition or Theory

Appetite stimulant, food uses, hypertension (high blood pressure), ischemia-reperfusion injury prevention.

DOSING
Adults (18 Years and Older)

- There is insufficient evidence to recommend a dose for malic acid.

Children (Younger than 18 Years)

- There is insufficient evidence to recommend a dose for malic acid in children.

SAFETY
Allergies

- Avoid in people with a known allergy or hypersensitivity to malic acid.

Side Effects and Warnings

- Reports of malic acid–related adverse effects are currently lacking. Although not well studied in humans, malic acid may irritate the skin and eyes when applied to the skin (topically). In a homeopathic pathogenetic trial of Acidum malicum 12 cH, no serious adverse reactions occurred. Use cautiously in patients with sensitive skin or eyes, or those with an allergy or sensitivity to malic acid.

Pregnancy and Breastfeeding

- Malic acid is not recommended in pregnant or breastfeeding women due to a lack of available scientific evidence.

INTERACTIONS
Interactions with Drugs

- Although not well studied in humans, malic acid may reduce blood pressure. Caution is advised in patients taking blood pressure–lowering agents.
- Chronic feeding of malic acid may increase weight gain and change eating habits. Although not confirmed in human studies, caution is advised when combining with weight loss agents due to conflicting effects.

Interactions with Herbs and Dietary Supplements

- Although not well studied in humans, malic acid may reduce blood pressure. Caution is advised in patients taking blood pressure–lowering herbs or supplements.
- Chronic feeding of malic acid may increase weight gain and change eating habits. Although not confirmed in human studies, caution is advised when combining with weight loss herbs or supplements due to conflicting effects.

For a complete list of references, please visit www.naturalstandard.com.

M

Mangosteen
(Garcinia mangostana)

RELATED TERMS

- Alpha-Mangostin, ambisiasin, anthocyanic glycosides, benzophenone, Best-Mangosteen, beta-mangostin, buah manggis (Malay), cay mang cut (Vietnamese), Clusiaceae, dao nian zi (Chinese), dulxanthone D, gamma-mangostin, garcinia (Italian), *Garcinia mangostana* Gaertn., *Garcinia mangostana* L., *Garcinia mangostana* Linn., garciniafuran, garcinone E, Guttiferae (family), king's fruit, maclurin, mang cut (Vietnamese), mang ko seu t'in (Korean), manggis (Dutch, Javanese, Malay, Tagalog), manggistan (Dutch, Malay), manggusta (Malay), mangkhut (Thai), mangkut (Thai), mangoosutin (Japanese), mangosta (Portuguese), mangostan (English, French), mangostán (Spanish), mangostana (Italian), Mangostanbaum (German), Mangostane (German), mangostanier (French), mangostannin, mangostano (Italian), mangostão (Portuguese), mangostenone C, mangostier (French), mangostin (German), mangosuchin (Japanese), mangosutin (Japanese), mangoustan (French), mangoustanier (French), mangoutse (French), mangoxanthone, manguita, mangushtanpazam, mangusta (Portuguese), mangustan (Russian), men-gu (Burmese), mesetor (Malay), pannerale, polysaccharides, prenylated xanthone, purple mangosteen, queen of fruits, sementah (Malay), semetah (Malay), shan zhu (Taiwanese), sugars, tannins, tavir, terpenoids, Thai-Go, xango, XanGo, xango juice, XanoMax, xanthones.

BACKGROUND

- Mangosteen is a tropical tree native to Asia. In southeast Asian traditional medicine, such as Thai indigenous medicine, the fruit hulls (pericarp) or rinds of mangosteen are used for many different conditions, including skin infections, wounds, and diarrhea. Other plant parts, such as the leaves, bark, and fruit pulp, are also used in traditional medicine.
- Mangosteen contains many active phytochemicals. One set of compounds, the prenylated xanthones, has been well researched; there are several laboratory studies showing antibacterial, anticancer, and anti-inflammatory effects, and studies in animals showing anti-inflammatory effects. However, currently there are no high-quality human trials supporting the effectiveness of mangosteen for any indication.

EVIDENCE

Uses Based on Scientific Evidence

No available studies qualify for inclusion in the evidence table.

Uses Based on Tradition or Theory

Abdominal pain, anaphylaxis, anthelminthic (expels worms), antibacterial, antifungal, anti-inflammatory, antimalarial, antioxidant, antiseptic, antiviral, cancer, cardiotonic, CNS stimulant, cystitis, depression, diabetes, diarrhea, dysentery, eczema, gonorrhea, immune system stimulant, leukorrhea (vaginal discharge), liver health (hydrocholeretic), osteoarthritis, skin infections, tuberculosis, ulcers, urinary tract infections, wound healing (infections).

DOSING
Adults (18 Years and Older)

- There is insufficient evidence to recommend a dose for mangosteen.

Children (Younger than 18 Years)

- There is insufficient evidence to recommend a dose for mangosteen, and use in children is not recommended.

SAFETY
Allergies

- Avoid in people with a known allergy or hypersensitivity to mangosteen.

Side Effects and Warnings

- No studies on the short- or long-term safety of mangosteen are currently available. When used as a food source, mangosteen seems to be well tolerated. However, there is some preliminary evidence that mangosteen extracts and constituents may cause cardiovascular, central nervous system, and musculoskeletal adverse effects. Based on this preliminary evidence, use cautiously in patients with cardiovascular disease or clotting disorders, or those using anticoagulation medicine. Also, use cautiously in patients using chemotherapeutic agents, as mangosteen may interact with chemotherapeutic agents (i.e., anthracyclines, platinum compounds, and alkylating agents) whose mechanism of action involves oxidation.

Pregnancy and Breastfeeding

- Medicinal use of mangosteen is not recommended in pregnant or breastfeeding women due to a lack of available scientific evidence.

INTERACTIONS
Interactions with Drugs

- Based on laboratory studies, mangosteen may increase the risk of bleeding. Some examples include aspirin, anticoagulants (blood thinners) such as warfarin (Coumadin) or heparin, antiplatelet drugs such as clopidogrel (Plavix), and nonsteroidal anti-inflammatory drugs such as ibuprofen (Motrin, Advil) or naproxen (Naprosyn, Aleve).
- Based on laboratory studies, mangosteen may have an antihistamine effect. Caution is advised in patients taking antihistamine medication.
- Due to antioxidant effects, mangosteen may interact with chemotherapeutic agents (i.e., anthracyclines, platinum compounds, and alkylating agents) whose mechanism of action involves oxidation.
- Based on laboratory study, mangosteen may inhibit phosphodiesterase. Caution is advised in patients taking phosphodiesterase inhibitors. Consult with a qualified health

care professional, including a pharmacist, before combining therapies.

- Mangosteen may block serotonin receptors. Caution is advised in patients taking selective serotonin reuptake inhibitor (SSRI) antidepressants. Dosing adjustments may be necessary.

Interactions with Herbs and Dietary Supplements

- Based on laboratory studies, mangosteen may increase the risk of bleeding when taken with herbs and supplements that are believed to increase the risk of bleeding. Multiple cases of bleeding have been reported with the use of *Ginkgo biloba*, and fewer cases with garlic and saw palmetto. Numerous other agents may theoretically increase the risk of bleeding, although this has not been proven in most cases.

For a complete list of references, please visit www.naturalstandard.com.

M

Marshmallow
(*Althaea officinalis*)

RELATED TERMS

- Althaea leaf, *Althaea officinalis* L. var robusta, *Althaea radix*, althaea root, Althaeae folium, althaeae radi, althea, althea leaf, althea root, Althea Rose of Sharon, altheia, apotheker-stockmalve (German), bismalva (Italian), buonvischio (Italian), cheeses, Eibischwurzel (German), Guimauve (French), gul hatem (Turkish), Herba Malvae, hitmi (Turkish), kitmi (Turkish), Mallards, Malvaceae (family), malvacioni (Italian), malvavisco (Spanish), malve, mortification root, mucilage, Racine De Guimauve, sweet weed, witte malve, wymote.
- **Note:** Not to be confused with mallow leaf and mallow flower. Not to be confused with confectionery marshmallows; although confectionery marshmallows were once made from the *Althaea officinalis* plant, they now contain mostly sugar.

BACKGROUND

- Both marshmallow *(Althaea officinalis)* leaf and root are used in commercial preparations. Herbal formulations are made from either the dried root or leaf (unpeeled or peeled). The actual mucilaginous content of the commercial product may vary according to the time of collection.
- There is a lack of available clinical trials assessing marshmallow alone for any specific health condition. Medicinal uses of marshmallow are supported mostly by traditional use and laboratory research. Limited human evidence is available studying the effects of marshmallow-containing combination products in skin conditions.
- Although clinically unproven, marshmallow may interfere with the absorption of medications taken by mouth. Therefore, ingestion of marshmallow several hours before or after other agents may be warranted.
- Marshmallow is "generally regarded as safe" (GRAS). However, the potential for marshmallow to cause allergic reactions or low blood sugar has been noted anecdotally.
- *Althaea* extract has been used to make pills. Marshmallow has also been used as an aid to X-ray exams of the esophagus.

EVIDENCE

Uses Based on Scientific Evidence	Grade
Inflammatory Skin Conditions (Eczema, Psoriasis) Marshmallow extracts have traditionally been used on the skin to treat inflammation. Several laboratory experiments, mostly in the 1960s, reported marshmallow to have anti-inflammatory activity, but limited human study is available. Safety, dosing, and effectiveness compared to other anti-inflammatory agents have not been examined.	C

Uses Based on Tradition or Theory
Abscesses (topical), antidote to poisons, aphrodisiac, arthritis, bee stings, boils (topical), bronchitis, bruises (topical), burns (topical), cancer, chilblains, colitis, congestion, constipation, cough, Crohn's disease, cystitis, diarrhea, diuretic, diverticulitis, duodenal ulcer, emollient, enteritis, expectorant, gastroenteritis, gum health, immunostimulant, impotence, indigestion, inflammation (small intestine), insect bites, irritable bowel syndrome, kidney stones, laxative, minor wounds, mouthwash, mucilage, muscular pain, Pap smear (abnormal), peptic ulcer disease, polyuria, skin ulcers (topical), soothing agent, sore throat, sprains, toothache, ulcerative colitis, urethritis, urinary tract infection, urinary tract irritation, varicose ulcers (topical), vomiting, whitening agent, whooping cough, wound healing.

DOSING

Adults (18 years and Older)

- Historically, 5-10 g of marshmallow in ointment or cream base or 5% powdered marshmallow leaf has been applied to the skin three times daily for skin inflammatory conditions. Daily oral doses of 5 g of marshmallow leaf or 6 g of marshmallow root have been suggested by mouth.
- A dose of 2 g of marshmallow in 1 cup of cold water, soaked for 2 hours and then gargled, has been used for oral and pharyngeal irritation, but it is not supported by scientific evidence.

Children (Younger than 18 Years)

- There is insufficient evidence to recommend marshmallow use in children.

SAFETY

Allergies

- Although there is a lack of known reports or studies about marshmallow allergy, allergic reactions to marshmallow may occur.

Side Effects and Warnings

- Historically, marshmallow is "generally regarded as safe" (GRAS) in healthy people. However, since studies have not evaluated the safety of marshmallow, proper doses and duration in humans are not known. Allergic reactions may occur.
- Based on animal study, marshmallow may lower blood glucose levels. Caution is advised in patients with diabetes or low blood sugar and in those taking drugs, herbs, or supplements that affect blood sugar levels. Serum glucose levels should be monitored closely, and medication adjustments may be necessary.

Pregnancy and Breastfeeding

- There is not enough scientific evidence to support the safe use of marshmallow during pregnancy or breastfeeding.

INTERACTIONS

Interactions with Drugs

- Based on animal studies, marshmallow may lower blood sugar levels. Caution is advised when using medications that may also lower blood sugar levels. A qualified health care professional should monitor patients taking drugs for diabetes by mouth or insulin closely. Medication adjustments may be necessary.

- Marshmallow may interfere with the absorption of other drugs and therefore should be taken 1 hour before or 2 hours after other drugs. It may also interact with topical steroids.

Interactions with Herbs and Dietary Supplements

- Based on animal studies, marshmallow may lower blood sugar levels. Caution is advised when using herbs or supplements that may also lower blood sugar levels. Blood glucose levels may require monitoring, and doses may need adjustment.
- Marshmallow may interfere with the absorption of other agents and therefore should be taken 1 hour before or 2 hours after other herbs and supplements.

For a complete list of references, please visit www.naturalstandard.com.

M

Mastic
(Pistacia lentiscus)

RELATED TERMS

- alpha-Pinene, alpha-terpineol, Anacardiaceae (family), arbre de mastic, beta-caryophyllene, beta-myrcene, beta-pinene, Chios tears, çori, evergreen pistache, germacrene D, legelt-xor, lentisc, lentisco, lentisco mastich, lentisk, lentisque, limonene, linalool, llentiscle, mastick, mastick tree, mastiek, mastiha, mastix, mastixpistazie, myrcene, *Pistacia lentiscus*, pinene, pistheqa-pesag, Saladin, schînos, schísei, trans-caryophyllene, verbenone.

BACKGROUND

- Mastic is the resin of *Pistacia lentiscus*, a shrub of the sumac family (Anacardiaceae) found in the Mediterranean regions of France, Spain, Portugal, Greece, Turkey, and Africa. Mastic has been used historically for the treatment of hypertension (high blood pressure) in the Mediterranean regions of Spain. It has also been used since the thirteenth century for the treatment of dyspepsia (upset stomach) and abdominal discomfort. Mastic has also been used in dentistry as a filling for cavities and in surgery as a varnish to cover wounds.
- Further trials are needed to confirm the anti-ulcer activity of mastic and to establish any benefit mastic may have over conventional pharmaceutical treatment for ulcer.

EVIDENCE

Uses Based on Scientific Evidence	Grade
Dental Plaque Mastic has shown antibacterial activity against *Helicobacter pylori in vitro*, therefore, mastic gum may reduce the amount of dental plaque in users. However, the comparative effectiveness of mastic remains unclear.	C
Duodenal Ulcer Mastic has been used by traditional Mediterranean healers to treat intestinal ulcers since the thirteenth century. Mastic has been shown to have antibacterial action against *Helicobacter pylori in vitro*, which may help to explain its ulcer-healing properties. However, the available evidence is not sufficient to support this use.	C
Gastric Ulcer Mastic may decrease the severity of induced gastric ulceration, but its exact mechanism of action is unknown. Additionally, mastic has been shown to have antibacterial action against *Helicobacter pylori in vitro*, which may help to explain its ulcer-healing properties. However, the available evidence is not sufficient to support this use.	C

Uses Based on Tradition or Theory
Abdominal pain, antibacterial, antifungal, antiseptic, antispasmodic, arthritis, astringent, bad breath, boils, bronchitis, catarrh, colds, cuts, cystitis, dental cavities (tooth fillings), diarrhea, diuretic, expectorant, flea control, gout, *Helicobacter pylori* infection, hemorrhoids, insect repellent, leukorrhea (vaginal discharge), lice, muscle aches, neuralgia, rheumatism, ringworm, scabies, sciatica, stimulant, urethritis (inflammation of the urethra), varicose veins, whooping cough, wounds.

DOSING

Adults (18 Years and Older)

- For duodenal or gastric ulcers, 1 g mastic powder has been taken by mouth daily, before breakfast, for a period of 2 weeks.

Children (Younger than 18 Years)

- There is insufficient evidence to recommend a dose for mastic in children.

SAFETY

Allergies

- Avoid in people with a known allergy or hypersensitivity to mastic, or members of the Anacardiaceae family, such as pistachio, terebinth, Chinese pistache, and *Schinus terebinthifolius* (Brazilian pepper).

Side Effects and Warnings

- In general, mastic was well tolerated when taken by mouth short-term to treat gastric or duodenal ulcer. There were no reports of adverse effects in 44 patients participating in the available human trials. No studies have evaluated the benefits or effects of mastic ingestion beyond 4 weeks and, as such, the long-term use of mastic cannot be recommended.
- Mastic may decrease blood pressure. People taking angiotensin-converting enzyme (ACE) inhibitors should use mastic with caution.

Pregnancy and Breastfeeding

- Mastic is not recommended in women who are pregnant or breastfeeding. In theory, mastic may cause fetal injury and death.

INTERACTIONS

Interactions with Drugs

- Mastic may have additive effects when taken with ACE inhibitors. Caution is advised.
- Extracts from *Pistacia lentiscus* may decrease blood pressure with no change in heart rate in normotensive patients. Caution is advised in those taking any medications that alter blood pressure. Consult with a qualified health care professional, including a pharmacist, before taking mastic.

Interactions with Herbs and Dietary Supplements

- Extracts from *Pistacia lentiscus* may decrease blood pressure with no change in heart rate in normotensive patients. Caution is advised in those taking any herbs and supplements that alter blood pressure. Consult with a qualified health care professional, including a pharmacist, before taking mastic.

For a complete list of references, please visit www.naturalstandard.com.

Meadowsweet
(Filipendula ulmaria)

RELATED TERMS

- Ascorbic acid, avicularin, bridewort, brideswort, chalcones, condensed tannins, coumarin, dolloff, dropwort, English meadowsweet, ethylsalicylate, European meadowsweet, *Filipendula occidentalis, Filipendula rubra, Filipendula ulmaria, Filipendula vulgaris,* flavonoids, gaultherin, hydrolyzable tannins, hyperoside, lady of the meadow, Mäde-süss (German), meadow queen, meadow sweet, meadow wart, meadow wort, meadsweet, methoxybenzaldehyde, methylsalicylate, monotropin, mountain spirea, mucilage, nature's aspirin, phenolic acids, phenolic glycosides, phenylcarboxylic acids, philipendula, plant heparin, pride of the meadow, queen of the forest, queen of the meadow, queen of the prairie, Rosaceae (family), rutin, salicin, salicylaldehyde, salicylates, salicylic acid, spiraea flos, spiraea herba, *Spiraea ulmaria* L., spiraein, spiraeoside, tannins, ulmaire (French), ulmaria (Spanish/Italian), vanillin, volatile oil.

- **Note:** Meadowsweet and its relatives (*Filipendula* spp.) are not related to water dropwort (*Oenanthe crocata*) even though members of both genera may be referred to as "dropworts." *Filipendula* spp. are members of the Rosaceae family, while the *Oenanthe* spp. are members of the Umbelliferae family.

BACKGROUND

- Meadowsweet *(Filipendula ulmaria)* is native to Europe and is found as an introduced plant in the northeastern region of the United States. Meadowsweet has historically been used in traditional medicine to treat symptoms of the common cold, stomach complaints, and inflammatory conditions. Herbalists recommend meadowsweet as one of the best digestive herbs for the treatment of ulcers and heartburn.

- Two prominent constituents of meadowsweet that are responsible for much of its pharmacological activity are salicylates and a plant heparin. Meadowsweet also contains high concentrations of phenolics, which are theoretically responsible for some of its antibacterial activity.

- Although meadowsweet shares chemistry, history, and proposed uses with the drug aspirin, its efficacy and place in pharmacotherapy compared to aspirin have not been evaluated in well-designed clinical studies.

EVIDENCE

Uses Based on Scientific Evidence

No available studies qualify for inclusion in the evidence table.

Uses Based on Tradition or Theory

Acne, analgesic (pain reliever), antacid, antibacterial, anticoagulation, anti-inflammatory, antineoplastic (tumor inhibiting), antioxidant, antiplatelet (blood thinning), antispasmodic, astringent, bladder inflammation, bronchitis, cellulitis (skin infection), cervical cancer, cervical dysplasia, common cold, congestion, cough, diabetes, diarrhea in children, diuretic (increasing urine flow), dyspepsia (upset stomach), fever, food use, gout (foot inflammation), headache, heart disease, heartburn, inflammation, influenza, intestinal disorders, kidney stones, menorrhagia (heavy menstrual bleeding), menstrual cramps, osteoarthritis, peptic ulcer disease, rheumatic disorders, rheumatoid arthritis, sedative, sinusitis (inflammation of sinuses), stomach disorders, toothache, ulcers, urinary retention (due to prostate enlargement), urinary tract infections, vaginitis (inflammation of vagina), water retention.

DOSING

Adults (18 Years and Older)

- There is insufficient evidence to recommend a dose for meadowsweet in adults. Traditionally, 2-3 (570-mg) capsules twice daily with water at mealtimes have been used as an antispasmodic, sedative, and anti-inflammatory treatment. One cup of tea (2.5-3.5 g, about 1-2 tsp dried flowers or 4-5 g of above-ground parts steeped in 150 mL boiling water for 10 minutes, then strained) ingested several times daily has been used. A liquid extract (1:1 in 25% alcohol) of 1.5-6 mL has been taken three times daily, as has 2-4 mL of tincture (1:5 in 45% alcohol) three times daily.

Children (Younger than 18 Years)

- There is insufficient evidence to recommend a dose for meadowsweet in children, and meadowsweet is not recommended. Meadowsweet should not be used in pediatric patients with fevers due to the risk of Reye's syndrome associated with the consumption of salicylates.

SAFETY

Allergies

- Avoid in people with a known aspirin allergy or a hypersensitivity to meadowsweet or salicylates. Meadowsweet may also exacerbate asthma. If this occurs, it may be due to the presence of the aspirin triad, a common co-occurrence of asthma, rhinitis, and aspirin allergy.

Side Effects and Warnings

- In general, there is very little scientific information about the adverse effects of meadowsweet. Care should be taken to ensure that only meadowsweet cultivated on land suitable for agriculture is consumed. Meadowsweet has been shown to be efficient in the uptake of the heavy metals zinc, copper, cadmium, and lead when grown in wetland areas contaminated with these metals. Most adverse effects are theoretical or based on expert opinion. Meadowsweet contains salicylate constituents, so adverse effects and toxicity normally associated with salicylates could occur.

- Meadowsweet may decrease vascular permeability, cause skin rash, increase uterine or intestinal tone, or cause gastrointestinal bleeding, nausea, vomiting, and other stomach complaints. Constituents found in meadowsweet may acidify the urine causing renal (kidney) irritation or nephrotoxicity (damage to the kidneys), or cause tinnitus (ringing in the ears). This herb may also induce muscle relaxation and decrease motor activity.

- Meadowsweet may increase bronchial tone or cause bronchospastic activity. It may also exacerbate asthma, especially if the aspirin triad (of asthma, rhinitis, and aspirin allergy) is present. In theory, meadowsweet may lower body temperature. However, hyperthermia could be a sign of salicylate toxicity.
- Avoid in patients who are allergic to aspirin or those who need to avoid aspirin due to other medications or medical conditions.
- Avoid in pediatric patients with fevers due to the risk of Reye's syndrome associated with the consumption of salicylates.
- Avoid use in patients with bleeding disorders, diabetes, and/ or compromised kidney or liver function due to salicylate content. Meadowsweet may increase the risk of bleeding. Caution is advised in patients taking agents that may increase the risk of bleeding. Dosing adjustments may be necessary.
- Use alcohol tinctures cautiously in patients with gastric ulcerations due to the alcohol content that may irritate the gut.

Pregnancy and Breastfeeding

- Avoid use during pregnancy. Meadowsweet may increase uterine tone and might stimulate uterine activity. Due to its salicylate content, meadowsweet taken during the third trimester theoretically may induce abnormalities in the fetus. Many tinctures contain high levels of alcohol and should be avoided during pregnancy.
- Meadowsweet is not recommended in breastfeeding women due to a lack of available scientific evidence.

INTERACTIONS
Interactions with Drugs

- Acetaminophen (Tylenol) or certain antibiotics such as tetracycline or penicillin may interact with meadowsweet and increase the risk of bleeding. The incidence of nephrotoxicity (kidney damage) may be augmented when acetaminophen and meadowsweet are used in combination due to salicylate content of meadowsweet. Meadowsweet may also increase the risk of bleeding when taken with drugs that increase the risk of bleeding. Some examples include aspirin, anticoagulants (blood thinners) such as warfarin (Coumadin) or heparin, antiplatelet drugs such as clopidogrel (Plavix), and nonsteroidal anti-inflammatory drugs such as ibuprofen (Motrin, Advil) or naproxen (Naprosyn, Aleve).
- Due to its salicylate content, meadowsweet may cause drug interactions similar to those of the salicylates or aspirin. The use of meadowsweet with other salicylates may potentiate both therapeutic and adverse effects. The adverse effects of salicylates may include impairing the effects of beta-adrenergic blockers, angiotensin-converting enzyme (ACE) inhibitors, loop diuretics, thiazide diuretics, probenecid, and sulfinpyrazone. High salicylate levels may increase the effects or toxicity of alcohol, anticoagulants, antiplatelet agents (e.g., ticlopidine, clopidogrel, and IIb/IIa antagonists), carbonic anhydrase inhibitors, heparin and low molecular weight heparins, methotrexate, older sulfonylureas (i.e., tolazamide, tolbutamide), and valproic acid.
- Antihistamines, such as diphenhydramine, chlorpheniramine, and brompheniramine, or intravenous nitroglycerin may interact with meadowsweet and decrease the anticoagulant effects in meadowsweet. Consult with a qualified health care professional, including a pharmacist, before combining any medications.
- Many tinctures contain high levels of alcohol and may cause nausea or vomiting when taken with metronidazole (Flagyl) or disulfiram (Antabuse). Also, a combination of alcohol with meadowsweet may increase risk of gastric mucosal damage. Caution is advised.
- Meadowsweet may induce muscle relaxation and potentiate narcotic effects. Caution is advised when taking with narcotics or other drugs with muscle relaxing effects.

Interactions with Herbs and Dietary Supplements

- Meadowsweet may increase the risk of bleeding when taken with herbs and supplements that are believed to increase the risk of bleeding. Multiple cases of bleeding have been reported with the use of *Ginkgo biloba*, and fewer cases with garlic and saw palmetto. Numerous other agents may theoretically increase the risk of bleeding, although this has not been proven in most cases.
- In theory, taking meadowsweet for more than 6 months may interfere with calcium absorption.
- Meadowsweet may induce muscle relaxation and potentiate narcotic effects. Caution is advised when taking with herbs or supplements with muscle-relaxing effects or narcotic effects.
- The use of meadowsweet with other herbs containing salicylate constituents could potentiate both therapeutic and adverse effects. Some of these herbs include black cohosh, poplar, sweet birch, white willow, and wintergreen. The adverse effects of high salicylate levels could include impairing the effects of herbs and supplements similar to beta-adrenergic blockers, angiotensin-converting enzyme (ACE) inhibitors, loop diuretics, thiazide diuretics, probenecid, and sulfinpyrazone.

For a complete list of references, please visit www. naturalstandard.com.

Melatonin

RELATED TERMS

- 5-Methoxy-N-acetyltryptamine, acetamide, beta-methyl-6-chloromelatonin, BMS-214778, luzindole, mel, MEL, melatonine, MLT, N-acetyl-5-methoxytryptamine, N-2-(5-methoxyindol-3-ethyl)-acetamide, Ramelteon (TAK-375), a selective MT1/MT2-receptor agonist.

BACKGROUND

- Melatonin is a hormone produced in the brain by the pineal gland, from the amino acid tryptophan. The synthesis and release of melatonin are stimulated by darkness and suppressed by light, suggesting the involvement of melatonin in circadian rhythm and regulation of diverse body functions. Levels of melatonin in the blood are highest prior to bedtime.
- Synthetic melatonin supplements have been used for a variety of medical conditions, most notably for disorders related to sleep.
- Melatonin possesses antioxidant activity, and many of its proposed therapeutic or preventive uses are based on this property.
- New drugs that block the effects of melatonin are in development, such as BMS-214778 or luzindole, and may have uses in various disorders.

EVIDENCE

Uses Based on Scientific Evidence	Grade
Jet Lag Several human trials suggest that melatonin taken by mouth, started on the day of travel (close to the target bedtime at the destination) and continued for several days, reduces the number of days required to establish a normal sleep pattern, diminishes the time it takes to fall asleep ("sleep latency"), improves alertness, and reduces daytime fatigue. Although these results are compelling, the majority of studies have had problems with their designs and reporting, and some trials have not found benefits. Overall, the scientific evidence does suggest benefits of melatonin in up to 50% of people who take it for jet lag. More trials are needed to confirm these findings, to determine optimal dosing, and to evaluate use in combination with prescription sleep aids.	A
Delayed Sleep Phase Syndrome (DSPS) Delayed sleep phase syndrome is a condition that results in delayed sleep onset, despite normal sleep architecture and sleep duration. Although these results are promising, additional research with larger studies is needed before a stronger recommendation can be made.	B
Insomnia in the Elderly Several human studies report that melatonin taken by mouth before bedtime decreases the amount of time it takes to fall asleep (sleep latency) in elderly people with insomnia. However, most studies have not been high quality in their designs, and some research has found limited or no benefits. The majority of trials have been brief in duration (several days long), and long-term effects are not known.	
Sleep Disturbances in Children with Neuro-Psychiatric Disorders There are multiple trials investigating melatonin use in children with various neuro-psychiatric disorders, including mental retardation, autism, psychiatric disorders, visual impairment, and epilepsy. Studies have demonstrated reduced time to fall asleep (sleep latency) and increased sleep duration. Well-designed controlled trials in select patient populations are needed before a stronger or more specific recommendation can be made.	B
Sleep Enhancement in Healthy People Multiple human studies have measured the effects of melatonin supplements on sleep in healthy people. A wide range of doses has been used, often taken by mouth 30-60 minutes prior to sleep time. Most trials have been small and brief in duration, and they have not been rigorously designed or reported. However, the weight of scientific evidence does suggest that melatonin decreases the time it takes to fall asleep (sleep latency), increases the feeling of "sleepiness," and may increase the duration of sleep. Better research is needed in this area.	B
Alzheimer's Disease (Sleep Disorders) There is limited research on melatonin for improving sleep disorders associated with Alzheimer's disease (including nighttime agitation or poor sleep quality in patients with dementia). It has been reported that natural melatonin levels are altered in people with Alzheimer's disease, although it remains unclear if supplementation with melatonin is beneficial. Further research is needed in this area before a firm conclusion can be reached.	C
Antioxidant (Free Radical Scavenging) There are well over 100 laboratory and animal studies of the antioxidant (free radical scavenging) properties of melatonin. As a result, melatonin has been proposed as a supplement to prevent or treat many conditions that are associated with oxidative damage. However, well-designed trials in humans are lacking.	C
Attention Deficit Hyperactivity Disorder (ADHD) There is limited research on the use of melatonin in children with ADHD both on the treatment of ADHD and insomnia in ADHD children. A clear conclusion cannot be made at this time	C

(Continued)

Uses Based on Scientific Evidence	Grade
Benzodiazepine Tapering A small amount of research has examined the use of melatonin to assist with tapering or cessation of benzodiazepines such as diazepam (Valium) or lorazepam (Ativan). Although preliminary results are promising, further studies are necessary before a firm conclusion can be reached.	C
Bipolar Disorder (Sleep Disturbances) There is limited research on melatonin given to patients with sleep disturbances associated with bipolar disorder (such as insomnia or irregular sleep patterns). No clear benefits have been reported. Further research is needed in this area before a clear conclusion can be reached.	C
Cancer Treatment There are several early-phase and controlled human trials of melatonin in patients with various advanced-stage malignancies, including brain, breast, colorectal, gastric, liver, lung, pancreatic, and testicular cancer, as well as lymphoma, melanoma, renal cell carcinoma, and soft-tissue sarcoma. Currently, no clear conclusion can be drawn in this area. There is not enough definitive scientific evidence to discern if melatonin is beneficial against any type of cancer, whether it increases (or decreases) the effectiveness of other cancer therapies, or if it safely reduces chemotherapy side effects.	C
Chemotherapy Side Effects Several human trials have examined the effects of melatonin on side effects associated with various cancer chemotherapies. Although these early reported benefits are promising, high-quality controlled trials are necessary before a clear conclusion can be reached in this area. It remains unclear if melatonin safely reduces side effects of various chemotherapies without altering effectiveness.	C
Circadian Rhythm Entraining (in Blind Persons) Limited human research is available in this area. Present studies and individual cases suggest that melatonin, administered in the evening, may correct circadian rhythm. Large, well-designed controlled trials are needed before a stronger recommendation can be made.	C
Depression (Sleep Disturbances) Depression can be associated with neuroendocrine and sleep abnormalities, such as reduced time before dream sleep (REM latency). Melatonin has been suggested for the improvement of sleep patterns in patients with depression, although research is limited in this area. Further studies are needed before a clear conclusion can be reached.	C
Glaucoma It has been theorized that high doses of melatonin may increase intraocular pressure and the risk of	C

glaucoma, age-related maculopathy and myopia, or retinal damage. However, there is preliminary evidence that melatonin may actually decrease intraocular pressure in the eye, and it has been suggested as a possible therapy for glaucoma. Additional research is necessary in this area. Patients with glaucoma taking melatonin should be monitored by a health care professional.

Headache Prevention Several small studies have examined the possible role of melatonin in preventing various forms of headache, including migraine, cluster, and tension-type headache (in people who suffer from regular headaches). Limited initial research suggests possible benefits in all three types of headache, although well-designed controlled studies are needed before a firm conclusion can be drawn.	C
High Blood Pressure (Hypertension) Several controlled studies in patients with high blood pressure report small reductions blood pressure when taking melatonin by mouth (orally) or inhaled through the nose (intranasally). Better-designed research is necessary before a firm conclusion can be reached.	C
HIV/AIDS There is a lack of well-designed scientific evidence to recommend the use of melatonin as a treatment for AIDS. Melatonin should not be used in place of more proven therapies, and patients with HIV/AIDS should be treated under the supervision of a medical doctor.	C
Inflammatory Bowel Disease (IBS) Based on preliminary studies, melatonin is a promising therapeutic agent for IBS. Further research is needed before a recommendation can be made.	C
Insomnia (of Unknown Origin in the Non-Elderly) Study results have been inconsistent, with some studies reporting benefits on sleep latency and subjective sleep quality, and other research finding no benefits. Most studies have been small and not rigorously designed or reported. Better research is needed before a firm conclusion can be drawn. Notably, several studies in elderly individuals with insomnia provide preliminary evidence of benefits on sleep latency (discussed previously).	C
Parkinson's Disease Due to very limited research to date, a recommendation cannot be made for or against the use of melatonin in parkinsonism or Parkinson's disease. Better-designed research is needed before a firm conclusion can be reached in this area.	C
Periodic Limb Movement Disorder There is very limited research to date for the use of melatonin as a treatment in periodic limb	C

(Continued)

Uses Based on Scientific Evidence	Grade
movement disorder. Better-designed research is needed before a recommendation can be made in this area.	
Preoperative Sedation/Anxiolysis Results are promising, with similar results reported for melatonin as for benzodiazepines such as midazolam (Versed), and superiority to placebo. There are also promising reports using melatonin for sedation/anxiolysis prior to magnetic resonance imaging (MRI). However, due to weaknesses in the design and reporting of the available research, better studies are needed before a clear conclusion can be drawn. Melatonin has also been suggested as a treatment for delirium following surgery, although there is little evidence in this area.	C
REM Sleep Behavior Disorder Limited case reports describe benefits in patients with REM sleep behavior disorder who receive melatonin. However, better research is needed before a clear conclusion can be drawn.	C
Rett Syndrome Rett syndrome is a presumed genetic disorder that affects female children, characterized by decelerated head growth and global developmental regression. There is limited study of the possible role of melatonin in improving sleep disturbance associated with Rett syndrome. Further research is needed before a recommendation can be made in this area.	C
Schizophrenia (Sleep Disorders) There is limited research on melatonin for improving sleep latency (time to fall asleep) in patients with schizophrenia. Further research is needed in this area before a clear conclusion can be reached.	C
Seasonal Affective Disorder (SAD) There are several small, brief studies of melatonin in patients with SAD. This research is not well designed or reported, and further studies are necessary before a clear conclusion can be reached.	C
Seizure Disorder (Children) The role of melatonin in seizure disorder is controversial. Better evidence is needed in this area before a clear conclusion can be drawn regarding the safety or effectiveness of melatonin in seizure disorder.	C
Sleep Disturbances Due to Pineal Region Brain Damage Several published cases report improvements in sleep patterns in young people with damage to the pineal gland area of the brain due to tumors or surgery. Due to the rarity of such disorders, controlled trials may not be possible. Consideration of melatonin in such patients should be under the direction of a qualified health care provider.	C

	Grade
Sleep in Asthma Based on preliminary study, melatonin may improve sleep in patients with asthma. Further studies looking into long-term effects of melatonin on airway inflammation and bronchial hyperresponsiveness are needed before melatonin can be recommended.	C
Smoking Cessation Although preliminary results are promising, due to weaknesses in the design and reporting of this research, further research is necessary before a firm conclusion can be reached.	C
Stroke At this time, the effects of melatonin supplements immediately after stroke are not clear.	C
Tardive Dyskinesia Tardive dyskinesia (TD) is a serious potential side effect of antipsychotic medications, characterized by involuntary muscle movements. Limited small studies of melatonin use in patients with TD report mixed findings. Additional research is necessary before a clear conclusion can be drawn.	C
Thrombocytopenia (Low Platelet Count) Increased platelet counts after melatonin use have been observed in patients with decreased platelets due to cancer therapies (several studies reported by the same author). Stimulation of platelet production (thrombopoeisis) has been suggested but not clearly demonstrated. Additional research is necessary in this area before a clear conclusion can be drawn.	C
Ultraviolet Light Skin Damage Protection It has been proposed that antioxidant properties of melatonin may be protective. Further research is necessary before a clear conclusion can be drawn about clinical effectiveness in humans.	C
Work Shift Sleep Disorder There are several studies of melatonin use in people who work irregular shifts, such as emergency room personnel. Results are mixed. Additional research is necessary before a clear conclusion can be drawn.	C

M

Uses Based on Tradition or Theory

Acetaminophen toxicity, acute respiratory distress syndrome (ARDS), aging, aluminum toxicity, asthma, beta-blocker sleep disturbance, cancer prevention, cardiac syndrome X, cognitive enhancement, colitis, contraception, critical illness/ICU sleep disturbance, depression, edema (swelling), duodenal ulcer, erectile dysfunction, fibromyalgia, gastroesophageal reflux disease (GERD), gentamicin-induced kidney damage, glaucoma, heart attack prevention, heart disease, hyperpigmentation, immunostimulant, interstitial cystitis, intestinal motility disorders, itching, kidney damage (amikacin-induced, cyclosporin-induced), lead toxicity, liver damage,

(Continued)

melatonin deficiency, memory enhancement, multiple sclerosis, neurodegenerative disorders, noise-induced hearing loss, pancreatitis, polycystic ovarian syndrome (PCOS), postmenopausal osteoporosis, postoperative adjunct, postoperative delirium, prevention of post-lung transplant ischemia-reperfusion injury, rheumatoid arthritis, sarcoidosis, sedation, sexual activity enhancement, schistosomiasis, sudden infant death syndrome (SIDS) prevention, tachycardia, tinnitus (ringing in the ears), tuberculosis, tuberous sclerosis, ulcerative colitis, wasting, withdrawal from narcotics, wound healing.

DOSING

Adults (18 Years and Older)

- Studies have evaluated 0.5-50 mg of melatonin taken nightly by mouth. Research suggests that quick-release melatonin may be more effective than sustained-release formulations for sleep-related conditions. Intramuscular injections of 20 mg of melatonin have also been studied.

- In studies of patients with melanoma, melatonin preparations have been applied to the skin. Patients are advised to discuss cancer treatment plans with an oncologist and pharmacist before considering use of melatonin either alone or with other therapies.

- Intranasal melatonin (1% solution in ethanol) at a dose of 2 mg/day for 1 week has also been studied for high blood pressure.

- There are other uses with limited study and unclear effectiveness or safety. Use of melatonin for any condition should be discussed with a primary health care provider, appropriate specialist, and pharmacist prior to starting and should not be substituted for more proven therapies.

Children (Younger than 18 Years)

- There is limited study of melatonin supplements in children, and safety is not established. Use of melatonin should be discussed with the child's physician and pharmacist prior to starting.

SAFETY

Allergies

- There are rare reports of allergic skin reactions after taking melatonin by mouth. Melatonin has been linked to a case of autoimmune hepatitis.

Side Effects and Warnings

- Based on available studies and clinical use, melatonin is "generally regarded as safe" (GRAS) in recommended doses for short-term use. Available trials report that overall adverse effects are not significantly more common with melatonin than placebo. However, case reports raise concerns about risks of blood clotting abnormalities (particularly in patients taking warfarin), increased risk of seizure, and disorientation with overdose.

- Commonly reported adverse effects include fatigue, dizziness, headache, irritability, and sleepiness, although these effects may occur due to jet lag and not to melatonin itself. Fatigue may particularly occur with morning use or high doses, and irregular sleep-wake cycles may occur. Disorientation, confusion, sleepwalking, vivid dreams, and nightmares have also been noted, with effects often resolving after cessation of melatonin. Due to risk of daytime sleepiness, those driving or operating heavy machinery should take caution. Headache has been reported. Ataxia (difficulties with walking and balance) may occur following overdose.

- It has been suggested that melatonin may lower seizure threshold and increase the risk of seizure, particularly in children with severe neurological disorders. However, multiple other studies actually report reduced incidence of seizure with regular melatonin use. This remains an area of controversy. Patients with seizure disorder taking melatonin should be monitored closely by a health care professional.

- Mood changes have been reported, including giddiness and dysphoria (sadness). Psychotic symptoms have been reported, including hallucinations and paranoia, possibly due to overdose. Patients with underlying major depression or psychotic disorders taking melatonin should be monitored closely by a health care professional.

- Melatonin should be avoided in patients using warfarin, and possibly in patients taking other blood-thinning medications or with clotting disorders.

- Melatonin may cause drops in blood pressure. Caution is advised in patients taking medications that may also lower blood pressure. Based on preliminary evidence, increases in cholesterol levels may occur. Caution is therefore advised in patients with high cholesterol levels or atherosclerosis, or those at risk for cardiovascular disease. Abnormal heart rhythms have been associated with melatonin.

- Elevated blood sugar levels (hyperglycemia) have been reported in patients with type 1 diabetes (insulin-dependent diabetes), and low doses of melatonin have reduced glucose tolerance and insulin sensitivity. Caution is advised in patients with diabetes or hypoglycemia, and those taking drugs, herbs, or supplements that affect blood sugar. Serum glucose levels may need to be monitored by a health care provider, and medication adjustments may be necessary.

- Hormonal effects are reported, including decreases or increases in levels of luteinizing hormone, progesterone, estradiol, thyroid hormone (T4 and T3), growth hormone, prolactin, cortisol, oxytocin, and vasopressin. Gynecomastia (increased breast size) has been reported in men, as well as decreased sperm count (both which resolved with cessation of melatonin). Decreased sperm motility has been reported in rats and humans.

- Mild gastrointestinal distress commonly occurs, including nausea, vomiting, or cramping. Melatonin has been linked to a case of autoimmune hepatitis and with triggering of Crohn's disease symptoms.

- It has been theorized that high doses of melatonin may increase intraocular pressure and the risk of glaucoma, age-related maculopathy and myopia, or retinal damage. However, there is preliminary evidence that melatonin may actually decrease intraocular pressure in the eye, and it has been suggested as a possible therapy for glaucoma. Patients with glaucoma taking melatonin should be monitored by a health care professional.

Pregnancy and Breastfeeding

- Melatonin supplementation should be avoided in women who are pregnant or attempting to become pregnant, based on possible hormonal effects. High levels of melatonin during pregnancy may increase the risk of developmental disorders. In animal studies, melatonin is detected in breast milk and therefore should be avoided during breastfeeding. In men, decreased sperm motility and decreased sperm count are reported with use of melatonin.

INTERACTIONS

Interactions with Drugs

- Melatonin is broken down (metabolized) in the body by liver enzymes. As a result, drugs that alter the activity of these enzymes may increase or decrease the effects of melatonin supplements.
- Increased daytime drowsiness is reported when melatonin is used at the same time as the prescription sleep-aid zolpidem (Ambien), although it is not clear that effects are greater than with the use of zolpidem alone. In theory, based on possible risk of daytime sleepiness, melatonin may increase the amount of drowsiness caused by some other drugs, for example, benzodiazepines such as lorazepam (Ativan) or diazepam (Valium), barbiturates such as phenobarbital, narcotics such as codeine, some antidepressants, and alcohol. Caution is advised while driving or operating machinery.
- Based on preliminary evidence, melatonin should be avoided in patients taking the blood-thinning medication warfarin (Coumadin) and possibly in patients using other blood thinners (anticoagulants) such as aspirin or heparin.
- Multiple drugs are reported to lower natural levels of melatonin in the body. It is not clear that there are any health hazards of lowered melatonin levels, or if replacing melatonin with supplements is beneficial. Examples of drugs that may reduce production or secretion of melatonin include nonsteroidal anti-inflammatory drugs (NSAIDs) such as ibuprofen (Motrin, Advil) or naproxen (Naprosyn, Aleve); beta-blocker blood pressure medications such as atenolol (Tenormin) or metoprolol (Lopressor, Toprol); and medications that reduce levels of vitamin B_6 in the body (e.g., oral contraceptives, hormone replacement therapy, loop diuretics, hydralazine, and theophylline). Other agents that may alter synthesis or release of melatonin include diazepam, vitamin B_{12}, verapamil, temazepam, and somatostatin.
- Based on preliminary evidence, melatonin should be avoided in patients taking anti-seizure medications. It has been suggested that melatonin may lower seizure threshold and increase the risk of seizure. However, multiple other studies actually report reduced incidence of seizure with regular melatonin use. This remains an area of controversy. Patients with seizure disorder taking melatonin should be monitored closely by a health care professional.
- Melatonin may increase or decrease blood pressure; study results conflict. Therefore it may interact with heart or blood pressure medications, making close monitoring necessary.
- It is not clear if caffeine alters the effects of melatonin supplements in humans. Caffeine is reported to raise natural melatonin levels in the body, possibly due to effects on liver enzymes. However, caffeine may also alter circadian rhythms in the body, with effects on melatonin secretion.
- Elevated blood sugar levels (hyperglycemia) have been reported in patients with type 1 (insulin-dependent) diabetes, and low doses of melatonin have reduced glucose tolerance and insulin sensitivity. Caution is advised in patients taking drugs for diabetes by mouth or insulin. Serum glucose levels may need to be monitored by a health care provider, and medication adjustments may be necessary.
- Alcohol consumption seems to affect melatonin secretion at night.
- Preliminary reports suggest that melatonin may aid in reversing symptoms of tardive dyskinesia associated with haloperidol use.
- Based on preliminary evidence, melatonin may increase the effects of isoniazid against *Mycobacterium tuberculosis*.
- Based on animal research, melatonin may increase the adverse effects of methamphetamine on the nervous system.
- Based on laboratory studies, melatonin may increase the neuromuscular blocking effect of the muscle relaxant succinylcholine, but not vecuronium.

Interactions with Herbs and Dietary Supplements

- Melatonin may increase daytime sleepiness or sedation when taken with herbs or supplements that may cause sedation.
- Elevated blood sugar levels (hyperglycemia) have been reported in patients with type 1 diabetes (insulin-dependent diabetes), and low doses of melatonin have reduced glucose tolerance and insulin sensitivity. Caution is advised when using herbs or supplements that may also raise blood sugar levels, such as arginine, cocoa, DHEA, and ephedra (when combined with caffeine).
- Based on preliminary evidence of an interaction with the blood-thinning drug warfarin and isolated reports of minor bleeding, melatonin may increase the risk of bleeding when taken with herbs and supplements that are believed to increase the risk of bleeding.
- It is not clear if caffeine alters the effects of melatonin supplements in humans. Caffeine is reported to raise natural melatonin levels in the body, possibly due to effects on liver enzymes. However, caffeine may also alter circadian rhythms in the body, with effects on melatonin secretion.
- Chasteberry (*Vitex agnus-castus*) may increase natural secretion of melatonin in the body, based on preliminary research.
- In animal study, DHEA and melatonin have been noted to stimulate immune function, with slight additive effects when used together. Effects of this combination in humans are not clear.
- Based on animal study, a combination of echinacea and melatonin may reduce immune function. Effects of this combination in humans are not clear.
- Severe folate deficiency may reduce the body's natural levels of melatonin, based on preliminary study.

For a complete list of references, please visit www. naturalstandard.com.

RELATED TERMS

- Acid esterase, aortic acid, aortic acid esterase, aortic acid extract, aortic acid mucopolysaccharides, aortic acid phosphatase, aortic extract, aortic GAGs, aortic glandular extract, aortic glycosaminoglycans, chondroitin, chondroitin polysulfate, chondroitin sulfate A, CSA, dermatan, GAGs, glycoproteins, glycosaminoglycans, heparinoid fraction, heparinoids, heparan sulfate, mesoglycan, mucopolysaccharide, sulfomucoploysaccharide.
- **Note:** This monograph does not include clinical information on chondroitin sulfate.

BACKGROUND

- Mesoglycan, also known as aortic acid, is a mucopolysaccharide extracted from the calf aorta. Interest in aortic acid began in the 1960s and focused on atherosclerosis (hardening of the arteries). This was a logical place to begin research, as aortic extract is usually manufactured from the hearts of animals, usually sheep, cows, or pigs. In this extract are many substances, including aortic acid, which is a broad term encompassing several constituents. Mesoglycan, a preparation of glycosaminoglycans, is the most studied of these constituents.
- Although mesoglycan is found in great quantities in the heart, it is found throughout the body, primarily in the cardiovascular system. It is in all three layers of blood vessels, and is responsible for maintaining vessel structure and flexibility. One of the glycosaminoglycans in mesoglycan is heparin sulfate, which may explain why mesoglycan has shown anticoagulation effects in some clinical studies.
- Because mesoglycan and aortic acid are extracted from the heart, preliminary studies have focused on cardiovascular disorders, such as atherosclerosis, deep vein thrombosis, lower limb ischemia, and cutaneous necrotizing venulitis. Mesoglycan has shown the most promise in treating chronic venous ulcers and intermittent claudication. Other areas of future interest may be hypercholesterolemia (high cholesterol), impaired fibrinolytic activity, and general wound healing. However, more high-quality research is needed in all of these areas.

EVIDENCE

Uses Based on Scientific Evidence	Grade
Chronic Venous Ulcers Mesoglycan, an aortic acid, is a structural component of blood vessels. In the case of venous ulcers, mesoglycan may be able to improve venous health.	B
Intermittent Claudication Intermittent claudication is part of late-stage atherosclerosis, and mesoglycan has shown some therapeutic ability in preliminary atherosclerosis studies in humans. In addition, mesoglycan is a heparin-like substance that has shown anticoagulation (blood-	B
thinning) properties in clinical studies. Additional studies are needed.	
Atherosclerosis Mesoglycan is a structural aspect of cardiovascular vessels and organs. Preliminary evidence indicates that mesoglycan may reduce blood vessel thickening; however, the overall evidence is not sufficient to support this use.	C
Cerebral Ischemia Mesoglycan has shown activity in anticoagulation (blood thinning) and increasing blood vessel health. Preliminary studies also indicate that it may be helpful in reducing recurring ischemic cerebral attacks and improving quality of life.	C
Vein Clots (Deep Vein Thrombosis) Currently, there is insufficient available evidence to recommend aortic acid for deep vein thrombosis.	C
Venous Disorders Mesoglycan has shown activity in anticoagulation (blood thinning) and increasing blood vessel health. Low-quality research shows that mesoglycan may be helpful in various venous disorders, including postphlebitic syndrome, venous insufficiency, and varicose syndrome. The overall evidence is not sufficient to support this use	C

Uses Based on Tradition or Theory

Acrocyanosis (lower limb ischemia), acquired immunodeficiency syndrome, allergies, angina (chest pain), anticoagulant (blood thinner), arthritis, autism, blood disorders (impaired plasma fibrinolytic activity), bursitis (inflamed bursa), cancer, circulatory disorders, dementia, gastrointestinal reflux disease, headaches, hemorrhoids, hypercholesterolemia (high cholesterol), immunomodulation, inflammation, kidney stones, macular degeneration (eye disease), obstetrical and gynecological disorders, pelvic inflammatory disease, peripheral obstructive arterial disease, skin conditions (cutaneous necrotizing venulitis), ulcerative colitis (inflammatory bowel disease), wound healing.

DOSING

Adults (18 Years and Older)

- Mesoglycan is likely safe when taken by mouth in doses less than or equal to 200 mg daily for 18 months. There is no proven effective dose. However, 96 or 100 mg mesoglycan daily by mouth for 6 months for cerebrovascular disease and hyperlipidemia (high cholesterol) has been used. For intermittent claudication (leg pain), one 24-mg mesoglycan tablet twice daily for 6 months has been used. For phlebitis, two 12-mg mesoglycan capsules three times daily for

30 days has been used. For postphlebitic syndrome, 50 mg mesoglycan twice a day for 3 months has been used.

- Mesoglycan is also likely safe when 90 mg is injected for 10 days under the supervision of a qualified health care professional, including a pharmacist.

Children (Younger than 18 Years)

- There is insufficient evidence to recommend a dose for mesoglycan in children.

SAFETY

Allergies

- There are currently no reported allergic reactions available. Due to the heparan sulfate content of mesoglycan, patients with an allergy to heparin or heparinoid derivatives should use caution.

Side Effects and Warnings

- Aortic acid, including mesoglycan, has been well tolerated for up to 18 months in the available human trials. However, the U.S. Food and Drug Administration (FDA) cautions against the consumption of any dietary supplement made from animal glands or organs, especially from cows and sheep from countries with known cases of bovine spongiform encephalitis (BSE, or "mad cow disease") or scrapie. It is thought that these extracts may contain viable prions that could infect humans. Currently, there are no available reports of transmission of BSE through aortic acid.
- Mesoglycan (injection or taken by mouth) has caused minor side effects, including diarrhea and headache.
- Use cautiously in patients with coagulation disorders or those taking anticoagulation therapy. Use cautiously in patients with an allergy to heparin or heparinoid derivatives.
- Use cautiously in patients with hypertension (high blood pressure) or those taking antihypertension drugs.

Pregnancy and Breastfeeding

- Aortic acid is not recommended in pregnant or breastfeeding women due to a lack of available scientific evidence. Although not well studied in humans, hormonal changes may affect aortic acid levels.

INTERACTIONS

Interactions with Drugs

- Aortic extract may inhibit vascularization, and caution is advised when taking aortic acid with any antiangiogenic drugs, which prevent new vessel growth.
- Aortic acid may increase the risk of bleeding when taken with drugs that increase the risk of bleeding. Some examples include aspirin, anticoagulants (blood thinners) such as warfarin (Coumadin) or heparin, antiplatelet drugs such as clopidogrel (Plavix), and nonsteroidal anti-inflammatory drugs (NSAIDs) such as ibuprofen (Motrin, Advil) or naproxen (Naprosyn, Aleve).
- Aortic acid may lower total cholesterol and very-low-density lipoprotein (VLDL)–triglyceride levels while raising high-density lipoprotein (HDL) cholesterol and lipoprotein lipase activity. Caution is advised in patients taking cholesterol-lowering medications, such as statins (simvastatin).
- Although not well studied in humans, aortic extract may alter blood pressure. Patients with high or low blood pressure or those taking blood pressure–lowering agents should use cautiously.
- Aortic extracts may inhibit the growth of tumors. In theory, aortic acid may have additive effects when used concomitantly with other antitumor agents. Consult with a qualified health care professional, including a pharmacist, to check for interactions.
- Cigarette smoke may reduce the activity of aortic acid.
- Mesoglycan may decrease fibrinogen concentration and regulate fibrinolysis. Caution is advised in patients taking any fibrinolytics agents, which act to dissolve blood clots.
- Although not well studied in humans, female sex hormones may affect aortic acid mucopolysaccharides' effect on atherosclerosis. Caution is advised in patients taking hormone replacement therapy or birth control pills.
- Mesoglycan may lower blood sugar levels. Caution is advised when using medications that may also lower blood sugar levels. Patients taking drugs for diabetes by mouth or insulin should be monitored closely by a qualified health care professional, including a pharmacist. Medication adjustments may be necessary.
- Bovine aorta extract may inhibit immune response. Caution is advised in patients taking any herbs or supplements with immunomodulating activity because in theory, there may be interactions.
- Thyroid drugs may affect aortic acid mucopolysaccharides' effect on atherosclerosis. In theory, combination of aortic acid with herbs or supplements used for thyroid disorders may cause an interaction.

Interactions with Herbs and Dietary Supplements

- Aortic acid may reduce the formation of blood clots, and mesoglycan may regulate fibrinolysis. In theory, aortic acid may interact with herbs with anticoagulating (blood thinning) effects. Multiple cases of bleeding have been reported with the use of *Ginkgo biloba*, and fewer cases with garlic and saw palmetto. Numerous other agents may theoretically increase the risk of bleeding, although this has not been proven in most cases.
- Aortic acid may lower total cholesterol and VLDL-triglyceride levels while raising HDL cholesterol and lipoprotein lipase activity. Caution is advised when taking aortic acid with herbs that have cholesterol-lowering effects, such as red yeast rice.
- Although not well studied in humans, aortic extract may alter blood pressure. Patients taking herbs for high blood pressure or patients with low blood pressure should use with caution.
- Aortic extracts may inhibit the growth of tumors. Caution is advised in patients taking any herb that has antitumor effects.
- Female sex hormones may affect aortic acid mucopolysaccharides' effect on atherosclerosis. Caution is advised in patients taking herbs or supplements with hormonal (estrogenic or progestic) effects.
- Mesoglycan may slightly lower blood sugar levels. Caution is advised when using herbs or supplements that may also lower blood sugar levels. Blood glucose levels may require monitoring, and doses may need adjustment.
- Bovine aorta extract may exert significant dose-dependent inhibition of lymphocyte response. Caution is advised when taking aortic extract in combination with other immunomodulating herbs or supplements.
- Thyroid drugs may affect aortic acid mucopolysaccharides' effect on atherosclerosis.
- Administration of vitamin C during copper deficiency may lead to an increase in aortic acid. However, copper deficiency itself may lead to an increase in aortic acid.

For a complete list of references, please visit www.naturalstandard.com.

M

Methylsulfonylmethane (MSM)

RELATED TERMS

- Crystalline DMSO, dimethyl sulfone, DMSO2, methyl sulfone, methyl sulfonyl methane, methyl-sulfonyl-methane, methylsulfonylmethane, OptiMSM, sulfonyl sulfur.

BACKGROUND

- Methylsulfonylmethane, or MSM, is a form of organic sulfur that occurs naturally in a variety of fruits, vegetables, grains, and animals. MSM is a normal oxidation product of dimethyl sulfoxide (DMSO). It arises from a series of reactions that begin on the surface waters of the ocean. MSM is a white, odorless, crystalline substance that is water-soluble and contains 34% element sulfur.

- No evidence suggests that MSM is a necessary part of a normal diet. Sulfur is considered an essential mineral, but no dietary requirement has been established for it. MSM as a vital source of dietary sulfur is unsupported by published research. The nutrient is generally well tolerated, but long-term effects of supplementation with MSM have not been examined.

- MSM seemed to improve symptoms of allergic rhinitis and osteoarthritis. However, more high-quality research using MSM is necessary to define its role in treating these conditions. Although the Arthritis Foundation reports that MSM is used for pain and inflammation, they do not recommend its use due to lack of clinical trials.

EVIDENCE

Uses Based on Scientific Evidence	Grade
Allergic Rhinitis Preliminary research suggests that MSM may reduce symptoms associated with seasonal allergic rhinitis (SAR). However, the overall evidence is not sufficient to support this use.	C
Osteoarthritis Preliminary research has used MSM, alone or in combination with glucosamine, in the treatment of osteoarthritis. The combination may provide pain relief and reduction in inflammation. Further studies on MSM and its effects on patients with osteoarthritis are warranted.	C

Uses Based on Tradition or Theory
Acne, analgesia, antiparasitic, antispasmodic, burns, cancer, cardiovascular (blood flow), connective tissue disorders, constipation, cramps, diabetes mellitus, drug hypersensitivity, eye disorders (inflammation), gastrointestinal disorders, headache, heartburn, immunostimulant, insect bites, interstitial cystitis (chronic inflammation of the bladder), liver disease, lupus erythematosus (autoimmune disorder with skin wounds), mood enhancement, obesity, periodontal disease, premenstrual syndrome (PMS), pulmonary conditions, radiation sickness, rheumatoid arthritis, scar prevention, scleroderma (chronic, degenerative disease that affects the joints, skin, and internal organs), sinusitis, skin conditions (stretch marks), snoring, synovitis (inflammation of the joint lining), tendonitis, wrinkle prevention.

DOSING

Adults (18 Years and Older)

- MSM comes in various dosages and is an ingredient in many products. Adult dosage may range from 500-8,000 mg daily with or after meals. For allergic rhinitis, 2,600 mg daily for up to 30 days has been used. For osteoarthritis, 500 mg daily for up to 12 weeks has been used.

Children (Younger than 18 Years)

- There is insufficient evidence to recommend a dose of MSM in children.

SAFETY

Allergies

- Avoid in people with a known allergy or hypersensitivity to MSM.

Side Effects and Warnings

- Studies have shown safety and tolerability of MSM products when taken by mouth in recommended doses. Minimal side effects, including mild gastrointestinal discomfort, have been associated with the use of MSM. No studies on the long-term effects of MSM have been conducted.

Pregnancy and Breastfeeding

- MSM is not recommended in pregnant or breastfeeding women due to a lack of available scientific evidence.

INTERACTIONS

Interactions with Drugs

- Although not well studied in humans, MSM may have anti-inflammatory and antioxidant activity. In theory, use of MSM with other anti-inflammatory or antioxidant agents may have additive effects.

Interactions with Herbs and Dietary Supplements

- Although not well studied in humans, MSM may have anti-inflammatory and antioxidant activity. In theory, use of MSM with other anti-inflammatory or antioxidant herbs or supplements may have additive effects.

For a complete list of references, please visit www.naturalstandard.com.

Milk Thistle
(*Silybum marianum*)

RELATED TERMS

- Bull thistle, cardo blanco, Cardui mariae fructus, Cardui mariae herba, *Cardum marianum* L., *Carduus marianus* L., Chardon-Marie, emetic root, flavonolignans, Frauendistel, Fructus Silybi mariae, fruit de chardon Marie, heal thistle, holy thistle, isosilibinin, isosilybin, kanger, kocakavkas, kuub, lady's thistle, Legalon, Marian thistle, mariana mariana, Mariendistel, Marienkrörner, Mary thistle, mild thistle, milk ipecac, natursil, natursilum, Our Lady's thistle, pig leaves, royal thistle, shui fei ji, silidianin, Silybi mariae fructus, silybin, silybinin, *Silybum marianum,* silychristin, silymarin, snake milk, sow thistle, St. Mary's thistle, thisylin, Venue thistle, variegated thistle, wild artichoke.

BACKGROUND

- Milk thistle has been used medicinally for over 2,000 years, most commonly for the treatment of liver and gallbladder disorders. A flavonoid complex called *silymarin* can be extracted from the seeds of milk thistle and is believed to be the biologically active component. The terms *milk thistle* and *silymarin* are often used interchangeably.
- Milk thistle products are popular in Europe and the United States for various types of liver disease. Although numerous human trials have been published, most studies have not been well designed or reported.

EVIDENCE

Uses Based on Scientific Evidence	Grade
Chronic Hepatitis (Liver Inflammation) Several studies of oral milk thistle for hepatitis caused by viruses or alcohol report improvements in liver tests. However, most studies have been small and poorly designed.	B
Cirrhosis Multiple studies from Europe suggest benefits of oral milk thistle for cirrhosis. In experiments up to 5 years long, milk thistle has improved liver function and decreased the number of deaths that occur in cirrhotic patients.	B
Acute Viral Hepatitis Research on milk thistle for acute viral hepatitis has not provided clear results, and milk thistle cannot be recommended for this potentially life-threatening condition.	C
***Amanita phalloides* Mushroom Poisoning** Milk thistle has been used traditionally to treat *Amanita phalloides* mushroom poisoning. However, there are not enough reliable studies in humans to support this use of milk thistle.	C
Cancer There are early reports from laboratory experiments that the chemicals silymarin and silibinin in milk thistle reduce the growth of human breast, cervical, and prostate cancer cells. There is also one report of a patient with liver cancer who improved following treatment with milk thistle. However, this research is too early to draw a firm conclusion, and effects have not been shown in high-quality human trials.	
Diabetes (in Patients with Cirrhosis) A small number of studies suggest possible improvements of blood sugar control in cirrhotic patients with diabetes. However, there is not enough scientific evidence to recommend milk thistle for this use.	C
Dyspepsia An herbal preparation containing milk thistle may be effective in decreasing symptoms of functional dyspepsia. However, milk thistle alone has not been researched thoroughly.	C
High Cholesterol Although animal and laboratory research suggests cholesterol-lowering effects of milk thistle, human studies have provided unclear results. Further studies are necessary before a firm recommendation can be made.	C
Liver Damage from Drugs or Toxins Several studies suggest possible benefits of milk thistle to treat or prevent liver damage caused by drugs or toxic chemicals. Results of this research are not clear, and most studies have been poorly designed. Therefore, there is not enough scientific evidence to recommend milk thistle for this use.	C
Menopausal Symptoms An herbal preparation containing milk thistle may be effective in decreasing menopausal symptoms. However, milk thistle alone has not been researched thoroughly.	C

Uses Based on Tradition or Theory

Acute liver injury, amiodarone toxicity reactions, antibacterial, asthma, bad breath, bleeding, bronchitis, constipation, diabetic nerve pain, eczema, fatty liver, gallbladder disease, gallstones, hangover, hemorrhoids, hyperthyroidism, immunomodulator, immunostimulant, inflammation, ischemic injury, liver protection, loss of appetite, malaria, menstrual problems, nutrition (dietary supplement), physical work capacity, plague, psoriasis, radiation toxicity, snakebites, spleen disorders, sunscreen, tumors, ulcers, varicose veins.

DOSING
Adults (18 Years and Older)

- Silymarin (Legalon) 230-600 mg may be taken daily in two to three doses.
- Silipide (IdB 1016) 160-480 mg in silybin equivalents may be taken daily.

Children (Younger than 18 Years)

- There is insufficient evidence to recommend milk thistle for use in children.

SAFETY
Allergies

- People with allergies to plants in the aster family (Compositae, Asteraceae) or to daisies, artichokes, common thistle, kiwi, or to any of milk thistle's constituents (silibinin, silychistin, silydianin, silymonin, siliandrin) may have allergic reactions to milk thistle. Anaphylactic shock (a severe allergic reaction) from milk thistle tea or tablets has been reported in several patients. Overall, silymarin has a good safety record with rare case reports of gastrointestinal disturbances and allergic skin rashes published.

Side Effects and Warnings

- Milk thistle appears to be well tolerated in recommended doses for up to 6 years. Some patients in studies have experienced stomach upset, headache, and itching. There are rare reports of appetite loss, gas, heartburn, diarrhea, joint pain, and impotence with milk thistle use. One person experienced sweating, nausea, stomach pain, diarrhea, vomiting, weakness, and collapse after taking milk thistle. This reaction may have been due to an allergic reaction, and improved after 24 hours. High liver enzyme levels in one person taking milk thistle returned to normal after the person stopped taking the herb.
- In theory, milk thistle may lower blood sugar levels. Caution is advised in patients with diabetes or hypoglycemia, and in those taking drugs, herbs, or supplements that affect blood sugar levels. Serum glucose levels may need to be monitored by a health care provider, and medication adjustments may be necessary.
- Theoretically, because milk thistle plant extract might have estrogenic effects, women with hormone-sensitive conditions should avoid milk thistle above-ground parts. Some of these conditions include breast, uterine, and ovarian cancers; endometriosis; and uterine fibroids. The more commonly used milk thistle seed extracts are not known to have estrogenic effects.
- Exacerbation of hemochromatosis has been associated with ingestion of milk thistle.

Pregnancy and Breastfeeding

- Milk thistle has been used historically to improve breast milk flow, and two brief studies of milk thistle in pregnant women reported no side effects. However, there is not enough scientific evidence to support the safe use of milk thistle during pregnancy or breastfeeding at this time.

INTERACTIONS
Interactions with Drugs

- Animal studies suggest that milk thistle may interfere with the way the body processes certain drugs using the liver's cytochrome P450 enzyme system. As a result, levels of these drugs may be increased in the blood and may cause increased effects or adverse reactions. Many types of drugs may be affected. Individuals should speak with a qualified health care provider to obtain a list of these drugs and their possible interactions. In theory, milk thistle may lower blood sugar levels. Caution is advised when using medications that may also lower blood sugar levels. Patients taking drugs for diabetes by mouth or insulin should be monitored closely by a qualified health care provider. Medication adjustments may be necessary.
- A possible interaction with phenytoin (Dilantin) has been reported with milk thistle. However, the facts are unclear.
- Milk thistle ingredients have been reported to prevent amiodarone toxicity in animal studies. Based on laboratory and animal studies, milk thistle may increase the effects of chemotherapy drugs like doxorubicin, cisplatin, and carboplatin. Milk thistle may interact with hormonal agents, alcohol, antiretroviral drugs, or indinivir.

Interactions with Herbs and Dietary Supplements

- Animal studies suggest that milk thistle may interfere with the way the body processes certain herbs or supplements using the liver's cytochrome P450 enzyme system. As a result, levels of other herbs or supplements may be too high in the blood. It may also alter the effects that other herbs or supplements have on the P450 system.
- Milk thistle may lower blood sugar levels. Caution is advised when using herbs or supplements that may also lower blood sugar levels. Blood glucose levels may require monitoring, and doses may need adjustment.
- Milk thistle may also interact with herbs and supplements with hormonal, antiretroviral, or antioxidant effects. Milk thistle may chelate iron and slow calcium metabolism.

For a complete list of references, please visit www.naturalstandard.com.

Mistletoe
(*Viscum album*)

RELATED TERMS

- ABNOBAviscum, Abnovaviscum Quercus (AQ), all-heal, American mistletoe, Australian mistletoe, avuscumine, bird's lime, birdlime mistletoe, devil's fuge, Drudenfuss, Eurixor, folia visci, galactoside-specfic lectin, golden bough, Helixor, herbe de qui (French), hexenbesen, Iscador QuFrF, Iscador Qu spezial, Isorel, lectine standard, Leim-mistel, Lektinol, *Lignum crusis* (Latin), Miselsenker, Mis-tlekraut (German), Mistletein, mistletoe of the appletree (*Malus*), mistletoe of the fir (*Abies*), mistletoe of the pine (*Pinus*), mistletoe extract PS76A2, mistletoe lectin (ML), mistrel, ML-1, mystyldene, *Phoradendron leucarpum*, *Phoradendron serotinum* (Raf.), *Phoradendron flavescens* (Pursh.) Nuttal, *Phoradendron macrophyllum*, *Phoradendron tomentosum* (DC) (American mistletoe), Plenosol, PS76A2, Syviman N (mistletoe and comfrey combination), Stripites Visci, Tallo de muerdago, VaQuFrF, Vischio (Italian), Visci, *Visci albi folia, Visci albi fructus, Visci albi herba, Visci albi stipites,* viscum, *Viscum album* Loranthaceae (family), *Viscum album coloratum* (Korean mistletoe), *Viscus album quercus* frischsaft [Qu FrF], *Viscum abietis, Viscum austriacum,* Viscum fraxini-2, viscumin, Vogelmistel, Vysorel, white mistletoe.

BACKGROUND

- Once considered a sacred herb in Celtic tradition, mistletoe has been used for centuries for conditions as diverse as high blood pressure, epilepsy, exhaustion, anxiety, arthritis, vertigo (dizziness), and degenerative inflammation of the joints.
- Beginning in the early twentieth century, mistletoe came into practice in Europe as an anticancer therapy. This remains a source of great popular interest. For example, in Norway, mistletoe has been considered a "non-proven therapy" or NPT but has been used as a popular method for healing.
- In the last 50 years, many laboratory, animal, and human studies have been conducted on potential anticancer effects thought to be caused by immunostimulatory effects of mistletoe.
- The most promising potential use is as a cancer therapy, but there is still insufficient clinical evidence to consider it a proven cancer therapy. Toxic effects seem to be rare but have been reported. The National Cancer Institute mono-graph "Mistletoe Extracts" provides a complementary and alternative medicine (CAM) information summary and overview of the use of mistletoe as a treatment for cancer, indicating that: [a] in animal studies mixed results have been obtained using mistletoe extracts for slowing tumor growth; [b] well-designed clinical trials using mistletoe or its components have not been sufficient to prove efficacy in the treatment of human cancer(s); [c] mistletoe plants and berries are toxic to humans and their extracts are not sold in the United States.

- Mistletoe is not commercially available in the United States, but two U.S. investigators currently have Investigational New Drug approval (IND) from the U.S. Food and Drug Administration (FDA) to study mistletoe.
- The German Commission E Monographs list mistletoe as a treatment for degenerative inflammation of the joints and as palliative therapy for malignant tumors.
- Two major types of mistletoe, European and American, contain very similar proteins and are reputed to have differ-ent uses. European mistletoe is believed to reduce blood pressure and act as an antispasmodic and calmative agent, while American mistletoe is believed to simulate smooth muscles, increase blood pressure, and trigger uterine and intestinal contractions. However, there is little research to substantiate any of these claims.

EVIDENCE

Uses Based on Scientific Evidence	Grade
Arthritis One retrospective case study documented potential benefits of mistletoe extract injection in the man-agement of arthritis. However, the clinical evidence is not sufficient to support the use of mistletoe in the treatment of this condition, for which other more proven treatments are available.	C
Cancer Mistletoe is one of the most widely used unconven-tional cancer treatments in Europe. Extracts have been studied for many types of human cancers, including bladder, breast, cervical, CNS, colorectal, head and neck, liver, lung, lymphatic, ovarian, and kidney cancers, as well as melanoma and leukemia. However, mistletoe has not been proven to be effective for any one type of cancer.	C
Hepatitis In a preliminary description in 1997, some patients achieved complete elimination of the virus after treatment with *Viscum album*, although these studies were not well designed. A small exploratory trial investigated the effects of mistletoe on liver function, reduction of viral load and inflammation, and maintenance of quality of life by the immuno-modulatory and/or cytotoxic actions of mistletoe extracts, but little effect was seen. The potential benefits of mistletoe remain uclear.	C
Humman Immunodeficiency Virus Treatment of humman immunodeficiency virus patients with mistletoe has been done in Europe	C

(Continued)

509

Uses Based on Scientific Evidence	Grade
since the beginning of the acquired immuno-deficiency syndrome epidemic based on proposed immunomodulatory effects. Treatment seems to be tolerable with minimal side effects reported. Mistletoe may assist in inhibiting progression, but not all mistletoe preparations have shown equal effects.	
Immunomodulation A few small trials found mistletoe to be promising as an immunostimulant in people with the common cold.	C
Respiratory Disease (Recurrent) Studies of Iscador (conducted by the same authors) document improved clinical symptoms and markers of immune function in children with recurrent respiratory disease (RRD) exposed to the Chernobyl nuclear accident. There is insufficient evidence to recommend mistletoe therapy for RRD in general.	C

Uses Based on Tradition or Theory

Abortion, abscesses, amenorrhea (lack of menstrual period), anxiety, arteriosclerosis, asthma, bleeding problems, blood disorders (malignant hematological disease), chorea, circulatory disorders, constipation, convulsions (infantile), degenerative joint disease/osteoarthritis, depression, diarrhea, dizziness, epilepsy, exhaustion, gallbladder disorders, gallstones, gastrointestinal disorders, gout, headaches, heart conditions, hemorrhoids, high blood pressure, hysteria, icterus, increased muscle mass (hypertonia), indigestion, infertility, jaundice, labor induction, liver disorders, low blood pressure, lymphatic disorders (malignant lymphatic disease), osteoporosis, ringing in the ears (tinnitus), skin conditions, sleep disorders, tachycardia, tranquilizer, ulcers, urinary disorders, varicose veins, vascular disorders, venous congestion, whooping cough.

DOSING
Adults (18 Years and Older)
- Traditionally, tea has been made with mistletoe leaves, hawthorn leaves and flowers, and lemon balm leaves in equal parts. Two cups daily has been prepared by infusing 2 tsp of the mixture for 5-10 minutes. Cold water infusions, dried aqueous extracts, and fluid extracts (1:1 in 25% alcohol) have been taken by mouth.
- Mistletoe has been studied in multiple injectable regimens (intravenous, subcutaneous, intrapleural) and given by a health care provider in a controlled setting. Sometimes therapy includes an induction phase and a maintenance phase. Mistletoe should only be given by a qualified health care professional. No standard dose can be recommended at this time. Further research is needed, as there are many potential side effects and interactions.

Children (Younger than 18 Years)
- Mistletoe has been studied in children for respiratory infections. Further research is needed before a recommendation can be made.

SAFETY
Allergies
- Avoid in people with a known allergy/hypersensitivity to mistletoe or to any of its constituents. A life-threatening allergic reaction, called anaphylaxis, occurred after injections of mistletoe.

Side Effects and Warnings
- Mistletoe is contraindicated in patients with protein hypersensitivity and/or chronic progressive infections (e.g., tuberculosis). Avoid use of mistletoe in patients with acute, highly febrile, inflammatory disease.
- Most clinical trials were performed with unfractionated extracts, which contain numerous components, and it is difficult to ascribe adverse effects to any component of the mistletoe extracts. Most of the injected administrations of mistletoe may be accompanied by mild manifestations of similar side effects, and most are transient.
- The most common reactions reported are erythema (reddening of the skin) and hyperemia (increased blood in an organ). Use of Iscador-M has resulted in grade 3-4 toxicities (e.g., anorexia, general malaise, depressive moods, fever, and swelling at the site of injection). Other side effects observed have included drug-related fever and pain at the site of injection. No drug-related discontinuation or toxic deaths occurred.
- Avoid the use of mistletoe with cardiovascular disease, as many adverse effects are possible.
- Dermatological (skin) adverse effects may include burning sensations, indurations, pruritus, swelling, urticaria, vasculitis, or allergic reactions such as delayed hypersensitivity.
- Avoid the use of mistletoe in active/uncontrolled hyperthyroid patients. The manufacturer of Isorel, Novipharm, notes that mistletoe may additionally activate the patient's already accelerated metabolism and cause overstimulation, thus worsening the patient's status. Also use cautiously in diabetics, as insulin levels may be altered.
- Congested intestine, diarrhea, gastroenteritis, nausea, and vomiting have been reported after mistletoe use. Moderate to mild flulike symptoms, transient exacerbation of gingivitis, and fever were observed in some patients with subcutaneous administration of mistletoe preparations. Hepatitis has been reported due to ingestion of herbal tablets containing mistletoe and other plant extracts. Elevations of liver enzymes have been reported with high doses of mistletoe.
- High urinary frequency/nocturia has been observed. Coma, delirium, fatigue, hallucinations, headaches, pain (generalized, bone, joint), abnormal blood cell counts, pancreas, and kidney damage have been reported, along with seizures and sleeplessness. In one clinical study, muscle contracture and muscular pain were reported. Ascites, slowed heart rates, cardiac arrest, dehydration, and high or low blood pressure have also been reported.
- Use cautiously in glaucoma patients or those on cholinergics. Mydriasis and myosis/myalgia has been reported in clinical study after mistletoe administration. One report exists of eye irritation after the ingestion of mistletoe.

Pregnancy and Breastfeeding
- Avoid use of mistletoe during pregnancy and breastfeeding due to the potential uterine stimulant activity of mistletoe.

INTERACTIONS
Interactions with Drugs

- Mistletoe may increase the effects of blood pressure–lowering medications or have other more serious adverse effects on the heart. Busulphan and mistletoe extract (Helixor) have been reported to cause organ fibrosis and death.
- Use of mistletoe with central nervous system (CNS) depressants may increase sedative effects.
- It is unclear if mistletoe interacts with drugs that affect blood sugar levels or drugs used to treat diabetes.
- Elevations of liver enzymes have been reported with high doses of mistletoe. Seizure risk may be increased. Seizures have been reported to poison control centers following the ingestion of crude mistletoe plant material. Immunomodulatory effects have also been proposed.
- Theoretically, concomitant use of mistletoe and monoamine oxidase inhibitors (MAOIs) may cause a hypertensive crisis due to mistletoe containing tyramine. Blood sugar levels may be altered by mistletoe. Mistletoe may have negative side effects on the eye and interact with eye drops.
- Avoid the use of mistletoe in patients with overactive thyroid glands (a condition called *hyperthyroidism*). Mistletoe may cause an inflammatory reaction when used in patients with untreated hyperthyroidism.

Interactions with Herbs and Dietary Supplements

- The use of garlic, lime tree *(Tilia platyphyllos)*, or hawthorn *(Crataegus oxyacantha)* with mistletoe may result in additive blood pressure–lowering action.
- European mistletoe can have cardiotoxic and negative effects on heartbeat strength, cause reflex bradycardia (slow heart rate), and depolarize cardiac muscle. Severe dehydration caused by mistletoe may lead to hypovolemic shock and cardiovascular collapse. Use cautiously with herbs or supplements that alter heart rhythm.
- Use of mistletoe with CNS depressants may enhance sedative effects.
- Use of mistletoe with cholinergic herbs or supplements may cause increased myosis due to additive adverse effects.
- Immunomodulatory effects have been proposed.
- Elevations of liver enzymes have been reported with high doses of mistletoe.
- Theoretically, the concomitant use of mistletoe and MAOIs may cause a hypertensive crisis due to mistletoe containing tyramine.
- It is unclear if mistletoe interacts with herbs or supplements that affect blood sugar levels or agents used to treat diabetes. Avoid the use of mistletoe in hyperthyroid patients. The manufacturer of Iscador noted that mistletoe may cause an inflammatory reaction when used during untreated hyperthyroidism.

For a complete list of references, please visit www.naturalstandard.com.

M

Modified Citrus Pectin (MCP)

RELATED TERMS

- Citrus pectin, depolymerized pectin, fractioned pectin, MCP, modified pectin, PectaSol, pH-modified pectin.

BACKGROUND

- Pectins are gel-forming polysaccharides from plant cell walls, especially apple and citrus fruits. Pectins are a type of viscous dietary fiber and vary in the length of their polysaccharide chains, from 300-1,000 monosaccharides. Although pectins are not digestible by humans, modified citrus pectin (MCP) is altered to increase their absorbability. Pectin from citrus rinds is depolymerized through a treatment with sodium hydroxide and hydrochloric acid. The resultant smaller molecule is composed predominantly of D-polygalacturonates and may be more easily absorbed by the human digestive system.
- Modified citrus pectin is most often used as an adjuvant to cancer therapy to prevent metastasis. Modified citrus pectin is still considered an experimental therapy for cancer and should be used as an adjuvant to standard cancer therapy under medical supervision. Pectins, including modified citrus pectin, have also been investigated for possible cardiovascular benefits, including lowering cholesterol and reducing atherosclerosis. Clinical studies are needed in these areas.
- Some experts caution that citrus pectin and all "modified" citrus pectins may not have the same effects as modified citrus pectin. Citrus pectin does not have the same short polysaccharide chains as modified citrus pectin, and "modified" pectin could indicate that the pectin has been altered in some way, but not necessarily have the shorter polysaccharide chains.

EVIDENCE

Uses Based on Scientific Evidence	Grade
Detoxification (Toxic Excretion) Modified citrus pectin may increase the excretion of metals, such as arsenic, cadmium, and lead. Additional studies are needed in this area before a firm recommendation can be made.	C
Prostate Cancer Modified citrus pectin may reduce the metastasis of certain types of cancers, including lung, prostate, and breast. More research is needed in this area, especially with other types of cancer and with other criteria for prostate cancer progression.	C

Uses Based on Tradition or Theory
Antithrombotic, atherosclerosis (hardening of the arteries), bulk laxative, chelating agent, diarrhea, hyperlipidemia (high cholesterol), immunostimulant, tonic (gastrointestinal).

DOSING

Adults (18 Years and Older)

- There is insufficient evidence to recommend a dose for modified citrus pectin. Although not well studied in human clinical trials, 6-30 g daily in divided doses, dissolved in a small amount of water, and diluted with juice, has been used. For capsules, a dose of 800 mg three times daily with meals has also been used. For biopsy and cancer, daily of 15 g daily (5 g three times daily) 1 week before procedure and 2 weeks after has been used. For toxic excretion, 15 g of MCP PectaSol (EcoNugenics Inc.) daily for 5 days and 20 g on day 6 has been used with some benefit.

Children (Younger than 18 Years)

- There is insufficient evidence to recommend a dose for modified citrus pectin in children, and use is not recommended.

SAFETY

Allergies

- Avoid in people with a known allergy or hypersensitivity to modified citrus pectin. Modified citrus pectin may cause gastrointestinal discomfort in patients who are allergic or sensitive to modified citrus pectin.

Side Effects and Warnings

- Modified citrus pectin is "generally regarded as safe" (GRAS) by the U.S. Food and Drug Administration (FDA), and few adverse effects have been reported in the available literature. Because it is a dietary fiber, modified citrus pectin may result in mild loose stools, but it should not cause other gastrointestinal problems in healthy patients. Theoretically, modified citrus pectin may cause fluid or electrolyte loss, constipation, or fecal impaction in some patients, especially geriatric patients, because it is a fiber.
- Use cautiously in patients taking chelating medications, as modified citrus pectin may significantly increase the urinary excretion of metals. Also, use cautiously in patients under treatment for cancer, as modified citrus pectin may inhibit tumor growth.

Pregnancy and Breastfeeding

- Modified citrus pectin is not recommended in pregnant or breastfeeding women due to a lack of available scientific evidence.

INTERACTIONS

Interactions with Drugs

- Modified citrus pectin may significantly increase the urinary excretion of metals. Caution is advised in patients taking chelating agents.
- Although not well studied in humans, pectin may lower cholesterol levels. Consult with a qualified health care professional, including a pharmacist, before combining modified citrus pectin with cholesterol-lowering agents.
- Based on animal research, modified citrus pectin may significantly inhibit carbohydrate-mediated tumor growth. Patients taking any agents for cancer should use modified citrus pectin with caution.

- Modified citrus pectin may slow or reduce the absorption of oral drugs. Caution is advised when taking medications by mouth.

Interactions with Herbs and Dietary Supplements

- Modified citrus pectin may significantly increase the urinary excretion of metals. Caution is advised in patients taking chelating agents.
- Although not well studied in humans, pectin may lower cholesterol levels. Consult with a qualified health care professional, including a pharmacist, before combining modified citrus pectin with cholesterol-lowering agents.

- Although not well studied in humans, modified citrus pectin may significantly inhibit carbohydrate-mediated tumor growth. Patients taking any herbs or supplements for cancer should use modified citrus pectin with caution.
- Modified citrus pectin may slow or reduce the absorption of oral agents. Caution is advised when taking herbs and supplements by mouth.

For a complete list of references, please visit www.naturalstandard.com.

M

Mugwort
(*Artemisia vulgaris*)

RELATED TERMS

- Ai ye, arbre aux cent gouts, armoise, armoise commune, artemisia, *Artemisia vulgaris*, *Artemisiae vulgaris* herba, *Artemisia vulgaris* L., *Artemisia vulgaris* pollen, *Artemisia vulgaris* R., *Artemisiae vulgaris* radix, Asteraceae (family), baru cina, bijvoet, borneol, Carline thistle, chernobyl, chornobyl, chrysanthemum weed, cineole, common mugwort, common wormwood, Douglas mugwort, felon herb, fuchiba, Gemeiner Beifuss, genje jawa, hierba de San Juan, hiyam, hydroxycoumarins, Japanese wormwood, linalool, lipohilic flavonoids, moxa, moxa rolls, nagadamni, pinene, polyn' obyknovennaya, prunasin, sailor's tobacco, St. John's plant, suket ganjahan, sundamala, thujone, triterpenes, tzu ai, vulgarin, wild wormwood, wormseed, yomogi, yomogiko.
- **Note:** Mugwort *(Artemisia vulgaris)* should not be confused with wormwood *(Artemisia absinthium)*, tarragon *(Artemisia dracunculus)*, or St. John's wort *(Hypericum perforatum* L.), despite similar names.

BACKGROUND

- Mugwort is a perennial herb native to Europe, Asia, and northern Africa. It pollinates mainly from July to September, although it may flower throughout the year, depending on the climate. The Chinese have used dried mugwort leaves (moxa) in moxibustion for centuries. Moxibustion is a method of heating specific acupuncture points on the body to treat physical conditions. Mugwort is carefully harvested, dried, and aged, and then it is shaped into a cigar-like roll. This "moxa" is burned close to the skin to heat the specific pressure points.
- Mugwort leaf and stem have been used medicinally to stimulate digestion and to promote menstruation. The nervine action of mugwort is thought to aid in depression and ease tension. Traditionally, mugwort was believed to provide protection from fatigue, sunstroke, wild animals, and evil spirits.
- No clinical studies have been performed on the use of mugwort as a medical treatment, although an extract from the related *Artemisia annua* suggests some promise in treating malaria. Dried mugwort (moxa) has been used in moxibustion to treat cancer, but there is no scientific evidence to support this use. Most research on mugwort has focused on its allergenic properties, as its pollen affects 10%-14% of the patients suffering from pollinosis in Europe.

EVIDENCE

Uses Based on Scientific Evidence

No available studies qualify for inclusion in the evidence table.

Uses Based on Tradition or Theory

Abortifacient (induces abortion), addiction (opium), anorexia, anthelminthic (expels worms), antidepressant, antifungal, antimicrobial, antioxidant, antiseptic, antispasmodic, anxiety, asthma, bowel cleansing, cancer, carminative (digestive aid), cathartic, cholagogue (stimulates bile flow), circulatory disorders, convulsions, diaphoretic (promotes sweating), digestion, emmenagogue (promotes menstruation), epilepsy, expectorant, fatigue, fever, food uses, gastric ulcers, gout, headaches, hysteria, infertility, insomnia, irritability, liver disorders, malaria, muscle spasm, nosebleeds, restlessness, rheumatic disorders, snakebites, stimulant, stress, sunstroke, tonic.

DOSING

Adults (18 Years and Older)

- There is insufficient evidence to recommend a dose for mugwort. Traditionally, 2 cups of mugwort tea (1 oz of fresh mugwort leaf infused 5-10 minutes, covered, in 1 pint boiling water) daily for 6 days has been used.

Children (Younger than 18 Years)

- There is insufficient evidence to recommend a dose for mugwort, and use in children is not recommended.

SAFETY

Allergies

- Avoid in people with a known allergy or hypersensitivity to mugwort, any of its constituents, or to other members of the Compositae/Asteraceae family, including ragweed, chrysanthemums, chamomile, marigolds, and daisies. Allergic responses have been associated with exposure to mugwort, including bronchoconstriction/asthma, upper and lower respiratory tract sensitization, seasonal allergic rhinitis, conjunctivitis, pollinosis, contact dermatitis, urticaria, and atopic eczema.
- Cross-reactivity has been noted between birch, cabbage, grass, hazelnut, olive pollen, honey, mustard, royal jelly, sage, sweet bell pepper pollen, and sunflower. Cross-reactivity has also been demonstrated between mugwort and kiwi, peach, mango, apple, celery, and carrots. A florist with a pre-existing sunflower allergy developed a life-threatening glottal edema after occupational contact with mugwort.

Side Effects and Warnings

- There is limited information regarding the adverse effects of mugwort. Mugwort has caused breathing difficulties and skin allergic responses, such as contact dermatitis, urticaria, conjunctivitis, atopic eczema, bronchoconstriction/asthma, upper and lower respiratory tract sensitization, seasonal allergic rhinitis, pollinosis, and anaphylaxis. According to traditional use and expert opinion, large doses of mugwort may cause abortion, nausea, vomiting, or damage to the nervous system.
- Mugwort is on the German Commission E (Germany's regulatory agency for herbs) list of unapproved herbs. Avoid if allergic to birch, grass, hazelnut, olive pollen, honey, mustard, royal jelly, sage, sweet bell pepper pollen, tobacco, and sunflower because cross-reactivity has been noted. Avoid with food allergies to kiwi, peach, mango, apple, celery, and carrots due to cross-reactivity.

Pregnancy and Breastfeeding

- Mugwort is not recommended in pregnant or breastfeeding women due to a lack of available scientific evidence. Mugwort is on the German Commission E (Germany's regulatory agency for herbs) list of unapproved herbs. Traditionally, mugwort has been used to induce abortion (abortifacient).

INTERACTIONS

Interactions with Drugs

- Mugwort contains coumarin derivatives, which may increase the risk of bleeding. Some examples include aspirin, anticoagulants (blood thinners) such as warfarin (Coumadin) or heparin, antiplatelet drugs such as clopidogrel (Plavix), and nonsteroidal anti-inflammatory drugs such as ibuprofen (Motrin, Advil) or naproxen (Naprosyn, Aleve).

Interactions with Herbs and Dietary Supplements

- Mugwort contains coumarin derivatives, which may increase the risk of bleeding. Caution is advised in patients with bleeding disorders or those taking herbs that may increase the risk of bleeding. Dosing adjustments may be necessary.

For a complete list of references, please visit www. naturalstandard.com.

M

Muira Puama
(*Ptychopetalum olacoides*)

RELATED TERMS

- Herbal vY, jarrow, lignum, marapama, marapuama, maripuama, muira-puama, muira puama wood, muira-puam, Muirae puama, muirapuamine, Olacaceae (family), olacoides, potency bark, potency wood, potenzholz, *Ptychopetali lignum*, ptychopetalum, *Ptychopetalum guyanna*, *Ptychopetalum olacoides* Bentham, *Ptychopetalum unicatum*, *Ptychopetalum uncinatum* Anselmino, *Ptychopetalum unicatum* Anselmino, *Ptychopetalum* spp., raiz del macho, Testor-plus.
- **Note:** Not to be confused with *Acanthea virilis* or *Liriosma ovata*, which are also called muira puama.

BACKGROUND

- Historically, all parts of the muira puama plant have been used medicinally, but the bark and roots are most highly utilized. Indigenous tribes in Brazil use the tea for treating neuromuscular problems, rheumatism, influenza, and cardiac and gastrointestinal asthenia, and to prevent baldness. In Europe, muira puama has a long history in herbal medicine as an anti-rheumatic, aphrodisiac, a tonic for the nervous system, and for the treatment of gastrointestinal disorders.
- Muira puama is included in combination products as a remedy for sexual impotence. Recent studies show promising evidence that it may increase sexual vitality and treat erectile dysfunction in males. Muira puama has also been used by bodybuilders and weight lifters to improve physical performance. This is due to proposed testosterone-like effects of muira puama.
- If buying preparations of muira puama, do so with caution, as *Liriosma ovata* and *Acanthea virilis* are commonly incorrectly sold as muira puama.

EVIDENCE

Uses Based on Scientific Evidence	Grade
Erectile Dysfunction Muira puama has long been used by Brazilian indigenous people as a treatment for impotence, and preliminary study has investigated muira puama's use for erectile dysfunction. However, clinical evidence is insufficient to support this use.	C
Sexual Dysfunction (Females) Muira puama has historically been recommended for enhancement of libido. However, clinical evidence is insufficient to support this use.	C

Uses Based on Tradition or Theory
Aging, alopecia (hair loss), Alzheimer's disease, analgesic (pain reliever), anxiety, aphrodisiac, appetite stimulation, ataxia (loss of coordination), atherosclerosis (hardening of the arteries), athletic performance enhancer, baldness, beriberi (vitamin deficiency), cancer, cardiac conditions (asthenia), central nervous system (CNS) stimulant, depression, diarrhea, dysentery (severe diarrhea), dysmenorrhea (painful menstruation), dyspepsia (upset stomach), energy, fatigue, gastric ulcers, gastrointestinal conditions (asthenia), hookworm, hypercalcemia (high calcium level), impotence, infertility, influenza, libido, memory improvement, menstrual cramps, menstrual irregularities, mental performance, nervous exhaustion, neuralgia (nerve pain), neurasthenia (nerve exhaustion), neuromuscular disorders, pain, paralysis, poliomyelitis (viral disease), premenstrual syndrome (PMS), rheumatism, stimulant, strength enhancement, stress, stroke, tonic, trauma.

DOSING

Adults (18 Years and Older)

- There is insufficient evidence to recommend a dose for muira puama. However, for erectile dysfunction, up to 2,580 mg of Herbal vY daily for 2 weeks has been used with minimal side effects.

Children (Younger than 18 Years)

- There is insufficient evidence to recommend a dose for muira puama in children.

SAFETY

Allergies

- Avoid in people with a known allergy or hypersensitivity to muira puama (*Ptychopetalum olacoides*), any of its constituents, or any related members of the Olacaceae family.

Side Effects and Warnings

- Muira puama is generally considered by experts to be a safe herb, and no serious adverse effects have been reported in the available scientific literature.
- Muira puama may raise blood pressure and CNS (central nervous system) stimulation, which may alter blood pressure, heart functions, and CNS effects on heart tissue. Muira puama may also have proposed testosterone-like proprieties, which may cause anabolic side effects, such as increases in energy, aggression, or appetite; changes in voice; or enlargement of genitalia.
- Use cautiously in patients taking steroidal drug therapy or in patients with hormone-sensitive conditions (e.g., breast cancer, endometriosis, ovarian cancer, prostate cancer).
- Use cautiously in patients with hypertension (high blood pressure) or cardiac disease, as muira puama may exacerbate these conditions.
- Use cautiously in patients taking CNS-acting medications, as muira puama may stimulate the CNS.

Pregnancy and Breastfeeding

- Avoid use during pregnancy due to reported idiosyncratic motor/sacral stimulant properties. Muira puama is not recommended in breastfeeding women due to a lack of available scientific data.

516

INTERACTIONS

Interactions with Drugs

- Although not well studied in humans, cross-tolerance with opioids may occur. Caution is advised when taking muira puama with other pain-relieving (analgesic) agents.
- Due to coumarin constituents of muira puama, the actions of warfarin and other anticoagulant and antiplatelet drugs may be potentiated. Caution is advised in patients with bleeding disorders or those taking drugs that may increase the risk of bleeding. Dosing adjustments may be necessary.
- Muira puama may increase blood pressure and central nervous system (CNS) stimulation, which may alter blood pressure, cardiac functions, and CNS effects on cardiac tissue.
- The combined use of muira puama with monoamine oxidase inhibitors (MAOIs) may potentiate the potential risk for hypertensive crisis.
- Due to serotonergic effects of muira puama, actions of antidepressants, such as selective serotonin reuptake inhibitors (SSRIs), may be altered.
- Due to proposed testosterone-like effects as well as positive or negative estrogenic effects, use of muira puama with testosterone or estrogen may result in additive or diminished effects.
- Combination use with sympathomimetics may lead to potentiation of sympathomimetic effects.

Interactions with Herbs and Dietary Supplements

- Although not well studied in humans, cross-tolerance with opioids may occur. Caution is advised when taking muira puama with other pain-relieving (analgesic) herbs or supplements.
- Due to coumarin constituents of muira puama, actions of anticoagulants and antiplatelets may be altered. Caution is advised in patients with bleeding disorders or those taking herbs or supplements that may increase the risk of bleeding. Dosing adjustments may be necessary.
- Due to proposed serotonergic effects of muira puama, the actions of antidepressant herbs may be altered.
- Muira puama may increase blood pressure and central nervous system (CNS) stimulation, which may alter blood pressure, cardiac functions, and CNS effects on cardiac tissue.
- The combined use of muira puama with monoamine oxidase inhibitors (MAOIs) may potentiate the potential risk for hypertensive crisis.
- Due to proposed testosterone-like effects of muira puama as well as positive or negative estrogenic effects, use of muira puama with testosterone or estrogen-like herbs may result in additive or diminished effects.
- Combination of muira puama with stimulant herbs may lead to potentiation of sympathomimetic effects.
- Hydroalcoholic extract of muira puama may potentiate yohimbine-induced toxicity.

For a complete list of references, please visit www.naturalstandard.com.

M

Mullein
(Verbascum thapsus)

RELATED TERMS

- Aaron's rod, Adam's flannel, beggar's blanket, beggar's flannel, beggar's stalk, big taper, blanket herb, blanket leaf, bullock's lungwort, candlewick plant, clot, clown's lungwort, common mullein, cuddy's lungs, duffle, feltwort, flannel plant, fluffweed, golden rod, great mullein, hag's taper, hare's taper, Jacob's staff, jupiter's staff, molene, mullein, mullein dock, old man's flannel, our lady's flannel, Peter's staff, rag paper, Scrophulariaceae (family), shepherd's club, shepherd's staff, torch, torches, velvet dock, velvet plant, *Verbascum densiflorum*, *Verbascum fruticulosum*, *Verbascum lychnitis*, *Verbascum macrurum*, *Verbascum nigrum*, *Verbascum nobile*, *Verbascum phlomoides*, *Verbascum sinaiticum*, *Verbascum songaricum*, *Verbascum thapsiforme*, *Verbascum thapsus*, *Verbascum undulatum*, white mullein, wild ice, wild ice leaf, woollen, wooly mullein, wooly mullin.
- **Note:** The common name *mullein* is associated with many different species. The following species are covered here: *Verbascum densiflorum*, *Verbascum fruticulosum*, *Verbascum lychnitis*, *Verbascum macrurum*, *Verbascum nigrum*, *Verbascum nobile*, *Verbascum phlomoides*, *Verbascum sinaiticum*, *Verbascum songaricum*, *Verbascum thapsiforme*, *Verbascum thapsus*, *Verbascum undulatum*.

BACKGROUND

- Mullein has been used in natural medicine for centuries and is among the oldest known medicinal plants. Mullein was brought to North America from Europe by settlers and was commonly used as a remedy for cough and diarrhea. It is found along roadsides, fields, and barren areas in the United States.
- Traditionally, a poultice made from mullein leaves has been applied to the skin to treat ulcers and hemorrhoids. Mullein is typically used for inflammation in various areas of the body. The most commonly reported use is for respiratory tract conditions such as bronchitis and asthma, and also for ear pain associated with earaches. The proposed mechanism of action is by reducing the amount of mucus formation and as an expectorant.
- Currently, there are no available scientific studies (animal or human) that examine the efficacy of mullein alone. As of July 2006, the U.S. Food and Drug Administration (FDA) reported that mullein flowers (*Verbascum phlomoides* L. or *Verbascum thapsiforme* Schrad.) are likely safe for use as natural flavoring substances and natural adjuvants in food in small amounts. However, mullein is categorized as a food additive for which a petition has been filed and a regulation issued. Further research is required before any recommendations can be made.

EVIDENCE

Uses Based on Scientific Evidence	Grade
Earache (Associated with Acute Otitis Media) There are some clinical studies using mullein *(Verbascum thapsus)* in combination with other herbal	C

products as an eardrop to treat otitis media. It is not clear what effect that mullein alone has on otitis media, as the product studied was a combination of different herbal products.

Uses Based on Tradition or Theory

Analgesic, antibacterial, anticancer, antihistamine, anti-inflammatory, antioxidant, antiseptic, antispasmodic, antitumor, antiviral, asthma, astringent, bronchitis, catarrh, colds, convulsions, cough (spasmodic), cramps, cystitis, deafness (prevention of), demulcent (soothes irritated tissue), diarrhea, diuretic, eczema (of the ear), estrogenic effects, expectorant, fungicide, hay fever, headache, hemorrhoids, herpes, hoarseness, influenza, nephritis (inflammation of the kidney), neuralgia (nerve pain), orchitis (inflammation of the testicle), pain relief (anodyne), pulmonary problems, pyelitis (inflammation of the renal pelvis), rheumatism, sedative, sore throat, sunburn, toothache, tuberculosis, ulcers, urinary irritation, warts, wound healing.

DOSING
Adults (18 Years and Older)

- There is insufficient evidence to recommend a dose for mullein in adults.

Children (Younger than 18 Years)

- There is insufficient evidence to recommend a dose for mullein, and use in children is not recommended.

SAFETY
Allergies

- Avoid in people with a known allergy or hypersensitivity to mullein *(Verbascum thapsus)*.

Side Effects and Warnings

- There is a discrepancy in the literature regarding the U.S. Food and Drug Administration's (FDA's) stance on the safety of mullein. As of July 2006, the FDA reported that mullein flowers (*Verbascum phlomoides* L. or *Verbascum thapsiforme* Schrad.) are likely safe for use as natural flavoring substances and natural adjuvants in food in small amounts. However, mullein is categorized as a food additive for which a petition has been filed and a regulation issued.
- There are reports of mullein containing coumarin derivatives, which may cause liver toxicity. This adverse effect, however, cannot be confirmed by current scientific research. There are also reports that mullein contains a sapotoxin called *rotenone*, which is an insecticide, but again human scientific evidence is lacking. Nonetheless, use cautiously in patients taking anticoagulants due to a theoretical additive effect from coumarins that may be contained in mullein.

Pregnancy and Breastfeeding

- Mullein is not recommended in pregnant or breastfeeding women due to a lack of available scientific evidence.

INTERACTIONS

Interactions with Drugs

- Mullein may contain coumarin and may increase the risk of bleeding when taken with drugs that increase the risk of bleeding. Some examples include aspirin, anticoagulants (blood thinners) such as warfarin (Coumadin) or heparin, antiplatelet drugs such as clopidogrel (Plavix), and non-steroidal anti-inflammatory drugs such as ibuprofen (Motrin, Advil) or naproxen (Naprosyn, Aleve).

Interactions with Herbs and Dietary Supplements

- Mullein may contain coumarin and may increase the risk of bleeding when taken with herbs and supplements that are believed to increase the risk of bleeding. Multiple cases of bleeding have been reported with the use of *Ginkgo biloba* and fewer cases with garlic and saw palmetto. Numerous other agents may theoretically increase the risk of bleeding, although this has not been proven in most cases.

For a complete list of references, please visit www.naturalstandard.com.

M

Neem
(Azadirachta indica)

RELATED TERMS

- *Azadirachta indica, Azadirachta indica* ADR, *Azadirachta indica* A. juss, azadirachtin, azadirachtin A, bead tree, beta-sitosterol, Bioneem, dogonyaro, holy tree, immobile, Indian lilac, isomeldenin, limonoids, margosa, margosa oil, Meliaceae (family), Neemix, neem flowers, neem-based pesticide, neem kernel powder (NP), neem leaf alcoholic extract (NLE), neem oil, neem seed kernel, neem seed oil, Nim, NIM-76, nimba, nimbandiol, nimbin, nimbinene, nimocinol, Persian lilac, Praneem polyherbal cream, Pride of China, quercetin, village of pharmacy.

BACKGROUND

- Neem has a long history of use in India. The leaf and bark extracts were recommended by herbal practitioners for gastrointestinal upsets, skin ulcers, infections, and malaria. Neem twigs were used regularly as toothbrushes, and the leaf gel was used to fight periodontal disease (inflammatory disease of the gum).

- The extracts from neem often have a pungent smell similar to garlic. This is because they contain sulfurous compounds. Neem has been reported to reduce plaque formation, act as a mosquito repellent, treat psoriasis vulgaris (chronic skin disease with reddened lesions covered by silvery scales), and aid in the healing of gastroduodenal ulcers. However, there is currently insufficient evidence to recommend these uses. In the United States, neem is used mainly for its antibacterial, antifungal, insect repellent, contraceptive, and hypothetical "life extension" qualities.

EVIDENCE

Uses Based on Scientific Evidence	Grade
Dental Plaque (Oral Bacteria) Neem has been found to have anti-plaque properties and antimicrobial activity against oral pathogens. Comparisons of neem to the prescription drug chlorhexidine have reported significant results. Further clinical evidence is needed.	C
Mosquito Repellent Neem oil and neem cream have showed protective effects against mosquito bites from various species. However, compared to other mosquito repellents, the comparative effectiveness of neem is unclear.	C
Psoriasis Vulgaris Limited human data is available, and early research suggests no benefit. Therefore, there is insufficient evidence to recommend the use of neem for the treatment of psoriasis vulgaris (chronic skin disease).	C

Ulcers (Gastroduodenal) Protective and healing effects on gastroduodenal ulcers have been reported in a preliminary human study. However, comparisons to other agents used for this purpose such as proton pump inhibitors or H2-antagonsits have not been conducted. Therefore, there is insufficient evidence to recommend the use of neem for gastroduodenal ulcers.	C

Uses Based on Tradition or Theory

Abortion, analgesic (pain reliever), antibacterial, antifertility, antifungal, anti-inflammatory, antimalarial, antimicrobial, antimutagenic, antiparasitic, antipyretic (fever-reducing), astringent, athlete's foot, cancer, cardiac arrhythmia (irregular heartbeat), cardiovascular disease (heart disease), colds/flu, conjunctivitis (pink-eye), contraception (before and/or after sexual intercourse), coronary artery disease, cystic fibrosis, diabetes, diarrhea, enhanced immune function, fever, gastric cancer, gastric ulcers (Type 2 diabetes–induced), gingivitis, glioblastoma (malignant brain tumor), human immunodeficiency virus/acquired immunodeficiency syndrome, hormonal effects (anti-androgen), hyperlipidemia (high cholesterol), hypertension (high blood pressure), insecticide (molluscicidal, nematicidal), insect repellent (sand fly), lice, life extension, liver protection, melanoma, periodontal disease (gum disease), polio virus, respiratory disorders, Reye's syndrome, scabies, sedative, sexually transmitted diseases (STDs), skin diseases, tonic, ulcers (chronic), virus (Dengue).

DOSING
Adults (18 Years and Older)

- There is insufficient evidence to recommend a dose for neem. The bark extract in a dose of 30-60 mg twice daily for 10 weeks by mouth has been used to treat gastroduodenal ulcers. A gel formulation containing neem extract twice a day, before bed and after breakfast, for 6 weeks has been used in the treatment of plaque and gingival condition. Neem cream or oil (2%-5% neem oil) has shown protective effects against mosquito bites.

Children (Younger than 18 Years)

- There is insufficient evidence to recommend a dose for neem in children, and use is not recommended.

SAFETY
Allergies

- Avoid in people with a known allergy or hypersensitivity to neem *(Azadirachta indica)*.

Side Effects and Warnings

- There are few scientific reports about the safety of the above-ground parts of neem. Nonetheless, several cases of death in children from neem oil poisoning have been reported. Other symptoms present in these children included vomiting, drowsiness, loose stools, metabolic acidosis, anemia, Reye-like syndrome, altered sensation and consciousness, seizures, decreased responsiveness, and liver enzyme increases with evidence of liver damage.

- Taking neem bark extract by mouth for up to 10 weeks appears well tolerated in adults, as well as neem leaf extract gel for use within the mouth for up to 6 weeks. A 5% neem cream or 0.5%-2% neem oil is also likely safe when applied on the skin as an insect repellent for up to 2 weeks.
- Ventricular fibrillation and cardiac arrest due to neem leaf poisoning has been reported. Neem leaf extract may also cause bradycardia (slowed heart rate), heart rate abnormalities, or low blood pressure.
- Although not well studied in humans, neem may cause increases in ammonia levels in the body or decreases in blood sugar. High concentrations of neem leaf extract may be inhibitory to thyroid function, particularly conversion of T3 and T4. Injections of neem oil may cause damage to the uterus and surrounding glands, mild transient eosinophilia (increased levels of white blood cells), and non-specific endometritis (inflammation of the lining of the uterus).
- Margosa oil causes toxic encephalopathy (degenerative brain disease), particularly in infants and young children. Drowsiness, seizures, lethargy, and extreme exhaustion followed with coma/hyporeactivity are also possible. Use cautiously in patients with liver disease.

Pregnancy and Breastfeeding

- Neem is not recommended in pregnant or breastfeeding women due to possible abortifacient (abortion-inducing) and anti-implantation effects observed in animal studies. However, teratogenic (causing malformations or defects to an embryo or fetus) effects have not been reported in animals.

INTERACTIONS
Interactions with Drugs

- Concomitant use of acetaminophen (Tylenol) and neem leaf extract may cause liver toxicity. Caution is advised in patients taking other agents that may cause liver toxicity.
- Due to possible hypotensive (blood pressure–lowering) effects, neem should be used cautiously with other hypotensive agents.
- Neem leaf extract may inhibit the clastogenic activity of cyclophosphamide (Cytoxan) and mitomycin C. Patients taking chemotherapy agents should use neem with caution.
- Neem may interfere with the way the body processes certain drugs using the liver's cytochrome P450 enzyme system. Neem has synergistic activity with dillapiol,

a cytochrome P450 3A4 inhibitor. Theoretically, neem may have synergistic activity with other cytochrome P450 3A4 inhibitors. Patients using any medications should check the package insert and speak with a qualified health care professional, including a pharmacist, about possible interactions.

- The combination of a low dose of neem leaf extract and a low dose of morphine produced an increased loss of pain sensation. Theoretically, neem and some opiate analgesics (pain relievers) may work together (synergistically) for a positive interaction, although a qualified health care professional, including a pharmacist, should be consulted before combining therapies.
- Neem may lower blood sugar levels. Caution is advised when using medications that may also lower blood sugar levels. Patients taking drugs for diabetes by mouth or insulin should be monitored closely by a qualified health care professional, including a pharmacist. Medication adjustments may be necessary.
- The use of neem extract and quinine hydrochloride has been reported to have positive (synergistic) effects in the spermicidal activity of these agents. Quinines are often used in the treatment of malaria.

Interactions with Herbs and Dietary Supplements

- Neem may lower blood sugar levels. Caution is advised in patients with diabetes (high blood sugar) or hypoglycemia (low blood sugar), and in those taking herbs or supplements that may also lower blood sugar levels. Serum glucose levels may need to be monitored by a health care provider, and medication adjustments may be necessary. Blood glucose levels may require monitoring, and doses may need adjustment.
- Neem may interfere with the way the body processes certain herbs or supplements using the liver's cytochrome P450 enzyme system. Neem has synergistic activity with dillapiol, a cytochrome P450 3A4 inhibitor. Theoretically, neem may have synergistic activity with other cytochrome P450 3A4 inhibitors. Patients using any medications should check the package insert and speak with a qualified health care professional, including a pharmacist, about possible interactions.
- Administration of garlic and neem leaf extracts may decrease the formation of lipid peroxides and enhance the levels of antioxidants and detoxifying enzymes in the stomach, as well as in the liver and circulation.
- Due to possible hypotensive (blood pressure–lowering) effects, neem should be used cautiously with other hypotensive herbs and supplements.

For a complete list of references, please visit www.naturalstandard.com.

Niacin

(Vitamin B$_3$, Nicotinic acid, Niacinamide)

RELATED TERMS

- 3-Pyridine carboxamide, anti-blacktongue factor, antipellagra factor, B-complex vitamin, benicot, Efacin, ENDUR-ACIN, Enduramide, Hexopal, NIAC, Niacor, Niaspan, Nicalex, nicamid, Nicamin, Nico-400, Nicobid, Nicolar, Nicotinex, nicosedine, Nico-Span, nicotinamide, nicotinic acid amide, nicotinic amide, nicotylamidum, Papulex, pellagra preventing factor, Slo-Niacin, Tega-Span, Tri-B3, Wampocap.

BACKGROUND

- Vitamin B$_3$ is made up of niacin (nicotinic acid) and its amide, niacinamide, and can be found in many foods, including yeast, meat, fish, milk, eggs, green vegetables, and cereal grains. Dietary tryptophan is also converted to niacin in the body. Vitamin B$_3$ is often found in combination with other B vitamins, including thiamine, riboflavin, pantothenic acid, pyridoxine, cyanocobalamin, and folic acid.

EVIDENCE

Uses Based on Scientific Evidence	Grade
High Cholesterol (Niacin) Niacin is a well-accepted treatment for high cholesterol. Multiple studies show that niacin (not niacinamide) has significant benefits on levels of high-density cholesterol (HDL or "good cholesterol"), with better results than prescription drugs such as statins like atorvastatin (Lipitor). There are also benefits on levels of low-density lipoprotein (LDL) cholesterol (also known as "bad cholesterol"), although these effects are less dramatic. Adding niacin to a second drug such as a statin may increase the effects on LDL cholesterol. 　The use of niacin for treating dyslipidemia associated with type 2 diabetes has been controversial because of the possibility of worsening glycemic control. Patients should check with a physician and pharmacist before starting niacin.	A
Pellagra (Niacin) Niacin (vitamin B$_3$) and niacinamide are FDA-approved for the treatment of niacin deficiency. Pellagra is a nutritional disease that develops from insufficient dietary amounts of vitamin B$_3$ or the chemical it is made from, tryptophan. Symptoms of pellagra include skin disease, diarrhea, dementia, and depression.	A
Atherosclerosis (Niacin) Niacin decreases blood levels of cholesterol and lipoprotein-a, which may reduce the risk of atherosclerosis ("hardening" of the arteries). However, niacin also can increase homocysteine levels, which may have the opposite effect. Overall, the scientific evidence supports the use of niacin in combination with other drugs (but not alone) to decrease cholesterol and slow the process of atherosclerosis.	B
Prevention of a Second Heart Attack (Niacin) Niacin decreases levels of cholesterol, lipoprotein-a, and fibrinogen, which can reduce the risk of heart disease. However, niacin also increases homocysteine levels, which can increase this risk. Numerous studies have looked at the effects of niacin, alone and in combination with other drugs, for the prevention of heart disease and fatal heart attacks. Overall, this research suggests benefits of niacin, especially when combined with other cholesterol-lowering drugs.	B
Alzheimer's Disease/Cognitive Decline Dementia can be caused by severe niacin insufficiency, but it is unclear whether variation in intake of niacin in the usual diet is linked to neurodegenerative decline or Alzheimer's disease (AD).	C
Osteoarthritis (Niacinamide) Preliminary human studies suggest that niacinamide may be useful in the treatment of osteoarthritis. However, the available evidence is not sufficient to support this use.	C

Uses Based on Tradition or Theory

Acne, age-related macular degeneration, alcohol dependence, anti-aging, anxiety, arthritis, Bell's palsy, blood circulation improvement, blood vessel spasms, bone marrow damage from chemotherapy, cancer prevention, cataract prevention, central nervous system disorders, cholera, chronic diarrhea, confusion, coronary heart disease (CHD), depression, diagnostic test for schizophrenia, digestion improvement, drug-induced hallucinations, ear ringing, edema, glucose intolerance, hearing loss, high blood pressure, human immunodeficiency virus prevention, hypothyroidism (reduced thyroid function), insomnia, intermittent claudication (painful legs from clogged arteries), ischemia-reperfusion injury prevention, kava-related skin disorders, leprosy, liver disease, low blood sugar, memory loss, Ménière's syndrome, migraine headache, motion sickness, multiple sclerosis, orgasm improvement, painful menstruation, peripheral vascular disease, photosensitivity, pregnancy problems, premenstrual headache prevention, premenstrual syndrome, prostate cancer, psoriasis, psychosis, Raynaud's phenomenon, schizophrenia, scleroderma, sedative, seizure, skin disorders, smoking cessation, stomach ulcer, tardive dyskinesia, taste disturbances (diminished/distorted sense of taste), tuberculosis, tumor detection, vertigo.

DOSING

Adults (18 Years and Older)

- Taking niacin with food may reduce stomach upset and the risk of stomach ulcer. Doses are usually started low and gradually increased to minimize the common side effect of skin flushing. Taking aspirin or nonsteroidal anti-inflammatory drugs (NSAIDs) at the same time during the first 1-2 weeks may reduce this flushing. Use of an antihistamine 15 minutes prior to a niacin dose may also be helpful. The flushing response may decrease on its own after 1-2 weeks of therapy. Extended release niacin products may cause less flushing than immediate release (crystalline) formulations but may have a higher risk of stomach upset or liver irritation. In general, not all niacin products are equivalent. Patients switching from one product to another may have an increase or decrease in side effects.

- The dietary reference intake established by the Food and Nutrition Board for niacin (in the form of niacin equivalents, 1 mg niacin = 60 mg tryptophan) ranges from 16-18 mg daily for adults, with a maximum intake of 35 mg daily. 50 mg-6 g has been taken in divided doses for other conditions based on physician and pharmacist recommendations.

Children (Younger than 18 Years)

- There is insufficient evidence to recommend the safe use of niacin or niacinamide in children. Niacinamide has been studied in children at daily doses of 150-300 mg per year of the child's age, or 25 mg/kg daily, for the prevention of type 1 diabetes mellitus in high-risk people. No serious side effects have been reported, although safety and effectiveness are not clear. Patients should speak with a qualified health care provider if considering this therapy.

SAFETY
Allergies

- Rarely, anaphylactic shock (severe allergic reaction) has been described after intravenous or oral niacin therapy.

Side Effects and Warnings

- Most people taking niacin experience skin flushing and a warm sensation, especially of the face, neck, and ears when they begin treatment or increase the dose. This reaction is usually mild but has been intolerable enough to cause up to half of participants in studies to stop therapy. Dry skin and itching is also commonly experienced. Taking aspirin or nonsteroidal anti-inflammatory drugs such as ibuprofen (Advil, Motrin), naproxen (Naprosyn), or indomethacin (Indocin) can reduce the flushing. Use of an antihistamine 15 minutes prior to a niacin dose may also be helpful. Slow-release niacin products may have less skin flushing than regular-release niacin preparations or may simply delay the appearance of flushing. The flushing response often decreases on its own after 1-2 weeks of therapy. Mild stomach upset, nausea, vomiting, and diarrhea also may occur when beginning niacin therapy and usually resolve with continued use.

- More serious side effects include liver toxicity, worsening of stomach ulcers, altered blood sugar or insulin levels, or altered uric acid concentrations. Numerous case reports describe liver toxicity, including increased liver enzyme levels in the blood, skin yellowing (jaundice), fluid in the abdomen (ascites), or liver failure. Monitoring of liver blood tests while using niacin is recommended. While slow-release niacin products may have less skin flushing than regular-release niacin preparations, they may worsen stomach and liver side effects. High doses of niacin may also cause low blood pressure.

- Lactic acidosis, muscle cell damage (myopathy), and increased blood levels of creatine kinase (a marker of muscle damage) have been reported in studies.

- Abnormal heart rhythms and heart palpitations have occurred in niacin studies. Based on human research, taking niacin alone or with colestipol may increase blood homocysteine levels. High levels of homocysteine have been associated with an increased risk of heart disease.

- Blood clotting problems have been reported during treatment with sustained-release niacin. Low white blood cell number (leukopenia) and slightly increased blood eosinophils have also been reported.

- Rarely reported side effects include headache, tooth or gum pain, dizziness, breathing difficulty, increased anxiety, panic attacks, and decreased thyroid function (hypothyroidism). There are published accounts of temporary side effects of the eye, including macular swelling and blurred vision as well as toxic amblyopia ("lazy eye"). These side effects resolved when niacin was stopped.

Pregnancy and Breastfeeding

- Use of niacin supplementation during pregnancy or breastfeeding is not recommended due to lack of sufficient research of safety and effectiveness.

INTERACTIONS
Interactions with Drugs

- In theory, there may be an increased risk of liver damage if niacin is taken with alcohol or drugs that are toxic to the liver. Niacin-induced flushing may be increased by simultaneous use of alcohol and nicotine.

- Based on human study, use of niacin with cholesterol-lowering drugs such as statins (3-hydroxy-3-methylglutaryl coenzyme A [HMG-CoA] reductase inhibitors), including lovastatin (Mevacor) or atorvastatin (Lipitor); bile acid sequestrants like cholestyramine; probucol; or antilipid agents like gemfibrozil may result in further reductions in cholesterol than caused by either agent alone. However, bile acid sequestrants cholestyramine and colestipol may reduce niacin absorption into the body. Use of niacin with HMG-CoA reductase inhibitors or gemfibrozil may increase the risk of serious side effects such as liver or muscle damage.

- Based on human research, niacin may increase blood sugar levels and may require dosing adjustments of insulin or prescription diabetes drugs. Caution is advised when using medications that may affect blood sugar levels.

- Antibiotics can lead to decreased amounts of B vitamins in the body. Conversely, based on animal research, pyrazinamide may increase niacin levels. Use of niacin with neomycin may add to the cholesterol-lowering effects of niacin. Based on laboratory research, niacinamide may interact with the antifungal drug griseofulvin (increases its solubility), with possible effects on its activity.

- In theory, niacin therapy may increase the risk of bleeding. There are published case reports of patients who developed reversible abnormal blood clotting (coagulopathy) conditions while taking sustained-release niacin. In addition, low blood platelet number (thrombocytopenia) has been observed in studies of niacin therapy. Some examples of drugs that may increase the risk of bleeding if taken with niacin include aspirin, and anticoagulants (blood thinners) such as warfarin (Coumadin).

N

- Based on animal research, use of niacinamide with seizure medications like diazepam (Valium), carbamazepine (Tegretol), or sodium valproate (Depakote) may increase their antiseizure action. In laboratory studies, niacinamide has interacted with diazepam (increases its solubility), with uncertain overall effects. If taken with blood pressure–lowering drugs, niacinamide may cause a greater lowering of blood pressure.
- Based on human research, niacin may alter thyroid hormones and thus may require dosing adjustment of thyroid medications. Based on laboratory research, niacinamide may interact with testosterone, estrogen, or progesterone. Use of birth control pills may increase the amount of niacin produced in the body, thus lowering the doses of niacin needed for treatment.

Interactions with Herbs and Dietary Supplements

- In theory, use of niacin or niacinamide with herbs or supplements that have potential to cause liver injury may cause greater risk of liver toxicity.
- Use of aspirin has been shown to reduce the tingling, itching, flushing, and warmth associated with oral niacin administration, an effect that may also result from use of possible salicylate-containing herbs like black cohosh, meadowsweet, poplar, sweet birch, willow bark, and wintergreen. However, levels of salicylates in herbs may vary or be too low to have this desired effect.
- Niacin may add to the effects of herbs that may lower blood cholesterol levels, including fish oil, garlic, or guggal. Based on human research, taking such combinations as chromium polynicotinate (niacin-bound chromium) with grape seed proanthocyanidin, or niacin with beta-sitosterol and dihydrositosterol, may result in greater improvements in cholesterol than either agent alone.
- Antioxidants may reduce niacin's beneficial effects on cholesterol levels and heart disease, possibly by interfering with niacin's effects on high-density cholesterol (HDL). Recent research suggests that the addition of antioxidants to a combination of niacin plus simvastatin (Zocor) reduced the benefit of niacin on heart blood vessel plaques, suggesting possible interference by antioxidants. In other research, use of niacin with vitamin A and vitamin E had greater effects on cholesterol levels than niacin alone. Vitamin E in combination with colestipol and niacin has also been associated with greater benefits on heart blood vessel plaques. This remains an area of controversy.
- Based on human research, niacin may increase blood sugar levels and may require dosing adjustments of hypoglycemic agents. In a study with children, use of niacinamide and insulin together has been shown to lead to a reduction in insulin dosage in patients with type 1 diabetes mellitus. Caution is advised when using herbs or supplements that may affect blood sugar levels.
- In theory, niacin therapy may increase risk of bleeding when taken with herbs and supplements that are believed to increase the risk of bleeding. There are published case reports of patients who developed reversible abnormal blood clotting (coagulopathy) conditions while taking sustained-release niacin. In addition, low blood platelet number (thrombocytopenia) has been observed in studies of niacin therapy. Multiple cases of bleeding have been reported with the use of *Ginkgo biloba*, and fewer cases with garlic or saw palmetto.
- Based on laboratory research, niacinamide may interact with herbs or supplements with estrogen-like properties and theoretically may increase the amount of niacin produced in the body (thus lowering the doses of niacin needed for treatment).
- Based on human research, niacin may interact with thyroid-active herbs or supplements such as bladderwrack and may alter thyroid hormone blood tests. Preliminary human research reports that zinc sulfate increases the amount of niacin breakdown products in the urine, suggesting a possible interaction between the two agents.

Interactions with Foods

- Hot beverages, when taken with niacin, may worsen niacin-induced skin flushing.

For a complete list of references, please visit www.naturalstandard.com.

Noni
(*Morinda citrifolia*)

RELATED TERMS

- Al, alizarin, alkaloids, americanin A, amino acids, anthraquinone, anthraquinone glycoside, asperuloside, asperulosidic acid, atchy (Hindi), beta-sitosterol, borreriagenin, cada pilva (Malay), caproic acid, caprylic acid, carotene, citrifolinin B epimer a, citrifolinin B epimer b, citrifolinoside, cytidine, deacetylasperuloside, dehydromethoxygaertneroside, d-glucose, dilo'k (Pijin), d-mannitol, epi-dihydrocornin, flavone glycosides, Indian mulberry, iridoid glycoside, kura (Fijian), kuti, ladda (Chamorro), L-asperuloside, linoleic acid, maddichettoo (Telugu), manja-pavattay, methyl alpha-D-fructofuranoside, methyl beta-D-fructofuranoside, molagha, *Morinda citrifolia*, morindacin, morindone, murier d'Inde, najalanun, nakura, narcissoside, nen (Chamorro), nicotifloroside, nolom, nono (Cook Islands Maori), nonu (Tongan, Wallisian, Futunian, Niuean, Tokelauan, Tuvaluan), nonu togi (Samoan), noona (Tamil), nordamnacanthal, nowoi (Bislama), octanoic acid, potassium, riro (Tok Pisin), proxeronine, Rubiaceae (family), rubiadin, rutin, scopoletin, te non (Gilbertese), terpenoids, TNJ, ursolic acid, vitamin A, vitamin C, yelotri.

BACKGROUND

- Noni (*Morinda citrifolia*) is a traditional folk medicinal plant that has been used for over 2,000 years in Polynesia. Traditionally, Polynesians had many medicinal uses for noni, including for fevers, headaches, malaria, bone fractures, dislocations, gastrointestinal disorders, urinary ailments, worms, wounds, rheumatism, and hypertension (high blood pressure). All parts of the noni plant were utilized.
- Although noni is a popular supplement, few clinical trials have been conducted on its uses. There is preliminary research supporting noni's popular use as an antioxidant, but more research is needed in this area to establish noni's effects.
- Based on scientific analysis and review of Tahitian Noni juice, the European Commission Health and Consumer Protection Directorate–General Scientific Committee on Food found that "although some nutritional benefits are claimed for *Morinda citrifolia* L. products, the data supplied and the information available to the Committee provided no evidence for special nutritional benefits of Tahitian Noni juice which go beyond those of other fruit juices."

EVIDENCE

Uses Based on Scientific Evidence	Grade
Antioxidant Laboratory studies indicated that Tahitian Noni juice (TNJ) may have greater antioxidant activity than some commonly used antioxidants. Although human research suggests that TNJ does have antioxidant effects, whether TNJ protects smokers from oxidative damage is yet to be proven.	C

Hearing Loss	C
Noni juice has been used for many years for a wide variety of indications in Southeast Asia, and noni juice may improve hearing in people with auditory dysfunction. Although results are promising, additional research is warranted.	

Uses Based on Tradition or Theory

Abscesses, addictions, allergies, analgesic (pain reliever), anthelminthic (kills intestinal/parasitic worms), antibacterial, antifungal, anti-inflammatory, antiviral, appetite stimulant, arthritis, asthma, atherosclerosis (hardened arteries), attention deficit and hyperactivity disorder (ADHD), boils, bone fractures, brain injuries, broken bones, bruises, burns, cancer, carbuncles (clusters of boils on the skin), cardiovascular disease, chemical sensitivities, chronic fatigue syndrome, chronic pain, colds, constipation, cuts, depression, diabetes, diarrhea, digestive problems, joint disorders (dislocation), ear infections, endometriosis (growth of endometrial tissue outside the uterus), energy, fever, fibromyalgia, food uses, gastric ulcers, gout (foot inflammation), headache, hemorrhoids, hernia, hypertension (high blood pressure), immune deficiency, infections, inflammation, inflammatory conditions, influenza, insect repellent, itching, intestinal worms, jaundice, jet lag, joint pain, laxative, lice, malaria, menstrual problems, mouth infections, multiple sclerosis, muscle aches, muscle pain, pregnancy (pain), rheumatism, scabies, senility, sinus disorders, sore throat, sores, sprains, sties, stiffness, stimulant (brain), stings (stonefish), stomachache, swelling (abdominal), toothaches, tuberculosis, ulcers, urinary tract disorders, vascular problems, veterinary medicine, viral infections (polio), vitamin A deficiency, weight loss, wounds.

DOSING
Adults (18 Years and Older)

- There is insufficient evidence to recommend a dose for noni in adults. However, 1 oz every 12 hours has been used. As an antioxidant 2 oz of Tahitian Noni juice twice daily for 30 days has been used; for hearing loss, 2 oz of noni juice twice daily (morning and evening) for 3 months has been used.
- Noni is likely safe when taken orally from preparations of fruits and leaves of the noni plant or when 10 g of ripe noni fruit extract is taken daily for up to 28 days. Noni is possibly unsafe when 10 g of ripe noni fruit extract is taken daily for more than 28 days.

Children (Younger than 18 Years)

- There is insufficient evidence to recommend a dose for noni in children.

SAFETY
Allergies

- Avoid in people with a known allergy or hypersensitivity to noni or its constituents.

N

Side Effects and Warnings

- Overall, noni has had very few reported side effects. Although noni roots are known to contain liver-damaging anthraquinones, recent research indicates that noni fruit also contains anthraquinones.
- There is one report of acquired coumarin resistance caused by increased vitamin K intake through ingestion of a noni juice product. However, the product appeared to be vitamin K fortified and contained >115 components from several plants. (Note: Noni juice/fruit itself is not a source of vitamin K; it would therefore be unsubstantiated to draw any conclusions concerning a potential warfarin/coumarin interaction with noni from this case report).
- Noni juice may cause elevated lactate dehydrogenase and elevated transaminases.
- Potassium concentrations of the noni juice samples were found to be similar to potassium levels in orange and tomato juice. Patients with kidney disease may wish to avoid noni products. Effects in people with normal kidney function are not known.
- Use cautiously in patients with injuries or postsurgery, as noni may have antiangiogenic properties (prevent new vessel growth).
- Avoid in patients with gastrointestinal disorders, as noni may decrease gastric transit time.

Pregnancy and Breastfeeding

- Noni is not recommended in pregnant or breastfeeding women due to a lack of available scientific evidence.

INTERACTIONS
Interactions with Drugs

- Noni may decrease gastric transit time, and patients taking any medication by mouth should consult with a qualified health care professional, including a pharmacist, to check for any interactions.
- Based on laboratory studies, noni may prevent new vessel growth. Caution is advised when taking noni with other antiangiogenic agents.
- Although not well studied in humans, a vitamin K–fortified juice product containing noni and >115 components from several other plants may have caused acquired coumarin resistance. Noni juice/fruit itself is not a source for vitamin K. It is unlikely that noni would interact with anticoagulants (blood thinners), although caution is advised.

- Although not well studied in humans, noni roots and various noni root extracts may lower blood pressure. Noni has also shown anti-inflammatory properties and may interact with other agents with similar effects.
- Noni may be hepatotoxic, and caution is advised when combining with other potentially liver-damaging agents. Studies have been inconclusive in this area, and clinical significance is currently unknown.
- Noni may stimulate the immune system. It may have either no effect or suppressive effects on human immunodeficiency virus. When taking with immune-enhancing or HIV medications, additive effects may occur, although this is not yet well proven.

Interactions with Herbs and Dietary Supplements

- Noni may decrease gastric transit time, and patients taking any herb or supplement by mouth should consult with a qualified health care professional, including a pharmacist, to check for any interactions.
- Based on laboratory studies, noni may prevent new vessel growth. Caution is advised when taking noni with other antiangiogenic agents.
- Although not well studied in humans, a vitamin K–fortified juice product containing noni and >115 components from several other plants may have caused acquired coumarin resistance. Noni juice/fruit itself is not a source of vitamin K. It is unlikely that noni would interact with other herbs with blood-thinning effects, although caution is advised.
- Although not well studied in humans, noni roots and various noni root extracts may lower blood pressure. Noni has also shown anti-inflammatory properties and may interact with other agents with similar effects.
- Noni may be hepatotoxic, and caution is advised when combining it with other potentially liver-damaging agents. Studies have been inconclusive in this area, and clinical significance is currently unknown.
- Noni may stimulate the immune system. It may have either no effect or suppressive effects on human immunodeficiency virus. When taking with immune-enhancing or HIV medications, additive effects may occur, although this is not yet well proven.
- Noni contains 56 mEq/L of potassium. In theory, noni juice may interact with other agents with high potassium content, such as orange and tomato juice.

For a complete list of references, please visit www.naturalstandard.com.

Nopal
(*Opuntia* spp.)

RELATED TERMS

- Alpha-pyrone glycoside, barbary fig, betalains, betanin, Blanca Cristalina, Cactaceae (family), cactus flowers, daucosterol, (E)-ferulic acid, Esmeralda, gracemere-pear, indicaxanthin, Naranjona, nopal cactus, nopal flour, nopales, nopalito, nopalitos, nopals, nopol, *Opuntia*, *Opuntia basilaris* (beavertail cactus), *Opuntia chlorotica* (pancake prickly pear), *Opuntia compressa* var. *humifusa* (eastern prickly pear), *Opuntia dillenii*, *Opuntia ectodermis*, *Opuntia elator*, *Opuntia engelmannii* (calico cactus, Engelmann prickly pear, Engelmann's pear), *Opuntia erinacea* (grizzly bear Opuntia, hedgehog prickly pear, porcupine prickly pear), *Opuntia ficus-indica* (Indian fig Opuntia), *Opuntia fragilis* (brittle cactus, little prickly pear), *Opuntia humifusa* (eastern prickly pear, low prickly pear, smooth prickly pear), *Opuntia hyptiacantha*, *Opuntia laevis*, *Opuntia lasciacantha*, *Opuntia leucotricha* (arborescent prickly pear, Aaron's beard cactus, duraznillo blanco, nopal blanco, semaphore cactus), *Opuntia lindheimeri* (Texas prickly pear), *Opuntia littoralis* (sprawling prickly pear), *Opuntia macrocentra* (black spine prickly pear, purple prickly pear), *Opuntia macrorhiza* (plains prickly pear, tuberous prickly pear), *Opuntia megacantha*, *Opuntia microdasys* (bunny ears), *Opuntia phaeacantha* (brown-spinded prickly pear, New Mexico prickly pear, purple-fruited prickly pear), *Opuntia polyacantha* (plains prickly pear), *Opuntia puberula*, *Opuntia pusilla* (creeping cactus), *Opuntia robusta*, *Opuntia rufida* (blind prickly pear), *Opuntia santa-rita* (Santa Rita prickly pear), *Opuntia spinosbacca* (spiny-fruited prickly pear), *Opuntia stricta* (coastal prickly pear, spineless prickly pear), *Opuntia strigil* (bearded prickly pear), *Opuntia velutina*, *Opuntia violacea* (purple prickly pear, Santa Rita prickly pear), opuntioside, opuntioside-I, penca, polyphenols, prickle pear cactus, prickly pear cactus, Sicilian cactus pear, tuna, tuna cardona, westwood-pear.

BACKGROUND

- Traditionally, nopal (also known as prickly pear cactus) has both food and medicinal uses. Nopal is common in North American deserts and are generally sold fresh, canned, or dried for use in the preparation of nopalitos a traditional Mexican dish made from nopal pads. They have a light, tart flavor. Nopals are commonly used in Mexican and New Mexican cuisine in dishes such as huevos con nopales (eggs with nopal) or tacos de nopales. The juice is used in jellies and candies. The fruit is also eaten fresh or used in pies, deserts, shakes, or spreads.
- Nopal is medicinally used as an anti-inflammatory antidiabetic or a laxative. More recently, nopal has been used in exercise recovery and in reducing the symptoms of alcohol hangovers. Nopal is the most commonly used substance for lowering blood sugar among people of Mexican descent.
- Nopal may offer benefits to people with alcohol-induced hangover, diabetes, or hyperlipidemia (high cholesterol). However, additional research is needed.

EVIDENCE

Uses Based on Scientific Evidence	Grade
Alcohol-Induced Hangover People who consume alcohol to the point of intoxication often experience what is known as a hangover, which can result in fatigue, headache, dizziness, and a general unpleasant feeling. Nopal may have hangover preventative effects, although more studies are needed to confirm this finding.	C
Diabetes Diabetes is a chronic health condition in which the body is unable to produce insulin and properly break down sugar (glucose) in the blood. Symptoms may include hunger, thirst, excessive urination, dehydration, and weight loss. Scientific studies suggest that nopal may decrease blood glucose levels in patients with type 2 diabetes.	C
Hyperlipidemia (High Cholesterol) Hyperlipidemia is described as excess levels of fats in the blood. Nopal may aid in reducing hyperlipidemia, although there is currently insufficient evidence to support this use.	C

Uses Based on Tradition or Theory

Acne, anti-inflammatory, antioxidant, antiviral, arthritis, astringent, benign prostate hypertrophy (enlarged prostate), burns, cardiovascular health, chest congestion, colitis, cuts, diarrhea, diuretic, exercise recovery, eye problems, hair tonic, hepatoprotection (liver protection), hypercholesterolemia (high blood cholesterol), hyperglycemia (high blood sugar), hyperlipidemia (high cholesterol), hypertension (high blood pressure), immunosuppression, insect bites, ischemic injury, laxative, obesity, platelet aggregation, rash, scrapes, skin irritations, skin toner, sunburn, ulcers, weight loss, wound healing.

DOSING

Adults (18 Years and Older)

- There is insufficient evidence to recommend a dose for nopal in adults.

Children (Younger than 18 Years)

- There is insufficient evidence to recommend a dose for nopal in children.

SAFETY

Allergies

- Avoid in people with a known allergy or hypersensitivity to nopal. Nasal inflammation or asthma has been reported due to allergy.

Side Effects and Warnings

- Nopal is likely safe when used in food amounts, as nopal is common in Mexican and southwestern American cuisine.
- Side effects associated with nopal may include mild diarrhea, nausea, abdominal fullness, headache, and increase in stool volume and frequency.
- Use cautiously in patients with diabetes or hypoglycemia (low blood sugar), high cholesterol, low blood pressure, or thyroid dysfunction.
- Use cautiously in people with rhinitis or asthma, as nopal may worsen symptoms.
- Avoid in patients with immunosuppression, as nopal may suppress the immune system.
- Avoid in patients with impaired liver function, as nopal may increase liver toxicity.

Pregnancy and Breastfeeding

- Nopal is not recommended in pregnant or breastfeeding women due to a lack of available scientific evidence.

INTERACTIONS

Interactions with Drugs

- When mixed with water or other fluids, nopal forms a sticky, slippery gel. Taking nopal by mouth could block the absorption of drugs, other supplements, and nutrients from foods that are taken at the same time. Traditionally, patients are advised to not eat meals or take medication within 2 hours of consuming nopal by mouth.
- Nopal may act as an acid absorber. Use cautiously with anti-ulcer medications.
- Use of nopal and chloropropamide concomitantly may increase the hypoglycemic (blood sugar–lowering) effect and levels of insulin in patients with type 2 diabetes. Broiled nopal stems (not crude stems), nopal extract, or dietary cactus ingestion may lower blood sugar levels. Consult with a qualified health care professional, as dosing may need to be adjusted.
- Large doses of nopal may cause adverse effects on the liver and spleen.
- Nopal may decrease lipids (fats) in the blood. Use cautiously in patients taking cholesterol-lowering medications due to possible additive effects.
- Use cautiously with blood pressure–altering medications.
- Although not well studied in humans, nopal may also interact with thyroid agents.

Interactions with Herbs and Dietary Supplements

- When mixed with water or other fluids, nopal forms a sticky, slippery gel. Taking nopal by mouth could block the absorption of drugs, other supplements, and nutrients from foods that are taken at the same time. Traditionally, patients are advised to not eat meals or take medication within 2 hours of oral consumption of nopal.
- Large doses of nopal may cause adverse effects on the liver and spleen. Use cautiously with herbs and supplements that may have similar effects.
- Broiled nopal stems (not crude stems), nopal extract, or dietary cactus ingestion may lower blood sugar levels.
- Nopal may decrease lipids (fats) in the blood. Use cautiously with cholesterol-lowering herbs and supplements due to possible additive effects.
- Use cautiously with blood pressure–altering herbs and supplements due to possible additive effects.
- Although not well studied in humans, nopal may also interact with thyroid agents. Use cautiously with herbs or supplements with similar or contradictory effects.

For a complete list of references, please visit www.naturalstandard.com.

Nux Vomica
(*Strychnos nux-vomica*)

RELATED TERMS

- Arabinose, Brechnuss, Brechnusssamen, brucine, brucine N-oxide, galactan, galactomannan, galactose, Loganiaceae (family), loganic acid, ma qian zi, noce vomica, noix vomique, nuez vomica, poison nut, Quaker buttons, rhamnose, shudha kupilu, slang nut, strychni semen, strychnine, *Strychnos nux-vomica*, strychnos seed, vishamushti.

BACKGROUND

- Nux vomica is the dried, ripe seed of *Strychnos nux-vomica* L., a native tree of Burma, China, eastern India, Thailand, and northern Australia. There are reports of toxic effects with traditional use of the seeds or fruit of *Strychnos nux-vomica* L.
- In homeopathy, nux vomica is used for allergies, back pain, colds, constipation, digestive problems, emotional stress, flu, hangovers, headaches, hemorrhoids, and menstrual problems. Nux vomica is also a polycrest, or a homeopathic remedy used to treat many ailments. As a polycrest, nux vomica's primary indication is for disorders related to abuse of narcotic drugs, alcohol, coffee, or tobacco; overindulgence of rich food and beverages; and mental strain from excessive work.
- Although nux vomica appeared as a treatment in nineteenth century medical publications, there is very little documentation on its therapeutic effectiveness in the scientific literature. However, because nux vomica is a common homeopathic medicine, research continues despite a lack of pharmacological basis for homeopathic concentrations, mostly in laboratory and animal studies. This remedy is in the category of unapproved herbs according to the German Commission E.

EVIDENCE

Uses Based on Scientific Evidence

No available studies qualify for inclusion in the evidence table.

Uses Based on Tradition or Theory

Abscesses, aging, alcohol abuse, allergies, analgesic (pain reliever), anemia (secondary), anthelminthic (expels worms), antibacterial, anti-inflammatory, antioxidant, anxiety, appetite stimulant, back pain, bubonic plague, cancer, cardiovascular disorders, colds, constipation, depression, drug abuse, eating disorders, encephalopathy (glycine), expectorant, eye diseases, neuralgia (facial nerve pain), gastrointestinal disorders, gout, hangovers, headaches, hemorrhoids, hysteria, impotence, indigestion, influenza, insomnia, irritable bowel syndrome, liver cancer, menstrual problems, menopausal symptoms, migraine, muscle spasm, myasthenia gravis, nerve disorders (paresthesia), rabies, Raynaud's disease, Reiter's syndrome, respiratory ailments, rheumatism, stress (emotional), substance abuse (coffee), substance abuse (tobacco), tonic.

DOSING
Adults (18 Years and Older)

- There is insufficient evidence to recommend a dose for nux vomica. As pills or powders, 0.3-0.9 g daily has traditionally been used.
- Homeopathic preparations are the most commonly used form, and nux vomica comes in several dilutions, including 6X, 12X, 30X, and 30C. Traditionally, sublingual doses are taken one-half hour before or after eating, brushing teeth, or drinking anything but water.

Children (Younger than 18 Years)

- There is insufficient evidence to recommend a dose for nux vomica, and use in children is not recommended due to potential toxicity. In children, as little as 50 mg of seed may cause intoxication or death.

SAFETY
Allergies

- Avoid in people with a known allergy or hypersensitivity to *Strychnos nux-vomica*.

Side Effects and Warnings

- In general, nux vomica has predominantly neurological effects and may cause painful seizures, spasms, difficulty breathing, dizziness, and confusion. Other adverse effects include muscle cramps, pain, and tenderness.
- Chest discomfort, tonic contractions of all limb muscles, carpopedal spasm, muscle pain, numbness, hyperventilation, confusion, hyperreflexia, nystagmus (rapid movement of the eyes), knee-jerks, tiredness, and seizure have been reported after taking a multi-herb concoction containing nux vomica. Seizures can occur within 15 minutes of ingestion (or 5 minutes of inhalation) and may result in hyperthermia, metabolic and respiratory acidosis, rhabdomyolysis, and myoglobinuric renal (kidney) failure. *Strychonos nux-vomica* fruit may also cause crampy abdominal and leg pain and tense thigh muscles with tenderness to touch.
- Avoid taking nux vomica seeds by mouth, as the seeds may contain toxic amounts of strychnine. Use cautiously in other forms due to potential toxicity from strychnine in nux vomica. Also use cautiously in patients with seizure disorders, as nux vomica has induced seizures.

Pregnancy and Breastfeeding

- Nux vomica should not be taken during pregnancy or breastfeeding due to risk of ingestion of toxic levels of strychnine. No safe internal dosage or maximum duration of homeopathic nux vomica during pregnancy or breastfeeding has been clinically established.

INTERACTIONS
Interactions with Drugs

- Antipsychotics and phenothiazines are contraindicated in people with symptoms of poisoning, as they may compound the symptoms exhibited by the patient. Use is not recommended with nux vomica.

- Strychnine in nux vomica can accumulate in the liver with extended administration, and especially in those with liver damage. Patients taking drugs that are potentially damaging to the liver should consult with a qualified health care professional, including a pharmacist.

Interactions with Herbs and Dietary Supplements

- Strychnine in nux vomica can accumulate in the liver with extended administration, and especially in those with liver damage. Patients taking herbs and supplements that are potentially damaging to the liver, such as kava, should consult with a qualified health care professional, including a pharmacist.

For a complete list of references, please visit www.naturalstandard.com.

Octacosanol

$(C_{28}H_{58}O)$

RELATED TERMS

- 1-octacosanol, (3)H-octacosanol, cluytyl alcohol, montanyl alcohol, n-octacosanol, octacosanoic acid, policosanol, *Suregada angustifolia* (Baill. ex Muell. Arg.), very long chain fatty alcohols.

BACKGROUND

- Policosanol is a mixture of very long chain alcohols that is purified from sugar cane wax. Approximately 67% of policosanol is octacosanol. Although some research has been conducted using policosanol, little research is currently available that focuses on octacosanol alone. One preliminary clinical study in amyotrophic lateral sclerosis (ALS or Lou Gehrig's disease, a chronic, progressive, neurological disease in which loss of nerve cells produces muscle paralysis) patients showed no measurable benefit from octacosanol. As octacosanol is the main component of policosanol, more research is needed to determine if octacosanol is the primary active component of policosanol.

EVIDENCE

Uses Based on Scientific Evidence	Grade
Amyotrophic Lateral Sclerosis (ALS) Amyotropic lateral sclerosis (ALS), or Lou Gehrig's disease, is a chronic, progressive, neurological disease in which loss of nerve cells produces muscle paralysis. Preliminary research does not show any clear evidence of benefit in neurological (brain) or pulmonary (lung) symptoms of ALS patients.	D

Uses Based on Tradition or Theory
Adrenoleukodystrophy (ALD, a rapidly progressive X-linked genetic degenerative disorder), antibacterial, antioxidant, atherosclerosis (hardening of the arteries), cardiovascular health, coronary heart disease, fatigue, granuloma annulare (chronic skin condition), hyperlipidemia (high cholesterol), hypertension (high blood pressure), intermittent claudication (muscle pain), ischemic heart disease, liver damage from drugs or toxins, neurological disorders (Sjögren-Larsson syndrome), osteoporosis (postmenopausal), Parkinson's disease, platelet aggregation inhibition (blood disorder), reactivity/brain activity, seizure disorder, stroke prevention.

DOSING

Adults (18 Years and Older)

- There is insufficient evidence to recommend a dose for octacosanol in adults.

Children (Younger than 18 Years)

- There is insufficient evidence to recommend a dose for octacosanol in children.

SAFETY

Allergies

- Avoid in people with a known allergy or hypersensitivity to octacosanol or policosanol.

Side Effects and Warnings

- Octacosanol is the main component of policosanol. Little research is currently available on octacosanol alone. Therefore, the safety information is based on research conducted on policosanol.
- Use octacosanol cautiously in patients taking nitrates.
- Use cautiously in patients who are taking other lipid-lowering drugs/herbs (e.g., acipimox, statins, bile acid sequestrants/resins) and cholesterol absorption inhibitors (e.g., ezetimibe, fish oil, plant stanols/sterols, polyphenols) as well as nutraceuticals (e.g., oat bran, psyllium, and soy proteins) due to potential additive blood cholesterol–lowering effects.
- Use cautiously in patients taking aspirin due to potential additive platelet inhibition and risk of bleeding.
- Use cautiously when using with drugs that lower blood pressure due to potential additive effects.

Pregnancy and Breastfeeding

- Octacosanol is not recommended in pregnant or breast-feeding women due to a lack of available scientific evidence.

INTERACTIONS

Interactions with Drugs

- Although not well studied in humans, octacosanol (the main component of policosanol) may increase the risk of bleeding when taken with drugs that increase the risk of bleeding. Some examples include aspirin, anticoagulants (blood thinners) such as warfarin (Coumadin) or heparin, antiplatelet drugs such as clopidogrel (Plavix), and non-steroidal anti-inflammatory drugs (NSAIDs) such as ibuprofen (Motrin, Advil) or naproxen (Naprosyn, Aleve). Octacosanol may also interact with aspirin.
- Octacosanol may alter blood sugar levels. Caution is advised when using medications that may also alter blood sugar levels. Patients taking drugs for diabetes by mouth or insulin should be monitored closely by a qualified health care professional, including a pharmacist. Medication adjustments may be necessary.
- In theory, octacosanol (the main component of policosanol) may lower blood pressure. Caution is advised in patients taking blood pressure medications due to possible additive effects.
- Although not well studied in humans, octacosanol (the main component of policosanol) may lower cholesterol. Caution is advised in patients taking cholesterol medications due to possible additive effects.
- Octacosanol (the main component of policosanol) may decrease blood pressure and may interact with beta-blockers. It may also interact with nitrates, but the effects in humans are unclear.

O

- Octacosanol may also have liver-damaging effects. Caution is advised in patients with liver disorders or those taking liver medications.

Interactions with Herbs and Dietary Supplements

- Although not well studied in humans, octacosanol (the main component of policosanol) may increase the risk of bleeding when taken with herbs and supplements that are believed to increase the risk of bleeding. Multiple cases of bleeding have been reported with the use of *Ginkgo biloba*, and fewer cases with garlic and saw palmetto. Numerous other agents may theoretically increase the risk of bleeding, although this has not been proven in most cases.
- Octacosanol may alter blood sugar levels. Caution is advised when using herbs or supplements that may also alter blood sugar levels. Blood glucose levels may require monitoring, and doses may need adjustment.
- In theory, octacosanol may lower cholesterol. Caution is advised in patients taking cholesterol-altering herbs and supplements due to possible additive effects.
- Octacosanol may be liver damaging. Caution is advised in patients taking herbs and supplements that may also damage the liver and in patients with liver disorders.
- Octacosanol may also lower blood pressure. Caution is advised in patients taking other blood pressure–altering herbs or supplements due to possible additive effects.
- Taking policosanol (which includes octacosanol) and omega-3 fatty acids or willow bark may have additive cholesterol-lowering effects and may also alter blood clotting.

For a complete list of references, please visit www.naturalstandard.com.

Oleander

(Nerium oleander, Thevetia peruviana)

RELATED TERMS

- Adelfa, adynerin, ahouai (Antilles), ahousin, Anvirzel, Apocyanaceae (family), ashwahan, ashwamarak (Sanskrit), be-still nuts (Hawaiian), betulin, betulinic acid, boissaisi (Haitian), cardenolides, cardiac glycosides, cascaveleira (Brazilian), *Cerebra thevetia* (Indian), cerebrine, cerebrose, common oleander, corrigen, dehydroadynerigen, digit-oxigenin, dogbane, exile, folinerin, horse poison, joro-joro (Dutch Guiana), karavira, karier, kohilphin, kokilpal (Indian), L-thevetose, laurier blane (Haitian), laurier bol, laurier desjundins, laurier rose, lorier bol, lucky seed (Jamaican), neriantin, neridiginoside, neridlenone A, nerii-folin, neriine, nerin, nerioside, neritaloside, *Nerium indicum*, *Nerium odorum*, nerizoside, NOAG-II, odoroside H, oleanderblatter, *Oleandri folium*, oleandrigenin, oleandrin, oleandrinogen, oleandroside, oleanolic acid, olinerin, peruvoside, pila kaner (Indian), pink oleander, rosa francesa, rosagenin, rosebay, rose laurel, rosen lorbeer, ruvoside, soland, strospeside, *Thevetia nerifolia*, *Thevetia neriifolia*, thevetin A, thevetin B, thevetine, thevetoxin, triterpenes, white oleander, yee tho (Thai), yellow oleander.

BACKGROUND

- The term *oleander* refers to two plant species, *Nerium oleander* (common oleander) and *Thevetia peruviana* (yellow oleander), which grow in temperate climates throughout the world. Both species contain chemicals called *cardiac glycosides* that have effects similar to the heart drug digoxin. Both species can be toxic when taken by mouth with many documented reports of deaths.

EVIDENCE

Uses Based on Scientific Evidence	Grade
Cancer Laboratory studies of oleander suggest possible anti-cancer effects, although reliable research in humans is not currently available. There are reports that long-term use of oleander may have positive effects in patients with leiomyosarcoma, Ewing's sarcoma, prostate cancer, or breast cancer.	C
Congestive Heart Failure The term *oleander* refers to two plants: *Nerium oleander* (common oleander) and *Thevetia peruviana* (yellow oleander). Both plants contain heart-active "cardiac glycoside" chemicals (similar to the prescription drug digoxin) and have been associated with serious side effects in humans, including death. The plants have been used to treat heart failure in China and Russia for decades, but scientific evidence supporting use is limited to small, poorly designed studies. Human research began in the 1930s but was largely abandoned due to serious gastrointestinal and heart toxicity.	C

It should be noted that the drug digoxin may improve symptoms of congestive heart failure but does not improve mortality (length of life).

Uses Based on Tradition or Theory

Abnormal menstruation, alcoholism, antifertility, antiparasitic, asthma, bacterial infections, cachexia (weight loss/wasting from some diseases), cardiac abnormalities, cathartic, corns, diuretic (increase urine flow), dysmenorrhea (painful menstruation), epilepsy (seizure), eye diseases, heart disease, hemorrhoids, indigestion, inflammation, insecticide, leprosy, loss of appetite, malaria, neurological disorders, pregnancy termination, psoriasis, psychiatric disorders, rat poison, sinus problems, skin diseases, skin eruptions, snake bites, swelling, venereal disease, vomiting, warts, weight gain.

DOSING

Adults (18 Years and Older)

- Safety has not been established for any dose of oleander. Peruvoside, a heart-active substance in yellow oleander kernels (similar to the drug digoxin), has been studied at 1.8-3.2 mg by mouth, as an initial dose, followed by an average daily dose of 0.6 mg/day for congestive heart failure.

Children (Younger than 18 Years)

- Oleander is not recommended for use in children due to risk of toxicity or death and lack of scientific data.

SAFETY

Allergies

- People with allergy/hypersensitivity to oleander or other cardiac glycosides such as digoxin or digitoxin may have reactions to oleander. Skin contact with sap from oleander leaves may cause rash.

Side Effects and Warnings

- Common oleander contains a strychnine-like toxin and a heart-active cardiac glycoside substance (similar to the prescription drug digoxin) that may cause the heart to beat rapidly or abnormally, or to stop beating. Common oleander has been used as rat poison, insecticide, and fish poison and is toxic to mammals, including humans. Animals (sheep) have died after eating as little as two to three leaves of *Nerium oleander* (common oleander). Children may die after eating a single leaf of common oleander. Eating the leaves, flowers, or bark of common oleander may cause nausea, vomiting, stomach cramps, pain, fatigue, drowsiness, unsteadiness, bloody diarrhea, abnormal heart rhythms, seizures, liver or kidney damage, or unconsciousness. Death may occur within 1 day. Reports of toxicity and deaths in children and adults have been reported for decades in Australia, India, Sri Lanka, and the United States.

O

- Fruits of *Thevetin peruviana* (yellow oleander) are thought to be even more toxic to mammals, including humans. Based on human studies of intentional overdose (suicide attempts), eating eight or more seeds of yellow oleander may be fatal. Additional side effects of oleander ingestion include irritation and redness of lips, gums, and tongue; nausea; vomiting; depression; irritability; fast breathing; sweating; stomach pain; diarrhea; headache; confusion; visual disturbances; and constricted pupils. Abnormal blood tests, including tests of liver and kidney function (potassium, bilirubin, creatinine, and blood urea), have been reported in humans.
- It is possible that plants grown in the same soil as oleander plants or in soil exposed to oleander may contain trace amounts of oleander.

Pregnancy and Breastfeeding

- Oleander is toxic and should be avoided by pregnant or breastfeeding women.

INTERACTIONS

Interactions with Drugs

- Based on animal and human studies, common oleander and yellow oleander contain cardiac glycoside heart-active substances similar to the drug digoxin. There may be an increased risk of unwanted side effects or damage to the heart if taken with other heart-active drugs such as digoxin (Lanoxin) or antiarrhythmics.
- Because oleander is similar to the drug digoxin, it may share some of the same interactions, although this has not been thoroughly studied.

- Low potassium levels in the blood may increase the dangerous side effects of oleander. Therefore, oleander should be used cautiously with drugs that may lower potassium levels, such as laxatives or some diuretics (drugs that increase urine flow).
- Oleander may interact with abortifacients, antibiotics, antidepressants, blood pressure–lowering drugs, antineoplastics, contraceptives, hormonal drugs, immunosuppressants, and neurological drugs.

Interactions with Herbs and Dietary Supplements

- Common oleander and yellow oleander contain cardiac glycoside heart-active substances and interact with other herbs and supplements with similar effects such as hawthorn. Notably, bufalin/Chan Suis is a Chinese herbal formula that has been reported as toxic or fatal when taken with cardiac glycosides.
- Toxic effects of oleander on the heart may be increased if used with calcium supplements or herbs that lower potassium levels, such as licorice. Potassium levels theoretically may be reduced by herbs and supplements with laxative properties such as senna or psyllium or by herbs and supplements with diuretic properties (increasing urine flow) such as artichoke, celery, or dandelion.
- Oleander may interact with abortifacients, antibiotics, antidepressants, blood pressure–lowering herbs and supplements, antineoplastics, contraceptives, hormonal herbs and supplements, immunosuppressants, and neurological herbs and supplements.

For a complete list of references, please visit www.naturalstandard.com.

Olive Leaf
(Olea europaea)

RELATED TERMS

- *Olea europae*, Oleaceae (family).

BACKGROUND

- Olive leaves come from the olive tree *(Olea europae)*, a native plant of the Mediterranean. Although olives and olive oil are used as foods, olive leaf is primarily used medicinally or as a tea.
- Laboratory studies indicate that olive leaf may be beneficial as an antibacterial, antifungal, antiviral, or antioxidant. However, there is insufficient evidence in humans to support the use of olive leaf for any indication.
- In the Middle East, olive leaf tea has been used for centuries to treat sore throat, coughs, fevers, high blood pressure, cystitis (bladder infection), and gout (foot inflammation), and to improve general health. Olive leaf poultices have been applied to the skin to treat dermatological conditions, such as boils, rashes, and warts.

EVIDENCE

Uses Based on Scientific Evidence

No available studies qualify for inclusion in the evidence table.

Uses Based on Tradition or Theory

Antibacterial, antifungal, antioxidant, antiviral, boils, common cold, conjunctivitis (pinkeye), controlling blood pressure, coughs, cystitis (inflamed bladder), ear infections, eye infections, fever, gout (inflamed foot), herpes simplex-1 virus, high blood pressure, human immunodeficiency virus/acquired immunodeficiency syndrome, impetigo (pus-filled blisters), influenza, mouth and throat infections, nose infection, parasites, rashes, skin conditions, sore throat, tonic, warts.

DOSING

Adults (18 Years and Older)

- There is insufficient evidence to recommend a dose for olive leaf in adults.

Children (Younger than 18 Years)

- There is insufficient evidence to recommend a dose for olive leaf in children.

SAFETY

Allergies

- Avoid in people with a known allergy or hypersensitivity to olive, olive leaf *(Olea europaea)*, its constituents, or related members of the Oleaceae family.

Side Effects and Warnings

- There are very few reports of olive leaf and its adverse effects. There is currently a lack of high-quality studies on the medicinal applications of olive leaf. Use cautiously in patients taking antiviral medications, as olive leaf may have antiviral properties.

Pregnancy and Breastfeeding

- Olive leaf is not recommended in pregnant or breastfeeding women due to a lack of available scientific evidence.

INTERACTIONS

Interactions with Drugs

- Although not well studied in humans, olive leaf water extract may have antibacterial, antioxidant, or antifungal properties. Caution is advised when taking olive leaf and other antifungal, antioxidant, or antibacterial agents due to potential additive effects.
- Based on preliminary research, olive leaf extracts may have antiviral effects and may aid in inhibiting human immunodeficiency virus-1 replication. Caution is advised when using olive leaf with antiviral agents or agents used for HIV.

Interactions with Herbs and Dietary Supplements

- Although not well studied in humans, olive leaf water extract may have antibacterial, antioxidant, or antifungal properties. Caution is advised when taking olive leaf and other antifungal, antioxidant, or antibacterial herbs or supplements due to potential additive effects.
- Taking elderberry extract and olive leaf extract may reduce viral loads. Although the interaction may be a positive one, caution is advised in patients taking elderberry or other herbs with potential antiviral effects, due to additive effects.

For a complete list of references, please visit www.naturalstandard.com.

O

Omega-3 fatty acids, fish oil, alpha-linolenic acid

RELATED TERMS

- Alpha-linolenic acid (ALA, C18:3n-3), alpha-linolenic acid, cod liver oil, coldwater fish, docosahexaenoic acid (DHA, C22:6n-3), eicosapentaenoic acid (EPA, C20:5n-3), fish oil fatty acids, fish body oil, fish extract, fish liver oil, halibut oil, long chain polyunsaturated fatty acids, mackerel oil, marine oil, menhaden oil, n-3 fatty acids, n-3 polyunsaturated fatty acids, omega fatty acids, omega-3 oils, polyunsaturated fatty acids (PUFA), salmon oil, shark liver oil, w-3 fatty acids.
- **Note:** Should not be confused with omega-6 fatty acids.

BACKGROUND

- Dietary sources of omega-3 fatty acids include fish oil and certain plant/nut oils. Fish oil contains both docosahexaenoic acid (DHA) and eicosapentaenoic acid (EPA), and some nuts (English walnuts) and vegetable oils (canola, soybean, flaxseed/linseed, olive) contain primarily alpha-linolenic acid (ALA). ALA is the parent compound to all omega-3 fatty acids; after it is ingested by animals, ALA is converted into DHA and EPA.
- There is evidence from multiple studies supporting that the intake of recommended amounts of DHA and EPA in the form of dietary fish or fish oil supplements lowers triglycerides; reduces the risk of death, heart attack, dangerous abnormal heart rhythms, and strokes in people with known cardiovascular disease; slows the buildup of atherosclerotic plaques ("hardening of the arteries"); and lowers blood pressure slightly. However, high doses may have harmful effects, such as an increased risk of bleeding. Although similar benefits are proposed for alpha-linolenic acid, scientific evidence is less compelling, and beneficial effects may be less pronounced.
- Some species of fish carry a higher risk of environmental contamination, such as with methylmercury.

EVIDENCE

Uses Based on Scientific Evidence	Grade
High Blood Pressure Multiple clinical trials report small reductions in blood pressure with intake of omega-3 fatty acids. DHA may have greater benefits than EPA. However, high intake of omega-3 fatty acids per day may be necessary to obtain clinically relevant effects, and at this dose level, there is an increased risk of bleeding. Therefore, a qualified healthcare provider should be consulted before starting treatment with supplements.	A
Hypertriglyceridemia (Fish Oil/EPA Plus DHA) There is strong scientific evidence from clinical trials that omega-3 fatty acids from fish or fish oil supplements (EPA and DHA) significantly reduce blood triglyceride levels. Benefits appear to be dose dependent. Fish oil supplements also appear to cause small improvements in high-density lipoprotein ("good cholesterol"); however, increases (worsening) in low-density lipoprotein levels (LDL/"bad cholesterol") are also observed.	A

It is not clear if alpha-linolenic acid significantly affects triglyceride levels, and there is conflicting evidence in this area.

The American Heart Association has published recommendations for EPA and DHA. Because of the risk of bleeding from omega-3 fatty acids, a qualified health care provider should be consulted before starting treatment with supplements.

There is growing evidence that reducing C-reactive protein (CRP) is beneficial toward favorable cardiovascular outcomes, although additional research is pending in this area. The data on fish oils and CRP levels are mixed.

	Grade
Secondary Cardiovascular Disease Prevention (Fish Oil/EPA Plus DHA) Several well-conducted randomized controlled trials report that in people with a history of heart attack, regular consumption of oily fish or fish oil/omega-3 supplements reduces the risk of non-fatal heart attack, fatal heart attack, sudden death, and all-cause mortality (death due to any cause). Most patients in these studies were also using conventional heart drugs, suggesting that the benefits of fish oils may add to the effects of other therapies.	A
Primary Cardiovascular Disease Prevention (Fish Intake) Several large studies of populations ("epidemiologic" studies) report a significantly lower rate of death from heart disease in men and women who regularly eat fish. Other epidemiologic research reports no such benefits. It is not clear if reported benefits only occur in certain groups of people, such as those at risk of developing heart disease. Overall, the evidence suggests benefits of regular consumption of fish oil. However, well-designed randomized controlled trials that classify people by their risk of developing heart disease are necessary before a firm conclusion can be drawn.	B
Protection from Cyclosporine Toxicity In Organ Transplant Patients There are multiple studies of heart transplant and kidney transplant patients taking cyclosporine (Neoral), who were administered fish oil supplements. The majority of trials report improvements in kidney function and less high blood pressure compared to patients not taking fish oil. Although several recent studies report no benefits on kidney function, the weight of scientific evidence favors the beneficial effects of fish oil.	B
Rheumatoid Arthritis (Fish Oil) Multiple randomized controlled trials report improvements in morning stiffness and joint tenderness with the regular intake of fish oil supplements for up to three months. Benefits have been reported as additive with anti-inflammatory medications such as NSAIDs (e.g., ibuprofen, aspirin). However, because	B

Uses Based on Scientific Evidence	Grade
of weaknesses in study designs and reporting, better research is necessary before a strong favorable recommendation can be made. Effects beyond three months of treatment have not been well evaluated.	
Angina Pectoris Preliminary studies report reductions in angina associated with fish oil intake. Better research is necessary before a firm conclusion can be drawn.	C
Asthma Several studies in this area do not provide enough reliable evidence to form a clear conclusion, with some studies reporting no effects and others finding benefits. Because most studies have been small without clear descriptions of design or results, the results cannot be considered conclusive.	C
Atherosclerosis Some research reports that regular intake of fish or fish oil supplements reduces the risk of developing atherosclerotic plaques in the arteries of the heart, whereas other research reports no effects. Additional evidence is necessary before a firm conclusion can be drawn in this area.	C
Bipolar Disorder Several studies in this area do not provide enough reliable evidence to form a clear conclusion.	C
Cancer Prevention Several population (epidemiologic) studies report that dietary omega-3 fatty acids or fish oil may reduce the risk of developing breast, colon, or prostate cancer. Randomized controlled trials are necessary before a clear conclusion can be drawn.	C
Cardiac Arrhythmias (Abnormal Heart Rhythms) There is promising evidence that omega-3 fatty acids may decrease the risk of cardiac arrhythmias. This is one proposed mechanism behind the reduced number of heart attacks in people who regularly ingest fish oil or EPA and DHA. Additional research is needed in this specific area before a firm conclusion can be reached.	C
Colon Cancer Omega-3 fatty acids are commonly taken by cancer patients. Although preliminary studies report that growth of colon cancer cells may be reduced by taking fish oil, effects on survival or remission have not been measured adequately.	C
Crohn's Disease It has been suggested that effects of omega-3 fatty acids on inflammation may be beneficial in patients with Crohn's disease when added to standard	C

therapy, and several studies have been conducted in this area. Results are conflicting, and no clear conclusion can be drawn at this time.

	Grade
Cystic Fibrosis A small amount of research in this area does not provide enough reliable evidence to form a clear conclusion.	C
Dementia Well-designed clinical trials are needed before omega-3 fatty acids can be recommended for the prevention of cognitive impairment or dementia.	C
Depression Several studies on the use of omega 3 fatty acids in depression, including positive results in postpartum depression, do not provide enough reliable evidence to form a clear conclusion or replace standard treatments. However, based on one recent study, omega-3 fatty acids may have therapeutic benefits in childhood depression. Promising initial evidence requires confirmation with larger, well-designed trials.	C
Dysmenorrhea (Painful Menstruation) There is preliminary evidence suggesting possible benefits of fish oil/omega-3 fatty acids in patients with dysmenorrhea. Additional research is necessary before a firm conclusion can be reached.	C
Eczema Several studies of EPA for eczema do not provide enough reliable evidence to form a clear conclusion.	C
Immunoglobulin A (IgA) Nephropathy There are conflicting results from several trials in this area.	C
Infant Eye/Brain Development Well-designed research is necessary before a clear conclusion can be reached.	C
Lupus Erythematosus There is not enough reliable evidence to form a clear conclusion in this area.	C
Nephrotic Syndrome There is not enough reliable evidence to form a clear conclusion in this area.	C
Preeclampsia Several studies of fish oil do not provide enough reliable evidence to form a clear conclusion in this area.	C
Prevention of Graft Failure After Heart Bypass Surgery There is limited study of the use of fish oils in patients after undergoing coronary artery bypass	C

O

(Continued)

Uses Based on Scientific Evidence	Grade
grafting (CABG). Additional evidence is necessary before a firm conclusion can be drawn in this area.	
Prevention of Restenosis After Coronary Angioplasty (PTCA) Several randomized controlled trials have evaluated whether omega-3 fatty acid intake reduces blockage of arteries in the heart after balloon angioplasty (percutaneous transluminal coronary angioplasty/PTCA). The evidence in this area remains inconclusive.	C
Primary Cardiovascular Disease Prevention (ALA) Additional research is necessary before a conclusion can be drawn in this area.	C
Psoriasis Several studies in this area do not provide enough reliable evidence to form a clear conclusion.	C
Schizophrenia There is promising preliminary evidence from several randomized controlled trials in this area. Additional research is necessary before a firm conclusion can be reached.	C
Secondary Cardiovascular Disease Prevention (ALA) Several randomized controlled trials have examined the effects of alpha-linolenic acid in people with a history of heart attack. Although some studies suggest benefits, others do not. Additional research is necessary before a conclusion can be drawn in this area.	C
Stroke Prevention Several large studies of populations ("epidemiologic" studies) have examined the effects of omega-3 fatty acid intake on stroke risk. Some studies suggest benefits, and others do not. Effects are likely on ischemic or thrombotic stroke risk, and very large intakes of omega-3 fatty acids ("Eskimo" amounts) may actually increase the risk of hemorrhagic (bleeding) stroke. At this time, it is unclear if there are benefits in people with or without a history of stroke or if effects of fish oil are comparable to other treatment strategies.	C
Ulcerative Colitis It has been suggested that effects of omega-3 fatty acids on inflammation may be beneficial in patients with ulcerative colitis when added to standard therapy, and several studies have been conducted in this area. Better research is necessary before a clear conclusion can be drawn.	C
Appetite/Weight Loss in Cancer Patients There is preliminary evidence that fish oil supplementation does not improve appetite or prevent weight loss in cancer patients. Further study is warranted.	D

	Grade
Diabetes The available scientific evidence suggests that there are no significant long-term effects of fish oil in patients with diabetes. Most studies in this area are not well designed.	D
Hypercholesterolemia Although fish oil is able to reduce triglycerides, beneficial effects on blood cholesterol levels have not been demonstrated. Fish oil supplements appear to cause small improvements in high-density lipoprotein ("good cholesterol"); however, increases (worsening) in low-density lipoprotein levels ("bad cholesterol") are also observed. Fish oil does not appear to affect C-reactive protein (CRP) levels.	D
Transplant Rejection Prevention (Kidney and Heart) There are multiple studies of heart transplant and kidney transplant patients taking cyclosporine (Neoral) who were administered fish oil supplements. The majority of trials report improvements in kidney function (glomerular filtration rate, serum creatinine) and less hypertension (high blood pressure) compared to patients not taking fish oil. However, several recent studies report no benefits on kidney function, and no changes have been found in rates of rejection or graft survival.	D

Uses Based on Tradition or Theory

Acute myocardial infarction (heart attack), acute respiratory distress syndrome (ARDS), age-related macular degeneration, aggressive behavior, agoraphobia, AIDS, allergies, Alzheimer's disease, anticoagulation, antiphospholipid syndrome, attention deficit hyperactivity disorder (ADHD), anthracycline-induced cardiac toxicity, bacterial infections, breast cysts, breast tenderness, chronic fatigue syndrome (postviral fatigue syndrome), chronic obstructive pulmonary disease, cirrhosis, common cold, congestive heart failure, critical illness, deficiency (omega-3 fatty acid), dermatomyositis, diabetic nephropathy, diabetic neuropathy, dyslexia, dyspraxia, endocrine disorders (glycogen storage diseases), exercise performance enhancement, fibromyalgia, gallstones, gingivitis, glaucoma, glomerulonephritis, gout, hay fever, headache, hepatorenal syndrome, hypoxia, ichthyosis (skin disorder), immunosuppression, inflammatory conditions (Behçet's syndrome), joint problems (cartilage repair), kidney disease prevention, kidney stones, leprosy, leukemia, malaria, male infertility, mastalgia (breast pain), memory enhancement, menopausal symptoms, menstrual cramps, methotrexate toxicity, multiple sclerosis, myopathy, nephritis (autoimmune), neuropathy, night vision enhancement, obesity, osteoarthritis, osteoporosis, otitis media (ear infection), panic disorder, peripheral vascular disease, pregnancy nutritional supplement, premature birth prevention, premenstrual syndrome, prostate cancer prevention, protection from isotretinoin drug toxicity, psychologic disorders (borderline personality disorder), Raynaud's phenomenon, Refsum's syndrome, retinitis pigmentosa, Reye's syndrome, seizure disorder, Sjögren's syndrome, suicide prevention, systemic lupus erythematosus, tardive dyskinesia, tennis elbow, ulcerative colitis, urolithiasis (bladder stones), vision enhancement, weight loss.

DOSING

Adults (18 Years and Older)

- **Average dietary intake of omega-3/omega-6 fatty acids**: Average Americans consume approximately 1.6 g of omega-3 fatty acids each day, of which about 1.4 g (~90%) comes from alpha-linolenic acid and only 0.1 to 0.2 g (~10%) from EPA and DHA. In Western diets, people consume roughly 10 times more omega-6 fatty acids than omega-3 fatty acids. These large amounts of omega-6 fatty acids come from the common use of vegetable oils containing linoleic acid (for example, corn oil, evening primrose oil, pumpkin oil, safflower oil, sesame oil, soybean oil, sunflower oil, walnut oil, wheatgerm oil). Because omega-6 and omega-3 fatty acids compete with each other to be converted to active metabolites in the body, benefits can be reached either by decreasing intake of omega-6 fatty acids or by increasing intake of omega-3 fatty acids.
- **Recommended daily intake of omega-3 fatty acids (healthy adults)**: For healthy adults with no history of heart disease, the American Heart Association recommends eating fish at least two times per week. In particular, fatty fish are recommended, such as anchovies, bluefish, carp, catfish, halibut, herring, lake trout, mackerel, pompano, salmon, striped sea bass, tuna (albacore), and whitefish. It is also recommended to consume plant-derived sources of alpha-linolenic acid, such as tofu/soybeans, walnuts, flaxseed oil, and canola oil. The World Health Organization and governmental health agencies of several countries recommend consuming 0.3 to 0.5 g of daily of EPA and DHA and 0.8 to 1.1 g daily of alpha-linolenic acid. A doctor and pharmacist should be consulted for dosing for other conditions.

Children (Younger than 18 Years)

- Omega-3 fatty acids are used in some infant formulas, although effective doses are not clearly established. Ingestion of fresh fish should be limited in young children because of the presence of potentially harmful environmental contaminants. Fish oil capsules should not be used in children except under the direction of a physician.

SAFETY

Allergies

- People with allergy or hypersensitivity to fish should avoid fish oil or omega-3 fatty acid products derived from fish. Skin rash has been reported rarely. People with allergy or hypersensitivity to nuts should avoid alpha-linolenic acid or omega-3 fatty acid products that are derived from the types of nuts to which they react.

Side Effects and Warnings

- The U.S. Food and Drug Administration classifies low intake of omega-3 fatty acids from fish as GRAS (generally regarded as safe). Caution may be warranted, however, in diabetic patients because of potential (albeit unlikely) increases in blood sugar levels, patients at risk of bleeding, or in those with high levels of low-density lipoprotein (LDL). Fish meat may contain methylmercury, and caution is warranted in young children and pregnant/breastfeeding women.
- Omega-3 fatty acids may increase the risk of bleeding, although there is little evidence of significant bleeding risk at lower doses. Very large intakes of fish oil/omega-3 fatty acids ("Eskimo" amounts) may increase the risk of hemorrhagic (bleeding) stroke. High doses have also been associated with nosebleed and blood in the urine. Fish oils appear to decrease platelet aggregation and prolong bleeding time, increase fibrinolysis (breaking down of blood clots), and may reduce von Willebrand factor.
- Potentially harmful contaminants such as dioxins, methylmercury, and polychlorinated biphenyls (PCBs) are found in some species of fish. Methylmercury accumulates in fish meat more than in fish oil, and fish oil supplements appear to contain almost no mercury. Therefore, safety concerns apply to eating fish but likely not to ingesting fish oil supplements. Heavy metals are most harmful in young children and pregnant/nursing women.
- Gastrointestinal upset is common with the use of fish oil supplements. Diarrhea may also occur, with potentially severe diarrhea at very high doses. There are also reports of increased burping, acid reflux/heartburn/indigestion, abdominal bloating, and abdominal pain. Fishy aftertaste is a common effect. Gastrointestinal side effects can be minimized if fish oils are taken with meals and if doses are started low and gradually increased.
- Multiple clinical trials report small reductions in blood pressure with intake of omega-3 fatty acids. Reductions of 2 to 5 mm Hg have been observed, and effects appear to be dose responsive (higher doses have greater effects). DHA may have greater effects than EPA. Caution is warranted in patients with low blood pressure or in those taking blood-pressure–lowering medications.
- Although slight increases in fasting blood glucose levels have been noted in patients with type 2 ("adult onset") diabetes, available scientific evidence suggests that there are no significant long-term effects of fish oil in patients with diabetes, including no changes in hemoglobin A1c levels. Limited reports in the 1980s of increased insulin needs in diabetic patients taking long-term fish oils may be related to other dietary changes or weight gain.
- Fish oil taken for many months may cause a deficiency of vitamin E, and therefore vitamin E is added to many commercial fish oil products. As a result, regular use of vitamin E–enriched products may lead to elevated levels of this fat-soluble vitamin. Fish liver oil contains the fat-soluble vitamins A and D, and therefore fish liver oil products (such as cod liver oil) may increase the risk of vitamin A or D toxicity.
- Increases (worsening) in LDL levels ("bad cholesterol") by 5%-10% are observed with the intake of omega-3 fatty acids. Effects are dose-dependent.
- Mild elevations in liver function tests (alanine aminotransferase) have been reported rarely.
- Skin rashes have been reported rarely.
- There are rare reports of mania in patients with bipolar disorder or major depression. Restlessness and formication (the sensation of ants crawling on the skin) have also been reported.

Pregnancy and Breastfeeding

- Potentially harmful contaminants such as dioxins, methylmercury, and PCBs are found in some species of fish and may be harmful in pregnant/nursing women. Methylmercury accumulates in fish meat more than in fish oil, and fish oil supplements appear to contain almost no mercury. Therefore, these safety concerns apply to eating fish but

O

likely not to ingesting fish oil supplements. However, unrefined fish oil preparations may contain pesticides.

- It is not known if omega-3 fatty acid supplementation of women during pregnancy or breastfeeding is beneficial to infants. It has been suggested that a high intake of omega-3 fatty acids, particularly DHA, during pregnancy may increase birth weight and gestational length. However, higher doses may not be advisable because of the potential risk of bleeding. Fatty acids are added to some infant formulas.

INTERACTIONS

Interactions with Drugs

- In theory, omega-3 fatty acids may increase the risk of bleeding when taken with drugs that increase the risk of bleeding. Some examples include aspirin, anticoagulants (blood thinners) such as warfarin (Coumadin) or heparin, anti-platelet drugs such as clopidogrel (Plavix), and non-steroidal anti-inflammatory drugs such as ibuprofen (Motrin, Advil) or naproxen (Naprosyn, Aleve).
- Based on clinical studies, omega-3 fatty acids may lower blood pressure and add to the effects of drugs that may also affect blood pressure.
- Fish oil supplements may lower blood sugar levels a small amount. Caution is advised when using medications that may also lower blood sugar levels. Patients taking drugs for diabetes by mouth or insulin should be monitored closely by a qualified health care provider. Medication adjustments may be necessary.
- Omega-3 fatty acids lower triglyceride levels but can actually increase (worsen) LDL ("bad cholesterol") levels by a small amount. Therefore, omega-3 fatty acids may add to the triglyceride-lowering effects of agents such as niacin/nicotinic acid, fibrates such as gemfibrozil (Lopid), or resins such as cholestyramine (Questran). However, omega-3 fatty acids may work against the LDL-lowering properties of "statin" drugs such as atorvastatin (Lipitor) and lovastatin (Mevacor).

Interactions with Herbs and Dietary Supplements

- In theory, omega-3 fatty acids may increase the risk of bleeding when taken with herbs and supplements that are believed to increase the risk of bleeding. Multiple cases of bleeding have been reported with the use of *Ginkgo biloba* and fewer cases with garlic and saw palmetto. Numerous other agents may theoretically increase the risk of bleeding, although this has not been proven in most cases.
- Based on clinical studies, omega-3 fatty acids may lower blood pressure and theoretically may add to the effects of agents that may also affect blood pressure.
- Fish oil supplements may lower blood sugar levels a small amount. Caution is advised when using herbs or supplements that may also lower blood sugar. Blood glucose levels may require monitoring, and doses may need adjustment.
- Omega-3 fatty acids lower triglyceride levels but can actually increase (worsen) LDL ("bad cholesterol") levels by a small amount. Therefore, omega-3 fatty acids may add to the triglyceride-lowering effects of agents such as niacin/nicotinic acid but may work against the potential LDL-lowering properties of agents such as barley, garlic, guggul, psyllium, soy, or sweet almond.
- Fish oil taken for many months may cause a deficiency of vitamin E, and therefore vitamin E is added to many commercial fish oil products. As a result, regular use of vitamin E–enriched products may lead to elevated levels of this fat-soluble vitamin. Fish liver oil contains the fat-soluble vitamins A and D, and therefore fish liver oil products (such as cod liver oil) may increase the risk of vitamin A or D toxicity. Since fat-soluble vitamins can build up in the body and cause toxicity, patients taking multiple vitamins regularly or in high doses should discuss this risk with their health care practitioners.

For a complete list of references, please visit www.naturalstandard.com.

Onion
(*Allium cepa*)

RELATED TERMS

- *Allium cepa, Allium cepa* L., allium vegetables, botanicals, Liliaceae (family), onion extract, onion juice, pickling onions, white onion.

BACKGROUND

- Onion (*Allium cepa* L.) is widely used around the world as a food product and has also been used for medicinal applications.
- Most of the available research has focused on scar prevention, but the results are mixed in this area. Onion has been used in the treatment of diabetes and alopecia areata (hair loss).
- As onion is a commonly consumed food, it is considered likely safe in smaller amounts, although there are reports of skin rash and gastrointestinal problems in sensitive individuals.

EVIDENCE

Uses Based on Scientific Evidence	Grade
Allergies Preliminary research suggests that application of an alcoholic onion extract on the skin may reduce allergic responses, such as wheals (hives) and flares.	C
Alopecia Areata (Hair Loss) Preliminary research using topical onion juice increased hair regrowth in alopecia areata (hair loss) patients, especially women.	C
Diabetes There is limited clinical evidence that fresh onion significantly decreased serum glucose (blood sugar) levels in diabetics.	C
Hypertension (High Blood Pressure) Onion–olive oil capsules may help lower blood pressure, although the evidence thus far has not been definitive.	C
Scar Prevention Several trials have been conducted using combination products that include an onion extract. These studies investigated onion's potential role in scar healing in adults and children, specifically due to injuries from laser tattoo removal or surgery. The overall results are mixed.	C

Uses Based on Tradition or Theory
Antibacterial, antifungal, antimicrobial, antioxidant, antiplatelet (blood thinning), arthritis, asthma, atherosclerosis (hardening of the arteries), cancer, cardiovascular (heart) disease, cataract, chilblains (inflammation of the hands and feet caused by exposure to cold and moisture), coronary heart disease, gastrointestinal disorders, hypercholesterolemia (high cholesterol), insecticidal, lung cancer, obesity, osteoporosis, prebiotic, splinters, stomach cancer, thrombosis (blood clot).

DOSING

Adults (18 Years and Older)

- There is insufficient evidence to recommend a dose of onion in adults. However, Mederma (Merz Pharmaceuticals, Greensboro, NC, USA) has been applied to the skin three times daily for 8 weeks. A topical onion gel extract applied three times a day for 1 month has also been used.

Children (Younger than 18 Years)

- There is insufficient evidence to recommend a dose of onion in children.

SAFETY

Allergies

- Avoid in people with a known allergy or hypersensitivity to onion (*Allium cepa*) or its constituents. In some people, handling onion bulbs has caused skin rash, painful tingling in the fingers, or a reddening of the skin.

Side Effects and Warnings

- Onion is likely safe when consumed in food amounts and when onion extract is applied to the skin for scar healing.
- Onion should be used cautiously in patients with hematological (blood) disorders or those taking anticoagulants or antiplatelets (blood thinners), patients with diabetes or hypoglycemia (high or low blood sugar), and patients with hypotension (low blood pressure).
- The primary adverse effects associated with onion are dermatological (pemphigus, a chronic blistering disease, and skin rash) and gastrointestinal (heartburn, dyspepsia [upset stomach], gastric acidity, and gastroesophageal reflux).
- In clinical studies, onion has been found to lower blood pressure in both patients with and without hypertension (high blood pressure).
- Avoid in patients who are allergic or hypersensitive to onion or plants in the Lilaceae family.

Pregnancy and Breastfeeding

- Onion, in medicinal amounts, is not recommended in pregnant or breastfeeding women due to a lack of available scientific evidence.

INTERACTIONS

Interactions with Drugs

- Cepae extract from onions, heparin, and allantoin may improve healing of injuries incurred during laser tattoo removal or surgery.
- Meals including onion have induced heartburn, dyspepsia (upset stomach), gastric acidity, and gastroesophageal reflux in clinical trials. Use onion cautiously with antacids.

O

541

- *Allium* plants, such as onion, may have antibiotic effects, and may have additive effects when used with other antibiotics.
- Onion may increase the risk of bleeding when taken with drugs that increase the risk of bleeding. Some examples include aspirin, anticoagulants (blood thinners) such as warfarin (Coumadin) or heparin, antiplatelet drugs such as clopidogrel (Plavix), and nonsteroidal anti-inflammatory drugs (NSAIDs) such as ibuprofen (Motrin, Advil) or naproxen (Naprosyn, Aleve).
- Onion may lower blood sugar. Caution is advised in patients with diabetes (high blood sugar) or hypoglycemia (low blood sugar), and in those taking drugs that affect blood sugar. Serum glucose levels may need to be monitored by a qualified health care professional, including a pharmacist, and medication adjustments may be necessary.
- Onion and onion essential oil may prevent fat-induced increases in serum cholesterol. Use cautiously with cholesterol-lowering medications.
- Onion or onion extract may have anticancer effects. Use cautiously when taken with medications to prevent or treat cancer.
- Onion may lower blood pressure; use cautiously with blood pressure medications.
- Onion may inhibit bone resorption; use cautiously with osteoporosis agents.

Interactions with Herbs and Dietary Supplements

- *Allium* plants, such as onion, may have antibiotic effects and may have additive effects when used with other antibiotic herbs.

- Onion may increase the risk of bleeding when taken with herbs and supplements that are believed to increase the risk of bleeding. Multiple cases of bleeding have been reported with the use of *Ginkgo biloba*, and fewer cases with garlic and saw palmetto.
- Onion may lower blood sugar. Caution is advised in patients with diabetes or hypoglycemia, and in those taking herbs or supplements that affect blood sugar. Serum glucose levels may need to be monitored by a qualified health care professional, including a pharmacist, and doses may need adjustment.
- Onion or onion extract may have anticancer effects. Use cautiously with herbs and supplements taken to prevent or treat cancer.
- Onion and onion essential oil may prevent fat-induced increases in serum cholesterol; use cautiously with herbs and supplements taken for cholesterol.
- Onion may decrease systolic and diastolic blood pressure; use cautiously if taking herbs or supplements for blood pressure.
- Onion may inhibit bone resorption; use cautiously with herbs or supplements taken for osteoporosis.

For a complete list of references, please visit www.naturalstandard.com.

Oregano
(Origanum vulgare)

RELATED TERMS

- Dostenkraut, Mediterranean oregano, mountain mint, oil of oregano, oregano oil, Origani vulgaris herba, origanum, wild marjoram, Zaatar.

BACKGROUND

- Oregano is a perennial herb. The leaves, stems, and flowers are used medicinally. Oregano has been recognized for its aromatic properties since ancient times. In ancient Greece, oregano was called "joy of the mountain" and was considered a symbol of joy and happiness. Ancient Egyptians considered *Origanum* species to be sacred to the god Osiris and wove it into crowns or wreaths worn during rituals.
- Oregano is commonly used as a food flavoring and preservative. Traditionally, oregano has been used to treat respiratory and gastrointestinal disorders and menstrual irregularities. Modern herbalists recommend topical application of oregano oil for the treatment of infection.
- Preliminary research suggests that oregano may have antiparasitic, antifungal, antioxidant, antibacterial, and insect repellent activities. There is limited scientific evidence to support any of these suggested uses for oregano.

EVIDENCE

Uses Based on Scientific Evidence	Grade
Parasites Preliminary research shows that taking oregano by mouth may help treat parasites. However, there is insufficient clinical evidence to support this use.	C

Uses Based on Tradition or Theory
Abortifacient (induces abortion), acne, antibacterial, antifungal, antimutagenic, antioxidant, antiparasitic, antithrombin, arthritis, asthma, athlete's foot (topically), bloating, bronchitis, canker sores (topically), carminative, colds, cough, croup, dandruff, diaphoretic, dysentery, dysmenorrheal (orally), dyspepsia, expectorant, flavoring, food preservative, gastrointestinal disorders, gum disease (topically), headaches (orally), heart conditions (orally), high blood sugar, increased insulin sensitivity, insect and spider bites, insect repellent menstrual stimulant (orally), menstrual irregularities, metorrhagia (painful menstruation), mild tonic (orally), muscle pain, phytoestrogenic, preservative, psoriasis, respiratory disorders, rheumatoid arthritis (orally), ringworm (topically), rosacea, seborrhea, superficial and systemic infections (topically), toothache, ulcers, urinary tract infections, varicose veins, warts.

DOSING

Adults (18 Years and Older)

- There is insufficient evidence to recommend a dose for oregano. Oregano has been taken in doses of 200 mg of emulsified oil three times daily with meals for 6 weeks for the treatment of enteric parasites. As a dietary supplement, two capsules (dose unknown) once or twice daily has been recommended with meals, or a few drops of oil of oregano can be added to milk or juice.
- Oregano oil has also been applied topically (on the skin), and shampoos and teas (gargle, mouthwash) are commercially available. For use as a bath additive, 100 g of dried oregano leaf may be steeped in 1L of water for 10 minutes, strained, and added to a full bath.

Children (Younger than 18 Years)

- There is insufficient evidence to recommend a dose for oregano in children.

SAFETY

Allergies

- Avoid in people with a known allergy or hypersensitivity to oregano. Possible cross-sensitivity exists with other herbs from the Lamiaceae family, including hyssop (*Hyssopus officinalis*), basil (*Ocicum basilicum*), marjoram (*Origanum majorana*), mint (*Mentha piperita*), sage (*Salvia officinalis*), and lavender (*Lavendula officinalis*).
- Itching and swelling of the lips and tongue, difficulty speaking and breathing, and face swelling have been reported following the ingestion of pizza containing oregano.

Side Effects and Warnings

- Based on historical use, it appears that oregano is well tolerated in recommended doses. However, there are no available reliable clinical trials demonstrating safety or efficacy of a particular dose or for a recommended treatment duration.
- Oregano may lower blood sugar levels. Caution is advised in patients with diabetes or hypoglycemia, and in those taking drugs, herbs, or supplements that affect blood sugar. Serum glucose levels may need to be monitored by a health care provider, and medication adjustments may be necessary.

Pregnancy and Breastfeeding

- Oregano is not recommended at doses above those normally found in food due to a lack of available scientific evidence. An herbal over-the-counter product called Carachipita that contains oregano, pennyroyal (*Mentha pulegium*), yerba de la perdiz (*Magiricarpus pinnaus*), and guaycuru (*Statice brasiliensis*) has been linked with case reports of induced abortion.

INTERACTIONS

Interactions with Drugs

- Oregano may lower blood sugar levels. Caution is advised when using medications that may also lower blood sugar levels. Patients taking drugs for diabetes by mouth or insulin should be monitored closely by a qualified health care professional, including a pharmacist. Medication adjustments may be necessary.
- Oregano may have phytoestrogenic effects. Interactions with hormonal agents are theoretically possible.

- Oregano may have antithrombin effects. Interactions with anticoagulants are theoretically possible.

Interactions with Herbs and Dietary Supplements

- Oregano may lower blood sugar levels. Caution is advised when using herbs or supplements that may also lower blood sugar levels. Blood glucose levels may require monitoring, and doses may need adjustment.

- Because oregano contains estrogen-like chemicals, the effects of other agents believed to have estrogen-like properties may be altered.
- Oregano may have antithrombin effects. Interactions with anticoagulants are theoretically possible.

For a complete list of references, please visit www.naturalstandard.com.

Pantethine

[D-bis-(N-Pantothenyl-B-aminoethyl)-disulfide]

RELATED TERMS

- Bile acid sequestrant, bis-pantothenamidoethyl disulfide, calcium pantothenate (CaP), coenzyme Q10, carnitine, cyproheptadine, cysteamine, D-pantethine, pantetheine, pantetheinase, Pantetina, panthenol, pantomin, pantosin, pantothenic acid, sulfopantetheine, vitamin B_5.

BACKGROUND

- Pantethine is a naturally occurring compound and the active form of pantothenic acid. Structurally, pantethine is a disulfide form of pantothenic acid; it is metabolized to coenzyme A. Pantethine received its name from the Greek word *pantos*, which means "everywhere" because it was in a wide variety of foods such as fish, legumes, organ meats, whole grains, and yogurt.
- Research has demonstrated that pantethine, when taken by mouth, can be used for lowering cholesterol. It is also used for lowering cardiovascular risk, improving energy, improving adrenal function, and preventing allergy symptoms in people allergic to formaldehyde. Reliable evidence on pantethine for enhancing exercise performance is lacking.
- Pantethine is believed to have lipid-modulating properties. It has been used to help convert fat and carbohydrates to energy. Pantethine has also been used to support adrenal function and act as an anti-stress aid.

EVIDENCE

Uses Based on Scientific Evidence	Grade
Hyperlipidemia (High Cholesterol) Numerous trials have examined the effects of pantethine taken by mouth on lipids. Reductions in total cholesterol, low-density lipoprotein (LDL), and triglycerides have occurred.	B
Ischemic Heart Disease Pantethine exhibits lipid-modulating effects; however, clinical evidence is insufficient to support this use.	C
Athletic Performance Overall evidence suggests that pantethine is helpful in athletic performance.	D
Cystinosis Cystinosis is a hereditary dysfunction of the renal (kidney) tubules characterized by the presence of carbohydrates and amino acids in the urine, excessive urination, and low blood levels of potassium ions and phosphates, and caused by the abnormal metabolism of cystine and the accumulation of cystine crystals in tissues. Preliminary research does not show any benefit for oral pantethine in the treatment of cystinosis.	D

Uses Based on Tradition or Theory

Adaptation to stress, adrenal cortex function, alcoholism and Parkinson's disease, anorexia, antianorectic activity, anticarcinogenic, anti-inflammatory, chronic hepatopathies (diseases of the liver), coronary disease, diabetic neuropathies (disease of the nervous system), infantile nephropathic cystinosis (autosomal recessive disorder), inhibition of lens opacification during the early stages of cataract formation, seborrheic states of the scalp.

DOSING

Adults (18 Years and Older)

- There is insufficient evidence to recommend a dose for pantethine. Pantethine is generally well tolerated. Most studies for hyperlipidemia (high cholesterol) have used doses of 600-900 mg daily by mouth. Up to 1,200 mg daily in divided doses has been taken by mouth.
- As an injection into the muscle, 400 mg/day has been given. Injections should only be given under the supervision of a qualified health care professional, including a pharmacist.

Children (Younger than 18 Years)

- There is insufficient evidence to recommend a dose for pantethine in children. However, for hypolipoproteinemia (low cholesterol), children have taken 900-1,200 mg daily for 3-6 months. Pantethine is generally well tolerated.

SAFETY

Allergies

- Avoid in people with a known allergy or hypersensitivity to pantethine or any component of the formulation.

Side Effects and Warnings

- Pantethine is generally well tolerated. It may cause mild gastrointestinal side effects such as nausea, heartburn, or diarrhea. There is some evidence that pantethine can decrease platelet aggregation, which may increase the risk of bleeding.

Pregnancy and Breastfeeding

- Pantethine is not recommended in pregnant or breastfeeding women due to a lack of available scientific evidence.

INTERACTIONS

Interactions with Drugs

- Theoretically, pantethine may increase the risk of bleeding when taken with drugs that increase the risk of bleeding. Some examples include aspirin, anticoagulants ("blood thinners") such as warfarin (Coumadin) or heparin, antiplatelet drugs such as clopidogrel (Plavix), and nonsteroidal anti-inflammatory drugs (NSAIDs) such as ibuprofen (Motrin, Advil) or naproxen (Naprosyn, Aleve).

P

- Taking probucol or cysteamine may cause additive lipid-lowering effects. Caution is advised.

Interactions with Herbs and Dietary Supplements
- In theory, pantethine may increase the risk of bleeding when taken with herbs and supplements that are believed to increase the risk of bleeding. Multiple cases of bleeding have been reported with the use of *Ginkgo biloba*, and fewer cases with garlic and saw palmetto. Numerous other agents may theoretically increase the risk of bleeding, although this has not been proven in most cases.
- Use of pantethine with other lipid-lowering agents, such as red yeast, may produce additive lipid-modulating effects. Caution is advised.

For a complete list of references, please visit www.naturalstandard.com.

Pantothenic acid

(vitamin B$_5$, dexpanthenol)

RELATED TERMS

- Calcii pantothenas, calcium pantothenate, $C_9H_{17}NO_5$, coenzyme A, D-calcium pantothenate, D (+)-*N*-(2,4-dihydroxy-3, 3-dimethylbutyryl)-beta-alanine, D-panthenol, D-pantothenic acid, D(+)-pantothenic acid, D-pantothenyl alcohol, dexpanthenol, dexpanthenolum, panthenol, pantoic acid, pantothenic, pantothenic acid, pantothenol, pantothenylol, vitamin B-5.

BACKGROUND

- Pantothenic acid (vitamin B$_5$) is an essential component of coenzyme A (CoA), a molecule that is necessary for numerous vital chemical reactions in cells. Pantothenic acid is essential to the metabolism of carbohydrates, proteins, and fats, as well as for the synthesis of hormones and cholesterol.

- The name pantothenic acid comes from the Greek word *pantos* (meaning "everywhere") in reference to its wide distribution in most plants and animals. Rich food sources include meats, liver, kidney, fish/shellfish, chicken, vegetables, legumes, yeast, eggs, and milk. However, freezing and canning may lead to a loss of much of the pantothenic acid content. Whole grains are also a good source, although refining may degrade much of the pantothenic acid content. In commercial supplement products, vitamin B$_5$ is available as D-pantothenic acid and as the synthetic products dexpanthenol (converted in the body to pantothenic acid) or calcium pantothenate. Pantothenic acid is frequently used in combination with other B vitamins in vitamin B complex formulations. Only the dextrorotatory (D) isomer of pantothenic acid possesses biological activity.

- Pantothenic acid deficiency is exceedingly rare and likely occurs only in cases of the most severe life-threatening malnutrition. Most people likely obtain sufficient amounts from dietary sources.

- Pantothenic acid has been used or studied for numerous health conditions but has not been clearly demonstrated as beneficial for any. Oral, topical (on the skin) or injected forms have been used.

EVIDENCE

Uses Based on Scientific Evidence	Grade
Pantothenic Acid Deficiency Pantothenic acid deficiency has been very rarely observed in humans. In cases of true pantothenic acid deficiency, oral pantothenic acid therapy is accepted as a treatment. It may also be merited as prevention in select patients at high risk for malnutrition. It should be included in tube feeds or parenteral (intravenous) nutrition formulas for patients unable to eat on their own.	A
Athletic Performance There is currently insufficient scientific evidence to support this use.	C
Attention Deficit Hyperactivity Disorder (ADHD) There is currently insufficient scientific evidence to support this use.	C
Burns Vitamin supplementation is often recommended in people who have sustained severe burns because of loss of nutrients and increased metabolic needs. It is unclear if vitamin B$_5$ has specific beneficial effects in burn healing beyond its usual functions in the body.	C
High Cholesterol Pantothenic acid itself has not been shown to have any cholesterol-lowering effects. However, a chemical derivative of pantothenic acid called *pantethine* has been studied for this purpose, with compelling preliminary evidence in humans.	C
Osteoarthritis There is currently insufficient scientific evidence to support this use.	C
Rheumatoid Arthritis It has been reported that pantothenic acid levels are lower in the blood of patients with rheumatoid arthritis compared to healthy people. However, it is not clear if this is a cause, effect, or a beneficial adaptive reaction.	C
Wound Healing In animal research, oral and topical pantothenic acid has been associated with accelerated skin wound healing. However preliminary clinical study results are conflicting.	C
Radiation Skin Irritation Based on one study, topical (skin) application of dexpanthenol, an analog of pantothenic acid, to areas of irradiated skin does not appear to reduce erythema, desquamation, itching, or pain following radiation treatment.	D

Uses Based on Tradition or Theory

Acne (topical dexpanthenol), adrenal gland stimulation, aging, alcoholism, allergies, alopecia, Alzheimer's disease, anxiety prevention, asthma, autism, burning feet syndrome, candidiasis, carpal tunnel syndrome, celiac disease, chronic fatigue syndrome, cold prevention, colitis, conjunctivitis (pinkeye), convulsions, cystitis, dandruff, dental conditions (bruxism), depression, diabetic neuropathy, diaper rash (topical dexpanthenol), eczema (topical dexpanthenol), glossitis, gray hair, headache, heart failure, hypertriglyceridemia,

(Continued)

P

Uses Based on Tradition or Theory—Cont'd

hypoglycemia, hypotension (low blood pressure), immune function enhancement, infection prevention, insect bites (topical), insomnia, irritability, itching (topical dexpanthenol), lupus, multiple sclerosis, muscle cramps, muscular dystrophy, neuralgia, obesity, Parkinson's disease, peripheral neuropathy, peristalsis stimulation (injected dexpanthenol), poison ivy (topical dexpanthenol), postoperative ileus (injected dexpanthenol), premenstrual syndrome (PMS), prostatitis, respiratory disorders, retarded growth, salicylate toxicity, shingles, skin disorders, stomatitis, streptomycin neurotoxicity, stress, thyroid therapy side effect prevention, ulcerative colitis (dexpanthenol enema), vertigo.

DOSING

Adults (18 Years and Older)

- Daily adequate intake (AI) of pantothenic acid levels have been established by the Food and Nutrition Board of the U.S. Institute of Medicine based on estimated dietary intakes in healthy populations. A Recommended Daily Allowance (RDA) has not been set because of insufficient available scientific evidence. For people 19 years and older, the daily AI is 5 mg daily. For pregnant women of any age, the daily AI is 6 mg daily; for breastfeeding women of any age the daily AI is 7 mg daily.
- As a dietary supplement, 5-10 mg of pantothenic acid has been used, although benefits have not been clearly demonstrated in healthy people. Pantothenic acid is frequently used in combination with other B vitamins in vitamin B complex formulations.
- Dexpanthenol 2% cream has been used on the skin for various conditions, applied once or twice daily.

Children (Younger than 18 Years)

- Daily adequate intake (AI) levels of pantothenic acid have been established by the Food and Nutrition Board of the U.S. Institute of Medicine based on estimated dietary intakes in healthy populations. A Recommended Daily Allowance (RDA) has not been set because of insufficient available scientific evidence. For infants ages 0-6 months old, the daily AI is 1.7 mg daily; for infants 7-12 months old, the daily AI is 1.8 mg daily; for children 1-3 years old, the daily AI is 2 mg daily; for children 4-8 years old, the daily AI is 3 mg daily; for children ages 9-13 years old, the daily AI is 4 mg daily; for adolescents ages 14-18 years old, the daily AI is 5 mg daily. For pregnant women of any age, the daily AI is 6 mg daily; for breastfeeding women of any age, the daily AI is 7 mg daily.
- There is insufficient evidence to recommend specific doses or supplementation in children, except in amounts found in foods or multivitamins.

SAFETY

Allergies

- Avoid if allergic to pantothenic acid or dexpanthenol. Use of dexpanthenol on the skin has been associated with skin irritation/contact dermatitis/eczema. Notably, dexpanthenol is found in many cosmetic products.

Side Effects and Warnings

- Pantothenic acid is likely safe when used orally in doses equivalent to the daily adequate intake (AI). Moderate doses have been ingested without significant reported adverse effects. Large amounts of pantothenic acid taken by mouth may cause diarrhea. In theory, nausea and heartburn may occur. It has been noted anecdotally that dexpanthenol may increase bleeding time and therefore potentially increase the risk of bleeding when combined with other agents with similar properties, but there is limited evidence in this area and this is generally not regarded as a serious potential risk.
- Use of dexpanthenol on the skin has been associated with skin irritation/contact dermatitis/eczema. Notably, dexpanthenol is found in many cosmetic products.
- Some authors advise against the use of injected dexpanthenol in patients with gastrointestinal obstruction.

Pregnancy and Breastfeeding

- Daily adequate intake (AI) levels of pantothenic acid have been established by the Food and Nutrition Board of the U.S. Institute of Medicine, based on estimated dietary intakes in healthy populations. Safety of doses beyond AI levels is not known and should be avoided.

INTERACTIONS

Interactions with Drugs

- It has been noted that dexpanthenol may increase bleeding time and therefore potentially increase the risk of bleeding when combined with other agents with similar properties. However, there is limited evidence in this area, and this is generally not regarded as a serious potential risk.
- In theory, pantothenic acid and dexpanthenol may increase the effects of cholinesterase inhibitor drugs (including multiple Alzheimer's drugs) by increasing production of acetylcholine, leading to potentially dangerous side effects. Examples of cholinesterase inhibitors include: donepezil (Aricept), rivastigmine (Exelon), galantamine (Reminyl), tacrine (Cognex), neostigmine (Prostigmin), edrophonium chloride (Tensilon), and pyridostigmine bromide (approved by the U.S. Food and Drug Administration [FDA] for use after exposure to the nerve gas Soman). Combining these agents should be avoided unless under strict medical supervision.
- Drugs containing estrogen and progestin may increase the daily requirement of pantothenic acid.

Interactions with Herbs and Dietary Supplements

- High doses of pantothenic acid may inhibit the absorption of biotin produced by microflora in the large intestine.
- It has been noted anecdotally that dexpanthenol may increase bleeding time and therefore potentially may increase the risk of bleeding when combined with other agents with similar properties. However, there is limited evidence in this area and this is generally not regarded as a serious potential risk. Multiple cases of bleeding have been reported with the use of *Ginkgo biloba* and fewer cases with garlic and saw palmetto. Numerous other agents may theoretically increase the risk of bleeding, although this has not been proven in most cases.
- Estrogen and progestin may increase the body's daily requirement for pantothenic acid.

For a complete list of references, please visit www.naturalstandard.com.

Passion Flower
(Passiflora incarnata)

RELATED TERMS

- Apigenin, apricot vine, banana passion fruit *(Passiflora mollissima)*, Calmanervin (combination product), chrysin, Compoz (combination product), corona de cristo, coumarin, cyanogenic glycosides, EUP, Euphytose (combination product), fleischfarbige, fleur de la passion, flor de passion, granadilla, grenadille, harmala alkaloids, harmaline, harmalol, harman, harmine, Jamaican honeysuckle *(Passiflora laurifolia)*, madre selva, maypops, Naturest, *Passiflora incarnata*, *Passiflora laurifolia*, *Passiflora mollissima*, pasipay, *Passiflora*, passionflower, passion vine, Passionsblume (German), purple passion flower, Sedacalm, umbeliferone, Valverde (combination product), vitexin, water lemon, wild passion flower.

BACKGROUND

- The dried aerial parts of passion flower *(Passiflora incarnata)* have historically been used as a sedative and hypnotic (for insomnia) and for "nervous" gastrointestinal complaints. However, there is a lack of clinical evidence supporting any therapeutic use. Preliminary evidence suggests that passion flower may have a benzodiazepine-like calming action.
- Evidence for significant side effects is also unclear and is complicated by the variety of poorly classified, potentially active constituents in different *Passiflora* species.
- Passion fruit *(Passiflora edulis* Sims), a related species, is used to flavor food.

EVIDENCE

Uses Based on Scientific Evidence	Grade
Congestive Heart Failure An extract containing passion flower and hawthorn has been studied as a possible treatment for shortness of breath and difficulty exercising in patients with congestive heart failure. Although the results are promising, the effects of passion flower alone are unclear.	C
Sedation (Agitation/Anxiety/Insomnia) Passion flower has a long history of use for symptoms of restlessness, anxiety, and agitation. Evidence from animal studies and weak human trials supports these uses.	C

Uses Based on Tradition or Theory
Alcohol withdrawal, antibacterial, antiseizure, antispasm, aphrodisiac, asthma, attention deficit hyperactivity disorder (ADHD), burns (skin), cancer, chronic pain, cough, drug addiction, Epstein-Barr virus, fungal infections, gastrointestinal discomfort (nervous stomach), *Helicobacter pylori* infection, hemorrhoids, high blood pressure, menopausal symptoms (hot flashes), nerve pain, pain (general), skin inflammation, tension, wrinkle prevention.

DOSING
Adults (18 Years and Older)

- There is insufficient evidence to recommend a dose of passion flower. Standard or well-studied doses of passion flower are currently lacking. Different preparations and doses have been used traditionally. Doses of 0.5-2 g of dried herb have been taken 3-4 times daily by mouth. Doses of 1- 4 mL of tincture (1:8) have been taken 3-4 times daily by mouth. Tea made from dried herb (4-8 g) has been taken daily. A dose of 2.5 g in an infusion has been used 3-4 times daily.

Children (Younger than 18 Years)

- There is insufficient evidence to recommend a dose of passion flower for use in children.

SAFETY
Allergies

- Few reports of allergic reactions, asthma, irritated sinuses, skin rashes, and skin blood vessel inflammation (vasculitis) have been reported in the available literature with the use of passion flower products. It is believed that some reactions may have been caused by impurities in combination products, not by passion flower itself.

Side Effects and Warnings

- Passion flower is generally considered to be a safe herb with few reported serious side effects. In cases of side effects, the products being used have rarely been tested for contamination, which may have been the cause. Cyanide poisoning has been associated with passiflora fruit, but this has not been proven in human studies.
- Rapid heart rhythm, nausea, and vomiting have been reported. Side effects may also include drowsiness/sedation and mental slowing. Patients should use caution if driving or operating heavy machinery.
- Passion flower may theoretically increase the risk of bleeding and affect blood tests that measure blood clotting (international normalized ratio or "INR").
- There is a case report of liver failure and death of a patient taking a preparation of passion flower with kava. Use cautiously with any kava-containing products, as kava has been associated with liver damage. It has been suggested that the cause of the liver damage is less likely related to the presence of passion flower.

Pregnancy and Breastfeeding

- There is not enough scientific evidence to recommend the safe use of passion flower in any dose during pregnancy or breastfeeding. During the 1930s, animal studies found uterine stimulant action in components of *Passiflora*.
- Many tinctures contain high levels of alcohol and should be avoided during pregnancy.

INTERACTIONS
Interactions with Drugs

- Certain substances (harmala alkaloids) with monoamine oxidase inhibitory (MAOI) action have been found in small amounts in some species of *Passiflora*. Although levels of these substances may be too low to cause noticeable effects, passion flower may theoretically increase the effects of MAOI drugs, such as isocarboxazid (Marplan), phenelzine (Nardil), and tranylcypromine (Parnate). Increased sedation or low blood pressure could also result from taking passion flower with tricyclic antidepressants such as amitriptyline (Elavil) and selective serotonin reuptake inhibitors (SSRIs) such as fluoxetine (Prozac).

- Based on animal research, use of passion flower with alcohol or other sedatives may increase the amount of drowsiness caused by some drugs. Examples include benzodiazepines, such as lorazepam (Ativan) or diazepam (Valium); barbiturates, such as phenobarbital; narcotics, such as codeine; some antidepressants; and alcohol. Caution is advised while driving or operating machinery.
- In theory, passion flower may increase the risk of bleeding when taken with drugs that increase the risk of bleeding. Some examples include aspirin, anticoagulants (blood thinners) such as warfarin (Coumadin) or heparin, antiplatelet drugs such as clopidogel (Plavix), and nonsteroidal anti-inflammatory drugs (NSAIDs) such as ibuprofen (Motrin, Advil) or naproxen (Naprosyn, Aleve).
- Many tinctures contain high levels of alcohol and may cause nausea or vomiting when taken with metronidazole (Flagyl) or disulfiram (Antabuse).
- Passion flower may also interact with anti-anxiety drugs, antibiotics, anticonvulsants, antifungals, antihistamines, anticancer drugs, antispasmodics, antitussives, caffeine, central nervous system (CNS) depressants, drugs broken down by the liver, flumazenil, naloxone, and other neurological agents.

INTERACTIONS WITH HERBS AND DIETARY SUPPLEMENTS

- Certain substances (harmala alkaloids) with monoamine oxidase inhibitory (MAOI) action have been found in small amounts in some species of *Passiflora*. Although levels of these substances may be too low to cause noticeable effects, in theory, use of passion flower with herbs or supplements with MAOI activity may cause additive effects. Kava *(Piper methysticum)* is believed to have weak monoamine oxidase inhibitor effects and may thus interact with passion flower. In addition, tricyclic antidepressants or selective serotonin reuptake inhibitors may lead to increased sedation or low blood pressure when taken with passion flower.
- Based on animal research, use of passion flower may increase the amount of drowsiness caused by some herbs or supplements, such as valerian and kava.
- Passion flower may have additive effects when taken with herbs or supplements that increase the risk of bleeding. Multiple cases of bleeding have been reported with the use of ginkgo *(Ginkgo biloba)*, and fewer cases with garlic and saw palmetto. Numerous other agents may theoretically increase the risk of bleeding, although this has not been proven in most cases.
- When taken with caffeine or herbs containing caffeine or caffeine-like compounds, passion flower may increase blood pressure.
- Passion flower contains lycopene and may have additive effects when taken with lycopene supplements.
- Passion flower may also interact with herbs or supplements taken for pain, anxiety, seizures, fungal infections, bacterial infections, or cancer. In addition, interactions with antihistamines, antispasmodics, antitussives, CNS depressants, herbs, and supplements broken down by the liver, and other neurological agents are possible.

For a complete list of references, please visit www.naturalstandard.com.

PC-SPES

RELATED TERMS

- **WARNING:** PC-SPES HAS BEEN RECALLED FROM THE U.S. MARKET AND SHOULD NOT BE USED.
- Baicalein, baicalin, *Chrysanthemum morifolium* (chrysanthemum, mum, Chu-hua); *Ganoderma lucidum* (reishi mushroom, Ling Zhi); *Glycyrrhiza glabra* (licorice); *Isatis indigotica* Fort (Da Qing Ye, dyer's wood); Oridonin, *Scutellaria baicalensis, Panax pseudo-ginseng* (San Qi); PC-CARE, Ponicidin, *Rabdosia rubescens* (rubescens, Dong Ling Cao); *Scutellaria baicalensis* (skullcap, Huang-chin); *Serenoa repens* (saw palmetto).
- Not to be confused with SPES (a different product), or with copycat products marketed with similar names.

BACKGROUND

- **WARNING:** THIS PRODUCT HAS BEEN RECALLED FROM THE U.S. MARKET AND SHOULD NOT BE USED.
- PC-SPES is an herbal combination product that was produced and marketed until early 2002 by BotanicLab, Inc. for the treatment of prostate cancer. The initials PC stand for "prostate cancer," and *"spes"* is the Latin word for "hope."
- Based on a Chinese herbal formula, PC-SPES saw palmetto (*Serenoa repens*), chrysanthemum (*Chrysanthemum morifolium*), reishi mushroom (*Ganoderma lucidum*), licorice (*Glycyrrhiza glabra*), dyer's wood (*Isatis indigotica*), san qi (*Panax pseudo-ginseng*), rubescens (*Rabdosia rubescens*), and Baikal skullcap (*Scutellaria baicalensis*). Diethylstilbestrol, indomethacin, warfarin, and several natural products have been found in some PC-SPES preparations.
- In low-quality studies, PC-SPES was observed to reduce serum prostate specific antigen (PSA) levels, reduce evidence of metastatic disease, diminish pain, and improve quality of life in patients with prostate cancer. This evidence was viewed as promising by major U.S. cancer centers.
- However, in early 2002, the FDA Safety Information and Adverse Event Reporting Program issued a warning to consumers to avoid using PC-SPES based on findings that the product contained the anticoagulant (blood thinner) warfarin. Bleeding disorders had previously been reported with PC-SPES. The manufacturer voluntarily recalled the product. Samples of PC-SPES were later found to contain variable amounts of the nonsteroidal anti-inflammatory drug indomethacin, the synthetic estrogen diethystilbesterol (DES), and the estrogen ethinyl estradiol.
- A study published in the September 2002 issue of the *Journal of the National Cancer Institute* analyzed lots of PC-SPES manufactured between 1996 and 2001. This evaluation found variable ingredients in PC-SPES between lots, with higher levels of indomethacin and DES after 1999. These post-1999 samples were found to have much greater estrogenic properties compared to earlier samples and to possess a higher level of activity against prostate cell lines in laboratory tests. After 2001, greater amounts of the natural constituents licochalcone A and baicalin, as well as warfarin, were found in samples. These results suggest that PC-SPES produced at different times may not be equivalent or comparable, and that the anticancer effects of PC-SPES

may have been due to undeclared prescription drug ingredients.
- Several other BotanicLab products have also been found to contain undeclared prescription drugs. It is not clear if these adulterants were present in raw materials obtained by BotanicLab from other sources or were added later in the manufacturing process.
- Since BotanicLab closed its doors, several products with similar names have been introduced on the market, but none has been evaluated scientifically to the same extent as PC-SPES. The National Center for Complementary and Alternative Medicine (NCCAM) has expressed willingness to support future research on formulations that are true to the claimed ingredients and proven not to be contaminated.

EVIDENCE

Uses Based on Scientific Evidence	Grade
Prostate Cancer Uncontrolled human studies of PC-SPES have reported improvements in patients with both androgen-dependent and androgen-independent prostate cancer. Overall, these studies found prostate-specific antigen (PSA) levels to fall by greater than 50% in most patients, improvements in bone scans and x-rays, reductions in pain scores, and improvements in quality of life. In a 2002 preliminary report (conference abstract) of a comparison between PC-SPES and diethylstilbestrol (DES) in patients with androgen-independent metastatic prostate cancer, patients treated with PC-SPES had a greater reduction in PSA levels. However, the later finding that undeclared amounts of DES are present in some PC-SPES samples clouds these results. Various explanations for the effectiveness of PC-SPES were initially proposed. Estrogen-like effects were reported prior to 1998. These may be due to herbs with estrogen-like effects or to undeclared estrogenic drugs. The constituent baicalin, a flavone found in *Scutellaria baicalensis*, was found in laboratory experiments to inhibit the enzymes 12-lipoxygenase, 5-alpha-reductase, and aromatase. In addition, PC-SPES extracts were reported to cause cell death (apoptosis) or to slow the growth of cancer cell lines. The recent finding that different lots of PC-SPES produced between 1996 and 2001 contained different ingredients from each other has raised questions about whether studies of PC-SPES can be compared with each other. The discovery of undeclared prescription drug ingredients including the nonsteroidal anti-inflammatory drug indomethacin, the synthetic estrogen diethystilbesterol (DES), the estrogen ethinyl estradiol, and the anticoagulant warfarin, make it unclear if these constituents may have caused the observed clinical effects.	C

(Continued)

Uses Based on Scientific Evidence	Grade
Because of these complicated circumstances, and the fact that PC-SPES has never been compared to placebo or standard cancer treatments in a well-reported study, the question of effectiveness remains unclear. Due to known and theoretical safety concerns, samples of PC-SPES that may be in the possession of patients should not be used.	

Uses Based on Tradition or Theory
Benign prostatic hypertrophy (BPH), breast cancer, breast enlargement, cancer prevention, colon cancer, leukemia, lymphoma, melanoma, pain, pancreatic cancer, prostate health, small cell lung carcinoma.

DOSING

Adults (18 Years and Older)

- Based on known safety concerns associated with PC-SPES, no dosing regimen is recommended. Samples of PC-SPES that may be in the possession of patients should not be used.

Children (Younger than 18 Years)

- Based on known safety concerns associated with PC-SPES, it should not be used in children.

SAFETY

Allergies

- In one human study, allergic reactions were reported in 2% of patients, and treatment was stopped in one case due to throat swelling and shortness of breath. It is not clear which ingredient in PC-SPES might have been responsible. Products containing herbs similar to PC-SPES should be avoided by people with allergies to any of the included herbs.

Side Effects and Warnings

- PC-SPES has been recalled and should *not* be used. Undeclared prescription drug ingredients have been found in samples of PC-SPES, including indomethacin, diethystilbesterol (DES), ethinyl estradiol, and warfarin.
- PC-SPES may increase the risk of blood clots. Several cases of blood clots, including life-threatening clots to the lungs, have been reported with PC-SPES use. In contrast, cases of bleeding have also been reported. These are theorized to be due to undeclared amounts of the prescription drug warfarin in some samples of PC-SPES, or to the presence of the PC-SPES ingredient saw palmetto, which is associated with one report of bleeding. This would add to the risk of bleeding in patients with bleeding disorders or those taking drugs that may increase the risk of bleeding. The bleeding disorder disseminated intravascular coagulation (DIC) which can include clotting, bleeding, or both, has also been reported.
- PC-SPES has also been associated with erectile dysfunction, loss of libido, hot flashes, breast/nipple tenderness, breast enlargement, water retention (edema), and leg cramps.
- Adverse effects associated with undeclared prescription drug ingredients in PC-SPES are possible, such as gastrointestinal distress from indomethacin.

Pregnancy and Breastfeeding

- PC-SPES has not been evaluated during pregnancy or breastfeeding and should be avoided. Estrogenic effects may be harmful. The undeclared prescription drug DES, discovered in some samples of PC-SPES, may increase the risk of reproductive tract abnormalities in daughters born to women taking this drug.

INTERACTIONS

Interactions with Drugs

- Based on reported cases of bleeding, and inclusion of undeclared amounts of the prescription blood thinner warfarin in some samples, PC-SPES may increase the risk of bleeding when taken with drugs that increase the risk of bleeding. Some examples include aspirin, anticoagulants (blood thinners) such as warfarin (Coumadin) or heparin, antiplatelet drugs such as clopidogrel (Plavix), and nonsteroidal anti-inflammatory drugs such as ibuprofen (Motrin, Advil) or naproxen (Naprosyn, Aleve). In contrast, PC-SPES has also been associated with an increased risk of blood clots, which may be due to estrogen-like effects. This would work against the action of blood-thinning medications.
- Based on the proposed antiandrogenic mechanism of action of saw palmetto, a major ingredient of PC-SPES, additive effects may occur with antiandrogen drugs such as the 5-reductase inhibitor finasteride (Proscar); the androgen receptor antagonists bicalutamide (Casodex), flutamide (Eulexin), and nilutamide (Nilandron); or the GnRH antagonists leuprolide (Lupron), goserelin (Zoladex), and histrelin (Supprelin). Similarly, this therapy may decrease the effectiveness of therapeutic androgens such as testosterone (Androderm, Testoderm), methyltestosterone (Android, Testred, Virilon), fluoxymesterone (Halotestin), nandrolone decanoate (Deca-Dubrolin), or stanozolol (Winstrol).
- PC-SPES may add to the estrogenic effects of other drugs, based on estrogen-like effects reported in studies, and the presence of undeclared amounts of prescription estrogen drugs in some samples of PC-SPES.
- PC-SPES may interfere with certain chemotherapy drugs such as paclitaxel. PC-SPES may affect the way the liver breaks down certain drugs.

Interactions with Herbs and Dietary Supplements

- Based on reported cases of bleeding and inclusion of undeclared amounts of the prescription blood thinner warfarin in some samples, PC-SPES may increase the risk of bleeding when taken with herbs and supplements that are believed to increase the risk of bleeding. Multiple cases of bleeding have been reported with the use of *Ginkgo biloba*, and fewer cases with garlic and saw palmetto. Numerous other agents may theoretically increase the risk of bleeding, although this has not been proven in most cases. In contrast, PC-SPES has also been associated with an increased risk of blood clots, which may be due to estrogen-like effects. This would work against the action of blood-thinning agents.
- PC-SPES may add to the estrogenic effects of other agents, based on estrogen-like effects reported in studies, and the presence of undeclared amounts of prescription estrogen drugs in some samples.
- PC-SPES may affect the way the liver breaks down certain herbs and supplements.

For a complete list of references, please visit www.naturalstandard.com.

Pennyroyal
(*Hedeoma pulegioides, Mentha pulegium*)

RELATED TERMS

- Aloe herbal horse spray, brotherwort, chasse-puces, churchwort, *Cunila pulegioides*, dictamne de Virginie, European pennyroyal, flea mint, fleabane, fretillet, *Hedeoma phlebitides*, herbal horsespray, herbe aux puces, herbe de Saint-Laurent, Labiatae (family), la menthe pouliot (French), Lamiaceae (family), Lurk-in-the-Ditch, *Melissa pulegioides*, mentha pouillot, Miracle Coat spray-on dog shampoo, mock pennyroyal, mosquito plant, Old World pennyroyal, pennyroyal essential oil, petit baume, piliolerial, poley, pouliot royal, pudding herb, pudding grass, pulegium, pulegium oil, *Pulegium regium*, *Pulegium vulgare*, puliollroyall, run-by-the-ground, squaw balm, squawmint, stinking balm, tickweed.

BACKGROUND

- American (false) pennyroyal (*Hedeoma pulegioides*) and European pennyroyal (*Mentha pulegium*) are distantly related plants in the mint (Lamiaceae) family with similar constituents and medicinal uses.
- The essential oil of pennyroyal is considered toxic. Death has been reported after the consumption of small amounts. A characteristic noted in most cases of pennyroyal overdose is a strong minty smell on the patient's breath.
- A possible role for N-acetylcysteine (NAC) in the management of pennyroyal overdose has been suggested. However, this application has not been confirmed by animal or human studies.
- The essential oil of pennyroyal may act as an emmenagogue (menstrual flow stimulant) and induce abortion. However, it may do so at lethal or near-lethal doses, making this action unpredictable and dangerous. Future research to determine the safety and efficacy of the less toxic parts of the pennyroyal plant on the menstrual cycle is needed before a recommendation can be made.

EVIDENCE

Uses Based on Scientific Evidence	Grade
Abortifacient (Uterus Contraction Stimulant/ Abortion Inducer) Folkloric use and several human case reports describe the use of the essential oil of pennyroyal to cause abortion. However, it may do so at deadly or toxic doses, making this an unpredictable and dangerous use.	C
Menstrual Flow Stimulant (Emmenagogue) Folkloric use and several human case reports describe the use of the essential oil of pennyroyal as an emmenagogue (menstrual flow stimulant). However, it may do so at lethal or near-lethal doses, making this action unpredictable and dangerous.	C

Uses Based on Tradition or Theory

Acaricidal (lethal to mites), acne, antiseptic, antispasm, anxiety, asthma, bruises and burns, cancer, chest congestion, colds, colic, cough, cramps, diarrhea, digestion, diuretic (increases urine flow), dizziness, dysentery, fever, flavoring agent, flea control, flu, fragrance (detergents, perfumes, soaps), fumigant, gallbladder disorders, gas, gout, hallucinations, headache, hysteria, immortality, indigestion, insect repellent, intestinal disorders, itchy eyes, joint problems, kidney disease, leprosy, liver disease, mouth sores, muscle pain, nosebleeds, pneumonia, potpourri, pregnancy, premenstrual syndrome, preparing the uterus for labor, purifier (water, blood), refrigerant, respiratory ailments, sedative, skin ailments (itching, burning, bruising), snake bites (venomous), stimulant, stomach pain, sunstroke, sweating, syncope, toothache, uterine fibroids, whooping cough.

DOSING
Adults (18 Years and Older)

- No safe dose of pennyroyal has been established. Extracts, oils, teas, and infusions have been taken by mouth, but may be toxic. Topical preparations have also been applied to the skin. Pennyroyal has been used as an herbal flea collar for animals by hanging a bag of pennyroyal from a regular collar or using a pennyroyal garland. Safety and effectiveness of these preparations have not been proven.

Children (Younger than 18 Years)

- Pennyroyal is not recommended in children due to insufficient evidence and known toxicity.

SAFETY
Allergies

- Allergic reactions, such as rash, to pennyroyal or to its components, including pulegone, may occur.

Side Effects and Warnings

- Pennyroyal herb and volatile oils have been associated with multiple reports of toxicity and adverse effects, including seizures, loss of consciousness, and death. In animals, pennyroyal (taken by mouth or placed on the skin) has been associated with liver, lung, and brain toxicity. Even small amounts of pennyroyal may be associated with death. Cases of human overdose and death have been reported in infants, children, and adults.
- Pennyroyal oil toxicity may cause nausea, vomiting, abdominal pain, burning in the throat, difficulty swallowing, diarrhea, excessive sweating, chills, fever, headache, ringing in the ears, dizziness, extreme thirst, muscle spasms, restlessness, tremor, excessive talkativeness, hallucinations, agitation, drowsiness, fatigue, confusion, mania, seizures, organ failure

(brain, liver, lung, kidney, heart), altered (low or high) heart rate, altered (low or high) blood pressure, slow breathing, coma, loss of consciousness, and death. Symptoms in pennyroyal overdose may mimic that of acetaminophen (Tylenol) overdose, and the use of N-acetylcysteine (an antidote used for acetaminophen toxicity) treatment may prove beneficial, although this is not well proven.

- Other side effects may include contact dermatitis, rash (when placed on the skin), malaise, lethargy, agitation, abnormal sensations, or change (increase or decrease) in pupil size. There are reports that pennyroyal may cause abortion. Pennyroyal has been used historically as an emmenagogue (menstrual stimulant) and may cause menstrual bleeding. There are reports that large amounts of pennyroyal may be irritating to the urinary tract. Pennyroyal may cause hypoglycemia (low blood sugar), hemolytic anemia (low red blood cell count due to destruction of cells), disseminated intravascular coagulation (widespread abnormal clotting and/or bleeding), and metabolic acidosis.

Pregnancy and Breastfeeding

- Pennyroyal should be avoided during pregnancy or breastfeeding, due to the risk of uterine contractions, stimulation of menstruation, and abortion.
- Many tinctures contain high levels of alcohol and should be avoided during pregnancy.

INTERACTIONS

Interactions with Drugs

- Pennyroyal may interact with hormonal drugs and decrease the effectiveness of fertility agents. Pennyroyal has been reported to cause uterine contractions, stimulation of menstruation, and abortion.
- In theory, the toxicity of pennyroyal may be increased when combined with acetaminophen (Tylenol). Pennyroyal may lower glutathione (a liver substance), which may increase the risk of acetaminophen toxicity. Pennyroyal may increase the risk of liver damage caused by other drugs.
- Pennyroyal may interfere with the way the body processes certain drugs using the liver's cytochrome P450 enzyme system. As a result, levels of these drugs may be increased in the blood and may cause increased effects or potentially serious adverse reactions. Patients using any medications should check the package insert and speak with a health care provider, including a pharmacist, about possible interactions.
- Pennyroyal may lower blood sugar levels. Caution is advised when using medications that may also lower blood sugar levels. Patients taking drugs for diabetes by mouth or insulin should be monitored closely by a qualified health care provider. Medication adjustments may be necessary.
- Pennyroyal may have antihistamine effects and may cause increased effects if combined with drugs that have antihistamine action, such as diphenhydramine (Benadryl), fexofenadine (Allegra), or loratidine (Claritin).
- Many tinctures contain high levels of alcohol and may cause nausea or vomiting when taken with metronidazole (Flagyl) or disulfiram (Antabuse).
- Pennyroyal may interact with drugs that lower the seizure threshold; use cautiously.

Interactions with Herbs and Dietary Supplements

- Pennyroyal may increase the risk of liver damage when combined with some herbs or supplements, such as kava.
- Pennyroyal has been found to inhibit the absorption of iron in meals.
- Pennyroyal may interfere with the way the body processes certain herbs or supplements using the liver's cytochrome P450 enzyme system. As a result, levels of these herbs or supplements may be increased in the blood and may cause increased effects or potentially serious adverse reactions. It may also alter the effects that other herbs or supplements possibly have on the P450 system, such as St. John's wort.
- Pennyroyal may lower blood sugar levels. Caution is advised when using herbs or supplements that may also lower blood sugar levels, such as American ginseng.
- Pennyroyal and black cohosh have been taken together to induce abortion, and this combination has been associated with toxicity and death.
- Pennyroyal and blue cohosh have traditionally been taken together to normalize the menstrual cycle in women. In theory, the combination of the two herbs may act together to increase menstrual flow. Notably, blue cohosh has been associated with multiple dangerous effects, including stroke.
- Severe psychotic episodes and seizures have been reported in a young pregnant woman after ingesting an unknown dose of pennyroyal and "Widow Welch's Female Pills," a combination of ferrous sulfate, sulfur, licorice (*Glycyrrhiza glabra*), and turmeric (*Curcuma longa*). The exact cause is unknown.

For a complete list of references, please visit www.naturalstandard.com.

Peony
(Paeonia spp.)

RELATED TERMS

- European peony, mudanpi (Chinese), *Paeonia, Paeonia emodi* Wall, *Paeonia* L., *Paeonia lactiflora, Paeonia lactiflora* Pallas, *Paeonia mascula, Paeonia officinalis, Paeonia radix, Paeonia rubra, Paeonia suffruticosa* Andrews, *Paeonia veitchii,* Paeoniaceae (family), paeoniae flos, paeoniflorgenin (PG), paeoniflorin, paeony, partially purified paeoniflorin (PF), peony flower, peony root, PG, PGG, phenolic glycoside, piney, Quilinggao, Ranunculaceae (family), red peony root, resveratrol, Shakuyaku, stilbenes, total glucosides of Peony (TGP), Unkei-to.

BACKGROUND

- Peony root has been used in traditional Chinese medicine (TCM) for centuries. Peony flowers are also used medicinally, for example, in cough syrups and in herbal teas. In combination with other herbs, peony has been used to treat a wide variety of health conditions, including menstrual problems, kidney problems, pulmonary heart disease, uterine fibroids, and pneumonia. Peony has been applied to the skin to prevent wrinkles and has been taken by mouth to treat pulmonary heart disease and liver problems caused by chronic hepatitis.
- There is good scientific evidence of an effect of peony in the treatment of pulmonary heart disease. There is also a growing body of research on TCM formulas containing peony for women's health conditions, including menstrual problems, uterine fibroids, hormone regulation, and heart disease prevention. Higher-quality studies are needed before a firm recommendation can be made.

EVIDENCE

Uses Based on Scientific Evidence	Grade
Heart Disease (Pulmonary) Pulmonary heart disease is a structural problem with the heart that is caused by a problem with the respiratory system. Studies suggest peony may benefit pulmonary heart disease.	B
Allergic Skin Disease Peony root may have beneficial effects on immune function. These effects may help decrease inflammation associated with allergic skin reactions. There is currently insufficient evidence to recommend the use of peony in allergic skin conditions.	C
Antioxidant Peony root may have antioxidant effects. However, there is currently insufficient evidence to recommend this use.	C
Heart Disease (Prevention) Peony may have positive effects on blood circulation and tone of the heart muscle; it has been used traditionally to prevent heart disease. The effectiveness of peony remains unclear for this use.	
Heart Disease (Treatment) Clinical studies suggest peony may help in the treatment of heart disease. However, further research is needed to define the effectiveness of peony in various forms of heart disease.	C
Hemolytic Disease of the Newborn Hemolytic disease of the newborn is a condition that occurs when the blood types of the mother and the newborn are incompatible. Studies in humans have used a traditional Chinese herbal medicine containing peony to prevent this condition. Thus far, the clinical evidence is not sufficient to support this use.	C
High Blood Pressure (During Pregnancy) Studies in humans have used peony for the treatment of high blood pressure that occurs during pregnancy. Thus far, the clinical evidence is not sufficient to support this use.	C
High Cholesterol Human studies in postmenopausal women suggest peony may have beneficial effects on cholesterol levels in the blood. Thus far, the clinical evidence is not sufficient to support this use.	C
Hormone Regulation Clinical studies have shown that peony may have hormonal activity. Thus far, the clinical evidence is not sufficient to support this use.	C
Kidney Problems (Crescentic Nephritis) Human studies suggest that patients with a type of kidney disease called *crescentic nephritis* may need less glucocorticoid medication with use of peony. Thus far, the clinical evidence is not sufficient to support this use.	C
Liver Inflammation (Cirrhosis) Peony has been used in traditional Chinese medicine (TCM) to treat liver disease. Thus far, the clinical evidence is not sufficient to support this use.	C
Lung Cancer Although not well-studied in humans, peony may have anticancer activity. Thus far, the clinical evidence is not sufficient to support this use.	C
Menstrual Problems Traditionally, peony was used to treat menstrual problems and lack of a menstrual period. Preliminary research suggests that peony may have hormonal	C

(Continued)

Uses Based on Scientific Evidence	Grade
effects. Thus far, the clinical evidence is not sufficient to support this use.	
Rheumatoid Arthritis Peony's anti-inflammatory effects may benefit patients with rheumatoid arthritis. There is currently not enough evidence for this use of peony.	C
Stomach Disorders (Campylobacter pyloridis) Peony root may have immune-stimulating properties. These effects may be of benefit in stomach disorders caused by *Campylobacter pyloridis* bacteria. Thus far, the clinical evidence is not sufficient to support this use.	C
Uterine Fibroids (Myomas) Peony may have hormonal activity that may have an effect on uterine fibroids. There is currently not enough evidence for this use of peony.	C
Wrinkle Prevention A compound found in peony may have antiaging properties. Thus far, the clinical evidence is not sufficient to support this use.	C

Uses Based on Tradition or Theory

Abortion inducing, anal fissures, anemia, anti-inflammatory, antimutagenic (inhibits mutations), antispasm, antiviral, blood clots, blood vessel dilation (relaxation), bowel disorders, cancer, chronic fatigue syndrome, circulation problems, common cold, cough, digestive system disorders, emetic (induces vomiting), epilepsy, gastritis (chronic), gout, gynecological disorders, heart disease, hepatitis B (hemolytic disease), herpes simplex virus, high blood sugar, human immunodeficiency virus, immune function, inflammation, leukemia, liver cancer, liver disease, menopausal disorders, menstruation pain, migraine headaches, nasal inflammation, nerve pain, nervous excitability, premenstrual syndrome (PMS), skin problems, stomach pain, sterility, tonic, upper respiratory infections, whooping cough.

DOSING
Adults (18 Years and Older)
- Various doses have been studied, and there is insufficient evidence to recommend a dose for peony. Typically, peony is consumed by mouth as a tea that is made by steeping 1 g peony flowers in 150 mL boiling water for 5-10 minutes.
- A preparation containing peony has been applied to the skin for 8 weeks for wrinkle prevention.

Children (Younger than 18 Years)
- There is insufficient evidence to recommend a dose for peony in children.

SAFETY
Allergies
- Avoid in people with a known allergy or sensitivity to peony.

Side Effects and Warnings
- Reported side effects of peony have included nausea, vomiting, hives, skin rash, breathing problems, and chest pain.
- Peony may increase the risk of bleeding. Caution is advised in patients with bleeding disorders or those taking drugs that may increase the risk of bleeding. Dosing adjustments may be necessary.
- Peony may have hormonal activity. Use with caution in women with estrogen-sensitive cancers or in patients taking hormonal agents such as birth control pills and hormone replacement therapy.

Pregnancy and Breastfeeding
- Peony is not recommended in pregnant or breastfeeding women due to a lack of available scientific evidence. Peony may have hormonal activity and has traditionally been used to induce menstruation or abortion.

INTERACTIONS
Interactions with Drugs
- Peony may increase the risk of bleeding when taken with drugs that increase the risk of bleeding. Some examples include aspirin, anticoagulants (blood thinners) such as warfarin (Coumadin) or heparin, antiplatelet drugs such as clopidogrel (Plavix), and nonsteroidal anti-inflammatory drugs such as ibuprofen (Motrin, Advil) or naproxen (Naprosyn, Aleve).
- Peony may interact with tamoxifen, drugs that decrease blood vessel growth, drugs that dilate or relax blood vessels, drugs used in the treatment of HIV, drugs with hormonal activity, drugs that affect the immune system, and drugs used to treat cancer, inflammation, viruses, high blood pressure, and high cholesterol.
- Peony may delay absorption of the anti-seizure drug phenytoin (Dilantin). Peony may decrease the need for steroid drugs in some patients.

Interactions with Herbs and Dietary Supplements
- Peony may increase the risk of bleeding when taken with herbs and supplements that are believed to increase the risk of bleeding. Multiple cases of bleeding have been reported with the use of *Ginkgo biloba*, and fewer cases have been reported with the use of garlic and saw palmetto. Numerous other agents may theoretically increase the risk of bleeding, although this has not been proven in most cases.
- Peony may interact with antioxidants; ferulic acid; resveratrol; herbs and supplements with hormonal activity; herbs and supplements that decrease blood vessel growth; and herbs and supplements that lower cholesterol, treat viruses, dilate or relax blood vessels, lower blood pressure, stimulate the immune system, or decrease inflammation.

For a complete list of references, please visit www.naturalstandard.com.

Peppermint
(Mentha x piperita)

RELATED TERMS

- Balm mint, black peppermint, brandy mint, curled mint, Feullis de menthe, Japanese peppermint, Katzenkraut (German), lamb mint, menta prima (Italian), *Mentha arvensis* L. var piperascens, *Menthae piperitae* aetheroleum (peppermint oil), *Menthae piperita* var officinalis, *Menthae piperitae* folium (peppermint leaf), *Menthe anglaise*, *Menthe poivre*, *Menthe poivree*, *Mentha piperita* var vulgaris, Our Lady's mint, pebermynte (Danish), peppermint oil, Pfefferminz (German), Porminzen, Schmecker, spearmint (*Mentha spicata* L.), water mint *(Mentha aquatica)*, white peppermint, WS(R) 1340.
- **Note:** *Mentha x villosa* L. is a different species of mint with a similar appearance, used primarily as a flavoring agent.

BACKGROUND

- Peppermint is a flowering plant that grows throughout Europe and North America. Peppermint is widely cultivated for its fragrant oil. Peppermint oil has been used historically for numerous health conditions, including common cold symptoms, cramps, headache, indigestion, joint pain, and nausea. Peppermint leaf has been used for stomach/intestinal disorders and for gallbladder disease.
- Mint plants such as peppermint and spearmint have a long history of medicinal use, dating to ancient Egypt, Greece, and Rome. The scientific name for peppermint *(Mentha x piperita)* is derived from the name Mintha, a Greek mythological nymph who transformed herself into the plant, and from the Latin piper meaning "pepper." Peppermint is a cross (hybrid) between spearmint (*Mentha spicata*) and water mint (*Mentha aquatica*).
- Peppermint oil is available in bulk herb oil, enteric-coated capsules, soft gelatin capsules, and in liquid form. In small doses, such as in tea or chewing gum, peppermint is generally believed to be safe in healthy, non-pregnant, non-allergic adults. The United States is a principal producer of peppermint, and the largest markets for peppermint oil are manufacturers of chewing gum, toothpaste, mouthwash, and pharmaceuticals.

EVIDENCE

Uses Based on Scientific Evidence	Grade
Antispasmodic (Colonic, Esophageal, Gastric Spasm) Peppermint oil may be beneficial in reducing intestinal spasm during and after endoscopic procedures.	B
Cough There is some evidence that peppermint may relieve cough, at least for a short duration. Although there is a lack of well-designed clinical trials showing the effectiveness of peppermint in managing cough, its historical use and known antispasmodic effects suggest that it is beneficial for this use.	B
Indigestion (Non-Ulcer Dyspepsia) There is preliminary evidence that a combination of peppermint oil and caraway oil may be beneficial for dyspepsia (heartburn) symptoms. It should be noted that heartburn can actually be a side effect of taking oral peppermint oil. Patients with chronic heartburn should be evaluated by a qualified health care provider.	B
Irritable Bowel Syndrome (IBS) Peppermint may improve irritable bowel syndrome (IBS) symptoms. Although the mechanism of action is not clear, preclinical studies suggest that the benefits may be due to smooth muscle relaxation and calcium antagonism.	B
Tension Headache Application of diluted peppermint oil to the forehead and temples has been tested in people with headache. It is not clear if this is an effective treatment, although benefits were observed.	B
Abdominal Distention There is not enough available scientific evidence to support this use of peppermint.	C
Asthma There is not enough available scientific evidence to support this use of peppermint.	C
Bad Breath Early research suggests that cleaning the mouth with an essential oil mixture of diluted tea tree, peppermint, and lemon may improve bad breath in intensive care unit patients.	C
Breast Tenderness (Preventing Cracked Nipples) Using peppermint gel during breastfeeding may help prevent cracked nipples. There is not enough available scientific evidence to support this use of peppermint.	C
Functional Bowel Disorders Early research suggests that peppermint oil taken by mouth may improve gastric emptying. Therefore, peppermint oil may help treat digestive disorders. There is not enough available scientific evidence to support this use of peppermint.	C
Nasal Congestion Menthol, a constituent of peppermint oil, is sometimes included in inhaled preparations for nasal congestion, including "rubs" that are applied to the skin and inhaled. High-quality research is lacking in this area.	C

(Continued)

P

Uses Based on Scientific Evidence	Grade
Nausea There is not enough evidence to recommend the use of peppermint oil in the treatment of nausea.	C
Post-Herpetic Neuralgia (Herpes Zoster Pain) There is currently insufficient research available to determine if there are benefits of peppermint oil in the treatment of post-herpetic neuralgia.	C
Stroke Recovery Aromatherapy with peppermint oil, lavender, and rosemary has been used to reduce shoulder pain and improve motor power in patients recovering from strokes. Although treatment appeared to have beneficial effects, it is unclear if this was caused by peppermint oil or the other two herbs. Additional studies using peppermint oil alone are needed.	C
Tuberculosis There is not enough available scientific evidence to support this use of peppermint.	C
Urinary Tract Infection Peppermint tea added to other therapies has been used in the treatment of urinary tract infections. It is not clear if this is an effective treatment, and it is not recommended to rely on peppermint tea alone to treat this condition.	C
Vigilance Improvement in Brain Injury (Aromatherapy) There is currently a lack of sufficient evidence to recommend the use of peppermint oil to affect vigilance following brain injuries.	C

Uses Based on Tradition or Theory

Anorexia, antacid, antiviral, arthritis, asthma, bile duct disorders, cancer, chicken pox, cholelithiasis (gallstones), common cold, cramps, dysmenorrhea (menstrual pain), enteritis, fever, fibromyositis, gallbladder disorders, gas (flatulence), gastritis, gonorrhea, ileus (postoperative), inflammation of oral mucosa, influenza, intestinal colic, lice, liver disorders, local anesthetic, morning sickness, motility disorders, mouth and throat inflammation, mosquito repellent, mouthwash, musculoskeletal pain, neuralgia (nerve pain), pruritus (itching), respiratory infections, rheumatic pain, sun block, tendonitis, toothache, tuberculosis, urticaria (hives), vomiting.

DOSING
Adults (18 Years and Older)
- Peppermint oil should be used cautiously, as doses of the constituent menthol over 1 g/kg of body weight may be deadly. For intestinal/digestion disorders, doses of 0.2-0.4 mL of peppermint oil in enteric-coated capsules, dilute preparations, or suspensions taken three times daily by mouth have been used or studied. Lozenges containing 2-10 mg of peppermint oil have been used. 10% peppermint oil (in methanol) has been applied to the skin (forehead and temples) multiple times per day for headache relief. Some sources recommend using peppermint oil preparations on the skin no more than 3-4 times per day. For inhalation, 3-4 drops of oil added to 150 mL of hot water and inhaled up to three times per day, or 1%-5% essential oil as a nasal ointment has been used to relieve congestion.
- As an infusion, 3-6 g of peppermint leaf has been used daily. Doses of other liquid preparations depend on concentration; for example, 2-3 mL of tincture (1:5 in 45% ethanol) three times daily or 1 mL of spirits (10% oil and 1% leaf extract, mixed with water) has been taken. Various doses of dried herb extract have also been used, ranging from 0.8 g/day up to 4 g taken three times daily, although safety is not clear.

Children (Younger than 18 Years)
- There is insufficient evidence to recommend the safe use of peppermint leaf or oil in children.

SAFETY
Allergies
- Allergic/hypersensitivity reactions may occur from using peppermint or menthol by mouth or on the skin, including throat closing (laryngeal spasm), breathing problems (bronchial constriction/asthma symptoms), or skin rash/hives/contact dermatitis. People with known allergy/hypersensitivity to peppermint leaf or oil should avoid peppermint products.

Side Effects and Warnings
- Peppermint oil may be safe in small doses, although multiple adverse effects are possible. When used on the skin, peppermint oil has been associated with allergic/hypersensitivity reactions, skin rash/hives/contact dermatitis, mouth ulcers/sores, chemical burn, and eye irritation. Lung injury has occurred following an injection of peppermint oil. Peppermint oil taken by mouth may cause headache, dizziness, heartburn, anal burning, slow heart rate, or muscle tremor. Very large doses of peppermint oil taken by mouth have resulted in muscle weakness, brain damage, and seizure.
- Peppermint oil should be used cautiously by people with G6PD deficiency or gallbladder disease. Use in infants or children is not recommended due to potential toxicity.
- Menthol, a constituent of peppermint oil that is included in mouthwashes, toothpastes, mentholated cigarettes, and decongestant "rubs" or lozenges, has been associated with multiple adverse effects, such as serious breathing difficulties, asthma, skin bruising (purpura), and mouth sores. Although small amounts may be safe in non-allergic adults, higher doses may be deadly in humans or cause brain damage. Use on the skin may also cause rash, severe skin damage (necrosis), or kidney damage (interstitial nephritis). Inhalation of large doses of menthol may lead to dizziness, confusion, muscle weakness, nausea, or double vision.

Pregnancy and Breastfeeding
- Peppermint oil and menthol should be avoided during pregnancy and breastfeeding due to insufficient information and potential for toxicity.

INTERACTIONS
Interactions with Drugs

- Peppermint oil by mouth may increase blood levels of the drugs felodipine (Plendil) and simvastatin (Zocor). Peppermint oil increases levels of cyclosporine in the blood. Peppermint oil used on the skin with 5-fluorouracil (5-FU) may increase the rate of absorption of 5-FU.
- Peppermint oil may interfere with the way the body processes certain drugs using the liver's cytochrome P450 enzyme system. As a result, levels of these drugs may be increased in the blood and may cause increased effects or potentially serious adverse reactions. Patients using these medications should check the package insert and speak with a qualified health care provider, including a pharmacist, about possible interactions.
- Peppermint may also interact with antacids, other calcium channel blockers, or drugs that lower high blood pressure. Caution is advised.

Interactions with Herbs and Supplements

- Peppermint oil may interfere with the way the body processes certain herbs or supplements using the liver's cytochrome P450 enzyme system. As a result, levels of other herbs or supplements may be too high in the blood. It may also alter the effects that other herbs or supplements possibly have on the P450 system. Patients using these medications should check the package insert and speak with a qualified health care provider, including a pharmacist, about possible interactions.
- Peppermint may also interact with herbs and supplements that raise or lower blood pressure or have antacid properties. Caution is advised.

For a complete list of references, please visit www.naturalstandard.com.

P

Perilla
(*Perilla frutescens*)

RELATED TERMS

- L-perillyl alcohol, alpha-linolenic acid, ao shiso, apigenin, baisu, ban tulsi (Bengali), beefsteak plant, bhanjira (Hindi), caffeic acid, Chinese basil, chi-ssu (Chinese), common perilla, d-limonene, dihydroperillic acid, egoma (Japanese), hung-sha-yao (Chinese), ji soo, kkaennip namul (Korean), Labiatae (family), Lamiaceae (family), limonene, luteolin, m-hydroxy-phenylpropionic acid, methyl caffeate, monoterpene, mono-terpene perillyl alcohol, perilla seed oil, perilla seed perillaldehyde, perilla oil, perillic acid, perilloside A, perilloside C, perillyl alcohol, *Perilla frutescens*, purple mint, purple perilla, rattlesnake weed, red perilla, rosmarinic acid, trans-caffeic acid, shiso (Japanese), shisonoha (Japanese, red leaved form), summer coleus, trans-carveol, trans-m-coumaric acid, ts'ao-t'ou (Chinese), tsu-shih ts'ao (Chinese), tzu ssu (Chinese), wild basil, wild coleus, wild red basil, yeh-ssu (Chinese), zisu.

BACKGROUND

- Perilla is a traditional crop of China, India, Japan, Korea, Thailand, and other Asian countries. In North America, it is occasionally called by its Japanese name, *shiso*. In North America, it is also known as purple mint, Chinese basil, or wild coleus. Perilla seed oil is used for cooking, as a drying oil, and as a fuel. Perilla seed oil is high in the omega-3 fatty acid, alpha-linolenic acid.
- Asian practitioners prescribe perilla for respiratory afflictions and prevention, pregnancy concerns, seafood poisoning, and "incorrect energy balance."
- Some evidence is available for the use of perilla oil for reduction in asthma symptoms, as well as use of perilla extract for seasonal allergies. Perillyl alcohol, isolated from the essential oil of perilla and several other plants, has been researched for potential anticancer properties. More clinical evidence is required before recommendations can be made for any clinical usage of perilla.

EVIDENCE

Uses Based on Scientific Evidence	Grade
Allergies Preliminary evidence suggests some benefit of perilla extract for seasonal allergies. However, the available clinical evidence is insufficient to support this use.	C
Aphthous Stomatitis (Mouth Ulcer or Canker Sore) Preliminary evidence suggests there is no benefit of perilla oil over soybean oil for aphthous stomatitis prevention. However, the available clinical evidence is insufficient to support this use.	C
Asthma Preliminary evidence suggests some benefit of perilla oil for symptoms of asthma. Further clinical trials are required before a firm recommendation can be made.	C

Uses Based on Tradition or Theory

Anti-inflammatory, antimicrobial, antioxidant, antiviral, arteriosclerosis (hardening of the arteries), atopic dermatitis, blood pressure control (lowering), brain function improvement, cancer, cardiovascular disease, colds, constipation, cough, Crohn's disease, dental caries (prevention), depression, diabetes, fever, hypercholesterolemia (high blood cholesterol), hypertriglyceridemia (high levels of triglycerides or fatty acid compounds in the blood), gastrointestinal disorders, immunomodulation, leukemia, lung conditions, memory, nausea and vomiting, obesity, osteoporosis, poisoning (seafood), pregnancy (morning sickness), pregnancy problems, respiratory tract infections, rosacea (skin condition characterized by red, oily skin and acne), schizophrenia, sedative, stress.

DOSING
Adults (18 Years and Older)

- There is insufficient evidence to recommend a dose for perilla. Traditionally, a tea (boiling water to ¼ cup dry herb, steep 10-15 minutes) consumed throughout the day has been used for colds, flu, sore throat, and congestion. For asthma, perilla seed oil for 4 weeks has been used. For seasonal allergic rhinoconjunctivitis, *Perilla frutescens* enriched with rosmarinic acid (200 mg or 50 mg) for 3 weeks has been used. Perilla has also been boiled and the steam has been inhaled to clear the sinuses.

Children (Younger than 18 Years)

- There is insufficient evidence to recommend a dose for perilla in children.

SAFETY
Allergies

- Avoid in people with a known allergy or hypersensitivity to perilla. Occupational allergic contact dermatitis from *Perilla frutescens* has been documented.

Side Effects and Warnings

- Perilla used in recommended doses is considered to be safe and well tolerated. In one study, patients reported no adverse events, and no significant abnormalities were detected in routine blood tests. However, occupational allergic contact dermatitis from *Perilla frutescens* has been documented.
- Use commercial perilla oil cautiously in patients with cancer, due to a mutagen formed in the oil, from omega-3 fatty acids.

Pregnancy and Breastfeeding

- Perilla is not recommended in pregnant or breastfeeding women due to a lack of available scientific evidence.

INTERACTIONS
Interactions with Drugs

- *Perilla frutescens* may contain sedative constituents. Drowsiness or sedation may occur. Use caution if driving or operating heavy machinery.

- Although not well studied in humans, perilla may lower HDL cholesterol levels. Caution is advised in patients with high cholesterol or those taking any cholesterol-lowering agents.
- Theoretically, perilla may suppress indomethacin-induced effects, due to a change in fatty acid and eicosanoid status. Caution is advised in patients taking indomethacin or other nonsteroidal anti-inflammatory drugs (NSAIDs).

Interactions with Herbs and Dietary Supplements

- *Perilla frutescens* may contain sedative constituents, and may interact with other herbs that have sedative properties. Drowsiness or sedation may occur. Use caution if driving or operating heavy machinery.

- Theoretically, the results from an animal study suggest that the combination of perilla and beta-carotene may reduce the risk of colon cancer.
- Theoretically, perilla may lower HDL cholesterol levels. Caution is advised in patients with high cholesterol or those taking any cholesterol-lowering agents, such as red yeast rice.
- Theoretically, use of fish oil or omega-3 fatty acid sources (flax oil, walnut oil, soybean oil) and perilla oil would increase omega-3 fatty acid status of blood and tissues to a greater effect than either alone. Caution is advised.

For a complete list of references, please visit www.naturalstandard.com.

P

Perillyl Alcohol

($C_{10}H_{16}O$)

RELATED TERMS

- L-perillyl alcohol, monoterpene, monoterpene perillyl alcohol, perilla, perillic acid, POH.

BACKGROUND

- Perillyl alcohol is isolated from the essential oils of several plants, including cherries, lavender, peppermint, spearmint, celery seeds, sage, cranberries, lemongrass, ginger grass, savin juniper, *Conyza newii*, caraway, perilla, and wild bergamot.
- Animal studies suggest that perillyl alcohol may help slow growth of pancreatic, mammary, and liver tumors. It may also help colon, lung, and skin cancer. Perillyl alcohol is under sponsorship from the National Cancer Institute (NCI) and is undergoing phase II clinical trials.

EVIDENCE

Uses Based on Scientific Evidence	Grade
Cancer Perillyl alcohol is used to treat cancer. However, strong scientific evidence is currently lacking. Further studies are ongoing.	C

Uses Based on Tradition or Theory
Antimicrobial, cardiovascular disease, chemotherapy support, glioblastoma, hypercholesterolemia, infection (protozoan), weight loss.

DOSING

Adults (18 Years and Older)

- There is insufficient evidence to recommend the use of perillyl alcohol in adults.

Children (Younger than 18 Years)

- There is insufficient evidence to recommend the use of perillyl alcohol in children.

SAFETY

Allergies

- Avoid in people with an allergy or hypersensitivity to perillyl alcohol. Allergic skin reaction to perillyl alcohol has been documented.

Side Effects and Warnings

- The main side effects associated with perillyl alcohol in patients with various types of tumors include gastrointestinal (reflux, nausea, vomiting, and diarrhea) and fatigue. Other gastrointestinal symptoms included loss of appetite, belching, abdominal bloating, constipation, and abdominal cramps.
- High blood pressure, hot flashes, unpleasant taste, satiety, mucositis, elevated liver enzymes, and headaches have been reported.
- Avoid use in the absence of medical supervision.

Pregnancy and Breastfeeding

- Elecampane is not recommended in pregnant or breast-feeding women due to a lack of available scientific evidence.

INTERACTIONS

Interactions with Drugs

- Perillyl alcohol may interact with chemotherapies, cholesterol-lowering drugs, phenothiazines, and other drugs use to control nausea and vomiting. Imatinib mesylate (Gleevec; STI571) may also interact with perillyl alcohol.

Interactions with Herbs and Dietary Supplements

- Herbs containing perillyl alcohol, including lavender, peppermint, spearmint, celery seeds, sage, lemongrass, ginger grass, savin juniper, *Conyza newii*, caraway, *Perilla frutescens*, and wild bergamot, may have additive effects.
- Perillyl alcohol may also interact with herbs and supplements used to control nausea and vomiting or that lower cholesterol; use cautiously.

For a complete list of references, please visit www.naturalstandard.com.

Peyote
(*Lophophora williamsii*)

RELATED TERMS

- Cactaceae (family), cactus methanolic extract, *Lophophora*, *Lophophora williamsii*, mescaline (3,4,5-trimethoxyphenethylamine).

BACKGROUND

- *Lophophora williamsii*, also known as peyote, is found primarily in dry regions from central Mexico to Texas, particularly in regions along the Rio Grande. Peyote is commonly used in rituals and as a hallucinogen (due to its mescaline content). In 1990, the U.S. Supreme Court ruled that states may prohibit the use of peyote for religious purposes. Although peyote is illegal, the Dona Ana cactus, *Coryphantha macromeris* (Engelm.) Br. and R. and its *runyonii* (Br. and R.) L. Benson variety have been promoted as natural and legal psychedelic agents with about one-fifth of the potency of peyote.
- To date, there are no available clinical trials investigating the use of peyote for any indication. However, preliminary research investigating peyote has not found long-term cognitive deficits, although more research is needed to make any firm conclusions about peyote's safety.
- Some experts believe that proper use of one psychoactive substance, such as peyote, within a spiritual or clinical context helps to free an individual from the adverse effects of their addiction to another substance and thus restores them as functioning members of their community or group.

EVIDENCE

Uses Based on Scientific Evidence

No available studies qualify for inclusion in the evidence table.

Uses Based on Tradition or Theory

Alcoholism, hallucinogenic, immunomodulator, tumor.

DOSING

Adults (18 Years and Older)

- There is insufficient evidence for peyote in adults.

Children (Younger than 18 Years)

- There is insufficient evidence to recommend a dose for peyote in children.

SAFETY

Allergies

- Avoid in people with a known allergy or hypersensitivity to peyote, mescaline, or members of the Cactaceae family.

Side Effects and Warnings

- There is limited available evidence describing the adverse effects of peyote. Due to the hallucinogenic activity of peyote, psychosis has been reported in case reports. Ritualistic use of peyote does not appear to cause long-term cognitive deficits, although more research is needed to clarify these findings.
- Use cautiously in patients with mental disorders, as peyote may induce psychotic episodes.
- Use cautiously in patients with high or low blood pressure, due to mescaline's potential to alter blood pressure.
- Avoid in patients who are pregnant or breastfeeding due to the potential of fetal abnormalities.

Pregnancy and Breastfeeding

- Peyote is not recommended in pregnant or breastfeeding women due to a lack of sufficient data in humans. Mescaline, a constituent of peyote, may cross the placenta and has been linked to congenital malformations.

INTERACTIONS

Interactions with Drugs

- The biochemical alkaloids common in the peyote cactus are thought to be pharmacologically similar to the neuroamine-derived alkaloids found in the brain during alcohol intoxication. Caution is advised when taking peyote with alcohol.
- Peyote extracts may regulate blood pressure, although the clinical significance of this is unknown. Caution is advised in patients taking agents that may also alter blood pressure.
- Peyote may stimulate lymphocytes and leukocytes. Caution is advised when taking peyote with immunomodulators due to possible additive effects.
- Chlorpromazine may affect the disposition of ^{14}C-labeled C-mescaline in fetal and maternal brain and liver. Caution is advised when taking peyote with phenothiazines.
- Due to peyote's hallucinogenic effects, combined use with other psychoactives may cause additive effects. Caution is advised in patients with mental disorders.
- Peyote may increase the amount of drowsiness caused by some drugs.

Interactions with Herbs and Dietary Supplements

- In theory, due to peyote's hallucinogenic effects, combined use with other psychoactive herbs or supplements may cause additive effects. Caution is advised in patients with mental disorders.
- Peyote extracts may regulate blood pressure, although the clinical significance of this is unknown. Caution is advised in patients taking herbs or supplements that may also alter blood pressure.
- Peyote may stimulate lymphocytes and leukocytes. Caution is advised when taking peyote with immunomodulator herbs or supplements due to possible additive effects.
- Peyote may increase the amount of drowsiness caused by some herbs or supplements.

For a complete list of references, please visit www.naturalstandard.com.

P

RELATED TERMS

- **Aluminum phosphate; calcium phosphate** (bone ash, bone phosphate, calcium orthophosphate, calcium phosphate dibasic anhydrous, calcium phosphate dibasic dihydrate, calcium phosphate tribasic, di-calcium phosphate, dicalcium phosphate, dicalcium phosphates, neutral calcium phosphate, precipitated calcium phosphate, tertiary calcium phosphate, tricalcium phosphate, whitlockite); **potassium phosphate** (dibasic potassium phosphate, dipotassium hydrogen orthophosphate, dipotassium monophosphate, dipotassium phosphate, monobasic potassium phosphate, potassium acid phosphate, potassium biphosphate, potassium dihydrogen orthophosphate), MCI-196 (colestilan), sevelamer (Renagel); **sodium phosphate** (anhydrous sodium phosphate, dibasic sodium phosphate, disodium hydrogen orthophosphate, disodium hydrogen orthophosphate dodecahydrate, disodium hydrogen phosphate, disodium phosphate, phosphate of soda, sodium orthophosphate).
- **Note on terminology:** The term *phosphates* in this monograph refers to anhydrous sodium acid phosphate, dibasic sodium phosphate, dipotassium phosphate anhydrous, monobasic potassium acid phosphate, monobasic sodium phosphate, phosphorus, potassium phosphate, sodium biphosphate, and sodium phosphate.
- **Caution:** Do not confuse phosphate salts with toxic substances such as organophosphates, or with tribasic sodium phosphates and tribasic potassium phosphates, which are strongly alkaline.

BACKGROUND

- Phosphorus is a mineral found in many foods, such as milk, cheese, dried beans, peas, colas, nuts, and peanut butter. Phosphate is the most common form of phosphorus. In the body, phosphate is the most abundant intracellular anion. It is critical for energy storage and metabolism, for the utilization of many B-complex vitamins, to buffer body fluids, for kidney excretion of hydrogen ions, for proper muscle and nerve function, and for maintaining calcium balance. Phosphorus is vital to the formation of bones and teeth, and healthy bones and soft tissues require calcium and phosphorus to grow and develop throughout life. Inadequate intake of dietary phosphate can lead to hypophosphatemia (low levels of phosphate in the blood), which can lead to long-term potentially serious complications. Conversely, excess phosphate intake can lead to hyperphosphatemia (high blood phosphorus levels), which can occur particularly in people with impaired kidney function and can lead to potentially serious electrolyte imbalances, adverse effects, or death.
- In adults, phosphorus makes up approximately 1% of total body weight. It is present in every cell of the body, although 85% of the body's phosphorus is found in the bones and teeth.
- Phosphates are used clinically to treat hypophosphatemia and hypercalcemia (high blood calcium levels), as saline laxatives, and in the management of calcium-based kidney stones. They may also be of some benefit to patients with vitamin D resistant rickets, multiple sclerosis, and diabetic ketoacidosis.

EVIDENCE

Uses Based on Scientific Evidence	Grade
Constipation Occasional constipation is a U.S. Food and Drug Administration (FDA)–approved use of phosphates in adults and children, both in oral form and as an enema (for example, Fleet Enema). Phosphates are also used to restore bowel activity after surgery.	A
Hypercalcemia (High Blood Calcium Levels) Phosphate salts (except for calcium phosphate) are effective in the treatment of hypercalcemia. However, intravenous phosphate for treating hypercalcemia is not recommended due to concerns about lowering blood pressure, excessively lowering calcium levels, heart attack, tetany, and kidney failure. Sudden hypotension (low blood pressure), kidney failure, and death have been reported after phosphate infusion.	A
Hypophosphatemia (Low Blood Phosphorus Levels) Phosphates are approved by the U.S. Food and Drug Administration (FDA) for treating hypophosphatemia in adults. Taking sodium phosphate or potassium phosphate is effective for preventing and treating most causes of hypophosphatemia and should be directed under medical supervision. The underlying cause of the hypophosphatemia should be identified and corrected whenever possible.	A
Kidney Stones (Calcium Oxalate Stones) Phosphates are approved by the FDA for treating kidney stones (nephrolithiasis) in adults. Taking potassium and sodium phosphate salts orally may help prevent kidney stones in patients with hypercalciuria (high urine calcium levels) and in patients with kidney stones made of calcium oxalate. However, phosphate administration when stones are composed of magnesium-ammonium–phosphate or calcium phosphate may increase the rate of stone formation.	A
Laxative/Bowel Preparation for Procedures Phosphates are approved by the FDA for use as a laxative in adults and children. Sodium phosphate taken orally or as an enema may be used for bowel cleansing in preparation for surgery, imaging studies, or endoscopy (for example, Fleet Phospho-soda, Fleet Enema). Phosphates appear to increase peristalsis and cause an influx of fluids into the intestine via osmotic action. Aluminum phosphate is used orally to neutralize gastric acid.	A

(Continued)

Uses Based on Scientific Evidence	Grade
Refeeding Syndrome Prevention After periods of severe malnutrition or starvation (for example, anorexia nervosa), intravenous phosphate may be necessary in order to prevent refeeding syndrome. Phosphate levels should be closely monitored in such patients.	B
Bone Density (Bone Metabolism) Early research shows that high amounts of phosphorus may have negative effects on bone density. This is because phosphorus decreases bone formation and increases bone resorption.	C
Burns Patients with serious burns may lose phosphates, and replacement may be necessary.	C
Diabetic Ketoacidosis The use of prophylactic phosphate therapy in diabetic ketoacidosis is controversial and may be considered, particularly in cases of low phosphate levels.	C
Hypercalciuria (High Urine Calcium Levels) Long-term, slow-release neutral potassium phosphate has been shown to reduce calcium excretion in subjects with absorptive hypercalciuria and appears to be well tolerated. This use of phosphates may be considered to prevent kidney stone formation.	C
Hyperparathyroidism This use of phosphates has not been clearly demonstrated as being beneficial in scientific studies.	C
Total Parenteral Nutrition (TPN) Critically ill patients receiving intravenous feedings often have low phosphate levels. Phosphate levels should be closely monitored in such patients, particularly if kidney function is impaired. Inorganic phosphates avoid incompatibility with calcium in TPN solutions. Addition of phosphate to TPN solutions should be under the supervision of a licensed nutritionist.	C
Vitamin D–Resistant Rickets This use of phosphates has not been clearly demonstrated as being beneficial in scientific studies.	C
Exercise Performance Several studies report that taking phosphates orally does not improve exercise performance.	D

Uses Based on Tradition or Theory

Cancer, clear cell carcinoma, depression, hypophosphatemic encephalopathy, multiple sclerosis, radioactive (thallium) parathyroid scanning enhancement, uterine papillary serous carcinoma.

DOSING
Adults (18 Years and Older)
- The National Academy of Sciences has recommended 700 mg of phosphorus daily in adults ages 18 years and older, including pregnant or breastfeeding women.
- The tolerable upper intake level (UL) for adults ages 19-70 years old is 4 g daily; for adults 70 years and older the UL is 3 g daily. The recommended UL in pregnant women is 3.5 g daily, and in breastfeeding women is 4 g daily. Phosphate salts should not be administered to patients with hyperphosphatemia and should be used cautiously in those with impaired kidney function.
- Doses typically range from 1-3 g of phosphorous (as a phosphate salt (sodium phosphate or potassium phosphate) or elemental phosphate) daily by mouth for the treatment of calcium oxalate kidney stones, hypercalcemia, or hypophosphatemia. Doses are usually divided and taken throughout the day.
- Fleet Enema (118 mL) can be used as a laxative when administered rectally. It should be administered as a single daily dose. Laxatives should not generally be used for more than 1 week. 4-8 g of sodium phosphate dissolved in water has also been used as a saline laxative (should be taken with plenty of water).
- Intravenous phosphate 50 mmol (sodium 81 mmol, potassium 9.5 mmol) over 24 hours has been used during refeeding syndrome when serum phosphate falls below 0.5 mmol/L. Phosphate blood levels should be closely followed.

Children (Younger than 18 Years)
- The recommended adequate intake in infants 0-6 months old is 100 mg daily (additional phosphorus may be added to infant formulas); the recommended adequate intake in infants 7-12 months old is 275 mg daily; the recommended daily intake in children ages 1-3 years old is 460 mg daily; the recommended daily intake in children ages 4-8 years old is 500 mg daily; the recommended daily intake in children ages 9-18 years old is 1,250 mg daily (including pregnant or breastfeeding women).
- The tolerable upper intake level (UL) for infants aged 0-12 months old is not clearly established, and the source of intake should be from food and formula only; for children 1-8 years old the UL is 3 g daily; for children 9-18 years old the UL is 4 g daily.
- Children under 12 years of age should not receive an adult size Fleet Enema. Children 2-12 years of age may receive a Fleet Ready-To-Use Enema for children in a single daily dose (2 fl oz). Laxatives should not generally be used for more than 1 week.
- Children 5-10 years old may receive 5 mL Fleet Phosphosoda and should not exceed 10 mL in a 24-hour period. Children between 10-12 years old may receive 10 mL and should not exceed 20 mL in a 24-hour period. Children over 12 years old may receive a dose of 20 mL and should not exceed 45 mL in a 24-hour period. Do not administer to children under 5 years of age.
- Children may also receive intravenous preparations, which should be given under the supervision of a licensed health care professional.

P

SAFETY
Allergies

- Avoid if allergic to any ingredients in phosphorus/phosphate preparations.

Side Effects and Warnings

- In general, sodium, potassium, aluminum, and calcium phosphates are likely safe when used orally in recommended doses for short-term periods by people without hyperphosphatemia, impaired kidney function, or other health conditions known to increase the risk of hyperphosphatemia. Sodium phosphate is likely safe when used rectally for short-term periods in otherwise healthy individuals with normal kidney function. Long-term use or high doses used orally or rectally require monitoring of serum electrolytes. Intravenous phosphate is likely safe when used as a U.S. Food and Drug Administration (FDA)–approved prescription drug under medical supervision in people without hyperphosphatemia, impaired kidney function, or other health conditions known to increase the risk of hyperphosphatemia.
- Excessive intake of phosphates can cause potentially serious or life-threatening toxicity. Intravenous, oral, or rectal/enema phosphates may cause electrolyte disturbances including hypocalcemia (low calcium blood levels), hypomagnesemia (low magnesium blood levels), hyperphosphatemia (high phosphorus blood levels), or hypokalemia (low potassium levels). Calcification of non-skeletal tissues (particularly in the kidneys), severe hypotension (low blood pressure), dehydration, metabolic acidosis, acute kidney failure, or tetany can occur. Death has been reported in infants or adults with oral, rectal, or intravenous phosphates, particularly in those at increased risk for electrolyte disturbances. Late symptoms may include abdominal pain, vomiting of phosphorescent materials, bloody vomiting and diarrhea, headache, limb aches, tongue coating, foul breath, weakness, and yellow conjunctivae (whites of the eyes). Rare complications may include confusion, convulsions (seizures), headache, dizziness, numbness, tingling, pain, weakness, anxiety, increased thirst, muscle cramps, or fatigue. Abnormal heart rhythms, shortness of breath, foot/leg swelling, and weight gain have been reported.
- Nausea or gastrointestinal irritation can occur. A reduction in dosage may be necessary to minimize diarrhea. Potassium acid phosphate may cause dyspepsia in patients with a history of peptic ulcer disease. Aluminum phosphate can cause constipation.
- Conditions that may be worsened with excessive phosphorus/phosphate supplementation include burns, heart disease, pancreatitis, rickets, osteomalacia (softening of bones), underactive parathyroid glands (with sodium phosphate or potassium phosphate), underactive adrenal glands (potassium phosphate may increase the risk of hyperkalemia), liver disease, and toxemia of pregnancy.

Pregnancy and Breastfeeding

- U.S. Food and Drug Administration (FDA) Pregnancy Category C.
- The tolerable upper intake level (UL) for phosphorus in pregnant women is 3.5 g daily, and in breastfeeding women it is 4 g daily. The recommended daily intake in pregnant or breastfeeding women 18 years and younger is 1,250 mg daily.

INTERACTIONS
Interactions with Drugs

- Antacids containing aluminum, calcium, or magnesium can bind phosphate in the gut and prevent its absorption, potentially leading to hypophosphatemia (low phosphate levels) when used chronically.
- Some anticonvulsants (including phenobarbital and carbamazepine) may lower phosphorus levels and increase levels of alkaline phosphatase.
- Bile acid sequestrants such as cholestyramine (Questran) and colestipol (Colestid) can decrease oral absorption of phosphate. Therefore, oral phosphate supplements should be administered at least 1 hour before or 4 hours after these agents.
- Corticosteroids may increase urinary phosphorus levels.
- Potassium supplements or potassium-sparing diuretics taken together with a phosphate may result in high blood levels of potassium (hyperkalemia).
- Alcohol (ethanol) may increase urinary phosphorus. Wine may enhance absorption of phosphorus (as well as calcium and magnesium).
- Medications that may affect electrolyte levels should be used cautiously with phosphates. Examples include: amiloride (Midamor); angiotensin-converting enzyme (ACE) inhibitors such as benazepril (Lotensin), captopril (Capoten), enalapril (Vasotec), fosinopril (Monopril), lisinopril (Zestril, Prinivil), quinapril (Accupril), or ramipril (Altace); cyclosporine; cardiac glycosides (Digoxin); heparins; anti-inflammatory drugs; potassium-containing agents; salt substitutes; spironolactone (Aldactone); and triamterene (Dyrenium).

Interactions with Herbs and Dietary Supplements

- Calcium may impair phosphates in the body and result in calcium deposits in tissues.
- Pumpkin seed may increase urine phosphates.
- Excessive doses of calcitriol, the active form of vitamin D (or its analogue) may result in hyperphosphatemia (high phosphate levels).

For a complete list of references, please visit www.naturalstandard.com.

Podophyllum
(*Podophyllum* spp.)

RELATED TERMS

- American mandrake, Araceae (family), bajiaolian, Berberidaceae (family), beta-peltatin, Condylox, devil's apple, diphyllin, duck's foot, *Dysosma pleianthum*, epipodophyllotoxin, etoposide 7a, etophos 7b, ground lemon, Hakkakuren, highly purified podophyllotoxin, Himalayan mayapple, hog apple, Indian apple, Indian podophyllum, kampherol, mandrake, mayapple, Podocon-25, podofilox, Podofin, podophylli pelati rhizome/resina, podophyllic acid, podophyllin, podophyllinic acid ethylhydrazide, podophyllotoxin, podophyllotoxin-beta-o-benzyliden-glucoside (SP-G), podophyllotoxin derivatives, *Podophyllum emodi*, *Podophyllum hexandrum*, *Podophyllum hexandrum* Royle, podophyllum lignan, *Podophyllum peltatum*, *Podophyllum peltatum* L., *Podophyllum pleianthum*, podophyllum resin, *Podophyllum versipelle*, Proresid, quercetin, raccoon berry, semisynthetic podophyllotoxin glycosides, *Sinopodophyllum emodi*, *Syngonium podophyllum*, umbrella plant, vegetable mercury, wild lemon, wild mandrake.
- **Note:** Podophyllum should not be confused with *Mandragora officinarum*, although both are commonly known as mandrake. Podophyllum is potentially toxic when orally ingested.

BACKGROUND

- Podophyllum is thus named from the Greek words *podos* and *phyllon*, meaning foot-shaped leaves. Podophyllum rhizomes have a long medicinal history among native North American tribes, who used a rhizome powder as a laxative or an agent that expels worms (anthelmintic). A poultice of the powder was also used to treat warts and tumorous growths on the skin.
- Podophyllotoxin is a plant-derived compound used to produce two cytostatic drugs, etoposide and teniposide. The substance has been primarily obtained from the American mayapple (*Podophyllum peltatum*). The Himalayan mayapple (*Podophyllum hexandrum* or *Podophyllum emodi*) contains this constituent in a much greater quantity but is endangered in the wild.
- Currently, extracts of the podophyllum plant are used in topical medications for genital warts, human immunodeficiency virus–related oral hairy leukoplakia, and some skin cancers. Preliminary research also shows that CPH 82, an oral form of *Podophyllum emodi* composed of two purified semisynthetic lignan glycosides, may be useful in treating rheumatoid arthritis. However, when used orally, podophyllum can be lethal and should be avoided. The drug etoposide (VePesid) is the semisynthetic derivative of podophyllotoxin and is approved by the U.S. Food and Drug Administration (FDA) for various types of cancer.

EVIDENCE

Uses Based on Scientific Evidence	Grade
Warts (Genital Warts, Plantar Warts) Podofilox, an active component of podophyllin resin, is marketed under the brand name Condylox	B

and is approved by the U.S. Food and Drug Administration (FDA) for the treatment of external genital warts and perianal warts. Preliminary study showed that podophyllum preparation was moderately effective in the treatment of genital warts. Additional study is needed before a firm conclusion regarding efficacy can be made.

Leukoplakia (HIV-Related) Oral hairy leukoplakia is an oral mucosal disease associated with the Epstein-Barr virus (EBV). Podophyllum and its derivatives are known to be active cytotoxic agents, which may be beneficial in the treatment of hairy leukoplakia. Additional study is needed before a firm conclusion regarding efficacy can be made.	C
Rheumatoid Arthritis Preliminary research suggests that podophyllum may be helpful for rheumatoid arthritis. Research is limited because of the possible adverse effects, such as severe diarrhea, associated with taking podophyllum by mouth. However, additional research is needed before a firm conclusion can be drawn.	C
Uterine Cancer Preliminary evidence suggests that podophyllum may inhibit the growth of cancer cells and may be beneficial as an adjunct to radiation for uterine cancer. Further research is needed before a strong recommendation can be made.	C

Uses Based on Tradition or Theory

Abortifacient (induces abortion), anthelmintic (expels parasitic worms), antibacterial, breast cancer, cathartic (relieves constipation), emetic (induces vomiting), fertility, fever, hepatitis, Hodgkin's disease, insecticide, jaundice, laxative, leukemia, liver disorders, mental disorders, non-Hodgkin's lymphoma, skin wounds, snake venom antidote, syphilis, tinea capitis (ringworm).

DOSING
Adults (18 Years and Older)

- Various doses have been studied with varying degrees of safety and efficacy. For rheumatoid arthritis, 300 mg of CPH 82, composed of two purified semisynthetic lignan glycosides of *Podophyllum emodi*, has been safely taken daily for up to 12 weeks.
- When used topically and appropriately, podophyllum has been used safely for up to 5 weeks. For genital warts, 5 mL of 0.5% podophyllin applied on the affected area twice daily, 3 days a week for 5 weeks has been used; a 2% podophyllin preparation has also been applied topically to the affected area twice daily, 3 days a week for 5 weeks.

P

For HIV-related hairy leukoplakia, topical podophyllum resin 25% solution for 30 days has been used.

Children (Younger than 18 Years)

- There is insufficient evidence to recommend a dose for podopyllum in children.

SAFETY
Allergies

- Avoid in individuals with a known allergy or hypersensitivity to podophyllum.

Side Effects and Warnings

- Podophyllum applied on the skin for genital warts and oral hairy leukoplakia appears to be well tolerated. Generally mild adverse effects include a burning sensation, bad or altered taste, and mild pain to severe irritation in topical application. Adverse effects from ingestion by mouth may include gastrointestinal discomfort (diarrhea and abdominal pain).
- Systemic absorption of podophyllum resin may result in tachycardia (increased heart rate), hypotension (low blood pressure), hallucinations, confusion, dizziness, and convulsions. These symptoms may be delayed in onset and prolonged in duration. Podophyllum may also cause nausea, vomiting, bloody-watery diarrhea, and a diminished number of neutrophils in the blood (neutropenia). Use cautiously in patients with Crohn's disease or irritable bowel syndrome (IBS).
- Podophyllum toxicity may cause muscle paralysis, ataxia (loss of coordination), urinary retention, renal (kidney) failure, and hypotonia (decreased muscle tone). Chronic use of podophyllum as a cathartic (relieves constipation) may cause abnormally low potassium concentrations in the blood (hypokalemia) and metabolic alkalosis.
- Podophyllotoxin solution (Wartec) may cause sweaty palms and feet or rash. Alopecia (hair loss) and gastrointestinal toxicity (nausea, vomiting, stomatitis) has occurred in about 20%-30% of patients given recommended dosages of etoposide, a semisynthetic derivative of podophyllotoxin. Patients receiving oral CPH 82 for rheumatoid arthritis reported gastrointestinal discomfort (diarrhea and abdominal pain).
- Use cautiously in patients with cardiovascular, muscular, and neurological disorders, renal (kidney) insufficiency, liver insufficiency, hypertension (high blood pressure), arrhythmia (abnormal heart rate), or psychosis.
- Avoid in patients with gallbladder disease or gallstones. Podophyllum is believed to stimulate the production of bile in the gallbladder.

Pregnancy and Breastfeeding

- Podophyllum is not recommended in pregnant or breastfeeding women because of a lack of available scientific evidence. Documented cases of birth defects and fetal deaths have been associated with podophyllum used during pregnancy.

INTERACTIONS
Interactions with Drugs

- Podophyllum toxicity may cause additive hypotension (low blood pressure) if administered with antihypertensive medications.
- Podophyllum interrupts cellular mitosis at metaphase. Podophyllum may interact with drugs that have a similar mechanism, such as paclitaxel or vincristine. Additionally, anticancer agents may cause neutropenia (diminished number of neutrophils in the blood). Concurrent use of podophyllum and antineoplastic agents may cause further bone marrow suppression.
- Podophyllum toxicity may cause a worsening of extrapyramidal symptoms that may occur with antipsychotic agents. Caution is advised when podophyllum is taken with other agents that could potentiate these symptoms.
- Although not well studied in humans, degenerative changes were observed in the liver after ingestion of podophyllum. Caution is advised when podophyllum is taken with other potentially liver-damaging agents because of the increased risk of liver damage.
- Podophyllum has been historically used as a laxative. Concurrent use of podophyllum and other laxatives may result in an additive effect and cause dehydration and electrolyte disturbances (usually fluid depletion and accumulation of electrolytes).

Interactions with Herbs and Dietary Supplements

- Podophyllum toxicity may cause additive hypotension (low blood pressure) if administered with antihypertensive (blood pressure–lowering) herbs and supplements.
- Podophyllum may interrupt mitosis and prevent cell division. Additionally, anticancer agents may cause neutropenia (shortage of white blood cells). Concurrent use of podophyllum and anticancer agents may cause an increase in neutropenia (shortage of white blood cells).
- Podophyllum toxicity may cause a worsening of extrapyramidal symptoms and neurological side effects that may occur with some antipsychotic agents. Caution is advised when podophyllum is taken with herbs or supplements that could potentiate these symptoms.
- Although not well studied in humans, degenerative changes were observed in the liver after ingestion of podophyllum. Caution is advised when podophyllum is taken with other potentially liver-damaging herbs because of the increased risk of liver damage.
- Podophyllum has been historically used as a laxative. Concurrent use of podophyllum and other laxatives may result in an additive effect and cause dehydration and electrolyte disturbances.

For a complete list of references, please visit www.naturalstandard.com.

Pokeweed
(Phytolacca americana)

RELATED TERMS

- American nightshade, American spinach, bear's grape, branching phytolacca, cancer jalap, chongras, coakum, coakum-chorngras, cokan, crowberry, endod, fitolaca, garget, hierba carmine, inkberry, jalap, kermesbeere, mitogenic lectins, monodesmosidic serjanic acid saponin, monodesmosidic spergulagenic acid saponin, phytolacain (G, R) *Phytolacca acinosa, Phytolacca acinosa* Esculenta, *Phytolacca americana,* phytolacca berry, *Phytolacca decandra, Phytolacca dioica, Phytolacca dodecandra* (Endod), *Phytolacca icosandra, Phytolacca octandra, Phytolacca rigida,* Phytolaccaceae (family), phytolaccagenin, phytolaccatoxin, phytolaccosides, pigeonberry, pocan, poke, poke root, poke salad, pokeberry, pokeweed antiviral protein (PAP), pokeweed berry, proteinaceous mitogens, raisin d'amérique, red-ink plant, red plant, red weed, resin, saponin glycosides, scoke, skoke, tannin, teinturiére, TXU-PAP, Virginian poke.

BACKGROUND

- In folk medicine, pokeweed leaves have been used for rheumatism, arthritis, emesis (vomiting), and purging. Unsubstantiated reports describe the toxicity of pokeweed root and berries, which may be due to the saponin content of the plant.
- Pokeweed antiviral protein (PAP), derived from the spring leaves of *Phytolacca americana,* shows promising therapeutic effects. Interest in PAP is growing due to its use as a potential anti–human immunodeficiency virus (HIV) agent. However, the clinical use of native PAP is limited because of inherent difficulties in obtaining sufficient quantities of homogeneously pure active PAP without batch-to-batch variation from its natural resource.
- The United Kingdom allows pokeweed in medicinal products where toxic constituents are absent and the product adheres to mandated limits. Ongoing research is investigating the use of pokeweed for the flu, herpes simplex virus (HSV)-1, and polio.

EVIDENCE

Uses Based on Scientific Evidence

No available studies qualify for inclusion in the evidence table.

Uses Based on Tradition or Theory

Abortifacient (induces abortion), abscesses (mammary), acne, anthrax, antimicrobial, antiviral, arthritis, cancer, contraception, dysmenorrhea (painful menstruation), earache, edema, emetic (induces vomiting), fatigue, fertility, food uses, gonorrhea, headache, human immunodeficiency virus, inflammation (upper and lower respiratory tract), intestinal worms, laryngitis, laxative, leeches, leukemia, lymphadenitis (inflammation of lymph nodes), mastitis (inflammation of the breast), pruritus (severe itching), purgative (laxative), rabies, rheumatism, ringworm, scabies, schistosomiasis (tropical parasitic infection), skin ailments (sycosis), skin disorders, stimulant (cardiac), syphilis (STD), tonsillitis.

DOSING

Adults (18 Years and Older)

- There is insufficient evidence to recommend a dose for pokeweed. Traditionally, 1 g of dried pokeweed root has been used as an emetic (induces vomiting) or purgative (laxative). For immune stimulation or rheumatism, 60-100 mg daily of the root and berries has been used.

Children (Younger than 18 Years)

- There is insufficient evidence to recommend a dose for pokeweed in children, and use is not recommended.

SAFETY

Allergies

- Avoid in individuals with a known allergy or hypersensitivity to pokeweed or its constituents.

Side Effects and Warnings

- All parts of the pokeweed plant are considered to be toxic. PAP appears to have fewer side effects, which include transient elevation of the liver enzyme alanine aminotransferase. Use PAP cautiously in patients with liver disorders. Use PAP cautiously and only under the guidance of a medical professional for HIV. Dosing and efficacy are unclear based on currently available literature.
- When taken by mouth, all parts of the pokeweed plant may cause nausea, vomiting, cramping, abdominal pain, diarrhea, hypotension (low blood pressure), blood abnormalities, burning sensations in the mouth and throat, weakness, bloody emesis (vomiting), bloody diarrhea, salivation, respiratory failure, difficulty breathing, tachycardia (fast heart rate), Mobitz type I heart block, transient blindness, urinary incontinence, spasm, convulsion, severe thirst, somnolence (sleepiness/drowsiness), or death.
- Protective gloves should be used to handle the plant because when the root comes in contact with broken skin or is ingested, pokeweed may cause changes in the blood. Use pokeweed cooked leaves cautiously in adult patients, as only cooked early spring leaves are considered nontoxic.

Pregnancy and Breastfeeding

- Pokeweed is not recommended in pregnant or breastfeeding women because of a lack of available scientific evidence. The berry may have uterine stimulant and abortifacient (abortion-inducing) effects.

INTERACTIONS

Interactions with Drugs

- Poke root may lower blood pressure and thus increase the action of antihypertensive agents. Patients taking blood pressure–lowering agents should consult with a qualified health care professional, including a pharmacist.

- Pokeweed root may have antiinflammatory effects and therefore may interact additively with antiinflammatory drugs.
- Pokeweed may have antiviral effects and therefore may interact with antiviral medications.
- Pokeweed may cause Mobitz type I heart block and may therefore interact with cardiac glycosides, such as digoxin or digitoxin.
- Theoretically, pokeweed may have diuretic activity and may interact additively with other diuretics. Caution is advised.
- Phytolaccosides from *Phytolacca americana* may increase the intestinal absorption of hydrophilic drugs or heparin, which may have difficulty crossing the intestinal epithelium. Consult with a qualified health care professional, including a pharmacist, for a full list of interactions.

Interactions with Herbs and Dietary Supplements

- Poke root may lower blood pressure and thus increase the action of antihypertensive herbs and supplements. Patients taking blood pressure–lowering herbs should consult with a qualified health care professional, including a pharmacist.
- Pokeweed root may have antiinflammatory effects and therefore may interact additively with herbs and supplements with antiinflammatory effects.
- Pokeweed may have antiviral effects and therefore may interact with antiviral herbs.
- Pokeweed may cause Mobitz type I heart block and may therefore interact with cardiac glycoside herbs, such as foxglove.
- Theoretically, pokeweed may have diuretic activity and may interact additively with other diuretics. Caution is advised.
- Phytolaccosides from *Phytolacca americana* may increase the intestinal absorption of hydrophilic herbs, which may have difficulty crossing the intestinal epithelium. Consult with a qualified health care professional, including a pharmacist, for a full list of interactions.

For a complete list of references, please visit www.naturalstandard.com.

Policosanol

$(CH_3\text{-}(CH_2)_n\text{-}CH_2OH)$

RELATED TERMS

- Hexacosanol, isopolicosanol, Octa-6, Octa-60, octacosanoic acid, octacosanol, policosanol, Ricewax, SCP, SFP, SFP winteriser cake, sugar cane policosanol, sunflower seed policosanols, triacontanol, wheat germ policosanol.

BACKGROUND

- Policosanol is a cholesterol-lowering natural mixture of primary alcohols, isolated and purified from sugar cane wax. Policosanol is safe and well tolerated, even in populations with high use of concomitant medications.
- Lipid profile improvements with the use of policosanol are seen in healthy volunteers, patients with type II hypercholesterolemia (high cholesterol), patients with type 2 diabetes and hypercholesterolemia, postmenopausal women with hypercholesterolemia, and patients with combined hypercholesterolemia and abnormal liver function tests. However, there is controversy in this based on recent negative evidence.
- Policosanol has performed equal to or better than simvastatin, pravastatin, lovastatin, probucol, or acipimox with fewer side effects in patients with type II hypercholesterolemia.
- Policosanol was approved for use in Cuba in 1991. Currently it is used in more than 25 countries throughout the world, mainly in South America and in the Caribbean region.

EVIDENCE

Uses Based on Scientific Evidence	Grade
Platelet Aggregation Inhibition Various studies have investigated the effect of policosanol on platelet aggregation. In general, studies suggest policosanol inhibits platelet aggregation induced by collagen and arachidonic acid.	A
Coronary Heart Disease (CHD) The effects of policosanol supplementation on exercise ECG testing responses have been studied in individuals with coronary heart disease (CHD). Beneficial changes were noted in functional capacity, rest and exercise angina (chest pain), cardiac events, and maximum oxygen uptake. Although this represents early compelling evidence, further research is necessary before a clear conclusion can be reached.	B
Intermittent Claudication (IC) There is limited study of the effects of policosanol supplementation on walking distance in individuals with IC. Additional human trials are necessary before a strong recommendation can be made.	B
High Cholesterol Policosanol has been used and recommended to treat high cholesterol levels (hypercholesterolemia). Many studies have tested the effects of policosanol on	C
cholesterol levels and have found benefits. However, some newer research suggests that policosanol may not be as beneficial as previously thought.	
Reactivity/Brain activity The effects of policosanol supplementation on reactivity and related brain activity have been examined. Although there is early compelling evidence, further research is necessary before a clear conclusion can be reached.	C

Uses Based on Tradition or Theory

Antiangiogenesis, antioxidant, atheroma (fatty material that builds up in the arteries and may lead to heart problems), atherosclerotic lesions (disease of arterial blood vessels), cerebral ischemia (lack of adequate blood flow to the brain), cerebrovascular disorders (disorders of the blood vessels in the brain), heart damage, high blood pressure, iatrogenic lipodystrophy (defective metabolism), liver damage, postmenopausal osteoporosis, stroke prevention, tumor (granuloma).

DOSING

Adults (18 Years and Older)

- Typical doses of policosanol are between 5-40 mg daily. Policosanol appears safe in these doses for up to 3 years. Based on the available evidence, this dose range is considered safe and effective in patients with coronary heart disease and for patients with type II hypercholesterolemia (high cholesterol). Doses as high as 80 g of policosanol have been taken daily for 12 weeks to treat high cholesterol. For platelet aggregation, 10-40 mg daily has been taken. For intermittent claudication, 10-20 mg has been used, and for hypertension (high blood pressure), a lower dose of 5-10 mg daily has been taken.

Children (Younger than 18 Years)

- There is insufficient evidence to recommend a dose for policosanol in children.

SAFETY

Allergies

- Avoid in individuals with a known allergy or hypersensitivity to policosanol.

Side Effects and Warnings

- Policosanol is generally regarded as safe and well tolerated. However, there are a few, minor, drug-related clinical or biochemical adverse effects observed in clinical trials. The death rate and the frequency of mild, moderate, and serious adverse events have been shown to be lower in diabetic and nondiabetic individuals taking policosanol compared with placebo.

- Policosanol may cause erythema (reddening of the skin), gum bleeding, headache, vertigo, or heartburn. Use cautiously in patients taking aspirin because of potential additive platelet inhibition and risk of bleeding. Also use caution in patients with high blood pressure or those taking agents to lower blood pressure because of a potential additive effect. Side effects of Octa-60 (a combination product including policosanol) may include skin rash and increased glucose and alanine aminotransferase levels.

Pregnancy and Breastfeeding

- Policosanol is not recommended in pregnant or breastfeeding women because of a lack of available scientific evidence. Although not well studied in humans, policosanol does not appear to affect reproductive performance, fetal/neonatal development, or breastfeeding. Additional study is needed in this area.

INTERACTIONS

Interactions with Drugs

- In theory, policosanol may interact additively with nicotinic acid (acipimox) or synthetic nicotinic acid because of acipimox's cholesterol-lowering activity. Caution is advised in patients taking other cholesterol-lowering agents. In theory, bile acid sequestrants/resins, ezetimibe (Zetia), or statins (lovastatin, atorvastatin, simvastatin, pravastatin) may have an additive cholesterol-lowering effect when given with policosanol.
- Policosanol may increase the risk of bleeding when taken with drugs that increase the risk of bleeding. Some examples include aspirin, antiplatelet drugs such as clopidogrel (Plavix), and nonsteroidal antiinflammatory drugs (NSAIDs) such as ibuprofen (Motrin, Advil) or naproxen (Naprosyn, Aleve). The addition of policosanol to warfarin therapy did not enhance the prolongation of the bleeding time induced by warfarin alone.
- Policosanol may decrease arterial pressure and thus may have additive effects with beta-blockers or other blood pressure–lowering agents. Medication adjustments may be necessary.

- Although not well studied in humans, a high dose of policosanol given to animals did not change the activity of nifedipine. There is no information regarding potential interactions with other calcium channel blockers.
- Because policosanol possesses an antioxidant effect and nitric oxide can be destroyed by oxygen-derived radicals, there is a theoretical interaction between policosanol and nitroprusside and other nitrates. Consult with a qualified health care professional, including a pharmacist, to check for any interactions.
- In theory, taking ticlopidine and policosanol together may cause an additive interaction.
- Although not well studied in humans, policosanol may also interact with agents broken down by the liver or agents taken for Alzheimer's disease, cardiovascular disorders, diabetes, or neurological disorders.

Interactions with Herbs and Dietary Supplements

- In theory, there may be an additive hypotensive (blood pressure–lowering) effect when policosanol is used with herbs that lower blood pressure.
- In theory, additive hypocholesterolemic (cholesterol-lowering) effects may occur when policosanol is used with herbs that decrease cholesterol levels, such as plant sterols, plant stanols, polyphenols, psyllium, soy proteins, soy isoflavones, red yeast, or garlic powder.
- Concurrent therapy with policosanol and omega-3 fatty acids may have an additive lowering effect on the lipid profile and platelet aggregation. Caution is advised.
- Although not well studied in humans, policosanol may also interact with herbs and supplements broken down by the liver or herbs and supplements taken for Alzheimer's disease, cardiovascular disorders, diabetes, or neurological disorders.

For a complete list of references, please visit www.naturalstandard.com.

Polypodium
(*Polypodium* spp)

RELATED TERMS

- Calaguala, calagualine, ferns, Polypodiaceae (family), *Polypodium cambricum*, *Polypodium decumanum*, *Polypodium leucotomus*, *Polypodium vulgare*, samambaia.

BACKGROUND

- Extracts of fern species (family Polypodiaceae) have been used traditionally for numerous indications, most commonly in South America and Europe.
- The South American species *Polypodium leucotomos* L. is commonly known as *calaguala*. Extracts of this species, called *anapsos*, have been marketed and used as a treatment for multiple indications. Although laboratory and animal studies have reported antiinflammatory, cytokine-suppressing, and leukotriene inhibitory properties, the small number of available human trials has not demonstrated efficacy for any specific indication.

EVIDENCE

Uses Based on Scientific Evidence	Grade
Atopic Dermatitis (Eczema) Laboratory and animal studies report that *Polypodium leucotomos* extract (anapsos) may reduce inflammation. However, there is little information about the effectiveness of anapsos taken by mouth in people with atopic dermatitis.	C
Dementia (Memory Loss, Disorientation), Alzheimer's Disease Limited scientific information is available about the effectiveness of polypodium in the treatment of dementia.	C
Psoriasis Extracts of *Polypodium leucotomos* (called *anapsos*) have been taken by mouth in Europe and South America for psoriasis since the 1970s. Poor quality human studies report that anapsos may improve skin appearance. However, there is currently little information supporting the use of *Polypodium leucotomos* for psoriasis. More research is needed in this area before a recommendation can be made.	C
Skin Damage Caused by the Sun Early study shows that polypodium may help to prevent sunburn, skin aging, and skin cancers resulting from uncontrolled overexposure of human skin to solar UV radiation (UVA and UVB). Further research is needed to confirm these results.	C
Vitiligo (Loss of Pigment in the Skin) A combination of polypodium and narrow-band UVB (NB-UVB) light therapy may help treat vitiligo, especially on the head and neck. However, clinical evidence is not sufficient to support this use.	C

Uses Based on Tradition or Theory

Antioxidant, arthritis, asthma, autoimmune diseases, cancer, diuretic, fever, high blood pressure, immune system stimulation, inflammation, neurodegenerative disorders, pertussis, rheumatism or joint diseases, tissue repair after brain damage, upper respiratory tract infection, vaccination in animals for *Fasciola hepatica*, water retention, whooping cough.

DOSING

Adults (18 Years and Older)

- For psoriasis, a dose of 120 mg of anapsos (*Polypodium leucotomos* extract), taken daily by mouth, has been used for short periods of time in limited research. For ultraviolet (UV) radiation, 7.5 mg/kg has been studied. For dementia, preliminary research reports using 360 mg daily for 4 weeks. Safety and effectiveness are not clear.
- No clear topical (on the skin) dosing regimen has been reported or established.
- For vitiligo, 250 mg of *Polypodium leucotomos* has been taken three times daily in combination with narrow-band UVB (NB-UVB) light therapy twice weekly for 25-26 weeks.

Children (Younger than 18 Years)

- There is insufficient evidence to recommend a dose of polypodium in children, and safety is not clear.

SAFETY

Allergies

- People with allergies to ferns (family Polypodiaceae) should avoid polypodium.

Side Effects and Warnings

- Isolated reports of itching or stomach upset have been published. Studies of a different fern species, *Polypodium vulgare*, report sedation, changes in heart function in animals, low blood pressure, and rapid heart rate. Avoid driving and use of heavy machinery when taking *Polypodium leucotomos* extract because of theoretical sedative effects. People with heart disease or those being treated for heart disorders or high blood pressure should use caution.

Pregnancy and Breastfeeding

- The use of polypodium during pregnancy or breastfeeding is not recommended because there is little information about its safety.

INTERACTIONS

Interactions with Drugs

- Polypodium may increase the amount of drowsiness caused by some drugs. Examples include benzodiazepines such as lorazepam (Ativan) or diazepam (Valium), barbiturates such as phenobarbital, narcotics such as codeine, some antidepressants, and alcohol. Use caution while driving or operating machinery.

P

- Most testing has been done with a related fern species, *Polypodium vulgare*. Animal studies show that this related plant can affect the function of the heart and lower blood pressure. In theory, the use of *Polypodium leucotomos* extract with medications that affect heart function or lower blood pressure may cause the effects of these drugs to increase. Use caution if combining polypodium with heart medications such as beta-blockers, calcium channel blockers, or digoxin.

Interactions with Herbs and Dietary Supplements

- In theory, polypodium may increase the amount of drowsiness caused by some herbs or supplements.
- In studies of a related fern species, *Polypodium vulgare*, animals treated with the herb developed low blood pressure and changes in heart function. In theory, the use of *Polypodium leucotomos* extract with herbs or supplements that lower blood pressure may cause the blood pressure to fall too low.
- For the same reason, be cautious if using *Polypodium leucotomos* extract with herbs or supplements that have possible cardiac glycoside ingredients that can affect the function of the heart. Notably, bufalin/chan suis is a Chinese herbal formula that has been reported as toxic or fatal when taken with cardiac glycosides.

For a complete list of references, please visit www.naturalstandard.com.

Pomegranate
(*Punica granatum*)

RELATED TERMS

- Ellagic acid, ellagitannins, Granada, Grenade, Grenadier, hydroalcoholic extract (HAE), PJ, polyphenols, POM Wonderful variety pomegranate juice, pomegranate extracts, POMx, *Punica protopunica*, Punicaceae (family), *Punica granatum*, Shi liu gen (Chinese), Shi liu gen pi (Chinese), Shi liu pi (Chinese), tannins.

BACKGROUND

- One pomegranate delivers approximately 40% of an adult's daily vitamin C requirement and is high in polyphenol compounds. These compounds are thought to reduce "silent inflammation," which is believed to be a contributing factor in diseases such as cancer, heart disease, and diabetes.
- Although pomegranate juice has been commonly consumed for atherosclerosis (hardening of the arteries), evidence of its effectiveness is inconclusive. Pomegranate juice may have antioxidant properties, but its effects have not been widely studied; more evidence is needed. More research is needed for the use of pomegranate as an antifungal agent before a firm recommendation can be made.
- Pomegranate has a long history of use as a food and medicine in Asia and South America. In the United States, pomegranate is typically juiced or the seeds are used as food. Pomegranate may have medicinal benefit as an anthelminthic (expels worms) and antidiarrheal agent, although reports conflict. The seeds may have phytoestrogenic qualities and may be used in hormonally related conditions such as menopause.

EVIDENCE

Uses Based on Scientific Evidence	Grade
Antifungal An extract of pomegranate was shown to be as effective as a commonly used oral (by mouth) gel when used topically (applied on the skin) to treat candidiasis (yeast infection) associated with denture stomatitis (mouth sores). However, there is insufficient clinical evidence to support this use.	C
Antioxidant Early studies suggest that pomegranate juice may have antioxidant properties, but the effects in humans are still unclear. Additional studies, including those in specific disease states in which free radical oxidation is prominent (such as diabetes and cancer), are warranted.	C
Atherosclerosis (Hardening of the Arteries) Preliminary research of pomegranate for atherosclerosis is mixed. Pomegranate juice may decrease serum angiotensin-converting enzyme (ACE) activity and lower blood pressure in elderly hypertensive (high blood pressure) patients.	C

	Grade
Dental Conditions Extracts from pomegranate fruits may be beneficial in dental plaque accumulation and gum disease. However, there is insufficient clinical evidence to support this use.	C
Erectile Dysfunction Pomegranate juice has been studied in the treatment of mild to moderate erectile dysfunction. Evidence remains unclear.	C
High Blood Pressure Pomegranate juice may lower blood pressure in patients with high blood pressure.	C
High Cholesterol Consumption of a juice containing a combination of fruits, including pomegranate, was found to have a beneficial effect on blood cholesterol levels. Additional studies in which pomegranate alone is used are needed.	C
Lung Disease (COPD, Chronic Obstructive Pulmonary Disease) It is unclear whether pomegranate juice is helpful for chronic obstructive lung disease. In theory, pomegranate may be beneficial because of its antioxidant effects, but studies in humans do not support this theory. However, there is insufficient clinical evidence to support this use.	C
Menopausal Symptoms There is currently not enough evidence to support the use of pomegranate in the reduction of menopausal symptoms.	C
Prostate Cancer Consumption of pomegranate juice may be beneficial to patients with prostate cancer. Although evidence study is promising, there is insufficient clinical evidence to support this use.	C
Sunburn Taking ellagic acid–rich pomegranate extract by mouth may reduce damage to the skin caused by exposure to ultraviolet (UV) rays. However, there is insufficient clinical evidence to support this use.	C

Uses Based on Tradition or Theory

Abortion, aging, anthelminthic (expels worms), astringent, bronchitis, colic, colitis (inflamed colon), diarrhea, dysentery (severe diarrhea), earache, headache, hemorrhoids, inflammatory bowel

P

(Continued)

DOSING
Adults (18 Years and Older)
- There is insufficient evidence to recommend a dose of pomegranate. Doses range from 50-1000 mL of pomegranate juice taken by mouth daily for 2-5 weeks. Pomegranate extracts with 100-200 mg of ellagic acid have also been taken. Pomegranate extracts in the form of gels and mouthwashes have also been used to treat dental conditions in the short-term.

Children (Younger than 18 Years)
- There is insufficient evidence to recommend a dose of pomegranate in children, and use is not recommended.

SAFETY
Allergies
- Avoid in individuals with a known allergy or hypersensitivity to pomegranate. There have been reports of cross-reactivity among pomegranate, hazelnut, and peanut.

Side Effects and Warnings
- Pomegranate root/stem bark should be used only under the direct supervision of an expert qualified in its appropriate use. In traditional Chinese medicine, pomegranate fruit husk is not recommended to be taken concurrently with oils or fats when used to treat parasites.
- Hypersensitivity reactions including pruritus (severe itching), angioedema (swelling), and bronchospasm have occurred with the ingestion of pomegranate fruit. Pomegranate is contraindicated in patients with known hypersensitivity to pomegranate and in patients with diarrhea. People with plant allergies seem to be at greater risk of allergic reactions to pomegranate. Use cautiously in patients with asthma.
- Dried pomegranate peel may contain aflatoxin, which is a potent hepatocarcinogen (may cause liver cancer) and toxin. Pomegranate root and stem contain pelletierine, and overdoses by mouth can cause strychnine-like effects in the form of reflex arousal that can escalate to paralysis. At high amounts, people may experience vomiting, including bloody emesis (vomit), followed by dizziness, chills, vision disorders, collapse, and possibly death due to respiratory failure. Avoid in patients with hypertension (high blood pressure) or hypotension (low blood pressure).
- Pomegranate has been reported to cause nausea, vomiting, transient total blindness, hypersensitivity characterized by urticaria (hives), rhinorrhea (nasal discharge), red itchy eyes, and dyspnea (difficulty breathing).
- In theory, the high tannin content may also cause liver toxicity or carcinogenicity. Use cautiously in patients with liver dysfunction and in patients taking hepatotoxic drugs.

Pregnancy and Breastfeeding
- Pomegranate is unsafe during pregnancy when taken by mouth. The bark, root, and fruit rind can stimulate menstruation or uterine contractions. There is insufficient reliable information available about the safety of applying pomegranate on the skin during pregnancy and breastfeeding.

INTERACTIONS
Interactions with Drugs
- Theoretically, concomitant use of pomegranate and other agents by mouth may cause precipitation of some drugs because of the high tannin content of pomegranate. Some experts recommend separating administration of oral drugs and tannin-containing herbs by the longest practical period of time.
- Pomegranate juice may have additive angiotensin-converting enzyme (ACE) inhibitor effects. Blood pressure and potassium levels should be monitored. ACE inhibitors include captopril (Capoten), enalapril (Vasotec), lisinopril (Prinivil, Zestril), ramipril (Altace), and others. Pomegranate juice was shown to decrease serum ACE activity and lower blood pressure in elderly hypertensive (high blood pressure) patients. Theoretically, concomitant use with pomegranate juice may cause additive antihypertensive (blood pressure–lowering) effects; use with caution.
- Pomegranate may affect the way in which the liver breaks down certain drugs.
- Pomegranate may increase the risk of harmful side effects with statin drugs such as rosuvastatin (Crestor), simvastatin (Zocor), and atorvastatin (Lipitor), which are taken to lower blood cholesterol levels.

Interactions with Herbs and Dietary Supplements
- The fruit husk and root/stem bark of pomegranate contain up to 28% and 25% tannins, respectively, compared with 12.9% in black tea and 22.2% in green tea. The tannin content of various herbs may interact with iron, forming nonabsorbable complexes. Some have concluded that if herbs containing tannins are consumed at mealtime, nonabsorbable complexes will form with iron, zinc, and copper. Concern has been raised that tannins may affect the administration of iron supplementation products. It is unknown to what extent the amount of tannin in pomegranate may affect iron absorption clinically. Until more is known, patients who need iron supplementation should be advised to separate administration times of these two compounds by 1-2 hours.
- Pomegranate juice may have antihypertensive (blood pressure–lowering) effects. Theoretically, concurrent use of pomegranate juice with other herbs and supplements that decrease blood pressure, such as danshen, ginger, and *Panax ginseng*, may increase the risk of hypotension (low blood pressure).
- Theoretically, herbs that contain high percentages of tannins (such as pomegranate) may cause precipitation of constituents of other herbs. Caution is advised.
- One pomegranate delivers approximately 40% of an adult's daily vitamin C requirement. In theory, large doses of pomegranate in combination with vitamin C supplements may result in additive effects or side effects.
- Pomegranate may affect the way in which the liver breaks down certain herbs and supplements.

For a complete list of references, please visit www.naturalstandard.com.

Probiotics

RELATED TERMS

- AB-yogurt, acidophilus, acidophilus milk, antibiophilus, *Bacillus*, bifidobacteria, *Bifidobacterium animalis* ssp. lactis (Bb-12), *Bifidobacterium* DN-173 010, *Enterococcus*, *Enterococcus faecium* M-74, *Escherichia*, fermented soymilk, flora, fructooligosaccharides (FOS), *Helicobacter pylori*, *Lactobacillus acidophilus* milk, *Lactobacillus acidophilus* yogurt, lactic acid bacteria, lactobacillus, Lactobacillaceae (family), lactobacilli, *Lactobacillus*, *Lactobacillus casei* DN-114001, *Lactobacillus casei* shirota, *Lactobacillus coryniformis* CECT5711, *Lactobacillus gasseri* CECT5714, *Lactobacillus johnsonii* LA1, *Lactobacillus rhamnosus* GR-1, *Lactobacillus paracasei* ssp. paracasei (CRL-431), *Lactobacillus reuteri* B-54 and RC-14, Lakcid L, oligofructose, oral bacteriotherapy, prebiotic, *Saccharomyces boulardii*, VSL#3, yogurt.
- **Note:** There are many other related terms that identify specific varieties or forms of probiotics. Many such terms are used in the naming of commercial probiotic products.
- Do not confuse probiotics with prebiotics (defined separately below).

BACKGROUND

- Probiotics are beneficial bacteria (sometimes referred to as *friendly germs*) that help to maintain the health of the intestinal tract and aid in digestion. They also help keep potentially harmful organisms in the gut (harmful bacteria and yeasts) under control. Most probiotics come from food sources, especially cultured milk products. Probiotics can be consumed as capsules, tablets, beverages, powders, yogurts, and other foods.
- *Pro*biotics should not be confused with *pre*biotics. Prebiotics are complex sugars (such as lactulose, lactitol, a variety of fructooligosaccharides, and inulin) that are used as fuel by the healthful bacteria to stimulate their growth and activity while suppressing the growth and activity of harmful organisms. Other foods that may support probiotic activity include Japanese miso, tempeh, kefir, raw milk, kombucha, bananas, garlic, and onions. When prebiotics and probiotics are combined in one product, it is called a *syn*biotic.
- Probiotics are thought to work by colonizing the small intestine and crowding out disease-causing organisms, thereby restoring proper balance to the intestinal flora. They compete with harmful organisms for nutrients and may also produce substances that inhibit growth of harmful organisms in the gut.
- Probiotic bacteria have been found to stimulate the body's immune system. They may also aid in several gastrointestinal illnesses such as inflammatory bowel diseases, antibiotic-related diarrhea, *Clostridium difficile* toxin–induced colitis, infectious diarrhea, hepatic encephalopathy, irritable bowel syndrome, and allergy.
- Probiotics have been found to enhance the digestion and absorption of proteins, fats, calcium, and phosphorus. They may help overcome lactose intolerance. Finally, they may help restore healthful bacteria after a course of antibiotic therapy has altered the normal gastrointestinal flora.

EVIDENCE

Uses Based on Scientific Evidence	Grade
Antibiotic (Probiotics to Reduce Related Adverse Effects) An increasing number of studies support the use of probiotics as a supplement to antibiotic therapy. Probiotic supplementation during a course of antibiotics may reduce the adverse effects of antibiotics in the intestinal environment. This includes reducing growth of *Clostridium difficile* bacteria, which can lead to colitis, a common complication of antibiotics, especially in the elderly. Some probiotics may also help prevent the development of antibiotic resistance. In acutely ill children, synbiotics have been linked to greater weight gain and fewer bacterial illnesses after antibiotics are ended. The evidence consistently supports supplementation of antibiotics.	A
Atopic Dermatitis (Eczema) Probiotics show promise for preventing atopic eczema/dermatitis syndrome in children. Infants benefit when their mothers take probiotics during pregnancy and breastfeeding. Direct supplementation of infants may reduce the incidence of atopic eczema by as much as half. It may also reduce cow's milk allergy and other allergic reactions during weaning. Probiotics may stabilize the intestinal barrier function and decrease gastrointestinal symptoms in children with atopic dermatitis. Children do differ, however, in their responsiveness to specific probiotics. The effectiveness of probiotics for the treatment of eczema is still under investigation.	A
Helicobacter pylori **Infection** Antibiotics are the main treatment to eradicate *Helicobacter pylori*, the cause of most stomach ulcers. Side effects commonly include bloating, diarrhea, and taste disturbances. Probiotics reduce these side effects and generally help people tolerate the treatment. They may also reduce levels of *Helicobacter pylori* in children and adults. Yogurt containing probiotics suppresses *Helicobacter pylori* infection and may lead to more complete eradication during antibiotic treatment.	A
Cirrhosis Liver cirrhosis may be accompanied by an imbalance of intestinal flora (bacteria). Probiotic supplementation in cirrhosis patients has been found to reduce the level of fecal acidity (pH) and fecal and blood ammonia, which are beneficial changes.	B

(Continued)

577

Uses Based on Scientific Evidence	Grade
Colon Cancer There is recent evidence that supplementation with *Lactobacillus casei* may help reduce the recurrence of colorectal tumors in patients who have previously undergone surgery for colon cancer.	B
Dental Caries Short-term consumption of probiotic-containing cheese may benefit dental caries. There is also evidence that the probiotic *Lactobacillus rhamnosus* GG, when added to milk, may help reduce dental carries in young children.	B
Diarrhea in Children (Nosocomial) *Lactobacillus* GG may reduce the risk of nosocomial (originating in a health care setting) diarrhea in infants, particularly cases caused by rotavirus gastroenteritis.	B
Diarrhea Prevention There is tentative support for probiotics to prevent diarrhea in adults and children. Supplementation may benefit human immunodeficiency virus–positive men, and yogurt containing *Lactobacillus casei* may help reduce incidence in healthy young adults. Children may benefit from *Bifidobacterium lactis* (strain Bb-12) added to their formula.	B
Diarrhea Treatment (Children) Probiotics may reduce the duration of diarrhea and related hospital stays in children. Fermented formula and formula supplemented with probiotics may reduce both the number and duration of episodes of diarrhea.	B
Growth There is evidence that young children (ages 6-36 months) who receive infant formula with bifidobacteria Bb12 supplementation may achieve faster growth than without the supplementation.	B
Immune Enhancement Research suggests that probiotics, especially those in milk or food, may help boost the immune system. However, commercially produced yogurt may not be as effective. More studies, particularly with yogurt, are needed to give recommendations.	B
Infections (Gastrointestinal/Respiratory) Limited evidence with day care children suggests supplementation with *Lactobacillus* GG may reduce the number of sick days, frequency of respiratory tract infections, and frequency of related antibiotic treatments. Fermented milk (with yogurt cultures and *Lactobacillus casei* DN-114001) may reduce the duration of winter infections (gastrointestinal and respiratory), as well as average body temperature, in elderly people.	B
Infectious Diarrhea Probiotics may reduce the duration of symptoms in adults and children with infectious diarrhea by 17-30 hours. Effective forms include *Lactobacillus* strain GG, *Lactobacillus reuteri*, combination *Lactobacillus rhamnosus* and *Lactobacillus reuteri*, and combination *Lactobacillus acidophilus* and *Lactobacillus bifidus*. More studies are needed to evaluate types, dosages, duration of treatment, and relationships to specific pathogens.	B
Irritable Bowel Syndrome (IBS) Many types of probiotics have been shown to moderately reduce symptoms of IBS, including pain, gas, bloating, and stool frequency. There is also some evidence that probiotics may reduce swelling and improve quality of life. However, not all studies show beneficial effects.	B
Pancreatitis (Acute) Supplementing with *Lactobacillus plantarum* 299 may help prevent pancreatic infection (sepsis), reduce the number of operations needed, and reduce the length of hospital stay in treatment of acute pancreatitis.	B
Radiation-Induced Colitis/Diarrhea Probiotics may help treat or prevent radiation-induced diarrhea in cancer patients.	B
Sinusitis (Hypertrophic) Use of probiotic *Enterococcus faecalis* bacteria in hypertrophic sinusitis (sinus inflammation) may reduce the frequency of relapses and the need for antibiotic therapy.	B
Ulcerative Colitis *Escherichia coli* Nissle 1917 (EcN) appears to be as effective as the drug mesalazine but is not currently available in the United States. A variety of Bifidophilus preparations have shown effects of preventing relapse or maintaining remission. These include Bifidophilus alone, Bifidophilus in fermented milk products, and a synbiotic preparation. A probiotic combination consisting of VSL#3 plus balsalazide may be more effective than balsalazide or mesalazine alone. More studies are needed to more clearly determine what outcomes can be expected.	B
Allergy There is promising early evidence that probiotics may help treat allergic conditions, especially allergic skin disorders in infants. Most studies have tested probiotics in children, teenagers, and young adults. Some evidence also suggests that probiotics help reduce swelling caused by allergies. However, study results are mixed for inhalant allergies, such as allergic rhinitis (nasal inflammation and discharge).	C

Uses Based on Scientific Evidence	Grade
Amoebiasis Combining a probiotic yeast (*Saccharomyces boulardii*) with antibiotics in the treatment of acute amoebiasis (amoebic dysentery) may decrease the duration of symptoms. More studies are needed to determine recommendations for probiotics in acute amoebiasis.	C
Asthma Laser acupuncture plus probiotics may help prevent asthma attacks in school-aged children with intermittent or mild persistent asthma. More research with probiotics alone is needed.	C
Bacterial Infection As a bacterial reservoir, the nose may harbor many varieties of potentially disease-causing bacteria. There is limited evidence that probiotic supplementation may reduce the presence of harmful bacteria in the upper respiratory tract. More studies are needed to establish this relationship and its implications for health.	C
Bacterial Vaginosis Vaginal suppositories containing probiotics may be effective in the treatment or prevention of bacterial vaginosis. Eating yogurt enriched with *Lactobacillus acidophilus* may also be beneficial. However, not all applications of probiotics show benefit. Additional research is necessary before firm conclusions can be reached regarding what probiotics and what methods can lead to reliable results.	C
Cardiovascular Disease There is limited evidence suggesting probiotics may help reduce low-density lipoprotein (LDL or "bad") cholesterol, a risk factor for cardiovascular disease, in overweight people. These findings are tentative, and more evidence is needed to arrive at firm conclusions.	C
Cardiovascular Risk Reduction (Smokers/ Atherosclerosis) One study suggests probiotic supplementation might reduce blood pressure and some biochemical risk factors for cardiovascular disease (leptin and fibrinogen). This implies a possible protective effect against atherosclerosis. However, more studies are needed to confirm such effects.	C
Colitis (Collagenous) There is not enough evidence on which to form conclusions for the use of probiotics in collagenous colitis.	C
Constipation Use of probiotics with constipation has had mixed results. Some research suggests that they may help reduce symptoms in patients with long-term constipation. However, another study did not show	C

effectiveness in young children. More studies are needed to determine what forms of probiotics might be effective for constipation.

Diarrhea (Acute) Probiotics may help treat acute diarrhea. *Saccharomyces boulardii* and a probiotic formula *Escherichia coli* Nissle 1917 (EcN) solution have been shown to moderately improve diarrhea in children. However, all probiotic preparations may not be effective.	C
Diarrhea (Antibiotic-Associated) Although some data support the use of probiotics for the treatment and prevention of antibiotic-associated diarrhea (AAD), other studies have found a lack of benefit. Although probiotics are considered a safe and reasonable approach for AAD, larger and better designed studies are needed for definitive recommendations.	C
Diarrhea (Chronic Bacterial Overgrowth– Related) There is limited evidence suggesting probiotics might help in the treatment of bacterial overgrowth–related chronic diarrhea. More studies are needed to provide guidelines for this use.	C
Diarrhea (*Clostridium difficile*) There is limited evidence suggesting that probiotics may reduce recurrence of *Clostridium difficile* after antibiotic therapy. However, more studies are needed to provide definitive guidelines about this use.	C
Ear Infections Probiotic capsules (containing *Lactobacillus rhamnosus* GG and LC705, *Bifidobacterium breve* 99 and *Propionibacterium freudenreichii* JS) did not protect against ear infections in children. More research is needed to confirm these findings.	C
Hepatic Encephalopathy (Confused Thinking Due to Liver Disorders) Initial studies in minimal hepatic encephalopathy are encouraging. Probiotics and prebiotics may lead to the improvement of symptoms and may be an alternative to lactulose for the management of this condition in people with cirrhosis. However, more studies are needed to determine the role of probiotics in this condition.	C
High Cholesterol There is conflicting evidence regarding the effects of probiotic-enriched dairy products on lowering blood levels of total cholesterol or low-density lipoprotein ("bad cholesterol"). More studies are needed.	C
Infections (Complications) Results are mixed regarding the ability of probiotics to reduce infective complications of medical treatment. Reduced incidence of infection has been seen	C

(Continued)

Uses Based on Scientific Evidence	Grade
in patients treated for brain injury, abdominal surgery, and liver transplantation. Other studies have shown no such reduction in elective abdominal surgery and critical care patients.	
Infections (Rotavirus, Nosocomial) Children receiving Bifidophilus-supplemented milk-based formula may be protected against rotavirus infection. *Lactobacillus* GG has shown mixed results, while early evidence suggests that *Lactobacillus rhamnosus* is not effective. Some studies suggest shorter duration of diarrhea, less chance of a protracted course, and faster discharge from the hospital with *Lactobacillus* GG, while others suggest it is ineffective compared with breastfeeding. More studies are needed to determine the optimal use of probiotics in rotavirus nosocomial infection.	C
Inflammatory Bowel Disease (IBD) It is unclear whether probiotics can help treat IBD. Study results are mixed. *Saccharomyces boulardii*, EcN, probiotics, yogurt, and high doses of probiotics have shown the most promise. More research is needed.	C
Lactose Intolerance Supplementation of infant formulas with probiotics is a potential approach for the management of cow's milk allergy, but there is conflicting evidence as to whether it improves digestion of lactose. More research is needed in this area before a conclusion can be drawn.	C
Necrotizing Enterocolitis (NEC) Prevention Little evidence is available on the effects of probiotics in the prevention of NEC. Study results conflict. Further studies are needed to determine the effectiveness of this application.	C
Nutrition Fermented milk containing the probiotic *Lactobacillus johnsonii* La1 may improve nutritional status in the elderly. More research is needed to confirm these results.	C
Peptic Ulcers Early research suggests that probiotics may help prevent peptic ulcers. However, more research is needed to determine whether this is an effective therapy.	C
Pneumonia There is insufficient evidence to draw any firm conclusions. More research is necessary.	C
Pouchitis Limited evidence suggests a probiotic preparation (VSL#3, containing lactobacilli, bifidobacteria, and *Streptococcus salivarius* subspecies *thermophilus*) may be effective in the prevention of pouchitis.	C
Notably, discontinuation appears to be followed by relapse, while continuation apparently maintains remission and better quality of life. *Lactobacillus* GG supplementation, however, has had conflicting results in preventing flare-ups. More studies are needed to arrive at concrete recommendations.	
Premature Labor Prevention There is not enough evidence to determine whether probiotics can help prevent preterm birth and its complications.	C
Rheumatoid Arthritis (RA) In a small study, *Lactobacillus* GG was associated with improved subjective well-being and trends in reduced symptoms, although these were not statistically significant. More studies on the effects of probiotics in RA are needed.	C
Supplementation in Preterm and Very Low Birth Weight Infants Probiotics, when added to formulas or breast milk, may foster better growth and higher counts of healthful bacteria in the gut of preterm infants. They may also boost the immune system and improve feeding tolerance. However, *Lactobacillus* GG may not be effective. More studies are needed to clarify specific guidelines for probiotics in preterm infant care.	C
Thrush Early research suggests that cheese-containing probiotics may help reduce the risk of a fungal mouth infection, called thrush, in the elderly. More research is needed in this area.	C
Urinary Tract Infection Studies of *Lactobacillus* preparations have had mixed results. Evidence suggests a combination of *Lactobacillus rhamnosus* GR-1 and *Lactobacillus fermentum* RC-14 may reduce potentially harmful vaginal bacteria and yeast in healthy women. Other studies have found no benefit for women or preterm infants. More studies are needed to determine the effectiveness of probiotics in urinary and urogenital tract infections.	C
Vaccine Adjunct *Lactobacillus fermentum* (CECT5716) may increase the protective effects of the flu vaccine. More research is needed.	C
Vaginal Candidiasis (Yeast Infection) Probiotics have not been adequately studied for the prevention or treatment of vaginal yeast infections. More research is needed in this area before a conclusion can be drawn.	C
Bacterial Infection (Translocation) Bacterial translocation (passage of bacteria from the gut to other areas of the body where they can cause	D

Uses Based on Scientific Evidence	Grade
disease) is of special concern in surgery. Limited evidence suggests that supplementation with probiotics may not reduce this problem.	
Diarrhea (HIV Patients Taking Antiretroviral Therapy) Probiotic therapy is well tolerated in HIV-infected patients taking antiretroviral therapy but may not be helpful for gastrointestinal symptoms.	D
Fertility Probiotics have been used in the vagina immediately after oocyte retrieval during in vitro fertilization (IVF), but they do not appear to have an effect on vaginal colonization or pregnancy rate in IVF cycles.	D

Uses Based on Tradition or Theory

Acne, antiinflammatory, asthma, bad breath, bone marrow transplantation, cancer, canker sores, colon cancer prevention, cystic fibrosis (respiratory and gastrointestinal problems), diaper rash, diverticulitis, *Escherichia coli* infection in cancer patients, fever blisters, gastroenteritis, heartburn, human immunodeficiency virus, hives, hormonal imbalances, indigestion, osteoporosis prevention, tuberculosis.

DOSING
Adults (18 Years and Older)

- Probiotics are commercially available as capsules, yogurts, powder, and dairy products. Various doses have been studied; however, additional study is needed to confirm the effectiveness of these doses. The most common probiotics are *Lactobacillus*, *Saccharomyces*, and *Bifidobacterium*.
- To reduce side effects when taking antibiotics, individuals have used 100 g of a probiotic drink containing *Lactobacillus casei*, *Lactobacillus bulgaricus*, and *Streptococcus thermophilus* twice daily in combination with antibiotics. The drink was continued for 1 week after the antibiotics were finished.

Children (Younger than 18 Years)

- Various doses and probiotic strains have been studied in children. Children (3-24 months of age) have taken *Saccharomyces boulardii* for 6 days for the treatment of diarrhea. Children (2-47 months old) have also taken *Escherichia coli* Nissle 1917 (EcN) solution daily. The specific dose of EcN depended on the child's weight. One capsule of *Lactobacillus rhamnosus* strain GG (Culturelle, ConAgra Foods, Omaha, Neb) has also been taken daily. Additional research is needed to confirm the effectiveness of these doses.

SAFETY
Allergies

- Probiotics are often found in yogurt, milk, and dairy products. Caution is advised in patients sensitive or intolerant to dairy products containing probiotics.

Side Effects and Warnings

- Probiotics are generally regarded as safe for human consumption. Long-term consumption of probiotics is considered safe. Few side effects have been reported in studies.
- Some people experience excessive production of gas due to the corrective activity of probiotics in the colon. This is patient specific and normally will decrease with use. Gradual increase of dosing over time is recommended to minimize this effect.
- Probiotics should not be taken in people who are allergic to any component of a probiotic-containing product. Lactose-sensitive people may develop abdominal discomfort from dairy products containing probiotics. Caution is advised when probiotics are used in neonates born prematurely or with immune deficiency.

Pregnancy and Breastfeeding

- Although probiotics (when consumed as dairy products or yogurt) appear safe during pregnancy and breastfeeding, additional study is needed to confirm these findings. Caution is advised when probiotics are used in neonates born prematurely or with immune deficiency.

INTERACTIONS
Interactions with Drugs

- Not enough evidence is available.

Interactions with Herbs and Dietary Supplements

- Not enough evidence is available.

For a complete list of references, please visit www.naturalstandard.com.

P

Probiotic yeast
(Saccharomyces boulardii)

RELATED TERMS

- Brewer's yeast, Florastor, Florastor Kids, Hansen CBS 5926, *Lactobacillus, Lactobacillus acidophilus, Lactobacillus bulgaricus, Lactobacillus gasseri,* Lactobacillus GG, *Lactobacillus plantarum,* Perenterol, probiotic, probiotic yeast, *Saccharomyces boulardii, Saccharomyces cerevisiae, Saccharomyces salivarius, Saccharomyces thermophilus,* Saccharomycetaceae (family), Ultra-Levure, yeast.
- **Note:** It was long debated as to whether *Saccharomyces boulardii* is a subspecies of *Saccharomyces cerevisiae* or a separate entity. Traditional techniques could distinguish the two, but manufacturers of *Saccharomyces boulardii* claimed that the two yeasts are separate species. Recent advances in DNA technology have confirmed that *Saccharomyces boulardii* is indeed a distinct species of yeast.

BACKGROUND

- *Saccharomyces boulardii* is a nonpathogenic yeast strain that has been used for treatment and prevention of diarrhea. *Saccharomyces boulardii* is classified as a "probiotic," or a microorganism that when ingested may have a positive influence on the host's health. Probiotics may exert their effects on the gastrointestinal system directly or may modulate the immune system in a larger scope.
- Human studies indicate that *Saccharomyces boulardii* may prevent antibiotic-associated diarrhea, *Clostridium difficile* diarrhea in combination with antibiotic therapy, diarrhea associated with tube feedings, and acute childhood diarrhea. Promising initial studies have shown that *Saccharomyces boulardii* may be beneficial in treating diarrhea associated with human immunodeficiency virus (HIV).
- The German Commission E has approved the use of *Saccharomyces boulardii* for symptomatic treatment of acute diarrhea, prophylactic and symptomatic treatment of diarrhea during travel, treatment of diarrhea occurring while tube feeding, use as an adjuvant for chronic acne, for a dietary supplementation, and for a source of B vitamins and protein.

EVIDENCE

Uses Based on Scientific Evidence	Grade
Diarrhea (Antibiotic Associated) There is good evidence that concurrent use of *Saccharomyces boulardii* with antibiotic therapy reduces the incidence of developing antibiotic-associated diarrhea (AAD) (*Clostridium difficile* and other). In general, positive results occur only when *Saccharomyces boulardii* is continued for several days to several weeks after the course of antibiotics is stopped.	A
Diarrhea in Children Several trials suggest efficacy of *Saccharomyces boulardii* in the treatment of diarrhea in childhood.	B
Further studies are still required. Use of *Saccharomyces boulardii* may be advantageous in both the reduction of stool frequency per day and the duration of diarrhea in this age group.	
Antibacterial (Amebiasis) Evidence from one clinical trial supports improvement of symptoms in patients with amebiasis treated with *Saccharomyces boulardii* in addition to standard therapy. Further clinical trials are warranted.	C
Crohn's Disease Evidence supports mild improvement of symptoms and quality of life in patients with Crohn's disease who use *Saccharomyces boulardii*. More clinical trials are warranted.	C
Diarrhea *(Clostridium difficile)* With the introduction of broad-spectrum antibiotics into clinical practice, *Clostridium difficile* infection has become a common cause of infectious diarrhea in hospitalized patients. For treatment of recurrent *Clostridium difficile*–associated diarrhea, *Saccharomyces boulardii* may decrease recurrence by about 50%, especially when combined with high-dose vancomycin. Clinical evidence is lacking, although anecdotal use seems to support this use.	C
Diarrhea (HIV-Associated) Although only small studies have been performed, treatment with *Saccharomyces boulardii* may improve quality of life for acquired immunodeficiency syndrome (AIDS) patients with chronic diarrhea. As fungemia has been associated with *Saccharomyces boulardii* administration in patients with central lines, care should be exercised in treating these patients.	C
Diarrhea (Prevention during Tube Feeding) Preliminary evidence supports the use of *Saccharomyces boulardii* for this indication. However, the role of antibiotics in the results is unclear.	C
Diarrhea (Traveler's) Although evidence supports the use of *Saccharomyces boulardii* for other forms of diarrhea, little evidence exists to support standard treatment with *Saccharomyces boulardii* for traveler's diarrhea.	C
Irritable Bowel Syndrome (IBS) Some evidence exists to support treatment with *Saccharomyces boulardii* for IBS. However, the available evidence has not been definitive.	C

(Continued)

Uses Based on Scientific Evidence	Grade
Nutritional Support (Premature Infants) One clinical trial exists investigating the addition of *Saccharomyces boulardii* to nutritional support for premature infants. No evidence was found for lipid gut absorption or increased weight gain. A benefit was noted on gut flora.	C

Uses Based on Tradition or Theory

Acne, aging, allergies, anorexia, autism, cancer, candidal infection, cholera, colitis (inflamed colon), constipation, cystic fibrosis, depression, diabetes, digestive disorders (Hirschsprung's disease), fatigue, fever, flatulence (gas), food allergies, *Helicobacter pylori* infection (children), herpes, hyperlipidemia (high cholesterol levels), lactose intolerance, mood changes (irritability), nutrition, osteoporosis (prevention), premenstrual syndrome (PMS), seborrheic dermatitis (inflamed skin), skin disorders, stress, ulcerative colitis, ulcers, urinary tract infections (UTIs), weight loss.

DOSING
Adults (18 Years and Older)

- In large multicenter trials, few (if any) side effects have been noted in patients taking *Saccharomyces boulardii* for up to 15 months. Regardless of diarrhea type, *Saccharomyces boulardii* is often taken in doses of 500–2000 mg in divided daily doses (three or four times daily). The brand name product, Ultra-Levure, has been studied in doses of two to four capsules daily for up to 8 months. For antibiotic-associated diarrhea, 1 g daily for 3 days following completion of antibiotics has been used. Two sachets per day containing 5 × 109 colony-forming units (CFU) per sachet has also been used for 4 weeks. One capsule twice daily has been used; duration was not noted. A range of 250–500 mg twice daily for up to 2 weeks following antibiotics has been used. Four capsules Ultra-Levure daily for 8 months has been used.

Children (Younger than 18 Years)

- The most commonly used dose of *Saccharomyces boulardii* in children for the treatment of diarrhea is 250–600 mg daily for up to 5 days. This has been given alone and in combination with antibiotics.

SAFETY
Allergies

- Avoid in individuals with a known allergy or hypersensitivity to yeast, *Saccharomyces boulardii*, *Saccharomyces cerevisiae*, or other species in the Saccharomycetaceae family. *Saccharomyces boulardii* use may be associated with itching, urticaria ("hives"), and generalized skin eruptions.

Side Effects and Warnings

- *Saccharomyces boulardii* has been generally well tolerated in human studies for treatment of various diarrheal disorders. Symptoms of *Saccharomyces cerevisiae* infection included septic shock in more than one patient and fever in another. Symptoms of sepsis (infection) included increased white blood cell count, abdominal meteorism (swelling from

gas), and respiratory insufficiency. In general, contamination occurred in patients with an indwelling vascular catheter.

- Constipation, increased thirst, flatulence (gas), and bloating have been associated with *Saccharomyces boulardii* use. Use cautiously in patients with constipation.
- *Saccharomyces boulardii* fungemia (fungal infection) has occurred. Avoid in patients with yeast infection. Symptoms included septic shock in more than one patient and fever in another. Symptoms of sepsis include white blood cell count increase, abdominal meteorism, and respiratory insufficiency. In general, contamination occurred in patients with an indwelling vascular catheter.
- *Saccharomyces boulardii* use may also cause Quincke's edema (swelling) or increases or decreases in blood pressure when used with monoamine oxidase inhibitors (MAOIs).

Pregnancy and Breastfeeding

- *Saccharomyces boulardii* is not recommended in pregnant or breastfeeding women because of a lack of available scientific evidence.

INTERACTIONS
Interactions with Drugs

- Concomitant antibiotic treatment may change gastrointestinal flora, subsequently increasing steady state levels of *Saccharomyces boulardii* in humans. According to various clinical trials, use of *Saccharomyces boulardii* in combination with antibiotics decreases the frequency and duration of diarrhea. Caution is also advised when *Saccharomyces boulardii* is taken with other antidiarrheal agents because of additive effects.
- Use of antifungal agents may result in decreased efficacy of *Saccharomyces boulardii*.
- Use of metronidazole plus iodoquinol plus *Saccharomyces boulardii* was more effective than metronidazole plus iodoquinol alone for reducing diarrhea associated with amebiasis (intestinal infection). Similarly, use of mesalamine plus *Saccharomyces boulardii* may be more effective than mesalamine alone for reducing diarrhea associated with Crohn's disease. These may be examples of positive interactions.
- *Saccharomyces boulardii* taken in combination with MAOIs may lower blood pressure.

Interactions with Herbs and Dietary Supplements

- Concomitant antibiotic treatment with herbs or supplements may change gastrointestinal flora, subsequently increasing steady state levels of *Saccharomyces boulardii* in humans. According to various clinical trials, use of *Saccharomyces boulardii* in combination with antibiotics decreases the frequency and duration of diarrhea.
- Caution is also advised when *Saccharomyces boulardii* is taken with other antidiarrheal herbs or supplements because of additive effects.
- Use of antifungal herbs or supplements may result in decreased efficacy of *Saccharomyces boulardii*.
- *Saccharomyces boulardii* taken in combination with herbs or supplements with MAOI-like activity may lower blood pressure.

For a complete list of references, please visit www.naturalstandard.com.

P

RELATED TERMS

- *Apis mellifera* L., bee glue, bee propolis, bee putty, Bienenharz (German), Brazilian green propolis, Brazilian propolis, Bulgarian propolis, caffeic acid phenethyl ester (CAPE), cera alba, Chizukit, cinnamic acid, flavonoids, galangin, Greek propolis, hive dross, Propolin H, propolis balsam, propolis resin, propolis wax, propolisina (Spanish), Russian penicillin, Taiwanese propolis, terpenes, water-soluble derivative of propolis (WSDP).

BACKGROUND

- Bees create propolis, a natural resin, to build their hives. Propolis is made from the buds of conifer and poplar trees, beeswax, and other bee secretions. Historically, propolis was used in Greece to treat abscesses. The Assyrians also used propolis to heal wounds and tumors, and the Egyptians used it for mummification. Today, propolis is commonly found in chewing gum, cosmetics, creams, lozenges, and skin creams. It is frequently used in foods and beverages with the claim that it can maintain or improve health.
- Propolis has shown promise in dentistry for dental caries and as a natural sealant and enamel hardener. The effectiveness of propolis against herpes simplex virus types 1 and 2 and parasitic infections has been demonstrated in early studies. However, well-designed studies are lacking, and further evidence is warranted to determine whether propolis is effective for any health condition.
- Numerous case reports have demonstrated propolis to be a potent allergen and sensitizing agent. Therefore, it should be used cautiously in allergic people. Toxicity with propolis is rare, although there are multiple case reports of skin irritation and itching, as well as blood vessel inflammation.

EVIDENCE

Uses Based on Scientific Evidence	Grade
Acute Cervicitis Several studies suggest that using propolis as a cream or ointment may help heal an inflamed cervix, the narrow passage at the lower end of the uterus. These studies, however, have been small, low quality, and not conclusive.	C
Burns Propolis may have a beneficial effect on the healing of minor burns. However, the available clinical evidence is not sufficient to support.	C
Canker Sores (Aphthous Ulcers) There is some evidence that propolis taken by mouth may help reduce outbreaks of canker sores. However, the available clinical evidence is not sufficient to support this use.	C
Colds (Prevention and Treatment) There is some evidence that propolis may help prevent infections with the virus that causes the	C

common cold. Propolis nasal sprays have been suggested as a treatment for runny nose, congestion, and fever in children with nose or throat infections. However, there is not enough clinical evidence to support this use of propolis.

Cornea Complications from Zoster Laboratory studies suggest that propolis has antiviral and antiinflammatory effects. There is limited research of propolis for the treatment of eye complications of *Varicella zoster*, the virus that causes chickenpox or shingles. Some evidence suggests that propolis may speed up healing and improve sight. However, the available clinical evidence is not sufficient to support this use.	C
Dental Pain There is some evidence suggesting that propolis (e.g., propolis gel) may reduce dental pain. However, the available clinical evidence is not sufficient to support this use.	C
Dental Plaque and Gingivitis (Mouthwash) Early studies suggest that using a propolis mouthwash may reduce plaque formation, reduce bacteria in the mouth, relieve dental pain and gum inflammation (periodontitis), be useful as a sealant after root canal surgery, and help heal dental wounds. Preliminary research using a gel prepared with propolis and caffeic acid phenethyl ester (CAPE) applied to the gums found that the gel provided comfort and was accepted by the volunteers. Although there has been promising research, particularly in the area of plaque reduction, most studies have been small, low quality, and not fully convincing.	C
Dental Wound Healing In animals, propolis helped the mouth heal after teeth were removed. However, the available clinical evidence is not sufficient to support this use.	C
Fungal Infections (of the Mouth) A Brazilian commercial ethanol propolis extract, formulated to ensure physical and chemical stability, was found to inhibit oral candidiasis, a fungal infection of the mouth. However, the available clinical evidence is not sufficient to support this use.	C
Genital Herpes Simplex Virus (HSV) Infection Laboratory studies report that propolis may have action against viruses, including herpes simplex virus types 1 and 2. Early results from poorly designed human studies suggest that propolis used on the skin may improve lesions from genital herpes virus infections. However, the available clinical evidence is not sufficient to support this use.	C

Uses Based on Scientific Evidence	Grade
Infections Animal and laboratory studies suggest that propolis may help treat various types of infections. Initial human research reports possible benefits against bacteria in the mouth, genital herpes, urine bacteria, intestinal giardia infections, or *Helicobacter pylori*. However, the available clinical evidence is not sufficient to support this use.	C
Legg-Calvé-Perthes Disease/Avascular Hip Necrosis These diseases are characterized by the death of bone at the hip joint (called the femoral head). Limited human research has tested propolis injections into the joint after hip replacement surgery for these conditions. However, the available clinical evidence is not sufficient to support this use.	C
Rheumatic Diseases Based on antiinflammatory effects observed in laboratory research, propolis has been proposed as a possible treatment for rheumatic and other inflammatory diseases. However, there is currently not enough scientific human study to make a clear recommendation.	C
Stomach Ulcers Caused by *Helicobacter pylori* Bacteria Some evidence suggests that propolis and some of its components may stop the growth of *Helicobacter pylori*, the bacterium that causes stomach ulcers. However, the available clinical evidence is not sufficient to support this use.	C
Vaginitis Propolis may be an effective treatment for vaginal inflammation. However, the available clinical evidence is not sufficient to support this use.	C

Uses Based on Tradition or Theory

Academic performance, acne, anticoagulant, antiinflammatory, antioxidant, antispasm, blood clots, bowel diseases, cancer, colorectal cancer, corneal regeneration, Crohn's disease, dermatitis, dilation of veins (vasorelaxant), diverticulitis, duodenal ulcers, eczema, human immunodeficiency virus, hyperglycemia (high blood sugar levels), immune stimulation, immunomodulatory, laryngitis, leukemia, liver protection, low blood pressure, nasopharyngeal carcinoma, osteoporosis, prostate carcinoma, pruritus (itching), psoriasis, rheumatoid arthritis, skin rejuvenator, thyroid disease, tissue healing after surgery (tissue regeneration), tuberculosis, ulcerative colitis, ultraviolet (UV)-induced erythema prevention/sunburn, wound healing.

DOSING
Adults (18 Years and Older)

- There is insufficient evidence to recommend a dose of propolis. However, a wide range of doses has been studied for various conditions. A 5% ointment/cream/aqueous solution of propolis applied in the form of vaginal dressings/douche daily has been used for 7-10 days for acute cervicitis or vaginitis. To treat recurring canker sores, a dose of 500 mg of propolis has been taken orally daily. A dose of 10 mL of 0.2%-10% propolis ethanol extract mouthwash (swished in the mouth for 60-90 seconds, then spit out) has been used once or twice daily for dental plaque. For genital herpes simplex virus infection, a 3% propolis skin cream (made from 75%-85% concentrated propolis extract) has been applied to the skin four times daily for 10 days. In cases of cervical or vaginal lesions, the same amount of ointment has been applied to the tip of a tampon and inserted vaginally four times daily for 10 days. Safety and effectiveness have not been established.

- A dose of two 250-mg propolis capsules has been taken by mouth three times daily for 3 days to treat bacteria in the urine. A 20%-30% propolis extract has been taken by mouth for 5 days to treat giardiasis (milligram dosing not clearly described). Safety and effectiveness have not been established.

- A dose of 2 mL of aqueous propolis extract has been injected every 14 days for up to 7 months for Legg-Calvé-Perthes disease/avascular necrosis of the hip. Effectiveness and safety have not been established, and dosing should only be under the supervision of a qualified health care professional.

Children (Younger than 18 Years)

- A 10% ethanol extract of propolis has been taken by mouth over 5 days for giardiasis (milligram dosing not established). Note that ethanol (alcohol) preparations should be used cautiously in children. Safety and effectiveness have not been established.

- A 0.5-mL propolis nasal spray (Nivcrisol) has been used once weekly for 5 months in preschool children (average age, 6 years) and school-age children (mean age, 9 years) over a 5-month period to treat respiratory infections. Safety and effectiveness have not been established. An herbal preparation (Chizukit) containing 50 mg/mL of echinacea, 50 mg/mL of propolis, and 10 mg/mL of vitamin C, or placebo (5 mL and 7.5 mL twice daily for ages 1-3 years and 4-5 years, respectively) has been used for 12 weeks. Currently there is not enough scientific evidence to support the use of propolis for respiratory tract infections.

SAFETY
Allergies

- Patients should avoid propolis if they have had allergic or hypersensitivity reactions to propolis, *Populus nigra* L. (black poplar), poplar bud, bee stings/bee products (including honey), or Balsam of Peru. There are multiple reports of swelling, fluid collection, redness, burning, eczema, swelling, fever, and other allergic reactions (including a severe allergic reaction called anaphylaxis) with repeated use of propolis on the skin. Propolis has been linked to several cases of contact dermatitis in beekeepers. Allergic contact stomatitis has been associated with the therapeutic use of propolis.

Side Effects and Warnings

- The safety of propolis has not been thoroughly studied. Although there are several case reports of allergic reactions to propolis, it is generally believed to be well tolerated in most adults. Allergic reactions may cause swelling, redness, eczema, or fever. Propolis may irritate the skin and may cause burning, peeling lips, irritation, lesions, itching, swelling, psoriasis, or eczema. Case reports of irritation in and around the mouth have occurred after use of propolis lozenges or extract taken by mouth.

- Toxicity data for propolis are limited. Early studies have found propolis to be relatively nontoxic. There has been one report of kidney failure with the ingestion of propolis that improved on discontinuing therapy and worsened with reexposure.

Pregnancy and Breastfeeding

- There is not enough scientific evidence to recommend the use of propolis during pregnancy or breastfeeding. Many tinctures contain high levels of alcohol and should be avoided during pregnancy.
- Propolis may protect against male infertility, although this use has not been thoroughly studied.

INTERACTIONS
Interactions with Drugs

- Many tinctures contain high levels of alcohol and may cause nausea or vomiting when taken with metronidazole (Flagyl) or disulfiram (Antabuse).

- Propolis may produce additive effects when taken with antimicrobial drugs.
- Propolis may interact with the following: anticoagulants, *Helicobacter pylori* agents, antibiotics, anticancer agents (antineoplastics), antifungals, antiinflammatory agents, infertility agents, anti–human immunodeficiency virus (HIV) agents (antiretrovirals), immunosuppressants, and osteoporosis agents.

Interactions with Herbs and Dietary Supplements

- Balsam of Peru and propolis are both known to cause allergic sensitization in some people and have multiple compounds in common, such as benzyl benzoate, benzyl cinnamate, benzyl alcohol, benzoic acid, cinnamic acid, caffeic acid, cinnamic alcohol, and vinillin. An increased risk of allergic sensitization may occur if both products are used together.
- Propolis may interact with the following herbs and supplements: anticoagulants (such as coumarin and licorice), antibacterials, anticancer agents (antineoplastics), antifungals, antiinflammatory agents, antioxidants, fertility agents, anti-HIV agents, immunostimulants, immunosuppressants, and osteoporosis agents.

For a complete list of references, please visit www.naturalstandard.com.

Protein-Bound Polysaccharide (PSK)
(*Coriolus versicolor*)

RELATED TERMS

- A beta-1,4-glucan, basidiomycetes, Basidiomycotinae, *Boletus versicolor*, BRM (biological response modifier), cloud mushroom, *Coriolus versicolor*, Kawaratake, Kayken Caps, Krestin, Polyporaceae, *Polyporus versicolor*, polysaccharide K, polysaccharide Kureha, *Polystictus versicolor*, protein-bound B-glucan, proteoglycans, PSP, *Saru-no-koshikake*, strain CM-101, turkey tail mushroom, *Trametes versicolor*, yun zhi.

BACKGROUND

- Protein-bound polysaccharide (PSK) has been used in traditional Chinese medicine (TCM) since the Ming Dynasty of China.
- In the 1980s, the Japanese government approved the use of PSK for treating several types of cancers. By 1984 it ranked nineteenth on the list of the world's most commercially successful drugs, with annual sales of $255 million.
- PSK is obtained from cultured mycelia of the *Coriolus versicolor*, a mushroom thought to have antimicrobial, antiviral, and antitumor properties.
- PSK extracts are available for clinical use in Japan, where it is widely used for cancer immunochemotherapy. In Japan, PSK is currently used as a cancer treatment, in conjunction with surgery, chemotherapy, and/or radiation. Its active ingredient can be administered as a tea or in oral capsule form. In the United States, a similar product is labeled simply *Coriolus versicolor* extract. *Coriolus versicolor* is available in limited supply in U.S. markets. In Japan, PSK is currently the best-selling cancer medicine.

EVIDENCE

Uses Based on Scientific Evidence	Grade
Colorectal Cancer (Adjuvant) PSK in addition to chemotherapy and surgery has been associated with an increased disease-free survival rate for patients with colorectal cancer in various clinical trials as opposed to using pharmaceutical drugs alone. Well-designed clinical trials are needed to confirm these results, along with optimal dosing regimens and optimal pharmaceutical combinations. PSK does not seem to affect the cure rate of colon cancer.	C
Esophageal Cancer (Adjuvant) A small number of clinical trials have examined the ability of PSK, in conjunction with chemotherapy and radiation, to increase survival time in esophageal cancer. Further well-designed trials are needed to fully understand PSK's potential therapeutic role in esophageal cancer.	C
Gastric Cancer (Adjuvant) Several clinical trials or case studies have investigated the use of PSK in combination with chemotherapy in the treatment of gastric cancer. Results from many of the clinical trials show that PSK administered along with chemotherapy is associated with increased 2- to 5-year survival rates. However, some trials found no significant effect on survival over this same period of time. No significant increase in survival has been shown in long-term (greater than 5 years) studies.	C
Leukemia (Adjuvant) One preliminary human trial in patients with acute leukemia suggests that adjunct PSK therapy may prolong duration of remission and survival time. In a second study in patients with acute nonlymphocytic leukemia, no significant increases in survival were found. Well-designed clinical trials are required to determine whether PSK therapy may in fact prolong remission and increase survival time in individuals with acute leukemia.	C
Liver Cancer (Adjuvant) Research using of PSK as an adjunct therapy for liver cancer yield mixed results. Well-designed clinical trials are needed to determine the role of PSK on survival time and remission in individuals with liver cancer.	C
Lung Cancer (Adjuvant) PSK has been studied as an adjuvant therapy in lung cancer patients. Further research is needed before a conclusion can be drawn.	C
Nasopharyngeal Carcinoma (Adjuvant) In preliminary human studies, PSK, used as adjuvant treatment to radiotherapy with or without chemotherapy, has been shown to increase the 5-year survival rate following treatment. Well-designed clinical trials, with larger patient numbers, are needed to confirm these results.	C
Non–Small Cell Lung Cancer (NSCLC) (Adjuvant) One controlled study supports the use of PSK after radiation therapy in patients with stages I, II, or III NSCLC. Further well-designed clinical trials are needed to confirm these results.	C
Breast Cancer (Adjuvant) The available evidence does not support the use of PSK, in conjunction with hormone therapy, chemotherapy, and/or surgery, to increase survival rates in breast cancer patients.	D

P

Uses Based on Tradition or Theory

Acquired immunodeficiency syndrome (AIDS), antibacterial, antifungal, antineoplastic, antioxidant, antiviral, atherosclerosis, cancer prevention, chemotherapy side effects, hepatic disorders, hepatitis, herpes, human immunodeficiency virus (HIV), immunomodulator, infections, kidney disease prevention, liver protection, pancreatic cancer, postsurgical recovery, radiation therapy side effects, stamina, strength.

DOSING

Adults (18 Years and Older)

- For antitumor effects, 1-3 g of PSK has been taken by mouth daily or every other day, either alone or with conventional therapy. PSK has also been administered at a dose of 2-3 g/m^2 daily in three divided doses for 1 month, and taken up to 3 years as a maintenance treatment.

Children (Younger than 18 Years)

- There is insufficient evidence to recommend a dose in children; use is not recommended.

SAFETY

Allergies

- Avoid in individuals with a known allergy or hypersensitivity to PSK, *Coriolus versicolor*, or any of its constituents.

Side Effects and Warnings

- PSK generally seems to have a low incidence of mild and tolerable side effects. In one report, three cases of toxicity were noted, and PSK was discontinued. PSK has been associated with side effects of gastrointestinal upset and darkening of the fingernails, but these effects have been limited; general safety has been demonstrated with daily oral doses for extended periods. Darkening of the fingernails and coughing have been reported during administration of powder drug.
- Low blood cell counts like leukopenia, thrombocytopenia, and albuminuria (protein in the urine) were observed in two clinical trials. It should be noted that patients also received chemotherapy in addition to PSK in these trials, which may have contributed.
- Use cautiously in patients with coronary artery disease because of antiangiogenic properties (inhibition of new blood vessel growth) in the heart.

Pregnancy and Breastfeeding

- Use is not recommended because of lack of sufficient data.

INTERACTIONS

Interactions with Drugs

- Liver function impairment and toxicity have been reported.
- Antiangiogenic properties (inhibition of new blood vessel growth) have been proposed. In theory, there could be an additive effect when PSK is taken in conjugation with other known antiangiogenic agents such as leflunomide.
- Thrombocytopenia (low blood platelet count) has been reported. Theoretically, this could increase the risk of bleeding. Leukopenia and albuminuria were also observed in two clinical trials. It should be noted that patients also received chemotherapy in addition to PSK in these trials. These effects may be attributed to either PSK or chemotherapy.
- Numerous animal and human studies have demonstrated that PSK improves survival time in patients with lung cancer, gastric cancer, stomach cancer, colon cancer, or leukemia when used in conjunction with chemotherapy.
- PSK in immunochemotherapy has been used in combination with hormone therapy to treat pancreatic cancer; therefore additive effects are possible.

Interactions with Herbs and Dietary Supplements

- Liver function impairment and toxicity have been reported.
- Antiangiogenic properties (inhibition of new blood vessel growth) have been proposed. In theory, there could be an additive effect when PSK is taken in conjugation with other known antiangiogenic herbs and supplements such as shark cartilage, horse chestnut, feverfew, and bilberry.
- Thrombocytopenia (low blood platelet count) has been reported. Theoretically, this could increase the risk of bleeding. Leukopenia and albuminuria were also observed in two clinical trials. It should be noted that patients also received chemotherapy in addition to PSK in these trials. These effects may be attributed to either PSK or chemotherapy.
- PSK in immunochemotherapy has been used in combination with hormone therapy to treat pancreatic cancer; therefore additive effects are possible.
- Theoretically, PSK may have a synergistic effect with other immunotherapeutic herbs and supplements. Numerous animal and human studies have demonstrated that PSK improves survival time in patients with lung cancer, gastric cancer, stomach cancer, colon cancer, or leukemia when used in conjunction with chemotherapy.

For a complete list of references, please visit www.naturalstandard.com.

Psyllium
(Plantago spp.)

RELATED TERMS

- Bran Buds cereal, Effersyllium, Fiberall, flea seed, Fybogel, Heartwise cereal, Hydrocil, I-so-gel, ispaghula, ispaghula husk, ispaghula seed, ispaghula, Konsyl, Lunelax, Metamucil, Minolest, natural vegetable laxative, Perdiem, *Plantago arenaria*, *Plantago psyllium*, Prodiem Plain, psyllion, psyllios, psyllium husk, psyllium seed, Regulan, Serutan, Vi-Siblin, Yerba Prima psyllium husk powder.

BACKGROUND

- Psyllium, also referred to as ispaghula, is derived from the husks of the seeds of *Plantago ovata*. Psyllium contains a high level of soluble dietary fiber, and is the chief ingredient in many commonly used bulk laxatives, including products such as Metamucil and Serutan.
- Psyllium has been studied as a "nonsystemic" cholesterol-lowering agent, with generally modest effects seen on total cholesterol and low-density lipoprotein levels. Several psyllium-containing cereals such as Heartwise and Bran Buds have appeared in the U.S. marketplace during the last 15 years and have been touted for their potential lipid-lowering and "heart health–promoting" effects.
- Allergic reactions, including anaphylaxis, have been reported, particularly in health care workers with previous experience preparing psyllium-containing bulk laxatives. Obstruction of the gastrointestinal tract by such laxatives has also been reported, particularly in patients with prior bowel surgeries or anatomical abnormalities or when mixed with inadequate amounts of water.

EVIDENCE

Uses Based on Scientific Evidence	Grade
High Cholesterol Psyllium is well studied as a lipid-lowering agent with generally modest reductions seen in blood levels of total cholesterol and low-density lipoprotein ("bad cholesterol"). Effects have been observed following 8 weeks of regular use. Psyllium does not appear to have significant effects on high-density lipoprotein ("good cholesterol") or triglyceride levels. Because only small reductions have been observed, people with high cholesterol should discuss the use of more potent agents with their health care provider. Effects have been observed in adults and children, although long-term safety in children has not been fully established.	A
Constipation Psyllium has long been used as a chief ingredient in "bulk laxatives." Generally, an increase in stool weight, an increase in bowel movements per day, and a decrease in total gut transit time has been observed in most studies.	B
Diarrhea Psyllium has been studied for the treatment of diarrhea, particularly in patients undergoing tube feeding. It has also been studied in addition to orlistat therapy in hopes of decreasing gastrointestinal effects (diarrhea and oily discharge) of this weight loss agent. An effective stool bulking effect has generally been found in scientific studies.	B
Anal Fissures (Tears or Cracks in the Anus) Psyllium may help to prevent or relieve anal fissures, which can result from constipation, diarrhea, inflammatory bowel disease, or irritable bowel syndrome. However, there is insufficient clinical evidence to support this use.	C
Colon Cancer According to preliminary research, diets that include psyllium may reduce the risk of colon cancer. It remain unclear whether it is effective for this use.	C
Colonoscopy Preparation Patients with new onset constipation or presumed hemorrhoid bleeding frequently require the use of both fiber supplements and diagnostic colonoscopy. Researchers have concluded that in nonconstipated patients, psyllium-based fiber supplementation should not be initiated in the few days before endoscopy using a polyethylene glycol preparation. Instructions given by the appropriate health care professional and pharmacist should be followed when preparing for colonoscopy.	C
Fat Excretion in Stool Preliminary research shows that dietary psyllium and chitosan supplementation may help to increase the excretion of fat in the stool.	C
Gas (Flatulence) Preliminary research suggests that diets high in fiber (such as psyllium) will increase gas production yet promote gas retention. The effect of psyllium on gas needs to be explored further.	C
Hemorrhoids Psyllium may reduce the symptoms of hemorrhoids, which can result from constipation. Further research is needed to determine whether psyllium can help relieve or prevent the symptoms of hemorrhoids.	C
Hyperglycemia (High Blood Sugar Levels) Several studies have examined the administration of psyllium with meals or just before meals to	C

(Continued)

Uses Based on Scientific Evidence	Grade
measure effects on blood sugar levels. Better evidence is necessary before a firm conclusion can be drawn.	
Induction of Labor/Abortion (Cervical Dilator) Preliminary research has examined whether a preparation made from psyllium could help dilate the cervix when labor or abortion is induced. Further research is needed to determine effectiveness.	C
Inflammatory Bowel Disease (Crohn's Disease, Ulcerative Colitis) There is limited and unclear evidence regarding the use of psyllium in patients with inflammatory bowel disease.	C
Irritable Bowel Syndrome Psyllium preparations have been studied for more than 20 years in the treatment of irritable bowel syndrome symptoms. Results of these trials have been conflicting. In some cases, insoluble fiber may worsen the clinical outcome.	C
Obesity The reviewed evidence seems to show that psyllium may improve blood sugar and lipid levels, which can be related to obesity in some children. However, further studies are needed to clarify its effects and the mechanisms involved. Body weight reduction has not been proven to be associated with psyllium use in adults.	C

Uses Based on Tradition or Theory

Abrasions, abscesses, atherosclerosis (hardening of the arteries), bladder disorders (cystitis), bleeding, blisters, boils, bronchitis, burns, cancer, cough, demulcent, diverticular disease, duodenal ulcer, dysentery, excessive menstrual bleeding, eyewash, fecal (stool) incontinence, gallbladder disease, gallstones, gout, hearing damage, heavy menstrual bleeding, high blood pressure, incontinence, insect bites and stings, intestinal ulcers, liver disorders, nose and throat irritation, parasites, poison ivy rash, psoriasis, radiation-induced colitis/diarrhea, skin soothing, sprains, stomach ulcer, urethritis, wound healing (used on the skin).

DOSING
Adults (18 Years and Older)

- Recommendations for dietary fiber intake for adults fall within the range of 20-35 g daily or 10-13 g per 1000 kilocalories ingested.
- It is important to take laxatives such as psyllium with sufficient amounts of water or liquid to reduce the risk of bowel obstruction. Doses ranging from 2.2-45 g by mouth daily in divided doses, often administered just before meals, have been used in studies.

Children (Younger than 18 Years)

- A range of 3.4-16 g by mouth daily has been studied, although more research is needed to establish benefits and long-term safety.

SAFETY
Allergies

- Serious allergic reactions including anaphylaxis, difficulty breathing/wheezing, skin rash, and hives have been reported after ingestion of psyllium products. Less severe hypersensitivity reactions have also been noted. Cross-sensitivity may occur in people with allergy to English plantain pollen (*Plantago lanceolata*), grass pollen, or melon.

Side Effects and Warnings

- Psyllium-containing laxatives, cereals, and other products are generally believed to be safe. Important exceptions include those with repeated psyllium exposure (such as health care workers frequently handling bulk laxatives who are at risk of hypersensitivity reactions) and patients with significant preexisting bowel abnormalities (such as gastrointestinal strictures or impaired motility) or prior bowel surgery.
- Obstruction of the gastrointestinal tract has been noted in numerous case reports of patients taking psyllium-containing laxatives, particularly in individuals with previous bowel surgery or problems and/or when the laxatives are mixed with inadequate amounts of water. Psyllium should be avoided by people who have throat problems or difficulty swallowing.
- Gastrointestinal side effects are generally mild and have not prompted discontinuation of psyllium in most clinical trials. Esophageal obstruction has been reported in a patient with Parkinson's disease.
- Because of potential reductions in blood sugar levels caused by psyllium, blood glucose levels in diabetic patients should be closely monitored.
- Immediate medical attention should be sought if any of these symptoms appear after taking psyllium: chest pain, vomiting, or difficulty swallowing or breathing.

Pregnancy and Breastfeeding

- Psyllium-containing laxatives are considered class C-2 drugs in pregnancy, meaning that they appear to be safe in all three trimesters, although studies in pregnant humans and animals have not been done. Psyllium-containing products are considered class 1 (apparently safe) during breastfeeding.

INTERACTIONS
Interactions with Drugs

- Psyllium-containing products may delay gastric emptying time and reduce the absorption of some drugs. It is advised that drugs be taken at separate administration times from psyllium to minimize potential interactions (e.g., 1 hour before or a few hours after taking psyllium).
- Although no effect on warfarin (Coumadin) levels with coadministration of psyllium was reported in one study, administration of these agents should be separated until better research is available.

- Because of potential reductions in blood sugar levels caused by psyllium, requirements for insulin or other diabetes drugs in diabetic patients may be reduced. Blood glucose levels should be closely monitored, and dosing adjustments may be necessary.
- Other drugs may be affected by psyllium, including anticoagulants, antidepressants, antigout agents, antiinflammatory agents, diuretics, salicylates, tetracyclines, nitrofurantoin, insulin, lithium (Lithobid, Eskalith), and digoxin (Lanoxin). People should speak with their health care providers before taking psyllium. Dosing adjustments may be necessary.

Interactions with Herbs and Dietary Supplements

- Psyllium-containing products may delay gastric emptying time and reduce the absorption of some herbs, supplements, vitamins, or minerals. Absorption of calcium, iron, zinc, and vitamin B_{12} may also be affected. Other agents should be taken 1 hour before or a few hours after psyllium to avoid potential interactions.

- Psyllium should be used cautiously with other laxatives, such as senna, because effects may be increased.
- Psyllium and chitosan together may increase fat excretion in the stool.
- Theoretically, psyllium may reduce the absorption of anticoagulant herbs and supplements. However, no effect on warfarin levels by coadministered psyllium was found in one study.
- Taking psyllium with herbs and supplements that alter blood sugar may increase the risk of hypoglycemia (lowered blood sugar). People using other herbs or supplements that may alter blood sugar levels, such as bitter melon (*Momordica charantia*), should be monitored closely by their health care provider while using psyllium. Dosing adjustments may be necessary.
- Psyllium may interact with herbs and supplements with antidepressant, antigout, antiinflammatory, and diuretic activities.

For a complete list of references, please visit www. naturalstandard.com.

P

Pycnogenol
(*Pinus pinaster* subsp. *atlantica*)

RELATED TERMS

- Cocklebut, condensed tannins, Evelle (vitamins C and E, carotenoids, selenium, zinc, amino acids, glycosaminoglycans, blueberry extract, Pycnogenol), French maritime pine bark extract, French Pinus maritime bark, grape marc extract, leucoanthocyanidins, *Pinus pinaster*, *Pinus maritima*, oligomeric proanthocyanidin complexes (OPCs), Pinaceae (family), proanthocyanidins, PYC, pygenol, stickwort, Zinopin (pycnogenol and standardized ginger root extract [SGRE]).

BACKGROUND

- Pycnogenol is the patented trade name for a water extract of the bark of the French maritime pine (*Pinus pinaster* ssp. *atlantica*), which is grown in coastal southwest France. Pycnogenol contains oligomeric proanthocyanidins (OPCs) as well as several other bioflavonoids: catechin, epicatechin, phenolic fruit acids (such as ferulic acid and caffeic acid), and taxifolin. Procyanidins are oligomeric catechins found at high concentrations in red wine, grapes, cocoa, cranberries, apples, and some supplements such as Pycnogenol.
- There has been some confusion in the U.S. market regarding OPC products containing Pycnogenol or grape seed extract (GSE) because one of the generic terms for chemical constituents ("pycnogenols") is the same as the patented trade name (Pycnogenol). Some GSE products were formerly erroneously labeled and marketed in the U.S. as containing "pycnogenols." Although GSE and Pycnogenol do contain similar chemical constituents (primarily in the OPC fraction), the chemical, pharmacological, and clinical literature on the two products is distinct. The term *Pycnogenol* should therefore only be used to refer to this specific proprietary pine bark extract. Scientific literature regarding this product should not be referenced as a basis for the safety or effectiveness of GSE.

EVIDENCE

Uses Based on Scientific Evidence	Grade
Asthma Pycnogenol may offer clinical benefit to both children and adults with asthma. Further research is needed to determine optimal dosing and safety.	B
Chronic Venous Insufficiency Chronic venous insufficiency (CVI) is a syndrome that includes leg swelling, varicose veins, pain, itching, skin changes, and skin ulcers. The term is more commonly used in Europe than in the United States. Pycnogenol used in people with chronic venous insufficiency is reported to reduce edema and pain. Pycnogenol may also be used in the management of other CVI symptoms.	B

ADHD (Attention Deficient Hyperactivity Disorder) Pycnogenol has been used in adult patients with ADHD to improve concentration but does not appear to be more effective than placebo.	C
Antioxidant Because of conflicting study results, it is unclear whether Pycnogenol has significant antioxidant effects in humans.	C
Cramps (Muscular Pain) Pycnogenol may effectively prevent cramps, muscular pain at rest, and pain after/during exercise in healthy people, in athletes prone to cramps, and in patients with venous disease, claudication, or diabetic microangiopathy.	C
Diabetes Supplementation of Pycnogenol with conventional diabetes treatment may lower glucose levels and improve endothelial function.	C
Diabetic Microangiopathy Supplementation with Pycnogenol may improve symptoms associated with diabetic microangiopathy.	C
Dysmenorrhea (Painful Menstruation) Preliminary clinical evidence shows that Pycnogenol may have a potential analgesic (pain-relieving) effect on menstrual pain.	C
Erectile Dysfunction Pycnogenol, in combination with L-arginine, may cause an improvement in sexual function in men with erectile dysfunction. It is not known what effect each of the individual compounds may have directly on this condition.	C
Gingival Bleeding/Plaque Chewing gum containing Pycnogenol is reported to minimize gingival bleeding and plaque formation. Pycnogenol has also been added to toothpaste for antioxidant effect.	C
High Blood Pressure Pycnogenol may reduce the need for nifedipine and decrease systolic blood pressure in patients with high blood pressure.	C
Platelet Aggregation Limited evidence suggests that Pycnogenol reduces platelet aggregation in smokers.	C

Uses Based on Scientific Evidence	Grade
Prevention of Blood Clots/Edema during Long Airplane Fights Pycnogenol treatment may be effective in decreasing the number of thrombotic events (deep venous thrombosis [DVT] and superficial vein thrombosis [SVT]) in moderate- to high-risk subjects during long-haul flights. Edema (swelling) may also be reduced. However, the evidence is insufficient to support this use.	C
Retinopathy Several studies report benefits of Pycnogenol in the treatment and prevention of retinopathy, including slowing the progression of retinopathy in diabetic patients. However, the evidence is insufficient to support this use.	C
High Cholesterol Pycnogenol may reduce low-density lipoprotein (LDL/"bad cholesterol") levels and increase high-density lipoprotein (HDL/"good cholesterol") levels. Evidence is conflicting.	C
Male Infertility Clinical studies report that Pycnogenol may improve sperm quality and function in subfertile men. However, the evidence is insufficient to support this use.	C
Melasma (Chloasma) Melasma (or chloasma) is a common disorder of hyperpigmentation of the skin predominately affecting sun-exposed areas in women. Formations of tan or brown patches/spots may occur. Pycnogenol has been reported to decrease the darkened area and the pigment intensity of melasma and improve symptoms of fatigue, constipation, body pains, and anxiety. However, the evidence is insufficient to support this use.	C
Sunburn Pycnogenol, taken by mouth, may reduce erythema (redness of the skin) caused by solar ultraviolet light. However, the evidence is insufficient to support this use.	C
Systemic Lupus Erythematosus (SLE) Pycnogenol may be useful as a second-line therapy to reduce inflammatory features of SLE. However, the evidence is insufficient to support this use.	C
Venous Leg Ulcers Pycnogenol may be useful for reduction of leg ulcers. However, the evidence is insufficient to support this use.	C

Uses Based on Tradition or Theory
ACE inhibitor activity, Alzheimer's disease, antihistamine, antimicrobial, antiparasitic, arthritis, atherosclerosis, autoimmune disorders, bleeding, bone marrow production, cancer prevention, cancer treatment, cardiac mitral valve prolapse, cardiovascular disease, cerebral ischemia, chemotherapy side effects, easy bruising, Ehlers-Danlos syndrome, exercise capacity, fat burning, glucose-6-phosphate dehydrogenase (G6PD) deficiency, gout prevention (xanthine oxidase and dehydrogenase inhibitor), hemorrhoids, immune enhancement, immune suppression, improving skin smoothness and elasticity, increased human growth hormone, inflammation, inflammatory bowel disease, inhibition of tumor necrosis factor (TNF)-alpha, joint hypermobility, leukemia, lung cancer, musculoskeletal problems, osteoporosis, periodontitis, poor tissue healing, premenstrual syndrome, macular degeneration, motion sickness, myalgia, myocardial ischemia/reperfusion injury, myopathy, neurodegenerative diseases, night vision, pelvic pain, prevention of fat formation, psoriasis, reducing scar formation, retinal protection, rheumatoid arthritis, sickle cell anemia, skin aging, skin disorders, spinal scoliosis, varicose veins, vascular problems, vasorelaxant, venous thromboembolism (VTE), wound healing.

DOSING
Adults (18 Years and Older)

- In general, 25-360 mg/day has been taken in divided doses by mouth. For gum health, 5 mg Pycnogenol in chewing gum for 14 days has been used.
- Pycnogenol appears to be absorbed into the bloodstream in about 20 minutes. Once absorbed, therapeutic effects are purported to last for approximately 72 hours, followed by excretion in the urine. Because of its astringent taste and occasional minor stomach discomfort, it may be best to take Pycnogenol with or after meals.

Children (Younger than 18 Years)

- There is insufficient evidence to recommend Pycnogenol use in children.

SAFETY
Allergies

- Individuals should not take Pycnogenol if allergic to it or any of its components.

Side Effects and Warnings

- Pycnogenol is generally reported as being well tolerated. Low acute and chronic toxicity with mild unwanted effects may occur in a small percentage of patients following oral administration. Because of its astringent taste and occasional minor stomach discomfort, it may be best to take Pycnogenol with or after meals. To date, no serious adverse effects have been reported in the available scientific literature, although systematic study of safety is not available.
- In theory, Pycnogenol may alter blood sugar levels. Caution is advised in patients with diabetes or hypoglycemia and in those taking drugs, herbs, or supplements that affect blood sugar. Serum glucose levels may need to be monitored by a health care provider, and medication adjustments may be necessary.
- In theory, Pycnogenol may increase the risk of bleeding. Caution is advised in patients with bleeding disorders or taking drugs that may increase the risk of bleeding. Dosing adjustments may be necessary.

Pregnancy and Breastfeeding

- Pycnogenol is not recommended during pregnancy or breastfeeding because of a lack of scientific evidence.

P

INTERACTIONS
Interactions with Drugs

- Pycnogenol may interact with other blood pressure–lowering medications, specifically angiotensin-converting enzyme inhibitors (ACE-I) such as benazepril (Lotensin), captopril (Capoten), enalapril (Vasotec), fosinopril (Monopril), lisinopril (Prinivil), moexipril (Univasc), perindopril (Aceon), quinapril (Accupril), ramipril (Altace), trandolapril (Mavik), or angiotensin-converting enzyme receptor blockers such as losartan (Cozaar), irbesartan (Avapro), candesartan cilexetil (Atacand), or valsartan (Diovan).
- Pycnogenol may lower blood sugar levels. Caution is advised when medications that may also lower blood sugar are used. Patients taking drugs for diabetes by mouth (such as metformin, glyburide, or glipizide) or using insulin should be monitored closely by a qualified health care provider. Medication adjustments may be necessary.
- Pycnogenol may increase the risk of bleeding when taken with drugs that increase the risk of bleeding. Some examples include aspirin, anticoagulants ("blood thinners") such as warfarin (Coumadin) or heparin, antiplatelet drugs such as clopidogrel (Plavix), and nonsteroidal antiinflammatory drugs such as ibuprofen (Motrin, Advil) or naproxen (Naprosyn, Aleve).
- Pycnogenol may interfere with immunosuppressant or immunostimulant drugs.
- In theory, Pycnogenol and antioxidants may have additive effects.

- Pycnogenol prevented fluoride-induced kidney damage.
- Pycnogenol may have protective effects against alcohol's effects on brain neurons, but further research is needed to confirm these results.

Interactions with Herbs and Dietary Supplements

- Although data have yet to confirm this claim, it has been proposed that Pycnogenol may increase vitamin C levels.
- Pycnogenol may lower blood sugar levels. Caution is advised when herbs or supplements that may also lower blood sugar are used. Blood glucose levels may require monitoring, and doses may need adjustment.
- Pycnogenol may increase the risk of bleeding when taken with herbs and supplements that are believed to increase the risk of bleeding. Multiple cases of bleeding have been reported with the use of *Ginkgo biloba*, and fewer cases have been reported with garlic and saw palmetto. Numerous other agents may theoretically increase the risk of bleeding, although this has not been proven in most cases.
- In theory, Pycnogenol may interact with herbs and supplements that effect blood pressure. Caution is advised.
- Pycnogenol may interfere with immunosuppressant or immunostimulant herbs and supplements.
- Pycnogenol and other antioxidants may have additive effects.

For a complete list of references, please visit www.naturalstandard.com.

Pygeum
(Prunus africanum, syn. Pygeum africanum)

RELATED TERMS

- African plum tree, African prune tree, African *Pygeum africanum* extract, alumty, iluo, kirah, Natal tree, Pigenil, Pronitol, Provol, prunier d'afrique, *Pygeum africanum*, Rosaceae (family), Tadenan, V1326, vla, wotangue.

BACKGROUND

- The *Pygeum africanum* (African plum) tree is a tall evergreen of the family Rosaceae found in central and southern Africa. Its bark has been used medicinally for thousands of years. Traditional African healers have used the bark to treat bladder and urination disorders, particularly symptoms associated with benign prostatic hypertrophy (BPH), which is an enlarged prostate. Historically, the bark was powdered and used to make a tea, which was taken by mouth for these conditions.
- The African plum tree has become endangered due to the demand for its bark to process *Pygeum africanum* extract.
- The majority of trials conducted since the 1970s report improvements in BPH symptoms with the administration of *Pygeum africanum* bark extract, including frequency of nighttime urination, urine flow rate, and leftover urine volume. This research has led some credibility to the common use of this agent in Europe for BPH. The herb is less commonly used in the United States, where prescription drugs or the herb saw palmetto is more commonly used.

EVIDENCE

Uses Based on Scientific Evidence	Grade
Benign Prostatic Hypertrophy/BPH Symptoms Pygeum (*Pygeum africanum* bark extract) has been observed to moderately improve urinary symptoms associated with enlargement of the prostate gland or prostate inflammation. Numerous human studies report pygeum to significantly reduce the number of nighttime urinary episodes, urinary hesitancy, urinary frequency, and pain with urination in men who experience mild-to-moderate symptoms. However, pygeum does not appear to reduce the size of the prostate gland or reverse the process of BPH. It is unclear how pygeum compares to the effectiveness or safety of other medical therapies, such as prescription drugs (e.g., alpha-adrenergic blockers or 5-alpha reductase inhibitors), surgical approaches, or other herbs or supplements such as saw palmetto. There is ongoing study in this area. Patients with urinary symptoms or BPH should speak with their health care professional about the various available treatment options.	B

Uses Based on Tradition or Theory

Aphrodisiac, bladder sphincter disorders, fever, impotence, inflammation, kidney disease, malaria, male baldness, partial bladder outlet obstruction, prostate cancer, prostatic adenoma, prostatitis, psychosis, sexual performance, stomach upset, urinary tract health.

DOSING
Adults (18 Years and Older)

- Capsules: For treating benign prostatic hypertrophy, 75-200-mg capsules of standardized pygeum extract have been taken daily by mouth either as a single dose or divided into two equal doses. One clinical human trial has shown that *Pygeum africanum* (25 mg) and stinging nettle (*Urtica dioica*) (30 mg), when used in combination, were efficient in treating BPH and its symptoms.

Children (Younger than 18 Years)

- There are not enough scientific data to recommend pygeum for use in children, and there are potential side effects.

SAFETY
Allergies

- People with known allergies to pygeum should avoid this herb.

Side Effects and Warnings

- Pygeum has been well tolerated in most studies, with adverse effects similar to placebo (sugar pill). Some people may experience stomach discomfort, including diarrhea, constipation, stomach pain, or nausea. Stomach upset is usually mild and does not typically cause people to stop using pygeum.
- Safety of use beyond 12 months has not been reliably studied.

Pregnancy and Breastfeeding

- Pygeum cannot be recommended during pregnancy or breastfeeding because of a lack of scientific information and possible hormonal effects.

INTERACTIONS
Interactions with Drugs

- Use of pygeum with other drugs commonly used to treat symptoms of prostate enlargement, called 5-alpha-reductase inhibitors, such as terazosin (Hytrin) or finasteride (Propecia, Proscar), may increase beneficial effects, although this is not well studied.

P

- In theory, pygeum may interact with estrogen or other hormones.

Interactions with Herbs and Dietary Supplements

- Pygeum may result in increased beneficial effects for the prostate if used with saw palmetto (*Serenoa repens*) or stinging nettle (*Urtica dioica*). Combination products are available containing both stinging nettle and pygeum.
- Pygeum may interact with herbs or supplements containing chemicals with estrogen-like effects ("phytoestrogens").

For a complete list of references, please visit www. naturalstandard.com.

Quassia
(*Quassia* spp.)

RELATED TERMS

- *Ailanthus,* amargo, bitter ash, bitter bark, bitterholz, bitterwood, bois amer, gorzkla, indaquassin, Jamaican quassia, Jamaica quassia extract, kvassia, kwassi, neoquassin, palo muneco, pau amarelo, pau quassia, pao tariri, *Picrasma*, quassia africana, *Quassia amara*, quassia bark, *Quassia bidwillii*, *Quassia indica*, *Quassia undulata*, quassia wood, quassin, quassinoids, ruda, samaderines, simarinolide, Simaroubaceae (family), Surinam quassia, Surinam wood.

BACKGROUND

- Quassia, a tree native to Jamaica and its neighboring islands, has traditionally been used as a remedy for roundworms, as an insecticide, and in brewing as a substitute for hops. It has also been used as a bitter digestive aid and a remedy for digestive disorders, parasites, and head lice.
- Several early studies performed on quassia verified its traditional use as a natural insecticide, documenting it as an effective treatment for head lice in humans. Because quassia has long been used for malaria in South America, researchers also studied this biological effect. One study showed strong antimalarial activity in mice.
- There is early evidence that quassia may be useful in the treatment of leukemia or gastric ulcers. Quassia may also have pain-relieving, muscle-relaxing, and sedating effects, but human clinical trials are currently lacking.

EVIDENCE

Uses Based on Scientific Evidence	Grade
Head Lice Early evidence suggests the effectiveness of quassia for head lice. More well-designed clinical trials are necessary to confirm these finding and make a firm conclusion regarding the safety and effectiveness for this condition.	C

Uses Based on Tradition or Theory
Amenorrhea (absence of menstruation), analgesic (reduces pain), anorexia (eating disorder), antibacterial, antifertility, antifungal, antimalarial, antivenom, antiviral, constipation, fever, flavoring agent, hepatoprotection (liver protection), hypoglycemic (blood sugar–lowering), indigestion, insecticide (larvae), kidney stones, laxative, leukemia, muscle relaxant, parasites, pesticides, salivary stimulant, sedative (causes drowsiness), tonic, ulcers, worms.

DOSING
Adults (18 Years and Older)

- There is insufficient evidence to recommend a dose for quassia in adults.

Children (Younger than 18 Years)

- There is insufficient evidence to recommend a dose for quassia in children. There is one report of death associated with quassia administered to a child via IV (through a vein).

SAFETY
Allergies

- Avoid in individuals with a known allergy or hypersensitivity to quassia or its constituents.

Side Effects and Warnings

- Quassia is likely safe when consumed in amounts found in foods and beverages. It has "generally recognized as safe" (GRAS) status in the United States.
- Quassia appears to have a very mild side effects profile. The most common side effects are nausea and vomiting, due to its bitter taste. There have also been reports of mucous membrane irritation.
- Quassia may cause drowsiness or sedation. Use cautiously if driving or operating heavy machinery. Long-term use of quassia may cause vision changes and blindness.
- Use cautiously with cardiac (heart) medications and blood thinners.
- Avoid in women who are pregnant; because of quassia's potential antifertility effects in males and females, avoid if trying to conceive.
- Avoid intravenous use in cardiomyopathy (heart disease) patients.

Pregnancy and Breastfeeding

- Avoid quassia if pregnant or breastfeeding because of a lack of available scientific evidence. Quassia may have antifertility effects in men and women.

INTERACTIONS
Interactions with Drugs

- Quassia may increase the risk of bleeding when taken with drugs that increase the risk of bleeding. Some examples include aspirin, anticoagulants ("blood thinners") such as warfarin (Coumadin) or heparin, antiplatelet drugs such as clopidogrel (Plavix), and nonsteroidal antiinflammatory drugs (NSAIDs) such as ibuprofen (Motrin, Advil) or naproxen (Naprosyn, Aleve).
- Quassia may interact with antacid medications and has been known to cause gastrointestinal adverse effects; use cautiously.
- Quassia may interact with heart medications. Use cautiously in patients with heart conditions or taking cardiac agents because of possible adverse effects.
- Quassia may interact with diuretics; use cautiously.
- Quassia may interact with hormonal agents. Use cautiously in male and female patients if couples are trying to conceive.
- Quassia may increase the amount of drowsiness caused by some drugs. Examples include benzodiazepines such as lorazepam (Ativan) or diazepam (Valium), barbiturates such as phenobarbital, narcotics such as codeine, some antidepressants, and alcohol. Use caution while driving or operating machinery.
- Quassia may interact with laxatives; use cautiously.

Interactions with Herbs and Dietary Supplements

- Quassia may increase the risk of bleeding when taken with herbs and supplements that are believed to increase the risk of bleeding.
- Quassia may interact with herbs and supplements taken to prevent or treat various heart conditions.
- Use cautiously with herbs and supplements with diuretic effects.
- Quassia may interact with hormonal agents. Use cautiously with herbs and supplements with known hormonal activity because of possible additive effects. Quassia may have negative effects on fertility in males and females.
- Theoretically, abuse of horsetail or licorice along with quassia might increase the risk of cardiac toxicity (heart damage).
- Quassia my increase the amount of drowsiness cause by some herbs or supplements. Use caution when driving or operating heavy machinery.
- Use cautiously with herbs or supplements with laxative effects.

For a complete list of references, please visit www.naturalstandard.com.

Quercetin

RELATED TERMS

- *Allium cepa*, American elder, apples, *Artemisia abrotanum* L., AS195 *Folia vitis viniferae* (red vine leaf extract), biflavonoids, bilberries, black currants, black tea, brassica vegetables (cabbage, broccoli, cauliflower, turnips, kale), buckwheat tea, citrus bioflavonoid, endive, flavones, flavonoids, flavonols, flavon(ol)-glycosides, *Ginkgo biloba* extract, ginkgo flavone glycosides, grapefruit, green tea, *Hypericum perforatum* L., isoflavones, isorhamnetin, isoquercitrin, kaemferol, meletin, Myrtaceae, naphthodianthrones, onion, parsley (*Petroselinum crispum* (Mill.) Nym.), phytodrug (QG-5), phytoestrogens, pine bark extract, polyphenol, *Psidium guajava* L. (Fam.), quercetin aglycone, quercetin chalcone, quercetin dimethyl ethers, quercetin glucoside, quercetin glucuronides, quercetin rutin, quercetin rutinoside, red vine leaf extract, red wine, red wine phenolics, rhamnose molecule, rutin, *Sambucus nigra* L., sophretin, St. John's wort, STW-3, Tycho, Venenkapseln, Venoruton (O-(beta-hydroxyethyl) rutosides (HR).

BACKGROUND

- Quercetin is a major flavonol, one of the almost 4,000 flavonoids (antioxidants) that occur in foods of plant origin, such as red wine, onions, green tea, apples, berries, and *Brassica* vegetables (cabbage, broccoli, cauliflower, turnips). Quercetin is also found in *Gingko biloba*, St. John's wort, and American elder.
- Quercetin and rutin (another flavonol) are used in many countries as vasoprotectants and are ingredients of numerous multivitamin preparations and herbal remedies. They occur mainly as glycosides, which means they are linked with various sugars. However, the ability of the body to absorb these compounds (bioavailability) is questionable.
- Quercetin and other flavonols have a wide variety of biological effects, but the scientific evidence for use in the prevention or treatment of disease is weak. Quercetin has been considered as a therapy for cardiovascular diseases, high cholesterol levels, diabetic cataracts, inflammation, ischemic injury, chronic prostatitis, chronic venous insufficiency, gastrointestinal ulceration, hepatitis, allergies, asthma, viral infections, and hay fever.
- Review of the literature shows that there have been several studies on the association of quercetin with risk reduction for coronary heart disease, stroke, and cancers and a few studies on other medical conditions. However, there is a lack of strong evidence to support any of these conditions.

EVIDENCE

Uses Based on Scientific Evidence	Grade
Cardiovascular Disease Several of the effects of flavonoids that have been observed in laboratory and animal studies suggest that they might be effective in reducing cardiovascular disease risk. Studies in humans using polyphenolic compounds from red grapes showed improvement in endothelial function in patients with coronary heart disease. Antioxidant and cholesterol-lowering effects are proposed.	C
Immune Function (after Intense Exercise) Quercetin does not appear to affect changes in the immune system caused by intense exercise. However, it reduced the number of respiratory tract infections in people who participated in intense cycling. More research is needed.	C
Pancreatic Cancer Prevention Some research suggests that quercetin may help prevent pancreatic cancer in smokers. However, quercetin did not have this effect in nonsmokers or former smokers. More research is needed to determine whether quercetin is beneficial.	C
Prostatitis/Chronic Pelvic Pain Syndrome There is some evidence that quercetin may be useful for the treatment of chronic prostatitis and chronic pelvic pain syndrome. Further research is needed to confirm these results.	C

Uses Based on Tradition or Theory

Allergic rhinitis, allergies, antihistamine, antiinflammatory, antioxidant, antispasmodic, antithrombotic, arthritis, antiviral, asthma, atherosclerosis (hardening of the arteries), autoimmune diseases, brain tumors, breast cancer prevention, cancer treatment, capillary fragility, cataract prevention, cerebrovascular disease, chronic venous insufficiency, coronary heart disease, cutaneous blood flux, diabetes mellitus, diarrhea (acute), depression, deoxyribonucleic acid damage, eczema, edema, fibromyalgia, gout, graft healing, hepatitis, herpes, high cholesterol levels, hives, ileostomy use, inflammation, interstitial cystitis, kidney toxicity, local anesthesia, macular degeneration, mucosal mast cell inhibition, peptic ulcers, platelet aggregation, prostate cancer prevention, protection against chemotherapy side effects, retinopathy, rheumatoid arthritis, schizophrenia, systemic lupus erythematosus (SLE), ulcers, vasoprotective, viral infections, vision problems (age-related).

DOSING

Adults (18 Years and Older)

- It has been suggested that quercetin should be taken 20 minutes before meals. Quercetin has been ingested from onions, juice, black tea, and red wine. Doses of 100-500 mg of quercetin have been taken two to three times daily. It is available in tablet, capsule, or softgel form. Intravenous and intramuscular forms have been injected by a health care provider.

Children (Younger than 18 Years)

- Insufficient evidence is available to recommend use of quercetin in children.

SAFETY

Allergies

- Avoid in individuals with a known allergy or hypersensitivity to quercetin by ingestion or skin contact. Eye, skin, gastrointestinal, and/or respiratory tract irritation is possible.

Side Effects and Warnings

- Being a common food component, quercetin is generally safe and well tolerated at usual dietary intake. However, it has been associated with headache, gastrointestinal effects, hematoma, and kidney toxicity.
- Intravenous injection has been associated with pain at the injection site that is dose related and can be controlled by reducing the rate of infusion. Intravenous administration of quercetin has also resulted in flushing, sweating, difficulty breathing (dyspnea), nausea, mild tingling of the extremities, lethargy, and vomiting.
- Concern had been expressed about the possible tumor-promoting effect of quercetin.
- Mild constipation and hair thinning were reported by two of 260 patients taking AS195, which contains red vine leaf extract, rich in quercetin.

Pregnancy and Breastfeeding

- Insufficient evidence is available.

INTERACTIONS

Interactions with Drugs

- Based on laboratory study, platelet aggregation may be inhibited, which may increase bleeding risk.

- Based on laboratory study, quercetin may enhance the effects of the cancer chemotherapy drug busulphan. Quercetin may decrease liver and kidney damage caused by the cancer chemotherapy drug cisplatin. Quercetin may also affect the levels of cyclosporine.
- Quercetin may increase the effects of steroids or interact with estradiol and nifedipine by interfering with the way that the liver breaks them down.
- Laboratory studies also suggest that quercetin may affect certain hormone levels.
- Quercetin may interact with quinolone antibiotics like ciprofloxacin or levofloxacin.
- Based on laboratory studies, short-term use of quercetin may result in higher uptake or influx of ritonavir and erythromycin. Quercetin may also inhibit cortisol.

Interactions with Herbs and Dietary Supplements

- Quercetin may interact with herbs or supplements that are broken down by the liver.
- Based on laboratory study, platelet aggregation may be inhibited, which may increase bleeding risk.
- Quercetin is found in elder, St. John's wort, parsley, green tea, and ginkgo; thus there may be additive effects if taken together. Consumption of black currants, lingonberries, and bilberries increases quercetin levels in the blood.
- Papain or bromelain may increase the absorption of quercetin. Vitamin C may enhance the antioxidant activity of quercetin. Consumption of rutin-containing herbs may cause additive effects because of quercetin content.

For a complete list of references, please visit www.naturalstandard.com.

Quinoa
(Chenopodium quinoa)

RELATED TERMS

- Amaranthaceae (family), bitter quinoa, *Chenopodium quinoa*, *Chenopodium quinoa* Willd., quinoa flour, quinoa seed, quinua, quinua flour, quinua seed, sweet quinoa.

BACKGROUND

- Quinoa has been cultivated by the Andes Incas for thousands of years. It has recently gained prominence around the world as a "super food" because of its high protein content. Although quinoa is high in protein content, it alone does not have enough protein to replace meat in the Western European diet because of current cultivation, technological, and processing restrictions. Quinoa is also used by some people as a substitute for wheat, especially those on a gluten-free diet because of celiac disease or other conditions.
- Other than its use as a food, there is insufficient evidence in humans to support the use of quinoa for any indication.

EVIDENCE

Uses Based on Scientific Evidence

No available studies qualify for inclusion in the evidence table.

Uses Based on Tradition or Theory

Antioxidant, celiac disease, food uses, hypertriglyceridemia (elevated level of fatty acid compounds in the blood).

DOSING

Adults (18 Years and Older)

- There is insufficient evidence to recommend a dose for quinoa in adults.

Children (Younger than 18 Years)

- There is insufficient evidence to recommend a dose for quinoa in children.

SAFETY

Allergies

- Avoid in individuals with a known allergy or hypersensitivity to quinoa (*Chenopodium quinoa*) or its constituents.

Side Effects and Warnings

- Quinoa is likely safe when quinoa seeds are used in food amounts, as quinoa has been used as a food for thousands of years. Quinoa is usually washed after harvest and before preparation to remove a natural coating of saponins on the seeds. Available reports of adverse effects related to quinoa are lacking.

Pregnancy and Breastfeeding

- Quinoa is not recommended in pregnant or breastfeeding women because of a lack of available scientific evidence.

INTERACTIONS

Interactions with Drugs

- Quinoa may have antioxidant properties. Caution is advised when quinoa is taken with other agents that have antioxidant properties.
- Quinoa may lower triglyceride concentrations compared with gluten-free bread and pasta. Caution is advised in patients taking triglyceride-lowering agents.

Interactions with Herbs and Dietary Supplements

- Quinoa may have antioxidant properties. Caution is advised when quinoa is taken with herbs and supplements that have antioxidant properties.
- Quinoa may lower triglyceride concentrations compared with gluten-free bread and pasta. Caution is advised in patients taking herbs or supplements that may lower triglycerides.

For a complete list of references, please visit www.naturalstandard.com.

Raspberry
(*Rubus idaeus*)

RELATED TERMS

- Alkalis, alpha-carotene, alpha-tocopherol, anthocyanin, aronia berry, ascorbic acid, berry phenolics, beta-carotene, calcium, casuarictin, copper, ellagic acid, ellagitannins, epicuticular wax, flavonoids, flavonol, framboise (French), furanones, hydroxycinnamate, iron, kaempferol, kaempferol 3-glucosides, linolenic acid, loratadine, lutein, magnesium, manganese, methyl gallate, miskominaga wunj (Ojibwe), omega 3, oo na joo kwa (Mohawk), omega 3, phosphorus, phytochemicals, phytonutrients, polyphenolic components, quercetin, quercetin glycosides, raspberry ketone, raspberry seed oil, raspberry leaf, raspberry leaf tea, red raspberry, resveratrol, Rosaceae (family), *Rubus, Rubus arcticus, Rubus arizonensis, Rubus deliciosus, Rubus discolor, Rubus idaeus, Rubus idaeus* ssp. *Strigosus, Rubus laciniatus, Rubus leucodermis, Rubus neomexicanus, Rubus occidentalis, Rubus parviflorus, Rubus spectabilis, Rubus strigosus, Rubus ursinus,* salicylates, sanguin H6, tannins, vitamin B, vitamin B_1, vitamin C, vitamin E, volatile compounds, western blackberry, xylitol, xyloside, zinc.

BACKGROUND

- Raspberry (*Rubus idaeus*) is cultivated and grows wild throughout temperate climates, including North America and Europe. For several centuries, midwives have used raspberry leaf to stimulate and ease labor. Tea made from raspberry leaves has been used for centuries as a folk medicine to treat wounds, diarrhea, and colic pain and as a uterine relaxant. In Bulgaria, the leaves were used for stomach bleeding, diarrhea, vomiting, menstrual problems, and respiratory diseases. In traditional Tibetan medical practices, the fruit and leaves of raspberry are made into an extract or decoction and used as a cure for emotional disturbances, exhaustion, irritability, and chronic infections.
- The raspberry fruit is also commonly eaten raw or used as a flavoring, coloring, or food, either fresh or processed into cordials, jams, or preserves. The fruit is also commonly consumed for its antioxidants. Raspberry flowers have also been used for pimples, hemorrhoids, and malaria and as a poultice for eye inflammations.
- Raspberry leaf is used during pregnancy and labor today, but there are few studies supporting this use. Raspberry may also be useful in cancer treatment or prevention or as an antimicrobial. More research is needed to confirm these findings.
- In the early 1990s, raspberries imported to the United States from Guatemala were infected with the *Cyclospora* parasite, which caused adverse effects such as fatigue, muscle aches, vomiting, and diarrhea. Periodic outbreaks of the *Cyclospora* parasite from imported raspberries continued throughout the next decade. In response to outbreaks, the Centers for Disease Control (CDC) placed periodic bans on imported raspberries.

EVIDENCE

Uses Based on Scientific Evidence	Grade
Antioxidant (Free Radical–Scavenging) Raspberry contains antioxidants and has antioxidant activity. Raspberry juice may have beneficial effects on exercise recovery. However, there is a lack of supportive clinical evidence.	C
Childbirth Raspberry leaf has been traditionally used during pregnancy and childbirth to improve labor. Early study shows that raspberry leaf may be safe for both mother and child. However, there is a lack of supportive evidence to recommend a dose.	C

Uses Based on Tradition or Theory

Acne, aging, alcohol intoxication (recovery), analgesic (pain reliever), anemia, antibacterial, antifungal, antimutagenic (inhibiting mutations), antiviral, anxiety, asthma, astringent, atherosclerosis, bile flow stimulation, bowel disorders (laxity), burns, cancer, cardiovascular disease, cardiovascular disorders, cleanser (blood), colic, diaphoretic (induces sweating), diarrhea, digestion, digestive disorders, diuretic, dysentery, dysmenorrhea (painful menstruation), exhaustion, expectorant, eye inflammation, fertility, fetal development (birth defects), fever, flavoring agent, food uses, galactagogue (promotes the flow of milk), gastric disorders (bleeding), gum disease, *Helicobacter pylori* infection, hemorrhage, herpes virus, infections (chronic), inflammation, influenza, irritability, laxative, malaria, measles, menorrhagia (heavy menstrual bleeding), menstrual cramps, menstrual problems, mental health, mental illness (neurosis), miscarriage prevention, muscle relaxant, nausea, nausea/vomiting (pregnancy), neurasthenia (nervous exhaustion), nutrition supplementation, obesity, osteoporosis prevention, pain, respiratory disease, respiratory disorders, rheumatism (chronic), sedative, skin inflammation, skin rash, snake bites, snoring, sore throat, stimulant, stomachache, thirst, urinary tract disorders, uterine tonic, varicose veins, viral infection (febrile stages), vomiting, weight loss, wounds.

DOSING
Adults (18 Years and Older)

- Based on scientific evidence, raspberry leaf tablets (2 × 1.2 g/day) have been used from 32 weeks' gestation until labor and appear safe for childbirth. Consult with a qualified health care professional, including a pharmacist, before making decisions about dosing.

- Traditionally, raspberry leaf tea (1 oz of the dried leaves infused in a pint of boiling water and gargled) has been used for sore mouth, sore throat, or wounds. Dehydrated raspberry fruit, crushed and made into a tea, has also been taken for viral infections. For diarrhea or dysentery, 1 cup of strong tea made of raspberry leaves or root at body temperature ingested every hour until symptoms decrease has been used.

Children (Younger than 18 Years)

- There is insufficient evidence to recommend a dose for raspberry, and use in children is not recommended.

SAFETY
Allergies

- Avoid in individuals with a known allergy to raspberry (*Rubus idaeus*). Occupational asthma (hay fever symptoms, wheezing, and shortness of breath) occurred in a 35-year-old after chewing gum coated with raspberry powder. Use cautiously in patients with asthma.

Side Effects and Warnings

- Side effects of raspberry appear to be minimal, although the lack of clinical trials investigating raspberry makes it difficult to assess its safety. Raspberries are likely safe when used in amounts normally found in food in healthy individuals.
- Most adverse effects appear to arise from contaminated fruits, which can cause gastrointestinal upset, vomiting, diarrhea, weight loss, paralyzing fatigue, and fever. Symptoms appear to come on suddenly, last up to a month, and resemble signs of severe stomach influenza. Cyclosporiasis associated with contaminated raspberries has been reported. Always thoroughly wash raspberries before ingestion.
- Contaminated raspberries may also carry Norwalk-like viruses (NLVs), estimated to be the most common causes of food-borne disease in the United States and accounting for two thirds of all food-related illnesses. NLVs are a principal cause of outbreaks of acute-onset vomiting and diarrhea in all age groups.
- Raspberry roots and leaves may be mild laxatives. They may also increase urine flow or have sedative effects. Methadone diluted with contaminated raspberry syrup may be a potential source of candidiasis in drug abusers.
- Raspberry leaf may induce labor. However, a clinical trial using raspberry leaf tablets reported no adverse effects.

Pregnancy and Breastfeeding

- Raspberry leaf may induce labor. However, a clinical trial using raspberry leaf tablets reported no adverse effects. More study is needed in this area before a recommendation can be made.

INTERACTIONS
Interactions with Drugs

- Raspberry may have antibiotic activity and interact additively with clarithromycin. Caution is advised. Consult with a qualified health care professional, including a pharmacist, before combining therapies.
- Raspberry contains antioxidants. Use with caution when taking other medications that also have antioxidant effects.
- Raspberry roots and leaves may be a mild diuretic and may increase the flow of urine. Patients taking medications that increase the flow of urine, such as bumetanide (Bumex) or chlorothiazide (Diuril), should use raspberry with caution. Raspberry may also have laxative properties, and care should be taken when it is used with other laxatives.
- Certain extracts of dried raspberry leaves may relax muscles. Use caution in patients taking medications that may have sedative, relaxing, or antispasmodic effects.
- Raspberries may contain salicylates. Caution is advised when medications are taken that contain high amounts of salicylates, such as aspirin.

Interactions with Herbs and Dietary Supplements

- Raspberry may have antibiotic activity. Raspberry also contains antioxidants. In theory, raspberry may interact additively with herbs and supplements that also have antibiotic or antioxidant effects. Caution is advised.
- Raspberry roots and leaves may be a mild diuretic and may increase the flow of urine. Patients taking herbs and supplements that increase the flow of urine should use raspberry with caution. Raspberry may also have laxative properties, and care should be taken with other herbs and supplement with these effects, such as psyllium.
- Certain extracts of dried raspberry leaves may relax muscles. Use caution in patients taking other herbs and supplements that may have sedative, relaxing, or antispasmodic effects.
- Raspberries may contain salicylates. Caution is advised when herbs and supplements are taken that contain high amounts of salicylates, such as willow bark.

For a complete list of references, please visit www.naturalstandard.com.

R

Red Clover
(Trifolium pratense)

RELATED TERMS

- Ackerklee (German), beebread, cow clover, genistein, isoflavone, isoflavone clover extract (ICE), meadow clover, phytoestrogen, Promensil, purple clover, Rimostil, Rotklee (German), trefle des pres (French), trefoil, *Trifolium pratense*, Trinovin, wild clover.

BACKGROUND

- Red clover is a legume that, similar to soy, contains phytoestrogens. Also known as isoflavones, phytoestrogens are plant-based chemicals that are similar to estrogen and may act in the body like estrogen or may actually block the effects of estrogen. Red clover was traditionally used to treat asthma, pertussis, cancer, and gout. In modern times, isoflavone extracts of red clover are most often used to treat menopausal symptoms, as an alternative hormone replacement therapy, for high cholesterol, or to prevent osteoporosis. However, at this time, there are no high-quality human studies supporting the use of red clover for any medical condition.

EVIDENCE

Uses Based on Scientific Evidence	Grade
Cardiovascular (Blood Flow) Red clover has been shown to improve the flow of blood through arteries and veins. However, there is limited study in this area, and more research is needed before a conclusion can be drawn.	C
Diabetes Red clover has been studied in patients with type 2 diabetes to determine potential benefits in diabetic complications such as high blood pressure and narrowing of the arteries and veins. However, the clinical evidence is insufficient to support this use.	C
High Cholesterol Red clover has not been clearly shown to have beneficial effects on blood cholesterol levels. However, study results are conflicting.	C
Hormone Replacement Therapy (HRT) Laboratory research suggests that red clover isoflavones have estrogen-like activity. However, there is no clear evidence that isoflavones share the possible benefits of estrogens (such as effects on bone density). In addition, hormone replacement therapy itself is a controversial topic, with recent research reporting that the potential harm may outweigh any benefits.	C
Menopausal Symptoms Red clover isoflavones are proposed to reduce symptoms of menopause (such as hot flashes) and	C

are popular for this use. Blood pressure and triglyceride levels may be lowered. However, most of the available human studies are poorly designed and short in duration (less than 12 weeks of treatment). The results of published studies are conflicting.

Osteoporosis It is not clear whether red clover isoflavones have beneficial effects on bone density. Most studies of isoflavones in this area have looked at soy, which contains different amounts of isoflavones, as well as other nonisoflavone ingredients.	C
Prostate Cancer Red clover isoflavones may have estrogen-like properties in the body and have been proposed as a possible therapy in prostate cancer and related hot flashes. Some isoflavones have also been shown in laboratory studies to have anticancer properties. However, there is a lack of clinical evidence to support this use.	C
Prostate Enlargement (Benign Prostatic Hypertrophy) There is only limited research examining red clover for benign prostatic hypertrophy.	C

Uses Based on Tradition or Theory
Acne, acquired immunodeficiency syndrome (AIDS), antibacterial, antioxidant, antispasm, appetite suppressant, arthritis, asthma, blood purification, breast cancer prevention, bronchitis, burns, cancer, cancer prevention, canker sores, cardiovascular disease, chronic skin diseases, cognitive function, cough, diuretic (increase urine flow), eczema, endocrine-responsive cancer, gout, increasing high-density lipoprotein (HDL) cholesterol levels, indigestion, mastalgia (breast pain), osteosarcoma, premenstrual syndrome, psoriasis, sexually transmitted diseases, skin ulcers/sores, sore eyes, tuberculosis, whooping cough (pertussis).

DOSING

Adults (18 Years and Older)

- Various doses of red clover isoflavones have been used to treat conditions. For instance, for benign prostatic hypertrophy, 40 mg of red clover isoflavones per day (Trinovin) has been studied. For breast cancer prevention, a red clover–derived isoflavone tablet containing 26 mg biochanin A, 16 mg formononetin, 1 mg genistein, and 0.5 mg of daidzein has been studied.
- For cardiovascular disease, 86 mg/day for 1 month has been studied. For diabetes, 50 mg/day and 86 mg/day of red clover isoflavones have been studied. For high

cholesterol levels, 28-86 mg of red clover isoflavones per day (Rimostil) or 80 mg of red clover isoflavones per day (Promensil) has been studied. For hormone replacement, 4-80 mg of red clover isoflavones per day (Promensil) has been studied.

- For menopausal symptoms 40 mg, 80 mg, or 160 mg of red clover isoflavones per day (Promensil) has been studied. Rimostil (57 mg of red clover) has also been used. For osteoporosis, 40 mg of red clover isoflavones per day (Promensil) has been studied.

Children (Younger than 18 Years)

- There is insufficient evidence to recommend use of red clover in children.

SAFETY
Allergies

- People with known allergies or reactions to products containing red clover or isoflavones should avoid taking red clover.

Side Effects and Warnings

- A small number of human studies using red clover extracts have all reported good tolerance without serious side effects after up to 1 year of treatment. In theory, based on the estrogen-like action of red clover seen in laboratory studies, side effects may include weight gain or breast tenderness, although these have not been reported clearly in humans. In theory, menstrual changes and increased uterine cell growth (endometrial hyperplasia) may also occur, although preliminary short-term studies (less than 6 months) have found no increases in uterine wall (endometrial) thickness with red clover. Red clover may affect hormonal levels of gonadotropin-releasing hormone (GrH), follicle stimulating hormone (FSH), and luteinizing hormone (LH), although early research has not found significant change in FSH or LH levels.
- In theory, red clover may increase the risk of bleeding. However, there are no reliable human reports of bleeding with red clover. Caution is advised in patients with bleeding disorders or taking drugs that may increase the risk of bleeding. Dosing adjustments may be necessary.
- Red clover has been studied for lowering blood sugar with inconclusive results. Caution is warranted until further research is available.

Pregnancy and Breastfeeding

- Red clover is not recommended during pregnancy and breastfeeding because of its estrogen-like activity. Red clover has been reported as a possible cause of infertility and abortion in grazing livestock.

INTERACTIONS
Interactions with Drugs

- Based on laboratory studies, red clover may interfere with the way the liver processes some drugs using an enzyme

called cytochrome P450 3A4. As a result, the levels of these drugs may be increased in the blood and may cause increased effects or potentially serious adverse reactions. Patients using any medications should check the package insert and speak with a health care professional or pharmacist about possible interactions.

- In theory, red clover may increase the risk of bleeding when taken with drugs that increase the risk of bleeding. Some examples include aspirin, anticoagulants ("blood thinners") such as warfarin (Coumadin) or heparin, antiplatelet drugs such as clopidogrel (Plavix), and nonsteroidal antiinflammatory drugs such as ibuprofen (Motrin, Advil) or naproxen (Naprosyn, Aleve).
- Red clover has been studied for lowering blood sugar with inconclusive results. Caution is warranted for people with diabetes or those taking other medications that may lower blood sugar until further research is available.
- In theory, red clover may interact with other estrogen-containing medications. Red clover contains phytoestrogens, which are plant-based chemicals that are similar to estrogen and that may act in the body like estrogen or may actually block the effects of estrogen.
- Because red clover contains estrogen-like chemicals, the effects of drugs with estrogen or estrogen-like properties may be altered, such as birth control pills or hormone replacement therapies like Premarin and Provera.

Interactions with Herbs and Dietary Supplements

- Based on laboratory studies, red clover may interfere with the way the liver processes some drugs using an enzyme called cytochrome P450 3A4. As a result, red clover may cause the levels of other herbs or supplements to be too high in the blood. It may also alter the effects that other herbs or supplements possibly have on the P450 system.
- In theory, red clover may increase the risk of bleeding when taken with herbs or supplements that increase the risk of bleeding. Multiple cases of bleeding have been reported with the use of *Ginkgo biloba*, fewer cases have been reported with garlic, and two cases have been reported with saw palmetto. Numerous other agents may theoretically increase the risk of bleeding, although this has not been proven in most cases.
- Because red clover contains estrogen-like chemicals, the effects of other agents believed to have estrogen-like properties may be altered.
- Red clover has been studied for lowering blood sugar with inconclusive results. Caution is warranted for people with diabetes or those taking other herbs or supplements that may lower blood sugar until further research is available.

For a complete list of references, please visit www.naturalstandard.com.

R

Red Yeast Rice
(*Monascus purpureus*)

RELATED TERMS

- Alkaloids, angkak, anka, ankaflavin, Asian traditional fermentation foodstuff, astaxanthin, beni-koju, ben-koji, Chinese red yeast rice (CRYR), citrinin, dehydromonacolin K, dietary red yeast, dihydromeyinolin, dihydromonacolin K, dihydromonacolin L, DSM1379, DSM1603, ergosterol, flavonoids, GABA, glycosides, HMG-CoA reductase inhibitors, hon-chi, hong qu, hongqu, hung-chu, hydroxymethylglutaryl coenzyme A reductase, KCCM11832, koji, linoleic acid, lovastatin, M9011, mevinolin, monacolin hydroxyacid, monacolin J, monacolin K, monacolin K (hydroxyl acid form), monacolin L, monacolin M, monacolin X, Monascaceae (yeast family), monascopyridine A, monascopyridine B, monascopyridine C, monascopyridine D, monascorubramine, monascorubrin, *Monascus*, *Monascus anka*, *Monascus purpureus* fermentate, *Monascus purpureus* HM105, *Monascus purpureus* NTU568, *Monascus purpureus* Went rice, *Monascus ruber*, oleic acid, orange anka pigment, palmitoleic acid, *Phaffia rhodozyma*, red fermented rice, red koji, red leaven, red mould rice, red rice, red rice yeast, red yeast, red yeast rice extract (RYRE), rice, RICE products, rubropunctamine, rubropunctatin, RYR, saponins, statins, stearic acid, xuezhikang, Xue Zhi Kang, yellow anka pigment, zhitai, Zhi Tai.

BACKGROUND

- Red yeast rice is the product of the yeast *Monascus purpureus* grown on rice and is served as a dietary staple in some Asian countries. It contains several compounds collectively known as monacolins, substances known to inhibit cholesterol synthesis. One of these, "monacolin K," is a potent inhibitor of 3-hydroxy-3-methylglutaryl coenzyme A (HMG-CoA) reductase and is also known as mevinolin or lovastatin (Mevacor, a drug produced by Merck & Co., Inc).
- Red yeast rice extract has been sold as a natural cholesterol-lowering agent in over-the-counter supplements, such as Cholestin (Pharmanex, Inc). However, there has been legal and industrial dispute as to whether red yeast rice is a drug or a dietary supplement, involving the manufacturer, the U.S. Food and Drug Administration (FDA), and the pharmaceutical industry (particularly producers of HMG-CoA reductase inhibitor prescription drugs or "statins").
- The use of red yeast rice in China was first documented in the Tang Dynasty in 800 A.D. A detailed description of its manufacture is found in the ancient Chinese pharmacopoeia, Ben Cao Gang Mu-Dan Shi Bu Yi, published during the Ming Dynasty (1368-1644). In this text, red yeast rice is proposed to be a mild aid for gastric problems (indigestion, diarrhea), blood circulation, and spleen and stomach health. Red yeast rice in a dried, powdered form is called Zhi Tai. When extracted with alcohol, it is called Xue Zhi Kang.

EVIDENCE

Uses Based on Scientific Evidence	Grade
High Cholesterol Since the 1970s, human studies have reported that red yeast lowers blood levels of total cholesterol, low-density lipoprotein (LDL, "bad cholesterol"), and triglyceride levels. Other products containing red yeast rice extract can still be purchased, mostly over the Internet. However, these products may not be standardized, and effects are not predictable. For lowering cholesterol levels, there is better evidence for using prescription drugs such as lovastatin.	A
Coronary Heart Disease Preliminary evidence shows that taking *Monascus purpureus* by mouth may result in cardiovascular benefits and may improve blood flow.	C
Diabetes Preliminary human evidence suggests the potential for benefits in patients with diabetes. Additional study is needed before a firm recommendation can be made.	C

Uses Based on Tradition or Theory
Acetaminophen toxicity, anthrax, antiinflammatory, antimicrobial, antioxidant, blood circulation problems, bruised muscles, bruises, cancer, colic in children, cuts, diarrhea, digestion, dysentery (bloody diarrhea), exercise performance enhancement, food additive (coloring), food preservative, hangover, high blood pressure, human immunodeficiency virus (HIV) (associated hyperlipidemia), immunosuppression, indigestion, liver disorders, metabolic disorders, obesity, ovarian cancer, postpartum problems, spleen problems, stomach problems, weight loss, wounds.

DOSING

Adults (18 Years and Older)

- A total of 1,200 mg of concentrated red yeast rice powder capsules has been taken two times daily by mouth with food.
- The average consumption of naturally occurring red yeast rice in Asia has been reported as 14-55 g daily.

Children (Younger than 18 Years)

- There is insufficient evidence to recommend red yeast rice for children.

SAFETY

Allergies

- There is one report of anaphylaxis (a severe allergic reaction) in a butcher who touched meat containing red yeast rice.

Side Effects and Warnings

- There is limited evidence on the side effects of red yeast rice. Mild headache and abdominal discomfort can occur. Side effects may be similar to those for the prescription drug lovastatin (Mevacor). Heartburn, gas, bloating, muscle pain or damage, dizziness, asthma, and kidney problems are possible. People with liver disease should not use red yeast products.
- In theory, red yeast rice may increase the risk of bleeding. Caution is advised in patients with bleeding disorders or taking drugs that may increase the risk of bleeding. Dosing adjustments may be necessary. A metabolite of *Monascus* called mycotoxin citrinin may be harmful.

Pregnancy and Breastfeeding

- Prescription drugs with similar chemicals as red yeast rice cannot be used during pregnancy. Therefore, it is recommended that pregnant or breastfeeding women not take red yeast rice.

INTERACTIONS

Interactions with Drugs

- There are not many studies of the interactions of red yeast rice extract with drugs. However, because red yeast rice extract contains the same chemicals as the prescription drug lovastatin, the interactions may be the same. Fibrate drugs or other cholesterol-lowering medications may cause additive effects or side effects when taken with red yeast rice. Alcohol and other drugs that may be toxic to the liver should be avoided with red yeast rice extract. Taking cyclosporine, ranitidine (Zantac), and certain antibiotics with red yeast rice extract may increase the risk of muscle breakdown or kidney damage.
- Certain drugs may interfere with the way the body processes red yeast using the liver's cytochrome P450 enzyme system. Inhibitors of cytochrome P450 may increase the chance of muscle and kidney damage if taken with red yeast rice.
- In theory, red yeast rice may increase the risk of bleeding when taken with drugs that increase the risk of bleeding. Some examples include aspirin, anticoagulants ("blood thinners") such as warfarin (Coumadin) or heparin, antiplatelet drugs such as clopidogrel (Plavix), and nonsteroidal antiinflammatory drugs such as ibuprofen (Motrin, Advil) or naproxen (Naprosyn, Aleve).
- Red yeast rice may produce gamma-aminobutyric acid (GABA) and therefore can have additive effects when taken with drugs that affect GABA such as neurontin (Gabapentin).
- Red yeast rice may also interact with digoxin, niacin, thyroid medications, and blood pressure–lowering medications. Caution is advised.
- Red yeast rice may alter blood sugar levels; patients taking drugs for diabetes by mouth or using insulin or blood sugar–lowering medications should consult with a qualified health care professional, including a pharmacist. Dosing adjustments may be necessary.

Interactions with Herbs and Dietary Supplements

- Red yeast rice may interact with products that cause liver damage or are broken down in the liver. Grapefruit juice may increase blood levels of red yeast rice. Milk thistle, St. John's wort, niacin, and vitamin A may interact with red yeast rice extract. Coenzyme Q10 levels may be lowered by red yeast rice extract. Cholesterol-lowering herbs and supplements such as guggul or fish oils may have increased effects when taken with red yeast rice. Although not well studied, red yeast rice may also interact with astaxanthin and zinc. Caution is advised.
- Certain herbs and supplements may interfere with the way the body processes red yeast rice using the liver's cytochrome P450 enzyme system. Inhibitors of cytochrome P450 may increase the chance of muscle and kidney damage if taken with red yeast rice.
- In theory, red yeast rice may increase the risk of bleeding when taken with herbs and supplements that are believed to increase the risk of bleeding. Multiple cases of bleeding have been reported with the use of *Ginkgo biloba*, and fewer cases have been reported with garlic and saw palmetto. Numerous other agents may theoretically increase the risk of bleeding, although this has not been proven in most cases.
- Red yeast rice may also interact with digitalis (foxglove) or herbs and supplements that affect the thyroid or blood pressure. It may also have antiinflammatory effects and should be used cautiously with other herbs or supplements that may have antiinflammatory effects.
- Red yeast rice may alter blood sugar levels, and patients with diabetes or those taking herbs and supplement to control blood sugar should use red yeast rice with caution.

For a complete list of references, please visit www.naturalstandard.com.

R

Rehmannia
(Rehmannia glutinosa)

RELATED TERMS

- Chinese foxglove, *Digitalis glutinosa*, di huang, dihuang, gan dihuang (dried rehmannia), Gesneriaceae (family), glutinous rehmannia, Gosha-jinki-gan, Hachimijio-gan, huaiqing dihuang, juku-jio (Chinese or Japanese steamed or processed root), Kan-jio (Korean or Japanese dried root), Liu Wei rehmannia oral liquid, *Rehmannia chinensis*, *Rehmannia glutinosa* Liboschitz, *Rehmannia glutinosa* Libosch. forma hueichingenis Hsiao (Kaikei-jio in Japanese), *Rehmannia glutinosa* Libosch. var. *purpurea* Makino, *Rehmannia glutinosa* steamed root (RGAE), Rehmannia polysaccharide (PRP), Rehmanniae radix, Rhizoma rehmanniae, saengjih-wang (Korean), Scrophulariaceae (family), sheng di huang (raw rehmannia), sho-jio (fresh root), shu di huang (cooked or cured rehmannia), sook-ji-whang, to-byun, (Akaya-jio in Japanese), xian dihuang (fresh rehmannia).

BACKGROUND

- Rehmannia has been used extensively in traditional Chinese medicine (TCM). Although thorough clinical trials are lacking, rehmannia has been used to treat rheumatoid arthritis, asthma, urticaria (hives), and chronic nephritis (kidney inflammation) in Chinese studies. Rehmannia may also be used to prevent the suppressive effects of corticosteroid (steroid) drugs.

- Rehmannia looks promising in treating aplastic anemia, mitigating side effects of chemotherapeutic agents and human immunodeficiency virus (HIV) medications, curing obdurate eczema (dry skin), relieving pain from lung or bone cancer or disk protrusion, and helping ameliorate lupus nephritis (kidney inflammation) and type 2 diabetes with hyperlipidemia (high cholesterol levels). However, presently, there are no high-quality, large randomized controlled trials supporting the efficacy of rehmannia for any of these indications.

- Rehmannia is in the *Pharmacopoeia of the People's Republic of China*. However, it is not on the United Kingdom's General Sale List and is not covered by a Commission E monograph in Germany. The U.S. Food and Drug Administration (FDA) has not granted "generalized recognized as safe" (GRAS) status to rehmannia; it is available in the United States as a dietary supplement under the Dietary Supplement Health and Education Act of 1994.

EVIDENCE

Uses Based on Scientific Evidence	Grade
Aplastic Anemia (Adjuvant) Rehmannia is frequently recommended to mitigate the duration and severity of aplastic anemia. Although preliminary results appear promising, additional study is needed to draw a firm recommendation.	C
Hypopituitarism (Sheehan's Syndrome) *Rehmannia glutinosa* has been used in the treatment of Sheehan's syndrome. However, the magnitude of therapeutic effects of rehmannia on Sheehan's syndrome remains unclear. More research is necessary in this area.	C

Uses Based on Tradition or Theory

Adrenal tonic, allergies, amenorrhea (absence of menstruation), anemia, antifungal, antiinflammatory, antipyretic (fever reducer), asthma, autoimmune diseases, blood clotting disorders, cancer pain (bone cancer), cataracts, central nervous system disorders, chemotherapy adverse effects, cognitive processing, coronary heart disease (postmenopausal symptoms), dementia, diabetes mellitus type 2, diuretic, dizziness, dysmenorrhea (painful menstruation), eczema (dry skin), fatigue, fever, gastric adenoma (benign tumor), hair tonic (premature graying), hearing damage (gentamicin-induced), hematopoiesis (stimulation of blood cell production), hematuria (blood in the urine), human immunodeficiency virus (medication side effects), hyperlipidemia (high cholesterol levels), hypertension (high blood pressure), hypotension (low blood pressure), hypoxia (very low oxygen levels, nocturnal), immunosuppression, laxative, liver protection, lumbar disk herniation (intervertebral disk protrusion), lung cancer, lupus nephritis, measles, menorrhagia (heavy menstrual bleeding), metrorrhagia (irregular uterine bleeding), nephritis (inflamed kidney, chronic), nosebleeds, rheumatoid arthritis, sarcomas (cancer of the bone, cartilage, fat, muscle, blood vessels, or other connective or supportive tissue), skin disorders, thirst, tinnitus (ringing in the ears), tonic, tranquilizer, urticaria (hives), vasoregulator, vasorelaxant, vertigo.

DOSING

Adults (18 Years and Older)

- There is insufficient evidence to recommend a dose for rehmannia. Herbal decoctions used in clinical trials have contained 12-30 g of rehmannia. For Sheehan's syndrome, 90 g of cleaned and finely chopped *Rehmannia glutinosa* root added to 900 mL of water and boiled down to 200 mL has been used in 3-day courses with an intermission of 3, 6, and 14 days. After a 1-month cessation, the second round of treatment commenced. Another dosing regimen used was 45-50 g of *Rehmannia glutinosa* daily in 5-day courses with an intermission of 5 days each time for 2-5 months.

Children (Younger than 18 Years)

- There is insufficient evidence to recommend a dose for rehmannia in children.

SAFETY

Allergies

- Avoid in individuals with a known allergy or hypersensitivity to rehmannia.

Side Effects and Warnings

- Rehmannia has been generally well tolerated in available research studies. It has been well tolerated for 20 days to 1.2 years in human trials. Rehmannia may cause palpitations, edema (swelling), gastrointestinal upset, infertility, dizziness, and lack of energy. Use cautiously in patients with diabetes, as rehmannia may lower blood sugar or additively

effect hypoglycemic (low blood sugar) agents. Avoid in patients with diarrhea and lack of appetite because of possible irritation of the gastrointestinal tract by rehmannia.
- Liu Wei Di Huang T'ang (decoction of rehmannia with six components) may lower blood pressure.
- Use cautiously in children younger than 2 years of age and in women who may be pregnant or breastfeeding.

Pregnancy and Breastfeeding

- Rehmannia is not recommended in pregnant or breastfeeding women because of a lack of available scientific evidence.

INTERACTIONS
Interactions with Drugs

- The concomitant use of aminoglycosides and rehmannia may decrease toxicity associated with aminoglycoside therapy.
- Man-Shen-Ling is a combination product that contains rehmannia, which may increase the risk of bleeding when taken with drugs that increase the risk of bleeding. Some examples include aspirin, anticoagulants ("blood thinners") such as warfarin (Coumadin) or heparin, antiplatelet drugs such as clopidogrel (Plavix), and nonsteroidal antiinflammatory drugs (NSAIDs) such as ibuprofen (Motrin, Advil) or naproxen (Naprosyn, Aleve).
- Rehmannia may interact with antihistamines.
- Although not well studied in humans, Liu Wei Di Huang T'ang (decoction of rehmannia with six components) may lower blood pressure. Caution is advised in patients with high blood pressure or taking any antihypertensive (blood pressure–lowering) agents.
- Rehmannia and corticosteroids (steroids) may result in a synergistic effect and the possibility of reduced side effects.
- Theoretically, rehmannia may decrease toxicity associated with chemotherapy. Shi-Quan-Da-Bu-Tang (SQT), which contains *Rehmannia glutinosa, Paeonia lactiflora, Liqusticum wallichii, Angelica sinensis, Glycyrrhiza uralensis, Poria cocos, Atractylodes macrocephala, Panax ginseng, Astragalus membranaceus,* and *Cinnamomum cassia,* was found to potentiate therapeutic activity of chemotherapy, radiotherapy, and prevent or minimize associated adverse events.
- Rehmannia may have an additive effect with diuretics.

- Rehmannia may interact additively with drugs that alter blood sugar because it can cause hypoglycemia (low blood sugar). Caution is advised in patients with diabetes or hypoglycemia and in those taking drugs that affect blood sugar. Serum glucose levels may need to be monitored by a health care provider, and medication adjustments may be necessary.
- The concomitant use of cholesterol-lowering drugs with rehmannia may result in additive effects.
- Rehmannia may have an additive effect with thyroid drugs. In a study on Sheehan's syndrome, *Rehmannia glutinosa* may have improved clinical symptoms and stimulated the hypothalamic–pituitary system.

Interactions with Herbs and Dietary Supplements

- Rehmannia may increase the risk of bleeding when taken with herbs and supplements that are believed to increase the risk of bleeding. Multiple cases of bleeding have been reported with the use of *Ginkgo biloba,* and fewer cases have been reported with garlic and saw palmetto. Numerous other agents may theoretically increase the risk of bleeding, although this has not been proven in most cases.
- Combination use of rehmannia with herbs or supplements that lower blood pressure may result in additive effects.
- Rehmannia and corticosteroids (steroids) may result in a synergistic effect, and there is a possibility of reduced side effects. Caution is advised in patients taking herbs with steroid-like effects.
- Rehmannia may have an additive effect with diuretics, such as astragalus.
- Rehmannia may interact additively with herbs that affect blood sugar because it may cause hypoglycemia (low blood sugar). Seishin-kanro-to, composed of rehmannia radix, may lower blood sugar levels. Caution is advised in patients with diabetes or hypoglycemia and in those taking herbs or supplements that affect blood sugar. Serum glucose levels may need to be monitored by a qualified health care provider, and medication adjustments may be necessary.
- The concomitant use of cholesterol-lowering herbs, such as red yeast rice, with rehmannia may result in additive effects.
- Rehmannia may have an additive effect with thyroid herbs.

For a complete list of references, please visit www.naturalstandard.com.

R

Reishi
(Ganoderma lucidum)

RELATED TERMS

- Chi zhi, Enhanvol, fungus, fu zhen herb, *Ganoderma tsugae* extract, Ganopoly, he ling zhi, holy mushroom, hong ling zhi, ling chi, ling chih, ling zhi (Chinese), ling zhi-8, Linzhi extract, Mannentake, mushroom, mushroom of immortality, mushroom of spiritual potency, polysaccharides peptide, rei-shi, shiitake, spirit plant, Sunrecome, triterpene, varnished polypore, young ji, zi zhi.

BACKGROUND

- Reishi mushroom (*Ganoderma lucidum*), also known as *ling zhi* in China, grows wild on decaying logs and tree stumps. Reishi occurs in six different colors, but the red variety is most commonly used and commercially cultivated in East Asia and North America.
- The reishi mushroom is a derivative of the Far East, with its usage dating back to ancient China. Royalty would utilize this precious mushroom in the hopes of obtaining immortality and promoting calmness and thought. Chinese medicine now includes therapy with reishi for fatigue, asthma, insomnia, and cough.
- *Ganoderma lucidum* has been used in traditional Chinese medicine for more than 4,000 years to treat liver disorders, high blood pressure, arthritis, and other ailments. In modern times, the available data from human trials together with evidence from animal studies suggest that *Ganoderma lucidum* may have some positive benefits for cancer and liver disease patients. However, the number and quality of trials is very limited. Other promising uses for which there is still inconclusive evidence include diabetes, heart disease, pain, *Russula subnigricans* poisoning (RSP), and proteinuria (protein in the urine). Reishi is also believed to reduce cholesterol levels and has an anticoagulant (blood-thinning) effect, which may make it useful in coronary heart disease prevention.
- Some experts believe that *Ganoderma lucidum* promotes longevity and maintains vitality of the human body. Reishi's major benefit appears to be its immunomodulating action, improvement of liver function, and improvement and restoration of the normal functions of the respiratory system. Antioxidant effects, which contribute to the overall well-being of patients, have been proposed. In the sixteenth century pharmacopeia *Ben Cao Gang Mu*, reishi was described as being able to affect the life energy, or qi, of the heart, repair the chest area, increase intellectual capacity, and banish forgetfulness.
- Reishi is currently regulated in the United States as a dietary supplement. It is also included in the 2000 *Pharmacopoeia of the People's Republic of China* as an agent approved for the treatment of dizziness, insomnia, palpitations, shortness of breath, cough, and asthma. At this time, high-quality clinical trials supporting the use of reishi mushroom are lacking. More proven therapies are recommended at this time.

EVIDENCE

Uses Based on Scientific Evidence	Grade
Arthritis A combination of reishi mushroom and San Miao San (a mixture of several Chinese herbs) may help reduce the pain of rheumatoid arthritis. These herbs did not reduce swelling. More research with reishi mushroom alone is needed.	C
Cancer Reishi has been shown to have antineoplastic and immunomodulatory effects in animal studies. One clinical trial and two case reports exist on patients with advanced cancer using Ganopoly, a *Ganoderma lucidum* polysaccharide extract. Results show improved quality of life and enhanced immune responses, which are typically reduced or damaged in cancer patients receiving chemotherapy and/or radiation therapy. It is important to note that these data were published by the same group of authors who are affiliated with the manufacturer of Ganopoly. Well-designed long-term studies are needed to confirm these results and potential side effects.	C
Chronic Hepatitis B Based on positive laboratory evidence, a clinical trial using Ganopoly or placebo was conducted in chronic hepatitis B patients. Ganopoly treatment decreased the level of hepatitis B virus (HBV) DNA. This virus is notoriously hard to clear from the body, and recurrence after treatment is common. Again, the affiliation of authors to the manufacturer of the drug is noteworthy. Independent evidence is warranted.	C
Coronary Heart Disease (CHD) A clinical trial was conducted to evaluate the effect of Ganopoly on coronary heart disease in humans. Ganopoly treatment improved the major symptoms (e.g., angina [chest pain], palpitations, and shortness of breath), decreased abnormal electrocardiographic (ECG) appearance, and decreased blood pressure and cholesterol levels in these patients. Long-term study is needed to evaluate the efficacy and safety of Ganopoly before it may be recommended for CHD. The authors are closely related to the manufacturer of Ganopoly.	C
Diabetes Mellitus Type 2 Based on animal studies that demonstrated the blood sugar and lipid-lowering activities of *Ganoderma lucidum* (ling zhi, reishi mushroom), a clinical	C

Uses Based on Scientific Evidence	Grade
study was conducted to evaluate the effect of Ganopoly versus placebo in diabetic patients. The treatment of Ganopoly slightly decreased the levels of plasma glucose and glycosylated hemoglobin and improved other markers for diabetes. Long-term studies with larger sample size are needed to evaluate the efficacy and safety of Ganopoly in treating diabetic patients. The authors are closely related to the manufacturer of Ganopoly.	
High Blood Pressure Ancient Chinese monks utilized the reishi mushroom to calm their minds for meditation. Theory would lead one to believe that the physiological effects of decreasing blood pressure may have lead to the calming effect precipitated by the ingested reishi. Preliminary data suggest that reishi may exert a blood pressure–lowering effect; however, the currently available evidence in this area is weak. Future studies are warranted to validate the results of these small studies and to prove the clinical usefulness of reishi as a possible treatment for high blood pressure.	C
Pain (Postherpetic) Reishi extract was effective in decreasing postherpetic pain (pain after herpes lesions heal) in one case series. Further research is needed to confirm these results.	C
Poisoning (*Russula subnigricans*) *Ganoderma lucidum* has shown a beneficial effect in treating RSP in one small trial. Further well-designed clinical trials are needed to confirm these results.	C
Proteinuria (Protein in the Urine) One clinical trial was conducted to evaluate the effect of *Ganoderma lucidum* in treating kidney disorder patients with persistent proteinuria resistant to steroids with or without immunosuppressants. *Ganoderma lucidum* treatment decreased proteinuria in the small number of patients in this study. This trial provides good preliminary data, but long-term studies with a larger amount of patients are needed to evaluate the effects of *Ganoderma lucidum* on proteinuria.	C

Uses Based on Tradition or Theory

Adaptogen, altitude sickness (treatment or prevention), antiaging, anticonvulsive, antiinflammatory, antioxidant, antiplatelet effects, antiviral, asthma, blood cleanser, bronchitis, cardiovascular disease, cough, Epstein-Barr virus, fatigue, herpes simplex virus infection, high cholesterol levels, high triglyceride levels, human immunodeficiency virus (HIV), immune system enhancement, insomnia, leukopenia, liver disorders, muscular dystrophy, myasthenia gravis, nephritis, neurasthenia (nerve weakness, nervous exhaustion), neuromuscular disorders, poisoning (general), tension, ulcers.

DOSING
Adults (18 Years and Older)

- Approximately 2-6 g daily of reishi as raw fungus or an equivalent dosage of concentrated extract has been taken with meals. In clinical trials studying cancer, chronic hepatitis B, coronary heart disease, or diabetes, doses of 600-1,800 mg have been taken three times daily. For high blood pressure, Linzhi extract (reishi) has been used in doses of 55 mg daily for 4 weeks. For pain management in herpes zoster, 36-72 g of dry weight per day for up to 10 days has been studied. Other doses used are 500-1,125 mg daily for the treatment of proteinuria (excess protein in the urine) or 100 g of reishi boiled in 600 mL water per dose for poisoning.

Children (Younger than 18 Years)

- Insufficient evidence is available to recommend the use of reishi mushroom in children.

SAFETY
Allergies

- Avoid in individuals with a known allergy or hypersensitivity to any constituents of *Ganoderma lucidum* or any member of its family. Skin reactivity to spore and whole body extracts have been reported. Hypersensitivity reactions to reishi and its derivatives may occur, including dry mouth, nosebleed, and nasal and throat dryness.

Side Effects and Warnings

- Acute and long-term studies have found *Ganoderma lucidum* to be generally well tolerated in recommended doses for up to 16 months. The most common adverse events reported are skin rash, dizziness, and headache.
- Use cautiously in patients who are taking diabetes or hypoglycemic drugs because reishi may lower blood sugar levels.
- Low blood pressure may occur with the utilization of reishi and its derivatives.
- Because of the blood thinning capabilities of reishi, gastric bleeding could result from its use. Reishi may prolong bleeding time, and caution is advised in those patients with bleeding disorders (ulcers, hemophilia) or taking anticoagulants. Diarrhea and bloody stools may occur with supplemental doses. Mild gastrointestinal discomfort including nausea and diarrhea has been found in a small percentage of cancer patients taking *Ganoderma lucidum* as Ganopoly.
- Severe liver inflammation that led to death has been linked to reishi mushroom powder.

Pregnancy and Breastfeeding

- Reishi mushroom is not recommended in pregnant or breastfeeding women because of a lack of sufficient data.

INTERACTIONS
Interactions with Drugs

- Reports have suggested that reishi may antagonize the effects of amphetamines.
- Reishi therapy may increase or decrease the activity of certain antibiotics such as ampicillin, cefazolin, oxytetracycline, and chloramphenicol.
- A study conducted on the antiherpetic activity of the acidic protein-bound polysaccharide (APBP) that was isolated from capophores of *Ganoderma lucidum* had synergistic

R

effects when administered with the prescription antiviral drug acyclovir.

- Reishi and anticoagulants or nonsteroidal antiinflammatory drugs (NSAIDs) may theoretically lead to additive effects or an increased risk of bleeding. Reishi may cause bleeding because of prolongation of prothrombin time. *Ganoderma lucidum* inhibits platelet aggregation.
- *Ganoderma lucidum* may cause additive blood pressure–lowering effects.
- Based on animal study, *Ganoderma lucidum* may cause an additive blood sugar–lowering effect.
- Reishi with 3-hydroxy-3-methylglutaryl coenzyme A (HMG-CoA) reductase inhibitor drugs ("statins") may result in additive effects.
- Theoretically, the use of reishi and protease inhibitors may result in additive effects.
- The risk of liver damage may increase when reishi mushroom powder is taken with drugs that are known to damage the liver.

Interactions with Herbs and Dietary Supplements

- Reishi and anticoagulant herbs and supplements may theoretically lead to additive effects, increasing bleeding risk.
- *Ganoderma lucidum* may cause additive blood pressure–lowering effects with herbs and supplements such as fish oil, coenzyme Q10, and ginseng.
- *Ganoderma lucidum* may cause additive blood sugar–lowering effects with herbs and supplements such as beta-glucan, bitter melon, ginseng, gymnema, and chromium.
- Theoretically, reishi may result in additive effects when taken with herbs and supplements like guggul, red yeast rice, or garlic.
- The risk of liver damage may increase when reishi mushroom powder is taken with herbs or supplements that are known to damage the liver.

For a complete list of references, please visit www.naturalstandard.com.

Resveratrol

$(C_{14}H_{12}O_3)$

RELATED TERMS

- Ban-ji-ryun, ban-zhi-lian, banjiryun, *Belamcanda chinensis*, bergenin, betulin, betulinic acid, cis-piceid, cis-resveratrol (cis-3,4′,5-trihydroxystilbene), *Cissus quadrangularis, Elephantorrhiza goetzei*, epsilon-viniferin (a dimer of resveratrol), *Erythrophleum lasianthum* (Caesalpinioideae, Leguminosae), flavonoid, French paradox, gnetin H (a resveratrol analog), *Gnetum montanum*, grape seed proanthocyanidin extract (GSPE), grape skin, heyneanol A (a resveratrol tetramer), hydroxystilbene, ko-jo-kon, Liliaceae, lyophilized grape powder (LGP), mangiferonic acid, nonflavonoid polyphenol, *Paeonia lactiflora* Pall. (Paeoniaceae), pallidol, parthenocissine A, phenolic antioxidant, phytoalexin, phytoantitoxin, phytoestrogens, phytohormones, phytostilbene, piceatannol, *Polygonum cuspidatum*, polyphenol, prenylflavanone, protykin, quadrangularin, red wine, red wine polyphenol, ResV, Resverol, resveratrol 3-O-beta-D-glucopyranoside, *Reynoutria japonica, Scutellaria barbata* D. Don (Lamiaceae), *Sophora moorcroftiana* Benth., *Sophora tomentosa* L., stilbene, stilbene derivative resveratrol, stilbene polyphenol, stilbenoid, suffruticosol B (a resveratrol analog), trans-3,4′,5-trihydroxystilbene, trans-piceid, trans-resveratrol, transhydroxystilbene, tyrphostin, vatdiospyroidol (a resveratrol tetramer), *Vatica pauciflora, Vatica rassak* (Dipterocarpaceae), vaticanol C (a resveratrol tetramer), vaticaphenol A, *Veratrum taliense*, viniferin (a resveratrol analog), *Vitis vinifera* L.

BACKGROUND

- Resveratrol is found in over 70 plant species, including nuts, grapes, pine trees, certain vines, and red wine. Some experts believe that resveratrol may be a factor in the French paradox that coronary heart disease mortality in France is lower than other similar industrialized countries because of the frequent consumption of red wine.
- Resveratrol has been shown in animal and laboratory studies to exhibit antioxidant, anticancer, antiproliferative, antifungal, antiviral, and antibacterial effects.
- At this time, there is a lack of clinical evidence supporting the efficacy of resveratrol for any indication. However, there are several observational studies that correlate the consumption of wine with a decrease in cancer and/or cardiovascular disease risk. There are multiple possible contributing factors to these conditions, and studies of resveratrol are difficult to design and implement. Too much alcohol intake may carry risks that potentially offset the benefits of red wine. Further research is needed before a firm recommendation can be made.

EVIDENCE

Uses Based on Scientific Evidence	Grade
Cancer The effects of resveratrol have not been thoroughly assessed from trials using foods, wine, or combination products containing resveratrol and other substances. Well-designed clinical trials of resveratrol alone are needed before a recommendation can be made in regard to cancer prevention and/or treatment.	C
Cardiovascular Disease The effects of resveratrol cannot be adequately assessed from trials using foods, wine, or combination products containing resveratrol and other substances. Well-designed clinical trials of resveratrol alone are warranted.	C
Longevity/Antiaging Resveratrol has been included in herbal products that are marketed to increase lifespan and prevent aging. Limited evidence shows a possible benefit for this use.	C

Uses Based on Tradition or Theory

Age-related macular degeneration, allergy, Alzheimer's disease, amyloidosis, amyotrophic lateral sclerosis, antifungal, antiinflammatory, antimicrobial, antioxidant, antiplatelet, antitumor agent, antiviral, atherosclerosis, bone density, cancer prevention, cerebral ischemia, chemoprotectant, chronic obstructive pulmonary disease (COPD), cognitive disorders, cosmetic, degenerative diseases, diabetic neuropathy, diabetic wound healing, edema, Epstein-Barr virus, hearing loss, *Helicobacter pylori* infection, herpes simplex virus types 1 and 2, human immunodeficiency virus, hormonal imbalances, hypercholesterolemia, immunomodulator, influenza, ischemia-reperfusion injury prevention, leukemia, medulloblastoma, menopausal symptoms, multiple sclerosis, nephrotoxicity, neuroblastoma, neuropathy, neuroprotection, pain, pancreatitis, Parkinson's disease, premature aging, renal impairment (protection), rheumatoid arthritis, seizure, skin disorders, spinal cord injury, stroke, vascular diseases, vasorelaxant, wound healing.

DOSING

Adults (18 Years and Older)

- There is insufficient evidence to recommend a dose of resveratrol in adults.

Children (Younger than 18 Years)

- There is insufficient evidence to recommend a dose of resveratrol in adults.

SAFETY

Allergies

- Avoid in individuals with a known allergy or hypersensitivity to resveratrol, grapes, red wine, or red wine polyphenols.
- Allergic contact dermatitis from pentylene glycol in an emollient cream, with possible cosensitization to resveratrol, has been reported.

Side Effects and Warnings

- Limited data in humans reveal that resveratrol seems quite safe. It is usually found as a component in food and beverages.

R

613

- There is limited long-term information regarding adverse effects associated with resveratrol supplements alone. The American Heart Association recommends limited consumption. Consumption of large quantities of red wine as a source of resveratrol is considered unsafe because of the alcohol content. Consuming large amounts of alcohol increases the risk of alcoholism, high blood pressure, obesity, stroke, breast cancer, suicide, and accidents. Drinking large quantities of red wine may also have adverse effects on the liver. Preliminary evidence suggests that resveratrol may weakly inhibit the way that the liver breaks down certain drugs, herbs, and supplements (inhibits multiple cytochrome P450 enzymes). Patients with a history of alcoholism should avoid red wine consumption.
- Use cautiously in patients taking anticoagulant/antiplatelet (blood-thinning) agents because of the potential for increased risk of bleeding.
- Patients taking blood pressure medications should use caution when taking large amounts of resveratrol.

Pregnancy and Breastfeeding

- According to the American College of Obstetricians and Gynecologists, red wine consumption is not recommended in pregnant women, as alcohol may affect the fetus and can lead to life-threatening damage.

INTERACTIONS
Interactions with Drugs

- Based on preliminary laboratory evidence, resveratrol may have additive effects when taken with antifungals, such as nystatin. There may be a protective effect of trans-resveratrol on side effects of some antibiotics, such as gentamicin-induced kidney toxicity.
- Laboratory evidence suggests that resveratrol has antiaggregating and antithrombin activity and may have additive effects when taken with other drugs with the same actions. Use of resveratrol with antiplatelet drugs like clodipogrel (Plavix), dipyridamole (Persantine), nonsteroidal antiinflammatory drugs (NSAIDs), and aspirin or anticoagulant drugs like warfarin (Coumadin) could cause increased risk of bleeding.
- Resveratrol may increase the effects of some antivirals, including antiretroviral human immunodeficiency virus (HIV) medications.
- Based on laboratory and animal evidence, the use of resveratrol with antihypertensive or cardiovascular drugs may result in additive effects.
- Based on laboratory evidence, resveratrol may sensitize or enhance the efficacy of anticancer drugs, such as paclitaxel or actinomycin D.
- Cholesterol levels have been lowered in rats, although the clinical significance is unknown in humans. In theory, resveratrol could increase the effects of cholesterol-lowering drugs such as 3-hydroxy-3-methylglutaryl coenzyme A (HMG-CoA) reductase inhibitors ("statins") or bile acid–sequestering agents (cholestyramine).
- Based on preliminary data, resveratrol may enhance the immune suppression caused by cyclosporin A.
- Drinking large quantities of red wine, which contains resveratrol, may have adverse effects on the liver. Preliminary evidence suggests that resveratrol may weakly inhibit the way that the liver breaks down certain drugs, herbs, and supplements (inhibits multiple cytochrome P450 enzymes).
- Based on resveratrol's chemical structure, which is similar to that of the synthetic estrogen agonist diethylstilbestrol, resveratrol may function as an estrogen agonist and exhibit an additive effect when taken in conjunction with estradiol. However, limited laboratory evidence has shown resveratrol acting as an estrogen antagonist. Resveratrol may have the potential to act as both an estrogen agonist or antagonist depending on a variety of factors.
- Based on preliminary evidence, resveratrol may interact with monoamine oxidase inhibitors (MAOIs) such as phenelzine (Nardil) and tranylcypromine (Parnate). This effect has not been confirmed in humans.
- Resveratrol may also interact with antiinflammatory agents, vasorelaxants, neurological agents, immune-enhancing agents, or agents that alter blood sugar levels.

Interactions with Herbs and Dietary Supplements

- Based on preliminary laboratory evidence resveratrol may have additive effects when taken with antifungal herbs and supplements.
- Laboratory evidence suggests that resveratrol has antiaggregating and antithrombin activity and may have additive effects when taken with other herbs and supplements with the same actions.
- Resveratrol may increase the effects of some antivirals.
- Theoretically, the use of resveratrol with blood pressure–lowering or cardiovascular herbs and supplements may result in additive effects.
- Cholesterol levels have been lowered in rats, although the clinical significance is unknown. In theory, resveratrol could increase the effects of herbs and supplements like garlic, guggul, red yeast rice, or niacin.
- Drinking large quantities of red wine, which contains resveratrol, may have adverse effects on the liver. Preliminary evidence suggests that resveratrol may weakly inhibit the way that the liver breaks down certain herbs and supplements (inhibits multiple cytochrome P450 enzymes).
- Based on resveratrol's chemical structure, resveratrol may function as an estrogen agonist. However, limited laboratory evidence has shown resveratrol acting as an estrogen antagonist. Resveratrol may have the potential to interact with phytoestrogens and supplements with hormonal effects, depending on a variety of factors.
- Based on preliminary evidence, resveratrol may interact with MAOIs such as St. John's wort. This effect has not been confirmed in humans.
- Based on laboratory evidence, resveratrol may increase inhibitory effects on carcinoma cells when combined with quercetin and rutin. Preliminary evidence also has shown that resveratrol may enhance the growth inhibitory effects of vitamin D.
- Resveratrol may also interact with antiinflammatory agents, vasorelaxants, neurological agents, immune-enhancing agents, or agents that alter blood sugar levels.

For a complete list of references, please visit www.naturalstandard.com.

Rhodiola
(Rhodiola rosea)

RELATED TERMS

- ADAPT-232, aliphatic alcohol, Arctic Root, benzyl alcohol, beta-sitosterol, caffeic acid, Chisan, cinnamyl glycoside, Crassulaceae (Family), daucosterol, *Eleutherococcus senticosus* Maxim., epigallocatechin, flavonoids, Full Spectrum Rhodiola Rosea Extract, gallic acid, galloylepigallocatechin, geraniol, geranyl acetate, geranyl formate, glucopyranoside, golden root, golden root tincture, goldenroot, goldroot, gossypetin, herbacetin, heterodendrin, hongjingtian, hydroquinone, jiangtian, kaempferol, linalool, lotaustralin, Mind Power Rx, monoterpene alcohols, monoterpene hydrocarbons, n-decanol, p-tyrosol, Passion Rx, phenylethyl alcohol, phenylpropamide, protocatechuic acid, queen's crown, REC-7004, rhamnopyranoside, rhizome, rhodakon, rhodalidin, rhodalin, rhodaxon, *Rhodiola alterna*, *Rhodiola brevipetiolata*, *Rhodiola crenulata*, *Rhodiola dumulosa*, Rhodiola Energy, Rhodiola Extended Release, Rhodiola Force, rhodiola herb, *Rhodiola heterodonta*, *Rhodiola imbricata* Edgew., *Rhodiola integrifolia* Raf., *Rhodiola kirilowii*, *Rhodiola quadrifida*, *Rhodiola rhodantha*, rhodiola root, *Rhodiola sachalinensis*, *Rhodiola sacra*, *Rhodiola semenovii*, *Rhodiola tibetica*, rhodiolgidin, rhodiolgin, rhodiolin, rhodionidin, rhodionin, rhodioniside, rhodiosin, rodia riza, rodiola, rosarin, rosavin, rose root, roseroot, roseroot stonecrop, rosin, rosiridin, rosiridol, Russian golden root, Russian root, SHR-5, salidroside, *Sedum rhodiola*, *Sedum rosea*, *Sedum rosea* (L.) Scop., *Sedum roseum* Scop., Siberian *Rhodiola rosea*, sitosterol, sterols, tannins, volatile oil, zolotoy koren.

BACKGROUND

- Rhodiola (*Rhodiola rosea*) grows in cold regions and at high altitudes in Europe and Asia, where its roots have traditionally been used to increase resistance to physical stress.
- Although there are more than 200 species of rhodiola, *Rhodiola rosea* is considered preferable because it contains rosavins. Supplements generally contain a minimum of 3% rosavins.
- Rhodiola has been used to prevent fatigue and enhance physical and mental performance. Rhodiola is considered an adaptogen, which is an agent that works in the cells to normalize function and stimulate healing.
- Rhodiola may provide benefit in bladder cancer, lung disease, and exercise and mental performance, but more studies are needed to confirm these findings.

EVIDENCE

Uses Based on Scientific Evidence	Grade
Bladder Cancer Preliminary evidence suggests that rhodiola may decrease the spread of cancer, increase survival rates, and provide benefit in bladder cancer. More evidence is needed.	C
Exercise Performance Enhancement There is promising preliminary evidence that rhodiola may improve exercise performance; however, the available evidence is limited.	C
Hypoxia (Lack of Oxygen) Although it has been suggested that rhodiola may protect against tissue damage caused by lack of oxygen, study results have not been sufficient to support this use.	C
Lung Disease (Acute Injury) Preliminary research suggests rhodiola may protect the lungs from acute injury. However, the available evidence is insufficient to support this use.	C
Mental Performance Preliminary clinical evidence suggests that rhodiola may benefit learning, memory, and mental performance. However, the available evidence is insufficient to support this use.	C

Uses Based on Tradition or Theory

Abnormal heart rhythm (arrhythmia), adrenal insufficiency, aging, allergy, altitude (mountain) sickness, amenorrhea (lack of menstrual period), antiinflammatory, antimicrobial, antioxidant, anxiety, appetite stimulant, autism, CNS stimulant, cancer, cancer (radiotherapy side effects), chelating agent (heavy metals), chronic fatigue syndrome, common cold, dementia, dental conditions, depression, diabetes, fatigue, fibromyalgia, flu, headaches, heart disease, hernia, high blood pressure, immune function, insomnia/sleep quality, leukorrhea (vaginal discharge), liver protection, lung infections, mania, memory, menopause, mood, myasthenia gravis, nerve disorders, obesity, ovarian cancer, pneumonia, quality of life, schizophrenia, seasonal affective disorder, sedation, sexual dysfunction, smoking cessation, stress, stroke, thyroid conditions, tonic.

DOSING
Adults (18 Years and Older)

- There is insufficient evidence to recommend a dose for rhodiola. Typically, 200-600 mg rhodiola has been used. High doses are considered to be 1,000 mg or more per day.
- *Rhodiola* extract (SHR-5) has been used in various doses, including one 200-mg dose, 100 mg/day for 20 days, and 100-555 mg for up to 20 days.
- Some sources suggest that rhodiola should be taken on an empty stomach and that individuals should take a break from rhodiola every 1-2 weeks.

Children (Younger than 18 Years)

- There is insufficient evidence to recommend a dose for rhodiola in children.

SAFETY
Allergies

- Avoid in individuals with a known allergy or sensitivity to rhodiola.

Side Effects and Warnings

- Rhodiola may lower blood sugar levels. Caution is advised in patients with diabetes or hypoglycemia and in those taking drugs, herbs, or supplements that affect blood sugar. Blood glucose levels may need to be monitored by a qualified health care professional, including a pharmacist, and medication adjustments may be necessary.
- Rhodiola may increase heart rate, irregular heart beats, restlessness, irritability, insomnia, and salivation, may alter blood pressure, and may have hormonal properties.

Pregnancy and Breastfeeding

- Rhodiola is not recommended in pregnant or breastfeeding women because of a lack of available scientific evidence.

INTERACTIONS
Interactions with Drugs

- Rhodiola may lower blood sugar levels. Caution is advised when drugs that may also lower blood sugar are used. Patients taking drugs for diabetes by mouth or injection should be monitored closely by a qualified health care professional. Dosing adjustments may be necessary.
- Rhodiola may alter blood pressure. Caution is advised in patients taking drugs that alter blood pressure.
- Rhodiola may have additive effects when taken with antianxiety, antibiotic, antidepressant, anticancer, antioxidant, central nervous system (CNS)-depressant, exercise performance–enhancing, immunosuppressant, neurological, and heart rate–regulating drugs, as well as certain pain drugs, such as nonsteroidal antiinflammatory agents (NSAIDs) and cyclooxygenase-2 (COX-2) inhibitors.
- Rhodiola may also interact with opiates, pentobarbital, hormonal agents, and drugs taken for erectile dysfunction.

Interactions with Herbs and Dietary Supplements

- Rhodiola may lower blood sugar levels. Caution is advised when herbs and supplements that may also lower blood sugar are used.
- Rhodiola may alter blood pressure. Caution is advised in patients taking herbs and supplements that alter blood pressure.
- Rhodiola may have additive effects when taken with adaptogen, antianxiety, antimicrobial, antiinflammatory, antidepressant, anticancer, antioxidant, CNS-depressant, exercise performance–enhancing, immune system–modulating, neurological, heart rate–regulating, and antiimpotence herbs and supplements.
- Rhodiola may also interact with cranberry extract, opiates, phytoestrogens, calcium pyruvate, chromium, *Cordyceps*, potassium phosphate, ribose, and sodium phosphate.

For a complete list of references, please visit www.naturalstandard.com.

Rhubarb
(*Rheum* spp.)

RELATED TERMS

- Amaro Medicinale Giuliani, anthraglycosides, anthranoids, anthranols, anthraquinone, anthraquinone glucoside, arabinose, Baoshen pill, bastard rhubarb, calcium oxalate, Canton rhubarb, catechin, Chinese rhubarb, chinesischer Rhabarber (German), chrysophanol, chong-gi-huang, common rhubarb, da-huang, dahuang liujingao, daio, danning pian, DHP-1, DHP-2, emodin, English rhubarb, extractum rhei liquidum, fatty acids, flavonoids, galactose, galacturonic acid, gallotannin, garden rhubarb, glucuronic acid, glucose, heterodianthrones, heteroglycans, Himalayan rhubarb, hydroxyanthracene derivatives, Indian rhubarb, Japanese rhubarb, jiang-zhi, Jiang-Zhi Jian-Fel Yao (JZJFY), jinghuang tablet, liujingao, lyxose, medicinal rhubarb, monoanthrones, naphthalene glucoside, O-glucosides, oxalates, oxalic acid, palmidin A, palmidin B, palmidin C, pectin, phenolic carboxylic acids, physcion, physcion monoglucoside, piceatannol, pie plant, pie rhubarb, Polygonaceae (family), procyanidin, qing shen tiao zhi (QSTZ), racine de rhubarbee (French), resin, Rhabarber (German), rhamnose, rhaponticin, rhapontigenin, rhapontin, rhei radix, rhei rhizoma, rheidin B, rheidin C, rhein, rhein-8-monoglucoside, rheinoside A, rheinoside B, rheinoside C, rheinoside D, rheirhubarbe de chine (French), rheum, *Rheum australe*, Rheum E, *Rheum emodi*, *Rheum emodi* Wall., *Rheum officinale* Baill., *Rheum rhabarbarum*, *Rheum rhaponticum*, *Rheum tanguticum* Maxim., *Rheum tanguticum* Maxim. ex. Balf., *Rheum tanguticum* Maxim L., *Rheum undulatum*, *Rheum webbianum*, rheum x cultorum, rhizoma, rhubarb extract tablet (RET), resin, rubarbo, ruibarbo (Spanish), rutin, sennidin C, sennoside A, sennoside B, shengxue, shenlong oral liquid, shenshi rhubarb, starch, stilbenes, sugars, sweet round-leaved dock, tai huang, tannins, Turkey rhubarb, Turkish rhubarb, volatile oil, wine plant, xin qin ning (XQN), xylose.
- **Note:** Garden (English) rhubarb (*Rheum rhabarbarum* or *Rheum rhaponticum*) is considered food rather than a medicinal herb and contains very small amount of anthraquinones.

BACKGROUND

- Chinese herbalists have utilized rhubarb rhizomes and roots for thousands of years. The rhizomes and roots contain powerful anthraquinones and tannins that act as stimulant laxatives and astringents, respectively. In traditional Chinese medicine, rhubarb is also used to treat gastric ulcers, chronic renal (kidney) failure, and pregnancy-induced hypertension (also known as preeclampsia) and eclampsia. European herbalists have recommended rhubarb as a laxative and a diuretic and to treat kidney stones, gout (foot inflammation), and liver diseases. Externally, it is recommended for healing skin sores and scabs.
- The current practice of using rhubarb to treat cancer (as an ingredient in the herbal Essiac formula) lacks the support of controlled clinical trials. However, rhubarb is being tested for multiple other conditions, including hyperlipidemia (high cholesterol levels) and obesity.

- Rhubarb's use for gingivitis, chronic renal failure, and upper gastrointestinal bleeding seems to be the most promising, although more research should be done in these areas, specifically with rhubarb as monotherapy.

EVIDENCE

Uses Based on Scientific Evidence	Grade
Bleeding (Upper Gastrointestinal) Rhubarb has been used in traditional Chinese medicine for many gastrointestinal disorders, including upper gastrointestinal bleeding. Preliminary evidence suggests that rhubarb may be beneficial in reducing upper gastrointestinal bleeding.	B
Gingivitis Pyralvex has been used for decades as a salve for gingivitis and the oral mucosa; Parodium was introduced more recently as a similar treatment. Their active components both include rhubarb extract. The results from several clinical studies investigating Pyralvex and Parodium indicate that these combination treatments may be beneficial in treating gingivitis.	B
Renal Failure (Chronic) A traditional Chinese medicine, rhubarb has shown positive effects on renal (kidney) failure in the laboratory and seems promising in human studies. In some studies, rhubarb is more effective than captopril, and rhubarb combined with captopril is more effective than either substance alone. Higher-quality studies are necessary to confirm this hypothesis.	B
Age-Associated Memory Impairment (AAMI) Preliminary study has investigated rhubarb along with other herbs in the treatment of AAMI. Studies of rhubarb alone are needed to discern rhubarb's effect on aging and memory.	C
Aplastic Anemia A combination mixture containing rhubarb seemed to alleviate aplastic anemia. However, the role of rhubarb in the treatment of this condition is still unclear, and additional study is needed.	C
Constipation (Chronic) Rhubarb has been used in multiple cultures as a laxative. Although preliminary evidence is promising, more studies using rhubarb alone are needed.	C
Fatty Liver (Nonalcoholic) A combination therapy, which included rhubarb, has been studied for nonalcoholic fatty liver disease. Because the therapy involved multiple herbs and other treatments, the effect of rhubarb on	C

(Continued)

R

Uses Based on Scientific Evidence	Grade
nonalcoholic fatty liver disease is difficult to discern. Additional study using rhubarb alone is needed in this area.	
Gastrointestinal Cancer Surgery Rhubarb has been used in traditional Chinese medicine for many gastrointestinal disorders. Currently, there is insufficient available evidence to recommend for or against the use of rhubarb for gastrointestinal cancer surgery.	C
Gastrointestinal Tract Disorders The herbal extract "Amaro Medicinale Giuliani" and its constituents, including rhubarb, has been studied as a treatment for mild gastrointestinal disturbances. Although the herbal extract and a combination of rhubarb and gentian seem promising, higher-quality studies with rhubarb as monotherapy are needed to discern rhubarb's effect on gastrointestinal disturbances.	C
Hemorrhagic Fever (Nephritic Syndrome) A combination of rhubarb and sanchi powder seems to reduce the hemorrhagic effects of nephritic syndrome more than dicynonum. However, the isolated effects of rhubarb remain unclear.	C
Hepatitis Studies have been conducted on rhubarb and its effects on hepatitis. In the case series, high doses of rhubarb decreased the symptoms and serum levels associated with hepatitis. However, the effectiveness remains unclear.	C
Herpes Topically applied rhubarb-sage extract cream may reduce the symptoms of herpes. However, the isolated effects of rhubarb remain unclear.	C
Hypercholesterolemia (High Cholesterol) A combination product containing rhubarb (*Rheum palmatum*) has been shown to lower cholesterol levels. Rhubarb (*Rheum rhabarbarum*) stalk fiber has also been shown to lower cholesterol levels. Further research is warranted.	C
Nasopharyngeal Carcinoma One clinical trial has looked at the effect of a combination therapy that includes rhubarb on nasopharyngeal carcinoma (cancer of the nasopharynx). However, the isolated effects of rhubarb remain unclear.	C
Nephritis (Midadvanced Crescentic) The combination therapy of decoction of qingre huoxue recipe (QHR), which contains less than 10% of rhubarb, may improve renal (kidney) function in patients with midadvanced crescentic nephritis. However, the isolated effects of rhubarb remain unclear.	C

	Grade
Obesity (Simple) Although the research indicates a positive effect of rhubarb compared with two other obesity treatments and a control group, more high-quality studies are needed to confirm rhubarb's effectiveness.	C
Preeclampsia Studies have examined rhubarb's effect on preeclampsia (a pregnancy disorder characterized by high blood pressure, swelling, and kidney malfunction) and indicate that it may be a helpful treatment. Further research is warranted.	C
Sepsis (Systemic Inflammation Reaction Syndrome [SIRS]) Some research indicates that rhubarb may be helpful in treating SIRS, and further research is warranted.	C

Uses Based on Tradition or Theory

Abortifacient (induces abortion), allergies, anal fissures, anthelmintic (expels worms), anticoagulation, antioxidant, antiparasitic, astringent, blood cleanser, blood disorders (disseminated intravascular coagulation), bruises, burns, cancer, conjunctivitis (pinkeye), constipation (acute), dental conditions (hypersensitive teeth), diarrhea, diuretic, dysentery (severe diarrhea), dyspepsia (upset stomach), fever, food uses, gastric ulcers, gastritis, gout (foot inflammation), headache, hemorrhoids, herpes simplex, hypertension (high blood pressure), immunomodulation, indigestion, jaundice, kidney stones, laxative, menstrual disorders, Oketsu syndrome, osteoarthritis, pregnancy-related complications (eclampsia), preparation for surgery (rectoanal), rheumatic pain, severe acute respiratory syndrome (SARS), skin sores, tonic, toothache, trauma, ulcer, uterine stimulant, wound healing.

DOSING
Adults (18 Years and Older)

- There is insufficient evidence to recommend a dose for rhubarb. Furthermore, there is no consensus about doses using rhubarb, and there is a wide range of doses and preparations that have been studied or used. Traditionally, rhubarb has been taken as a decoction, tincture, tea, or powdered root for conditions such as constipation, diarrhea, or upset stomach in doses ranging from 0.1-4.0 g daily. Enemas using 10 g of rhubarb powder have also been used twice daily for up to 7 days in chronic renal (kidney) failure patients.
- Rhubarb is possibly safe when used short-term (less than 8 days) in lower doses. For upper gastrointestinal bleeding, 3 g alcoholic extract tablets or powder or 6 mL of rhubarb syrup has been taken two to four times daily for up to 2 weeks. For gonorrhea, seven to eight tablets of rhubarb (dose not specified) has been taken three times daily for 4 days.
- Rhubarb is often taken in large doses when using the crude material (root or stalk), and up to 50 g of *Rheum officinale* decocted in 200 mL of liquid ingested once daily for 16 days has been used for hepatitis. For hypercholesterolemia (high cholesterol levels), 27 g of ground rhubarb fiber stalk has been taken daily for 4 weeks. Lower doses have been

studied in chronic renal failure patients: 6-9 g of rhubarb daily for 6-22 months with an initial dose of 1 g daily; 0.5 g daily with maximum doses of 3 g daily for 4 weeks has been used; 1-3 g of rhubarb extract daily for 6-48 months, with an average of 18.9 months.

- For preeclampsia, 0.75 g of rhubarb taken by mouth daily for 9-10 weeks, from the 28th week of pregnancy until delivery, has been used.

Children (Younger than 18 Years)

- There is insufficient evidence to recommend a dose for rhubarb in children. According to traditional use, when rhubarb is used in older children or elderly individuals older than 65 years, lower-strength preparations should be used. In case reports, rhubarb has caused neonatal jaundice.
- For the treatment of hepatitis, 25-30 g of *Rheum officinale* decocted in 200 mL of liquid has been taken once daily for 16 days, with a 1-day break every six treatments. For simple obesity, 5 tablets of 2.5-3.75 g of refined rhubarb extract have been taken every night for 1 week.

SAFETY
Allergies

- Avoid in individuals with a known allergy or hypersensitivity to rhubarb or its constituents. Anaphylaxis and rash have been reported.

Side Effects and Warnings

- Rhubarb leaves contain poisonous oxalic acid. Oxalic acid may form insoluble calcium oxalate crystals in the blood that may be deposited in the kidneys, leading to kidney stones. Excessive consumption of rhubarb leaves may cause abdominal pain, electrolyte loss (especially potassium), hyperaldosteronism (overproduction of the hormone aldosterone), edema (swelling), burning of the mouth and throat, arrhythmias (irregular heartbeat), cardiac toxicity, diarrhea, seizures, bone deterioration, muscular weakness, nausea, vomiting, seizures, and death.
- Rhubarb may cause bright yellow or red urine. Chronic use of rhubarb stalk or root may cause dependence with possible need for increased doses. It may also lead to electrolyte depletion (especially potassium), hyperaldosteronism, accelerated bone deterioration, edema, inhibition of gastric motility, pseudomelanosis coli, intestinal griping, colic, melanosis coli, and atonic colon. Avoid using rhubarb for more than 2 weeks. Although not well studied in humans, rhubarb anthraquinones may cause nephrotoxicity (kidney damage).
- Short-term use of rhubarb may cause uterine contraction, hematuria (blood in the urine), elevations of serum alanine aminotransferase (ALT) levels, spasmodic cramps, watery diarrhea, impaired hemostasis, hemorrhaging, and neonatal jaundice. High tannin levels of rhubarb root may increase the chance of hepatic necrosis (death of liver cells). Increased gurgling sounds, abdominal discomfort, increased stool passage, mild abdominal pain before defecation, nausea, and vomiting has occurred with short-term use of rhubarb. The adverse effects of short-term use of Pyralvex (contains rhubarb) include abdominal pain, slight burning, and dark discoloration of the gums. Use of rhubarb during menstruation may impair hemostasis.
- Handling rhubarb leaves may cause a rash.

- Use cautiously in patients with bleeding disorders or those using coagulation therapy, as rhubarb leaves may impair hemostasis; there was report of one patient having severe hemorrhaging because of a respiratory tract infection and fever.
- Use cautiously in patients with preeclampsia; rhubarb may interact with preeclampsia drugs.
- Use cautiously in patients with constipation because the astringent effects of rhubarb may exacerbate the condition.
- Use cautiously in patients with hemorrhoids because of the potential for inducing or aggravating hemorrhoidal thrombosis or prolapse.
- Avoid using rhubarb if fever, inflammation, and abdominal pain of unknown origin are present or in cases of appendicitis because of possible rupture of inflamed viscus, such as the appendix.
- Avoid using rhubarb with intestinal obstruction or ileus because of cathartic effects of anthraquinone derivatives, rhein, and the sennosides.
- Avoid using rhubarb with diarrhea because of the chance of electrolyte disturbances.
- Avoid using rhubarb in patients with Crohn's disease, ulcerative colitis, colitis, and irritable bowel syndrome (IBS), as rhubarb may have irritating effects.
- Avoid in patients with insufficient liver function, as rhubarb may be hepatotoxic (liver damaging).

Pregnancy and Breastfeeding

- Rhubarb is not recommended in pregnant or breastfeeding women because of a lack of available scientific research. In theory, rhubarb may have uterine stimulant effects. Because of anthraquinone alkaloids, which are potentially mutagenic and genotoxic, rhubarb may be risky during breastfeeding. In case reports, rhubarb has also caused neonatal jaundice. Pregnant women considering taking rhubarb should consult with a qualified health care professional, including a pharmacist, to check for interactions.

INTERACTIONS
Interactions with Drugs

- Rhubarb root contains tannins that may possess inhibitory activity against angiotensin-converting enzyme (ACE). Caution is advised in patients with high blood pressure or those taking ACE inhibitors or other blood pressure–lowering agents.
- If taken within 1 hour, antacids may decrease the effectiveness of rhubarb.
- Overuse of rhubarb may cause potassium depletion, increasing the risk of toxicity of other antiarrhythmic agents (for treatment of irregular heartbeat), such as quinidine. It may also increase the risk of digoxin toxicity.
- Rhubarb and low doses of antipsychotic drugs reduced the need for higher doses of antipsychotic drugs in schizophrenic patients.
- In clinical trials, rhubarb has shown a synergistic effect with captopril to reduce serum creatinine levels.
- Rhubarb may reduce gingivitis when used with chlorhexidine.
- Although not well studied in humans, the combination of cisplatin and rhubarb may reduce the lethal toxicity and renal (kidney) toxicity of cisplatin, a common chemotherapeutic agent. The combination does not appear to interfere with the chemotherapeutic effect of cisplatin.

R

- Rhubarb may increase potassium loss, thus aggravating electrolyte imbalance (e.g., with steroids). Concomitant use of rhubarb with other laxatives may increase electrolyte and fluid loss, potentiating their effect.
- The high tannin level of rhubarb root may increase the chance of hepatic necrosis (liver death). Caution is advised when rhubarb is taken with other potentially liver-damaging agents because of the increased risk of liver damage.
- Although not well studied in humans, the anthraquinones present in rhubarb may increase the risk of nephrotoxicity (kidney damage). Consult with a qualified health care professional, including a pharmacist, to check for interactions with other kidney-damaging agents.
- Rhubarb enhanced nifedipine's antipreeclampsia effects.
- Rhubarb's laxative effects may reduce the absorption of other drugs taken by mouth because of a reduction in gastrointestinal transit time.

Interactions with Herbs and Dietary Supplements

- Rhubarb is frequently used as a small component in multiherb traditional Chinese medicine decoctions. Examples of herbs that have been combined with rhubarb include *Alismatis orientalis*, sanchi powder, and sage.
- Because of rhubarb's potential to deplete potassium, concomitant use of rhubarb may increase cardiac toxicity of cardiac glycoside–containing herbs. An increase in potassium depletion and severe cardiac toxicity may be caused by concomitant use of rhubarb with cardioactive herbs, such as calamus, ginger, and *Panax ginseng*.

- Rhubarb may enhance the effects of some herbs or supplements, such as the laxative effects of Glauber's salt. Rhubarb used with leech therapy reduced the need for antipsychotic drugs in schizophrenic patients.
- The high tannin level of rhubarb root may increase the chance of hepatic necrosis (liver cell death).
- The action of jimsonweed may be increased in chronic use or abuse of rhubarb.
- Concomitant use of rhubarb and licorice or horsetail may cause potassium depletion. Although not well studied in humans, diuretic properties that may be in rhubarb may compound diuretic-induced potassium loss. Rhubarb is also proposed to cause bowel movements and may cause potassium depletion when used with other laxatives. Rhubarb may also increase potassium loss when used with steroids.
- Although not well studied in humans, the anthroquinones present in rhubarb taken with other potentially nephrotoxic (kidney-damaging) herbs may increase the risk of kidney damage.
- Concomitant use of rhubarb with other herbs taken by mouth may reduce their absorption because of reduction in gastrointestinal transit time. Rhubarb may also decrease mineral absorption. Its oxalate content may bind multivalent metal ions in the gastrointestinal tract and decrease their absorption.

For a complete list of references, please visit www.naturalstandard.com.

Riboflavin
(Vitamin B$_2$)

RELATED TERMS

- 7,8-Dimethyl-10 (1'-D-ribityl) isoalloxazine, B-complex vitamin, Dolo-Neurotrat, flavin, flavine, lactoflavin, riboflavine, vitamin B$_2$, vitamin G.

BACKGROUND

- Riboflavin is a water-soluble vitamin that is involved in vital metabolic processes in the body and is necessary for normal cell function, growth, and energy production. Small amounts of riboflavin are present in most animal and plant tissues.
- Healthy individuals who eat a balanced diet rarely need riboflavin supplements. Especially good dietary sources of riboflavin are milk (and other dairy products), eggs, enriched cereals/grains, meats, liver, and green vegetables (such as asparagus or broccoli). Intake may be lower in vegetarians compared with nonvegetarians.
- Riboflavin is often used as a tracer of medication compliance in the treatment of patients with alcohol dependence, mental disorders, and other conditions. Urinary riboflavin levels may be measured to determine the level of compliance.
- **Supplements**: The most common forms of riboflavin available in supplements are riboflavin and riboflavin 5'-monophosphate. Riboflavin is most commonly found in multivitamin and vitamin B–complex preparations.

EVIDENCE

Uses Based on Scientific Evidence	Grade
Neonatal Jaundice Riboflavin supplementation is included in the treatment of neonatal jaundice with phototherapy.	A
Riboflavin Deficiency (Ariboflavinosis) Studies suggest that riboflavin is beneficial in patients with riboflavin deficiency (ariboflavinosis). Ariboflavinosis may cause weakness, throat swelling/soreness, glossitis (tongue swelling), angular stomatitis/cheilosis (skin cracking or sores at the corners of the mouth), dermatitis (skin irritation), or anemia. Particular groups may be especially susceptible to riboflavin deficiency, including the elderly, those with chronic illnesses, the poor, and those with alcohol dependency. Patients with suspected riboflavin deficiency should be evaluated by a qualified health care professional.	A
Anemia Some research suggests that riboflavin may play an adjunct role in the treatment of iron deficiency anemia and sickle cell anemia; levels of riboflavin may be low in these conditions. Correction of riboflavin deficiency in individuals who are both riboflavin deficient and iron deficient appears to improve response to iron therapy.	C
Anorexia/Bulimia Levels of important nutrients are often low in individuals with anorexia or bulimia, with up to 20%-33% of patients deficient in vitamins B$_2$ (riboflavin) and B$_6$ (pyridoxine). Dietary changes alone, without additional supplements, can often bring vitamin B levels back to normal. However, extra B$_2$ and B$_6$ may be required. Nutritional and medical guidance for such patients should be under the direction of a qualified health care professional.	C
Cataracts It has been suggested that low riboflavin levels may be a risk factor for developing cataracts or that riboflavin supplementation may be beneficial for prevention. Additional evidence is needed.	C
Cognitive Function Adequate nutrient supplementation with riboflavin may be required for the maintenance of adequate cognitive function. Treatment with B vitamins including riboflavin has been reported to improve scores of cognitive function in patients taking tricyclic antidepressants. This may be related to tricyclic-caused depletion of riboflavin levels.	C
Depression Treatment with B vitamins, including riboflavin, has been reported to improve depression scores in patients taking tricyclic antidepressants. This may be related to tricyclic-caused depletion of riboflavin levels.	C
Esophageal Cancer (Prevention and Treatment) Riboflavin supplementation has been studied in the prevention and treatment of esophageal cancer, mostly in China, with mixed results.	C
Ethylmalonic Encephalopathy Although the exact pathogenesis of this disorder is unknown, some research suggests that riboflavin may lead to slight improvements in motor function, cognitive behavior, and diarrhea.	C
Malaria It remains unclear how riboflavin supplementation may affect malarial infections.	C
Migraine Headache Prevention Several studies suggest benefits of high-dose riboflavin in preventing migraine headaches, although the effectiveness remains unclear.	C
Preeclampsia Limited research has reported an association between low riboflavin levels and an increased risk	C

R

(Continued)

Uses Based on Scientific Evidence	Grade
of preeclampsia (high blood pressure in pregnancy). However, it is not clear whether low riboflavin levels are a cause or consequence of this condition or whether additional supplementation is warranted in pregnant women at risk of preeclampsia/eclampsia (beyond the routine use of prenatal vitamins).	

Uses Based on Tradition or Theory

Acne, aging, alcohol dependence, ataxia, atherosclerosis, athletic performance, burning eyes, burning feet syndrome, burns, canker sores, carpal tunnel syndrome, cervical cancer, colon cancer, congenital methemoglobinemia, Crohn's disease, excess tearing, dementia, dermatitis, diabetes, digestive disorders, eczema, eye disorders, eye strain/fatigue, fatigue, glaucoma, glossitis (tongue inflammation), growth disorders, healthy hair, human immunodeficiency virus (HIV), hypertension (high blood pressure), immune system function, lactic acidosis, leg cramps, liver disease, memory loss, mitochondrial disorders, mood disorders, mouth cancer, multiple acyl coenzyme A dehydrogenase deficiency, multiple sclerosis (MS), neural tube defects, pain, peptic ulcer disease (PUD), postoperative muscle cramps, red blood cell aplasia, reproductive disorders, rheumatoid arthritis, skin disorders, stress, stroke, ureteral colic pain, vitality problems.

DOSING
Riboflavin Deficiency

- The U.S. Recommended Dietary Allowance (RDA) for riboflavin was revised in 1998, with the goal to prevent riboflavin deficiency. Clinical signs of deficiency in humans may appear at intakes less than 0.5-0.6 mg daily, and excess urinary excretion of riboflavin can be seen at intake levels of approximately 1 mg daily. Riboflavin deficiency (ariboflavinosis) can be associated with weakness, throat soreness/swelling, tongue swelling (glossitis), angular stomatitis/cheilosis (skin cracking or sores at the corners of the mouth), dermatitis (skin irritation), and anemia. Good dietary sources of riboflavin are milk (and other dairy products), eggs, enriched cereals/grains, meats, liver, and green vegetables (such as asparagus or broccoli). Riboflavin is easily destroyed by exposure to light (e.g., riboflavin in milk stored in clear glass bottles).
- Particular groups of people may be particularly susceptible to riboflavin deficiency, including the elderly, those with chronic illnesses, the poor, and those with alcohol dependence.

Adults (18 Years and Older)

- The U.S. RDA for adults (by mouth) is 1 mg for female adolescents (14-18 years old); 1.3 mg for male adolescents (14-18 years old); 1.1 mg for female adults (older than 18 years); 1.3 mg for male adults (older than 18 years); 1.4 mg for pregnant women (any age); and 1.6 mg for breastfeeding women (any age).

Children (Younger than 18 Years)

- The U.S. RDA for infants and children (by mouth) is 0.3 mg for 0-6 months old; 0.4 mg for 7-12 months old; 0.5 mg for 1-3 years old; 0.6 mg for 4-8 years old; 0.9 mg for 9-13 years old; 1 mg for female adolescents (14-18 years old); and 1.3 mg for male adolescents (14-18 years old).

SAFETY
Allergies

- Riboflavin supplementation has been associated with rare reports of allergy and anaphylaxis.

Side Effects and Warnings

- In general, the limited capacity of human adults to absorb orally administered riboflavin limits its potential for harm. Riboflavin intake many times higher than the RDA is apparently without demonstrable toxicity. Nevertheless, the photosensitizing (sensitivity to light) properties of riboflavin raise the possibility of some potential risks. Other possible reactions to very high doses include itching, numbness, burning/prickling sensations, and yellow discoloration of the urine.
- Very low birth weight infants who receive preterm infant formulas (PIF) augmented to provide riboflavin at levels five times that in term infant formulas have demonstrated high plasma levels of riboflavin and urinary riboflavin concentrations; lower doses can be considered in this setting.

Pregnancy and Breastfeeding

- Riboflavin is generally regarded as being safe during pregnancy and breastfeeding.

INTERACTIONS
Interactions with Drugs

- There are numerous drugs that may alter the amount of riboflavin in the body or alter the intended effect of riboflavin supplementation. Examples include anticholinergic drugs, doxorubicin (Adriamycin), methotrexate, phenobarbital, phenothiazine antipsychotic medications (e.g., chlorpromazine), probenecid, thiazide diuretics, and tricyclic antidepressants.
- Low riboflavin levels have been associated with antimalarial effects, and antiriboflavin therapies were proposed in the 1980s, although more recent evidence has challenged this proposed association.
- Early reports suggested that women taking high-dose birth control bills developed diminished riboflavin nutritional status, but when investigators controlled for dietary riboflavin intake, no impact was found.
- There is preliminary evidence suggesting that postmenopausal breast cancer patients with low riboflavin levels will normalize their levels following treatment with tamoxifen. However, the cause of their baseline low riboflavin is unclear and may be related to prior treatment with doxorubicin chemotherapy, a suspected cause of low riboflavin levels (which would likely recover with or without tamoxifen).
- Riboflavin either alone or in combination with other B vitamins should be taken at different times from the antibiotic

tetracycline. In addition, long-term use of antibiotics can deplete vitamin B levels in the body (particularly B_2, B_9, B_{12}, and biotin).

Interactions with Herbs and Dietary Supplements

- Severe riboflavin deficiency may impact multiple enzyme systems in the body because of involvement in the metabolism of other vitamins including B_6 (pyridoxine), B_3 (niacin), and folate.
- Although not well studied in humans, herbs and supplements with anticholinergic, antimalarial, hormonal, antipsychotic, diuretic, or antidepressant activity should be used cautiously with riboflavin.

For a complete list of references, please visit www.naturalstandard.com.

R

Rooibos

(Aspalathus linearis, syn. *Borbonia pinifolia)*

RELATED TERMS

- Aspalathin, *Aspalathus acuminatus, Aspalathus contaminata, Borbonia pinifolia*, chrysoeriol, Fabaceae/Leguminosae (family), hyperoside, isoorientin, isoquercitrin, isovitexin, Kaffree tea, long life tea, luteolin, orientin, *Psoralea linearis*, quercetin, red bush tea, redbush tea, red tea, rutin, vitexin.

BACKGROUND

- An increasingly popular beverage, rooibos tea originates from the leaves and stems of the indigenous South African plant *Aspalathus linearis*. It has gained much attention for clinical purposes in the case of nervous tension, allergies (dermatitis), and various digestive problems. Rooibos tea contains a large amount of flavonoids and acts as a potent antioxidant. In Africa, it has been used to treat malignancies and inflammatory disorders.
- Rooibos (pronounced ROY-boss) is not a natural source of caffeine and is low in tannins. Rooibos tea may be preferred by people who cannot tolerate either the caffeine effects or astringency of *Camellia sinensis* teas.

EVIDENCE

Uses Based on Scientific Evidence

No available studies qualify for inclusion in the evidence table.

Uses Based on Tradition or Theory

Allergic dermatitis, allergies, antioxidant, asthma, cancer, colic, diaper rash, digestive problems, eczema, headache, hepatoprotection (in liver disease), human immunodeficiency syndrome/acquired immuno-deficiency syndrome (HIV/AIDS), hypertension (high blood pressure), infections, insomnia, kidney stones, nervousness, vascular disorders (blood vessel disorders, prevention in diabetic patients).

DOSING

Adults (18 Years and Older)

- There is insufficient evidence to recommend a dose of rooibos. Traditionally, 1 teabag or teaspoon to 8 oz of hot water has been used.

Children (Younger than 18 Years)

- There is insufficient evidence to recommend a dose of rooibos in children.

SAFETY

Allergies

- Avoid in individuals with a known allergy or hypersensitivity to *Aspalathus linearis*, its constituents, or related members of the Fabaceae/Leguminosae family. Other members of this family include peas, soybeans, clover, and peanuts.

Side Effects and Warnings

- Little evidence is available to describe the adverse effects of rooibos. Rooibos is likely safe when ingested as a tisane (herbal infusion) in food amounts. However, use cautiously in patients taking drugs or herbs metabolized by cytochrome P450 enzymes, as there is unclear evidence regarding whether rooibos affects these enzymes.

Pregnancy and Breastfeeding

- Rooibos is not recommended in pregnant or breastfeeding women because of a lack of available scientific evidence.

INTERACTIONS

Interactions with Drugs

- There is mixed evidence on whether rooibos affects P450 metabolism. In theory, rooibos may interfere with the way the body processes certain drugs using the liver's cytochrome P450 enzyme system. As a result, the levels of these drugs may be increased in the blood and may cause increased effects or potentially serious adverse reactions. Patients taking any medications should check the package insert and speak with a qualified health care professional, including a pharmacist, about possible interactions.

Interactions with Herbs and Dietary Supplements

- There is mixed evidence on whether rooibos affects P450 metabolism. In theory, rooibos may interfere with the way the body processes certain herbs or supplements using the liver's cytochrome P450 enzyme system. As a result, the levels of other herbs or supplements may be too high in the blood. It may also alter the effects that other herbs or supplements possibly have on the P450 system, such as bloodroot, cat's claw, or chamomile. Patients taking any medications should check the package insert and speak with a qualified health care professional, including a pharmacist, about possible interactions.

For a complete list of references, please visit www. naturalstandard.com.

Rosemary
(Rosmarinus officinalis Linn.)

RELATED TERMS

- Albus (cultivar), Arp (cultivar), Aureus (cultivar), Benenden Blue (cultivar), Blue Boy (cultivar), caffeic acid, carnosol, carnosic acid, compass plant, compass-weed, dew of the sea, diterpenes, epirosmanol, Fierabras, Golden Rain (cultivar), Herbor 025, Hungary water, Incensier (cultivar), Irene (cultivar), Ken Taylor (cultivar), Labiatae (family), Lamiaceae (family), Lockwood de Forest (cultivar), Majorica Pink (cultivar), methanol (MeOH), Miss Jessop's Upright (cultivar), phenols, pilgrim's flower, Pinkie (cultivar), polar plant, polyphenolic compounds, Prostratus (cultivar), Pyramidalis (cultivar), Queen of Hungary water, romero (Spanish), Roseus (cultivar), rosmanol, Rosmanox, Rosmarini folium, rosmarinic acid, *Rosmarinus officinalis*, Severn Sea (cultivar), Suffolk Blue (cultivar), Tuscan blue (cultivar).

BACKGROUND

- Rosemary (*Rosmarinus officinalis* Linn.) is a common, dense, evergreen, aromatic shrub grown in many parts of the world. Historically, rosemary has been used as a medicinal agent to treat renal colic and dysmenorrhea (painful menstruation). It has also been used to relieve symptoms caused by respiratory disorders and to stimulate the growth of hair. Traditionally, rosemary has been used for improving memory and has been a symbol of remembrance and friendship for centuries. In Morocco, rosemary has been used to treat diabetes and hypertension (high blood pressure).
- The most researched constituents of rosemary are caffeic acid and its derivative rosmarinic acid. These compounds are thought to have antioxidant effects and are being studied as potential therapies for cancer, hepatotoxicity (liver toxicity), and inflammatory conditions.
- Currently, available studies show some promise for rosemary in the treatment of anxiety/stress (aromatherapy) and alopecia (hair loss). Current cosmetic uses of rosemary include treating cellulite and wrinkles and normalizing excessive oil secretion of the skin. Germany's Commission E has approved rosemary leaf for treatment of dyspepsia and rosemary oil (used externally) for joint pain and poor circulation.

EVIDENCE

Uses Based on Scientific Evidence	Grade
Alopecia Areata (Hair Loss) Rosemary oil is reported to increase circulation and possibly promote hair growth in patients with alopecia areata. Additional research is warranted to confirm these findings.	C
Anxiety/Stress Rosemary extract is frequently used in aromatherapy for treatment of a variety of conditions, including anxiety, mood enhancement, alteration of pain	C

perception, and to increase alertness. Preliminary research has shown benefit in reducing stress levels and increasing alertness.

Uses Based on Tradition or Theory

Abortifacient, air purifier, analgesic (pain reliever), anthelmintic (expels worms), antiaging, antibacterial, anticoagulant (blood-thinning), antifungal, antioxidant, antispasmodic, appetite stimulation, atherosclerosis (hardening of the arteries), baldness, bronchial asthma, cancer prevention, cataracts, colic, dandruff, diaphoretic (promotes sweating), diuretic, drug withdrawal (morphine), dysmenorrhea (painful menstruation), dyspepsia (upset stomach), gout, hepatoprotection (liver protection), human immunodeficiency virus (HIV) infection, hypercholesterolemia (high cholesterol levels), hyperglycemia, hypertension (high blood pressure), immunostimulation, inflammation, ischemic heart disease, joint pain, lice, liver cirrhosis, memory enhancement, muscle relaxant (smooth muscle), nerve regeneration, osteoporosis, paralysis, peptic ulcer disease, peripheral vascular disease, photoprotection, poor circulation, preservative, quality of life, renal colic, respiratory disorders, rheumatism, skin care (cosmetic), skin conditions (excessive oil secretion of the skin, cellulite), sperm motility, tonic, wound healing, wrinkle prevention.

DOSING
Adults (18 Years and Older)

- There is insufficient evidence to recommend a dose for rosemary. Rosemary has been used in aromatherapy. Rosemary essential oil should not be used internally.

Children (Younger than 18 Years)

- There is insufficient evidence to recommend a dose for rosemary, and use in children is not recommended.

SAFETY
Allergies

- Avoid in individuals with a known allergy or hypersensitivity to rosemary. Contact dermatitis has been reported in a small number of people exposed to rosemary. A 56-year-old man reacted to carnosol, the main constituent of Rosmanox, which is made from the leaves of rosemary (*Rosmarinus officinalis*). A 23-year-old woman using a cleansing gel containing rosemary leaf extract developed an itchy erythema on her face. Occupational asthma has also been reported.

Side Effects and Warnings

- In general, rosemary appears well tolerated with few documented cases of adverse events. Rosemary is likely safe when taken by mouth in amounts commonly found in foods. It is possibly safe when rosemary and rosemary extracts are taken by mouth and used appropriately in medicinal

R

amounts or when used topically in medicinal amounts for up to 7 months.

- Allergic contact dermatitis, occupational asthma, and chelitis have occurred in some individuals. Ingestion of rosemary oil can be toxic.

- In large doses, rosemary may be irritating to the mucosa of the intestinal tract and may cause nausea and cramping. Also, rosemary has been shown to decrease iron absorption. Although not well studied, the volatile oil of rosemary leaves may have musculoskeletal effects. Rosemary may also increase the rate at which the liver deactivates estrogen, which may lead to estrogen-deficient conditions. Rosemary may also cause hypotension (low blood pressure). In theory, it may also stimulate hair growth, and hirsutism may occur.

- Although not well studied in humans, rosemary leaf volatile oil may increase blood sugar levels. Caution is advised in patients with diabetes or hypoglycemia and in those taking drugs, herbs, or supplements that affect blood sugar. Serum glucose levels may need to be monitored by a health care provider, and medication adjustments may be necessary.

- Rosemary may increase the effects of furosemide (Lasix). Diuretic properties of rosemary have not been established, but it is possible that electrolyte changes may occur. Aqueous extracts of rosemary may increase urinary excretion of sodium, potassium, and chloride and decrease creatinine clearance.

- Use cautiously in patients with peptic ulcer disease, low blood pressure, coagulation disorders, or iron deficiency anemia.

Pregnancy and Breastfeeding

- Based on its traditional use for abortion, the risk of abnormalities caused by altered hormone levels, and preliminary evidence showing embryotoxic effects, rosemary should not be used by pregnant women or women who wish to become pregnant. Rosemary is not recommended in breastfeeding women because of a lack of available scientific evidence.

INTERACTIONS
Interactions with Drugs

- Rosemary may increase the risk of bleeding when taken with drugs that increase the risk of bleeding. Some examples include aspirin, anticoagulants ("blood thinners") such as warfarin (Coumadin) or heparin, antiplatelet drugs such as clopidogrel (Plavix), and nonsteroidal antiinflammatory drugs such as ibuprofen (Motrin, Advil) or naproxen (Naprosyn, Aleve).

- Water extracts of rosemary may inhibit angiotensin I–converting enzyme (ACE). This may cause low blood pressure. Caution is advised in patients taking medications that also can reduce blood pressure, such as ACE inhibitors.

- Rosemary may have antiinflammatory, antispasmodic, antifungal, and antibacterial activity. Patients taking any medications with similar effects should use rosemary cautiously.

- Rosemary and its various constituents have been noted for their high antioxidant properties, including carnosol, carnosic acid, rosmanol, epirosmanol, and hesperidin.

- Alcohol extracts of rosemary may have antitumorigenic activity. Rosemary may increase the accumulation of commonly used chemotherapeutic agents, including doxorubicin and vinblastine, in cancer cells that express P-glycoprotein. However, rosemary extract probably does not affect accumulation or efflux of doxorubicin in cells that lack P-glycoprotein. Use cautiously in patients taking agents for cancer or chemotherapy drugs.

- Constituents in rosemary extract may inhibit cholesterol oxidation product formation. Caution is advised in patients taking cholesterol-lowering medications.

- Rosemary may interfere with the way the body processes certain drugs using the liver's cytochrome P450 enzyme system. As a result, the levels of these drugs may be decreased in the blood and may reduce the intended effects. Patients taking any medications should check the package insert and speak with a qualified health care professional, including a pharmacist, about possible interactions.

- Rosemary has been shown to increase the effects of furosemide (Lasix), which belongs to the class of loop diuretics. Patients taking medications that increase the flow of urine should consult with a qualified health care professional, including a pharmacist, before combining therapies.

- Rosemary may precipitate lithium toxicity because of its diuretic properties. Caution is advised in patients with bipolar disorder or those taking medications containing lithium. Medication adjustments may be necessary.

- Rosemary extract may increase blood sugar levels in both diabetic and nondiabetic patients. Caution is advised when medications that may lower blood sugar are used. Patients taking drugs for diabetes by mouth or using insulin should be monitored closely by a qualified health care provider. Medication adjustments may be necessary.

- In theory, rosemary, rosemary essential oil, and its components may inhibit bone resorption. Theoretically, there may be additive effects. Patients taking medications for osteoporosis should consult with a qualified health care professional, including a pharmacist.

- Although not well-studied, rosemary may also interact with peptic ulcer disease drugs and estrogen-containing medications such as birth control pills.

Interactions with Herbs and Dietary Supplements

- Rosemary may increase the risk of bleeding when taken with herbs and supplements that are believed to increase the risk of bleeding. Multiple cases of bleeding have been reported with the use of *Ginkgo biloba*, and fewer cases have been reported with garlic and saw palmetto. Numerous other agents may theoretically increase the risk of bleeding, although this has not been proven in most cases.

- Water extracts of rosemary may inhibit ACE. This may cause low blood pressure. Caution is advised in patients taking herbs or supplements that can also reduce blood pressure.

- Rosemary may have antispasmodic, antifungal, antibacterial, and antiinflammatory effects. Patients taking any herbs or supplements with similar effects should use rosemary cautiously.

- Rosemary and its various constituents have been noted for their high antioxidant properties, including carnosol, carnosic acid, rosmanol, epirosmanol, and hesperidin. Combination with lycopene may increase rosemary's antioxidative effects. Consult with a qualified health care professional, including a pharmacist, before making decisions about therapies.

- Alcohol extracts of rosemary may have antitumorigenic activity. Use caution in patients taking herbs or supplements that may be used for cancer because of possible additive effects.

- Constituents in rosemary extract may inhibit cholesterol oxidation product formation. Caution is advised in patients taking cholesterol-lowering herbs and supplements, such as red yeast rice.
- Rosemary may interfere with the way the body processes certain herbs or supplements using the liver's cytochrome P450 enzyme system. As a result, the levels of other herbs or supplements may become too low in the blood. It may also alter the effects that other herbs or supplements potentially may have on the P450 system.
- Rosemary may enhance the effects of herbal agents used to increase the flow of urine.
- Although not well studied, rosemary may enhance the liver's rate of deactivating estrogen in the body. Caution is advised when combining rosemary with other herbs and supplements that contain phytoestrogens.
- Rosemary extract may increase blood sugar levels in both diabetic and nondiabetic patients. Caution is advised when agents that may lower blood sugar are used. Patients taking herbs or supplements for diabetes by mouth or using insulin should be monitored closely by a qualified health care provider. Medication adjustments may be necessary.
- Rosemary may decrease iron absorption. Caution is advised in patients taking iron supplements or multivitamins.

For a complete list of references, please visit www.naturalstandard.com.

Rutin
($C_{27}H_{30}O_{16}$)

RELATED TERMS

- Alpha-glycosylrutin, ascorutin, benzopyrone, Birutan Forte, buckwheat (*Fagopyrum esculentum*), dihydroxyethylrutoside, eldrin, Ercevit fort, ergot compound, essaven, flavonoid, Fleboside, Globulariacitrin, glucopyranoside, hydrolytic enzymes (HE), hydroxyethylrutoside (HR), hydroxyethylrutosiden, ilixanthin, melin, myrticolorin, paliuroside, Paroven (United Kingdom, South Africa, Australasia), paveron 75, phlebolanspray, phlebotropic drugs, phytomelin, Q1, quercetin, quercetin rutinoside, Relvene (France), Rexiluven (DRA 363, Sandoven), ritmilen, rutabion, rutin trihydrate, rutinic acid, rutinion acid, rutosid, rutoside, rutozyd, sandoven, sophorin, tanrutin, tetrahydroxyethyl-quercetin, tetrahydroxyethyl-rutoside, tri-(hydroxyethyl)-rutin, trihydroxyethylrutoside (Varemoid), trioxyethylrutin, troxerutin (CAS 7085-55-4), trypsin, Venoruton (most of continental Europe), Venoruton 1000, Venoruton Forte, Vicalin, violaquercitrin, vitamin P.

BACKGROUND

- Rutin is a yellow crystalline flavonol glycoside ($C_{27}H_{30}O_{16}$) that occurs in various plants (rue, tobacco, buckwheat, etc.). On hydrolysis (a chemical reaction that uses water to break down a compound), rutin yields quercetin and rutinose.
- Rutin is used in many countries as a vasoprotectant and is an ingredient in numerous multivitamin preparations and herbal remedies. The rutosides are naturally occurring flavonoids that have documented effects on capillary permeability and edema (swelling) and have been used for the treatment of disorders of the venous and microcirculatory systems.
- There is some evidence for the use of rutin for chronic venous insufficiency, edema, hemorrhoids, microangiopathy (disease of small blood vessels), varicosis, and venous disorders. Well-presented clinical trials are required in these fields before solid recommendations can be made.
- Formulations, mainly consisting of the trihydroxyethyl derivative of rutin, are used in Europe, Mexico, and other Latin American countries for the treatment of such venous disorders as varicose veins and hemorrhoids. The generic name for these formulations is troxerutin. Troxerutin has been widely used in Europe since the mid-1960s.

EVIDENCE

Uses Based on Scientific Evidence	Grade
Chronic Venous Insufficiency Overall, the results suggest a benefit for O-(beta-hydroxyethyl)-rutoside in chronic venous insufficiency.	B
Edema Overall, the results suggest a benefit for various rutin compounds in reducing edema and flight edema.	B
Hemorrhoids Preliminary evidence suggests that O-(beta-hydroxyethyl) rutoside and trihydroxyethylrutoside may be safe and effective treatments for hemorrhoids. Studies investigating the effect of rutin in different populations, as well as efficacy on third- or fourth-degree hemorrhoids, are warranted in the future.	C
Ménière's Syndrome Some clinical evidence supports the use of O-(beta-hydroxyethyl)-rutoside for reduction of symptoms associated with Ménière's syndrome. Additional study is warranted.	C
Microangiopathy Overall, the results suggest a benefit for O-(beta-hydroxyethyl)-rutoside in microangiopathy (disease of the small blood vessels). However, the results have not been conclusive.	C
Retinal Vein Occlusion Some clinical research has been conducted in the area of retinal vein occlusion. However, the available evidence is not sufficient to support this use.	C
Retinopathy Preliminary evidence does not suggest that tri-(hydroxyethyl)-rutin offer benefits to retinopathy patients.	C
Schizophrenia One well-designed study suggests that O-(beta-hydroxyethyl)-rutoside may offer benefit in cases of schizophrenia.	C
Skin Conditions In one clinical trial, O-(beta-hydroxyethyl)-rutoside offered benefit in terms of skin irritation to individuals with breast cancer undergoing radiation treatment.	C
Thrombosis Superficial vein thrombosis (SVT) is a common complication of varicose veins. One clinical trial suggests that Venoruton, in combination with elastic compression or thrombectomy, offers benefit as compared with these treatments alone.	C
Varicose Leg Ulcers Rutin, in combination with compression, appears to have benefit over compression alone in the treatment of varicose leg ulcers. However, results are conflicting.	C

Uses Based on Scientific Evidence	Grade
Varicose Veins Overall, the evidence suggests a benefit of troxerutin or O-(beta-hydroxyethyl) rutoside for varicosis. However, the available evidence has not been conclusive.	C
Venous Hypertension Overall, the results suggest a benefit of hydroxyethyl-rutoside for venous hypertension (high blood pressure). However, the available evidence has not been conclusive.	C

Uses Based on Tradition or Theory

Anticoagulant (dicoumarin damage), antioxidant, arrhythmia (cardiac rhythm abnormalities), atherosclerosis (arterial insufficiency), blood circulation (hemodynamic effects), brain injuries (cerebral function disorders), breast disease (mastopathy), common cold, coronary heart disease (CHD), deafness (sudden), dental procedures, eye diseases (euthyroid endocrine ophthalmopathy), gastric ulcer, Graves' disease (orbitopathy), immunomodulation, inflammation (oral, radiogenic sialadenitis and mucositis), mucositis, multiple sclerosis, musculoskeletal conditions (orthopedics), neck pain (cervical syndrome), nutritional deficiencies (trophic complications), osteoarthritis, pain, platelet aggregation (inhibition), postoperative pain, recovery after surgery (recovery from hemorrhoidectomy), sepsis, surgical uses, trauma.

DOSING
Adults (18 Years and Older)

- There are various preparations of rutin used in clinical trials, including capsules, sachets, and injections. Various dosages of hydroxyethylrutoside (HR) have been used, including 500 mg twice daily and 250-300 mg three to four times daily for 28 days. The most commonly used dose by mouth is 1-2 g of rutin daily in divided doses for 4 weeks. However, up to 3500 mg has been studied in clinical trials. Rutin has also been taken as trihydroxyethylrutoside (troxerutin) and oxerutin. Brand name products studied include Venoruton and Paroven.
- Venoruton 1 g three times daily is a commonly used dose in combination with elastic compression for 8 weeks to treat superficial vein thrombosis or flight edema.
- Troxerutin is typically taken in higher doses of 3500-7000 mg daily in divided doses for up to 4 months. To treat venous insufficiency in premenstrual and pregnant women, 4 g daily troxerutin has been given for 4 months.
- One 300-mg tablet of trihydroxyethylrutoside twice daily for up to 4 weeks has been used for hemorrhoids. However, 500-4000 mg HR given by mouth twice daily in the treatment of first-, second-, or third-degree hemorrhoids is more commonly used.
- For schizophrenia, 3 g/day of a mixture of O-(beta-hydroxyethyl)-rutosides (Paroven/Venoruton) for 3 months has been used.
- A single injection of 1000 mg HR followed by 500 mg three times daily by mouth for 4 weeks has been used for chronic venous insufficiency. Injections should be given only under the supervision of a qualified health care professional, including a pharmacist.

Children (Younger than 18 Years)

- There is insufficient evidence to recommend a dose of rutin in children.

SAFETY
Allergies

- Avoid in individuals with a known allergy or hypersensitivity to O-(beta-hydroxyethyl)-rutoside or plants that rutin is commonly found in, such as rue, tobacco, or buckwheat. One case of leg dermatitis was noted in an elderly patient taking O-(beta-hydroxyethyl)-rutoside.

Side Effects and Warnings

- Rutins, oxerutins, and troxerutins have been used effectively and safely in several clinical and equivalence trials. Numerous reports have reported no adverse side effects with rutin treatment. Laboratory findings were noted as unchanged. Few adverse effects have been reported, most of which were mild or transient. Rutin is possibly unsafe when taken in very high doses for long periods of time.
- Adverse effects reported while taking O-(beta-hydroxyethyl)-rutoside have included monocytosis, eosinophilia (increased white blood cell count), deep vein thrombosis, superficial thrombophlebitis, skin rash, hair loss, gastritis (stomach inflammation), vomiting, diarrhea, constipation, dry mouth, abdominal pain, headache, acute brain syndrome, dizziness, sleeping problems, tiredness, swelling, muscle stiffness, and upper respiratory tract infection.
- Use cautiously in elderly patients; most adverse effects have been reported in elderly populations.
- Use cautiously in individuals with skin conditions; dermatitis has been noted with use.

Pregnancy and Breastfeeding

- Rutin supplements have been safely used during pregnancy to treat venous insufficiency, hemorrhoids, and varicose veins. Consult with a qualified health care professional, including a pharmacist, before taking rutin to make sure that the benefits of rutin supplementation outweigh the risks in each individual. Rutin is not recommended in breastfeeding women because of a lack of available scientific evidence.

INTERACTIONS
Interactions with Drugs

- Rutin is often used in combination with coumarin. Caution is advised in patients with bleeding disorders or taking drugs that may increase the risk of bleeding. Dosing adjustments may be necessary.
- Phlogenzym tablets (a combination product containing rutin) have been used with antibiotics. In theory, rutin should be safe to combine with antibiotics.
- Theoretically, rutin may have additive effects when used in combination with benzopyrones, antiedema drugs, Wobenzym (contains rutin), Dicynone, or Reparil.
- Intramuscular administration of the fixed combination of troxerutin and carbazochrome has been well tolerated in improving hemorrhoidal and postsurgical symptoms during the 5 days following surgery. Injections should be given only under the supervision of a qualified health care professional, including a pharmacist.

R

- Theoretically, rutin may have additive effects when used in combination with diuretics. Caution is advised.
- Taking hydroxyethylrutoside by mouth may counteract docetaxel fluid retention.
- N-acetylcysteine (NAC) in combination with rutin may reduce ethane and malondialdehyde (MDA) concentrations and increase the glutathione (GSH) concentration; this combination may be efficient in protecting the lungs of patients with adult respiratory distress syndrome.
- High doses of O-(beta-hydroxyethyl)-rutoside may counteract the unwanted activity of birth control pills on venous function.
- Theoretically, rutin may competitively inhibit action of quinolone antibiotics, which are used in the treatment of malaria.

Interactions with Herbs and Dietary Supplements

- Oxerutins may have an additive effect when used concomitantly with horse chestnut extract.

- Rutosid enzyme is often used in combination with bromelain and trypsin. Based on early evidence, troxerutin appears safe for use with *Gingko biloba* for the treatment of hemorrhoids.
- NAC in combination with rutin may reduce ethane and MDA concentrations and increase the GSH concentration; this combination may be efficient in protecting the lungs of patients with adult respiratory distress syndrome.
- Rutin supplements may have an additive effect with quercetin supplements because quercetin is a flavonoid derived from rutin.
- Theoretically, rutin may increase absorption of vitamin C. Rutin is found in buckwheat herb tea and thus may have an additive effect when taken concomitantly.

For a complete list of references, please visit www.naturalstandard.com.

Safflower
(Carthamus tinctorius)

RELATED TERMS

- American saffron, Asteraceae (family), bastard saffron, *Carthamus tinctorius*, *Carthamus tinctorius* L., Compositae (family), dyer's saffron, EH0202, fake saffron, false saffron, high oleic acid safflower oil, hing hua, honghua, Intralipid, kinobeon A, linoleate, linoleic acid, Liposyn, Liposyn II, Modified Liposyn, Microlipid, monounsaturated fatty acids (MUFA), n-6, n-6 polyunsaturated fatty acid, n-6 rich vegetable oils, nonesterified fatty acid (NEFA), N-(p-coumaroyl) serotonin, oleate, omega 6, polyunsaturated fat, polyunsaturated fatty acids (PUFA), polyunsaturated fat (PSF), SAF, safflower injection, safflower meal, safflower oil, safflower oil cake, safflower oil emulsion, safflower oil esters, safflower oil-based lipid emulsion, safflower petals, safflower seeds, safflower yellow, safloroil, Safola, tocopherols, triglyceride, US, zaffer, zafran.

BACKGROUND

- Two parts of the safflower are primarily used: the flower itself and safflower seeds. There are two types of safflower oil with corresponding types of safflower varieties: those high in monounsaturated fatty acid (oleic) and those high in polyunsaturated fatty acid (linoleic). Currently, the seed varieties that produce oil high in oleic acid and very low in saturated fatty acids predominate in the United States market. High oleic safflower oil is lower in saturates and higher in monounsaturates than olive oil.
- In the U.S. diet, safflower oil has been frequently substituted for oils with higher saturated fat content because monounsaturated fat may have a beneficial effect on the risk of coronary heart disease.
- Some clinical studies have shown that safflower oil supplementation may be helpful in patients with cystic fibrosis, Friedreich's ataxia, and neurotoxicity from lithium. However, more study is needed in these areas before a firm conclusion can be drawn.
- In traditional Chinese medicine, safflower is used to invigorate the blood and dissipate stasis, amenorrhea (absence of menstruation), pain, and traumatic injuries. It is also used to "calm" a live fetus and abort a dead fetus; therefore it should be used cautiously during pregnancy.

EVIDENCE

Uses Based on Scientific Evidence	Grade
Deficiency (Fatty Acid) Fatty acid intake is required for many physiological processes, including cellular maintenance, skin repair, and production of prostaglandins. Safflower oil may improve fatty acid deficiency, especially oleic acid, linoleic acid, and archadonic acid levels.	B
Angina Pectoris/Coronary Artery Disease Safflower yellow injection has been used to improve symptoms for angina pectoris and coronary artery disease in both western and traditional Chinese	C

medicine. However, safety and effectiveness have not been conclusively demonstrated.

Atherosclerosis (Lipid Peroxidation) Limited available evidence suggests that safflower oil may increase oxidation of low-density lipoproteins (LDL) and lower levels of thiobarbituric acid reactive substances (TBARS) when compared with fish oil.	C
Cardiovascular Disorders (Chronic Cor Pulmonale) Safflower oil has lowered high blood pressure and coagulation in patients with chronic cor pulmonale, although there is limited available evidence.	C
Chronic Hepatitis (Hepatitis C) EH0202 is a traditional Japanese Kampo therapy containing safflower seed extract and is used for immunostimulation. EH0202 may decrease hepatitis C virus ribonucleic acid (RNA) levels in patients with high viral titers. The direct effects of safflower remain unclear.	C
Cystic Fibrosis Cystic fibrosis patients are frequently deficient in fatty acids because of reduced absorption of nutrients. Results from studies using safflower oil supplements are mixed.	C
Diabetes Mellitus Type 2 Lipid (fat) abnormalities are commonly associated with diabetes, and complications of atherosclerotic disease are frequently associated with diabetes. Safflower oil may negatively affect glucose metabolism because of the extra intake of energy or fat, but these effects may be less pronounced than in fish oil.	C
Familial Hyperlipidemia Ingestion of certain lipids is known to affect various serum lipid levels. Preliminary evidence suggests that ingestion of safflower oil may reduce serum cholesterol levels. Additional study is needed.	C
Friedreich's Ataxia Friedreich's ataxia is a genetic neurodegenerative disease. There is some clinical evidence that safflower may decrease deterioration caused by Friedreich's ataxia. Rigorous clinical evidence is lacking.	C
Hypercholesterolemia Ingestion of certain lipids is known to affect various serum lipid levels. In the case of safflower oil, results are conflicting. More study is needed before a firm conclusion can be drawn.	C
Hypertension (High Blood Pressure) Based on preliminary evidence, safflower oil may be involved in synthesis of prostaglandins, which are	C

(Continued)

S

631

Uses Based on Scientific Evidence	Grade
responsible for vascular regulation and inflammatory responses and may affect hypertension (high blood pressure). However, there is conflicting evidence that safflower oil ingestion decreases or does not affect blood pressure.	
Kidney Disorders (Type II Nephritic Syndrome) There is currently insufficient available evidence to recommend for or against the use of safflower in the treatment of type II nephritic syndrome.	C
Malnutrition (Protein-Energy) Safflower oil has been used in patients with protein-energy malnutrition to promote balance in their nutritional intake. Although the patients improved, the effect cannot be isolated to safflower oil intake because of the many other nutrients the patients were ingesting.	C
Nutritional Supplement (Infant Formula) Infants require higher fat intake to support their rapid growth and brain development. Infant formula supplemented with safflower oil may increase the energy density of formula for very-low-birth-weight neonates. Although preliminary research is promising, strong clinical evidence is lacking.	C
Skin Conditions (Phrynoderma) Preliminary evidence looks promising for the use of safflower oil in the treatment of phrynoderma, a rough, dry skin generally associated with a vitamin A deficiency.	C
Total Parenteral Nutrition (TPN) Parenteral nutrition requires a certain percentage of fats to provide full nutrition. Various sources of fats have been used, including safflower oil. Overall, clinical trials have shown safflower oil TPN to be safe when used at the doses in the trials. However, more studies should be conducted to see whether safflower oil is superior to other sources of TPN lipids.	C
Toxicity (Lithium) Based on preliminary study, safflower oil may effectively remit the symptoms of neurotoxicity from lithium.	C

Uses Based on Tradition or Theory

Abortifacient (induces abortion), Alzheimer's disease prevention, amenorrhea (absence of menstruation), antiaging, anticoagulant (blood-thinning), antiinflammatory, antioxidant, antiperspirant, appetite suppressant, blood stagnation, bronchial irritation, cardiovascular, cathartic, circulatory/blood flow disorders (hyperemia in women), cognition, constipation, cosmetic coloring, cough, diaphoretic (promotes sweating), dysmenorrhea (painful menstruation), emmenagogue (stimulates menstruation), expectorant, fabric dyes, fever, food uses, hair growth, human immunodeficiency virus (HIV), immunomodulation, inflammation after tooth extraction (dry socket), laxative, memory, neuromuscular disorders (essential tremor), pain, paint solvent, prostate cancer, stimulant, trauma, tumors, uterine stimulant, vaginal dryness (lubricant), venous disorders (phlebitis).

DOSING
Adults (18 Years and Older)

- Safflower oil has been used in varying doses in numerous clinical trials, and there is no proven effective dose. However, Liposyn is possibly safe when used for up to 10 days to prevent essential fatty acid deficiency. When administered to patients undergoing operations, 10%-20% safflower oil emulsions as 30%-50% of total caloric intake were found to be safe as a major component of adult parenteral nutrition for up to 42 days, including cardiopulmonary bypass patients and in children for up to 2 weeks.
- For high blood pressure, 1-6 g safflower oil daily for up to 8 weeks has been used, as has 23 g daily of linoleic acid or oleic acid (constituents of safflower seed oil) for 4 weeks. As an anticoagulant (blood thinner), 60 mL daily of safflower oil for 2 weeks has been used. For atherosclerosis (lipid peroxidation), 15 g of safflower oil daily has been used in postmenopausal women. Higher doses of safflower oil (102-132 mg/kg) daily have been studied for 6 weeks for cystic fibrosis.
- Ethyl ester of safflower oil and linoleic acid have also been taken by mouth. Continued topical application of safflower oil (60%-70% linoleic acid) for at least 21 days has been used for fatty acid deficiency.

Children (Younger than 18 Years)

- Safflower oil has been used primarily in neonatal total parenteral nutrition. Brands studied include Liposyn and Modified Liposyn. Both 10% and 20% Liposyn are equally safe and effective components of a parenteral nutrition program for children. Examples of other doses studied in clinical trials include 1.0 g/kg of safflower oil emulsion for 4 hours; 0.34-0.68 g/kg of Liposyn daily for 5 days in preterm infants; 0.68 g/kg of Modified Liposyn daily for 5 days in preterm infants; 23 g of Liposyn 20%, 25 g of Modified Liposyn 20%, or 50 g of safflower oil-based lipid emulsion daily for up to 7 days.

SAFETY
Allergies

- Avoid in individuals with a known allergy or hypersensitivity to safflower. Safflower is a member of the daisy family (Asteraceae/Compositae) and may cause allergic reactions in patients sensitive to daisies. Other members of this family include ragweed, chrysanthemums, marigolds, and many other plants. A case of contact dermatitis from safflower has been reported.

Side Effects and Warnings

- In several clinical trials, 10%-20% safflower oil emulsions were found to be safe and effective as a major component of adult parenteral nutrition. Both 10% and 20% Liposyn are equally safe and effective components of a parenteral nutrition program for children. The most common adverse effects of safflower oil are cardiovascular, including increased serum lipids, and gastrointestinal, including diarrhea and loose stools.
- Intravenous fat emulsion in newborns may cause hyperlipemia (high cholesterol) if serum triglyceride and free fatty acid levels are not monitored.
- Belching, loose stools, nausea, vomiting, and diarrhea have been reported in patients taking safflower oil daily. Ingestion of high doses of safflower oil per day may decrease blood pressure. Use cautiously in patients with hypotension

(low blood pressure), as safflower oil may cause a modest fall in blood pressure.

- Adverse effects reported in neonates taking Modified Liposyn include tachycardia (increased heart rate) and tachypnea (rapid breathing). Patients taking Microlipid, a safflower oil emulsion taken by mouth, have reported a feeling of fullness, nausea, loss of appetite, bad aftertaste, stomach cramps, and diarrhea.

- Other possible side effects of safflower supplementation that have been noted in clinical trials include cardiac arrhythmia (altered heart rate), diarrhea, angina (chest pain), death, increase in acne, development of diabetes, and development of necrotizing enterocolitis (intestinal illness in babies). These adverse effects are rare, and it is unclear whether they can be solely attributed to safflower or whether another study drug caused these side effects. Use cautiously in patients with diabetes, as safflower oil may adversely affect glycemic control in type 2 diabetes patients.

- Eosinophilia (increased number of white blood cells) developed in three newborn infants administered parenteral safflower oil emulsion for 2 weeks. Hypertriglyceridemia (elevated level of triglycerides and fatty acid compounds) has been reported during the intravenous infusion (injection) of a safflower oil-based fat emulsion. Elevation of serum triglyceride and liver enzyme concentrations occurred in some patients administered Liposyn. Use safflower oil and parenteral safflower oil emulsions cautiously in patients with inadequate liver function, as they have been associated with elevation of liver enzyme concentrations.

- Use parenteral safflower oil emulsions cautiously in newborns, as serum triglyceride and free fatty acid levels must be monitored to avoid the complications of iatrogenic hyperlipemia (high cholesterol levels) and intolerance. Use cautiously in patients with hypercoagulability, as safflower oil infusion may increase this condition.

- Use cautiously in patients with skin pigmentation conditions, as kinobeon A, a rose-colored pigment found in safflower tissue, has demonstrated potent tyrosinase activity.

Pregnancy and Breastfeeding

- Safflower flower is possibly unsafe in pregnant women, as *Carthamus tinctorius* may have stimulating action on the uterus. However, safflower oil is likely safe when used in food amounts in healthy patients. Soybean/safflower lipid-based emulsions are likely safe when administered to pregnant patients. Safflower oil is likely safe when used in breastfeeding women, although there is rapid transfer of dietary fatty acids into human milk.

INTERACTIONS
Interactions with Drugs

- In children with cystic fibrosis, ingestion of safflower oil, antacids, cimetidine, and pancreatic capsules caused greater increases in plasma linoleic acid levels.

- Safflower may increase the risk of bleeding. Caution is advised in patients with bleeding disorders or taking drugs that may increase the risk of bleeding. Some examples include aspirin, anticoagulants ("blood thinners") such as warfarin (Coumadin) or heparin, antiplatelet drugs such as clopidogrel (Plavix), and nonsteroidal antiinflammatory drugs (NSAIDs) such as ibuprofen (Motrin, Advil) or naproxen (Naprosyn, Aleve). Dosing adjustments may be necessary.

- Safflower may prohibit platelet aggregation and anticoagulation and may promote microcirculation. Caution is advised when safflower is taken with calcium channel blockers (verapamil). However, results are conflicting because safflower oil has also been documented to cause hypercoagulation. Check with a qualified health care professional before combining therapies.

- Ingestion of safflower oil may decrease serum total cholesterol, high-density lipoprotein (HDL), low-density lipoprotein (LDL), apolipoprotein B, and malondialdehyde-LDL levels. Results are conflicting; nonetheless, caution is advised in patients taking cholesterol-lowering agents in combination with safflower oil.

- Safflower oil may alter blood sugar levels; however, clinical relevance is unclear. Caution is advised when medications that may lower blood sugar are used. Patients taking drugs for diabetes by mouth or using insulin should be monitored closely by a qualified health care professional, including a pharmacist. Medication adjustments may be necessary.

- Safflower oil may cause a modest fall in blood pressure and interact additively with hypotensive (blood pressure–lowering) agents. However, several other clinical studies have shown no effect on blood pressure.

- Safflower oil may have immunostimulation properties. Although clinical relevance is unknown, caution is advised when immunostimulating agents and safflower oil are combined.

- Although not well studied in humans, safflower oil may remit the symptoms of low-dose lithium neurotoxicity. This appears to be a positive interaction, although more study is needed to clarify this finding.

- Safflower oil may increase pentobarbital-associated mortalities.

- Kinobeon A, a rose-colored pigment found in safflower tissue, demonstrated potent tyrosinase activity. Caution is advised when safflower oil is taken with tyrosinase inhibitors.

Interactions with Herbs and Dietary Supplements

- In children with cystic fibrosis, ingestion of safflower oil, antacids, cimetidine, and pancreatic capsules caused greater increases in plasma linoleic acid levels. In theory, safflower oil may interact with herbs or supplements with antacid effects.

- Safflower may increase the risk of bleeding. Caution is advised in patients with bleeding disorders or taking herbs or supplements that are believed to increase the risk of bleeding.

- Safflower oil may interact additively with fish oil to reduce C-reactive protein and interleukin-6. However, results are unclear. Caution is advised when fish oil is combined with safflower oil.

- Ingestion of safflower oil may decrease serum total cholesterol, HDL, LDL, apolipoprotein B, and malondialdehyde-LDL. Results are conflicting; nonetheless, caution is advised in patients taking cholesterol-lowering agents, such as red yeast rice, in combination with safflower oil.

- Safflower oil may alter blood sugar levels. Caution is advised when herbs or supplements that may lower blood sugar are used. Blood glucose levels may require monitoring, and doses may need adjustment.

- Safflower oil may cause a modest fall in blood pressure and interact additively with hypotensive (blood pressure–

lowering) agents. However, several other clinical studies have shown no effect on blood pressure.

- Safflower may interact when taken with safflower-containing products, such as Renal Disease Basic-prescription (RDBP) and EH0202 (pumpkin seed extract, safflower seed extract, Asian plantain seed extract, and Japanese honeysuckle flower extract). Safflower oil may also interact with calcium.

For a complete list of references, please visit www.naturalstandard.com.

Sage
(Salvia officinalis)

RELATED TERMS

- Black sage, broad-leafed sage, common sage, dalmatian sage, east Mediterranean sage, edelsalbei, feuilles de sauge (French), garden sage, gartensalbei, Greek sage, Herba salviae, kitchen sage, Labiatae (former family name), Lamiaceae (family), meadow sage, Newe Ya'ar No. 4, oleoresin sage, quinines, red sage, royleanones, salbeiblatter, *Salvia fruticosa*, *Salvia hispanorum* Lag., *Salvia officinalis* Lavandulaefolia, *Salvia officinalis* Lavandulaefolia Vahl., *Salvia libanotica*, *Salvia mellifera*, *Salvia officinalis*, *Salvia officinalis* L. "Desislava," *Salvia officinalis* var. purpurea, *Salvia officinalis* x *Salvia fruticosa*, *Salvia reflexa* Hornem., *Salvia triloba*, Salvin, sawge, scarlet sage, Spanish sage, true sage.
- **Note:** This monograph does not contain information on clary sage (*Salvia sclarea*), red or Chinese sage (danshen or *Salvia miltiorrhiza*), prairie sage (*Artemisia ludoviciana*), white sage (*Salvia apiana*), or Jerusalem sage (*Phlomis fruticosa*).

BACKGROUND

- Sage has been used in Europe for centuries as a spice and a medicine. There are many different species of sage, with some reports describing more than 500 species. However, *Salvia officinalis* is more commonly used medicinally, horticulturally, and commercially. Many cultivars of *Salvia officinalis* have been developed, such as *Salvia officinalis* lavandulaefolia (characterized by small leaves).
- Sage is a popular European treatment for inflammations of the mouth and throat, upset stomach, and excessive sweating, in addition to other uses. An extract of sage (*Salvia libanotica*) native to the Mediterranean region has been noted as a popular plant remedy used by Middle Eastern people as a soporific and antimicrobial and to treat colds, influenza, abdominal pain, headaches, heart disorders, and gallstones. Sage has a long history of use against inflammation of the oral cavity and throat when used as a mouthwash or gargle, especially in Europe.
- The strongest evidence for the use of sage comes from clinical trials conducted with sage for Alzheimer's disease, menopausal discomfort, pharyngitis, herpes infections, and to improve mood, cognition, and memory. Potential uses of sage include decreasing menopausal symptoms and for lung cancer prevention.

EVIDENCE

Uses Based on Scientific Evidence	Grade
Cognitive Improvement Sage has long been suggested to improve memory. Several trials provide evidence for the use of sage. Additional study is needed to confirm these findings and determine the best dose.	A
Mood Enhancement Sage has long been suggested to improve mood. Several trials provide evidence for the use of sage.	A
Additional study is needed to confirm these findings and determine the best dose.	
Acute Pharyngitis Sage mouthwashes and gargles have been approved for use against sore throat in Germany by the German Commission E for many years. Additional study is needed comparing sage with standard therapies.	B
Alzheimer's Disease Alzheimer's disease is characterized by memory loss that interferes with social and occupational functioning. Early evidence suggests that sage oil may be useful for treating Alzheimer's disease.	B
Herpes Early evidence suggests that sage extracts may be useful for treating herpes skin manifestations.	B
Menopausal Symptoms Sage has been tested against menopausal symptoms with promising results.	B
Lung Cancer Prevention Sage used daily as a spice in foods has been associated with a lower risk of lung cancer in the Mediterranean diet.	C

Uses Based on Tradition or Theory

Abdominal pain, aging, antibacterial, antifungal, antiinflammatory, antimicrobial, antioxidant, antiseptic, antitumor, appetite stimulant, asthma, bad breath, baldness, bleeding gums, bloating, bone loss, bronchitis, coagulation disorders, colds, diabetes, dyspepsia (upset stomach), estrogenic effects, food uses, *Helicobacter pylori* gastric infection, hemorrhoids, inflammation (intestinal, skin), insect bites, lactation suppression, liver diseases, memory enhancement, periodontitis/gingivitis (gum disease), sedative, sexually transmitted disease, sore throat, stomachic, sweating (excessive), urinary tract infection, venereal disease.

DOSING
Adults (18 Years and Older)

- Doses of 25-50 mcL of the essential oil have been taken by mouth one to three times daily. Single daily doses of 60 drops of an ethanolic extract of *Salvia officinalis* were used in a clinical study with benefit. A combination of 120 mg of sage extract and 60 mg of alfalfa extract (*Medicago sativa*) has been used daily for up to 3 months to alleviate symptoms of menopause. Dried sage leaf, 300 or 600 mg, in single daily doses has been used. A 15% spray containing 140 mcL of *Salvia officinalis* extract per dose has been applied to the skin six to nine times daily for 3 days.

Children (Younger than 18 Years)

- There is insufficient evidence to recommend a dose for sage in children. However, secondary sources note that children have safely eaten sage as a spice in foods for many centuries.

SAFETY
Allergies

- Avoid in individuals with a known allergy or hypersensitivity to sage species, their constituents, or to members of the Lamiaceae family. Systemic allergic reactions relating to cross-sensitivity have been noted.
- Dust from sage plants may contain airborne microorganisms that may induce allergic reactions in farm workers and herb processors.
- Sage powder should not be used for asthma. Although some formulations of sage have been reported to be useful in asthma, sage powder is not appropriate for use in asthmatic patients because it can cause bronchial reactions.

Side Effects and Warnings

- Sage (*Salvia officinalis*) is uncontrolled in the United States. This means all parts of the plant and its extracts are legal to cultivate, buy, possess, and distribute (sell, trade, or give) without a license or prescription. If sold as a supplement, sales must conform to U.S. supplement laws. If sold for consumption as a food or drug, the U.S. Food and Drug Administration (FDA) regulates sales. Sage is approved for food use as a spice or seasoning in the United States and appears on the FDA's list of substances "generally recognized as safe" (GRAS).
- Skin rash may occur in some patients who are exposed to the leaves.
- Sage is likely safe when included in the preparation of foods as a spice or for upset stomach because of a long history of use around the world. Sage is also likely safe when used in moderate amounts as a cream applied to the skin for herpes infections.
- Certain medicinal preparations or high doses of sage have been documented to induce seizures. Large amounts or prolonged use of sage leaf or ingestion of sage oil may cause restlessness, vomiting, dizziness, rapid heart beats, tremors, seizures, and kidney damage.
- Some patients may exhibit increases in blood pressure during sage essential oil therapy.
- When a 15% spray containing sage extract was used for 3 days, minor dry pharynx or mild burning of the throat was reported in some patients. Other side effects may include cheilitis (cracking and drying of the lips), stomatitis (mouth sores), dry mouth, and local irritation.
- A plant preparation that is not sterile and not free of particles should not be used in the eye because these preparations may damage the cornea.
- Sage powder should not be used for asthma because sage powder can cause asthmatic attacks.

Pregnancy and Breastfeeding

- Because of a lack of available scientific evidence, women should avoid sage supplementation during pregnancy and breastfeeding. Hormonal effects are possible and could be dangerous.

INTERACTIONS
Interactions with Drugs

- Sage essential oil and tinctures may increase the effects of drugs used for treating Alzheimer's disease.
- Sage extracts may have antimicrobial effects.
- Sage may lower blood sugar levels. Caution is advised when medications that may also lower blood sugar are used. Patients taking drugs for diabetes by mouth or using insulin should be monitored closely by a qualified health care professional, including a pharmacist. Medication adjustments may be necessary.
- Sage may have antiinflammatory activity. Use cautiously with antiinflammatory medications because of possible additive effects.
- Sage may have antioxidant activity.
- Use cautiously with benzodiazepines or drugs broken down by the liver. Sage may increase sedation.
- Sage essential oil and tinctures can induce seizures and may enhance the ability of some drugs to induce seizures.
- Sage essential oil may have estrogenic activity. Extracts of the leaves of sage may abolish hot flashes and night sweating in some menopausal women.
- Use cautiously with thyroid hormones because of possible additive effects.

Interactions with Herbs and Dietary Supplements

- Sage may increase the effects of alfalfa (*Medicago sativa*) on the reduction of menopausal symptoms, including hot flashes, insomnia, nocturnal sweating, dizziness, headaches, and palpitations.
- Sage essential oil and tinctures may increase the anticholinergic effects of herbs and medications used for treating Alzheimer's disease.
- Sage extracts may have antimicrobial effects.
- Some species of sage may cause convulsions. Theoretically, this might interfere with anticonvulsant drug therapy.
- Sage may have antiinflammatory activity. Caution is advised when other antiinflammatory herbs or supplements are taken because of possible additive effects.
- Based on laboratory studies, sage may have antioxidant activity.
- Sage may interact with therapies that are broken down by the liver.
- Sage may lower blood sugar levels. Caution is advised when herbs or supplements that may also lower blood sugar are used. Blood glucose levels may require monitoring, and doses may need adjustment.
- Sage essential oil may have estrogenic activity. In addition, extracts of the leaves of sage may abolish hot flashes and night sweating in some menopausal women. Caution is advised in patients taking phytoestrogens.
- Sage may increase the amount of drowsiness caused by some herbs or supplements.
- Sage may induce a significant increase in thyroid-stimulating hormone and interact with other herbs and supplements that affect the thyroid.

For a complete list of references, please visit www.naturalstandard.com.

Salvia
(Salvia divinorum)

RELATED TERMS

- Diviner's mint, diviner's sage, hardwickiic acid, hierba Maria (Spanish), hojas de la pastora (Spanish), hojas de Maria pastora (Spanish), la hembra (Spanish), la Maria (Spanish), Lamiaceae (family), loliolide, magic mint, María pastora, Mexican mint, mint plant, neoclerodane diterpene, neoclerodane diterpenoids, presqualene alcohol, sage of the seers, Sally-D, salvia, salvinorinyl-2-heptanoate, shepherdess's herb, ska Maria pastora (Mazatec), ska pastora (Mazatec), the female, yerba de Maria (Spanish), yerba Maria (Spanish).

BACKGROUND

- Salvia (*Salvia divinorum*) is a hallucinogenic plant that is traditionally used by the Mazatec culture in central Mexico. It is grown in California and other parts of the United States where it is used as a legal hallucinogen and is becoming popular with teenagers and young adults. Laws in Finland, Denmark, and Australia prohibit cultivating, consuming, or dealing with salvia.
- Most studies have investigated salvia's active constituent, salvinorin A. Currently, there are no high-quality trials investigating salvia's therapeutic uses. Animal studies of salvia have not shown any toxicity even at high doses, but use of salvia can cause central nervous system (CNS) and psychiatric effects because of its hallucinogenic properties. Some researchers believe that salvinorin A may show promise as a psychotherapeutic compound for diseases manifested by perceptual distortions (e.g., schizophrenia, dementia, and bipolar disorders).

EVIDENCE

Uses Based on Scientific Evidence

No available studies qualify for inclusion in the evidence table.

Uses Based on Tradition or Theory

Alzheimer's disease, bipolar disorder, cardiovascular disease, dementia, depression, diarrhea, drug abuse (stimulant), gastrointestinal motility, hallucinogenic, pain, pruritus (severe itching), schizophrenia.

DOSING

Adults (18 Years and Older)

- There is insufficient evidence to recommend a dose for salvia in adults.

Children (Younger than 18 Years)

- There is insufficient evidence to recommend a dose for salvia in children.

SAFETY

Allergies

- Avoid in individuals with a known allergy or hypersensitivity to salvia.

Side Effects and Warnings

- Salvia may cause decreased heart rate, increased perspiration, changes in body temperature, chills, inability to control muscles, inability to maintain balance, loss of coordination, and short-term effects on motor control. The effects of salvia are typically short lived.
- Salvia may induce hallucinations and psychedelic-like changes in visual perception and mood. Visual hallucinations may include perception of bright lights and vivid colors and shapes, as well as body movements and body or object distortions.
- Dizziness, slurred speech, nausea, awkward sentence patterns, and general change in consciousness have been reported.
- Use cautiously in patients with psychiatric disorders, including depression, because of salvia's ability to induce hallucinations and other mood changes.

Pregnancy and Breastfeeding

- Salvia is not recommended in pregnant or breastfeeding women because of a lack of available scientific evidence.

INTERACTIONS

Interactions with Drugs

- Salvia may have hallucinogenic effects. Salvia may also have additive effects with other opioid drugs, and caution is advised when certain pain-relieving agents are taken. Consult with a qualified health care professional before taking salvia with opioids.

Interactions with Herbs and Dietary Supplements

- Salvia may have hallucinogenic effects. Salvia may also have additive effects with other opioids, and caution is advised when certain pain-relieving agents are taken. Consult with a qualified health care professional before taking salvia with opioids.

For a complete list of references, please visit www.naturalstandard.com.

RELATED TERMS

- Alpha-santalol, beta-santalol, East Indian sandalwood, sandal, sandalwood oil, Santalaceae (family), *Santalum album*, white sandalwood.
- **Note**: This monograph does not include false sandalwood (*Myoporum sandwicense*) or red sandalwood (*Pterocarpus santalinus*).

BACKGROUND

- Endemic in Indonesia, Australia, and the Indian peninsula, the *Santalum album* tree is the primary source of sandalwood and sandalwood oil. Both are used in Hindu religious ceremonies. In Ayurvedic medicine, East Indian sandalwood is an important remedy for both physical and mental disorders. Sandalwood is also a popular fragrance for incense and perfumes.
- There is insufficient evidence in humans to support the use of sandalwood for any indication. However, preliminary aromatherapy studies with sandalwood have indicated that it may have anxiolytic (anxiety-reducing) and stimulating properties.

EVIDENCE

Uses Based on Scientific Evidence	Grade
Alertness Preliminary evidence indicates that sandalwood oil may increase alertness; however, more research is needed.	C
Anxiety Sandalwood is frequently used in incense and aromatherapy. Preliminary research indicates that sandalwood may reduce anxiety in palliative patients. However, clinical evidence is insufficient to recommend this use.	C

Uses Based on Tradition or Theory
Antifungal, insect repellent.

DOSING

Adults (18 Years and Older)

- There is insufficient evidence to recommend a dose for sandalwood.

Children (Younger than 18 Years)

- There is insufficient evidence to recommend a dose for sandalwood in children.

SAFETY

Allergies

- Avoid in individuals with a known allergy or hypersensitivity to sandalwood (*Santalum album*) or its constituents. There are reports of sandalwood causing dermatitis and sandalwood oil causing photoallergy.

Side Effects and Warnings

- There are very few reports available of sandalwood and related adverse effects. Of the available literature, there are a few cases of allergic reactions that document dermatitis and photoallergy. Sandalwood is likely safe when 1% sandalwood oil in sweet almond carrier oil is applied to the skin during massage in nonallergic people.

Pregnancy and Breastfeeding

- Sandalwood is not recommended in pregnant or breastfeeding women because of a lack of available scientific evidence.

INTERACTIONS

Interactions with Drugs

- Although not well studied in humans, the sandalwood constituent alpha-santalol may induce apoptosis (cell death), and thus may interact with anticancer agents. Sandalwood may also have antifungal properties, and caution is advised in patients taking antifungal agents.
- Based on preliminary human study, application of the sandalwood oil constituent alpha-santalol on patients' skin may have a relaxing/sedative effect. Combined use of anxiolytics with sandalwood may result in additive effects.

Interactions with Herbs and Dietary Supplements

- Although not well studied in humans, the sandalwood constituent alpha-santalol may induce apoptosis (cell death) and thus may interact with anticancer agents. Sandalwood may also have antifungal properties, and caution is advised in patients taking antifungal agents.
- Based on preliminary human study, application of the sandalwood oil constituent alpha-santalol on patients' skin may have a relaxing/sedative effect. Combined use of anxiolytics with sandalwood may result in additive effects.

For a complete list of references, please visit www.naturalstandard.com.

Sanicle
(*Sanicula europaea*)

RELATED TERMS

- Acylated triterpenoid saponins, Apiaceae (family), caffeic acid, chlorogenic acid, European sanicle, flavonoids, glucopyranosyl rosmarinic acid, neochlorogenic acid, oleanane-type triterpenoid saponins, phenolic acids, phenols, poolroot, quercetin, rosmarinic acid, saccharose, sandrosaponin, *Sanicula aqua*, *Sanicula elata*, *Sanicula elata* Ham. var. *chinensis* Makino, *Sanicula graveolens*, *Sanicula* L., saniculae herba, saniculasaponins, saniculoids, Saniculoideae (Apiaceae subfamily), saniculoside N, saponins, self-heal, triterpene saponin glycosides, triterpenoid saponins, Umbelliferae (family), wood sanicle.
- **Note**: Sanicle has been called "self-heal," which is the common name for *Prunella vulgaris* L., a member of the Lamiaceae family. Sanicle products have been reported to be contaminated with drooping bittercress (*Cardamine enneaphyllos*) and great masterwort (*Astrantia major*).

BACKGROUND

- Sanicle (*Sanicula europaea*) is a perennial plant in the Apiaceae family that is found in woodlands across Europe, Asia, and Africa. Sanicle products are generally made from the aerial plant parts.
- Sanicle has been used for mild lung inflammation and congestion, cough, and bronchitis. Early study has investigated the potential antifungal, antioxidant, antiviral, and anti-HIV effects of sanicle. Sanicle has also been studied for its use in ear infections, atopic eczema, and asthma.

EVIDENCE

Uses Based on Scientific Evidence	Grade
Asthma Sanicle has been studied for use in asthma, although the evidence thus far has not been sufficient to support this use.	C
Ear Infection (Otitis Media) Sanicle may help recurrent ear infections. However, the evidence thus far has not been sufficient to support this use.	C
Skin Problems (Atopic Eczema) Sanicle has been studied for use in atopic eczema. However, the evidence thus far has not been sufficient to support this use.	C

Uses Based on Tradition or Theory

Antifungal, antioxidant, antiviral, bronchitis, cough (suppression or loosening of mucus), flu, hemorrhoids, HIV, lung inflammation, nerve disorders, wounds.

DOSING
Adults (18 Years and Older)

- From 4-6 g of dried or aerial parts of sanicle has been taken by mouth.

Children (Younger than 18 Years)

- There is insufficient evidence to recommend a dose for sanicle, and use in children is not recommended.

SAFETY
Allergies

- Avoid in individuals with a known allergy or hypersensitivity to sanicle. Skin rash has been reported with sanicle.

Side Effects and Warnings

- Use with caution in people taking blood pressure–lowering or diuretic drugs. Avoid in people with gastrointestinal problems because of the risk of stomach upset, nausea, vomiting, and irritation.

Pregnancy and Breastfeeding

- Sanicle is not recommended in pregnant or breastfeeding women because of a lack of available scientific evidence.

INTERACTIONS
Interactions with Drugs

- Sanicle may have additive effects when taken with antifungal, antioxidant, antiretroviral, antiviral, diuretic, and blood pressure–lowering drugs. Sanicle may also add to the effects of drugs that thin mucus.

Interactions with Herbs and Dietary Supplements

- Sanicle may have additive effects when taken with antifungal, antioxidant, antiviral, diuretic, and blood pressure–lowering herbs and supplements. Sanicle may also add to the effects of herbs or supplements that thin mucus.

For a complete list of references, please visit www.naturalstandard.com.

S

Sassafras

(Sassafras spp.)

RELATED TERMS

- Brazilian sassafras, Chinese sassafras, Lauraceae (family), *Ocotea pretiosa*, red sassafras, *Sassafras albidum* (Nutt.) Nees, *Sassafras randaiense* (Hayata) Rehd., *Sassafras tzumu* (Hemsl.) Hemsl., silky sassafras, Taiwan sassafras, tzumu (Chinese), white sassafras.

BACKGROUND

- The genus *Sassafras* contains two main species, *Sassafras albidum* (Nutt.) Nees and *Sassafras tzumu* (Hemsl.) Hemsl. *Sassafras albidum* is found in eastern North America, and *Sassafras tzumu* is found in Asia, primarily in China.
- Although sassafras was used originally in Native American medicine, sassafras should not be used internally, as safrole found in sassafras oil and tea is carcinogenic (cancer causing). Increased incidence of esophageal cancer has been noted in areas with habitual sassafras consumption. In addition, safrole is hepatotoxic and may cause liver damage.
- Sassafras root was used to flavor root beer until it was banned by the U.S. Food and Drug Administration in 1960.
- There is insufficient evidence in humans to support the use of sassafras for any indication.

EVIDENCE

Uses Based on Scientific Evidence

No available studies qualify for inclusion in the evidence table.

Uses Based on Tradition or Theory

Anticoagulant (blood thinner), antifungal, diaphoretic (promotes sweating).

DOSING

Adults (18 Years and Older)

- Because of known toxicity, sassafras should not be used in adults.

Children (Younger than 18 Years)

- Because of known toxicity, sassafras should not be used in children.

SAFETY

Allergies

- Avoid in individuals with a known allergy or hypersensitivity to *Sassafras* species, their constituents, or members of the Lauraceae family.

Side Effects and Warnings

- Safrole found in sassafras oil and tea is carcinogenic (cancer causing). Increased incidence of esophageal cancer has been noted in areas with habitual sassafras consumption. In addition, safrole is hepatotoxic (liver damaging) and may inhibit some cytochrome P450 pathways. Sassafras may also have a diaphoretic (promotes sweating) side effect.
- Use cautiously in patients taking drugs or herbs metabolized by the cytochrome P450 pathways, as safrole may be a potent inhibitor of several of these pathways.
- Avoid in patients with compromised liver function.

Pregnancy and Breastfeeding

- Avoid sassafras tea and oil if pregnant or breastfeeding, as they are considered carcinogenic (cancer causing).

INTERACTIONS

Interactions with Drugs

- Although not well studied in humans, the aryl-sulfonamide compounds found in safrole may induce platelet aggregation. Caution is advised in patients with bleeding disorders and in those taking agents to either clot or thin the blood.
- Safrole may interfere with the way the body processes certain drugs using the liver's cytochrome P450 enzyme system. As a result, the levels of these drugs may be increased in the blood and may cause increased effects or potentially serious adverse reactions. Patients using any medications should check the package insert and speak with a qualified health care professional, including a pharmacist, about possible interactions.

Interactions with Herbs and Dietary Supplements

- Although not well studied in humans, the aryl-sulfonamide compounds found in safrole may induce platelet aggregation. Caution is advised in patients with bleeding disorders and in those taking herbs or supplements that may either clot or thin the blood.
- Safrole may interfere with the way the body processes certain herbs or supplements using the liver's cytochrome P450 enzyme system. As a result, the levels of other herbs or supplements may become too high in the blood. It may also alter the effects that other herbs or supplements possibly have on the P450 system.

For a complete list of references, please visit www. naturalstandard.com.

Saw Palmetto
(Serenoa repens)

RELATED TERMS

- American dwarf palm tree, Arecaceae (family), cabbage palm, dwarf palm, Elusan Prostate, IDS 89, lipidosterolic extract of *Serenoa repens* (LSESR), PA 109, Palmae (family), palmetto scrub, palmier de l'amerique du nord (French), palmier nain (French), Permixon, Prostagutt, Prostaserine, *Sabal*, sabalfruchte (German), *Sabal fructus*, savpalme (Danish), saw palmetto berry, *Serenoa*, *Serenoa repens*, *Serenoa serrulata* Hook F., SG 291, Strogen, WS 1473, Zwegpalme.

BACKGROUND

- Saw palmetto (*Serenoa repens*, *Sabal serrulata*) is used popularly in Europe for symptoms associated with benign prostatic hypertrophy (enlargement of the prostate). Although not considered standard care in the United States, it is the most popular herbal treatment for this condition.
- Historical use of saw palmetto can be traced in the Americas to the Mayans, who used it as a tonic, and to the Seminoles, who took the berries as an expectorant and antiseptic.
- Saw palmetto was listed in the United States Pharmacopeia from 1906 to 1917 and in the National Formulary from 1926 to 1950. Saw palmetto extract is a licensed product in several European countries.
- Multiple mechanisms of action have been proposed, and saw palmetto appears to possess 5-alpha-reductase inhibitory activity (thereby preventing the conversion of testosterone to dihydrotestosterone). Hormonal or estrogenic effects have also been reported, as well as direct inhibitory effects on androgen receptors and antiinflammatory properties.

EVIDENCE

Uses Based on Scientific Evidence	Grade
Enlarged Prostate (Benign Prostatic Hypertrophy [BPH]) Numerous human trials report that saw palmetto improves symptoms of BPH such as nighttime urination, urinary flow, and overall quality of life, although it may not greatly reduce the size of the prostate. The effectiveness may be similar to the medication finasteride (Proscar) with fewer side effects. Although the quality of these studies has been variable, overall they suggest effectiveness. Saw palmetto has not been thoroughly compared with other types of drugs used for BPH, such as doxazosin (Cardura) or terazosin (Hytrin). Most available studies have assessed the standardized saw palmetto product Permixon. Although a 2003 study by Willetts et al. reported no difference over a 12-week period and a 2006 well-designed study by Bent et al. reported no difference over a 12-month period, overall the weight of available scientific evidence favors the effectiveness of saw palmetto over placebo.	A

Male Pattern Hair Loss It has been suggested that saw palmetto may block some effects of testosterone and therefore reduce male pattern hair loss, similar to the medication finasteride (Propecia). However, clinical evidence is not sufficient to support this use.	C
Prostate Cancer There is not enough scientific evidence to recommend the product PC-SPES (which contains saw palmetto) for prostate cancer. PC-SPES also contains seven other herbs (*Chrysanthemum morifolium*, *Isatis indigotica*, *Glycyrrhiza glabra*, *Ganoderma lucidum*, *Panax pseudoginseng*, *Rabdosia rubescens*, and *Scutellaria baicalensis*). It has been a popular treatment for prostate cancer, but the U.S. Food and Drug Administration (FDA) has issued a warning not to use PC-SPES because it contains the anticoagulant chemical warfarin and may cause bleeding.	C
Prostatitis/Chronic Pelvic Pain Syndrome (CP/CPPS) A prospective, randomized, open label, one-year study was designed to assess the safety and efficacy of saw palmetto and finasteride in the treatment of men diagnosed with category III chronic prostatitis/chronic pelvic pain syndrome (CP/CPPS). CP/CPPS treated with saw palmetto had no appreciable long-term improvement. In contrast, patients treated with finasteride had significant and durable improvement in multiple parameters except for voiding.	C
Underactive Bladder There is currently little information on the effectiveness of saw palmetto for the treatment of bladder disorders.	C

Uses Based on Tradition or Theory
Acne, aphrodisiac, asthma, bladder inflammation, breast enlargement or reduction, breastfeeding, bronchitis, cancer, catarrh, cough, cystitis, diabetes, diarrhea, digestive aid, diuretic, dysentery, Epstein-Barr virus, excess hair growth, expectorant, high blood pressure, hormone imbalances (estrogen or testosterone), immune stimulation, impotence, indigestion, inflammation, laryngitis, menstrual pain, migraine headache, muscle or intestinal spasms, ovarian cysts, performance enhancement, polycystic ovarian syndrome, postnasal drip, reproductive organ problems, sedation, sexual vigor, sore throat, sperm production, testicular atrophy, upper respiratory tract infection, uterine or vaginal disorders.

S

DOSING
Adults (18 Years and Older)

- For enlarged prostate (benign prostatic hypertrophy), a dose of 320 mg daily, in one dose or two divided doses (80%-90% liposterolic content), has been used in numerous studies. Reports suggest that 160 mg once daily may be as effective as twice daily.
- Traditional or other suggested doses that are less studied include 1-2 g of ground, dried, or whole berries daily; 2-4 mL of tincture (1:4) three times daily; 1-2 mL fluid extract of berry pulp (1:1) three times daily; or tea (2 teaspoons dried berry with 24 oz water, simmered slowly until liquid is reduced by half) taken as 4 oz three times daily. Teas prepared from saw palmetto berries are potentially not as effective because the active ingredients may not dissolve in water. Some experts believe that a preparation called lipidosterolic extract of *Serenoa repens* (LSESR) may cause fewer side effects.

Children (Younger than 18 Years)

- There is insufficient evidence to recommend the use of saw palmetto in children.

SAFETY
Allergies

- Few allergic symptoms have been reported with saw palmetto. A study of people taking the combination product PC-SPES (no longer commercially available), which includes saw palmetto and seven other herbs, reports that 3 of 70 people developed allergic reactions. In one case, the reaction included throat swelling and difficulty breathing.

Side Effects and Warnings

- Few severe side effects of saw palmetto are noted in the published scientific literature. The most common complaints involve the stomach and intestines, and include stomach pain, nausea, vomiting, bad breath, constipation, and diarrhea. Stomach upset caused by saw palmetto may be reduced by taking it with food. Some reports suggest that there may be less abdominal discomfort with the preparation LSESR. A small number of reports describe ulcers or liver damage and yellowing of the skin (jaundice), but the role of saw palmetto is not clear in these cases. Similarly, reports of headache, dizziness, insomnia, depression, breathing difficulties, muscle pain, high blood pressure, chest pain, abnormal heart rhythm, and heart disease have been reported but are not clearly caused by saw palmetto. People with health conditions involving the stomach, liver, heart, or lungs should use caution.
- Caution is advised in people scheduled to undergo some surgeries or dental work, who have bleeding disorders, or who are taking drugs that may increase the risk of bleeding. Dosing adjustments may be necessary.
- Some men using saw palmetto report difficulty with erections, testicular discomfort, breast tenderness or enlargement, and changes in sexual desire. Saw palmetto may have effects on the body's response to the sex hormones estrogen and testosterone, but no specific effect has been well demonstrated in humans. Men or women taking hormonal medications (such as finasteride [Proscar, Propecia] or birth control pills) or who have hormone-sensitive conditions should use caution. Tinctures may contain high

levels of alcohol; avoid when driving or operating heavy machinery.
- In theory, prostate-specific antigen (PSA) levels may be artificially lowered by saw palmetto, based on a proposed mechanism of action of saw palmetto (inhibition of 5-alpha-reductase). Therefore, there may be a delay in diagnosis of prostate cancer or interference with following PSA levels during treatment or monitoring in men with known prostate cancer.
- The combination product PC-SPES, which contains saw palmetto and seven other herbs, has been found to contain prescription drugs including warfarin, a "blood thinner." The U.S. Food and Drug Administration (FDA) has issued a warning not to use PC-SPES for this reason, and it is no longer commercially available.

Pregnancy and Breastfeeding

- Because of possible hormonal activity, saw palmetto extract is not recommended for women who are pregnant or breastfeeding. Many tinctures contain high levels of alcohol and should be avoided during pregnancy.

INTERACTIONS
Interactions with Drugs

- Saw palmetto may increase the risk of bleeding when taken with drugs that increase the risk of bleeding. Some examples include aspirin, anticoagulants (blood thinners) such as warfarin (Coumadin) or heparin, antiplatelet drugs such as clopidogrel (Plavix), and nonsteroidal antiinflammatory drugs such as ibuprofen (Motrin, Advil) or naproxen (Naprosyn, Aleve). Some batches of the discontinued combination herbal preparation PC-SPES, which contains saw palmetto and seven other herbs, have been found to contain several medications including the blood thinner warfarin.
- Saw palmetto should not be taken with drugs that affect the levels of androgens (male sex hormones), such as finasteride (Proscar, Propecia) or flutamide (Eulexin). In theory, saw palmetto may interfere with birth control pills or hormone replacement therapy in women. Tinctures may contain high levels of alcohol and may cause nausea or vomiting when taken with metronidazole (Flagyl) or disulfiram (Antabuse).
- Study in normal volunteers reveals no effects of saw palmetto on cytochrome P450 3A4 or 2D6 activity.

Interactions with Herbs and Dietary Supplements

- Based on at least two reports of serious bleeding, saw palmetto may increase the risk of bleeding when taken with herbs and supplements that are believed to increase the risk of bleeding. Multiple cases of bleeding have been reported with the use of *Ginkgo biloba*, and fewer cases have been reported with garlic. Numerous other agents may theoretically increase the risk of bleeding, although this has not been proven in most cases.
- Because saw palmetto may have activity on the body's response to estrogen, the effects of other agents believed to have estrogen-like properties may be altered.
- Tannins in saw palmetto may prevent iron absorption.

For a complete list of references, please visit www.naturalstandard.com.

Scotch Broom
(Cytisus scoparius)

RELATED TERMS

- Bannal, basam, Besenginaterkraut, besom, bissom, bream, broom, broom tops, broomtops, browme, brum, common broom, Cystisi scoparii flos, *Cytisus scoparius*, English broom, European broom, Fabaceae (family), genet a balais, *Genista andreana*, *Genista scoparius* (Lam.), Ginsterkraut, green broom, herba spartii scoparii, herbe de genet a balais, herbe de genistae scopariae, herbe de hogweed, hogweed, Irish broom, Irish tops, Leguminosae (family), Papilionaceae (family), sarothamni herb, *Sarothamnus scoparius* (Koch), *Sarothamnus vulgaris*, scoparii cacumina, scoparii herba, scotch broom top, scotchbroom, sparteine, *Spartium scoparium* Linn.
- **Note:** Scotch Broom should not be confused with Spanish broom (*Spartium junceum*), which has been associated with severe toxicity, or Butcher's broom (*Ruscus aculeatus*).

BACKGROUND

- Scotch broom (*Cytisus scoparius*), also referred to as broom, is a perennial woody plant native to Europe. The species was introduced as a garden ornamental to North America and now is common across western Canada and California. Scotch broom plants grow up to 10 feet tall with sharply angled branches off the main stem, trifoliate leaves, and small, bright yellow flowers. Scotch broom spreads quickly and aggressively at the expense of other plants and trees and is often considered a pest.
- Both the flower and herb of scotch broom have been used medicinally. There is very little available scientific evidence about the efficacy or safety of this plant, and most conclusions come from knowledge of its constituents or from traditional use. There is particular concern about the potential toxicity of scotch broom due to the presence of small amounts of the toxic alkaloids sparteine and isosparteine, which are found in both the flowers and herb (above-ground parts). Sparteine has known effects on the electrical conductivity of heart muscle and can potentially cause dangerous heart rhythms or interact with cardiac drugs. Sparteine is also known to cause uterine contractions and should be avoided during pregnancy. Life-threatening adverse effects have been associated with sparteine; therefore scotch broom should be used only under strict medical supervision.

EVIDENCE

Uses Based on Scientific Evidence	Grade
Cardiovascular Conditions Scotch broom herb has been taken by mouth traditionally for a variety of conditions related to the heart or blood circulation. These include abnormal heart rhythms (arrhythmias), fast heart rate (tachycardia), swelling in the legs (peripheral edema), water in the lungs (pulmonary edema, congestive heart failure), and low blood pressure (hypotension).	C

Scotch broom flower has been taken by mouth traditionally for tachycardia and to reduce leg swelling by increasing urination (diuretic), as well as for damage to the heart muscle (cardiomyopathy) and for poor circulation.

There is a scientific basis for some of these uses because of the presence of small amounts of the alkaloid sparteine in scotch broom herb and flower. Sparteine may affect the electrical conductivity of heart muscle (similar to type 1A antiarrhythmic drugs such as quinidine). However, there is limited evidence in humans, and it is not clear whether sparteine found in the plant form has clinically meaningful effects. These potential properties of scotch broom may be dangerous in individuals with heart disease or in those taking cardiac medications. People with cardiovascular disorders should be evaluated and supervised by a licensed health care professional.

Diuretic (Increased Urine Flow) Scotch broom preparations, particularly those made from the flower, have been used traditionally as diuretics (to increase urination). Diuretic effects have been attributed by some to the constituent scoparin or scoparoside. There is insufficient scientific evidence at this time to form clear conclusions about safety or efficacy in humans.	C
Labor Induction (Oxytocic) Scotch broom herb has been used historically to stimulate uterine contractions at birth and to reduce postpartum hemorrhage (bleeding after birth). There is a scientific basis for this use because of the presence in scotch broom of small amounts of the alkaloid sparteine, which was studied and used through the 1970s as an oxytocic drug (to induce labor). This use was discontinued because of serious toxicities associated with sparteine. Currently, other drugs such as oxytocin (Pitocin) are used for this purpose. The safety and efficacy of scotch broom preparations in labor are not well studied or established. Women who may require labor induction should be evaluated and supervised by a physician.	C

Uses Based on Tradition or Theory

Abscess, angina, astringent, beer flavor, bladder disorders, bleeding gums, blood cleansing, bronchitis, cancer, cathartic, coagulation (bleeding) disorders, congestive heart failure, diphtheria, emetic (vomiting inducer), euphoria (when smoked in cigarettes), food flavoring, gallstones, gout, hemophilia, hypertension, inflammation, intoxication, jaundice, kidney inflammation, kidney stones, lice, liver disorders, menorrhagia (excessive menstruation), muscle ache, nausea, postpartum hemorrhage, relaxation (when smoked in cigarettes), rheumatic disorders, sciatica, splenomegaly (enlarged spleen), snake bite, toothache.

DOSING
Adults (18 Years and Older)

- There is insufficient evidence to recommend a dose of scotch broom, and use should be under medical supervision only. Storage of the flower or herb should be in a cool, dry location.
- A juice has been made by pressing the bruised, fresh tops and adding one-third volume alcohol, allowing it to sit for 7 days, followed by filtration, and taken daily as needed. An infusion has been made by adding 1 oz of dried tops to a pint of boiling water (or 1 teaspoon in 200 mL boiling water) and taken as a cupful once or twice daily, as needed.
- As a tea, 1-2 g (1 level teaspoon) of herb can be steeped in 150-200 mL of boiling water, then strained after 5-10 minutes and taken as a cupful, up to three times daily as needed. As a decoction, 1-2 g of herb has been used in preparations. As a liquid extract, a 1:1 preparation in 25% ethanol (v/v) has been prepared and taken as 1-2 mL, as needed. As a tincture, a 1:5 preparation in 45% ethanol (v/v) has been taken at a dose of 0.5-2 mL daily. The herb may also be available as an aqueous ethanol preparation (1:1:5) or as an aqueous essential oil extract.

Children (Younger than 18 Years)

- Avoid in children because of potentially life-threatening toxicity.

SAFETY
Allergy

- Avoid if hypersensitive to scotch broom or any of its constituents, including sparteine.

Side Effects and Warnings

- Scotch broom contains sparteine, an alkaloid with antiarrhythmic properties and potential cardiac toxicity (reported as similar to class 1A antiarrhythmics such as quinidine). Blood pressure changes and circulatory collapse may occur with large doses taken in any form, including by mouth or smoked in cigarettes. There is a possibility of abnormal heart rhythms, heart attack, and worsening of heart failure. Therefore, use of this herb should be under medical supervision only, and extreme caution is warranted in individuals with a history of heart disease, abnormal heart rhythms, high blood pressure, or those taking heart medications.
- High doses of scotch broom taken by mouth may cause toxic symptoms including dizziness, headache, weakness, fatigue, sleepiness, blurry vision, sweating, nausea, vomiting, gastrointestinal distress, diarrhea, and confusion. When smoked in cigarette form, headache, confusion, relaxation, and euphoria may occur. Driving or operating heavy machinery should be avoided. Smoking cigarettes containing scotch broom carries a risk of inhalation of fungal contaminants *(Aspergillus)*, with a possibility of resulting fungal pneumonia.
- Topical (skin) use may cause irritation due to the presence of saponins.

Pregnancy and Breastfeeding

- Scotch broom should be avoided during pregnancy. Scotch broom contains the alkaloid sparteine, which is known to cause uterine contractions, and carries a risk of inducing abortion (abortifacient properties).
- Scotch broom should be avoided during breastfeeding because of insufficient evidence and a hypothetical risk of serious toxicity.

INTERACTIONS
Interactions with Drugs

- Scotch broom contains the alkaloid sparteine, which may affect cardiac conductivity. Use in individuals taking other heart medications that affect heart rhythm such as digoxin, beta-blockers, calcium channel blockers, or other antiarrhythmics may be hazardous and should be avoided unless under strict medical supervision.
- Scotch broom contains the alkaloid sparteine, which can potentially increase (or decrease) blood pressure. Use is not recommended in patients with a history of abnormal blood pressure or in those taking blood pressure medications.
- Scotch broom contains the toxic alkaloid sparteine, which is metabolized (broken down) by the liver's cytochrome P450 2D6 (CYP2D6) isoenzyme system. Therefore, drugs that inhibit CYP2D6 can increase the potential toxicity of scotch broom, including a risk of life-threatening adverse events such as cardiovascular collapse. This includes the drugs amiodarone, celecoxib, chlorpheniramine, cimetidine, clomipramine, cocaine, doxorubicin, halofantrine, haloperidol, methadone, mibefradil, moclobemide, nefazodone, quinidine, ranitidine, ritonavir, terbinafine, venlafaxine, and multiple antidepressants in the selective serotonin reuptake inhibitor (SSRI) class, particularly fluoxetine and paroxetine. In particular, the drug haloperidol (Haldol) has been shown to increase blood levels of sparteine.
- Scotch broom contains small amounts of tyramine, which can lead to hypertensive crisis in individuals taking monoamine oxidase inhibitor (MAOI) drugs. Therefore, this combination should be avoided. MAOI drugs include isocarboxazid (Marplan), phenelzine (Nardil), and tranylcypromine (Parnate).

Interactions with Herbs and Dietary Supplements

- Scotch broom contains the alkaloid sparteine, which can potentially decrease or increase blood pressure. Use is not recommended in patients with a history of abnormal blood pressure or taking agents with significant effects on blood pressure.
- Herbs with potential effects on heart rhythm similar to digoxin may pose a risk of heart block or abnormal cardiac rhythms when used with scotch broom, which contains the cardioactive constituent sparteine.
- Scotch broom contains the toxic alkaloid sparteine, which is metabolized (broken down) by the liver's CYP2D6 isoenzyme system. Therefore, herbs that inhibit CYP2D6 can increase the potential toxicity of scotch broom, including a risk of life-threatening adverse events such as cardiovascular collapse.
- Scotch broom contains small amounts of tyramine, which can lead to hypertensive crisis in individuals taking MAOI agents. Therefore, this combination should be avoided.

For a complete list of references, please visit www.naturalstandard.com.

Sea Buckthorn
(Hippophae rhamnoides)

RELATED TERMS

- Aekol, argasse, argousier (French), artificial sea-buckthorn oil, buckthorn, carotenoids, common sea-buckthorn, dharbu (Lao [Sino-Tibetan]), dhurchuk (Hindi), Elaeagnaceae (family), *Elaeagnus rhamnoides* (L.) A. Nelson, espino amarillo, espino falso, finbar (Swedish), flavonol aglycones, flavonols, grisset, *Hippophae angustifolia* Lodd., *Hippophae littoralis* Salisb., *Hippophae rhamnoides*, *Hippophae rhamnoides* cv. Indian Summer, *Hippophae rhamnoides* oil, *Hippophae rhamnoides* Saint-Lager, *Hippophae sibirica* Lodd., *Hippophae stourdziana* Szabó, isorhamnetin, meerdorn, oblepiha, oleum hippophae, *Osyris rhamnoides* Scop., Prielbrusie, pulp oil, purging thorn, *Rhamnoides hippophae* Moench., rokitnik, sallow thorn, sanddorn, sandthorn, sceitbezien, sea-buckthorn, sea-buckthorn oil, seabuckthorn, seabuckthorn oil, seabuckthorn powder, seed oil, Seedorn (German), seed residues of *Hippophae rhamnoides* L, shaji (Chinese), star-bu (Lao [Sino-Tibetan]), tindved (Danish), total flavones of *Hippophae rhamnoides* L. (TFH).
- **Note:** Sea buckthorn (*Hippophae rhamnoides*) should not be confused with alder buckthorn (*Rhamnus frangula*), common buckthorn (*Rhamnus cathartica*), or cascara/California buckthorn (*Rhamnus purshiana*), although these plants have similar common names.

BACKGROUND

- Sea buckthorn (*Hippophae rhamnoides*) is found throughout Europe and Asia, particularly eastern Europe and central Asia. The plant's orange fruit and the oil from its pulp and seeds have been used traditionally for skin conditions, coughing, phlegm reduction, and digestive disorders.
- Sea buckthorn has been used for centuries in Mongolia, China, and Tibet. In Tibet, sea buckthorn is recommended for pulmonary disorders, cough, colds, fever, inflammation, abscesses, toxicity, constipation, tumors, and gynecological diseases. According to the Chinese Pharmacopeia, internal use of sea buckthorn is recommended as a pain reliever, cough suppressant, expectorant, digestive tonic, and blood flow promoter. In traditional Chinese medicine (TCM), sea buckthorn is used mainly as an expectorant and demulcent (soothing agent).
- In Russia, sea buckthorn seed and fruit oil have been used topically for eczema, psoriasis, burns, frostbite, lupus, and cervical erosion and internally for blood clots as well as eye disorders. In Tajikistan, sea buckthorn flowers are used to soften the skin. In other parts of central Asia, the leaves are used internally for gastrointestinal and skin disorders and topically for rheumatoid arthritis. In India, sea buckthorn fruit is used to treat lung, gastrointestinal, heart, blood, liver, and metabolic disorders.

EVIDENCE

Uses Based on Scientific Evidence	Grade
Atopic Dermatitis (Skin Rash) Study results are mixed. The available evidence is insufficient to support this use.	C
Burns *Hippophae rhamnoides* oil is a traditional Chinese medicine (TCM) preparation derived from the fruits of sea buckthorn. In one clinical trial, application of *Hippophae rhamnoides* oil seemed to help skin burns. However, stronger evidence is needed to support this use.	C
Cardiovascular Disease *Hippophae rhamnoides* may help to improve cardiovascular conditions. The available evidence is insufficient to support this use.	C
Cirrhosis Sea buckthorn extract may improve liver health in people with cirrhosis. Although the results are intriguing, stronger evidence is needed to support this use.	C
Gastric Ulcers There is some (although weak) evidence that *Hippophae* oil may be beneficial when added to other therapies for gastric ulcer.	C
Hypertension (High Blood Pressure) Limited research has evaluated the use of sea buckthorn in patients with high blood pressure.	C
Pneumonia Limited research has been conducted in children, but the available evidence is not sufficient to support this use.	C

Uses Based on Tradition or Theory

Abscesses, ACE inhibitor activity, aging, analgesic (pain-reliever), angina (chest pain), anthelmintic (expels worms), antibacterial, antiinflammatory, antioxidant, antiplatelet, antitussive (cough suppressant), arthritis, asthma, astringent, atherosclerosis (hardening of the arteries), bedsores, blood flow enhancement, cancer, chemotherapy adjuvant, colds, colitis (inflammation of the colon), cosmetics, demulcent (soothing agent), diarrhea, digestive stimulant, digestive tonic, dry skin, ear infections, eczema, enteritis (inflammation of the small intestine), expectorant, fatigue, fever, food uses, frostbite, gastroesophageal reflux disease (GERD), gastrointestinal disorders, gout, gynecological disorders, *Helicobacter pylori* infection, hepatoprotection (liver protection), hyperlipidemia (high cholesterol levels), immunomodulation, infections, laxative, leukemia, lupus, metabolic disorders, nasopharyngitis, night vision enhancement, nutrition, ocular (eye) disorders, periodontitis/gingivitis, postpartum hyperpigmentation, psoriasis (chronic skin disease), pulmonary (lung) conditions, radiation injuries, radiation therapy side effects, scurvy, senility, skin eruptions, skin irritation, skin ulcers, stomachache, stress (due to cold conditions), stroke

(Continued)

Uses Based on Tradition or Theory—Cont'd

prevention, sunscreen, swollen mucous membranes, thrombosis (blood clots in the heart), tonic, toxicity, ulcers (gastroduodenal), vision improvement, wound healing.

DOSING

Adults (18 Years and Older)

- According to secondary sources, 1-2 cups of sea buckthorn leaf tea has been consumed daily. One to three seed oil capsules (500 mg per capsule) have been used three times daily. A range of 3-5 mL sea buckthorn seed oil has been used three times daily. Up to 2 "droppersful" of sea buckthorn berry oil have been used three times daily.

Children (Younger than 18 Years)

- There is insufficient evidence to recommend a dose for sea buckthorn in children.

SAFETY

Allergies

- Avoid in people with a known allergy or hypersensitivity to sea buckthorn or its constituents.

Side Effects and Warnings

- Sea buckthorn is likely safe when used in food amounts, according to secondary sources.
- Use cautiously in patients taking blood pressure medications such as angiotensin-converting enzyme (ACE) inhibitors.
- Use cautiously in patients taking blood thinners, as sea buckthorn may decrease platelet aggregation.
- Use cautiously in patients taking antineoplastics (anticancer agents), as extracts of sea buckthorn may have additive effects.
- Use cautiously in patients taking cyclophosphamide or epirubicin (Farmorubicin), as sea buckthorn oil may significantly decrease their action.
- Avoid higher doses than food amounts in people who are pregnant or breastfeeding because of a lack of clinical data.

Pregnancy and Breastfeeding

- Sea buckthorn is not recommended in pregnant or breastfeeding women because of a lack of available scientific evidence.

INTERACTIONS

Interactions with Drugs

- Sea buckthorn may interact with antibiotics or blood pressure medications such as ACE inhibitors.
- Sea buckthorn may increase the risk of bleeding when taken with drugs that increase the risk of bleeding. Some examples include aspirin, anticoagulants ("blood thinners") such as warfarin (Coumadin) or heparin, antiplatelet drugs such as clopidogrel (Plavix), and nonsteroidal antiinflammatory drugs (NSAIDs) such as ibuprofen (Motrin, Advil) or naproxen (Naprosyn, Aleve).
- Sea buckthorn may lower blood sugar levels. Caution is advised when medications that may also lower blood sugar are used. Patients taking drugs for diabetes by mouth or using insulin should be monitored closely by a qualified health care professional, including a pharmacist. Medication adjustments may be necessary.
- Use cautiously if taking cholesterol-altering medications because of the risk of additive effects.
- The antioxidant activity of sea buckthorn is unclear. Use cautiously with antioxidant drugs because of possible additive effects.
- Sea buckthorn oil may significantly reduce ulcer formation. Use cautiously with antiulcer medications because of possible additive effects.
- Sea buckthorn oil may significantly affect the action of some immunosuppressants and chemotherapies.
- Sea buckthorn may interact with herbs and supplements that are broken down by the liver.
- Sea buckthorn may have immunomodulatory activity. Use cautiously with immunosuppressants because of possible additive effects.

Interactions with Herbs and Dietary Supplements

- Sea buckthorn may have antibiotic properties. Use cautiously with herbs and supplements with antibacterial activity because of possible additive effects.
- Sea buckthorn may increase the risk of bleeding when taken with herbs and supplements that are believed to increase the risk of bleeding. Multiple cases of bleeding have been reported with the use of *Ginkgo biloba*, and fewer cases have been reported with garlic and saw palmetto.
- Sea buckthorn may lower blood sugar levels. Caution is advised when herbs or supplements that may also lower blood sugar are used. Blood glucose levels may require monitoring, and doses may need adjustment.
- Sea buckthorn may have additive effects with cholesterol-altering herbs and supplements.
- Use cautiously in patients with cancer or taking herbs or supplements for cancer, as there may be additive effects and side effects.
- Use cautiously with other antioxidant herbs and supplements because of possible additive effects.
- Sea buckthorn oil may significantly reduce ulcer formation and have additive effects with antiulcer therapies.
- Sea buckthorn may interact with cardioactive herbs and supplements. Caution is advised.
- Sea buckthorn may interact with other herbs and supplements that are broken down by the liver.
- Sea buckthorn may have immunomodulatory activity. Caution is advised when other herbs or supplements with immunomodulatory activity are taken because of possible additive or competing effects.

For a complete list of references, please visit www.naturalstandard.com.

Seaweed
(Fucus vesiculosus)

RELATED TERMS

- Black-tang, bladder, bladder fucus, bladderwrack, Blasentang, brown algae, common seawrack, cut weed, Dyers fucus, edible seaweed, fucoidan, fucoxanthin, *Fucus vesiculosis*, green algae, Hai-ts'ao, kelp, kelpware, knotted wrack, *Laminaria* spp., Meereiche, Quercus marina, popping wrack, red algae, red fucus, rockrack, rockweed, schweintang, sea kelp, sea oak, seetang, seaware, seaweed, sea wrack, swine tang, tang, Varech vesiculeux, vraic, wrack.

BACKGROUND

- *Fucus vesiculosus* is a brown seaweed that grows on the northern coasts of the Atlantic and Pacific oceans and the North and Baltic seas. Its name is sometimes used for *Ascophyllum nodosum*, which is another brown seaweed that grows alongside *Fucus vesiculosus*. These species are often included in kelp preparations along with other types of seaweed.
- Asian populations consume seaweed as food in various forms: raw in a salad and as a vegetable, pickled with sauce or with vinegar, as a relish or in sweetened jellies, and also cooked for vegetable soup. As an herbal medicine, seaweed has been used for traditional cosmetics, treatments for cough, asthma, hemorrhoids, boils, goiters, stomach ailments, and urinary diseases, and for reducing the incidence of tumors, ulcers, and headaches. Vietnam has an abundance of algae flora with a total number of species estimated to be nearly 1000, of which there are 638 species of marine algae identified.

EVIDENCE

Uses Based on Scientific Evidence	Grade
Antibacterial/Antifungal Laboratory study suggests antifungal and antibacterial activity of bladderwrack. However, there is insufficient clinical evidence to support its use as an antibacterial or antifungal agent.	C
Anticoagulant (Blood Thinner) Laboratory study has found anticoagulant properties in fucans or fucoidans, which are components of brown algae such as bladderwrack. However, there is insufficient clinical evidence to support this use.	C
Antioxidant Laboratory study suggests antioxidant activity in fucoidans, which are components in some brown algae. However, there is a lack of high-quality human studies available to support its use as an antioxidant.	C
Cancer Several brown algae, including bladderwrack (*Fucus vesiculosus*), appear to suppress the growth of various cancer cells in animal and laboratory studies. However, currently there is insufficient clinical evidence to support its use in cancer.	C
Diabetes On the basis of animal research, extracts of bladderwrack may lower blood sugar levels. However, there is insufficient clinical evidence to support its use in diabetes.	C
Goiter (Thyroid Disease) Bladderwrack contains variable levels of iodine. As a result, it has been used to treat thyroid disorders, such as goiters, although the clinical evidence is insufficient to support its use.	C
Weight Loss Bladderwrack and other seaweed products are often marketed for weight loss. However, its safety and effectiveness have not been well studied in humans.	C

Uses Based on Tradition or Theory

Antiviral, arthritis, atherosclerosis (hardening of the arteries), benign prostatic hypertrophy (BPH or enlarged prostate), bladder inflammatory disease, eczema, edema, enlarged glands, fatigue, hair loss, heart disease, heartburn, herpes simplex virus, high cholesterol levels, kidney disease, laxative, lymphoma, malnutrition, menstruation irregularities, orchitis (swollen or painful testes), parasites, psoriasis, radiation protection, rheumatism, sore throat, stomach upset, stool softener, ulcer, urinary tract tonic.

DOSING
Adults (18 Years and Older)

- Soft capsules (alcohol extract) in doses of 200-600 mg daily have been taken by mouth. Tablets have also been used, initially taken three times per day and gradually increased to 24 tablets per day. Sixteen grams of bruised plant mixed with 1 pint of water has been used, administered in 2 fl oz doses three times per day or in an alcoholic liquid extract in a dose of 4-8 mL before meals.
- Topical (on the skin) bladderwrack and seaweed patches are sold commercially as weight loss products, although there is a lack of commonly accepted or well tested doses.

Children (Younger than 18 Years)

- There is not enough scientific evidence to recommend the safe use of bladderwrack in children. Because of the iodine content and potential for contamination with heavy metals, it may be inadvisable for use in children.

SAFETY
Allergies

- Avoid in individuals with an allergy or hypersensitivity to *Fucus vesiculosus*, any of its components, or iodine, as sensitivity may occur.

Side Effects and Warnings

- Most adverse effects appear related to the high iodine content, heavy metal, or other contamination of bladderwrack preparations, rather than to the seaweed itself. Because of the potential contamination of bladderwrack with heavy metals, its consumption should always be considered potentially unsafe.
- Based on the known effects of iodine toxicity and case reports, the high iodine content in bladderwrack may lead to abnormal thyroid conditions. In theory, bladderwrack may increase or decrease blood thyroid hormone levels. In addition, acne-type skin lesions may occur, and there are reports of severe acne exacerbations with the use of kelp. Iodine may also cause a brassy taste, increased salivation, and stomach irritation.
- Reports of kidney and nerve toxicity have occurred in persons taking seaweed/kelp and have been attributed to high levels of arsenic. Abnormal bleeding and reduced blood platelet count were attributed to contaminants in a kelp product. Bladderwrack may contain vitamins and minerals, calcium, magnesium, potassium, and sodium and may increase blood levels.
- Extracts of bladderwrack may cause lowered blood sugar levels. Caution is advised in patients with diabetes or hypoglycemia and in those taking drugs, herbs, or supplements that affect blood sugar. Serum glucose levels may need to be monitored by a health care provider, and medication adjustments may be necessary.
- Bladderwrack may have blood-thinning (anticoagulant) properties. Abnormal bleeding, petechiae, and autoimmune thrombocytopenic purpura with dyserythropoiesis have been reported. Caution is advised in patients with bleeding disorders or taking drugs that may increase the risk of bleeding. Dosing adjustments may be necessary.
- Laxative properties have traditionally been attributed to chronic use of bladderwrack and other brown seaweeds and may be due to the component alginic acid, present in many laxative agents.

Pregnancy and Breastfeeding

- Bladderwrack is not recommended during pregnancy or lactation because of a lack of reliable scientific information and because of the presence of high levels of iodine and possible heavy metal contamination.

INTERACTIONS
Interactions with Drugs

- In theory, the high iodine content of bladderwrack may interfere with the function of drugs that act on the thyroid such as levothyroxine (Synthroid, Levoxyl). Use of bladderwrack and amiodarone may alter thyroid function because of high iodine levels in both agents. Use of iodine-containing agents such as bladderwrack or kelp may alter thyroid function when used with lithium. Other endocrine hormones, estrogen levels, and progesterone levels may be affected; therefore, bladderwrack may interact with hormonal drugs.

- Extracts of bladderwrack may cause lowered blood sugar. Caution is advised when using medications that may also lower blood sugar. Patients taking drugs for diabetes by mouth or using insulin should be monitored closely by a qualified healthcare provider. Medication adjustments may be necessary.
- Bladderwrack may have blood-thinning (anticoagulant) properties. Therefore, bladderwrack may increase the risk of bleeding when taken with drugs that increase the risk of bleeding. Some examples include aspirin, anticoagulants ("blood thinners") such as warfarin (Coumadin) or heparin, antiplatelet drugs such as clopidogrel (Plavix), and nonsteroidal antiinflammatory drugs such as ibuprofen (Motrin, Advil) or naproxen (Naprosyn, Aleve).
- Laxative properties have traditionally been attributed to chronic use of bladderwrack and other brown seaweeds and may be due to the component alginic acid, present in many laxative agents. Combination with laxatives may cause an additive effect. In theory, because of thyroid stimulant properties, bladderwrack may cause additive effects if taken with stimulants. The presence of heavy metal contaminants in bladderwrack preparations, including arsenic, cadmium, chromium, or lead, may increase the risk of kidney toxicity if taken with drugs that cause kidney damage. Bladderwrack may interact with diuretics.

Interactions with Herbs and Dietary Supplements

- Extracts of bladderwrack may lower blood sugar levels. Caution is advised when herbs or supplements that may also lower blood sugar are used. Blood glucose levels may require monitoring, and doses may need adjustment.
- Bladderwrack may increase the risk of bleeding when taken with herbs and supplements that are believed to increase the risk of bleeding. Multiple cases of bleeding have been reported with the use of *Ginkgo biloba*, and fewer cases have been reported with garlic and saw palmetto. Numerous other agents may theoretically increase the risk of bleeding, although this has not been proven in most cases.
- Laxative properties have traditionally been attributed to the chronic use of bladderwrack and other brown seaweeds and may be due to the component alginic acid, present in many laxative agents. Combination with laxatives may cause an additive effect.
- In theory, because of thyroid stimulant properties, bladderwrack may cause additive effects if taken with herbs or supplements with stimulant-type activity, such as caffeine, guarana, or ephedra (ma huang). The presence of heavy metal contaminants in bladderwrack preparations, including arsenic, cadmium, chromium, or lead, may increase the risk of kidney toxicity if taken with herbs or supplements that can cause kidney damage.
- In theory, bladderwrack may decrease iron absorption, especially if ingested over a prolonged period of time. Bladderwrack preparations contain variable levels of calcium, magnesium, potassium, sodium, vitamins, and minerals and may therefore increase corresponding blood levels. Bladderwrack may interact with diuretics.

For a complete list of references, please visit www.naturalstandard.com.

Selenium (Se)

RELATED TERMS

- Adrusen zinco, atomic number 34, DL-selenomethionine, high-selenium yeast, L-selenium methionine, L-selenomethionine, Na_2SeO_3, pea selenium, Se, Se-EMP, Selen, selenate, selenious acid, selenite, selenite-exchangeable metabolic pool, selenium dioxide, selenium disulfide, selenium sulfide, selenium supplementation, selenium-enriched wheat, selenium-enriched yeast, selenium-rich pea flour, selenium-zinc, selenized yeast, seleno yeast, selenocysteine, selenoenzymes, selenomethionine, selenoproteins, selenous acid, Sele-Pak, Selepen, Selmevit, Se-malt, Seme, SeMet, Se-methylselenocysteine (SeMCYS), SeO_3^{2-}, SeO_4^{2-}, SeS, Se-spirulina, Se-yeast, sodium selenite, Spirulin-Sochi-Selen, wheat selenium.

BACKGROUND

- Selenium is a trace mineral found in soil, water, and some foods. It is an essential element in several metabolic pathways.
- Selenium deficiency can occur in areas where the soil content of selenium is low, and it may affect thyroid function and cause conditions such as Keshan disease. Selenium deficiency is also commonly seen in patients receiving total parenteral nutrition (TPN) as their sole source of nutrition. Gastrointestinal disorders may decrease the absorption of selenium, resulting in depletion or deficiency. Selenium may be destroyed when foods are refined or processed.
- Specific dietary sources of selenium include brewer's yeast, wheat germ, butter, garlic, grains, sunflower seeds, Brazil nuts, walnuts, raisins, liver, kidney, shellfish (lobster, oyster, shrimp, scallops), and fresh-water and salt-water fish (red snapper, salmon, swordfish, tuna, mackerel, halibut, flounder, herring, smelts). Selenium is also found in alfalfa, burdock root, catnip, fennel seed, ginseng, raspberry leaf, radish, horseradish, onion, chives, medicinal mushrooms (reishi, shiitake), and yarrow.
- The role of selenium in cancer prevention has been the subject of recent study and debate. Initial evidence from the Nutritional Prevention of Cancer (NPC) trial suggests that selenium supplementation reduces the risk of prostate cancer among men with normal baseline PSA (prostate-specific antigen) levels and low selenium blood levels. However, in this study, selenium did not reduce the risk of lung, colorectal, or basal cell carcinoma of the skin and actually *increased* the risk of squamous cell skin carcinoma. The ongoing Selenium and Vitamin E Cancer Prevention Trial (SELECT) aims to definitively address the role of selenium in prostate cancer prevention.

EVIDENCE

Uses Based on Scientific Evidence	Grade
Antioxidant Selenium is a component of glutathione peroxidase, which possesses antioxidant activity and demonstrates antioxidant properties in humans. Long-term clinical benefits remain controversial.	B
Keshan Disease Keshan disease is a cardiomyopathy (heart disease) restricted to areas of China in people having an extremely low selenium status. Prophylactic administration of sodium selenite has been shown to significantly decrease the incidence of this disorder. Organic forms of selenium (such as selenized yeast or Se-yeast) may have better bioavailability than selenite and thus may be better preventative treatments for Keshan disease. Selenium is used to treat and prevent selenium deficiency (e.g., in those with human immunodeficiency virus [HIV] or those receiving enteral feedings).	B
Prostate Cancer Prevention Initial evidence has suggested that selenium supplementation reduces the risk of developing prostate cancer in men with normal baseline prostate-specific antigen (PSA) levels and low selenium blood levels. This is the subject of large well-designed studies, including the Nutritional Prevention of Cancer (NPC) trial and the ongoing Selenium and Vitamin E Cancer Prevention Trial (SELECT), as well as prior population and case-control studies. The NPC was conducted in 1312 Americans and reported that daily selenium reduces the overall incidence of prostate cancer. However, these protective effects occurred only in men with baseline PSA levels less than or equal to 4 nanograms per milliliter and those with low baseline blood selenium levels. The NPC trial was primarily designed to measure the development of nonmelanoma skin cancers, not other types of cancers; therefore these prostate cancer results cannot be considered definitive. To settle this question, further study is under way. The SELECT trial is in progress, with a goal to include 32,400 men with serum PSA levels less than or equal to 4 nanograms per milliliter. SELECT was started in 2001, with results expected in 2013. Laboratory studies have reported several potential mechanisms for selenium's beneficial effects in prostate cancer, including decreases in androgen receptors and PSA production, antioxidant effects, angiogenesis inhibition, or apoptosis. It is not known whether selenium is helpful in men who already have been diagnosed with prostate cancer to prevent progression or recurrence of the disease. It does appear that selenium may not be beneficial in those with elevated PSA levels or with normal to high selenium levels. It remains unclear whether men at risk (or all men) should have their serum selenium values measured; results of the SELECT study may provide additional guidance. There is evidence that low selenium levels are associated with an increased risk of prostate cancer, and several mechanisms for the beneficial	B

(Continued)

S

Uses Based on Scientific Evidence	Grade
effects of selenium supplementation have been suggested. In the NPC trial, no benefits were seen in reducing the risk of colorectal or lung cancers. Although an overall reduction in cancer risk was observed, it is not clear what specific types of cancer, besides prostate cancer, may be prevented by selenium supplementation.	
Asthma Preliminary research suggests that selenium supplementation may help improve asthma symptoms. However, the available evidence is insufficient to support this use.	C
Blood Disorders Selenium supplementation may offer benefits in patients with glucose-6-phosphate dehydrogenase (G-6-PD) deficiency and chronic hemolysis. Selenium supplementation may also affect platelet function and coagulation.	C
Bronchitis Because selenium is proposed to have a role in immune function, selenium supplementation has been studied in patients with various infections. Some evidence suggests that selenium may promote recovery from bronchitis and pneumonia caused by respiratory syncytial virus (RSV). Although selenium may correct selenium deficiency in patients with bronchitis, it remains unclear whether it is effective.	C
Cancer Prevention Several studies suggest that low levels of selenium may be a risk factor for developing cancer, particularly gastrointestinal, gynecological, lung, colorectal, and esophageal cancer. Studies have shown significantly reduced risk of some (but not all) cancers in subjects taking selenium supplements. Selenium supplementation may reduce cancer incidence in men more than in women. Ongoing trials are examining the precise role of selenium in reducing cancer risk.	C
Cancer Treatment Several studies suggest that low levels of selenium (measured in the blood or in tissues such as toenail clippings) may be a risk factor for developing cancer, particularly prostate, gastrointestinal, gynecological, and colorectal cancer. Population studies suggest that people with cancer are more likely to have low selenium levels than healthy matched individuals, but in most cases it is not clear whether the low selenium levels are a cause or merely a consequence of disease. It remains unclear whether selenium is beneficial in the treatment of any type of cancer.	C
Cardiomyopathy Low selenium levels have been associated with the development of cardiomyopathy, and selenium supplementation is likely of benefit in such cases (e.g.,	C

in Keshan disease and Chagas' disease). However, most cases of cardiomyopathy are not due to low selenium levels; therefore selenium may not be helpful.

It has been suggested that low selenium levels may be a risk for coronary heart disease, although this remains unclear.

Cardiovascular Disease (Prevention) Despite the documented antioxidant and chemopreventive properties of selenium, studies of the effects of selenium intake and supplementation on cardiovascular disease yield inconsistent findings. Stronger evidence is needed to support this use.	C
Central Nervous System Disorders Studies have consistently shown that antioxidants have no clinical benefits in motor neuron diseases such as amyotrophic lateral sclerosis (ALS). Although the research thus far does not discourage selenium supplementation in patients, more research is needed before selenium is recommended as a treatment for central nervous system disorders.	C
Chemotherapy Side Effects Study results of selenium supplementation during chemotherapy are mixed. General concern has been raised that antioxidants may interfere with radiation therapy or some chemotherapy agents, which themselves can depend on oxidative damage to tumor cells for anticancer activity. Therefore, patients undergoing cancer treatment should speak with their oncologist and pharmacist before taking selenium supplements.	C
Critical Illness Selenium is known to play important roles in human health. Although some studies have produced promising results, many showed no evidence that selenium can improve health or decrease mortality in critically ill patients. Research is ongoing, although presently there is not enough evidence to recommend the use of selenium therapy in critical illnesses.	C
Cystic Fibrosis Preliminary research of selenium supplementation in cystic fibrosis patients yields indeterminate results. Further research is needed in this area before a conclusion can be drawn.	C
Dandruff Evidence suggests that selenium-containing shampoos may help improve dandruff, and selenium is included in some commercially available products.	C
Dialysis The benefits of selenium supplementation in dialysis patients remain unclear. Some methods of dialysis may lower plasma selenium levels.	C

Uses Based on Scientific Evidence	Grade
Eye Disorders Although selenium appears to be involved in cataract development and uveitis (eye inflammation), it is not known whether selenium supplements may affect the risk of developing these disorders. Research in this area is warranted.	C
Fatigue Evidence of benefit is inconclusive in this area.	C
High Blood Pressure Some studies have reported that low serum selenium levels may be related to increased blood pressure. Furthermore, known antihypertensive therapies (such as angiotensin-converting enzyme [ACE] inhibitors) do not appear to affect the activity of serine-dependent enzymes.	C
HIV/AIDS Selenium supplementation has been used to treat or prevent selenium deficiency in HIV/AIDS patients, and some reports associate low selenium levels with complications such as cardiomyopathy. It remains unclear whether selenium supplementation is beneficial in patients with HIV, particularly during antiretroviral therapy.	C
Infection Prevention Preliminary research suggests that selenium can be beneficial in the prevention of several types of infection, including recurrence of erysipelas (bacterial skin infection associated with lymphedema), sepsis, or *Mycoplasma* pneumonia. Selenium may help prevent infection by stimulating immune function.	C
Infertility Selenium supplementation has been studied for male infertility and sperm motility with mixed results. Evidence is lacking regarding the potential effects on female infertility.	C
Intracranial Pressure Symptoms Preliminary research shows a decrease of symptoms of elevated intracranial pressure (headaches, nausea, vomiting, vertigo, unsteady gait, speech disorders, and seizures).	C
Liver Disease Selenium supplementation has been studied in various liver disorders, including hepatitis, cirrhosis, and liver cancer, with mixed results.	C
Longevity/Antiaging Because antioxidant supplements are thought to slow aging and prevent disease, selenium supplementation may increase longevity. However, results from clinical trials are mixed, and it is still unclear whether selenium supplementation can affect mortality in healthy individuals.	C

	Grade
Low Birth Weight Selenium supplementation has been studied in low birth weight infants. Additional evidence is warranted in this area before a clear conclusion can be drawn.	C
Malabsorption Low selenium status has been demonstrated in several malabsorptive syndromes and in some digestive and gastrointestinal allergic conditions. There is some evidence that children with food allergies have a higher risk of selenium deficiency. There is no clear benefit of selenium supplementation as a therapy for malabsorptive syndromes, although vitamin supplementation in general may be warranted.	C
Pancreatitis There is inconclusive evidence regarding the use of selenium in pancreatitis.	C
Physical Endurance The antioxidant effects of selenium have been suggested to improve physical endurance. However, the available evidence suggests that selenium supplementation does not affect physical performance or endurance training.	C
Postoperative Recovery There is some evidence that selenium may aid postoperative recovery and reduce edema (swelling) after surgery. Patients with severe inflammation resulting from surgeries or extensive burns may benefit from supportive selenium therapy. More studies are needed to determine whether selenium is a suitable addition to postoperative therapy and care.	C
Preeclampsia Preliminary research in women with pregnancy-induced hypertension has reported reduced edema, without significant impact on birth outcomes.	C
Quality of Life Studies of selenium supplementation for mood elevation and quality of life yield mixed results.	C
Radiation Side Effects Selenium supplementation has been used as an adjunct therapy to treat radiation side effects. The effectiveness remains unclear.	C
Rheumatoid Arthritis Selenium supplementation has been studied in rheumatoid arthritis patients with mixed results.	C
Seizures It is unclear whether serum selenium levels are related to seizures in patients with epilepsy or brain tumors.	C
Sepsis (Severe Bacterial Infection in the Blood) Study results of selenium supplementation in septic patients are mixed.	C

S

(Continued)

Uses Based on Scientific Evidence	Grade
Skin Disorders Taking selenium by mouth has been studied for its effects on psoriasis and lesions induced by arsenic or the human papilloma virus (HPV). Selenium has also been used to treat eczema and to increase the rate of burn wound healing. Although some results appear promising, the overall results are mixed.	C
Sunburn Prevention Photoprotection was initially observed in preliminary research using selenium supplementation and other antioxidants, although there is some evidence of ineffectiveness in preventing light-induced erythema (skin redness).	C
Thyroid Conditions Thyroid function is thought to depend on selenium, and thyroid problems are common in patients with selenium deficiency. Selenium has been suggested to improve goiter, as well as inflammatory activity in chronic autoimmune thyroiditis or Graves' disease.	C
Trauma Because selenium levels and thyroid hormones are disrupted in trauma patients, selenium supplementation has been suggested as a treatment for critically injured patients. Presently, there is not enough evidence to recommend the use of selenium therapy in severe injuries.	C
Yeast Infections Commercially available 1% selenium sulfide shampoo has been reported as equivalent to sporicidal therapy in the adjunctive treatment of tinea capitis and tinea versicolor infections, although further high-quality evidence is warranted.	C
Arthritis (Osteoarthritis, Rheumatoid Arthritis) Selenium-ACE, a formulation containing selenium with three vitamins, has been promoted for the treatment of arthritis. Research has failed to demonstrate significant benefits, with a possible excess of side effects compared with placebo.	D
Diabetes (Prevention) Some studies have suggested that selenium supplementation may help prevent type 2 diabetes by improving glucose metabolism. However, results from the Nutritional Prevention of Cancer (NPC) trial showed increased rates of type 2 diabetes in subjects taking selenium supplements. Although diabetes was not the primary focus of this study, these results indicate a potential risk of selenium supplementation that needs further examination.	D
Kashin-Beck Osteoarthropathy Kashin-Beck disease is an osteoarthropathy endemic in selenium- and iodine-deficient areas. Preliminary	D

evidence suggests that selenium supplementation does not significantly improve this disease.

	Grade
Muscle and Joint Disorders Selenium and vitamin supplementation has been studied in patients with Duchenne muscular dystrophy (DMD), myotonic dystrophy, and exercise-induced muscle injury. However, selenium does not appear to improve muscle strength or motor performance in patients with myotonic dystrophy. Despite promising early evidence, selenium supplementation does not appear to affect muscle strength or disease progression in muscular dystrophy.	D
Skin Cancer (Nonmelanoma) Prevention Results from the Nutritional Prevention of Cancer (NPC) trial, conducted among 1312 Americans over a 13-year period, suggested that selenium supplementation given to individuals at high risk of nonmelanoma skin cancer is ineffective at preventing basal cell carcinoma and actually *increases* the risk of squamous cell carcinoma and total nonmelanoma skin cancer. Therefore, selenium supplementation should be avoided in individuals at risk or with a history of nonmelanoma skin cancer.	D

Uses Based on Tradition or Theory

Abnormal pap smears, acne, alcoholism, allergic rhinitis, altitude sickness, anemia, arsenic poisoning, atherosclerosis (hardening of the arteries), bone density, burns, cardiac arrhythmia, celiac disease, childhood growth promotion, cognitive dysfunction, colitis, depression, diabetic retinopathy, Down's syndrome, gray hair, growth disorders (growing pains), helminth reinfection, hypersensitivity to electricity, inflammation, inflammatory bowel disease, lupus, macular degeneration, menopausal symptoms, metabolic enhancement, miscarriage prevention, non-Hodgkin's lymphoma, organ dysfunction, Osgood-Schlatter disease, otitis media, pain, phenylketonuria, poor elasticity, poison prophylaxis, Raynaud's phenomenon, sleep apnea, stroke, sudden infant death syndrome (SIDS), ulcerative colitis, vaccine adjunct, vasculitis.

DOSING
Adults (18 Years and Older)
- The U.S. Recommended Dietary Allowance (RDA) for adults is 80-200 mcg taken by mouth, specifically, 55 mcg for female adults; 70 mcg for male adults; 40-70 mcg for adolescent males, 45-55 mcg for adolescent females; 65 mcg for pregnant females; and 75 mcg for breastfeeding females.
- Some forms of selenium, such as organic L-(+) selenomethionine, may have better bioavailability than selenite and selenate. Bioavailability may also be affected by vitamin C. Selenium absorption may be lower in those adapted to low selenium diets.
- A common dosing range studied is 80-200 mcg daily. However, these doses have not been proven effective. The dose of selenium associated with a reduced risk of prostate

cancer in the NPC trial is 200 mcg daily. Although the maximum daily dose recommended is 200 mcg, other trials have used 200, 400, or 800 mcg of selenized yeast in the prevention of prostate cancer. Selenized yeast (200 or 800 mcg daily) is being tested as a treatment for prostate cancer.

- Intravenous doses have been given but should be used only under the direction of a qualified health care professional.
- Selenium sulfide (1%-2.5% lotion or shampoo) has been used to treat dandruff and yeast infections.

Children (Younger than 18 Years)

- The U.S. RDA for infants and children is 10 mcg taken by mouth daily for ages 0-6 months; 15 mcg daily for ages 6-12 months; 20 mcg for ages 1-6 years; 30 mcg for ages 7-10 years; 45 mcg for ages 11-14 years; and 50 mcg for ages 5-18 years. Adequate intake for infants up to 6 months old may be 2.1 mcg/kg/day, and for infants 7-12 months old it may be 2.2 mcg/kg/day.
- The maximum daily dose recommended is 45 mcg for ages 0-6 months; 60 mcg for ages 7-12 months; 90 mcg for ages 1-3 years; 150 mcg for ages 4-8 years; and 280 mcg for ages 9-13 years.
- Intravenous doses have been given but should be used only under the direction of a qualified health care professional.

SAFETY
Allergies

- Selenium is a trace element, and hypersensitivity is unlikely. Avoid in individuals with a known allergy or hypersensitivity to products containing selenium.

Side Effects and Warnings

- The level of selenium exposure that will cause chronic toxicity is not known. Selenium toxicity may cause gastrointestinal symptoms (nausea, vomiting, abdominal pain, diarrhea, garlic-like breath odor, and metallic taste), neuromuscular-psychiatric disturbances (weakness/fatigue, lightheadedness, irritability, hyperreflexia, muscle tenderness, tremor, and peripheral neuropathy), dermatological changes (skin rash/dermatitis/flushing, fingernail loss/thickening/blotching/streaking/paronychia, and hair changes/loss), liver dysfunction, kidney dysfunction, thrombocytopenia (low blood platelets), immune alterations (natural killer cell impairment), thyroid dysfunction (decreased triiodothyronine [T_3]), reduced sperm motility, or growth retardation.
- Acute selenium poisoning may cause fever, gastrointestinal symptoms (nausea, vomiting, pain, anorexia), liver or kidney functional impairment, respiratory distress, cardiac complications (electrocardiographic [ECG] changes, increased creatine kinase levels, heart damage), and even death if levels are high enough. Other symptoms similar to chronic selenium toxicity may also occur.
- Chronic low selenium levels are associated with the development of cardiomyopathy and possibly with coronary artery disease. Selenium supplementation in selenium-deficient rats may lead to increased serum homocysteine, which is linked to cardiovascular disease. However, human studies suggest that this does not occur in healthy humans.
- There have been numerous reports of adverse reactions to shampoos and lotions containing 2.5% selenium sulfide. Selenium applied topically apparently is not absorbed significantly into the bloodstream.
- In animals, selenium deprivation can result in cataracts. Cataracts can be induced by administering selenium in

doses several hundred times higher than the daily requirement. At present, there is not enough human evidence that selenium supplementation beyond the normal dietary requirement will affect the rate of cataract formation.

- Results from the NPC trial, conducted among 1312 Americans over a 13-year period, suggest that selenium supplementation given to individuals at high risk of non-melanoma skin cancer is ineffective at preventing basal cell carcinoma and actually *increases* the risk of squamous cell carcinoma and total nonmelanoma skin cancer. Therefore, selenium supplementation should be avoided in individuals at risk or with a history of nonmelanoma skin cancer.
- Researchers have reported high levels of selenium in children with behavioral problems, although causality has not been established.

Pregnancy and Breastfeeding

- No pregnancy category has been established for supplemental selenium intake, although it is generally believed to be safe during pregnancy when consumed in amounts normally found in foods. Studies suggest that a daily intake of 50-75 mcg is adequate during lactation.
- Animal research reports that large doses of selenium may contribute to birth defects.
- Selenium is excreted in breast milk, but it is generally believed to be safe to consume during lactation in amounts commonly found in foods. Studies have shown that different types of selenium consumed may have varying affects on the selenium content of breast milk. For example, selenomethionine appears to increase milk selenium concentrations more significantly than selenium-enriched yeast.

INTERACTIONS
Interactions with Drugs

- Agents that alter the pH of the stomach may decrease the absorption of selenium.
- Concern has been raised that antioxidants may interfere with radiation therapy or some chemotherapy agents (such as alkylating agents, anthracyclines, or platinums), which themselves can depend on oxidative damage to tumor cells for antitumor effects. Studies of the effects of antioxidants on cancer therapies yield mixed results, with some reporting antagonistic effects (interference), others noting synergism (benefit), and most suggesting no significant interaction. This remains an area of study and controversy. In particular, selenium may reduce toxic side effects associated with chemotherapy drugs including cisplatin, doxorubicin, irinotecan (Camptosar), or bleomycin. However, until better evidence is available, selenium supplementation is not recommended during chemotherapy or radiation therapy because of potential interference. Patients considering the use of selenium during chemotherapy or radiation therapy should discuss this choice with their medical and radiation oncologists.
- High-dose steroid therapy may decrease plasma selenium levels.
- Selenium has been suggested to increase the effects of erythropoietin in hemodialysis patients.
- Chronic high selenium levels may decrease sperm motility, although effects on fertility are not known.
- Taking selenium in combination with beta-carotene and vitamins C and E appears to decrease the effectiveness of the combination of simvastatin (Zocor) and niacin, although long-term effects are not known. This may be

S

due to antioxidant effects associated with selenium use. Theoretically, selenium could reduce the effectiveness of other 3-hydroxy-3-methylglutaryl coenzyme A (HMG-CoA) reductase inhibitors such as atorvastatin (Lipitor), fluvastatin (Lescol), lovastatin (Mevacor), and pravastatin (Pravachol).

- Selenium levels may vary in the female life cycle and may be related to estrogen status. Selenium levels may be increased in patients taking birth control pills.

Interactions with Herbs and Dietary Supplements

- Selenium is a component of glutathione peroxidase, which possesses antioxidant activity and demonstrates antioxidant properties in humans. Long-term clinical benefits remain controversial. Selenium may add to the effects of other antioxidants in the body, such as vitamins A, C, and E, lycopene, green tea, soy, grape seed extract, or melatonin. The antioxidant activity of selenium may be affected by n-3 polyunsaturated fatty acids (n-3 PUFA).

- There is preliminary evidence that vitamin C may be necessary for maintaining selenium levels in the body. Vitamin C appears to increase the absorption of natural selenium (found in foods) but not sodium selenate (found in supplements).

- Selenium supplementation may affect the absorption of calcium and magnesium.

For a complete list of references, please visit www.naturalstandard.com.

Shark Cartilage

RELATED TERMS

- AE-941, Arthrovas, cartilage, *Cephaloscyllium ventriosum*, chondroitin sulfate, chondrosine, Haifischknorpel (German), Houtsmuller diet, *Mustelus californicus*, Neoretna, Neovastat, octasaccharides, polar shark cartilage, Psovascar, shark, shark fin soup, smooth-hound shark, *Sphyrna lewini* (hammerhead shark), squalamine, *Squalus acanthias* (spiny dogfish shark), swell shark, U-955.
- **Note**: The product Catrix is made from cow cartilage, not shark cartilage.

BACKGROUND

- Shark cartilage is one of the most popular supplements in the United States, with more than 40 brand name products sold in 1995 alone. Primarily used for cancer, its use became popular in the 1980s after several poor-quality studies reported "miracle" cancer cures.
- Laboratory research and animal studies of shark cartilage or the shark cartilage derivative product AE-941 (Neovastat) have demonstrated some anticancer (antiangiogenic) and antiinflammatory properties. However, there is currently not enough reliable clinical evidence to recommend shark cartilage for any condition. There are several ongoing cancer studies. Many trials are supported by manufacturers of shark cartilage products, which raises questions about impartiality.
- Commercial shark cartilage is primarily composed of chondroitin sulfate (a type of glycosaminoglycan), which is further broken down in the body into glucosamine and other end products. Although chondroitin and glucosamine have been extensively studied for osteoarthritis, there is a lack of evidence supporting the use of unprocessed shark cartilage preparations for this condition. Shark cartilage also contains calcium. Manufacturers sometimes promote its use for calcium supplementation.
- Shark cartilage supplements at common doses can cost as much as $700-$1000 per month.

EVIDENCE

Uses Based on Scientific Evidence	Grade
Arthritis Chondroitin sulfate, a component of shark cartilage, has been shown to benefit patients with osteoarthritis. However, the concentrations of chondroitin in shark cartilage products may be too small to be helpful. The ability of shark cartilage to block new blood vessel growth or reduce inflammation is proposed to be helpful in rheumatoid arthritis. However, there is limited research in these areas, and clinical evidence is insufficient to support this use.	C
Cancer For several decades, shark cartilage has been proposed as a cancer treatment. Studies have shown shark cartilage or the shark cartilage product AE-	C

941 (Neovastat) to block the growth of new blood vessels, a process called antiangiogenesis, which is believed to play a role in controlling the growth of some tumors. There have also been several reports of successful treatments of end-stage cancer patients with shark cartilage, but these have not been well-designed or included reliable comparisons to accepted treatments.

Many studies have been supported by shark cartilage product manufacturers, which may influence the results. In the United States, shark cartilage products cannot claim to cure cancer, and the U.S. Food and Drug Administration (FDA) has sent warning letters to companies not to promote products in this way. Without further evidence from well-designed human trials, it remains unclear whether shark cartilage is of any benefit in cancer, and patients are advised to check with their doctor and pharmacist before taking shark cartilage.

	Grade
Macular Degeneration It is proposed that shark cartilage or the shark cartilage product AE-941 (Neovastat) may be helpful in patients with macular degeneration. A small amount of research suggests possible benefits, but clinical evidence is insufficient to support this use.	C
Pain Based on laboratory studies, shark cartilage may reduce inflammation. However, it is unclear whether shark cartilage is a safe or helpful treatment for pain in humans.	C
Psoriasis Shark cartilage products have been tested by mouth or on the skin in people with psoriasis. However, no clear benefits have been shown.	C

Uses Based on Tradition or Theory

Allergic skin rashes, atherosclerosis (clogged arteries), bacterial infections, degenerative diseases (chronic), diabetic retinopathy, diarrhea, fungal infections, glaucoma, immune system stimulant, intestinal disorders, Kaposi sarcoma, kidney disease, kidney stones, nervous system disorders, osteoporosis, Reiter's syndrome, sarcoidosis, scar healing, Sjögren's syndrome, skin rash, systemic lupus erythematosus (SLE), wound healing, wrinkle prevention.

DOSING

Adults (18 Years and Older)

- Studies have used doses of 0.2-2.0 g/kg of body weight taken by mouth daily in two to three divided doses.
- A range of 80-100 g of ground shark cartilage extract has been taken by mouth daily, divided into two to four doses. Doses of the shark cartilage derivative AE-941 (Neovastat), available in clinical trials, have ranged from 30-240 mL/day taken by mouth or 20 mg/kg taken twice daily. Rectal

doses of 15 g/day or 0.5-1.0 g/kg of body weight per day in two to three divided doses (prepared as an enema) have also been studied.

- Creams applied to the skin with 5%-30% shark cartilage are available and have been recommended by some practitioners for the treatment of psoriasis alone or with shark cartilage by mouth, for 4-6 weeks. Studies have used 5%-10% preparations applied daily.

Children (Younger than 18 Years)

- Shark cartilage is not recommended in children because of a lack of scientific study and a theoretical risk of blocking blood vessel growth. There is one report of a 9 year-old child with a brain tumor treated with shark cartilage who died 4 months later.

SAFETY
Allergies

- Allergic reactions to shark cartilage or to any of its ingredients are possible, although there is limited human information in this area. Caution should be used in patients with a sulfur allergy because products may be sulfated.

Side Effects and Warnings

- A limited amount of published research suggests that shark cartilage is well tolerated in most people at recommended doses. The most common adverse effects reported are mild-to-moderate stomach upset and nausea. In several studies, patients stopped taking shark cartilage because of gastrointestinal distress, cramping, or bloating. Liver damage and taste alteration has been reported.
- Uncommon side effects reported in studies or historically include confusion, decreased muscle strength, decreased sensation, weakness, dizziness, fatigue, increased or decreased blood sugar levels, and low blood pressure. Shark cartilage products may contain high levels of calcium, which may be harmful to patients with kidney disease, abnormal heart rhythms, those with a tendency to form kidney stones, and those with cancers that raise calcium levels. In theory, because of the blocking of new blood vessel growth, shark cartilage may be harmful in people with heart disease or narrowed blood vessels of the legs (peripheral vascular disease). In theory, wound healing and recovery from surgery or trauma may be reduced.
- One case report implicates inhaled shark cartilage dust in an asthma exacerbation and resulting death of a 38-year-old male.

Pregnancy and Breastfeeding

- Shark cartilage is not recommended in pregnant or breastfeeding women. Shark cartilage may block the growth of new blood vessels and drugs with similar properties, such as thalidomide, can cause birth defects. There is limited study of shark cartilage in these areas.

INTERACTIONS
Interactions with Drugs

- Shark cartilage products may contain high doses of calcium and may cause dangerously high blood calcium levels when taken with drugs known to increase blood calcium. Examples include long-term use of thiazide diuretics such as chlorothiazide (Diuril) and antacids such as Tums. In theory, shark cartilage may add to the effects of drugs and experimental agents that block new blood vessel growth. Based on one animal study, the cancer drug cisplatin and shark cartilage may act together against tumors, although there is a lack of reliable human supportive evidence.
- Limited evidence suggests that shark cartilage may lower blood sugar levels. Caution is advised when medications that may also lower blood sugar are used. Patients taking drugs for diabetes by mouth or using insulin should be monitored closely by a qualified health care provider. Medication adjustments may be necessary.

Interactions with Herbs and Dietary Supplements

- Shark cartilage products may contain high doses of calcium and may cause dangerously high calcium levels in the blood when taken with calcium supplements or antacids. Chondroitin sulfate and glucosamine may have additive effects when taken with shark cartilage.
- Limited evidence suggests that shark cartilage may lower blood sugar levels. Caution is advised when herbs or supplements that may also lower blood sugar are used. Blood glucose levels may require monitoring, and doses may need adjustment.
- Trace elements that are found in shark cartilage in higher amounts than those in other fish or animal bones include iron, zinc, selenium, manganese, copper, molybdenum, titanium, and strontium.

For a complete list of references, please visit www.naturalstandard.com.

Shea
(Butyrospermum parkii)

RELATED TERMS

- *Butyrospermum paradoxum* (C.F. Gaertn.), *Butyrospermum parkii* (G. Don) Kotschy, catechin, epicatechin, epicatechin gallate, epigallocatechin, epigallocatechin gallate, gallic acid, gallocatechin, gallocatechin gallate, oleic acid, phenolics, quercetin, saturated fatty acids, shea butter seed husks, shea kernels, shea nut butter, shea tree, stearic acid, sterols, stigmasterol, tocopherol, trans-cinnamic acid, triglycerides, triterpene alcohol, unsaturated fatty acids, *Vitellaria paradoxa* (C.F. Gaertn.).

BACKGROUND

- Shea butter comes from the nut of the shea tree (*Butyrospermum parkii*), which grows in West Africa. It has been used for centuries in Africa for various skin-protecting effects.
- Shea butter has been marketed as a skin and hair moisturizer and as a treatment for a variety of skin conditions, including acne, burns, chapped lips, dry skin, eczema, psoriasis, scars, stretch marks, and wrinkles. It has also been used as a cream to relieve arthritis and rheumatism and to heal bruises and muscle soreness; however, there is questionable evidence to support these uses of shea butter.
- Based on clinical research, shea butter may be effective for relief of nasal congestion, lowering of cholesterol levels, and for blood thinning.

EVIDENCE

Uses Based on Scientific Evidence	Grade
Anticoagulant (Blood Thinner) In clinical trials, shea butter was shown to reduce blood clotting after meals. However, the clinical use of shea requires further scientific evidence.	C
Decongestant (Nasal) Limited evidence suggests that shea butter may relieve nasal congestion.	C
Lipid-Lowering Effects (Cholesterol and Triglycerides) In clinical trials, shea butter was shown to lower increases in lipids after eating. However, there is not enough strong evidence to support its use for lipid disorders.	C

Uses Based on Tradition or Theory
Acne, allergic skin reactions, anti-inflammatory, antioxidant, arthritis, bruising, burns, chapped lips, dandruff, diarrhea, dry skin, headache, inflammation, jaundice, muscle soreness, rash, rheumatic diseases, scar prevention, skin conditions, skin inflammation, stomach ache, stretch marks, wound healing, wrinkle prevention.

DOSING
Adults (18 Years and Older)

- For lipid-lowering and blood-thinning effects, a diet consisting of shea butter has been used.
- For nasal congestion, shea butter has been applied to the skin.

Children (Younger than 18 Years)

- There is insufficient evidence to recommend a dose in children.

SAFETY
Allergies

- Avoid with a known allergy or sensitivity to shea butter. People with latex allergies should ask about the presence of latex in some shea butter formulations.

Side Effects and Warnings

- Shea butter may increase the risk of bleeding. Caution is advised in patients with bleeding disorders or those taking drugs, herbs, or supplements that may increase the risk of bleeding. Dosing adjustments may be necessary.

Pregnancy and Breastfeeding

- Avoid in patients who are pregnant or breastfeeding because of lack of safety evidence.

INTERACTIONS
Interactions with Drugs

- Shea butter may increase the risk of bleeding when taken with drugs that increase the risk of bleeding. Some examples include aspirin, anticoagulants (blood thinners) such as warfarin (Coumadin) or heparin, anti-platelet drugs such as clopidogrel (Plavix), and non-steroidal anti-inflammatory drugs such as ibuprofen (Motrin, Advil) or naproxen (Naprosyn, Aleve).
- Shea butter may add to the effects of anti-inflammatory drugs, antirheumatic drugs, lipid-lowering drugs, and nasal decongestants.

Interactions with Herbs and Dietary Supplements

- Shea butter may increase the risk of bleeding when taken with herbs and supplements that are believed to increase the risk of bleeding. Multiple cases of bleeding have been reported with the use of *Ginkgo biloba* and fewer cases with garlic and saw palmetto. Numerous other agents may theoretically increase the risk of bleeding, although this has not been proved in most cases.
- Shea butter may add to the effects of anti-inflammatory herbs or supplements, antirheumatic herbs or supplements, lipid-lowering herbs or supplements, and nasal decongestants.

For a complete list of references, please visit www.naturalstandard.com.

S

RELATED TERMS

- Basidiomycete, beta-glucan, black forest mushroom, *Copri-nopsis cinerea*, D-glucopyranose, forest mushroom, ha gu, hua gu, king of mushrooms, *Lentinula edodes* (Berk. Pegler), lenthionine, lentiane, *Lentinus edodes*, lentin, lentinan (LNT), lentinan edodes, *Lentinula*, *Lentinula edodes*, *Lycoriella mali* Fitch, monarch of mushrooms, mycelia, mycelium, pasania fungus, *Phanerochaete chrysosporium*, polyphenols, Polyporaceae (family), polysaccharide L-II, shiitake, shiitake mushroom extract (SME), snake butter, *Tricholomopsis edodes*, xylanase enzymes.

BACKGROUND

- Shiitake mushrooms were originally cultivated on natural oak logs and grown only in Japan but are now available in the United States. These mushrooms are large, black-brown, and have an earthy rich flavor. This fungus is consumed in foods such as stir-fries, soups, and as a meat substitute.
- Shiitake contains proteins, fats, carbohydrates, soluble fiber, vitamins (A, B, B_{12}, C, D, niacin), and minerals. Commercial preparations often use the powdered mycelium of the mushroom before the cap and stem grow. This preparation is called *Lentinus edodes* mycelium extract (LEM). LEM is rich in polysaccharides and lignans.
- Shiitake has been taken by mouth for boosting the immune system, decreasing cholesterol levels, and for antiaging. Lentinan, derived from shiitake (*Lentinus edodes*), has been injected as an adjunct treatment for cancer and human immunodeficiency virus (HIV) infection, although currently high-quality human scientific evidence is lacking for many proposed indications. Purified lentinan is considered a drug in Japan.

EVIDENCE

Uses Based on Scientific Evidence	Grade
Cancer (Chemotherapy Adjunct) Laboratory, animal, and human studies of lentinan have shown positive results in cancer patients when used in addition to chemotherapy drugs. Further well-designed clinical trials on all types of cancer are required to confirm these results. Shiitake mushroom extract (SME) used alone did not show benefit in prostate cancer patients in one study. Please check with a medical oncologist and pharmacist before taking any therapies.	C
Genital Warts (Condyloma Acuminatum) Based on preliminary study, lentinan could modulate the immune function and reduce the recurrence rate of genital warts. Further well-designed studies are needed to confirm these results. Currently, more proven therapies are recommended.	C
HIV (Adjunct Therapy) Based on preliminary studies, lentinan may increase CD4 counts and may qualify in future multidrug studies in HIV patients. Further well-designed studies are needed to confirm these results. Side effects have been reported, and more proven therapies are recommended at this time.	C
Immunomodulator Currently, there is a lack of available human evidence supporting the role of lentinan and shiitake as an immunomodulator. Additional research is needed.	C

Uses Based on Tradition or Theory

Antiaging, antifungal, antimicrobial, aphrodisiac, atherosclerosis (hardening of the arteries), blood disorders, cancer prevention, cavities, chronic fatigue syndrome (CFS), common cold, coronary artery disease, diabetes, heart disease, hepatitis, herpes simplex virus type 1, high blood pressure, high cholesterol levels, infection, kidney protection, liver protection, stimulant, stroke prevention, tonic, worms.

DOSING
Adults (18 Years and Older)

- There is insufficient evidence to recommend a dose for shiitake. Traditionally, 6-16 g of the whole, dried shiitake mushroom has been ingested daily. It is typically eaten in soups or taken as a decoction (i.e., boiled for 10-20 minutes, cooled, strained, and consumed). A dose of 1-3 g of LEM has been taken two to three times per day. Shiitake-containing capsules have been taken three times daily for 6 months. A dose of 4 g of shiitake powder has also been taken daily for 10 weeks.
- Injections should be given only by a qualified health care provider.
- Intranasal application of lentinan has been studied at a dose of 1 mg/kg, used three times at 2-day intervals. Safety and effectiveness have not been conclusively demonstrated.

Children (Younger than 18 Years)

- There is insufficient evidence to recommend the use of shiitake in children.

SAFETY
Allergies

- Avoid in individuals with a known allergy or hypersensitivity to shiitake mushrooms. Rash, toxic epidermal necrolysis, and photodermatitis may occur from contact or ingestion. Allergic contact dermatitis has been induced by shiitake hyphae (filaments). Mushroom workers exposed to shiitake spores by inhalation have experienced hypersensitivity pneumonitis. A case report exists of an anaphaylactoid (life-threatening) reaction in a patient with HIV who was taking lentinan.

Side Effects and Warnings

- Most minor adverse effects are believed to be caused by lentinan, the polysaccharide derivative of shiitake. There has been one report each of depression, rigor, fever, chills, and abnormal blood cell counts (granulocytopenia); elevated liver enzymes were reported in one study following treatment with lentinan in cancer patients.
- Shiitake can cause abdominal discomfort and abnormal blood cell counts (eosinophilia) when taken by mouth. Abdominal obstruction and death was reported due to the ingestion of a whole shiitake mushroom. Temporary diarrhea and abdominal bloating may occur after taking high amounts of shiitake.
- Mushroom workers exposed to shiitake spores by inhalation have experienced hypersensitivity pneumonitis (lung inflammation).
- Rapid intravenous infusion of lentinan, the polysaccharide derivative of shiitake, to advanced cancer patients was reported to cause anterior chest depression and dryness of the throat in one study; slow infusion relieved these symptoms.
- Back pain and leg pain has been reported following the administration of lentinan in cancer patients.
- Shiitake can cause "shiitake" dermatitis and possibly photosensitivity when taken by mouth. Allergic contact dermatitis has been induced by shiitake hyphae (filaments).

Pregnancy and Breastfeeding

- Shiitake mushroom is not recommended in pregnant or breastfeeding women in medicinal amounts because of a lack of available scientific evidence.

INTERACTIONS

Interactions with Drugs

- Although not well studied in humans, lentinan and shiitake extracts may interact with antifungals, antivirals, antioxidants, and immunomodulators. Caution is advised.
- Lentinan has been used as an adjunct with cancer therapies to prolong survival time and increase quality of life.
- Based on preliminary animal study, shiitake may reduce blood levels of free cholesterol, triglycerides, and phospholipids.

- In a laboratory study, essential oil from shiitake inhibited platelet aggregation and therefore may increase the risk of bleeding when taken with drugs that also increase bleeding risk like warfarin (Coumadin) or ibuprofen (Advil, Aleve). Lentinan, the polysaccharide derivative of shiitake, may cause mildly abnormal blood cell counts (thrombocytopenia).
- *Lentinus edodes* has been shown to inhibit cyclooxygenase activity in laboratory study and therefore may interact with drugs like acetaminophen (Tylenol) or celecoxib (Celebrex).
- Mushroom polysaccharides, especially beta-glucans such as lentinan from *Lentinus edodes*, may interfere with the way the liver breaks down certain drugs (through the suppression of cytochrome P450 1As [CYP1As]). Consult a qualified health care professional, including a pharmacist, to check for interactions.
- Taking didanosine (ddI, Videx), the nucleoside reverse transcriptase inhibitor (NRTI) antiretroviral drug for HIV, with lentinan (the polysaccharide derivative of shiitake) may help to increase CD4 levels in HIV-positive patients.
- Lentinan may cause increased sun sensitivity that can be worsened by drugs like tretinoin (Retin-A) and tetracycline antibiotics.

Interactions with Herbs and Dietary Supplements

- Although not well studied in humans, lentinan and shiitake extracts may interact with antifungals, antivirals, antioxidants, and immunomodulators. Caution is advised.
- Based on preliminary animal study, shiitake may reduce blood levels of free cholesterol, triglycerides, and phospholipids.
- In a laboratory study, essential oil from shiitake inhibited platelet aggregation and therefore may increase the risk of bleeding when taken with herbs or supplements that also increase bleeding risk like garlic or saw palmetto. Lentinan, the polysaccharide derivative of shiitake, may cause mildly abnormal blood cell counts (thrombocytopenia).
- Mushroom polysaccharides, especially beta-glucans such as lentinan from *Lentinus edodes*, may interfere with the way the liver breaks down certain herbs and supplements (through suppression of CYP1As). Please check with a doctor and pharmacist to screen for potential interactions.
- Lentinan may cause increased sun sensitivity that can be worsened by herbs and supplements like St. John's wort or capsaicin.

For a complete list of references, please visit www.naturalstandard.com.

Skullcap
(*Scutellaria* spp.)

RELATED TERMS

- Apigenin, baicalin, ban-ji-ryun (Korean), banjiryun (Korean), ban-zhi-lian (Chinese), barbatin A, barbatin B, barbatin C, benzyaldehyde, berberine, carthamidin, flavonoidglycoside, flavonoids, Herba Scutellariae barbatae, hexahydrofarnesylacetone, isocarthamidin, Lamiaceae (family), luteolin, menthol, neo-clerodane diterpenoids, PC-SPES, pheophorbide A, resveratrol, SBJ, scutebarbatine B, scutellarein, *Scutelleria baicalensis*, *Scutellaria baicalensis* Georgi, *Scutellaria barbata* D. Don, *Scutellaria lateriflora*, *Scutellaria macrantha*, *Scutellaria rivularis* Wall., scutellarin, wogonin.
- **Note:** Baikal skullcap (*Scutellaria baicalensis*), barbat or Chinese skullcap (*Scutellaria barbata*), and North American skullcap (*Scutellaria lateriflora*) have overlapping uses in traditional herbal medicine. The efficacy in treating various conditions may vary significantly among different species of *Scutellaria*.

BACKGROUND

- Barbat or Chinese skullcap (*Scutellaria barbata*) is a plant native to southern China and all of Korea. In traditional Chinese medicine (TCM), it is used as an anti-inflammatory, diuretic, and antitumor agent, especially in liver diseases such as hepatitis and liver cancer. Baikal skullcap (*Scutellaria baicalensis*) is perhaps best known as an ingredient in PC-SPES. High quality human study is lacking,
- WARNING: PC-SPES HAS BEEN RECALLED FROM THE U.S. MARKET AND SHOULD NOT BE USED.
- There is little safety information available from clinical trials using Baikal skullcap. However, BZL101 (an aqueous Baikal skullcap extract) administered short term to patients with advanced breast cancer showed no serious side effects other than nausea, diarrhea, headache, flatulence, vomiting, constipation, and fatigue.

EVIDENCE

Uses Based on Scientific Evidence	Grade
Cancer Although the outcomes of early studies are promising, high-quality clinical studies are needed in this area before a recommendation can be made.	C

Uses Based on Tradition or Theory
Allergies, anemia, antibacterial, antifungal, anti-inflammatory, antioxidant, antiviral, diuretic, hepatitis, high cholesterol, liver diseases, liver protection, myocardial ischemia (insufficient blood flow to the heart), neurological trauma, sedative, stroke.

DOSING

Adults (18 Years and Older)

- There is insufficient evidence to recommend a dose for skullcap in adults. As a sole cancer therapy, 350 mL of BZL101 (an extract of Baikal skullcap) has been used.

Children (Younger than 18 Years)

- There is insufficient evidence to recommend a dose for skullcap in children.

SAFETY

Allergies

- Avoid in people with a known allergy or hypersensitivity to plants in the genus *Scutellaria*, their constituents, or members of the Lamiaceae family.

Side Effects and Warnings

- Baikal skullcap is an ingredient in PC-SPES, a product that has been recalled from the U.S. market and *should not be used*.
- Adverse effects may include nausea, diarrhea, flatulence, vomiting, constipation, fatigue, and headache.
- Use cautiously in patients taking sedatives and/or operating heavy machinery.
- Use cautiously in patients taking therapies for cancer, especially cyclophosphamide.
- Use cautiously in patients taking therapies broken down by the liver.
- Avoid in patients who are pregnant or breastfeeding, due to a lack of scientific evidence.

Pregnancy and Breastfeeding

- Skullcap is not recommended in pregnant or breastfeeding women due to a lack of available scientific evidence.

INTERACTIONS

Interactions with Drugs

- Skullcap extract may help treat 5-fluorouracil-induced bone marrow damage.
- Caution is advised in patients taking antibiotics, antifungals, antihistamines, antiviral agents, and anti-inflammatory medications, due to possible additive effects.
- Skullcap extract may increase or decrease serum lipid levels. Use cautiously with cholesterol-lowering medications due to possible additive effects.
- Caution is advised in patients with cancer or taking anti-cancer medications due to possible additive effects.
- Skullcap may have antioxidant activity. Caution is advised in patients taking antioxidant agents due to possible additive effects.
- Skullcap may interact with drugs that are broken down by the liver.
- Skullcap is used in traditional Chinese medicine (TCM) as a diuretic.
- Skullcap may cause drowsiness and may have additive effects with other sedatives.

Interactions with Herbs and Dietary Supplements

- Use cautiously with herbs and supplements with antibacterial activity, antifungal activity, antihistamine activity, anti-inflammatory activity, antioxidant activity, and antiviral activity due to possible additive effects.
- Skullcap extract may increase or decrease cholesterol levels. Use cautiously with cholesterol-lowering herbs and supplements due to possible additive effects.

- Use cautiously in patients with cancer and in those taking herbs or supplements to treat cancer.
- Skullcap may reduce the berberine content in berberine-containing herbs.
- Skullcap may interact with herbs and supplements that are broken down by the liver.
- Skullcap is used in traditional Chinese medicine (TCM) as a diuretic.
- Skullcap dry extract and baicalin may interact with hematological (blood) agents.

- Skullcap and *Oldenlandia diffusa* in combination exhibit additive antimutagenic effects.
- PC-SPES contains Baikal skullcap, and thus additive effects may occur in theory.
- Skullcap may cause additive drowsy effects when taken with sedatives. Caution is advised if driving or operating machinery.

For a complete list of references, please visit www.naturalstandard.com.

S

Skunk Cabbage
(*Symplocarpus foetidus*)

RELATED TERMS

- Alkaloids, Araceae (family), caffeic acid, calcium oxalate, col apestosa, *Dracontium*, *Dracontium foetidum* L., eastern skunk cabbage, fatty oil, flavonol glycosides, Indian potato, meadow cabbage, N-hydroxytryptamine, narcotic, *Orontium*, phenolic compounds, pole-cat cabbage, polecatweed, *Spathyema foetida*, swamp cabbage, *Symplocarpus*, *Symplocarpus foetidus*, *Symplocarpus renifolia*, tannin.
- **Note:** This monograph covers only eastern skunk cabbage (*Symplocarpus foetidus*), not western skunk cabbage (*Lysichiton americanus*) or plants of the genus *Veratrum* (also commonly known as skunk cabbage).

BACKGROUND

- Eastern skunk cabbage (*Symplocarpus foetidus*), or skunk cabbage, is closely related to western skunk cabbage (*Lysichiton americanus*). Although very similar, these swamp-growing plants do not belong to the same genus. Skunk cabbage is predictably named for the foul-smelling oil produced by the plant. Care must be taken in preparation of skunk cabbage, as the large amounts of calcium oxylate in all parts of the plant may cause excruciating pain on ingestion.
- Skunk cabbage is used to promote labor and treat dropsy (edema). The flower essence of the plant is also indicated to "move stagnated energy." In addition to its medicinal properties, skunk cabbage is boiled and eaten by Native Americans as a famine food.
- Currently, there is a lack of available scientific evidence supporting the use of skunk cabbage for any indication.

EVIDENCE

Uses Based on Scientific Evidence

No available studies qualify for inclusion in the evidence table.

Uses Based on Tradition or Theory

Antispasmodic, asthma, bleeding, bronchitis, bruises, cancer, catarrh (inflammation of the mucous membrane), chorea (involuntary muscle movement), convulsions, cough, dental caries, diaphoretic (promotes sweating), diuretic, dropsy (swelling), edema, emetic (induces vomiting), epilepsy, expectorant, fever, food uses, hay fever, headache, hemorrhage (bleeding), hysteria, insecticide, labor induction, narcotic, parasites and worms, rheumatism, ringworm, scabies, skin sores, snakebite, stimulant (gastrointestinal), swelling, toothache, vertigo, whooping cough, wounds.

DOSING

Adults (18 Years and Older)

- There is insufficient evidence to recommend a dose for skunk cabbage. Traditionally, 0.5-1 mg of powdered rhizome/root has been taken three times daily. A liquid extract (1:1 in 25% alcohol) 0.5-1 mL or tincture (1:10 in 45% alcohol) 2-4 mL has been used three times daily.

Children (Younger than 18 Years)

- There is no proven safe or effective dose for skunk cabbage in children, and use is not recommended.

SAFETY

Allergies

- Avoid in individuals with a known allergy or hypersensitivity to skunk cabbage (*Symplocarpus foetidus*) or any of its constituents. When applied on the skin, the fresh plant may cause severe itching, inflammation, and blistering. Skin hives, rash, and itchy or swollen skin have been reported.

Side Effects and Warnings

- Skunk cabbage is possibly safe when used as food and taken by mouth as boiled leaves, roots, and stalks.
- Large amounts of skunk cabbage taken by mouth may cause nausea, vomiting, headache, vertigo, and dimness of vision. It may aggravate gastrointestinal ulcers or gastrointestinal inflammation or cause irritation, abdominal cramps, burning, blistering in the mouth and throat, colic, and watery or bloody diarrhea. When applied on the skin, the fresh plant may cause severe itching, inflammation, and blistering. Skin hives, rash, and itchy or swollen skin have been reported. Skunk cabbage may alter the menstrual cycle; uterine contractions due to irritant properties have been reported. Breathing problems, tightness in the throat or chest, and chest pain have also been reported with the use of skunk cabbage.
- Skunk cabbage should be used cautiously in individuals with a history of oxalate kidney stones, as the calcium oxalate in the plant may irritate the kidney or promote kidney stones in sensitive individuals. Also use cautiously in patients with gastrointestinal ulcers, inflammation, or irritation, as skunk cabbage may aggravate these conditions.

Pregnancy and Breastfeeding

- Skunk cabbage is not recommended in pregnant or breastfeeding women because of a lack of available scientific evidence. Skunk cabbage may alter the menstrual cycle; uterine contractions may occur because of irritant properties.

INTERACTIONS

Interactions with Drugs

- Skunk cabbage may cause drowsiness or increase the risk of drowsiness caused by some drugs. Examples include benzodiazepines such as lorazepam (Ativan) or diazepam (Valium), barbiturates such as phenobarbital, narcotics such as codeine, some antidepressants, and alcohol. Use caution while driving or operating machinery.

Interactions with Herbs and Dietary Supplements

- Because of the oxalate content of skunk cabbage, concomitant use may reduce mineral absorption of iron, calcium, or zinc. Caution is advised.
- Skunk cabbage may cause drowsiness or increase the amount of drowsiness caused by some herbs or supplements. Use caution while driving or operating machinery.

For a complete list of references, please visit www.naturalstandard.com.

Slippery Elm
(*Ulmus rubra* syn. *Ulmus fulva*)

RELATED TERMS

- Indian elm, moose elm, red elm, rock elm, slippery elm, sweet elm, Ulmaceae (family), Ulmi rubrae cortex, *Ulmus fulva* Michaux, *Ulmus rubra*, winged elm.

BACKGROUND

- The slippery elm is native to eastern Canada and the eastern and central United States, where it is found mostly in the Appalachian Mountains. Its name refers to the slippery consistency that the inner bark assumes when it is chewed or mixed with water. Slippery elm inner bark has been used historically as a demulcent, emollient, nutritive, astringent, antitussive, and vulnerary. It is included as one of four primary ingredients in the herbal cancer remedy, Essiac, and in a number of Essiac-like products such as Flor-Essence.
- There is a lack of scientific research evaluating the common uses of this herb, but because of its high mucilage content, slippery elm bark may be a safe herbal remedy to treat irritations of the skin and mucus membranes.
- Although allergic reactions after contact have been rarely reported, there is no known toxicity with typical dosing when products made only from the inner bark are used. Inner bark of slippery elm should not be confused with the whole bark, which may be associated with significant risk of adverse effects. Bark of Californian slippery elm (*Fremontia californica*) is often used similarly medicinally, but it is not botanically related.

EVIDENCE

Uses Based on Scientific Evidence	Grade
Cancer Slippery elm is found as a common ingredient in a purported herbal anticancer product called Essiac and a number of Essiac-like products. These products contain other herbs such as rhubarb, sorrel, and burdock root. Currently, there is not enough evidence to recommend the use of this herbal mixture as a therapy for any type of cancer.	C
Diarrhea Traditionally, slippery elm has been used to treat diarrhea. Although theoretically the tannins found in the herb may decrease water content of stool and mucilage may act as a soothing agent for inflamed mucous membranes, there is insufficient scientific evidence to support this indication.	C
Gastrointestinal Disorders Slippery elm is traditionally used to treat inflammatory conditions of the digestive tract such as gastritis, peptic ulcer disease, or enteritis. It may be taken alone or in combination with other herbs. Clinical evidence is insufficient to support this use.	
Sore Throat Slippery elm is commonly used to treat sore throats, most typically taken as a lozenge. Supporting evidence is largely based on traditional evidence and the fact that the mucilages contained in the herb appear to possess soothing properties. Clinical evidence is insufficient to support this use.	C

Uses Based on Tradition or Theory

Abortifacient, abrasions, abscesses, acidity, anal fissures, anthelmintic (expels worms), antioxidant, boils, bronchitis, burns, carbuncles, cold sores, colitis, congestion, constipation, cough, cystitis, demulcent, diuretic, diverticulitis, dysentery, emollient, eruptions, esophageal reflux, expectorant, gout, gynecological disorders, heartburn, hemorrhoids, herpes, immunomodulation, inflammation, laxative, lung problems, milk tolerance, pleurisy, psoriasis, rheumatism, swollen glands, synovitis, syphilis, toothache, typhoid fever, ulcerative colitis, vaginitis, varicose ulcers, wounds.

DOSING

Adults (18 Years and Older)

- There is insufficient evidence to recommend a dose for slippery elm in adults. Slippery elm could theoretically slow down or decrease absorption of other oral medications because of hydrocolloidal fibers, although there is a lack of actual interactions reported. Teas, decoctions, liquid extracts, powdered inner bark preparations, and capsules/tablets are all commercially available.
- Slippery elm bark 400-500-mg tablets or capsules have been taken three or four times daily, although strengths may vary because of lack of standardization. Lower doses of 200-mg capsules have been taken twice or three times daily for bronchitis.
- Slippery elm has been applied on the skin for wound care and inflammation. Typically, the coarse powdered inner bark is mixed with boiling water to make a paste. Various concentrations and application schedules have been used.

Children (Younger than 18 Years)

- Traditionally, it has been accepted that slippery elm can be used safely in children complaining of stomach upset and diarrhea. However, there is insufficient evidence to recommend a dose in children.

S

SAFETY

Allergies

- Known allergy or hypersensitivity such as hives (urticaria) has been reported with slippery elm; some persons may have contact sensitivity to elm tree pollen (or sensitivity when breathing it in), but allergic reactions to medicinal use of elm bark products are extremely rare.

Side Effects and Warnings

- Contact dermatitis and urticaria have been reported after exposure to slippery elm or an oleoresin contained in the slippery elm bark. Based on historical accounts, whole bark of slippery elm (but not inner bark) may possess abortifacient properties.

Pregnancy and Breastfeeding

- Avoid during pregnancy because of the risk of contamination with slippery elm whole bark, which may increase the risk of miscarriage.

INTERACTIONS

Interactions with Drugs

- Slippery elm could theoretically slow down or decrease the absorption of other oral medications because of hydrocolloidal fibers, although there is a lack of actual interactions reported. Slippery elm contains tannins, which could theoretically decrease the absorption of nitrogen-containing substances such as alkaloids, although there is a lack of actual interactions reported.

Interactions with Herbs and Supplements

- Slippery elm could theoretically slow down or decrease the absorption of other herbs or supplements taken by mouth because of hydrocolloidal fibers, although there is a lack of actual interactions reported. Slippery elm contains tannins, which could theoretically decrease the absorption of nitrogen-containing substances such as alkaloids, although there is a lack of actual interactions reported.

For a complete list of references, please visit www.naturalstandard.com.

Sorrel
(Rumex acetosa)

RELATED TERMS

- Acedera, acid sorrel, aglycones, aloe-emodin, aloe-emodin acetate, anthracene derivatives, anthranoids, ascorbic acid, azeda-brava, buckler leaf, cigreto, common sorrel, cuckoo sorrow, cuckoo's meate, dock, dog-eared sorrel, emodin, FE, field sorrel, flavonoids, French sorrel, garden sorrel, gowke-meat, greensauce, green sorrel, herba acetosa, keme-kulagi, oxalates, phenylpropanoid, physcion, Polygonaceae (family), quinoids, red sorrel, red top sorrel, rhein, round leaf sorrel, *Rumex scutatus*, *Rumex acetosa* L., *Rumex acetosella* L., sheephead sorrel, sheep sorrel, sheep's sorrel, sorrel dock, sour dock, sour grass, sour sabs, sour suds, sour sauce, Wiesensauerampfer, wild sorrel.
- **Note:** Sorrel *(Rumex acetosa)* should not be confused with shamrock (*Oxalis hedysaroides*, also redwood sorrel, sorrel, violet wood sorrel) or roselle (*Hibiscus sabdariffa*, also Guinea sorrel, Jamaican sorrel).

BACKGROUND

- Historically, sorrel has been used as a salad green, spring tonic, diarrhea remedy, weak diuretic, and soothing agent for irritated nasal passages. Sorrel has been used with other herbs to treat bronchitis and sinus conditions in Germany since the 1930s. The possible benefit of the multiingredient product Sinupret has recently been supported by clinical studies. Sorrel is also found in the proposed herbal cancer remedy, Essiac, but effectiveness has not been proven.
- Sorrel contains oxalate (oxalic acid), which is potentially toxic in large doses. Organ damage and death were reported following ingestion of a concentrated sorrel soup. Other adverse and drug or herb interactions are possible.

EVIDENCE

Uses Based on Scientific Evidence	Grade
Allergies (Allergic Rhinitis) There is insufficient evidence to recommend sorrel for allergies.	C
Antibacterial There is insufficient evidence to recommend sorrel for its antibacterial properties.	C
Bronchitis Sorrel, in combination with other herbs, may have beneficial effects for acute bronchitis, but it is not clear what dose is safe or effective. Sorrel alone has not been studied thoroughly for this indication.	C
Cancer Early evidence suggests that herbal formulations containing sorrel, such as Essiac, do not shrink tumor size or increase life expectancy in patients with cancer. However, currently there is a lack of studies that look at sorrel as the sole treatment for cancer.	
Quality of Life (Cancer) Essiac is a popular therapy for cancer. It is unclear whether Essiac is helpful in increasing quality of life in women with breast cancer.	C
Sinusitis Research suggests that an herbal combination preparation containing sorrel called Sinupret may have beneficial effects in improving symptoms of sinus infection when used with antibiotics. It is not clear whether these same effects would be seen with sorrel alone or what dose may be safe and effective.	C

Uses Based on Tradition or Theory

Acne, anemia, antimicrobial, antiviral, appetite stimulant, asthma, astringent, bleeding, boils, constipation, diarrhea, diuresis (urine production), fever, gonorrhea, human immunodeficiency virus (HIV), infection, inflammation, itching, jaundice, kidney stones, nasal inflammation, nettle rash, parasites, rash, respiratory disease, respiratory inflammation, ringworm, skin cancer, sore throat, stomach problems, ulcerated bowel, ulcers (gastrointestinal), vitamin C deficiency (scurvy), wound healing.

DOSING
Adults (18 Years and Older)

- There is a lack of established dosages for sorrel taken alone. In small doses, sorrel is likely safe. However, because of reports of significant oxalate toxicity when taken in larger doses, caution is advised.
- Sorrel is most often used medicinally as a part of combination formulas. For cancer, a dose of 30 mL (two tablespoons) of Essiac tea has been taken one to three times daily. For sinus infections, one to two tablets of the combination product Sinupret taken by mouth one to three times daily for 2 weeks has been studied. Sinupret is a combination product containing sorrel, gentian root, European elderflower, verbena, and cowslip flower. Fifty drops of an alcohol-based (19%) Sinupret tincture has also been taken by mouth three times daily.

Children (Younger than 18 Years)

- There is insufficient evidence to recommend sorrel for use in children, and sorrel is not recommended because of potential side effects and toxicity.

SAFETY

Allergies

- People should avoid sorrel if they have known allergies to sorrel (*Rumex acetosa*) or any member of the Polygonaceae family. Sorrel's pollen is a potential respiratory allergen and may trigger allergic reactions or bronchial asthma. Signs of allergy include rash, itching, and shortness of breath.

Side Effects and Warnings

- There is limited evidence for the safety of sorrel consumed alone. Sorrel seems to be well tolerated by most people. Some people may experience stomach pain or cramping, vomiting, nausea, and diarrhea. Other side effects may include difficulty breathing or skin irritation caused by sorrel allergies. Rarely, kidney stones or kidney damage may occur, causing either frequent urination or lack of urination. Low levels of calcium in the blood may also occur, which can lead to muscle spasms. Dizziness, gastrointestinal tract damage, and liver disease are also possible side effects. Many tinctures contain high levels of alcohol; avoid when driving or operating heavy machinery. Large doses of sorrel should be avoided; they have been associated with reports of toxicity and death, possibly caused by oxalates found in sorrel.
- The combination formula Sinupret, which contains sorrel in combination with gentian root, European elderflower, verbena, and cowslip flower, is reported to be well tolerated but has been associated with infrequent cases of gastrointestinal upset. Essiac, an herbal combination product that contains sorrel, has also caused minor side effects.
- Caution should be used among patients with kidney or stomach conditions.
- Sorrel is possibly unsafe in children because of its oxalic acid content; ingestion of rhubarb leaves, another source of oxalic acid, is reported to have caused death in a 4-year-old child.

Pregnancy and Breastfeeding

- There is not enough scientific evidence to recommend using sorrel during pregnancy or breast-feeding. Many tinctures contain high levels of alcohol and should be avoided during pregnancy. Sinupret did not increase the risk of birth defects in one study.

INTERACTIONS

Interactions with Drugs

- In general, prescription drugs should be taken 1 hour before or 2 hours after sorrel to reduce the likelihood of drug interactions. Many tinctures contain high levels of alcohol and may cause nausea or vomiting when taken with metronidazole (Flagyl) or disulfiram (Antabuse).
- In theory, herbs with high tannin content, such as sorrel, should not be used in combination with alkaloid agents, such as atropine, galantamine, scopolamine (Transderm-Scop), or vinblastine.
- Use of the antibiotic doxycycline with Quanterra Sinus Defense or Sinupret may have a positive interaction and improve outcomes in patients with acute bacterial sinusitis.
- Sorrel is popularly taken in Essiac as a cancer therapy. In theory, sorrel and sorrel combination products (e.g. Essiac, Flor-Essence) may interact with other cancer therapies.
- Excessive urination has been reported with the use of sorrel, and sorrel may add to the effects of diuretics, such as hydrochlorothiazide or furosemide (Lasix).
- In large amounts, ingestion of sorrel may lead to kidney stones, kidney damage, or liver damage and should be avoided with agents that are toxic to the kidney or liver.
- Sorrel may also interact with antivirals or gastrointestinal drugs.

Interactions with Herbs and Dietary Supplements

- In theory, sorrel should be administered separately from other herbs or supplements, especially alkaloid agents, such as belladonna. Sorrel may impair absorption of calcium, iron, and zinc supplements.
- Excessive urination has been reported with the use of sorrel. Sorrel may add to the effects of diuretic herbs such as artichoke, celery, or dandelion.
- In large amounts, ingestion of sorrel may lead to kidney stones, kidney damage, or liver damage and should be avoided with agents that are toxic to the kidney or liver.
- Rhubarb and shamrock are sources of oxalate and may add to the toxic effects of oxalate in sorrel.
- Sorrel may also interact with antibacterial, anticancer, antiviral, and gastrointestinal herbs and supplements.

For a complete list of references, please visit www.naturalstandard.com.

Soy
(*Glycine max*)

RELATED TERMS

- Coumestrol, daidzein, edamame, frijol de soya, genistein, greater bean, haba soya, hydrolyzed soy protein, isoflavone, isoflavonoid, legume, natto, phytoestrogen, plant estrogen, shoyu, soja, sojabohne, soya, soya protein, soybean, soy fiber, soy food, soy product, soy protein, Ta-tou, texturized vegetable protein.

BACKGROUND

- Soy is a subtropical plant native to southeastern Asia. This member of the pea family (Fabaceae) grows from 1-5 feet tall and forms clusters of three to five pods that each contain two to four beans. Soy has been a dietary staple in Asian countries for at least 5000 years. During the Chou dynasty in China (1134-246 B.C.), fermentation techniques were discovered that allowed soy to be prepared in more easily digestible forms such as tempeh, miso, and tamari soy sauce. Tofu was invented in second century China.
- Soy was introduced to Europe in the 1700s and to the United States in the 1800s. Large-scale soybean cultivation began in the United States during World War II. Currently, midwestern U.S. farmers produce about half of the world's supply of soybeans.
- Soy and components of soy called "isoflavones" have been studied for many health conditions. Isoflavones (such as genistein) are believed to have estrogen-like effects in the body, and as a result, they are sometimes called "phytoestrogens." In laboratory studies, it is not clear whether isoflavones stimulate or block the effects of estrogen or both (acting as "mixed receptor agonists/antagonists").

EVIDENCE

Uses Based on Scientific Evidence	Grade
Dietary Source of Protein Soy products, such as tofu, are high in protein and are an acceptable source of dietary protein.	A
High Cholesterol Numerous human studies report that adding soy protein to the diet can moderately decrease blood levels of total cholesterol and low-density lipoprotein ("bad" cholesterol). Small reductions in triglycerides may also occur, but high-density lipoprotein ("good" cholesterol) does not seem to be significantly altered. Some scientists have proposed that specific components of soybean, such as the isoflavones genistein and daidzein, may be responsible for the cholesterol-lowering properties of soy. However, this has not been clearly demonstrated in research and remains controversial. It is not known whether products containing isolated soy isoflavones have the same effects as regular dietary intake of soy protein.	A

Dietary soy protein has not been proven to affect long-term cardiovascular outcomes, such as heart attack or stroke.

Diarrhea (Acute) in Infants and Young Children Numerous studies report that infants and young children (2-36 months old) with diarrhea who are fed soy formulas experience fewer daily bowel movements and fewer days of diarrhea. This research suggests that soy has benefits over other types of formula, including cow's milk–based solutions. The addition of soy fiber to soy formula may increase the effectiveness. Better quality research is needed before a strong recommendation can be made. Parents are advised to speak with qualified health care providers if their infants experience prolonged diarrhea, become dehydrated, develop signs of infections (such as fever), or have blood in the stool. A health care provider should be consulted for current breastfeeding recommendations and to suggest long-term formulas that provide enough nutrition.	B
Menopausal Symptoms Overall, evidence suggests that soy products containing isoflavones may help reduce menopausal symptoms, such as hot flashes.	B
Breast Cancer Prevention Several large population studies have asked women about their eating habits and reported that higher soy intake (such as dietary tofu) is associated with a decreased risk of developing breast cancer. However, other research suggests that soy does not have this effect. Until better research is available, it remains unclear whether dietary soy or soy isoflavone supplements increase or decrease the risk of breast cancer.	C
Cancer Treatment Genistein, an isoflavone found in soy, has been found in laboratory and animal studies to have anticancer effects, such as blocking new blood vessel growth (antiangiogenesis), acting as a tyrosine kinase inhibitor (a mechanism of many new cancer treatments), or causing cancer cell death (apoptosis). In contrast, genistein has also been reported to *increase* the growth of pancreas tumor cells in laboratory research. Until reliable human research is available, it remains unclear whether dietary soy or soy isoflavone supplements are beneficial, harmful, or neutral in cancer patients.	C
Cardiovascular Disease Dietary soy protein has not been shown to affect long-term cardiovascular outcomes, such as heart	C

(Continued)

S

Uses Based on Scientific Evidence	Grade
attack or stroke. Research does suggest cholesterol-lowering effects of dietary soy, which, in theory, may reduce the risk of heart problems. Soy has also been studied for blood pressure–lowering and blood sugar–reducing properties in people with type 2 diabetes, although the evidence is not definitive in these areas.	
Cardiac Ischemia Cardiac ischemia occurs when blood flow to the heart is blocked. In women with suspected cardiac ischemia, high levels of the soy isoflavone genistein have been associated with blood vessel problems. Until more research is done, it is unknown whether soy plays a role in cardiac ischemia.	C
Cognitive Function It is unclear whether soy isoflavone supplementation in postmenopausal women can improve cognitive function. Results from studies are mixed.	C
Colon Cancer Prevention There is not enough scientific evidence to determine whether dietary intake of soy affects the risk of developing colon cancer. Study results are mixed.	C
Crohn's Disease Because of limited human research, there is not enough evidence to recommend for or against the use of soy as a way to prevent Crohn's disease.	C
Cyclical Breast Pain It has been theorized that the "phytoestrogens" (plant-based compounds with weak estrogen-like properties) in soy may be beneficial to premenopausal women with cyclical breast pain. However, because of limited human research, there is not enough evidence to recommend for or against the use of dietary soy protein as a therapy for this condition.	C
Diarrhea in Adults Because of limited human study, there is not enough evidence to recommend for or against the use of soy-polysaccharide/fiber in the treatment of diarrhea.	C
Endocrine Disorders (Metabolic Syndrome) Soy nuts may help reduce inflammation, improve blood sugar control, and improve lipid profiles in postmenopausal women with metabolic syndrome. More research is needed in this area.	C
Endometrial Cancer Prevention There is not enough scientific evidence to determine whether dietary intake of soy affects the risk of developing endometrial cancer.	C
Exercise Capacity Improvement (Spinal Cord Injury Patients) Soy appears to be less effective than whey protein at improving caloric expenditure and the distance and length of time that patients with spinal cord injuries are able to walk before feeling tired. More research is needed in this area.	C
Gallstones (Cholelithiasis) Because of limited human research, there is not enough evidence to recommend for or against the use of soy as a therapy in cholelithiasis. Further research is needed before a strong recommendation can be made.	C
High Blood Pressure There is limited human research on the effects of dietary soy on blood pressure. Some research suggests that substituting soy nuts for non-soy protein may help improve blood pressure. Further research is needed before a firm recommendation can be made.	C
Kidney Disease (Chronic Renal Failure, Nephrotic Syndrome, Proteinuria) Because of limited human study, there is not enough evidence to recommend for or against the use of soy in the treatment of kidney diseases, such as nephrotic syndrome. People with kidney disease should speak with their health care providers about the recommended amounts of dietary protein because soy is a high-protein food.	C
Menstrual Migraine A phytoestrogen combination may help prevent menstrual migraine attacks. Further research is needed before a strong recommendation can be made.	C
Obesity/Weight Reduction Some research suggests that soy might be as effective as skim milk and more effective than a low-calorie diet alone in reducing weight. Other research has reported conflicting results. Further research is needed before a strong recommendation can be made.	C
Osteoporosis, Postmenopausal Bone Loss It has been theorized that phytoestrogens in soy (such as isoflavones) may increase bone mineral density in postmenopausal women and reduce the risk of fractures. However, more research is needed before a conclusion can be made.	C
Prostate Cancer Prevention Early research has tested the effects of dietary soy intake on prostate cancer development in humans, but the results have not been conclusive. Better research is needed before a recommendation can be made.	C
Skin Aging It is unclear whether aglycones, a form of soy isoflavone, can improve aged skin in middle-aged women when it is taken by mouth. More research is needed.	C

Uses Based on Scientific Evidence	Grade
Skin Damage Caused by the Sun	C
A soy moisturizing cream may help improve signs of sun damage, including discoloration, blotchiness, dullness, fine lines, and overall texture. Because the cream contained other ingredients besides soy, more research with soy alone is needed.	
Stomach Cancer	C
Early research suggests that intake of soy products may be associated with a reduced risk of death from stomach cancer. Further investigation is needed before a conclusion can be drawn.	
Thyroid Disorders	C
Early research suggests that soy supplements do not affect thyroid function. More research is needed.	
Tuberculosis	C
It has been suggested that soy may be beneficial for tuberculosis when taken with standard medications. According to early research, soy may improve the process of detoxification, have positive effects on the liver, reduce cell damage, and decrease inflammation. Therefore, soy supplements may allow patients to safely take higher doses of antimicrobial drugs that are used to treat tuberculosis.	
Type 2 Diabetes	C
Several small studies have examined the effects of soy products on blood sugar levels in people with type 2 (adult-onset) diabetes. Results are mixed, with some research reporting decreased blood glucose levels and other trials noting no effects. Overall, research in this area is not well designed or reported, and better information is needed.	

Uses Based on Tradition or Theory

Anemia, anorexia, antifungal, antioxidant, antithrombotic (preventing clots), atherosclerosis (hardening of the arteries), attention deficit hyperactivity disorder (ADHD), autoimmune diseases, breast enlargement, cystic fibrosis, diabetic neuropathy, fever, gastrointestinal motility, headache, hepatitis (chronic), inflammation, insect repellant, lymphoma, memory enhancement, nosebleed (chronic), osteosarcoma, ovarian disorders (premature ovarian failure), pancreatic cancer, respiratory problems (cough, phlegm), rheumatoid arthritis, urinary tract cancer, vaginitis, vasoregulator.

DOSING
Adults (18 Years and Older)

- Soy is typically consumed as a protein drink, soy flour, isolated soy protein (e.g., Supro), extract, fiber/cereal, or milk beverage. Studies have examined the effects of 10-80 g of soy with an isoflavone content of about 40-120 mg taken daily for up to 6 months by mouth.
- A dose of 25-50 g of soy protein taken daily by mouth has been studied in people with high cholesterol levels. Isoflavone content has ranged from 60-90 mg daily. Cholesterol

and low-density lipoprotein levels have been reduced in people using 28 g daily of soy protein with a high isoflavone content, or with Abacor, a brand that contains 26 g of soy protein. There is limited study of soy milk (400 mL daily) in premenopausal women, with reported benefits on cholesterol levels. Additional doses have been studied but are not recommended because of a lack of available scientific evidence.

Children (Younger than 18 Years)

- Because of potential safety concerns, a qualified health care provider should be consulted regarding the choice of infant formula.

SAFETY
Allergies

- Soy may act as a food allergen. Symptoms of an allergic reaction range from a runny nose to a sudden drop in blood pressure.

Side Effects and Warnings

- Soy has been a dietary staple in many countries for more than 5000 years, and it does not appear to cause long-term toxicity. Aside from allergic reactions, limited side effects have been reported in infants, children, and adults.
- Soy protein taken by mouth has been associated with stomach and intestinal difficulties, such as bloating, nausea, and constipation. More serious intestinal side effects have been uncommonly reported in infants fed soy protein formula, including vomiting, diarrhea, growth failure, and damage/bleeding of the intestine walls. People who experience intestinal irritation (colitis) from cow's milk may also react to soy formula.
- Based on human case reports and animal research, soy may affect thyroid hormone levels in infants. There have been rare reports of goiters (enlarged neck due to increased thyroid size). Hormone levels became normal again after stopping soy. Infants fed soy or cow's milk formula may also have higher rates of atopic eczema than infants who are breastfed.
- Acute migraine headache has been reported with the use of a soy isoflavone product. Based on animal research, damage to the pancreas may theoretically occur from regularly eating raw soybeans or soy flour/protein powder made from raw, unroasted, or unfermented beans.
- The use of soy is often discouraged in patients with hormone-sensitive cancers, such as breast, ovarian, or uterine cancer because of concerns about possible estrogen-like effects (which theoretically may stimulate tumor growth). Other hormone-sensitive conditions, such as endometriosis, may also theoretically be worsened. In laboratory studies, it is not clear whether isoflavones stimulate or block the effects of estrogen or both (acting as a receptor agonist/antagonist). Until additional research is available, patients with these conditions should be cautious and speak with a qualified health care practitioner before starting use.
- It is not known whether soy or soy isoflavones share the same side effects as estrogens, such as increased risk of blood clots. Early studies suggest that soy isoflavones, unlike estrogens, do not cause the lining of the uterus (endometrium) to build up.
- There has been a case report of vitamin D deficiency rickets in an infant nursed with soybean milk (not specifically designed for infants). Patients should consult their qualified

S

health care practitioners for current breastfeeding recommendations and use formulas with adequate nutritional value.

Pregnancy and Breastfeeding

- Soy as a part of the regular diet is traditionally considered to be safe during pregnancy and breastfeeding, although scientific research is limited in these areas. The effects of high doses of soy or soy isoflavones in humans are not clear and therefore are not recommended.
- Recent study demonstrates that isoflavones, which may have estrogen-like properties, are transferred through breast milk from mothers to infants. High doses of isoflavones given to pregnant rats have resulted in tumors in female offspring, although this has not been tested in humans.
- In one human study, male infants born to women who ingested soy milk or soy products during pregnancy experienced more frequent hypospadias (a birth defect in which the urethral meatus, the opening from which urine passes, is abnormally positioned on the underside of the penis). However, other human and animal studies have examined males or females fed soy formula as infants and have not found abnormalities in infant growth, head circumference, height, weight, occurrence of puberty, menstruation, or reproductive ability.
- Research in children during the first year of life has found that the substitution of soy formula for cow's milk may be associated with significantly lower bone mineral density. Parents considering the use of soy formula should speak with qualified health care practitioners to make sure the appropriate vitamins and minerals are provided in the formula.

INTERACTIONS
Interactions with Drugs

- Soy contains phytoestrogens (plant-based compounds with weak estrogen-like properties), such as isoflavones. It is not clear whether isoflavones stimulate or block the effects of estrogen or both (acting as a receptor agonist/antagonist). It is not known whether taking soy or soy isoflavone supplements increases or decreases the effects of estrogen on the body, such as the risk of blood clots. It is unclear whether taking soy alters the effectiveness of birth control pills containing estrogen.
- It is not known what the effects of soy phytoestrogens are on the antitumor effects of selective estrogen receptor modulators (SERMs) such as tamoxifen. The effects of aromatase inhibitors such as anastrozole (Arimidex), exemestane (Aromasin), or letrozole (Femara) may be reduced. Because of the potential estrogen-like properties of soy, people receiving these drugs should speak with their oncologists before taking soy in amounts greater than normally found in the diet.
- Soy protein may interact with warfarin (Coumadin), although this potential interaction is not well-characterized. Patients taking warfarin should check with a doctor and pharmacist before taking soy supplementation.

Interactions with Herbs and Dietary Supplements

- The effects of soy protein or flour on iron absorption are not clear. Studies in the 1980s reported decreases in iron absorption, although more recent research has noted no effects or increased iron absorption in people taking soy. People using iron supplements as well as soy products should consult their qualified health care practitioners to follow blood iron levels. Calcium and phosphate levels may be altered.
- Some experts believe that there may be a potential interaction between soy extract and *Panax ginseng*, although this possible interaction is not well understood.
- Prebiotics (complex sugars) do not appear to affect how the body absorbs soy. It is unclear whether probiotics (commonly found in cultured milk products like yogurt) affect the absorption of soy.

For a complete list of references, please visit www.naturalstandard.com.

Spirulina
(*Arthrospira* spp.)

RELATED TERMS

- *Aphanizomenon flos-aquae* (AFA), *Arthrospira platensis*, blue-green algae (BGA), calcium, copper, cyanobacteria, cyanobacterium, dihe, free fatty acids, iron, Immulina, klamath, magnesium, manganese, *Microcystis aeruginosa*, *Microcystis wesenbergii*, monogalactosyl monoacylglycerols, Multinal, nickel, *Nostoc* spp., lead, phosphatidylglycerols, phycocyanin, phytoplankton, plant plankton, pond scum, prokaryotic cyanobacterium, Selen-Spirulina, *Spirulina fusiformis*, *Spirulina maxima*, *Spirulina platensis*, Spiruline, tecuitlatl, sulfoquinovosyl diacylglycerols, zinc.
- **Note:** The cyanobacteria commonly know as *spirulina* were once classified in the genus *Spirulina* but are now known to be a separate genus. However, they are still known as *spirulina*. Nonspirulina species, such as *Anabaena* species, *Aphanizomenon* species, and *Microcystis* species are possibly unsafe because they are usually harvested naturally and may be subject to contamination.

BACKGROUND

- The term *spirulina* refers to a large number of cyanobacteria or blue-green algae, which includes *Aphanizomenon* spp., *Microcystis* spp., *Nostoc* spp., and *Spirulina* spp. Most commercial products contain *Aphanizomenon flos-aquae*, *Arthrospira maxima*, and/or *Arthrospira platensis*. These algae are found in the warm, alkaline waters of the world, especially in Mexico and Central Africa. *Arthrospira* spp. are most often grown under controlled conditions and are subject to less contamination than the nonspirulina species that are harvested naturally.
- Spirulina is a rich source of nutrients, containing up to 70% protein, B-complex vitamins, phycocyanin, chlorophyll, beta-carotene, vitamin E, and numerous minerals. In fact, spirulina contains more beta-carotene than carrots. Spirulina has been used since ancient times as a source of nutrients and has been said to possess a variety of medical uses, including as an antioxidant, antiviral, antineoplastic, weight loss aid, and lipid-lowering agent. Preliminary data from animal studies demonstrate effectiveness for some conditions as well as safety, although human evidence is lacking. Based on available research, no recommendation can be made for or against the use of spirulina for any indication.

EVIDENCE

Uses Based on Scientific Evidence	Grade
Allergic Rhinitis (Nasal Allergies) Antiinflammatory properties of spirulina may improve certain aspects of nasal allergies. However, further high-quality studies are needed to confirm these findings.	C
Arsenic Poisoning Spirulina extract plus zinc may be useful for the treatment of arsenic poisoning. Additional research is needed to confirm these findings.	C
Diabetes In people with type 2 diabetes mellitus spirulina may reduce fasting blood sugar levels after 2 months of treatment. However, evidence is not sufficient to support this use.	C
Eye Disorders (Blepharospasm) Super blue-green algae may decrease eyelid spasms, but additional high-quality research is warranted.	C
High Cholesterol In animal studies, spirulina has been found to lower blood cholesterol and triglyceride levels. Preliminary poor-quality studies in humans suggest a similar effect.	C
Malnutrition Spirulina has been studied as a food supplement in infant malnutrition, but results have been mixed.	C
Oral Leukoplakia (Precancerous Mouth Lesions) Preliminary research has not clearly shown benefits of spirulina in the treatment of oral leukoplakia.	C
Weight Loss Spirulina is a popular therapy for weight loss and is sometimes marketed as a "vitamin-enriched" appetite suppressant. However, little scientific information is available on the effect of spirulina on weight loss in humans.	C
Chronic Fatigue Syndrome There is currently inadequate evidence to recommend the use of spirulina in chronic fatigue syndrome.	D
Chronic Viral Hepatitis Preliminary research of spirulina for chronic viral hepatitis shows negative results.	D

Uses Based on Tradition or Theory

Anaphylaxis (severe allergic reaction) prevention, anemia, antibacterial, antifungal, antiinflammatory, antioxidant, antiviral, anxiety, arthritis, atherosclerosis (hardening of the arteries), attention deficit hyperactivity disorder (ADHD), autoimmune disorders, bowel health, brain damage, cancer prevention, cancer treatment, cirrhosis, colitis, cytomegalovirus infection, depression, digestion, doxorubicin cardiotoxicity, energy booster, fatigue, fatty liver, fibromyalgia, hair loss, heart disease, *Helicobacter pylori* infection, herpes simplex-1 virus (HSV-1), high blood pressure, human immunodeficiency virus (HIV), immune system enhancement, infectious disease, influenza, iron deficiency, ischemic injury (ischemic reperfusion injury), kidney disease, lead-induced organ damage, leukemia, liver protection, measles, memory

S

(Continued)

Uses Based on Tradition or Theory—Cont'd

improvement, mood stimulant, mumps, nerve damage, obstetric and gynecological disorders, Parkinson's disease, pneumonia, premenstrual syndrome, radiation sickness, radiation-induced damage, skin disorders, stomach acid excess, stress, ulcers, vitamin and nutrient deficiency, warts, wound healing, yeast infection.

DOSING
Adults (18 Years and Older)

- Spirulina has typically been taken by mouth two to three times daily with meals in doses of 1-1.4 g for diabetes mellitus (type 2), high cholesterol levels, or oral leukoplakia (precancerous mouth lesions). For weight loss, 200 mg of spirulina tablets by mouth three times daily, taken just before eating, has been studied. In addition, 2 g of spirulina has been used for nasal allergies. For arsenic poisoning, twice-daily doses of 250 mg of spirulina extract plus 2 mg of zinc may be helpful.

Children (Younger than 18 Years)

- Not enough scientific information is available to advise the safe use of spirulina in children.

SAFETY
Allergies

- Avoid use in individuals with known allergy to spirulina, blue-green algae species, or any of their constituents.

Side Effects and Warnings

- Few side effects have been reported with spirulina use. The most frequently reported adverse effects are headache, muscle pain, flushing of the face, sweating, and difficulty concentrating. These have been described in people taking 1 g of spirulina by mouth daily. Skin reactions have also been reported.
- Blue-green algae, especially types that are usually harvested in uncontrolled settings (*Anabaena* spp., *Aphanizomenon* spp., and *Microcystis* spp.), may be contaminated with heavy metals. Liver damage, diarrhea, and vomiting have been reported.

- The amino acid phenylalanine in blue-green algae may cause an adverse reaction in people with the genetic condition phenylketonuria (PKU) and should be used cautiously.

Pregnancy and Breastfeeding

- There is not enough information to recommend the safe use of spirulina during pregnancy or breastfeeding. In mice, diets containing up to 30% spirulina are not reported to cause harmful effects to either the mother or the offspring. However, reliable human studies addressing safety during pregnancy or breastfeeding are not available.

INTERACTIONS
Interactions with Drugs

- Spirulina may interact with certain drugs taken for immune system disorders, high blood pressure (angiotensin-converting enzyme [ACE] inhibitors), inflammation, diabetes, high cholesterol levels, neurological conditions, and viruses and may also interact with blood thinners and antihistamines.
- Spirulina may also interact with drugs taken for weight loss, cancer, heart disorders, and osteoporosis. There is a possible interaction when taking spirulina with drugs that are potentially toxic to the kidney.

Interactions with Herbs and Dietary Supplements

- Small increases in calcium levels have been reported, although it is unclear whether this is due to the effects of spirulina alone. Use of spirulina and calcium supplements together may further increase calcium levels.
- Spirulina may increase levels of protein, iron, gamma-linolenic fatty acid, carotenoids, vitamin B_1, vitamin B_2, vitamin B_{12}, and vitamin E.
- Spirulina may interact with certain dietary supplements taken for immune system disorders, high blood pressure, cancer, weight loss, heart disorders, inflammation, diabetes, high cholesterol levels, neurological conditions, blood clots, and viruses. Use cautiously with antihistamines or any herb or supplement that is potentially toxic to the kidney.

For a complete list of references, please visit www.naturalstandard.com.

Spleen Extract

RELATED TERMS

- Bovine spleen, predigested spleen extract, raw spleen, spleen, spleen concentrate, spleen factors, spleen peptides, spleen polypeptides, splenopentin, tetrapeptide tuftsin, tuftsin, tuftsin (L-prolyl-L-arginine), tuftsin (Thr-Lys-Pro-Arg), water-soluble spleen extract.

BACKGROUND

- The spleen is a fist-sized organ located under the lower left side of the rib cage that removes worn-out red blood cells and platelets, produces certain types of white blood cells, and destroys bacteria and cellular debris. Spleen extract primarily comes from the spleens of cows or pigs.
- The primary use of spleen extracts is after a splenectomy, or removal of the spleen. Preliminary studies indicate that spleen extract may stimulate the immune system in conditions such as human immunodeficiency virus/acquired immunodeficiency syndrome (HIV/AIDS), leukemia, leprosy, Crohn's disease, and sickle cell disease. However, there are no high-quality clinical trials currently available on the use of spleen extract.
- Some concern has been raised about the safety of spleen extract, as it is made of animal spleens, which may be infected with prion (proteinaceous infectious protein) diseases. Although there are currently no available reports of diseases such as bovine spongiform encephalitis (BSE, or "mad cow disease") attributed to the consumption of spleen extract, the U.S. Food and Drug Administration (FDA) still cautions against use of any animal organ extract. It is not clear how the processing of spleen extract affects the transmission of these diseases.

EVIDENCE

Uses Based on Scientific Evidence

No available studies qualify for inclusion in the evidence table.

Uses Based on Tradition or Theory

Antibacterial, antifungal, antimicrobial, antioxidant, bleeding disorders, cancer, celiac disease, common cold, Crohn's disease, dermatitis herpetiformis, emotional disorders, fatigue, glomerulonephritis (inflammation of the kidney), graft-versus-host disease (prevention), HIV/AIDS, Hodgkin's disease, immunomodulation, influenza, leprosy, leukemia, pulmonary (lung) conditions, quality of life in HIV patients, radiation side effects, rheumatoid arthritis, sarcoidosis, sickle cell disease, spleen disorders (lymphoproliferative diseases), supplementation in preterm and very low birth weight infants, systemic lupus erythematosus (autoimmune disease), thrombocytopenia (low platelet count), ulcerative colitis (inflammatory bowel disease), vasculitis (inflamed blood vessels).

DOSING

Adults (18 Years and Older)

- There is insufficient evidence to recommend a dose for spleen extract. Nonetheless, 150-300 mg two or three times daily has been used.

Children (Younger than 18 Years)

- There is insufficient evidence to recommend a dose for spleen extract, and use in children is not recommended.

SAFETY

Allergies

- Avoid in individuals with a known allergy or hypersensitivity to spleen extract or its components, including tuftsin.

Side Effects and Warnings

- In general, there is insufficient available evidence on the adverse effects of spleen extract. The U.S. FDA cautions against the consumption of any dietary supplement made from animal glands or organs, especially from cows and sheep from countries with known cases of BSE (mad cow disease) or scrapie. It is thought that these extracts may contain viable prions that could infect humans. Currently, there are no available reports of transmission of BSE through spleen extract.
- Spleen extract is possibly unsafe when used in patients with bleeding disorders or immune system disorders. It is also possibly unsafe when used from countries where BSE (mad cow disease) has been reported.
- Tuftsin, a component of spleen extract, has low toxicity. However, it may enhance the perception of pain. Tuftsin in spleen extract may also enhance immune function and thus provide overly optimistic results of spleen functioning.
- Tuftsin deficiency may cause impaired immunity and/or recurrent and severe infections of the respiratory system, skin, and lymph nodes, especially in symptomatic HIV-positive individuals. Tuftsin deficiency may be due to splenectomy, splenic hypofunction, or familial tuftsin deficiency syndrome.

Pregnancy and Breastfeeding

- Spleen extract is not recommended in pregnant or breastfeeding women because of a lack of available scientific evidence.

INTERACTIONS

Interactions with Drugs

- Tuftsin may enhance the perception of pain. Patients taking analgesics or other pain-reducing medication should consult with a qualified health care professional, including a pharmacist.
- Based on laboratory study, the tuftsin in spleen extract may behave as a carrier of antibiotics in intracellular infections, and simultaneous administration of antibiotics and spleen

S

extract may have a synergistic quality on this class of herbs and supplements. Caution is advised.

- Tuftsin, found in spleen extract, may increase the risk of bleeding when taken with herbs and supplements that increase the risk of bleeding.
- Although not well studied in humans, spleen extract may interact with antifungal drugs, psychotropic drugs, immunomodulators, or immunostimulants (such as bestatin). Spleen extract should also be used cautiously in patients taking medication for Hodgkin's disease, systemic lupus erythematosus, cancer, or leukemia.

Interactions with Herbs and Dietary Supplements

- Tuftsin may enhance the perception of pain. Patients taking analgesics or other pain-reducing herbs or supplements should consult with a qualified health care professional, including a pharmacist.
- Based on a laboratory study, the tuftsin in spleen extract may behave as a carrier of antibiotics in intracellular

infections, and simultaneous administration of antibiotics and spleen extract may have a synergistic quality on this class of drugs.

- Tuftsin, found in spleen extract, may increase the risk of bleeding when taken with drugs that increase the risk of bleeding. Some examples include aspirin, anticoagulants (blood thinners) such as warfarin (Coumadin) or heparin, antiplatelet drugs such as clopidogrel (Plavix), and nonsteroidal antiinflammatory drugs such as ibuprofen (Motrin, Advil) or naproxen (Naprosyn, Aleve).
- Although not well studied in humans, spleen extract may interact with herbs and supplements with antifungal, psychotropic, immunomodulating, or immunostimulating effects. Spleen extract should also be used cautiously in patients taking herbs and supplements for Hodgkin's disease, systemic lupus erythematosus, cancer, or leukemia.

For a complete list of references, please visit www.naturalstandard.com.

Squill
(*Urginea maritima,* syn. *Scilla maritima*)

RELATED TERMS

- Basal tal-ghansar, bulbo de escila, *Charybdis maritima, Drimia maritima,* European squill, ghansar, Indian squill, maritime squill, Mediterranean squill, Meerzwiebel, methylproscillaridin, pharmacist's squill, proscillaridine A, red squill, scilla, *Scilla maritima, Scilla maritima* (Linn.), *Scilla urginea,* scille, sea onion, sea squill, sea squill bulb, *Urginea indica, Urginea maritima, Urginea maritima* Baker, white sea onion, white squill.

BACKGROUND

- About twenty-five species of squill have been described. Red squill and white squill varieties are distinguished by herbalists. No essential difference exists in the medicinal properties of the two kinds. The bulb has been used mainly as a stimulant, expectorant, and diuretic. The fresh bulb is slightly more active medicinally than the dried bulb, but it also contains a sticky acrid juice that can cause skin inflammations.
- Squill seems to have cardiac effects similar to digoxin, although to a lesser degree because of its poor absorption. Therefore, serious caution is indicated before its use.

EVIDENCE

Uses Based on Scientific Evidence	Grade
Coronary Artery Disease Currently, there is insufficient available evidence to recommend for or against the use of squill for coronary artery disease.	C

Uses Based on Tradition or Theory
Abortifacient (induces abortion), arrhythmia (abnormal heart rhythms), arthritis, asthma (with bronchitis), cancer, cardiotonic, catarrh (inflammation of the mucous membrane), chronic bronchitis, croup (laryngitis in infants), dandruff, diuretic, dropsy (swelling), dropsy (cardiac), edema (swelling), emetic (induces vomiting), expectorant, hair tonic, heart conditions, kidney disease, poisoning (rat), renal impairment, seborrhea, venous disorders, whooping cough.

DOSING
Adults (18 Years and Older)

- There is insufficient evidence to recommend a dose for squill. Traditionally, extracts, syrups, tinctures, and vinegar preparations have been taken by mouth. Squill has also been studied for its cardiovascular effects using 1 mg of an intravenous (injected) dose of methylproscillaridin (a cardiac glycoside of squill). Injections should be given only under the supervision of a qualified health care professional.

Children (Younger than 18 Years)

- There is insufficient evidence to recommend a dose for squill in children, and use is not recommended.

SAFETY
Allergies

- Avoid in individuals with a known allergy or hypersensitivity to squill (*Urginea maritima*).

Side Effects and Warnings

- Because of its cardiac glycoside constituents, squill has similar adverse effects as digitalis (a drug that regulates the rate and strength of the heartbeat), including arrhythmia (abnormal heart rate) and atrioventricular block. Other common adverse effects include abdominal pains, vomiting, blood in the vomit, nausea, and seizures. Death has been reported. When rubbed on the skin, irritation, including skin eruption, may occur.
- Recurrent fever, arthralgia (joint pain), myalgia (muscle pain), leukocytosis (high white blood cell count), and lymphopenia (loss of lymphocytes, a type of white blood cell) have occurred after ingestion of Venocuran. Venocuran was taken off of the market in 1975, and it is not clear whether it was the *Urginea maritima* or another constituent that caused the adverse effects.
- Avoid using squill in patients with heart, stomach, or intestinal problems, including second- or third-degree atrioventricular block, hypertrophic cardiomyopathy (enlarged heart), carotid sinus syndrome, ventricular tachycardia, thoracic aortic aneurysm, or Wolff-Parkinson-White syndrome. Also avoid in patients with low potassium or high calcium levels.

Pregnancy and Breastfeeding

- Squill is not recommended for use in pregnant or breastfeeding women because of a lack of available scientific evidence. Squill may have abortifacient (abortion-inducing) effects.

INTERACTIONS
Interactions with Drugs

- Squill (*Urginea maritima*) has shown toxic effects similar to cardiac glycoside toxicity. In theory, squill may have additive toxic effects when used with cardiac glycosides, such as digoxin or digitoxin.
- Concomitant use with corticosteroids (steroids) may increase effects and adverse effects of long-term corticosteroid use. Caution is advised.
- When combined with quinidine (Quinidex, Quinora) or calcium, squill may increase the risk of cardiac toxicity and adverse effects. Laxatives and diuretics may deplete

S

potassium and increase the risk of cardiac toxicity when taken with squill. Consult with a qualified health care professional, including a pharmacist, before combining therapies.

Interactions with Herbs and Dietary Supplements

- Squill (*Urginea maritima*) has shown toxic effects similar to cardiac glycoside toxicity. In theory, squill may have additive toxic effects when used with cardiac glycosides, such as foxglove.
- When combined with calcium, squill may increase the risk of cardiac toxicity and adverse effects. Laxatives, diuretics, and licorice all may deplete potassium and increase the risk of cardiac toxicity when taken with squill.

For a complete list of references, please visit www. naturalstandard.com.

Star Anise
(Illicium verum)

RELATED TERMS

- Anice stellato, anis de la Chine (French), anis estrellado, anise étoilé (French), anise stars, aniseed, Anisi stellati fructus, ba chio, badain, badaine, badian, badiana, ba(ht) g(h) ok, bart gok, bunga lawang, Chinese anise, Chinese star anise, eight-horned anise, eight horns, *Illicium anisatum*, *Illicium anisatum L.* (Japanese star anise), *Illicium religiosum*, *Illicium verum*, *Illicium verum* Hook f, pa-chiao, pak kok, peh kah, star anise, sternanis, Tamiflu.

BACKGROUND

- Chinese star anise *(Illicium verum)* should not be confused with anise *(Pimpinella anisum)*, a member of the carrot family, or with Japanese star anise *(Illicium anisatum)*. Chinese star anise (star anise) is native to China and Vietnam and has been used for its carminative (gas-reducing), stomachic (digestive aid), stimulant, and diuretic medicinal properties. Star anise is used by the Malays for stomachaches due to the accumulation of intestinal gas, headaches, and the promotion of vitality.
- Shikimic acid extracted from the pods (which wrap the seeds) of star anise is the starting material of Tamiflu. Tamiflu (Roche Laboratories) is an antiviral drug that has gained popularity with the recent spread of pandemic influenza strains. Roche Laboratories and its partners mainly use the shikimic acid extracted from Chinese star anise. However, they are developing new technologies that use an *Escherichia coli* bacteria that produces shikimic acid when overfed glucose.
- In September 2003, the U.S. Food and Drug Administration (FDA) advised consumers not to consume teas containing star anise. Such teas have been linked with serious neurological effects such as seizures, vomiting, jitteriness, and rapid eye movement. Some reports have found Chinese star anise *(Illicium verum)* to be contaminated with Japanese star anise *(Illicium anisatum)*, which is a known neurotoxin. Chinese star anise is recognized as safe for food use by the FDA, as acknowledged in the FDA's advisory. Chinese star anise is believed to help with colic in infants; however, the FDA is unaware of scientific evidence to support this claim. In addition, the FDA has not identified the specific type of star anise associated with the adverse effects. Similar reports of adverse effects have been found in Florida, Illinois, New Jersey, and Washington in the United States as well as in The Netherlands, Spain, and France.

EVIDENCE

Uses Based on Scientific Evidence

No available studies qualify for inclusion in the evidence table.

Uses Based on Tradition or Theory

Analgesia (inability to feel pain), antibacterial, antimicrobial (bacteria, yeast, fungus), appetite stimulant, arthritis, bronchitis, childbirth, cough, cramps (intestinal), digestive aid, diuretic, emmenagogue (promotes menstruation), flatulence (gas), flavoring agent, galactogogue (promotes lactation), gastrointestinal distress, indigestion, insecticide, libido, male climacteric symptoms, paralysis (facial), respiratory congestion (inhaled), respiratory tract infections, rheumatism, stimulant, stomachache.

DOSING

Adults (18 Years and Older)

- There is insufficient evidence to recommend a dose for star anise. Products containing 5%-10% of essential oil have been inhaled. Typical doses of star anise may include 1 cup of tea or 0.5-1 g of the coarsely ground seed boiled in 150 mL water for 120 minutes and then strained. Ground star anise has been taken in a dose of 3 g daily. Use of the essential oil of star anise in a dose of 300 mg daily has also been reported.

Children (Younger than 18 Years)

- There is insufficient evidence to recommend a dose for star anise in children, and use is not recommended. There have been many case reports of neurological and gastrointestinal toxic effects in infants with home administration of star anise tea. In some of the cases, adulteration or contamination of Chinese star anise with Japanese star anise may have caused the poisoning. Avoidance or extreme caution is recommended before using Chinese star anise to treat infant colic because of the possible contamination with Japanese star anise.

SAFETY

Allergies

- Avoid in individuals with a known allergy or hypersensitivity to Chinese star anise. There are reports of allergy to star anise and its constituents (anethole, alpha-pinene, limonene, and safrole); patients have had positive skin patch tests to star anise.

Side Effects and Warnings

- Chinese star anise is recognized by the U.S. FDA as "generally recognized as safe" (GRAS); however, patients should be cautious when using Chinese star anise as a tea and should verify its contents. In 2003, the FDA issued a consumer warning about consumption of teas containing Chinese star anise *(Illicium verum)* because of reports of contamination with the toxic Japanese star anise *(Illicium anisatum)*. There are reports of allergy to star anise and its constituents (anethole, alpha-pinene, limonene, and safrole). Nausea, vomiting, tremors, spasms, hypertonia (muscle tension), seizures, convulsions, rapid eye movement, general malaise, and hypothermia have been reported after taking star anise herbal tea. It is not clear whether these toxic effects are caused by Chinese star anise or Japanese star anise, which may contaminate some of the herbal teas.
- In patients with convulsive disorders, such as epilepsy, Chinese star anise should be avoided based on its theoretical convulsive effects.

- Star anise may increase the risk of bleeding. Caution is advised in patients with bleeding disorders or taking agents that may increase the risk of bleeding. Dosing adjustments may be necessary.

Pregnancy and Breastfeeding

- Star anise is not recommended in pregnant or breastfeeding women because of a lack of available scientific evidence.

INTERACTIONS
Interactions with Drugs

- Star anise may increase the risk of bleeding when taken with drugs that increase the risk of bleeding. Some examples include aspirin, anticoagulants ("blood thinners") such as warfarin (Coumadin) or heparin, antiplatelet drugs such as clopidogrel (Plavix), and nonsteroidal antiinflammatory drugs (NSAIDS) such as ibuprofen (Motrin, Advil) or naproxen (Naprosyn, Aleve).

Interactions with Herbs and Dietary Supplements

- Star anise may increase the risk of bleeding when taken with herbs and supplements that are believed to increase the risk of bleeding. Multiple cases of bleeding have been reported with the use of *Ginkgo biloba*, and fewer cases have been reported with garlic and saw palmetto. Numerous other agents may theoretically increase the risk of bleeding, although this has not been proven in most cases.

For a complete list of references, please visit www.naturalstandard.com.

Stevia
(Stevia rebaudiana)

RELATED TERMS

- Alpha-monoglucosylstevioside, alpha-monoglucosylrebaudioside A, Asteraceae, azucacaa, candyleaf, capim doce, Compositae, dihydroisosteviol (DHISV), dihydropseudoivalin, dihydrosteviol A, ent-kaurenoic acid, epidihydropseudoivalin, erva doce, glucosyl stevioside, isosteviol, ka'a he'e, kaa he-he, kaa jhee, NPI-028, octaacetylombuoside, ombuine, ombuoside, Paraguayan sweet herb, rebaudioside A (RA), rebaudioside F, retusine, roninowa, ronion, sacharol, SE, *Stevia connata*, *Stevia eupatoria*, stevia glycosides, *Stevia lita*, *Stevia pilosa*, *Stevia rebaudiana* (SR), *Stevia rebaudiana* Bertoni (SrB), *Stevia rebaudiana* standardized extracts (SSEs), *Stevia salicifolia*, *Stevia subpubescens*, *Stevia tomentosa*, *Stevia triflora* DC, *Stevia viscida*, steviol (SV), steviolbioside, stevioside (SVS), stevisalioside A, Stevita, sweet serb, sweetleaf, yerba dulce.
- **Note:** Do not confuse *Stevia rebaudiana* with *Stevia salicifolia*, also called ronion or roninowa. *Stevia salicifolia* contains the bitter glycoside stevisalioside.

BACKGROUND

- Extracts of leaves from *Stevia rebaudiana* Bertoni have been used for many years in traditional treatment of diabetes in South America. Paraguay's rural and indigenous populations have used *Stevia rebaudiana* for the control of fertility.
- *Stevia rebaudiana* standardized extracts are used as natural sweeteners or dietary supplements in different countries for their content of stevioside or rebaudioside A. These compounds possess up to 250 times the sweetness intensity of sucrose and do not have any calories. Stevioside, a natural plant glycoside isolated from the plant *Stevia rebaudiana*, has been commercialized as a noncaloric sweetener in Japan for more than 20 years.
- The stevia extract rebaudioside A (rebiana) is was approved by the U.S. Food and Drug Administration (FDA) as a sweetener; however, the whole stevia plant (and other constituents) are not "generally recognized as safe" (GRAS) nor approved as food additives by the FDA. Stevia may be imported only if "explicitly labeled as a dietary supplement or for use as a dietary ingredient in a dietary supplement." Although stevia may be marketed as a dietary supplement or an ingredient of a dietary supplement under the Dietary Supplement Health and Education Act (DSHEA), products that are labeled as using stevia plant parts or extracts as flavoring agents, sweeteners, or for other food additive purposes are deemed as "unsafe" because "available toxicological information on stevia is inadequate to demonstrate its safety." Regulatory agencies in Canada and Europe also have not approved use of stevia as a food additive.

EVIDENCE

Uses Based on Scientific Evidence	Grade
Hyperglycemia Stevia has been widely used for diabetes in South America, and animal studies have had promising results. Studies report decreases in plasma glucose levels when stevia was taken by healthy volunteers, but there is currently a lack of conclusive evidence of effectiveness when used for diabetes.	B
Hypertension (High Blood Pressure) Stevioside is a natural plant glycoside isolated from the plant *Stevia rebaudiana*, which has demonstrated blood pressure–lowering effects. Despite evidence of benefits in some human studies and support from laboratory and animal studies, more research is warranted to compare stevia's effectiveness with the current standard of care and make a firm recommendation. Stevia appears to have no major side effects.	B

Uses Based on Tradition or Theory

Alcohol abuse, antibacterial, antiinflammatory, antimicrobial, antimutagenic, antitumor, antiviral (human rotavirus activity), contraceptive (birth control), digestive aid, immunomodulation, obesity.

DOSING
Adults (18 Years and Older)

- For hyperglycemia (high blood sugar), 1 g of stevioside has been taken with meals to lower blood sugar levels in patients with type 2 diabetes. Water extracts of 5 g of leaves have also been used at regular 6-hour intervals for 3 days to increase glucose tolerance.
- For hypertension (high blood pressure), stevioside (250-500 mg) capsules given three times daily decreased systolic and diastolic blood pressure after 3 months of therapy and have been studied for up to 2 years. Despite early evidence that this may be an effective dose, a recent study did not find any benefit of crude steviosides (up to 15 mg/kg taken twice daily) for 2 years.

Children (Younger than 18 Years)

- There is insufficient evidence to recommend a dose for stevia, and use in children is not recommended.

SAFETY
Allergies

- Avoid in individuals with a known allergy or hypersensitivity to stevia or the daisy family (Asteraceae or Compositae). Other members of the daisy family include ragweed, chrysanthemums, marigolds, and many other herbs.

Side Effects and Warnings

- Stevioside may lower blood glucose levels. Caution is advised in patients with diabetes or hypoglycemia (low blood sugar levels) and in those taking drugs, herbs, or supplements that affect blood sugar. Serum glucose levels may need to be monitored by a health care provider, and medication adjustments may be necessary.

- Myalgia (muscle pain), muscle weakness, dizziness, asthenia (loss of strength), nausea, and abdominal fullness have been reported after taking stevioside. These effects resolved after the first week of treatment. Stevia may also lower systolic and diastolic blood pressure in patients with high blood pressure. Use cautiously in patients with hypotension (low blood pressure) or those taking hypotensive drugs because various human and animal studies have shown that stevioside may significantly decrease systolic and diastolic blood pressure.
- Higher doses of stevia may affect renal activity and perfusion, sodium excretion, and urinary flow. Avoid using stevia therapeutically in patients with impaired kidney function or other kidney diseases until human safety data are available.

Pregnancy and Breastfeeding

- Stevia is not recommended in pregnant or breastfeeding women because of a lack of available scientific evidence.

INTERACTIONS
Interactions with Drugs

- Stevia may lower blood sugar levels. Caution is advised in patients with diabetes or hypoglycemia (low blood sugar levels) and in those taking drugs that affect blood sugar. Serum glucose levels may need to be monitored by a health care provider, and medication adjustments may be necessary.
- Based on clinical observations in humans, stevioside may decrease systolic and diastolic blood pressure. Caution is advised in patients taking blood pressure–lowering medications.

- Although not well-researched, stevia may also interact with monoketocholate (a substance that may affect glucose and lipid levels), diuretics (medications that increase urine flow), or hypocalcemic agents. Caution is advised.
- Steviol is a vasodilator (medication that causes the blood vessels to dilate or expand). Caution is advised when stevia is taken with other vasodilators. Consult with a qualified health care professional, including a pharmacist, before combining therapies.
- Verapamil is a calcium antagonist and may exhibit additive effects with stevioside. In an animal study, verapamil tended to increase the renal (kidney) and systemic effects of stevioside. Caution is advised.

Interactions with Herbs and Dietary Supplements

- Although not well-researched, stevia may also interact with monoketocholate, diuretics (herbs and supplements that increase urine flow), or hypocalcemic agents. Caution is advised.
- Stevia may lower blood sugar levels. Caution is advised when herbs or supplements that may also lower blood sugar are used. Blood glucose levels may require monitoring, and doses may need adjustment.
- Stevioside may decrease systolic and diastolic blood pressure. Caution is advised in patients taking blood pressure–lowering herbs and supplements.
- Steviol is a vasodilator. Caution is advised when stevia is taken with other herbs and supplements that are vasodilators. Consult with a qualified health care professional, including a pharmacist, before combining therapies.

For a complete list of references, please visit www.naturalstandard.com.

Stinging Nettle
(Urtica dioica)

RELATED TERMS

- Bazoton, big string nettle, Brennessel (German), bull nettle, chichicaste, common nettle, dog nettle, extract of radix urticae (ERU), Fragdor, garden nettle, gerrais, grand ortie (French), grande ortie, great stinging nettle, great nettle, greater nettle, gross d'ortie, Hostid, isirgan, kazink, Kleer, nabat al nar, Nessel (German), nettle, nettles, ortic (Italian), ortie, ortiga (Spanish), pokrywa grosse brennessel, Prostaforton, Prostagalen, racine d'ortie, small nettle (*Urtica urens*), stingers, *Urtica, Urtica dioica, Urtica dioica* agglutinin (UDA), Urticae herba/folium (dried leaves or aerial parts of *Urtica dioica* and *Urtica urens*), *Urtica major*, Urticae radix (root), Urticaceae, urtiga, zwyczajna (Polish).

BACKGROUND

- The genus name *Urtica* comes from the Latin verb *urere* meaning, "to burn" because of its urticate (stinging) hairs that cover the stem and underside of the leaves. The species name *dioica* means "two houses" because the plant usually has male or female flowers.
- The most common uses for stinging nettle are treatment of benign prostatic hyperplasia (BPH, enlarged prostate), arthritis, allergies and pain, cough, tuberculosis, and urinary tract disorders, as an astringent and expectorant, and externally as a hair and scalp remedy for oily hair and dandruff. It is also frequently used as a diuretic to increase the flow of urine. There are some data supporting the use of nettle in the treatment of symptoms of BPH, but solid clinical data are lacking for other indications.
- Nettle is generally regarded as safe because the plant is also used as a green, leafy vegetable. Other than urticaria ("hives") from contacting the stinging hairs, gastrointestinal discomfort is the only reported adverse effect.

EVIDENCE

Uses Based on Scientific Evidence	Grade
Allergic Rhinitis For many years, a freeze-dried preparation of *Urtica dioica* has been prescribed by physicians and sold over-the-counter for the treatment of allergic rhinitis. However, there is insufficient evidence to support the use of nettle in the treatment of allergic rhinitis.	C
Arthritis Nettle is widely used as a folk remedy to treat arthritic and rheumatic conditions throughout Europe and in Australia. Preliminary evidence suggests that certain constituents in the nettle plant have anti-inflammatory and/or immunomodulatory activity.	C
Benign Prostatic Hypertrophy (BPH) Stinging nettle is used rather frequently in Europe in the treatment of symptoms associated with benign prostatic hyperplasia (enlarged prostate). Early evidence suggests an improvement in symptoms, such as the alleviation of lower urinary tract symptoms associated with stage I or II BPH, as a result of nettle therapy.	
Insect Bites Preliminary study has examined the effect of a combination product containing nettle applied on the skin. Preliminary results do not appear to confirm nettle as an effective therapy for itching caused by insect bites.	C
Joint Pain Nettle has historically been used in several different forms to treat pain of varying origins. However, there is a lack of available scientific evidence to support this use.	C
Plaque/Gingivitis One study has examined the effect of a mouthwash containing nettle on plaque and gingivitis in healthy adults and did not find any benefit. Further studies are required before a strong recommendation can be made.	C

Uses Based on Tradition or Theory

Abortion, aging, allergies, alopecia (hair loss), anaphylactic shock, anemia, angina pectoris (chest pain), animal bites, anthelmintic (expels worms), antidote to poisons (hemlock and henbane), antifungal, antihypertensive (blood pressure–lowering), antiinflammatory, antiviral, aphrodisiac, asthma, astringent, biliary colic, bladder disturbances, bleeding, blood purification, breast milk stimulation, bruises, burns, cancer, cardiac abnormalities, chickenpox, childbirth facilitation/induction, cholera, colitis (inflammation of the colon), coma, cough, cutaneous (skin) disorders, dandruff, diabetes, diarrhea, diuretic, dysentery (severe diarrhea), eczema, edema (swelling), exhaustion, expectorant, food uses, gangrene, gastric secretory inhibition, goiter (enlarged thyroid), gout (inflammation of the foot), hair tonic, hemorrhage, hemorrhoids, herpes (sexually transmitted disease [STD]), immunostimulation, insect repellant, iron deficiency, kidney disorders, kidney or bladder stones, labor induction, laxative, menorrhagia (excessive menstruation), mouth sores, muscle aches, nasal polyposis (growths), nephritis (inflammation of the kidney), neuralgia (nerve pain), nosebleeds, paralysis, parasitic worm infections, poor circulation, pregnancy problems, promotion of menstruation, pulmonary conditions, rash, renal impairment, rheumatism, scabies, sciatica (leg pain), scurvy, seborrhea (inflammation near the oil glands), shivering, shortness of breath, skin eruptions, snakebites, sore throat, spleen disorders, splenomegaly (enlarged spleen), sprains, stiff joints, stings (scorpion), stomachache, swelling, systemic lupus erythematosus (autoimmune disease in which the body's immune

(Continued)

Uses Based on Tradition or Theory—Cont'd

system attacks cells and tissue), tendonitis (inflamed tendon), tonic, tuberculosis, typhus (disease transmitted by lice or fleas), urinary tract infection (UTI), uterine bleeding (after childbirth), venous disorders, wheezing, wound healing.

DOSING
Adults (18 Years and Older)

- Various doses of nettle have been used in clinical trials; however, none have been proven effective. For BPH (enlarged prostate), one to two capsules of Bazoton containing 300 mg extract of Radix urticae (ERU) has been taken twice daily for up to 6 months. Bazoton Liquidum has also been studied in doses of 3 mL twice daily for 3 months. For allergic rhinitis, 600 mg freeze-dried nettle at the onset of symptoms for 1 week has been used. As an extract, nettle has traditionally been given in doses of 30-150 drops daily for 6 months.

Children (Younger than 18 Years)

- There is insufficient evidence to recommend a dose for nettle in children.

SAFETY
Allergies

- Avoid in individuals with a known allergy or hypersensitivity to nettle, the Urticaceae family, or any constituent of nettle products. Two patients taking a freeze-dried preparation of *Urtica dioica* for the treatment of allergic rhinitis had intensification of allergy symptoms.

Side Effects and Warnings

- Nettle therapy was generally well-tolerated for up to 2 years in available human trials. However, contact with the hairs of the nettle plant may cause short-lived whealing (hives), burning, itching, localized rash, and a prolonged tingling sensation. Other reported side effects include continual pain in the gastrointestinal tract, hyperperistalsis (excessive rapidity of the passage of food through the stomach and intestine), and mild gastric discomfort when the medication was taken on an empty stomach. Patients taking Bazoton capsules have experienced side effects such as constipation, diarrhea, and gastric disorder.
- The nettle plant contains a substance that is a coumarin derivative. Nettle may increase the risk of bleeding. Caution is advised in patients with bleeding disorders or taking drugs that may increase the risk of bleeding. Dosing adjustments may be necessary.
- Although not well studied in humans, nettle may increase blood glucose levels but not likely by enough to be of clinical concern. Nonetheless, use cautiously in patients with diabetes mellitus because of potential increased glycemia. Monitor blood glucose levels.
- Although not well-studied in humans, nettle may cause diuresis (water loss, excessive urination), uterine contractions, or low blood pressure. Use with caution in patients with hyponatremia (low sodium levels in the blood) as nettle has a synergistic diuretic effect. Monitor sodium levels.

- Elderly persons should use nettle cautiously for a possible hypotensive (decreased blood pressure) crisis that might be affected by nettle. Nettle should not be administered to children, as it has not been studied.

Pregnancy and Breastfeeding

- Nettle is not recommended in pregnant or breastfeeding women because of a lack of available scientific evidence. In theory, nettle may induce uterine stimulation.

INTERACTIONS
Interactions with Drugs

- Alpha blockers are typically given to treat high blood pressure (hypertension) and to treat BPH (enlarged prostate). Coadministration of nettle and alpha blockers may theoretically have an additive blood pressure–lowering effect. Caution is advised.
- Administration of nettle may also theoretically have an additive effect with antihypertensive (blood pressure–lowering) agents.
- Nettle root contains a coumarin constituent, and nettle leaves contain vitamin K. Thus, nettle may increase the risk of bleeding when taken with drugs that increase the risk of bleeding. Some examples include aspirin, anticoagulants ("blood thinners") such as warfarin (Coumadin) or heparin, antiplatelet drugs such as clopidogrel (Plavix), and nonsteroidal antiinflammatory drugs (NSAIDS) such as ibuprofen (Motrin, Advil) or naproxen (Naprosyn, Aleve).
- Nettle leaves have been used with diclofenac in the treatment of acute arthritis.
- Although not well-studied in humans, administration of nettle may theoretically have an additive effect on diuretics, resulting in dehydration and abnormally low potassium concentrations in the blood (hypokalemia).
- Finasteride, a 5-alpha-reductase inhibitor, is used in the treatment of benign BPH. Coadministration of finasteride and nettle may have additive effects. Caution is advised.
- Although not well-studied in humans, nettle may increase blood sugar levels. Caution is advised when medications that may alter blood sugar are used. Patients taking drugs for diabetes by mouth or using insulin should be monitored closely by a qualified health care professional, including a pharmacist. Medication adjustments may be necessary.

Interactions with Herbs and Dietary Supplements

- Theoretically, nettle may cause diuresis (increased flow of urine). Caution is advised when nettle is taken with other herbs that have a similar effect.
- Although not well-studied in humans, nettle may increase the risk of bleeding. Multiple cases of bleeding have been reported with the use of *Ginkgo biloba*, and fewer cases have been reported with garlic and saw palmetto. Numerous other agents may theoretically increase the risk of bleeding, such as kava, dong quai, horse chestnut, and niacin, although this has not been proven in most cases. Nettle leaves may also theoretically have an additive effect with other antiinflammatory agents.
- Theoretically, nettle may increase blood glucose levels. Caution is advised when herbs or supplements that may alter blood sugar are used. Blood glucose levels may require

monitoring, and doses may need adjustment. Theoretically, nettle may lower blood pressure levels.

- Saw palmetto and pygeum are used to treat BPH (enlarged prostate) and may have additive therapeutic effects with nettle.

- Soy isoflavones appear to inhibit type II 5α-reductase and may have additive effects with nettle.

For a complete list of references, please visit www.naturalstandard.com.

St. John's Wort
(Hypericum perforatum)

RELATED TERMS

- Amber touch-and-heal, balm-of-warrior's wound, balsana, bassant, Blutkraut, bossant, corazoncillo, dendlu, devil's scourge, Eisenblut, flor de Sao Joao, fuga daemonum, goatweed, hartheu, heofarigo on, herba de millepertius, herba hyperici, herrgottsblut, hexenkraut, hierba de San Juan, hipericao, hiperico, hipericon, HP, isorhamnetin, Jarsin, Johanniskraut, klamath weed, Liebeskraut, LI 160, lord God's wonder plant, millepertius pelicao, perforate, pinillo de oro, PM235, pseudohypericin, rosin rose, tenturotou, Teufelsflucht, touch and heal, Walpurgiskraut, wicher's herb, WS 5572.

BACKGROUND

- Extracts of *Hypericum perforatum* L. (St. John's wort) have been recommended traditionally for a wide range of medical conditions. The most common modern-day use of St. John's wort is for the treatment of depression. Numerous studies report St. John's wort to be more effective than placebo and equally effective as tricyclic antidepressant drugs in the short-term treatment of mild-to-moderate major depression (1-3 months). It is not clear whether St. John's wort is as effective as selective serotonin reuptake inhibitor (SSRI) antidepressants such as sertraline (Zoloft).

- Recently, controversy has been raised by two high-quality trials of St. John's wort for major depression that did not show any benefits. However, because of problems with the designs of these studies, they cannot be considered definitive. Overall, the scientific evidence supports the effectiveness of St. John's wort in mild-to-moderate major depression. The evidence in severe major depression remains unclear.

- St. John's wort can cause many serious interactions with prescription drugs, herbs, or supplements. Therefore, people using any medications should consult their health care providers, including their pharmacist, before starting therapy.

EVIDENCE

Uses Based on Scientific Evidence	Grade
Depressive Disorder (Mild-to-Moderate) St. John's wort has been extensively studied in Europe over the last 2 decades, with more recent research in the United States. Short-term studies (1-3 months) suggest that St. John's wort is more effective than placebo (sugar pill) and equally effective as tricyclic antidepressants (TCAs) in the treatment of mild-to-moderate major depression. Comparisons with the more commonly prescribed selective serotonin reuptake inhibitor (SSRI) antidepressants, such as fluoxetine (Prozac) or sertraline (Zoloft), are more limited. However, other data suggest that St. John's	A
wort may be just as effective as SSRIs with fewer side effects. Safety concerns exist, as with most conventional and complementary therapies.	
Anxiety Disorder Overall, there is currently not enough evidence to recommend St. John's wort for the primary treatment of anxiety disorders.	C
Atopic Dermatitis Preliminary, research of hypericum cream in the topical treatment of mild to moderate atopic dermatitis shows positive results.	C
Depressive Disorder (Severe) Studies of St. John's wort for severe depression have not provided clear evidence of effectiveness.	C
Obsessive-Compulsive Disorder (OCD) There are a few reported cases of possible benefits of St. John's wort in patients with obsessive–compulsive disorder (OCD). Currently, there is not enough scientific evidence to recommend St. John's wort for this condition.	C
Perimenopausal Symptoms There is currently not enough scientific evidence to recommend St. John's wort for this indication.	C
Premenstrual Syndrome (PMS) There is currently not enough scientific evidence to recommend St. John's wort for this indication.	C
Seasonal Affective Disorder (SAD) Despite some promising early data, there is currently not enough evidence to recommend St. John's wort for depressive disorder with seasonal pattern or seasonal affective disorder (SAD).	C
Human Immunodeficiency Virus (HIV) Antiviral effects of St. John's wort have been observed in laboratory studies but were not found in clinical research thus far. Multiple reports of significant adverse effects and interactions with drugs used for HIV/AIDS, including protease inhibitors (PIs) and nonnucleoside reverse transcriptase inhibitors (NNRTIs), suggest that patients being treated for HIV/AIDS should avoid this herb. Therefore, there is evidence to recommend against using St. John's wort in the treatment of patients with HIV/AIDS.	D
Social Phobia Results of preliminary research fail to provide evidence for the efficacy of St. John's wort in social phobia.	D

Uses Based on Tradition or Theory

Abdominal discomfort or irritation, alcoholism, allergies, anti-inflammatory, antiviral, athletic performance enhancement, bacterial skin infections (topical), bedwetting, benzodiazepine withdrawal, bruises (topical), burns (topical), cancer, chronic bowel irritation, chronic ear infections, dental pain, diarrhea, diuretic (increases urine flow), Epstein-Barr virus infection, fatigue, glioma, heartburn, hemorrhoids, herpes virus infection, influenza, insomnia, joint pain, liver protection from toxins, malaria treatment, menstrual pain, nerve pain, pain relief, rheumatism, skin scrapes, snakebites, sprains, ulcers, wound healing (topical).

DOSING
Adults (18 Years and Older)

- Clinical trials have used a range of doses, including 0.17-2.7 mg of hypericin by mouth and 900-1800 mg of St. John's wort extract daily by mouth.
- For treatment of atopic dermatitis, 1.5% hyperforin (verum) has been applied to the skin.

Children (Younger than 18 Years)

- There is insufficient evidence to recommend St. John's wort in children.

SAFETY
Allergies

- Infrequent allergic skin reactions, including rash and itching, have been reported in human studies.

Side Effects and Warnings

- In published studies, St. John's wort has generally been well-tolerated at recommended doses for up to 1-3 months. The most common adverse effects include gastrointestinal upset, skin reactions, fatigue/sedation, restlessness or anxiety, sexual dysfunction (including impotence), dizziness, headache, and dry mouth. Several recent studies suggest that side effects occur in 1%-3% of patients taking St. John's wort and that the number of adverse events may be similar to placebo (and less than standard antidepressant drugs). Animal toxicity studies have found only nonspecific symptoms such as weight loss. Elevated thyroid-stimulating hormone (TSH) levels have been associated with taking St. John's wort.
- It has been reported that St. John's wort may cause psychiatric symptoms such as suicidal and homicidal thoughts.
- Delayed ejaculation has been reported in animal studies.

Pregnancy and Breastfeeding

- There are insufficient data available at this time to recommend use during pregnancy or breastfeeding.

INTERACTIONS
Interactions with Drugs

- St. John's wort interferes with the way the body processes many drugs using the liver's cytochrome P450 enzyme system. As a result, the levels of these drugs may be increased in the blood in the short-term (causing increased effects or potentially serious adverse reactions) and/or decreased in the blood in the long-term (which can reduce the intended effects). Examples of medications that may be affected by St. John's wort in this manner include carbamazepine, cyclosporine, irinotecan, midazolam, nifedipine, birth control pills, simvastatin, theophylline, tricyclic antidepressants, warfarin, or human immunodeficiency virus (HIV) drugs such as nonnucleoside reverse transcriptase inhibitors (NNRTIs) or protease inhibitors (PIs). The U.S. Food and Drug Administration suggests that patients with HIV/AIDS taking protease inhibitors or NNRTIs avoid taking St. John's wort.
- Case reports exist of significant reductions in cyclosporine, tacrolimus, and mycophenolic acid drug levels and possible organ rejections in people with transplants who are taking St. John's wort. Reports also exist of altered menstrual flow, bleeding, and unwanted pregnancies in women taking birth control pills and St. John's wort at the same time. St. John's wort may interact with digoxin or digitoxin, resulting in a decrease in digoxin blood concentration. In general, individuals should check the package insert and speak with a qualified health care professional including a pharmacist about possible interactions with St. John's wort.
- Taking St. John's wort with other antidepressants may lead to increased side effects, including serotonin syndrome and mania. Serotonin syndrome is a condition defined by muscle rigidity, fever, confusion, increased blood pressure and heart rate, and coma. Mania is defined by symptoms of elevated or irritable mood, rapid speech or thoughts, increased activity, and decreased need for sleep. These interactions may occur in people taking St. John's wort with SSRI antidepressants such as fluoxetine (Prozac) or sertraline (Zoloft) or with monoamine oxidase inhibitors (MAOIs) such as isocarboxazid (Marplan), phenelzine (Nardil), or tranylcypromine (Parnate). Using St. John's wort with MAOIs may also increase the risk of severely increased blood pressure.
- St. John's wort may lead to increased risk of sun sensitivity when taken with other drugs such as antibiotics or birth control pills. St. John's wort may interact with anesthetic drugs. A possible interaction with loperamide (Imodium) has been reported; confusion and agitation occurred in one patient taking St. John's wort, loperamide, and the herb valerian (*Valeriana officinalis*). St. John's wort may interact with triptan-type headache medications. Examples include naratriptan (Amerge), rizatriptan (Maxalt), sumatriptan (Imitrex), and zolmitriptan (Zomig). In theory, St. John's wort may also interact with certain chemotherapy drugs such as anthracyclines. St. John's wort may increase antiinflammatory effects of COX-2 inhibitor drugs like rofecoxib (Vioxx) or nonsteroidal antiinflammatory drugs (NSAIDS) like ibuprofen (Motrin).
- St John's wort may increase imatinib clearance. Thus patients taking imatinib should avoid taking St John's wort. Concomitant use of enzyme inducers, including St John's wort, may necessitate an increase in the imatinib dose to maintain effectiveness.
- In higher doses, St. John's wort has been shown to decrease the blood concentrations of omeprazole, tolbutamide, caffeine, dextromethorphan, fexofenadine, carbamazepine, and cimetidine, among other medications. No relevant interactions have been seen with alprazolam, caffeine, tolbutamide, and digoxin after treatment with a low-hyperforin St. John's wort extract.
- Coadministration of St. John's wort leads to a short-term but clinically irrelevant increase followed by a prolonged

extensive reduction in voriconazole exposure. St. John's wort might put certain individuals at highest risk of potential voriconazole treatment failure.

- Although cases of interaction are rare, caution is advised when St. John's wort is taken with coumarin-type anticoagulants.
- Caution is also advised when benzodiazepine tranquilizers, opioids, or P-glycoprotein–regulated drugs are taken. In general, individuals should check the package insert and speak with a qualified health care professional, including a pharmacist, about possible interactions with St. John's wort.

Interactions with Herbs and Dietary Supplements

- St. John's wort may interfere with the way the body processes certain herbs and supplements using the liver's cytochrome P450 enzyme system. As a result, the levels of these drugs may be increased in the blood in the short-term, causing increased effects or potentially serious adverse reactions, or decreased in the blood in the long-term, which can reduce the intended effects.
- Taking St. John's wort with herbs or supplements with antidepressant activity may lead to increased side effects, including serotonin syndrome, mania, or a severe increase in blood pressure. There is a particular risk of these interactions occurring with agents that possess possible MAOI properties.
- St. John's wort may lead to increased risk of sun sensitivity when taken with capsaicin or other photosensitizing products. St. John's wort may interact with herbs that also possess cardiac glycoside properties and decrease blood levels.
- A possible interaction with the herb valerian (*Valeriana officinalis*) has been reported: confusion and agitation occurred in one patient taking St. John's wort, loperamide (Imodium), and valerian. However, St. John's wort and valerian are often used together, with few reported of adverse events. In theory, because of the presence of tannins, St. John's wort may inhibit the absorption of iron.
- Although cases of interaction are rare, caution is advised when St. John's wort is taken with coumarin-type anticoagulants.
- Caution is also advised when red yeast rice or any herb or supplements that is P-glycoprotein–regulated is taken. In general, individuals should speak with a qualified health care professional, including a pharmacist, about possible interactions with St. John's wort.

For a complete list of references, please visit www.naturalstandard.com.

Strawberry
(*Fragaria* spp.)

RELATED TERMS

- Allstar, Annapolis, Earliglow, Evangeline, *Fragaria chiloensis* ssp. Chiloensis, *Fragaria* x *ananassa* Duch., *Fragaria* x *ananassa* Duchesne, garden strawberry, Jewel, Mesabi, Rosaceae (family), Sable, Sparkle, woodland strawberry.

BACKGROUND

- Strawberry (*Fragaria* spp.) is predominantly known for its bright red, edible fruit covered in small seeds. The fruit is fragrant and high in fiber, vitamin C, folate, potassium, and antioxidants. Retrospective, epidemiological studies indicate that strawberry ingestion may reduce the risk of colorectal cancer. Preliminary research also indicates that strawberry may be useful as an antiinflammatory and may help enhance iron absorption. Further research is needed to confirm these results.
- Strawberry represents a valuable contrasting source of potentially healthy compounds and can represent an important component of a balanced diet if an individual is not allergic.

EVIDENCE

Uses Based on Scientific Evidence	Grade
Antioxidant Laboratory studies suggest that strawberry has antioxidant properties. However, the clinical effects are unclear. Further study is needed to define strawberry's effectiveness in humans.	B
Colorectal Cancer Prevention Strawberry and other fruits may reduce the risk of adenoma (noncancerous tumor) with mild dysplasia (abnormal growths) in women. However, the evidence is insufficient to support this use.	C

Uses Based on Tradition or Theory
Antiaging, antibacterial, anticoagulant (blood thinner), antiinflammatory, cancer, cancer (antiangiogenesis, destruction of blood vessels), food uses, iron absorption enhancement, leukemia, malnutrition, scurvy (vitamin C deficiency).

DOSING

Adults (18 Years and Older)

- There is insufficient evidence to recommend a dose for strawberry.

Children (Younger than 18 Years)

- There is insufficient evidence to recommend a dose for strawberry in children.

SAFETY

Allergies

- Avoid in individuals with a known allergy or hypersensitivity to strawberry (*Fragaria* spp.) or its constituents. Hypersensitivity to strawberry is fairly common, especially among children, although there are only a few cases of patients with adverse reactions to strawberry listed in the currently available literature compared with other Rosaceae fruit. There is some evidence that some proteins in strawberries are homologues for birch pollen and stone and pome fruit allergens, which may explain the prevalence of strawberry sensitivity. There also seems to be a connection between acetylsalicylic acid intolerance and strawberry sensitivity.

Side Effects and Warnings

- Strawberries are likely safe when used in food amounts in healthy patients. Strawberry extract or very large amounts of strawberries may be unsafe if consumed by pregnant patients because of insufficient available evidence. In sensitive subjects, strawberry has caused contact urticaria (hives) and pruritic dermatoses (eczema and neurodermatitis). Strawberries, especially fresh ones, may be contaminated with bacteria, pesticides, or fungi and should be thoroughly washed before consuming.
- Use cautiously in patients with hematological (blood) disorders or in patients taking anticoagulants or antiplatelet agents (blood thinners).
- Use cautiously in patients with iron-absorption disorders.

Pregnancy and Breastfeeding

- Based on traditional use as a food, strawberry in food amounts seems safe. Larger amounts and strawberry extract are not recommended in pregnant or breastfeeding women because of a lack of available scientific evidence.

INTERACTIONS

Interactions with Drugs

- Individual compounds in strawberries have demonstrated anticancer activity in several different studies. Caution is advised when strawberry is taken with anticancer agents.
- Strawberry may have blood-thinning properties. Caution is advised in patients with bleeding disorders or taking drugs that may increase the risk of bleeding. Dosing adjustments may be necessary.
- Strawberry may have antioxidant, antiinflammatory, and antibacterial properties. Caution is advised when strawberry is taken with agents with similar effects.
- Although not well-studied in humans, strawberry extract may interfere with gastrointestinal absorption of drugs taken by mouth. Strawberry (*Fragaria* spp.) may have a mild to moderate enhancing effect on iron absorption.
- Based on tests performed in allergic patients, there may be a connection between acetylsalicylic acid intolerance and strawberry sensitivity.

S

Interactions with Herbs and Dietary Supplements

- Individual compounds in strawberries have demonstrated anticancer activity in several different studies. Caution is advised when strawberry is taken with herbs and supplements with anticancer effects.
- Strawberry may have blood-thinning properties. Caution is advised in patients with bleeding disorders or taking herbs or supplements that may increase the risk of bleeding. Multiple cases of bleeding have been reported with the use of *Ginkgo biloba*, and fewer cases have been reported with garlic and saw palmetto.
- Strawberry may have antioxidant, antiinflammatory, and antibacterial properties. Caution is advised when strawberry is taken with herbs and supplements with these properties.
- Although not well-studied in humans, strawberry extract may interfere with gastrointestinal absorption of herbs and supplements taken by mouth. Strawberry (*Fragaria* spp.) may have a mild to moderate enhancing effect on iron absorption.
- Based on tests performed in allergic patients, there may be a connection between acetylsalicylic acid intolerance and strawberry sensitivity.

For a complete list of references, please visit www.naturalstandard.com.

Sweet Almond
(*Prunus amygdalus dulcis*)

RELATED TERMS

- Almendra, Almendra dulce, almond beta-galactosidase, almond beta-glucosidase, almond glycopeptidase, almond oil, amande, amande douce, amandel, amendoa, amendoa doce, amigdalo, *Amygdala dulcis*, *Amygdalus communis*, arginine, aspartic acid, B-complex vitamins, badam, badami, badamo, badamshirin, bedamu, bian tao, bilati badam, cno ghreugach, daucosterol, emulsion, expressed almond oil, fixed almond oil, galactosidase, glucosidase, glutamic acid, harilik mandli-puu, Jordan almond, lawz, lozi, mandel, mandla, mandorla, mandorla dulce, mandula, mangel, mannosidase, mantelli, migdal, migdala, migdalo, mindal, prunasin, Prunoideae (sub-family), *Prunus communis dulcis*, *Prunus dulcis* var. dulcis, Rosaceae (family), sladkiy mindal, sötmandel, süßmandel, sweet almond oil, tatli badem, tian wei bian tao, tian xing ren, vaadaam, vadumai, vitamin A, vitamin E, zoete amandel.
- **Note:** Sweet almond should not be confused with bitter almond, which contains amygdalin and can be broken down into the poisonous substance hydrocyanic acid (cyanide).

BACKGROUND

- The almond is closely related to the peach, apricot, and cherry (all classified as drupes in the genus *Prnus*). Unlike the others, however, the outer layer of the almond is not edible. The edible portion of the almond is the seed. Sweet almonds and bitter almonds belong to the same species; a compound called amygdalin differentiates the bitter almond from the sweet almond.
- Sweet almonds are a popular nutritious food. Researchers are especially interested in their level of monounsaturated fats, as these appear to have a beneficial effect on blood lipids.
- Almond oil is widely used in lotions and cosmetics.

EVIDENCE

Uses Based on Scientific Evidence	Grade
High Cholesterol (Whole Almonds) Preliminary studies in humans and animals report that whole almonds may lower levels of total cholesterol and low-density lipoprotein (LDL/"bad" cholesterol) and raise levels of high-density lipoprotein (HDL/"good" cholesterol). It is not clear what dose may be safe or effective.	B
Anxiety (in Palliative Care Patients) It is unclear whether sweet almond improves anxiety in palliative care patients, but more research investigating sweet almond as the active treatment is needed to make a firm recommendation.	C
Radiation Therapy Skin Reactions (Used on the Skin) In preliminary study, an ointment made of sweet almond has not shown a benefit when applied to the skin of patients treated with radiation.	D

Uses Based on Tradition or Theory

Antibacterial, aphrodisiac, bladder cancer, breast cancer, chapped lips, colon cancer, dilution of injected medications, heart disease, increasing sperm count, mild laxative, mouth and throat cancers, plant-derived estrogen, skin moisturizer, uterine cancer.

DOSING
Adults (18 Years and Older)

- Studies have used 84-100 g of whole almonds daily by mouth with no reported side effects to treat high cholesterol levels. As a laxative, 30 mL of sweet almond oil daily by mouth has been used.

Children (Younger than 18 Years)

- Little information is available for the use of sweet almonds in children, aside from the amounts normally eaten in the diet.

SAFETY
Allergies

- Allergies to almonds are common and can lead to severe reactions, including oral allergic syndrome (OAS), swelling of the lips and face, and closure of the throat. People who are allergic to one type of nut may also be allergic to other nuts. Avoid use in anyone with a known allergy to almonds, almond products, or other nuts.

Side Effects and Warnings

- In most reports, sweet almond is generally considered to be safe when taken by mouth. Sweet almond may lower blood sugar levels. Caution is advised in patients with diabetes or hypoglycemia and in those taking drugs, herbs, or supplements that affect blood sugar. Serum glucose levels may need to be monitored by a health care provider, and medication adjustments may be necessary.
- Sweet almond may have estrogen-like activity. A study in mice reports hair loss and inflammation in the leg joints. There is a report of a fat embolism (fat bubbles traveling through the bloodstream, which is potentially dangerous) due to injection of almond oil into the penis.
- Theoretically, increased intake of almonds (and therefore increased intake of unsaturated fat) can lead to weight gain. However, one study reports that consuming approximately 320 calories of almonds daily for 6 months does not lead to statistically or biologically significant average changes in body weight and does increase the consumption of unsaturated fats.

Pregnancy and Breastfeeding

- There is little information about the use of sweet almond during pregnancy or breastfeeding. It appears that almonds in regular dietary intake are safe for most nonallergic individuals.

S

INTERACTIONS
Interactions with Drugs

- Based on animal studies, sweet almond may lower blood sugar levels. Caution is advised when medications that may also lower blood sugar are used. Patients taking drugs for diabetes by mouth or using insulin should be monitored closely by a qualified health care provider. Medication adjustments may be necessary.
- Theoretically, almonds and cholesterol-lowering agents may have additive effects when taken together. Sweet almond may also interact with drugs taken for cardiovascular conditions, fertility, or estrogen activity.

Interactions with Herbs and Dietary Supplements

- Based on animal studies, sweet almond may lower blood sugar levels. Caution is advised when herbs or supplements that may also lower blood sugar are used. Blood glucose levels may require monitoring, and doses may need adjustment.
- Theoretically, almonds may add to the effects of herbs or supplements that lower blood cholesterol levels, such as fish oil, garlic, guggul, or niacin.
- Sweet almond may also interact with agents taken for cardiovascular conditions, fertility, or estrogen activity.

For a complete list of references, please visit www. naturalstandard.com.

Sweet Annie
(*Artemisia annua*)

RELATED TERMS

- Arteannuin-B, arteether, artemether, artemetin, *Artemisia annua*, *Artemisia annua* essential oil, *Artemisia apiacea*, artemisia ketone, *Artemisia lancea*, artemisinic acid, artemisinin, artemotil, artenimol, artesunate, artemisinin, beta-caryophyllene, beta-selinene, camphor, Chinese wormwood, deoxyartemisinin, dihydroartemisinin, dihydroqinghaosu, endoperoxide sesquiterpene lactone artemisinin, friedelin, germacrene D, oriental wormwood, qing hao (Chinese), qing hao su (Chinese), qinghaosu (Chinese), quinghao (Chinese), sodium artesunate, stigmasterol, sweet wormwood, thanh hao (Vietnamese), trans-pinocarveol, yin-chen.
- **Note**: This monograph does not include information on wormwood (absinthe, *Artemisia absinthium*) or mugwort (*Artemisia vulgaris*).

BACKGROUND

- Sweet Annie (*Artemisia annua*) is also known as Chinese wormwood or sweet wormwood. Although it is in the same genus as both wormwood (absinthe, *Artemisia absinthium*) and mugwort (*Artemisia vulgaris*), each of these herbs has different uses and should not be confused.
- For more than 1500 years, sweet Annie tea was used in traditional Chinese medicine (TCM) to treat fevers, although the herb fell out of favor for a few centuries. In 1970, a TCM handbook from the fifth century was discovered and stimulated interest in sweet Annie. Although originally used to treat fevers, sweet Annie was not used specifically for malaria.
- Sweet Annie's main active constituent is artemisinin, which has shown rapid antimalarial activity in humans, especially when used as an adjuvant with standard antimalarial drugs. Considered a weed by some, the plant can be grown in many climates, and a simple and effective preparation of *Artemisia annua* could be a much-needed, inexpensive, and convenient weapon against malaria. In addition to sweet Annie's promise in treating malaria, preliminary evidence indicates that it may have potential as an anticancer agent and an antiviral.

EVIDENCE

Uses Based on Scientific Evidence	Grade
Cancer Certain constituents found in sweet Annie show promise when used in combination with standard chemotherapy. However, currently there is not enough scientific evidence in humans to make a strong recommendation for this use.	C
Malaria Malaria is a serious health concern in many poorer parts of the world where modern antimalarial drugs may not be available. Although there has been some interest in using sweet Annie as an antimalarial, and the constituent artemisinin is widely used for treating malaria, there is currently not enough clinical evidence to support the use of the herb.	C

Uses Based on Tradition or Theory

Antibacterial, antioxidant, antiparasitic, antiviral, fever, immunosuppression, leukemia, melanoma, neonatal jaundice.

DOSING
Adults (18 Years and Older)

- There is insufficient evidence to recommend a dose for sweet Annie in adults.

Children (Younger than 18 Years)

- There is insufficient evidence to recommend a dose for sweet Annie in children.

SAFETY
Allergies

- Avoid in individuals with a known allergy or hypersensitivity to sweet Annie or members of the Asteraceae/Compositae family such as dandelion, goldenrod, ragweed, sunflower, and daisy.

Side Effects and Warnings

- Certain constituents in sweet Annie (artemisinin and artesunate) have been well-tolerated when taken by mouth with no reported adverse effects. However, there is a lack of available information on the safety of sweet Annie, and caution is advised.
- Use cautiously in patients with compromised heart or brain function, as a related species has shown potential toxicity.
- Use cautiously in patients who are pregnant or recovering from surgery or other wounds.
- Use cautiously in patients with compromised immune function, as sweet Annie may have immunomodulatory activity.

Pregnancy and Breastfeeding

- Sweet Annie is not recommended in pregnant or breastfeeding women because of a lack of available scientific evidence. Sweet Annie may inhibit angiogenesis, which is the development of new blood vessels.

INTERACTIONS
Interactions with Drugs

- Sweet Annie may inhibit angiogenesis, which is the development of new blood vessels. Caution is advised in patients taking agents that affect angiogenesis.
- Although not well studied in humans, sweet Annie may also inhibit bacterial and fungal growth. Thus, patients taking antibiotics and antifungals should be aware that additive effects might occur.
- Artesunate, a constituent found in sweet Annie, may be incompatible with quinolines, which are used as food preservatives and in making antiseptics. These should not be confused with quinolones, which are a family of broad-spectrum antibiotics.

- Sweet Annie has been studied for its antimalarial and anti-cancer effects, and use with other antimalarial or anticancer agents may have additive effects.
- Sweet Annie may have antioxidant and immunomodulatory activity. Consult with a qualified health care professional, including a pharmacist, to check for possible interactions.

Interactions with Herbs and Dietary Supplements

- Sweet Annie may inhibit angiogenesis, which is the development of new blood vessels. Caution is advised in patients taking herbs or supplements that affect angiogenesis.
- Although not well-studied in humans, sweet Annie may also inhibit bacterial and fungal growth. Thus, patients taking antibiotics and antifungals should be aware that additive effects might occur.
- Sweet Annie has been studied for its antimalarial and anti-cancer effects, and use with other antimalarial or anticancer herbs or supplements may have additive effects.
- Sweet Annie may have antioxidant and immunomodulatory activity. Consult with a qualified health care professional, including a pharmacist, to check for possible interactions with herbs or supplements with these effects.

For a complete list of references, please visit www.naturalstandard.com.

Sweet Basil
(Ocimum basilicum)

RELATED TERMS

- Apigenin, basil, citral, common basil, estragole, eugenol, geraniol, Lamiaceae (family), linalol, linolen, methylchavikol, methylcinnamate, *Ocimum*, *Ocimum basilicum*, *Ocimum basilicum* var. citratum, rosmarinic acid, Thai basil, ursolic acid.

BACKGROUND

- Sweet basil (*Ocimum basilicum*) is a commonly used medicinal herb in Thailand, India, and Turkey and has been used as a spice in cooking. The constituent, estragole, is naturally found in sweet basil and is used in fragrances and flavorings. Although laboratory study has found that estragole may be associated with cancer, human study is lacking.
- Laboratory studies have investigated sweet basil for its antiviral, anticancer, and antibacterial effects. However, currently, there is not enough clinical evidence to support the use of sweet basil for any indication. Side effects are rarely reported, aside from allergy and contamination. Sweet basil appears safe in food amounts.

EVIDENCE

Uses Based on Scientific Evidence

No available studies qualify for inclusion in the evidence table.

Uses Based on Tradition or Theory

Acne, aging, antibacterial, antiinflammatory, antimicrobial, antioxidant, antiviral, cancer, cardiovascular risk reduction, chronic bronchitis, dental conditions, human immunodeficiency virus/acquired immunodeficiency syndrome (HIV/AIDS), spermicide (kills sperm).

DOSING

Adults (18 Years and Older)

- There is insufficient evidence to recommend a dose for sweet basil in adults; sweet basil is generally considered safe in amounts found in food after proper washing.

Children (Younger than 18 Years)

- There is insufficient evidence to recommend a dose for sweet basil in children; sweet basil is generally considered safe in amounts found in food after proper washing.

SAFETY

Allergies

- Avoid in individuals with a known allergy or hypersensitivity to sweet basil, its constituents, or members of the Lamiaceae/Labiatae family, such as hyssop, marjoram, mint, sage, lavender, oregano, or thyme.

Side Effects and Warnings

- Sweet basil is likely safe when used in amounts commonly found in foods in nonallergic people. However, fresh basil may carry pathogens; fresh sweet basil should always be washed before use.
- Based on laboratory study, estragole, a constituent of sweet basil, may cause liver damage.
- Cow's urine concoction (CUC) is prepared from leaves of tobacco, garlic, basil, lemon juice, rock salt, and bulbs of onion and is thought to be toxic.
- Use cautiously in patients who are pregnant or breastfeeding, as amounts higher than food amounts have not been fully investigated.

Pregnancy and Breastfeeding

- Sweet basil is not recommended in pregnant or breastfeeding women because of a lack of available scientific evidence in amounts higher than those found in food. Based on laboratory study, sweet basil may be a potent spermicide (kills sperm) in humans.

INTERACTIONS

Interactions with Drugs

- Sweet basil may have additive effects with antibiotics.
- Sweet basil may have antioxidant effects, anticancer activity, and antiviral activity; use cautiously.
- Sweet basil may interfere with drugs broken down by the liver.

Interactions with Herbs and Dietary Supplements

- Sweet basil may have antibacterial effects, antioxidant effects, anticancer activity, and antiviral effects. Use cautiously with herbs and supplement with similar effects.
- Sweet basil may interact with herbs and supplements broken down by the liver.

For a complete list of references, please visit www.naturalstandard.com.

Tamanu
(Calophyllum inophyllum)

RELATED TERMS

- Alexandrian laurel, ati tree, bioflavonoids, brasiliensic acid, calaustralin, calophyllolide, *Calophyllum inophyllum* L., calophyllic acid, calophynic acid, caloxanthone A, Clusiaceae (family), delta-tocotriene, dilo, dipyranocoumarin, dolno, fatty acids, feta'u, fetau, Foraha oil, Guttiferae (family), hydrocyanic acid, Hypericaceae (family), inocalophyllin A, inocalophyllin B, inophylloidic acid, inophyllum B, inophyllum C, inophyllum E, kamani, kamanu, linoleic fatty acid, nambagura, ndamanu, oleic fatty acid, palmitic fatty acid, poon, punnai, punnakkai, saponins, stearic fatty acid, sterols, temanu, ti, tocopherol, tocotriene, tree of a thousand virtues, triterpenes, undi, xanthone.

BACKGROUND

- Tamanu is a large tropical tree native to Polynesia and Southeast Asia. In Chinese and Tahitian traditional medicine, tamanu is used for abrasions, acne, anal fissures, blisters, burns (boiling water, sun, x-rays), cuts, diabetic ulcers, dry skin, eczema, herpes sores, insect bites and stings, psoriasis, scars, sore throat, foot and body odor, and for pain from muscle, nerve, shingles, leprous neuritis (inflammation associated with leprosy), or rheumatological etiologies.
- The phytochemistry of tamanu has been well-established, and there are several laboratory and animal trials showing effectiveness of tamanu as an antibacterial, anticancer, antiinflammatory, and antiviral agent. There is limited evidence from human clinical trials, however, about its safety or effectiveness.

EVIDENCE

Uses Based on Scientific Evidence

No available studies qualify for inclusion in the evidence table.

Uses Based on Tradition or Theory

Abrasions, acne, age spots, anal fissures, analgesia (inability to feel pain), anthelmintic (expels worms), antibacterial, anticoagulant, antiinflammatory, antiviral, athlete's foot, bed sores, blisters, burns (boiling water, sun, x-rays), cancer, cicatrizant (scar tissue formation), constipation, cuts, diabetic ulcers, diaper rash, dry skin, dysentery (severe diarrhea), eczema, eye disorders (sore eyes), eyewash, gout, hemorrhage (internal bleeding), herpes, insect bites and stings, leprosy, molluscicidal (kills mollusks), neuralgia (nerve pain), pain, psoriasis, rheumatism, ringworm, scabies, sedative, skin conditions, sore throat, stretch marks, wound care.

DOSING
Adults (18 Years and Older)

- There is insufficient evidence to recommend a dose for tamanu. For wound healing, tamanu oil has been applied "liberally" to cuts and other wounds.

Children (Younger than 18 Years)

- There is insufficient evidence to recommend a dose for tamanu in children, and use is not recommended.

SAFETY
Allergies

- Avoid in individuals with a known allergy or hypersensitivity to tamanu or its constituents. Allergic dermatitis has been reported.

Side Effects and Warnings

- There are very few reports of tamanu and its adverse effects. Allergic dermatitis has been reported. Although not well studied in humans, tamanu may cause central nervous system depression (e.g., sedation) and increase prothrombin and bleeding time. Caution is advised in patients with bleeding disorders or taking drugs that may increase the risk of bleeding. Dosing adjustments may be necessary.

Pregnancy and Breastfeeding

- Tamanu is not recommended in pregnant or breastfeeding women because of a lack of available scientific evidence.

INTERACTIONS
Interactions with Drugs

- Although not well studied in humans, xanthone compounds from tamanu may potentiate ether anesthesia. Consult with a qualified health care professional, including a pharmacist, before combining therapies.
- Tamanu may increase the risk of bleeding when taken with drugs that increase the risk of bleeding. Some examples include aspirin, anticoagulants ("blood thinners") such as warfarin (Coumadin) or heparin, antiplatelet drugs such as clopidogrel (Plavix), and nonsteroidal antiinflammatory drugs such as ibuprofen (Motrin, Advil) or naproxen (Naprosyn, Aleve).
- Xanthone compounds from tamanu may increase the amount of drowsiness caused by some drugs. Examples include benzodiazepines such as lorazepam (Ativan) or diazepam (Valium), barbiturates such as phenobarbital, narcotics such as codeine, some antidepressants, and alcohol. Use caution while driving or operating machinery.

Interactions with Herbs and Dietary Supplements

- Tamanu may increase the risk of bleeding when taken with herbs and supplements that are believed to increase the risk of bleeding. Multiple cases of bleeding have been reported with the use of *Ginkgo biloba*, and fewer cases have been reported with garlic and saw palmetto. Numerous other agents may theoretically increase the risk of bleeding, although this has not been proven in most cases.
- Xanthone compounds from tamanu may increase the amount of drowsiness caused by some herbs or supplements.

For a complete list of references, please visit www.naturalstandard.com.

Tamarind

(Tamarindus indica)

RELATED TERMS

- Ambilis, amli, asam, asam jawa, Caesalpiniaceae (subfamily), chintachettu, chintapandu, da ma lin, daaih mah lahm, demirhindi, glyloid, glyloid sulphate 4324, imlee, imli, Indian date, indijska tamarinda, loh fong ji, loh mohng ji, luo huang zi, luo wang zi, ma-gyi-thi, puli, Pulpa tamarindorum, sampalok, sbar, siyambala, swee boey, tamalen, tamar hindi, tamarin, tamarind brown, tamarind flour, tamarind gum, tamarind kernel powder, tamarind nutshell activated carbon, tamarind seed polysaccharide, tamarind seed powder, tamarind seed xyloglucan (XG), tamarinde, tamarindienal, tamarindipuu, tamarindo, *Tamarindus* amyloid, *Tamarindus indica L., Tamarindus indica Linn., Tamarindus indica* seed, tamarynd, tamr al-hindi, tamre hendi, tentuli, teteli, tintiri, tintul, titri, TS-polysaccharide, ukwaju, xyloglucan.
- **Note:** *Tamarindus indica* should not be confused with the dried fruit rind of *Garcinia cambogia*, also known as Malabar tamarind.

BACKGROUND

- Tamarind is native to tropical Africa and grows wild throughout the Sudan. It was introduced to India thousands of years ago. In Jordan and other middle eastern countries, tamarind juice from the tamarind tree is made into a drink prepared by infusing dried tamarind pulp. It has also been used for the preservation of food products. Tamarind may be used as a paste and sauce and included in recipes. Tamarind is also used in India as part of Ayurvedic herbal medicine.
- In animal studies, tamarind has been found to lower serum cholesterol and blood sugar levels. Because of a lack of available human clinical trials, there is insufficient evidence to recommend tamarind for the treatment of hypercholesterolemia (high cholesterol levels) or diabetes.
- Based on clinical evidence, tamarind intake may delay the progression of fluorosis by enhancing excretion of fluoride. However, additional research is needed to confirm these results.

EVIDENCE

Uses Based on Scientific Evidence	Grade
Bone Diseases (Skeletal Fluorosis Prevention) Preliminary research has examined the use of tamarind for fluorosis prevention. Although beneficial outcomes have been reported, the available evidence is not conclusive.	C

Uses Based on Tradition or Theory
Anthelmintic (expels worms), antimicrobial, antiseptic, antiviral, asthma, astringent, bacterial skin infections (erysipelas), boils, chest pain, cholesterol metabolism disorders, colds, colic, conjunctivitis (pink eye), constipation (chronic or acute), diabetes, diarrhea (chronic), dry eyes, dysentery (severe diarrhea), eye inflammation, fever, food preservative, food uses (coloring), gallbladder disorders, gastrointestinal disorders, gingivitis, hemorrhoids, indigestion, insecticide, jaundice, keratitis (inflammation of the cornea), leprosy, liver disorders, nausea and vomiting (pregnancy-related), paralysis, poisoning (*Datura* plant), rash, rheumatism, saliva production, skin disinfectant/sterilization, sore throat, sores, sprains, sunscreen, sunstroke, swelling (joints), urinary stones, wound healing (corneal epithelium).

DOSING

Adults (18 Years and Older)

- There is insufficient evidence to recommend a dose of tamarind. However, 10 g daily for up to 3 weeks has been used to delay the progression of fluorosis by enhancing excretion of fluoride. As a laxative, 10-50 g of tamarind paste as fermented fruit cubes has been used.

Children (Younger than 18 Years)

- There is insufficient evidence to recommend a dose of tamarind in children. However, 10 g daily for up to 3 weeks has been used to delay the progression of fluorosis by enhancing excretion of fluoride.

SAFETY

Allergies

- Avoid in individuals with a known allergy or hypersensitivity to tamarind or its constituents.

Side Effects and Warnings

- Based on the available research, it appears that tamarind is well tolerated in recommended doses. Tamarind is "generally recognized as safe" (GRAS) in the United States when used orally and appropriately in food amounts, at a maximum use of 0.81% of dietary intake.
- There is one reported outbreak of weaver's cough associated with tamarind seed powder. Dust exposure to tamarind flours may also induce chronic changes in lung function. Additionally, tamarind seed preparations have been linked to acute respiratory reactions. Be aware that tamarind candy has been associated with lead poisoning and death. Use cautiously in patients with diabetes because of its possible glucose-lowering effects.

Pregnancy and Breastfeeding

- Tamarind is not recommended in pregnant or breastfeeding women because of a lack of available scientific evidence. Avoid using in amounts greater than those found in foods.

INTERACTIONS

Interactions with Drugs

- Tamarind may increase the risk of bleeding when taken with drugs that increase the risk of bleeding. Some examples include aspirin, anticoagulants ("blood thinners") such as warfarin (Coumadin) or heparin, antiplatelet drugs such as clopidogrel (Plavix), and nonsteroidal antiinflammatory

T

drugs (NSAIDS) such as ibuprofen (Motrin, Advil) or naproxen (Naprosyn, Aleve).

- Although not well studied in humans, tamarind may lower blood sugar levels. Caution is advised in patients with diabetes or hypoglycemia (low blood sugar levels) and in those taking drugs that affect blood sugar. Serum glucose levels may need to be monitored by a health care provider, and medication adjustments may be necessary.
- The fruit pulp may have mild laxative properties, but heat may cause loss of this effect. Caution is advised when tamarind is combined with other laxatives because of additive effects.
- Concurrent use of tamarind and topical ophthalmic (eye) antibiotics may result in a synergistic effect. Consult with a qualified health care professional, including a pharmacist, to check for interactions.
- Taking vasoconstrictors and tamarind together may cause a potential additive interaction. Caution is advised.

Interactions with Herbs and Dietary Supplements

- Tamarind may increase the risk of bleeding when taken with herbs and supplements that are believed to increase the risk of bleeding. Multiple cases of bleeding have been reported with the use of *Ginkgo biloba*, and fewer cases have been reported with garlic and saw palmetto. Numerous other agents may theoretically increase the risk of bleeding, although this has not been proven in most cases.
- Although not well studied in humans, tamarind may lower blood sugar levels. Caution is advised in patients with diabetes or hypoglycemia (low blood sugar levels) and in those taking herbs or supplements that affect blood sugar. Serum glucose levels may need to be monitored by a health care provider, and medication adjustments may be necessary.
- The fruit pulp may have mild laxative properties, but heat may cause loss of this effect. Caution is advised when tamarind is combined with other laxatives because of additive effects.
- Taking vasoconstrictors and tamarind together may cause a potential additive interaction. Caution is advised when herbs or supplements with similar effects are taken.

For a complete list of references, please visit www. naturalstandard.com.

Tangerine
(*Citrus reticulata*)

RELATED TERMS

- Beta-carotene, beta-cryptoxanthin, carotenoids, Citri Reticulatae Viride Pericarpium, *Citrus reticulata*, *Citrus reticulata* Blanco, Citrus reticulate, Dancy tangerine (*Citrus tangerina*), folate, grapefruit (*Citrus paradisi*), limonin, limonoid glucoside mixture, limonoids, lutein, magnesium, mandarin (*Citrus reticulata* Blanco), nomilin, orange (*Citrus sinensis*), polyphenols, Rutaceae (family), tangeretin, tangerine juice, vitamin C, xanthophyll esters, zeaxanthin.

BACKGROUND

- Tangerine (*Citrus reticulata*) is a citrus fruit that is well-known for being sweet and easy to peel. The name tangerine comes from Tangier, Morocco, the port from which the first tangerines were shipped to Europe. Tangerine contains vitamin C, folate, and beta-carotene. In Korea, tangerine peel has traditionally been used to promote liver qi activity and the function of the digestive system.
- Tangerine may have antioxidant and anticancer properties. It is also a good source of vitamin C. However, there is currently a lack of clinical evidence to support the use of tangerine for any medical indication.

EVIDENCE

Uses Based on Scientific Evidence

No available studies qualify for inclusion in the evidence table.

Uses Based on Tradition or Theory

Antibacterial, antiinflammatory, antioxidant, atherosclerosis (hardening of the arteries), cancer, cancer prevention, cardiovascular disease, chemotherapeutic adjunct, gastrointestinal disorders, *Helicobacter pylori* infection, leukemia, scurvy.

DOSING

Adults (18 Years and Older)

- There is insufficient evidence to recommend a dose for tangerine in adults.

Children (Younger than 18 Years)

- There is insufficient evidence to recommend a dose for tangerine in children.

SAFETY

Allergies

- Avoid in individuals with a known allergy or hypersensitivity to tangerine or other citrus fruits. The essential oil of tangerine in a fragrance has been associated with skin rash.

Side Effects and Warnings

- There are few reports of adverse effects associated with tangerine. However, skin rash has been associated with tangerine essential oil, and bowel obstructions have been reported.
- Use cautiously in patients with gastrointestinal disorders, as tangerine has been associated with intestinal obstructions.
- Use cautiously in patients taking agents for cancer. Also, use cautiously in patients taking agents metabolized by cytochrome P450, as tangerine may stimulate cytochrome P450 3A4. Consult with a qualified health care professional, including a pharmacist, to check for interactions.

Pregnancy and Breastfeeding

- Tangerine is not recommended in pregnant or breastfeeding women in amounts higher than those found in foods because of a lack of available scientific evidence.

INTERACTIONS

Interactions with Drugs

- Although not well studied in humans, tangerine may inhibit *Helicobacter pylori*. Use cautiously with other antibiotics because of possible additive effects. Preliminary evidence also suggests that tangerine may have antioxidant properties.
- Tangerine juice may lower cholesterol and triglyceride levels. Use cautiously with high or low cholesterol levels or if taking cholesterol-altering medications.
- In theory, constituents found in citrus fruits, including tangerine, may have additive effects with other antiinflammatory agents.
- Although not well studied in humans, tangerine peel or its extracts may have anticancer activity. In addition, tangerine and other Chinese medicinal herbs may decrease the toxic effects of chemotherapy.
- Tangerine juice may interfere with the way the body processes certain drugs using the liver's cytochrome P450 enzyme system. As a result, the levels of these drugs may be decreased in the blood and the intended effects may be reduced. Patients taking any medications should check the package insert and speak with a qualified health care professional, including a pharmacist, about possible interactions.

Interactions with Herbs and Dietary Supplements

- Although not well studied in humans, tangerine may inhibit *Helicobacter pylori*. Caution is advised in patients taking other herbs or supplements with antibacterial activity because of possible additive effects. Preliminary evidence also suggests that tangerine may have antioxidant properties.
- Tangerine juice may also lower cholesterol and triglyceride levels. Use cautiously with high or low cholesterol levels or if taking cholesterol-altering herbs or supplements.
- In theory, constituents found in citrus fruits, including tangerine, may have additive effects with other herbs with antiinflammatory effects.
- Although not well studied in humans, tangerine peel or its extracts may have anticancer activity. In addition, tangerine and other Chinese medicinal herbs may decrease the toxic effects of chemotherapy.

T

697

- Tangerine juice may interfere with the way the body processes certain herbs or supplements using the liver's cytochrome P450 enzyme system. As a result, the levels of other herbs or supplements may become too low in the blood. It may also alter the effects that other herbs or supplements potentially may have on the P450 system.

For a complete list of references, please visit www.naturalstandard.com.

Taurine
(2-Aminoethanesulfonic acid)

RELATED TERMS

- Acamprosate, glycochenodeoxycholic acid, glycocholic acid, taltrimide, taurochenodeoxycholic acid, taurocholic acid, tauro-UDCA, tauroursodeoxycholic acid (TUDCA), ursodeoxycholic acid.

BACKGROUND

- Taurine, or 2-aminoethanesulfonic acid, was originally discovered in ox (*Bos taurus*) bile and was named after taurus, or bull. A nonessential amino acid-like compound, taurine is found in high abundance in the tissues of many animals, especially sea animals, and in much lower concentrations in plants, fungi, and some bacteria. As an amine, taurine is important in several metabolic processes of the body, including stabilizing cell membranes in electrically active tissues, such as the brain and heart. It also has functions in the gallbladder, eyes, and blood vessels and may have some antioxidant and detoxifying properties.

- Taurine is a constituent of some energy drinks, including Red Bull. Numerous clinical trials suggest Red Bull and similar energy drinks may be effective in reducing fatigue and improving mood and endurance. However, these drinks contain other ingredients, which may also offer benefit in these areas, including caffeine and glucuronolactone. The effect of taurine alone in energy drinks has not been studied. Thus, the effectiveness of taurine in energy drinks is unclear, and further research is still required.

- Several taurine derivatives are being investigated for medical use, such as taltrimide as an antiepileptic drug. Other taurine derivatives in various stages of development include acamprosate (antialcoholic), tauromustine (anticancer), and tauroursodeoxycholic acid (liver disorders).

- The efficacy of taurine has been investigated for diabetes, hypertension (high blood pressure), cystic fibrosis, liver disorders, cardiovascular disorders, and nutritional support. Although promising in many fields, taurine needs additional study before a firm recommendation can be made for these indications. Taurine is added to many infant formulas based on the decreased ability to form taurine from cysteine in this population.

EVIDENCE

Uses Based on Scientific Evidence	Grade
Nutritional Supplement (Infant Formula) Early evidence suggests that taurine supplementation may aid in auditory maturation, fatty acid absorption, and increased serum taurine levels. However, additional study is needed in this area.	B
Congestive Heart Failure (CHF) Preliminary study suggests that taurine may be beneficial as an adjunct to traditional medications for symptoms of CHF. Taurine may be superior to coenzyme Q10, although further study is warranted to confirm these findings.	C
Cystic Fibrosis The interest in taurine for individuals with cystic fibrosis is based on its potential to increase effects of ursodeoxycholic acid (UDCA), as well as its potential to increase nutritional status. However, results are mixed. More study is needed to draw a firm recommendation in this area.	C
Diabetes Mellitus (Type 2) It has been proposed that diabetes patients have decreased taurine levels. Currently, there is limited available evidence to recommend for or against the use of taurine in the treatment of diabetes.	C
Energy Energy drinks containing taurine, along with other ingredients such as caffeine and glucuronolactone, have been available for about a decade. Overall these drinks have been suggested to decrease sleepiness associated with driving, increase concentration, mood, and memory, and positively affect well-being and vitality. Further study is required to examine the effect of taurine alone.	C
Epilepsy (Seizure) Preliminary evidence suggests that taurine may be beneficial in epileptic patients. However, additional study is needed in this area.	C
Hypercholesterolemia (High Cholesterol) Taurine may offer benefit to individuals fed a high fat and high cholesterol diet. More study is needed to make a firm recommendation.	C
Hypertension (High Blood Pressure) Preliminary results suggest that taurine may be beneficial in lowering blood pressure in individuals with borderline hypertension. Additional study is needed before a firm recommendation can be made.	C
Iron Deficiency Anemia Preliminary study suggests that taurine aids in the ability of iron supplements to increase hemoglobin, red blood cell count, and serum ferritin. Additional study is needed before a firm recommendation can be made.	C
Liver Disease Currently, the evidence in support of taurine in liver disease is minimal, and additional study with positive results is needed before a firm recommendation can be made.	C
Myotonic Dystrophy Preliminary study indicates that taurine supplementation may result in improvements in myotonic	C

T

(Continued)

Uses Based on Scientific Evidence	Grade
complaints. Although promising, these findings need additional study before they can be confirmed.	
Nutritional Support (Total Parenteral Nutrition [TPN]) The use of taurine has been examined in TPN in various patient groups (trauma, cancer, and long-term TPN patients). Preliminary research is promising.	C
Obesity Currently, there is insufficient available evidence to recommend for or against the use of taurine in the treatment of obesity.	C
Surgery (Coronary Bypass) Taurine may act as an antioxidant. The results from preliminary research are encouraging.	C
Vaccine Adjunct Currently, there is insufficient available evidence to recommend for or against the use of taurine as a vaccine adjunct.	C
Vision Problems (Fatigue) Taurine supplementation may reduce visual fatigue due to visual display terminals. However, clinical evidence thus far is not sufficient to support this use.	C

Uses Based on Tradition or Theory

Aerobic fitness, alcohol dependence, alertness, Alzheimer's disease, antioxidant, attention deficit hyperactivity disorder (ADHD), autism, bile secretion problems (biliary atresia), bipolar disorder, breast cancer, cardiac abnormalities (cardiac contractility), cardiomyopathy (dilated, hypertrophic), cardiovascular health (myocardial revascularization), cholestasis (stoppage of bile flow), cirrhosis (liver disease), concentration enhancement, depression, diabetes (prevention), digestive aid (fat absorption), Down's syndrome, exercise performance enhancement, fatigue, fatty liver, Huntington's chorea/disease, hypertriglyceridemia (elevated level of fatty acid compounds in the blood), ischemic heart disease, macular degeneration, malnutrition, memory enhancement, mental performance, mood stabilization, muscle atrophy (myotonia), myocarditis/endocarditis (acute viral), nervous system function (neurobehavioral development), nutritional supplement (amino acid supplementation), platelet aggregation inhibition, quality of life, retinitis pigmentosa (eye disease), steatorrhea (excess fat in the stool), thalassemia (inherited blood disorder), tinnitus (ringing in the ears), trauma, weight loss.

DOSING

Adults (18 Years and Older)

- Taurine is likely safe when taken by mouth by adults in doses up to 3 g daily for up to 1 year.
- Up to 9 g/day has been studied, but there is currently no proven effective dose for any indication. Nonetheless, for congestive heart failure, 3-6 g of taurine has been taken by mouth daily for up to 1 year. The same dose has been

studied for up to 2 months for high blood pressure. For diabetes mellitus type 2, 1000-1500 mg daily in divided doses for 30-90 days has been used. For hypercholesterolemia, 6 g of taurine powder daily for 3 weeks has been used. For iron deficiency anemia, 1000 mg of taurine per day has been used for 20 weeks, and for liver disease, 4 g has been used three times daily for 6 weeks. For visual fatigue, 3 g/day for 12 days has been used. As a vaccine adjuvant, 9 g taurine on the same day and 1 day before influenza vaccine administration has been used. For obesity, 3 g daily for 7 weeks has been used.

- Injections of taurine have been used in the treatment of epilepsy, as a nutritional supplement, and for coronary bypass surgery. Injections should be given only under the supervision of a qualified health care professional.

Children (Younger than 18 Years)

- Taurine is possibly safe in children when taken by mouth at 30 mg/kg body weight daily for up to 4 months.
- Other doses have been studied but are not necessarily safe or effective. For cystic fibrosis, 30-40 mg/kg body weight daily for 7 days to 6 months has been used. As a fortified infant formula, 470 micromoles/L of taurine has been taken by mouth daily for 6 days in preterm and full term infants; 45 micromoles/L of taurine added to Similac Special Care formula in low-birth-weight infants has also been taken by mouth until release from hospital or the infant attained a weight of 2500 g. As parenteral nutrition, 10.8 mg/kg daily during the first 10 days of life has been used.

SAFETY

Allergies

- Taurine is an amino acid, and it is unlikely that there are allergies related to this constituent. However, allergies may occur from multiingredient products that contain taurine.

Side Effects and Warnings

- Taurine is an amino acid, and oral (by mouth) supplementation has been well tolerated for up to 1 year.
- Taurine supplementation may reduce blood pressure in individuals with high blood pressure. Use cautiously in individuals with a history of low blood pressure because of the potential for increased hypotensive (blood pressure–lowering) effects.
- In human infants, taurine-supplemented formula increased absorption of fat, particularly saturated fat. The same was observed in cystic fibrosis patients supplemented with taurine.
- Taurine was found to reduce platelet aggregation and may increase the risk of bleeding. Caution is advised in patients with bleeding disorders or taking drugs that may increase the risk of bleeding. Dosing adjustments may be necessary.
- Use cautiously in patients with epilepsy, as taurine derivatives, specifically taltrimide, may increase seizure frequency. Taurine may also cause drowsiness and ataxia.
- An energy drink containing taurine, caffeine, glucuronolactone, B vitamins, and other ingredients (Red Bull Energy Drink) caused mania in a stable bipolar man. It is not known if this effect is related to taurine itself. Deaths following Red Bull Energy Drink have also been reported and are likely a result of dehydration because of the combined effects of caffeine and alcohol and/or exercise.

- Use cautiously in patients with high levels of very low density lipoprotein (VLDL) cholesterol because of potential for further increases. Also use cautiously in individuals taking hypolipidemic (cholesterol-lowering) medications because of potential for antagonistic effects. Patients with hypertriglyceridemia should also use with caution because of potential for increased levels of triglycerides.

Pregnancy and Breastfeeding

- Taurine supplementation is not recommended in pregnant or breastfeeding women because of a lack of available scientific evidence, although taurine is a natural component of breast milk.

INTERACTIONS
Interactions with Drugs

- Caution is advised in patients taking anesthetics because injections of taurine may decrease plasma malondialdehyde (MDA) and glutathione peroxidase in erythrocyte lysate and plasma.
- Taurine may reduce platelet aggregation and may increase the risk of bleeding when taken with drugs that increase the risk of bleeding. Some examples include aspirin, anticoagulants ("blood thinners") such as warfarin (Coumadin) or heparin, antiplatelet drugs such as clopidogrel (Plavix), and nonsteroidal antiinflammatory drugs (NSAIDS) such as ibuprofen (Motrin, Advil) or naproxen (Naprosyn, Aleve).
- Based on studies in cystic fibrosis patients, preterm infants, and biliary surgical patients, taurine may increase the absorption of fat and decrease fatty acid excretion. Patients taking antihyperlipidemic agents should use taurine with caution because of possible additive effects.
- Taurine may suppress the sympathetic nervous system and may decrease blood pressure. Caution is advised in patients taking antihypertensive (blood pressure–lowering) agents.
- A mixture of taurine, diltiazem, and vitamin E may have a beneficial effect on the progression of visual field loss in retinitis pigmentosa patients.
- Taurine may lower blood sugar levels. Caution is advised when medications that may also lower blood sugar are used. Patients taking drugs for diabetes by mouth or using insulin should be monitored closely by a qualified health care professional, including a pharmacist. Medication adjustments may be necessary.
- Taltrimide is a taurine derivative with potent anticonvulsant activity. The combination of taurine and taltrimide may result in increased seizure frequency. Taltrimide may also increase phenytoin concentrations and decrease serum carbamazepine concentrations. Furthermore, a potential exists for taurine or its metabolites to antagonize the effects of anticonvulsant therapy.
- Tamoxifen is often used as an adjuvant in patients with advanced breast cancer. Taking taurine with tamoxifen may reduce the tamoxifen-induced hepatotoxicity (liver toxicity). Consult with a qualified health care professional, including a pharmacist, before combining therapies.

Interactions with Herbs and Dietary Supplements

- Taurine may reduce platelet aggregation and may increase the risk of bleeding when taken with herbs and supplements that are believed to increase the risk of bleeding. Multiple cases of bleeding have been reported with the use of *Ginkgo biloba*, and fewer cases have been reported with garlic and saw palmetto. Numerous other agents may theoretically increase the risk of bleeding, although this has not been proven in most cases.
- Based on studies in cystic fibrosis patients, preterm infants, and biliary surgical patients, taurine may increase the absorption of fat and decrease fatty acid excretion. Patients taking antihyperlipidemic herbs, such as red yeast, should use taurine with caution because of possible additive effects.
- Taurine may suppress the sympathetic nervous system and may decrease blood pressure. Caution is advised in patients taking antihypertensive (blood pressure–lowering) herbs or supplements.
- An energy drink containing taurine, caffeine, glucuronolactone, glucose, sucrose, and B vitamin complex may reduce sleepiness and lane drifting while driving after sleep restriction or increase readiness potential after exhaustive exercise. In theory, these energy drinks may have antagonistic effects when used with herbs with sedative effects. When these energy drinks are taken with other supplements included in the drinks, such as B vitamin complex, additive effects may occur.
- Taurine may lower blood sugar levels. Caution is advised when herbs or supplements that may also lower blood sugar are used. Blood glucose levels may require monitoring, and doses may need adjustment.
- Taurine may also increase the absorption of iron or reduce tyrosine levels. Ingestion of glutamine may increase plasma taurine levels.
- A mixture of taurine, diltiazem, and vitamin E may have a beneficial effect on the progression of visual field loss in retinitis pigmentosa patients.

For a complete list of references, please visit www.naturalstandard.com.

T

Tea tree

(Melaleuca alternifolia)

RELATED TERMS

- Australian tea tree oil, Bogaskin (veterinary formulation), breathaway, Burnaid, cymene, malaleuca, *Malaleuca alternifolia*, *Malaleuca alternifolia* Cheel, Melaleuca Alternifolia Hydrogel (burn dressing), melaleuca oil, melaleucae, oil of mela-leuca, oleum, *Oleum melaleucae*, T36-C7, tea tree oil, Tebodont, Teebaum, terpinen, terpinen-4-ol, terpinenol-4, ti tree, TTO.
- **Note:** Should not be confused with cajeput oil, niauouli oil, kanuka oil, or manuka oil obtained from other *Melaleuca* species. Tea tree (*Melaleuca alternifolia*) is distinct from the *Camellia sirensis* plant, which is used to make the beverage tea.

BACKGROUND

- Tea tree oil is obtained by steam distillation of the leaves of *Melaleuca alternifolia*. Tea tree oil is purported to have antiseptic properties and has been used traditionally to prevent and treat infections. While numerous laboratory studies have demonstrated antimicrobial properties of tea tree oil (likely due to the compound terpinen-4-ol), only a small number of high-quality trials have been published. Human studies have focused on the use of topical tea tree oil for fungal infections (including fungal infections of the nails and athlete's foot), acne, and vaginal infections. However, there is a lack of definitive available evidence for the use of tea tree oil in any of these conditions, and further study is warranted.
- Tea tree oil should not be used orally; there are reports of toxicity after consuming tea tree oil by mouth. When applied to the skin, tea tree oil is reported to be mildly irritating and has been associated with the development of allergic contact dermatitis, which may limit its potential as a topical agent for some patients.

EVIDENCE

Uses Based on Scientific Evidence	Grade
Acne Vulgaris Although available in many products, little information is available from human studies to evaluate the benefit of tea tree oil used on the skin for the treatment of acne. Tea tree oil may reduce the number of inflamed and non-inflamed lesions.	C
Allergic Skin Reactions Preliminary studies show that tea tree oil applied to this skin may reduce histamine-induced inflammation. The evidence of benefit is not entirely clear.	C
Athlete's Foot (Tinea Pedis) Early studies report that tea tree oil may have activity against several fungal species. However, at this time there is not enough information to recommend topical tree oil for this condition.	C

	Grade
Bad Breath Tea tree oil is used in mouthwash for dental and oral health. However, there is currently insufficient evidence in humans to recommend for or against this use of tea tree. Tea tree oil can be toxic when taken by mouth and therefore should not be swallowed.	C
Dandruff Preliminary research suggests that the use of 5% tea tree oil shampoo on mild-to-moderate dandruff may be effective and well tolerated.	C
Dental Plaque/Gingivitis Study results on the effects of tea tree oil mouthwash on gum inflammation and plaque are mixed.	C
Eye Infections (Ocular Parasitic Mites) Preliminary studies have shown that tea tree oil may help rid the eye area of the mite infection caused by ocular parasitic mites.	C
Fungal Nail Infection (Onychomycosis) Although tea tree oil is thought to have activity against several fungus species, there is not enough information to make recommendations for or against the use of tea tree oil on the skin for this condition.	C
Genital Herpes Laboratory studies show that tea tree oil has activity against some viruses, and it has been suggested that a tea tree gel may be useful as a treatment on the skin for genital herpes. However, there is currently not enough information to recommend this use of tea tree oil.	C
Lice Preliminary studies have found that tea tree alone or in combination with other agents may be effective against lice.	C
Methicillin-Resistant *Staphylococcus aureus* (MRSA) Chronic Infection (Colonization) Laboratory studies report that tea tree oil has activity against methicillin-resistant *Staphylococcus aureus* (MRSA). It has been proposed that using tea tree oil ointment in the nose and a tea tree wash on the body may treat colonization by these bacteria. However, there is currently not enough information from human studies to make recommendations for this use of tea tree oil.	C
Thrush (*Candida albicans* of the Mouth) In laboratory studies, tea tree oil has been shown to kill fungus and yeast such as *Candida albicans*. However, at this time, there is not enough information available from human studies to make recommendations for this use of tea tree oil. Tea tree oil can be	C

Uses Based on Scientific Evidence	Grade
toxic when taken by mouth and therefore should not be swallowed.	
Vaginal Infections (Yeast and Bacteria) In laboratory studies, tea tree oil has been shown to kill yeast and certain bacteria. However, at this time there is not enough information available from human studies to make recommendations for this use of tea tree oil for vaginal infections. Although tea tree oil may reduce itching caused by yeast or bacteria, it may cause itching from dry skin or allergy.	C

Uses Based on Tradition or Theory

Abscesses (prostatic), anti-inflammatory, antihistamine, antioxidant, antiseptic, body odor, boils, bone diseases (osteomyelitis), bronchial congestion, bruises, burns, canker sores, carbuncles, colds, chronic venous insufficiency, contraction cessation, corns, cough, dermatitis, eczema, furuncles, gangrene, immune system deficiencies, impetigo, insect bites/stings, leg ulcers, lung inflammation, melanoma, mouth sores, muscle and joint pain, nose and throat irritation, pressure ulcers, psoriasis, ringworm, root canal treatment, rosacea, scabies, sinus infections, skin ailments/infections, solvent, sore throat, swelling, tonsillitis, vulvovaginitis, warts, wound healing.

DOSING
Adults (18 Years and Older)

- Although there is insufficient evidence to recommend a dose, a common dose studied in trials is 5% to 10% tea tree oil in gel or shampoo form applied on the skin daily for up to four weeks. While 100% tea tree oil is sometimes used for certain conditions, such as fungal nail infections, it is often diluted with inactive ingredients. Because of reports of severe side effects after tea tree oil ingestion, it is strongly recommended that tea tree oil not be taken by mouth. Although tea tree oil solution has been used as a mouthwash, it should not be swallowed.

Children (Younger than 18 Years)

- There is insufficient evidence to recommend the safe use of tea tree oil in children.

SAFETY
Allergies

- There are many reports of allergy to tea tree oil when taken by mouth or used on the skin. Skin reactions range from mild contact dermatitis to severe blistering rashes. People with a history of allergy to tea tree oil (*Melaleuca alternifo-*

lia) or any of its components; plants that are members of the myrtle (Myrtaceae) family; balsam of Peru; or benzoin should not use tea tree oil. Use cautiously if allergic to eucalyptol as many tea tree preparations contain eucalyptol.

Side Effects and Warnings

- Tea tree oil taken by mouth has been associated with potentially severe reactions, even when used in small quantities. Several reports describe people using tea tree oil by mouth who developed severe rash, reduced immune system function, abdominal pain, diarrhea, lethargy, drowsiness, inflammation of the corners of the mouth, slow or uneven walking, confusion, or coma. There have also been reports of nausea, unpleasant taste, burning sensation, and bad breath associated with tea tree oil use. Many tea tree preparations contain large volumes of alcohol.

- When used on the skin, tea tree oil may cause allergic rash, redness, blistering, and itching. This may be particularly severe in people with pre-existing skin conditions such as eczema. Use of tea tree oil inside of the mouth or eyes can cause irritation. Animal research suggests that tea tree oil used on the skin in large quantities can cause serious reactions such as difficulty walking, weakness, muscle tremor, slowing of brain function, and poor coordination. When applied in the ears of animals, 100% tea tree oil has caused reduced hearing, although a 2% solution has not led to lasting changes in hearing. The effect of tea tree oil on hearing when used in the ears of humans is not known.

Pregnancy and Breastfeeding

- Not enough scientific information is available to recommend tea tree oil during pregnancy or breastfeeding. Animal studies suggest caution in the use of tea tree oil during childbirth because tea tree oil has been reported to decrease the force of spontaneous contractions, which theoretically could put the baby and mother at risk. Women who are breastfeeding should not apply tea tree oil to the breast or nipple since it may be absorbed by the infant.

INTERACTIONS
Interactions with Drugs

- Skin products containing tea tree oil may dry the skin and may worsen the dryness caused by skin treatments such as tretinoin (Retin-A), benzoyl peroxide, salicylic acid, or isotretinoin (Accutane, taken by mouth).
- Tea tree oil may interact with anti-inflammatory, antibiotic, antifungal, and anti-cancer drugs.

Interactions with Herbs and Dietary Supplements

- Tea tree oil may interact with anti-inflammatory, antibacterial, antifungal, and anti-cancer herbs or supplements as well as insect repellants.

For a complete list of references, please visit www.naturalstandard.com.

Thiamin (thiamine), vitamin B$_1$

RELATED TERMS

- Aneurine, aneurine HCl, aneurine mononitrate, antiberiberi factor, antiberiberi vitamin, antineuritic factor, antineuritic vitamin, anurine, B complex vitamin, beta-hydroxy-ethylthiazolium chloride, thiamin, thiamin chloride, thiamin diphosphate, thiamin HCl, thiamin hydrochloride, thiamin monophosphate (TMP), thiamin nitrate, thiamin pyrophosphate (TPP), thiamin triphosphate (TTP), thiamine, thiamine chloride, thiaminium chloride HCl, thiaminium chloride hydrochloride.

BACKGROUND

- Thiamin (also spelled "thiamine") is a water-soluble B-complex vitamin, previously known as vitamin B$_1$ or aneurine. Thiamin was isolated and characterized in the 1920s, and thus was one of the first organic compounds to be recognized as a vitamin.
- Thiamin is involved in numerous body functions, including: nervous system and muscle functioning; flow of electrolytes in and out of nerve and muscle cells (through ion channels); multiple enzyme processes (via the coenzyme thiamin pyrophosphate); carbohydrate metabolism; and production of hydrochloric acid (which is necessary for proper digestion). Because there is very little thiamin stored in the body, depletion can occur as quickly as within 14 days.
- Severe chronic thiamin deficiency (beriberi) can result in potentially serious complications involving the nervous system/brain, muscles, heart, and gastrointestinal system.
- Dietary sources of thiamin include beef, brewer's yeast, legumes (beans, lentils), milk, nuts, oats, oranges, pork, rice, seeds, wheat, whole grain cereals, and yeast. In industrialized countries, foods made with white rice or white flour are often fortified with thiamin (because most of the naturally occurring thiamin is lost during the refinement process).

EVIDENCE

Uses Based on Scientific Evidence	Grade
Metabolic Disorders (Subacute Necrotizing Encephalopathy, Maple Syrup Urine Disease, Pyruvate Carboxylase Deficiency, Hyperalaninemia) Taking thiamin by mouth helps to temporarily correct some complications of metabolic disorders associated with genetic diseases including subacute necrotizing encephalopathy (SNE, Leigh's disease), maple syrup urine disease (branched-chain aminoacidopathy), and lactic acidosis associated with pyruvate carboxylase deficiency and hyperalaninemia. Long-term management should be under strict medical supervision.	A
Thiamin Deficiency (Beriberi, Wernicke's Encephalopathy, Korsakoff's Psychosis, Wernicke-Korsakoff Syndrome) Humans are dependent on dietary intake to fulfill their thiamin requirements. Because there is very	A

little thiamin stored in the body, depletion can occur as quickly as within 14 days. Severe chronic thiamin deficiency can result in potentially serious complications involving the nervous system/brain, muscles, heart, and gastrointestinal system. Patients with thiamin deficiency or related conditions should receive supplemental thiamin under medical supervision.

Acute Alcohol Withdrawal Patients with chronic alcoholism or alcohol withdrawal are at risk of thiamin deficiency and its associated complications and should be administered thiamin.	B
Total Parenteral Nutrition (TPN) Thiamin should be added to TPN formulations for patients who are unable to receive thiamin through other sources (such as a multivitamin) for more than seven days.	B
Alzheimer's Disease Because thiamin deficiency can result in a form of dementia (Wernicke-Korsakoff syndrome), its relationship to Alzheimer's disease and other forms of dementia has been investigated. Whether thiamin supplementation is of benefit in Alzheimer's disease remains controversial. Further evidence is necessary before a firm conclusion can be reached.	C
Atherosclerosis: Prevention in Patients with Acute Hyperglycemia, Impaired Glucose Tolerance (IGT), and Diabetes Mellitus Patients with diabetes are at risk of developing hardened arteries (called *atherosclerosis*). This happens when cholesterol and other substances build up and clog the arteries. Thiamin has been studied as a way to help widen arteries that are too narrow. Regular intake of thiamin might help slow the progression of atherosclerosis. However, additional research is needed.	C
Athletic Performance There is inconclusive scientific evidence to support this use.	C
Cancer Thiamin deficiency has been observed in some cancer patients, possibly due to increased metabolic needs. It is not clear if lowered levels of thiamin in such patients may actually be adaptive (beneficial). Currently, it remains unclear if thiamin supplementation plays a role in the management of any particular type(s) of cancer.	C
Cataract Prevention Preliminary evidence suggests that high dietary thiamin intake may be associated with a decreased risk of cataracts.	C

Uses Based on Scientific Evidence	Grade
Coma/Hypothermia of Unknown Origin Administration of thiamin is often recommended in patients with coma or hypothermia of unknown origin, owing to the possible diagnosis of Wernicke's encephalopathy.	C
Crohn's Disease Decreased serum thiamin levels have been reported in patients with Crohn's disease. It is not clear if routine thiamin supplementation is beneficial in such patients generally.	C
Didmoad (Wolfram) Syndrome Didmoad (Wolfram) syndrome is a rare autosomal recessive inherited disease that results in diabetes mellitus, optic atrophy, diabetes insipidus, sensorineural deafness, and occasionally megaloblastic anemia. The defect is believed to cause a decrease in the enzyme that converts thiamin to its active form. Management, including thiamin supplementation, should be under strict medical supervision.	C
Heart Failure (Cardiomyopathy) Chronic severe thiamin deficiency can cause heart failure (wet beriberi), a condition that merits thiamin supplementation. It is not clear that thiamin supplementation is beneficial in patients with heart failure due to other causes. However, it is reasonable for patients with heart failure to take a daily multivitamin including thiamin because they may be thiamin deficient. Diuretics may lower thiamin levels. Since diuretics are commonly administered to patients with heart failure, patients taking diuretics are at an increased risk of thiamin deficiency. This area remains controversial.	C
Leg Cramps (During Pregnancy) Vitamin B supplements have been used to treat leg cramps during pregnancy. However, additional studies are needed to determine if it is effective.	C
Pyruvate Dehydrogenase Deficiency (PDH) There is preliminary evidence of clinical improvements in children with PDH following thiamin administration.	C
Subclinical Thiamin Deficiency in the Elderly While typically asymptomatic, the elderly have been found to have lower thiamin concentrations than younger people. There is limited evidence that thiamin supplementation may be beneficial in people with persistently low thiamin blood levels.	C
Fractures (Hip) Preliminary evidence shows that supplemental thiamin is not beneficial for hip fractures.	D

Uses Based on Tradition or Theory

Age-related lens opacification, Bell's palsy, brain damage (ifosfamide-induced encephalopathy), canker sores, chronic diarrhea, circulation improvement, depression, diabetes, diabetic nephropathy, dysmenorrhea (painful menstruation), epilepsy, erectile dysfunction, fibromyalgia, gastrointestinal disorders, high blood pressure, HIV support, insect repellant, learning, loss of appetite, low back pain, megaloblastic anemia, memory enhancement, myelodysplastic syndrome, optic nerve dysfunction (optic neuropathy), multiple sclerosis, radiation-induced damage (protection from genetic changes), tissue healing after surgery, ulcerative colitis.

DOSING
Adults (18 Years and Older)

- The U.S. Recommended Daily Allowance (RDA) for adults ages 19 years and older is 1.2 mg daily for males and 1.1 mg daily for females, taken by mouth. The RDA for pregnant or breastfeeding women of any age is 1.4 mg/day, taken by mouth. As a dietary supplement in adults, 1 to 2 mg daily is sometimes used. Thiamin is also used to treat thiamin deficiency, metabolic/genetic enzyme deficiency disorders, neuropathy, and Wernicke's encephalopathy (prevention/treatment) under medical supervision.

Children (Younger than 18 Years)

- The adequate intake (AI) for infants ages 0 to 6 months is 0.2 mg; for infants 7 to 12 months the AI is 0.3 mg; for children ages 1 to 3 years the U.S. Recommended Daily Allowance (RDA) is 0.5 mg; for children ages 4 to 8 years the RDA is 0.6 mg; for children ages 9 to 13 years the RDA is 0.9 mg; for males ages 14 to 18 years the RDA is 1.2 mg; and for females ages 14 to 18 years the RDA is 1 mg, taken by mouth. The RDA for pregnant or breastfeeding women of any age is 1.4 mg daily, taken by mouth. Thiamin is also used to treat thiamin deficiency/beriberi under medical supervision.

SAFETY
Allergies

- Rare hypersensitivity/allergic reactions have occurred with thiamin supplementation. A small number of life-threatening anaphylactic reactions have been observed with large parenteral (intravenous, intramuscular, subcutaneous) doses of thiamin, generally after multiple doses.
- Skin irritation, burning, or itching may rarely occur at injection sites.
- Contact dermatitis may occur with occupational exposure and may cause sensitization and lead to dermatitis-type reactions after subsequent oral or injected administrations.

Side Effects and Warnings

- Thiamin is generally considered safe and relatively nontoxic, even at high doses. No clear tolerable upper level (UL) of intake has been established. Dermatitis or more serious hypersensitivity reactions occur rarely.
- Large doses may cause drowsiness or muscle relaxation.

T

- Injections of thiamin may cause burning. Reactions can often be avoided by slow administration into larger veins.

Pregnancy and Breastfeeding

- U.S. Food and Drug Administration Pregnancy Category C.

INTERACTIONS

Interactions with Drugs

- Reduced levels of thiamin in blood and cerebrospinal fluid have been reported in people taking phenytoin (Dilantin) for extended periods of time.
- Antacids may lower thiamin levels in the body by decreasing absorption and increasing excretion or metabolism.
- Barbiturates may lower thiamin levels in the body by decreasing absorption and increasing excretion or metabolism.
- Loop diuretics, particularly furosemide (Lasix), have been associated with decreased thiamin levels in the body by increasing urinary excretion (and possibly by decreasing absorption and increasing metabolism). Examples of other loop diuretics include bumetanide (Bumex), ethacrynic acid (Edecrine), and torsemide (Demadex). Theoretically, this effect may also occur with other types of diuretics, including thiazide diuretics such as chlorothiazide (Diuril), chlorthalidone (Hygroton, Thalidone), hydrochlorothiazide (HCTZ, Esidrix, HydroDIURIL, Ortec, Microzide), indapamide (Lozol), and metolazone (Zaroxolyn), or potassium-sparing diuretics, such as amiloride (Midamor), spironolactone (Aldactone), and triamterene (Dyrenium). Effects may be most pronounced with larger doses taken over extended periods of time.
- Tobacco use decreases thiamin absorption and may lead to decreased levels in the body.
- Effects of neuromuscular blocking agents (NMBAs) may be enhanced with concomitant (simultaneous) use of thiamin.
- Some antibiotics destroy gastrointestinal flora (normal bacteria in the gut), which manufacture some B vitamins. In theory, this may decrease the amount of thiamin available to humans, although the majority of thiamin is obtained through the diet (not via bacterial production).
- Oral contraceptives (birth control pills/OCPS) may decrease levels of some B vitamins, vitamin C, and zinc in the body.
- People receiving fluorouracil-containing chemotherapy regimens may be at risk for developing symptoms and signs of thiamin deficiency.
- In theory, metformin may reduce thiamine activity, and based on animal research, taking thiamin and metformin together may contribute to the risk of lactic acidosis.
- Thiamin has been shown to improve vasodilation (the widening of blood vessels) in patients with high blood sugar levels or diabetes. This response was not seen in patients with normal blood sugar levels. Therefore, thiamin may increase the effects of vasodilators in these patients.

Interactions with Herbs and Dietary Supplements

- Consumption of betel nuts (*Areca catechu* L.) may reduce thiamine activity owing to chemical inactivation and may lead to symptoms and signs of thiamin deficiency.
- Horsetail (*Equisetum arvense* L.) contains a thiaminase-like compound that can destroy thiamine in the stomach and theoretically causes symptomatic thiamine deficiency. Horsetail products are available without this property and, for example, the Canadian government requires that horsetail products be certified free of thiaminase activity.
- In theory, diuretic herbs may decrease thiamin levels in the body by increasing urinary excretion.
- Thiamin has been shown to improve vasodilation (the widening of blood vessels) in patients with high blood sugar levels or diabetes. This response was not seen in patients with normal blood sugar levels. Therefore, thiamin may increase the effects of vasodilators in these patients.

For a complete list of references, please visit www.naturalstandard.com.

Thyme
(*Thymus* spp.)

RELATED TERMS

- Common thyme, common garden thyme, English thyme, farigola, folia thymi, French thyme, garden thyme, Gartenthymian, herba thymi, herba timi, Labiatae (family), Lamiaceae (family), mother of thyme, red thyme, rubbed thyme, serpyllium, shepherd's thyme, Spanish thyme, ten, thick leaf thyme, time, timo, thym, thyme aetheroleum, thyme oil, thymi herba, Thymian, *Thymus serpyllum, thymus zygis* L., wild thyme, white thyme oil.
- **Note:** There are up to 400 subspecies of thyme; common thyme *(Thymus vulgaris)* and Spanish thyme *(Thymus zygis)* are often used interchangeably for medicinal purposes. Not to be confused with calamint (calamintha ascendens, basil thyme) or with Spanish origanum oil *(Thymus capitatus,* Sicilian thyme, Spanish thyme).

BACKGROUND

- Thyme has been used medicinally for thousands of years. Beyond its common culinary application, it has been recommended for a myriad of indications, based upon proposed antimicrobial, antitussive, spasmolytic, and antioxidant activity. To date, there is insufficient clinical evidence to support thyme monotherapy for use in humans.
- Thymol, one of the constituents of thyme, is contained in antiseptic mouthwashes. However, there are limited clinical studies in the available literature to verify its efficacy as a monotherapy in dental outcomes, such as reductions in plaque formation, gingivitis, and caries.
- Traditional uses of thyme include for coughs and upper respiratory congestion; it continues to be one of the most commonly recommended herbs in Europe for these indications. The German Commission E (expert panel) has approved thyme for symptoms of bronchitis, whooping cough, and catarrh (inflammation of upper respiratory tract mucous membranes).
- Experts have recommended the use of thymol in treatment of actinomycosis (lumpy jaw disease), onycholysis (separation or loosening of a fingernail or toenail from its nail bed), and paronychia (inflammation of the tissue surrounding a fingernail or toenail) because of to its antifungal properties.

EVIDENCE

Uses Based on Scientific Evidence	Grade
Alopecia Areata (Hair Loss) There is currently insufficient information to recommend for or against the use of topical thyme oil for alopecia areata.	C
Bronchitis/Cough Thyme has traditionally been used for the treatment of respiratory conditions including cough and bronchitis. The German Commission E (expert panel), has approved thyme for use in bronchitis. However,	C
there is a lack of clinical research examining thyme alone.	
Dental Plaque One of thyme's main constituents, thymol, has antibacterial effects. Thymol is included as one of several ingredients in antiseptic mouthwashes such as Listerine. Clinical studies have reported efficacy of Listerine in decreasing plaque formation and gingivitis, although human evidence for thymol alone is limited.	C
Inflammatory Skin Disorders Historically, thyme has been used topically for a number of dermatologic (skin) conditions. Results are mixed.	C
Paronychia/Onycholysis/Antifungal Thyme essential oil and thymol have antifungal effects. Topical thymol has been used traditionally in the treatment of paronychia (skin infection around a fingernail or toenail) and onycholysis (separation/loosening of the nail from the nail bed). Currently, there is insufficient evidence to recommend thyme/thymol as a treatment for fungal infections.	C

Uses Based on Tradition or Theory

Abscess, acne, appetite stimulant, antioxidant, anxiety, arthritis, asthma, burns, cancer, cellulitis (skin inflammation), depression, gastritis (inflammation of the stomach), colic, cystitis (bladder infection), dermatitis, dermatomyositis (muscle inflammation), diarrhea, diuresis (increased urine production), dysmenorrhea (painful menstruation), dyspepsia (upset stomach), dyspnea (difficulty breathing), eczema, edema (swelling), enuresis (bed wetting), epilepsy, fever, flatulence (gas), flu, gingivitis, gout (foot inflammation), *H. pylori*, halitosis (bad breath), headache, heartburn, hookworms, indigestion, inflammation of the colon, insect bites, insomnia, intestinal parasites, laryngitis, lice, methicillin-resistant *Staphylococcus aureus* (MRSA), neuralgia (nerve pain), nightmares, obesity, pertussis (whooping cough), pruritus (severe itching), rheumatism, roundworms, scabies, scleroderma (chronic degenerative disease that affects the joints, skin, and internal organs), sinusitis, sore throat, spasms, sprains, stomach cramps, stomatitis (mouth sores), tonsillitis, urethritis, upper respiratory tract infection, urinary tract infection, vaginal irritation, warts, wound healing.

DOSING
Adults (18 Years and Older)

- There is insufficient evidence to recommend a dose for thyme or thymol. Teas, liquid extracts, oils, ointments, compresses, and combination products are all commercially available. Thyme oil is considered to be highly toxic and should not be taken internally. Combination products

T

studied in available trials include Bronchipret (Primulae radis and thyme) and Listerine (containing thymol, a constituent of thyme).

- For alopecia areata (hair loss), 2 to 3 drops of an essential oil combination (thyme, lavender, rosemary, and cedarwood added to grapeseed and jojoba oil) massaged into the scalp every night for seven months has been studied. For paronychia (skin infection around a fingernail or toenail), 1 drop of 1% to 2% thymol in chloroform to the affected area three times daily, or 1 drop of 4% thymol in chloroform has been applied to a chronically affected area three times daily. Diluted thyme oil has been applied as needed in 1% to 2% ointments for a variety of skin disorders. Safety and efficacy have not been proven, and thyme oil is considered to be highly toxic.
- As a compress for rheumatic diseases, bruises, and miscellaneous skin disorders, 5 g of dried leaf per 100 ml boiling water for 10 minutes and strain has been used in compress form.

Children (Younger than 18 Years)

- There is insufficient evidence to recommend a dose for thyme in children, and use is not recommended. However, for prevention of periodontal infections, a combination product containing 1% chlorhexidine/thymol varnish (Cervitec) was tolerated in 110 healthy children, ages 8 to 10 years, when taken three times within two weeks.

SAFETY
Allergies

- Avoid in people with a known allergy or hypersensitivity to members of the Lamiaceae (mint) family or to any component of thyme, or to rosemary (*Rosmarinus officinalis*).
- Cross-reactions to birch pollen, celery, oregano, and to other species in the Lamiaceae/Labiatae (mint) family may occur. Symptoms of allergy may include nausea, emesis (vomiting), pruritus (severe itching), angioedema (swelling under the skin), dysphagia (difficulty swallowing), dysphonia (altered voice), hypotension (low blood pressure), and progressive respiratory difficulty. Occupational asthma has been reported.

Side Effects and Warnings

- Although not well studied in humans, thyme flowers and leaves appear to be safe in culinary and in limited medicinal use. Caution is warranted with the use of thyme oil, which should not be taken by mouth and should be diluted when applied on the skin because of potentially toxic effects.
- Side effects of thyme taken by mouth may include headache, dizziness, hypotension (low blood pressure), bradycardia (slowed heart rate), heartburn, nausea, vomiting, diarrhea, gastrointestinal irritation, muscle weakness, and

exacerbated inflammation associated with urinary tract infections. Use cautiously in patients with gastrointestinal irritation or peptic ulcer disease.
- Taking thyme oil by mouth may also cause seizure, coma, cardiac arrest, or respiratory arrest. High doses of thyme or thyme oil may elicit tachypnea (rapid breathing). Inflammation of the eye and nasal mucosa has also been reported with exposure to thyme dust.
- Topical application of Listerine antiseptic solution to a chronic parenchyma of the toe has caused inflammation of the skin. Avoid topical preparations in areas of skin breakdown or injury, or in atopic patients. As an ingredient in toothpaste, cases of inflamed lips and tongue have been attributed to thyme oil.
- Although not well studied in humans, *Thymus serpyllum*, a related species to *Thymus vulgaris*, has been shown to exert effects on the thyroid. Use cautiously in patients with thyroid disorders. Estradiol and progesterone receptor-binding activity has also been demonstrated.

Pregnancy and Breastfeeding

- Thyme is not recommended in pregnant or breastfeeding women because of a lack of available scientific evidence. Thyme may act as an emmenagogue (promotes menstruation) and abortifacient (promotes abortion).

INTERACTIONS
Interactions with Drugs

- Theoretically, thyme may decrease levels of thyroid hormone. Patients taking thyroid replacement therapy or anti-thyroid agents should use cautiously. Monitoring may be necessary.
- Although not well studied in humans, thyme may interact with agents with estrogen or progesterone receptor activity. Examples of agents that may be affected include hormone replacement therapies and birth control pills.
- Topical (applied on the skin) thymol may increase the absorption of 5-fluorouracil. Caution is advised in chemotherapy patients, as 5-fluorouracil is often used in cancer chemotherapy. Consult with a qualified healthcare professional, including a pharmacist, to check for interactions.

Interactions with Herbs and Dietary Supplements

- Although not well studied in humans, thyme may interact with herbs with estrogen or progesterone receptor activity. Caution is advised when combining thyme with other herbs and supplements with proposed hormonal effects, such as black cohosh.

For a complete list of references, please visit www.naturalstandard.com.

Thymus extract

RELATED TERMS

- Aqueous calf thymus extract, bovine thymic extract, calf thymus, calf thymus acid lysate, calf thymus extract, calf-thymus lysate, calf thymus nuclear extract, Complete Thymic Formula, CSFa, CSFb, CTE, facteur thymique serique, fetal thymus, fraction V, FTS, glandular therapy, hormonal thymic factor, IFX, immunophan, Leucotrofina, leucotrofina-L (Timolimfotropina-T), leukotrophin, oligopeptide (fractionV), organotherapy, peptide thymosin alpha 1, polypeptides, polypeptide thymus extract, rabbit thymus, RTE, serum thymic factor, tactivin, T-activin, taktivin, Talpha1, TFX, TFX-JELFA ini., Thymalfasin (thymosin alpha1, Talpha1, Zadaxin, SciClone Pharmaceuticals, Inc.), thymalin, thymex L, thymex-L, thymic calf extract (leucotrofina), thymic extract, thymic factor, thymic factor X, thymic hormones, thymic humoral factor, thymic peptides, Thymoject, thymomodulin, thymomodulins, thymopoietin, thymosin, thymosin alpha, thymosin alpha 1, thymosin fraction 5, thymosin fraction V, thymostimulin (TS, TST, Tp-1, Serono, bovine thymic extract), thymsin (TP-1), thymulin, thymus extract (TFX-JELFA ini.), Thymus Extract Mulli, thymus gland, TP1, TP-1, Tp-1 Serono, TS, TST, ubiquitin, umoral factor, vilozen, whole calf thymus extract (TFX-Polfa), Zadaxin.

BACKGROUND

- The thymus is a lobular gland located under the breastbone near the thyroid gland. It reaches its maximum size during early childhood and plays a large role in immune function. The thymus is responsible for the production of T-lymphocytes, as well as the production of various hormones including thymosin, thymopoietin, thymulin, thymic humoral factor, and serum thymic factor. These hormones may be involved in the increase in lymphokines (interleukin 2, interferon, colony stimulating factor), increase of interleukin 2 receptors, and regulation of weight. With age, the thymus is replaced by fat and connective tissue.
- According to legend, glandular or organotherapy, which refers to the use of animal tissues or cell preparations to improve physiologic functioning and support the natural healing process, first gained popularity in the early to mid 1900s. The idea of homeopathic glandular therapy was first introduced almost 200 years ago.
- Thymus extracts for nutritional supplements are usually derived from young calves (bovine). Bovine thymus extracts are found in capsules and tablets as a dietary supplement.
- Thymus extract is commonly used to treat primary immunodeficient states, bone marrow failure, autoimmune disorders, chronic skin diseases, recurrent viral and bacterial infections, hepatitis, allergies, chemotherapy side effects, and cancer. Most basic and clinical research involving oral and injectable thymus extract has been conducted in Europe.
- Clinical trials in humans suggest promising results in terms of allergies, asthma, cancer, chemotherapeutic side effects, cardiomyopathy, chronic obstructive pulmonary disease, HIV/AIDS, immunostimulation, liver disease, respiratory tract infections, systemic lupus erythematosus, and tuberculosis. However, not all study results agree, and properly randomized, double-blind clinical trials are still needed in many fields.
- Future areas of research include (but are not limited to) rheumatoid arthritis, warts, urinary tract infections (UTIs), psoriasis, eczema, alopecia (hair loss), and appendicitis.

EVIDENCE

Uses Based on Scientific Evidence	Grade
Allergy Preliminary evidence suggests that thymus extract may be useful for allergy symptom reduction. More clinical trials are required before recommendations can be made involving thymus extract for this use.	C
Alopecia Preliminary evidence suggests that thymus extract may be useful for hair regrowth. More clinical trials are required before recommendations can be made involving thymus extract for this use.	C
Anxiety/Stress Thymus extract has been investigated for use in immune-modulating acute stress and adaptive disorders. More clinical trials are required before recommendations can be made involving thymus extract for this use.	C
Arthritis From the available evidence, any potential benefit of thymus extract is unclear. More clinical trials are required before recommendations can be made involving thymus extract for this use.	C
Asthma Preliminary evidence suggests that thymus extract may be useful for asthma symptom reduction. More clinical trials are required before recommendations can be made involving thymus extract for this use.	C
Burns Thymus extract may be useful for reducing infections, septicemia, and mortality. However, the evidence is mixed. More clinical trials are required before recommendations can be made involving thymus extract for this use.	C
Cancer Preliminary evidence suggests that thymus extract may increase disease-free survival and immunological improvement. Early studies have investigated thymus extract for the treatment of hematopoietic cancer, histiocytosis X, larynx and oropharyngeal cancer, and skin cancer, among others. Additional research is needed in this area.	C

(Continued)

Uses Based on Scientific Evidence	Grade
Cancer (Chemotherapy Adjunct) Preliminary evidence suggests that thymus extract may reduce side effects and infection rates associated with chemotherapy and may increase disease-free survival.	C
Cancer (Radiotherapy Side Effects) Preliminary evidence suggests that intramuscular thymus extract may help treat immunodeficiency associated with radiotherapy.	C
Cardiomyopathy Preliminary evidence suggests that thymus extract may increase left ventricular function, exercise tolerance, and survival.	C
Chronic Obstructive Pulmonary Disease Preliminary evidence suggests that thymus extract may be useful for reducing disease exacerbations and hospital admission.	C
Dermatomyositis Thymus extract is of interest for treatment of dermatomyositis (inflammation of the muscles) because of its role in immunostimulation. However, clinical evidence is insufficient to support this use.	C
Diabetes Preliminary evidence in conventionally treated patients with type I diabetes suggests that a combination of azathioprine and thymostimulin increased remission. Thymostimulin alone had no effect.	C
Eczema Preliminary evidence suggests that thymus extract has no clinical effect in patients with atopic eczema, despite anecdotal evidence suggesting the use of thymus extract for dermatological uses.	C
Encephalitis Preliminary evidence suggests that thymus extract has no clinical effect in patients with subacute sclerosing panencephalitis.	C
Gastritis Preliminary evidence suggests that thymus extract speeds healing of gastric lesions.	C
Glaucoma Well-designed clinical trials are required before thymus extract can be recommended in the treatment of glaucoma.	C
HIV/AIDS Preliminary evidence found no improvement in HIV progression to AIDS or immunostimulation, although some immunological activity was noted in a non-randomized controlled trial. Additional research is needed in this area.	C
Human Papilloma Virus (HPV) Thymus extract is of interest in the treatment of human papillomavirus because of its role in immunostimulation. Preliminary positive results were found in five cases.	C
Immunostimulation Preliminary evidence suggests that thymus extract increases T- and B-lymphocyte counts, the number of rosette-forming cells, and response of T-lymphocytes. Also, in cancer patients, T-activin significantly increases the number of natural killer cells (CD16+).	C
Keratitis Preliminary evidence suggests that thymus extract, in addition to local treatment, reduces the recurrence rate of keratitis.	C
Liver Disease Preliminary evidence suggests that thymus extract may offer benefit to people with HIV/AIDS and human papillomavirus. Also, thymus extract is of interest because of its role in immunostimulation. More well-designed clinical trials are required in the area of non-hepatitis B and hepatitis B liver disorders before recommendations can be made involving thymus extract for this use.	C
Myelodysplastic Syndrome Thymus extract is of interest in the treatment of myelodysplastic syndrome because of its role in immunostimulation *in vitro* and in human and animal studies.	C
Psoriasis Preliminary results suggest that the combination of an intravenous thymus extract plus selenium and fumaric acid may increase healing rate.	C
Respiratory Tract Infections Preliminary evidence suggests that both intramuscular and oral thymus extract may be useful for reducing the presence of respiratory tract symptoms.	C
Skin Conditions Despite use of thymus extracts for dermatological conditions, there is currently inconclusive evidence recommending thymus extract for use in skin conditions.	C
Systemic Lupus Erythematosus Preliminary results indicate that articular and cutaneous symptoms associated with systemic lupus erythematosus can be improved with thymus extract use.	C
Tuberculosis Although inconclusive, preliminary evidence suggests that thymus extract may improve effectiveness of antibacterial therapy in patients with tuberculosis. Well-designed clinical trials are required before recommendations can be made.	C

Uses Based on Scientific Evidence	Grade
Urinary Tract Infection Preliminary evidence from a controlled trial suggests that thymus extract reduces re-infection frequency and infection persistence.	C
Warts Preliminary evidence suggests that thymus extract increased T cell count and activation in patients with warts.	C

Uses Based on Tradition or Theory

Aging, allergic rhinitis, anemia (chronic autoimmune hemolytic), anemia (thalassemia), angina (chest pain), antifungal (adjuvant), antimicrobial (adjuvant), antiparasitic, antiviral, aphthous stomatitis (RAS, mouth sores), atopic dermatitis, autoimmune disorders (hemolytic anemias), bacterial infection (severe diarrhea due to *Shigella* infection), bone disorders (bone marrow protection), bronchitis (asthma), cardiac bypass, cardiac (heart) disease, chicken pox, cirrhosis (liver disease), colorectal cancer, connective tissue disorders (mixed connective tissue disease), Crohn's disease (refractory), depression (short-term), diabetic retinopathy (eye disease), fatigue, food allergy diagnosis/treatment, gastrointestinal inflammation (appendicitis), hepatitis (acute, chronic, cholestatic, B, C), herpes simplex (cold sores), herpes simplex labialis (recurrent), herpes zoster, Hodgkin's disease, immune system deficiencies (hereditary and nonhereditary), infections (including postoperative), inflammation (maxillofacial), ischemic heart disease, leukemia (chronic), leukopenia (abnormally low white blood cell count), liver disease (echinococciasis), lymphedema, lymphoma, male infertility, multiple myeloma, multiple sclerosis, otitis media (middle ear infection), pre-eclampsia, rheumatoid arthritis, sarcoidosis (intrathoracic lymph node sarcoidosis), sepsis, sinusitis, skin conditions, surgery (abdominal, orthopedic), surgery (colorectal), viral myocarditis, weight loss (wasting or catabolic), wound healing, yeast infections.

DOSING

Adults (18 Years and Older)

- There is insufficient evidence to recommend a dose for thymus extract. Thymus extract is typically given as an injection, although thymomodulin 80 mg has been taken by mouth daily for up to 90 days for the treatment of asthma. Injections have been given for the treatment of arthritis, breast cancer, burns, cancer, chronic obstructive pulmonary disease, HIV/AIDS, human papillomavirus infections, immunostimulation, male infertility, psoriasis sinusitis, and systemic lupus erythematosus. A number of doses have been used, but none has been standardized. Injections should be given only under the supervision of a qualified health care professional, including a pharmacist.

Children (Younger than 18 Years)

- There is no proven effective dose for thymus extract in children. A thymus extract has been taken by mouth for three months for the treatment of bronchial asthma. Injections have also been given. For example, thymostimulin 1.5 to

3 mg/kg has been injected into the muscle daily for up to 30 days. Injections should be given only under the supervision of a qualified health care professional, including a pharmacist.

SAFETY
Allergies

- Avoid in people with a known allergy or hypersensitivity to thymus extracts. A severe anaphylactic reaction to injected thymostimulin has been documented in a case report. Allergy to thymic extracts has not been demonstrated in currently available clinical trials.

Side Effects and Warnings

- Use bovine thymus extract supplements cautiously because of potential for exposure to the virus that causes "mad cow disease."
- Avoid use in patients with an organ transplant or other forms of allografts or xenografts because of the possibility of thymus extract stimulating an immune response, and thus transplant rejection.
- Patients receiving immunosuppressive therapy should not use thymus extract because of the potential for immunostimulation.
- Use of thymus extract is not recommended in patients with myasthenia gravis, untreated hypothyroidism, or thymic tumors because of inadequate available safety information.
- Avoid use in patients on hormonal therapy because of preliminary evidence suggesting thyroid extract may alter levels of certain hormones. Also, avoid in patients with a known allergy to thymus or those who are pregnant or breastfeeding.

Pregnancy and Breastfeeding

- Thymic extract increases human sperm motility and progression. Avoid use during pregnancy or breastfeeding because of inadequate available safety information.

INTERACTIONS
Interactions with Drugs

- Preliminary evidence in humans suggests that thymus extract may have additive effects with antibiotics. Also, the use of thymus extract may decrease infections and thus the need for antibiotics.
- In humans, a combination of azathioprine and thymostimulin may be beneficial in the management of type I diabetes. Caution is advised when using medications that may alter blood sugar. Patients taking drugs for diabetes by mouth or insulin should be monitored closely by a qualified healthcare professional, including a pharmacist. Medication adjustments may be necessary.
- Thymus extract may reduce the frequency of acute allergic episodes. Thus, thymus extracts and antihistamines may have additive effects.
- In humans, thymus extracts and chemotherapeutic agents have shown additive effects. Thymus extracts may also offer protective effects in terms of reduced side effects associated with chemotherapy.
- Thymus extract may play a role in immunological disorders associated with stress and anxiety. Caution is advised in patients taking anxiolytics because of possible additive effects.

T

- Thymus extract may improve symptoms associated with asthma. Thus, thymus extracts and bronchodilators may have additive effects.
- In humans, thymomodulin had an additive effect on conventional medications for cardiomyopathy. Caution is advised in patients with heart problems.
- Although not well studied in humans, thymic extract may reduce the dose of corticosteroids required. Caution is advised in patients taking corticosteroids because of possible additive effects.
- Although not well studied in humans, a combination of thymus extract, selenium, and fumaric acid may be beneficial for psoriasis.
- Preliminary evidence in humans suggests thyroid extract can improve alopecia (hair loss). It is possible that thyroid extract is able to offer other hormonal effects and have additive effects.
- In humans, T-activin has immunomodulatory effects. Caution is advised when taking with other agents that affect the immune system.
- Preliminary evidence suggests that thyroid extracts offer benefits to patients with systemic lupus erythematosus (SLE). Thus, use in combination with medications for SLE, such as methylxanthines, may have additive effects.
- Thymus extract may increase the amount of drowsiness caused by some drugs. Examples include benzodiazepines such as lorazepam (Ativan) or diazepam (Valium), barbiturates such as phenobarbital, narcotics such as codeine, some antidepressants, and alcohol. Caution is advised while driving or operating machinery.
- Although not well studied in humans, purified thymus gland extract may decrease average thyroid gland weights and serum T3 serum levels and significantly decrease serum T4 levels. It is not clear what effect thymus gland extract would have on external thyroid hormones.

Interactions with Herbs and Dietary Supplements

- Preliminary evidence in humans suggests that thymus extract may have additive effects to antibiotics. Use of thymus extract may decrease infections and thus the need for antibiotics.
- In humans, a combination of azathioprine and thymostimulin may be beneficial in the management of type I diabetes. Caution is advised when using herbs or supplements that may alter blood sugar. Blood glucose levels may require monitoring, and doses may need adjustment.
- In humans, thymus extracts and chemotherapeutic agents have additive effects. Caution is advised when taking thymus extract with other herbs or supplements used in chemotherapy.
- Thymus extract may play a role in immunological disorders associated with stress and anxiety. Caution is advised in patients taking herbs or supplements with anxiolytic activity because of possible additive effects.
- Thymus extract improves symptoms associated with asthma. Thus, thymus extracts and agents that act as bronchodilators may have additive effects.
- In humans, thymomodulin had an additive effect on conventional medications for cardiomyopathy. Thymomodulin may also have additive effects on herbal agents that act in a similar manner. Caution is advised in patients with heart problems.
- In patients with complicated liver echinococciasis, the combined use of phospholipids and T-activin normalized hepatic liver function and immunity and reduced the incidence of postoperative complications.
- Although not well studied in humans, a combination of thymus extract, selenium, and fumaric acid may be beneficial for psoriasis. Fumaric acid is found in some dietary supplements; caution is advised because of possible additive effects.
- Preliminary evidence in humans suggests thyroid extract can improve alopecia (hair loss). It is possible that thyroid extract is able to offer other hormonal effects and have additive effects with agents that alter hormone levels in the body.
- In humans, T-activin has immunomodulatory effects. Caution is advised when taking with other agents that affect the immune system.
- Thymus extract may increase the amount of drowsiness caused by some herbs or supplements. Caution is advised while driving or operating machinery.
- Although not well studied in humans, purified thymus gland extract may insignificantly decrease average thyroid gland weights and serum T3 levels and significantly decrease serum T4 levels. It is not clear what effect thymus gland extract would have on external thyroid hormone-like herbs or supplements.

For a complete list of references, please visit www.naturalstandard.com.

Tribulus
(*Tribulus terrestris*)

RELATED TERMS

- Abrojos, al-Gutub, bullhead, calthrops, caltrop, cat's-head, common dubbletjie, devil's-thorn, devil's-weed, espigon, goathead, gokhru, Gokshura, Mexican sandbur, nature's Viagra, puncture vine, puncture weed, qutiba, Texas sandbur, tribule terrestre, *Tribulus terrestris*, Trilovin.

BACKGROUND

- *Tribulus terrestris* has a long history of use for a variety of conditions. It has been suggested that it was used in ancient Greece and India as a physical rejuvenation tonic. In China, it is used as a component of therapy for conditions affecting the liver, kidney, cardiovascular system, and immune system. It has also been used in Eastern European folk medicine for increased muscle strength and sexual potency. Despite its history of use, there is limited human data available in order to evaluate its clinical effectiveness.
- Tribulus has been studied as a non-steroidal alternative to treatment of infertility. Although the results of the few studies done with the combination product Tribestan are promising, more studies are needed in order to further evaluate its clinical effectiveness. Preliminary research with tribulus also suggests that it may be useful in treating coronary heart disease, but additional studies are needed.

EVIDENCE

Uses Based on Scientific Evidence	Grade
Coronary Artery Disease Preliminary research suggests that tribulus may be beneficial to patients with coronary heart disease. Additional study is needed to further evaluate its clinical effectiveness.	C
Exercise Performance Enhancement Preliminary studies suggest that tribulus may enhance body composition or exercise performance in resistance trained males.	C
Infertility (Female) Although the results of one study investigating the effects of *Tribulus terrestris* are encouraging, larger studies of better design are needed in order to evaluate the effectiveness of Tribestan for treating female infertility.	C
Infertility (Male) Although Tribestan seems to increase sperm count and viability and increase libido, its effectiveness in the treatment of male infertility remains inconclusive, owing to a lack of well-designed clinical trials.	C

Uses Based on Tradition or Theory

Abortifacient (induces abortion), anemia, angina pectoris (chest pain), anthelminthic (expels worms), aphrodisiac, appetite stimulant, astringent, atopic dermatitis, body tone improvement, breast milk stimulant, Bright's disease, cancer, childbirth, chronic fatigue syndrome, colic, cough, digestion, diuretic, dysuria (painful urination), flatulence (gas), gonorrhea (STD), headache, hepatitis, high cholesterol, hypertension (high blood pressure), immune enhancement, inflammation, kidney stones, leprosy, menopausal symptoms, mood stimulant, neurasthenia (nervous exhaustion), pain relief, premenstrual syndrome (symptoms), psoriasis (chronic skin disease), rheumatism (painful disorder of the joints, muscles, or connective tissues), scabies, sore throat, spermatorrhea (excessive ejaculation), stomatitis (mouth sores), tonic, tumors (nasal), vertigo.

DOSING

Adults (18 Years and Older)

- There is insufficient evidence to recommend a dose for tribulus; 85 to 250 mg of 40% furostanol saponins extract in three divided doses with meals has been used. For exercise performance enhancement, 3.21 mg/kg of tribulus for eight weeks has been used.

Children (Younger than 18 Years)

- There is insufficient evidence to recommend a dose for tribulus in children.

SAFETY

Allergies

- Avoid in people with a known allergy or hypersensitivity to *Tribulus terrestris* or its constituents.

Side Effects and Warnings

- *Tribulus terrestris* appears to be generally safe with a few adverse events of insomnia and menorrhagia (heavy menstrual bleeding) occurring. Use cautiously in patients with menstrual disorders. One case of pneumothorax (air between the lungs and the lining of the chest cavity) upon digestion of the fruit has been reported. In another case report, the patient developed a polyp in the lobar bronchus of the right interior lobe due to the presence a tribulus fruit spine. In a case report, gynecomastia (excessive development of male breasts) was observed in a weight trainer taking an herbal supplement containing tribulus.
- Most adverse effects reported, such as exceptionally strong libido, general excitation, and insomnia have been from use of the combination product Tribestan. However, these adverse effects cannot be solely attributed to tribulus, because of the other ingredients in this product.

T

- Although not well studied in humans, a saponin from tribulus may reduce levels of glucose and total cholesterol. Use cautiously in patients with diabetes (high blood sugar) or using hypoglycemic (blood sugar–altering) medication, as tribulus may decrease blood sugar levels.
- Although not well studied in humans, tribulus may increase prostate weight. Use cautiously in patients with benign prostatic hyperplasia (enlarged prostate) or prostate cancer.

Pregnancy and Breastfeeding

- Tribulus is not recommended in pregnant or breastfeeding women because of a lack of available scientific evidence. Traditionally, tribulus has been used as an abortifacient (induces abortion).

INTERACTIONS
Interactions with Drugs

- Tribulus may add to calcium channel blocker or beta-blocker effects because of its negative chronotropic activity in cardiac muscle.
- Tribulus may exacerbate digoxin effects. Caution is advised.
- Tribulus may exhibit diuretic effects (increases urine flow). Caution is advised when used with other drugs that have diuretic effects.
- Tribulus may lower blood glucose levels. Caution is advised when using medications that may also lower blood sugar levels. Patients taking drugs for diabetes by mouth or insulin should be monitored closely by a qualified healthcare professional, including a pharmacist. Medication adjustments may be necessary.
- Tribulus has been found to have blood pressure–lowering effects and may affect patients taking drugs that also alter blood pressure.
- Based on preliminary study and studies of combination products containing tribulus, tribulus may increase levels of steroid hormones.

Interactions with Herbs and Dietary Supplements

- Tribulus may exacerbate the effects of cardiac glycoside herbs.
- Tribulus may exhibit diuretic effects (increase urine flow). Caution is advised when used with other herbs that have diuretic effects.
- Tribulus may lower blood glucose levels. Caution is advised when using herbs or supplements that may also lower blood sugar levels. Blood glucose levels may require monitoring, and doses may need adjustment.
- Tribulus has been found to have blood pressure–lowering effects and may affect patients taking herbs that also alter blood pressure.
- Based on preliminary study and studies of combination products containing tribulus, tribulus may increase levels of steroid hormones.

For a complete list of references, please visit www.naturalstandard.com.

Turmeric
(*Curcuma longa*)

RELATED TERMS

- Amomoum curcuma, anlatone (constituent), ar-tumerone, CUR, *Curcuma*, *Curcuma aromatica*, *Curcuma aromatica* salisbury, *Curcuma domestica*, *Curcuma domestica* valet, *Curcuma longa*, *Curcuma longa* Linn, *Curcuma longa* rhizoma, curcuma oil, curcumin, diferuloylmethane, E zhu, Gelbwurzel, gurkemeje, haldi, Haridra, Indian saffron, Indian yellow root, jiang huang, kunir, kunyit, Kurkumawurzelstock, kyoo, NT, number ten, Olena, radix zedoaria longa, rhizome de curcuma, safran des Indes, sesquiterpenoids, shati, turmeric, tutmeric oil, turmeric root, tumerone (constituent), Ukon, yellowroot, zedoary, Zingiberaceae (family), zingiberene, Zitterwurzel.

BACKGROUND

- The rhizome (root) of turmeric (*Curcuma longa* Linn.) has long been used in traditional Asian medicine to treat gastrointestinal upset, arthritic pain, and low energy. Laboratory and animal research has demonstrated anti-inflammatory, antioxidant, and anti-cancer properties of turmeric and its constituent curcumin. Preliminary human evidence, albeit poor quality, suggests possible efficacy in the management of dyspepsia (heartburn), hyperlipidemia (high cholesterol), and scabies (when used on the skin).

EVIDENCE

Uses Based on Scientific Evidence	Grade
Blood Clot Prevention Preliminary research suggests that turmeric may prevent the formation of blood clots.	C
Cancer Several preliminary animal and laboratory studies report anti-cancer (colon, skin, breast) properties of curcumin. Many mechanisms have been considered, including antioxidant activity, anti-angiogenesis (prevention of new blood vessel growth), and direct effects on cancer cells. Currently it remains unclear if turmeric or curcumin has a role in preventing or treating human cancers. There are several ongoing studies in this area.	C
Cognitive Function Curcumin has been shown to have antioxidant and anti-inflammatory properties and to reduce beta-amyloid and plaque burden in lab studies. However, there is currently not enough evidence to suggest the use of curcumin for cognitive performance.	C
Dyspepsia (Heartburn) Turmeric has been traditionally used to treat stomach problems (such as indigestion from a fatty meal). There is preliminary evidence that turmeric may offer some relief from these stomach problems. However,	C

at high doses or with prolonged use, turmeric may actually irritate or upset the stomach.

Gallstone Prevention/Bile Flow Stimulant It has been said that there are fewer people with gallstones in India, which is sometimes credited to turmeric in the diet. Preliminary studies report that curcumin, a chemical in turmeric, may decrease the occurrence of gallstones. However, reliable human studies are lacking in this area. The use of turmeric may be inadvisable in patients with active gallstones.	C
High Cholesterol Preliminary studies suggest that turmeric may lower levels of low-density lipoprotein ("bad" cholesterol) and total cholesterol in the blood.	C
HIV/AIDS Several laboratory studies suggest that curcumin, a component of turmeric, may have activity against HIV.	C
Inflammation Laboratory and animal studies show anti-inflammatory activity of turmeric and its constituent curcumin. Reliable clinical research is lacking.	C
Irritable Bowel Syndrome (IBS) Irritable bowel syndrome (IBS) is a common functional disorder for which there are limited reliable medical treatments. One study investigated the effects of *Curcuma xanthorriza* on IBS and found that treatment did not show any therapeutic benefit over placebo.	C
Liver Protection In traditional Indian Ayurvedic medicine, turmeric has been used to tone the liver. Preliminary research suggests that turmeric may have a protective effect on the liver.	C
Oral Leukoplakia Results from lab and animal studies suggest that turmeric may have anticancer effects. Clinical evidence is insufficient.	C
Osteoarthritis Turmeric has been used historically to treat rheumatic conditions. Laboratory and animal studies show anti-inflammatory activity of turmeric and its constituent curcumin, which may be beneficial in people with osteoarthritis. Reliable human research is lacking.	C
Peptic Ulcer Disease (Stomach Ulcer) Turmeric has been used historically to treat stomach and duodenal ulcers. However, at high doses or with	C

(Continued)

T

715

Uses Based on Scientific Evidence	Grade
prolonged use, turmeric may actually further irritate or upset the stomach. Currently, there is not enough clinical evidence to support this use.	
Rheumatoid Arthritis Turmeric has been used historically to treat rheumatic conditions and based on animal research may reduce inflammation. Currently, there is no clinical evidence to support this use.	**C**
Scabies Historically, turmeric has been used on the skin to treat chronic skin ulcers and scabies. It has also been used in combination with neem (*Azadirachta indica*).	**C**
Uveitis (Eye Inflammation) Laboratory and animal studies show anti-inflammatory activity of turmeric and its constituent curcumin. Limited evidence suggests a possible benefit of curcumin in the treatment of uveitis.	**C**
Viral Infection Evidence suggests that turmeric may help treat viral infections. However, there is not enough human evidence in this area.	**C**

Uses Based on Tradition or Theory
Abdominal bloating, Alzheimer's disease, antibacterial, antifungal, antimicrobial, antispasmodic, anti-venom, appetite stimulant, asthma, boils, breast milk stimulant, bruises, cataracts, chemoprotective, contraception, cough, cystic fibrosis, diabetes, diarrhea, dizziness, epilepsy, flavoring agent, gas, gonorrhea, heart damage from doxorubicin (Adriamycin, Doxil), *Helicobacter pylori* infection, hepatitis, high blood pressure, histological dye, human papillomavirus (HPV), hypoglycemic agent (blood sugar lowering), infections (methicillin-resistant *Staphylococcus aureus*), insect bites, insect repellent, jaundice, kidney disease, kidney stones, leprosy, liver damage from toxins/drugs, male fertility, menstrual pain, menstrual period problems/lack of menstrual period, multidrug resistance, neurodegenerative disorders, pain, parasites, ringworm, scarring, scleroderma, weight reduction.

DOSING
Adults (18 Years and Older)

- Doses used range from 450 mg of curcumin capsules to 3 g of turmeric root daily, divided into several doses, taken by mouth. As a tea, 1 to 1.5 g of dried root may be steeped in 150 ml of water for 15 minutes and taken twice daily. Average dietary intake of turmeric in the Indian population may range between 2 and 2.5 g, corresponding to 60 to 200 mg of curcumin daily. A dose of 0.6 ml of turmeric oil has been taken three times daily for one month and a dose of 1 ml in three divided doses has been taken for two months.
- One reported method for treating scabies is to cover affected areas once daily with a paste consisting of a 4:1 mixture of *Azadirachta indica* ADR ("neem") to turmeric,

for up to 15 days. Scabies should be treated under the supervision of a qualified healthcare professional.

Children (Younger than 18 Years)
- There is insufficient evidence to recommend a dose of turmeric in children.

SAFETY
Allergies
- Allergic reactions to turmeric may occur, including contact dermatitis (an itchy rash) after skin or scalp exposure. People with allergies to plants in the *Curcuma* genus are more likely to have an allergic reaction to turmeric. Use cautiously in people allergic to turmeric or any of its constituents (including curcumin), to yellow food colorings, or to plants in the Zingiberaceae (ginger) family.

Side Effects and Warnings
- Turmeric may cause an upset stomach, especially in high doses or if given over a long period of time. Heartburn has been reported in patients being treated for stomach ulcers. Since turmeric is sometimes used for the treatment of heartburn or ulcers, caution may be necessary in some patients. Nausea and diarrhea have also been reported.
- Based on laboratory and animal studies, turmeric may increase the risk of bleeding. Caution is advised in patients with bleeding disorders or those taking drugs that may increase the risk of bleeding. Dosing adjustments may be necessary. Turmeric should be stopped prior to scheduled surgery.
- Limited animal studies show that a component of turmeric, curcumin, may increase liver function tests. However, one human study reports that turmeric has no effect on these tests. Turmeric or curcumin may cause gallbladder squeezing (contraction) and may not be advised in patients with gallstones. In animal studies, hair loss (alopecia) and lowering of blood pressure have been reported. In theory, turmeric may weaken the immune system and should be used cautiously in patients with immune system deficiencies.
- Turmeric should be used with caution in people with diabetes or hypoglycemia or people taking drugs or supplements that lower blood sugar.

Pregnancy and Breastfeeding
- Historically, turmeric has been considered safe when used as a spice in foods during pregnancy and breastfeeding. However, turmeric has been found to cause uterine stimulation and to stimulate menstrual flow and caution is therefore warranted during pregnancy. Animal studies have not found turmeric taken by mouth to cause abnormal fetal development.

INTERACTIONS
Interactions with Drugs
- Based on laboratory and animal studies, turmeric may inhibit platelets in the blood and increase the risk of bleeding caused by other drugs. Some examples include aspirin, anticoagulants (blood thinners) such as warfarin (Coumadin) or heparin, anti-platelet drugs such as clopidogrel (Plavix), and non-steroidal anti-inflammatory drugs such as ibuprofen (Motrin, Advil) or naproxen (Naprosyn, Aleve).
- Based on animal data, turmeric may lower blood sugar and therefore may have additive effects with diabetes medications.

- In animals, turmeric protects against stomach ulcers caused by non-steroidal anti-inflammatory drugs (NSAIDs) such as indomethacin (Indocin) and against heart damage caused by the chemotherapy drug doxorubicin (Adriamycin).
- Turmeric may lower blood pressure levels and may have an additive effect if taken with drugs that also lower blood pressure.
- Turmeric may lower blood levels of low-density lipoprotein (LDL or "bad" cholesterol) and increase high-density lipoprotein (HDL or "good" cholesterol). Thus, turmeric may increase the effects of cholesterol-lowering drugs such as lovastatin (Mevacor) or atorvastatin (Lipitor).
- Based on animal studies, turmeric may interfere with the way the body processes certain drugs using the liver's cytochrome P450 enzyme system. As a result, levels of these drugs may be increased in the blood and may cause increased effects or potentially serious adverse reactions. Patients using any medications should check the package insert and speak with a healthcare professional or pharmacist about possible interactions.
- When taken with indomethacin or reserpine, turmeric may help reduce the number of stomach and intestinal ulcers normally caused by these drugs. However, when taken in larger doses or when used for long periods of time, turmeric itself can cause ulcers.

Interactions with Herbs and Dietary Supplements

- Based on animal studies, turmeric may increase the risk of bleeding when taken with herbs and supplements that are believed to increase the risk of bleeding. Multiple cases of bleeding have been reported with the use of *Ginkgo biloba*, some cases with garlic, and fewer cases with saw palmetto.
- Based on animal data, turmeric may lower blood sugar. Individuals taking other herbs or supplements or diabetes medications should speak with a healthcare professional before starting turmeric.
- Turmeric may lower blood levels of low-density lipoprotein (LDL or "bad" cholesterol) and increase high-density lipoprotein (HDL or "good" cholesterol). Thus, turmeric may increase the effects of cholesterol-lowering herbs or supplements such as fish oil, garlic, guggul, or niacin.
- Based on animal studies, turmeric may interfere with the way the body processes certain herbs or supplements using the liver's cytochrome P450 enzyme system. As a result, levels of other herbs or supplements may become too high in the blood. It may also alter the effects that other herbs or supplements possibly have on the P450 system.
- Turmeric may lower blood pressure and may therefore have an additive effect if taken with herbs that also lower blood pressure.

For a complete list of references, please visit www.naturalstandard.com.

T

Tylophora
(*Tylophora* spp.)

RELATED TERMS

- Anta-mul (Hindi), Indian ipecac, Indian ipecacuahna, Jangli-pikavan, *Tylophora asthmatica*, *Typhora indica*, *Tylophora pubescens*, *Tylophora vomitoria*.

BACKGROUND

- Tylophora is a climbing perennial plant that grows in India. The leaves of tylophora have been traditionally used for treating asthma, earning the name of *Tylophora asthmatica*. In folk medicine, it has been used for other respiratory problems such as allergies, bronchitis, and the common cold. It is also believed by some to have laxative and other purgative properties. Additionally, it has been employed to treat dysentery and joint pain.
- Clinical trials have examined the effectiveness of tylophora in bronchial asthma. To date, there is insufficient research examining its effectiveness in treating other conditions.
- The occurrence of adverse events that occur when the leaf of tylophora is taken orally seems to be reduced when the leaves are taken in capsule form instead of chewing.

EVIDENCE

Uses Based on Scientific Evidence	Grade
Asthma Available studies of tylophora for asthma show conflicting results, and therefore efficacy remains unproven.	C

Uses Based on Tradition or Theory
Adrenal support, allergies, antispasmodic, bronchitis, colds, dermatitis, diaphoretic, dysentery, expectorant, inflammation, joint pain, laxative, rheumatism.

DOSING

Adults (18 Years and Older)

- There is insufficient evidence to recommend a dose for tylophora. Traditionally, doses of 250 mg one to three times daily, standardized to 0.1% of tylophorine per dose, and doses of 30 to 60 mg twice daily, standardized to 0.15% of tylophorine have been used. One clinical trial reports using 350 mg of tylophora leaf placed in a capsule and given once daily for seven days. Some experts have used tylophora leaf taken in the amount of 200 to 400 mg dried herb daily. A clinical trial reports the use of one tylophora leaf taken orally daily in the morning for six days. One clinical trial reports the use of 40 mg of alcoholic extract of *Tylophora indica* daily for six days.
- There are reports using 400 to 500 mg of alkaloid tylophora in powder form given once daily to asthmatic patients for six days. Another trial used one leaf of tylophora daily for up to 12 days in asthmatic patients.

Children (Younger than 18 Years)

- There is insufficient evidence to recommend a dose for tylophora in children.

SAFETY

Allergies

- Avoid in people with a known allergy or hypersensitivity to tylophora.

Side Effects and Warnings

- Tylophora has been reported to cause infrequent nausea, vomiting, change in taste perception, and mouth soreness. Rare instances of drowsiness and respiratory distress have also been reported.
- Use cautiously in patients with diabetes, congestive heart failure, arrhythmia, hypertension, and edema.
- Avoid in patients with serious infections, organ transplantation, major systemic disease, or major recent surgery.

Pregnancy and Breastfeeding

- Tylophora is not recommended in pregnant or breastfeeding women because of to a lack of available scientific evidence. *Tylophora asthmatica* has been reported to have abortion-inducing properties. Many tinctures contain high levels of alcohol and should be avoided during pregnancy.

INTERACTIONS

Interactions with Drugs

- Tylophora was found to have central nervous system (CNS) depressant effects in high doses. Caution is advised when taking tylophora with antidepressants or other CNS stimulants.
- Tylophora may increase bronchodilation, and caution is advised when taking with bronchodilators.
- Although not well studied in humans, tylophora may antagonize dextramethasone/hypophysectomy-induced suppression of the pituitary. Caution is advised when taking tylophora with corticosteroids (steroids).
- Tylophora leaf extract of *Tylophora conspicua* may exhibit dose-dependent inhibition of indomethacin-induced gastric ulceration, possibly through gastric acid inhibition. Use caution when taking with indomethacin or other antacids.
- Many tinctures contain high levels of alcohol and may cause nausea or vomiting when taken with metronidazole (Flagyl) or disulfiram (Antabuse).

Interactions with Herbs and Dietary Supplements

- Tylophora leaf extract of *Tylophora conspicua* exhibits dose-dependent inhibition of indomethacin-induced gastric ulceration, possibly through gastric acid inhibition. Use caution when taking with other antacids.
- Tylophora was found to have central nervous system (CNS) depressant effects in high doses. Caution is advised when

taking tylophora with herbs or supplements with antidepressant or CNS stimulant effects.

- Although not well studied in humans, tylophora may antagonize dextramethasone/hypophysectomy-induced suppression of the pituitary. Caution is advised when taking tylorphora with herbs or supplements with corticosteroid-like effects.

For a complete list of references, please visit www.naturalstandard.com.

Usnea
(*Usnea* spp.)

RELATED TERMS

- Ab-Solution plus, ascorbic acid, atranorin, barbatic acid, binan, depsides, depsidones, diffractaic acid, dihydrousnic acid, evernic acid, glutinol, isoanhydromethyldihydrousnic acid, isodihydrousnic acid, isolichenin, isomethoxide, lichen, Lipokinetix, longissiminone A, longissiminone B, methylusnic acid, oak moss extract, old man's beard, parmeliaceae, raffinose, sodium usnate, sodium usnic acid, tree's dandruff, tree moss, woman's long hair, *Usnea amblyoclada, Usnea barbata, Usnea complanta, Usnea dasypoga, Usnea diffracta, Usnea fasciata, Usnea florida, Usnea ghattensis, Usnea hirta, Usnea longissima, Usnea rubiginea, Usnea siamensis, Usnea subfloridana,* Usneaceae (family), usnic acid, usno, Zeta-N.

BACKGROUND

- Species in the genus *Usnea* are classified as fruticose lichens, which are a symbiosis of fungus and algae. Usnea grows on the bark and wood of coniferous (e.g., spruces, firs, and pines) and deciduous hardwood (e.g., oak, hickory, walnut, apple, and other fruit trees) host trees throughout the northern hemisphere in Asia, Europe, and North America.
- Usnea has been used as a therapeutic agent in traditional Chinese medicine (TCM) for thousands of years. *Usnea longissima* is traditionally taken by mouth for lung and upper respiratory infections, and applied on the skin to treat surface infections or external ulcers. It is still used today in TCM in liquid extract and tincture form to treat tuberculosis lymphadenitis.
- Usnic acid is a secondary metabolite uniquely found in all lichens. Usnea or usnic acid has been used as a human papillomavirus (HPV) treatment and as an oral hygiene agent, with limited effectiveness.
- Usnic acid is also found in various oral (by mouth) dietary supplements, including Lipokinetix, marketed as a weight loss agent. However, Lipokinetix may not be safe and may cause liver damage. Lipokinetix, now withdrawn from the market, contained phenylpropanolamine (PPA), caffeine, yohimbine hydrochloride, diiodothyronine, and usnic acid.

EVIDENCE

Uses Based on Scientific Evidence	Grade
Human Papillomavirus Usnea and usnic acid both are reported in laboratory studies to have antiviral activity. A combination of usnic acid and zinc sulfate may help treat human papillomavirus. However, clinical evidence is insufficient to support this use.	C
Oral Hygiene Usnea has been used historically as an oral antibacterial agent, and animal and laboratory studies support this. However, there is currently insufficient clinical evidence to recommend the use of mouthwashes or rinses containing usnea extracts or usnic acid for oral hygiene.	C

Uses Based on Tradition or Theory

Analgesic (pain reliever), antibacterial, anticoagulant (blood thinning), antifungal, anti-inflammatory, antioxidant, antiparasitic, antipyretic (fever reducer), antiviral, cancer, deodorant, gastric ulcers, headache, lupus, oral hygiene, sunscreen, sunstroke, tetanus, tuberculosis, weight loss, wound healing.

DOSING

Adults (18 Years and Older)

- There is insufficient evidence to recommend a dose. However, the German Commission E has approved 1 usnea lozenge (equivalent of 100 mg powdered usnea lichen) 3 to 6 times daily for mouth irritation. Usnea has also been taken by mouth as a powder (100 mg three times daily), tea, or tincture (3 to 4 ml three times daily). Usnea has also been applied on the affected area(s) of the skin two or three times daily.

Children (Younger than 18 Years)

- There is insufficient evidence to recommend a dose for usnea in children, and use is not recommended.

SAFETY

Allergies

- Avoid in people with a known allergy or hypersensitivity to usnea, its constituents, or related lichens. Usnea and its constituents have been reported to cause allergic reactions, such as skin rash, in individuals handling usnea, or using usnic acid vaginally. Deodorant sprays containing usnic acid have been linked to allergic contact eczema.

Side Effects and Warnings

- It appears that usnea is not well tolerated in humans except when applied on the skin or used as a homeopathic agent. The chemical constituent usnic acid has been reported in laboratory studies to be toxic, and dietary supplement products containing usnic acid have been reported to cause liver damage. Based on available research, only preparations of homeopathic usnea are recommended for oral (taken by mouth) use at this time.
- Usnea and usnic acid may cause contact dermatitis that may lead to a hypersensitivity reaction, including urticaria (hives), rhinitis (runny or congested nose), asthma, or photoallergic contact dermatitis.
- Although not well studied in humans, usnic acid may increase the risk of bleeding. Caution is advised in patients with bleeding disorders or those taking drugs that may increase the risk of bleeding. Dosing adjustments may be necessary.

Pregnancy and Breastfeeding

- Usnea or usnic acid is not recommended in pregnant or breastfeeding women based on a lack of available scientific evidence.

INTERACTIONS

Interactions with Drugs

- Usnea may increase bleeding time by inhibition of platelet aggregation. Caution is advised in patients with bleeding disorders or those taking drugs that may increase the risk of bleeding. Some examples of drugs that increase the risk of bleeding include aspirin, anticoagulants (blood thinners) such as warfarin (Coumadin) or heparin, anti-platelet drugs such as clopidogrel (Plavix), and non-steroidal anti-inflammatory drugs such as ibuprofen (Motrin, Advil) or naproxen (Naprosyn, Aleve). Dosing adjustments may be necessary.
- Usnea may interfere with the way the body processes certain drugs using the liver's cytochrome P450 enzyme system. As a result, levels of these drugs may be decreased in the blood and reduce the intended effects. Patients taking any medications should check the package insert and speak with a qualified healthcare professional, including a pharmacist, about possible interactions.

Interactions with Herbs and Dietary Supplements

- Usnea may increase the risk of bleeding when taken with herbs and supplements that are believed to increase the risk of bleeding. Multiple cases of bleeding have been reported with the use of *Ginkgo biloba* and fewer cases with garlic and saw palmetto. Numerous other agents may theoretically increase the risk of bleeding, although this has not been proven in most cases.
- Usnea may interfere with the way the body processes certain herbs or supplements using the liver's cytochrome P450 enzyme system. As a result, levels of other herbs or supplements may become too low in the blood. It may also alter the effects that other herbs or supplements potentially may have on the P450 system.

For a complete list of references, please visit www.naturalstandard.com.

Uva ursi
(*Arctostaphylos uva-ursi*)

RELATED TERMS

- Arberry, arbusier (French), arbutin, *Arbutus uva ursi*, arctostaphylos, *Arctostaphylos adenotricha*, *Arctostaphylos coactilis*, *Arctostaphylos coactylis*, *Arctostaphylos uva-ursi*, arctuvan, barentraube (German), bearberry, bear grape, bear's grape, bearsgrape, beerendruif (Holland), bousserole (French), common bearberry, common beargrape, coralillo (Spanish), creeping manzanita, crowberry, Cystinol akut, Dunih'tan (Carrier people), Ericaceae (family), foxberry, gayuba (Spanish), hog berry, hydroquinone, kanya'ni, kwica (American Indian), kinnikinnick (American Indian), macnicy (Polish), manzanita, mealberry, mehlberre (German), melbaerblad (Norweigan), melbarrisblade (Danish), methyl arbutin, mjolonrisblad (Swedish), mossberre (German), mountain box, mountain cranberry, phenolic glycoside, ptarmigan berry, raisin d'ours (French), redberry, red bearberry, rock berry, rockberry, sagsckhomi (American Indian), sand berry, sandberry, Solvefort, s'qaya'dats, tannin, toloknianka (Russian), upland cranberry, Uroflux, uva d'orso (Italian), UVA-E, Uvae ursi folium, Uvalyst, uva-ursi, uva ursi leaf, whortle berry, wilder Buchsbaum (German), Wolfstraube (German).

BACKGROUND

- Uva ursi (bearberry) is described as a small evergreen shrub with clusters of small white or pink bell-shaped flowers and dull orange berries. Although the berries do not seem to possess any medicinal benefits, the leaves have been used traditionally as an herbal remedy for mild, uncomplicated cystitis (inflammation of the bladder).
- Grown throughout Asia, North America, and Europe, uva ursi has a long history of medicinal use dating back to the thirteenth century. The leaves have been used worldwide as a diuretic, astringent, antiseptic, and a treatment for urinary tract infections (UTIs). A tea brewed with the leaves has also been used as a laxative.
- Arbutin, the main chemical constituent of uva ursi, is a phenolic glycoside that becomes hydrolyzed to hydroquinone. Both chemicals contribute to the antiseptic effects in the urinary tract. Arbutin alone has been reported to relieve pain from kidney stones, cystitis (bladder infection), and nephritis (kidney inflammation). However, due to its high tannin content, uva ursi may cause acute nausea and intestinal irritation.
- Uva ursi leaf was listed on the U.S. National Formulary as a urinary antiseptic from 1820 to 1950, but it is no longer listed in the United States Pharmacopoeia. The European Scientific Cooperative on Phytotherapy (ESCOP) lists uva ursi as a treatment for uncomplicated cystitis where antibiotics are not warranted. The German Commission E Monographs recommend it for inflammatory conditions of the lower urinary tract.

EVIDENCE

Uses Based on Scientific Evidence	Grade
Hyperpigmentation The chemical constituents of the herbal product uva ursi have been used for a variety of conditions such as chloasma, a skin condition that appears as a blotchy, brownish discoloration on the skin, especially the face. Females are usually targeted for the condition because it occurs as a result of oral contraception use, or during pregnancy or menopause. The clinical usefulness of uva ursi has not been well established in the current literature.	C
Urinary Tract Infection (UTI) Uva ursi has long been used as a folk remedy to treat urinary tract infection. The active ingredients in the herb are believed to be ursolic acid and isoquercitrin. Clinical evidence is insufficient to support this use.	C

Uses Based on Tradition or Theory

Allergic reactions, antimicrobial, antiseptic, arthritis, astringent, benign prostate hyperplasia (enlarged prostate), bronchitis, childbirth cramps, catarrh (inflammation of the mucous membrane), cystitis (chronic), dermatitis, diabetes, diuretic, dysentery (severe diarrhea) (astringent), dysmenorrhea (painful menstruation), flavoring agent, gonorrhea (antiseptic), hematuria (blood in the urine), hypertension (high blood pressure), incontinence (mild), kidney disease, kidney infection (pyelonephritis), kidney stones (pain), kidney stone prevention, laxative, leukorrhea (vaginal discharge) (antiseptic), menorrhagia (heavy menstrual bleeding), menopause (tension, edginess), nephritis (inflammation of the kidney), postpartum hemorrhage, prostatitis (inflammation of the prostate), tonic, urethritis (inflammation of the urethra), vaginal ulceration (antiseptic), weight loss.

DOSING

Adults (18 Years and Older)

- There is insufficient evidence to recommend a dose for uva ursi. Cystinol akut is one brand that has been studied. A typical dose taken by mouth is 3 g of uva ursi (or 400 to 800 mg of hydroquinone derivatives) steeped in water and taken as a tea, or taken in powder form, four times a day for inflammatory conditions. For urinary tract infection (UTI), 250 to 500 mg of uva ursi powdered extract (20% arbutin) has been taken three times a day (for no more than four days). When applied on the skin, a 2% or 5% hydroquinone cream has been used for hyperpigmentation. A topical preparation containing 3% arbutin (glycoside in uva ursi) has been used over a 12-week period.

Children (Younger than 18 Years)

- There is insufficient evidence to recommend a dose of uva ursi in children, and use is not recommended.

SAFETY

Allergies

- Avoid in people with a known allergy or hypersensitivity to *Arctostaphylos uva-ursi* or its constituents.

Side Effects and Warnings

- Uva ursi is generally well tolerated in short-term, traditional doses, but clinical evidence is limited. Uva ursi may cause tachycardia (fast heartbeat), cardiac arrhythmias (abnormal heart rate), skin irritations, nausea, vomiting, diarrhea, stomach upset, greenish-brown urine color, irritation and inflammation of the urinary tract mucous membranes, hepatotoxicity (liver damage), insomnia, convulsions, seizures, irritability, motor restlessness, cyanosis (bluish skin discoloration due to lack of oxygen in the blood), headaches, shortness of breath, or tinnitus (ringing in the ears).
- Long-term ingestion of uva ursi has caused bilateral bull's-eye maculopathy and may be considered a potential retinal toxic herb. Use cautiously in patients with renal (kidney) or hepatic (liver) dysfunction, because of risk of inflammation of the urinary tract and hepatotoxicity. Avoid in patients with kidney disease. Use cautiously in patients with gastrointestinal distress because the preparation can be irritating to the mucous membrane of the stomach and the intestine because of high amounts of tannins. Use cautiously in patients taking diuretics, which may promote electrolyte imbalance. Use cautiously in patients suffering from gallstones.

Pregnancy and Breastfeeding

- Uva ursi is not recommended in pregnant or breastfeeding women because of a lack of sufficient available evidence. Large amounts of uva ursi may induce labor.

INTERACTIONS
Interactions with Drugs

- Uva ursi may increase the inhibitory effect of prednisolone on swelling. The arbutin in uva ursi may potentiate the effects of prednisolone and dexamethasone on contact dermatitis. Caution is advised when using uva ursi with corticosteroids (steroids).
- Uva ursi may increase urine flow and may interact with other agents that increase urine flow (diuretics).
- The arbutin in uva ursi may increase the anti-inflammatory activity of indomethacin on contact dermatitis, hypersensitivity, and arthritis. Caution is advised when taking uva ursi with non-steroidal anti-inflammatory drugs (NSAIDs) because of theoretical interactions.
- Concomitant use of uva ursi and urine acidifiers may result in decreasing the effects of uva ursi.
- Concomitant use of uva ursi and products that can alkalinize the urine can enhance the antibacterial activity of uva ursi.

Interactions with Herbs and Dietary Supplements

- Combination of uva ursi and aloesin inhibits tyrosinase activity in a synergistic manner by combined mechanisms of noncompetitive and competitive inhibitions.
- Herbs containing arbutin, a constituent of uva ursi, may result in increases in serum and urinary levels of hydroquinone and its metabolites. Arbutin is found in sweet marjoram, damiana, and other herbs.
- Uva ursi may increase urine flow and may interact with other herbs and supplements with diuretic effects.
- Concomitant use of uva ursi and products that can acidify the urine (e.g., vitamin C) can potentially reduce the antibacterial activity of uva ursi.
- Concomitant use of uva ursi and products that can alkalinize the urine may enhance the antibacterial activity of uva ursi.

For a complete list of references, please visit www.naturalstandard.com.

U

Valerian
(Valeriana officinalis)

RELATED TERMS

- All-heal, amantilla, balderbrackenwurzel, baldrian, baldrianwurzel, baldrion, Belgian valerian, blessed herb, capon's tail, common valerian, English valerian, fixed valerian-hops extract combination Ze91019, fragrant valerian, garden heliotrope, garden valerian, German valerian, great wild valerian, heliotrope, herba benedicta, Indian valerian, Jacob's ladder, Japanese valerian, katzenwurzel, laege-baldrian, Li 156, Mexican valerian, Nervex, Neurol, Orasedon, pacific valerian, phu, phu germanicum, phu parvum, pinnis dentatis, racine de valèriane, radix valerian, red valerian, Sanox-N, Sedonium, setewale capon's tail, setwall, setwell, tagara, theriacaria, Ticalma, *Valeriana edulis, Valeriana faurieri, Valeriana foliis pinnatis, Valeriana jatamansi, Valeriana radix, Valeriana sitchensis, Valeriana wallichii,* valeriana, Valerianaceae (family), Valerianaheel, valeriane, Valmane, vandal root, Vermont valerian, wild valerian.

BACKGROUND

- Valerian is an herb native to Europe and Asia that currently grows in most parts of the world. The name is believed to come from the Latin word *valere* meaning to be healthy or strong. The root of the plant is believed to contain its active constituents. Use of valerian as a sedative and anti-anxiety treatment has been reported for more than 2,000 years. For example, in the second century AD, Galen recommended valerian as a treatment for insomnia. Related species have been used in traditional Chinese and Indian Ayurvedic medicine. Preparations for use on the skin have been used to treat sores and acne, and valerian by mouth has been used for other conditions such as digestive problems, flatulence (gas), congestive heart failure, urinary tract disorders, and angina (chest pain).
- Valerian extracts became popular in the United States and Europe in the mid-1800s and continued to be used by both physicians and the lay public until it was widely replaced by prescription sedative drugs. Valerian remains popular in North America, Europe, and Japan and is widely used to treat insomnia and anxiety. Although the active ingredients in valerian are not known, preparations are often standardized to the content of valerenic acid.

EVIDENCE

Uses Based on Scientific Evidence	Grade
Anxiety Disorder Several studies of valerian have reported benefits in reducing non-specific anxiety symptoms. Valerian has also been given in combination with other herbs, such as passionflower and St. John's wort, to treat anxiety. However, there is a lack of conclusive clinical evidence to support this use.	C
Depression There is not enough available scientific evidence in this area.	C
Insomnia Several studies in adults suggest that valerian improves the quality of sleep and reduces the time to fall asleep (sleep latency) for up to four to six weeks. Ongoing nightly use may be more effective than single-dose use, with increasing effects over four weeks. Better effects have been found in poor sleepers. However, most studies have not used scientific ways of measuring sleep improvements, such as sleep pattern data in a sleep laboratory.	C
Menopausal Symptoms There is not enough available scientific evidence in this area.	C
Sedation Although valerian has not been studied specifically as a sedative, evidence from studies conducted for other purposes suggests that valerian may not have significant sedative effects when used at recommended doses. Therefore, even though valerian could be helpful as a sleep aid, it does not appear to cause sedation.	C

Uses Based on Tradition or Theory

Acne, amenorrhea (lack of menstruation), angina (chest pain), anorexia, anti-seizure, antiperspirant, antiviral, arthritis, asthma, bloating, bronchospasm, congestive heart failure, constipation, cough, cramping (abdominal, pelvic, menstrual), digestive problems, diuretic (increase urine flow), dysmenorrhea (pain with menstrual cycle), emmenagogue (stimulation of menstrual blood flow), epilepsy, fatigue, fever, flatulence (gas), hangovers, headache, heart disease, heartburn, high blood pressure, HIV, hot flashes, hypochondria, irritable bowel syndrome, liver disorders, measles, memory enhancement, migraine, mood enhancement, muscle pain/spasm/tension, nausea, nerve pain, pain relief, restlessness, stomach ulcers, premenstrual syndrome (PMS), restless leg syndrome, rheumatic pain, skin disorders, stress, urinary tract disorders, vaginal infections, vertigo, viral gastroenteritis, vision problems, withdrawal from tranquilizers.

DOSING
Adults (18 Years and Older)

- Studied doses range from 400 to 900 mg of an aqueous or aqueous-ethanolic extract (corresponding to 1.5 to 3 g of herb) taken 30 to 60 minutes before going to bed. Valerian has historically been used in the form of a tea (1.5 to 3 g root steeped for 5 to 10 minutes in 150 ml boiling water), although this formulation has not been studied. Doses of 300 to 1,800 mg of valerian have also been taken by mouth in capsule form.

Children (Younger than 18 Years)

- There is insufficient evidence to recommend the use of valerian in children.

SAFETY
Allergies

- People with allergies to plants in the Valerianaceae family may be allergic to valerian.

Side Effects and Warnings

- Studies report that valerian is generally well tolerated for up to four to six weeks in recommended doses. Valerian has occasionally been reported to cause headache, excitability, stomach upset, uneasiness, dizziness, unsteadiness (ataxia), and low body temperature (hypothermia). Chronic use (longer than two to four months) may result in insomnia. Slight reductions in concentration or complicated thinking may occur for a few hours after taking valerian. Use caution if driving or operating heavy machinery. Some research suggests that valerian may not cause sedation.
- A drug "hangover" effect has been reported in people taking high doses of valerian extracts. "Valerian withdrawal" may occur if you stop using valerian suddenly after chronic high-dose use, including confusion (delirium) and rapid heartbeat. These symptoms may improve with the use of benzodiazepines such as lorazepam (Ativan). Although unknown, valerian may have similar brain activity as benzodiazepines (which are commonly used to treat anxiety and insomnia) through effects on the brain chemical gamma-amino-butyric acid (GABA).
- Valerian has been on the U.S. Food and Drug Administration's (FDA's) GRAS (Generally Regarded as Safe) list, and no deaths due to overdose have been reported.
- Liver toxicity has been associated with some multi-herb preparations that include valerian. However, the contribution of valerian itself is not clear because of the potential liver toxicity of other included ingredients and the possibility of contamination with unlisted herbs.

Pregnancy and Breastfeeding

- Because there is limited human safety data, valerian use during pregnancy and breastfeeding is not recommended. There are theoretical concerns over the adverse effects of chemical components that are toxic in laboratory studies.

INTERACTIONS
Interactions with Drugs

- Based on animal and human studies, valerian may increase the amount of drowsiness caused by some drugs, although this is an area of controversy. Examples include benzodiazepines such as lorazepam (Ativan) or diazepam (Valium), barbiturates such as phenobarbital, narcotics such as codeine, some antidepressants, and alcohol. Caution is advised while driving or operating machinery. In one human study, a combination of valerian and the beta-blocker drug propranolol (Inderal) reduced concentration levels more than valerian alone. A brief episode of confusion was reported in one patient using valerian with loperamide (Imodium) and St. John's wort (*Hypericum perforatum* L.).
- An episode of agitation, anxiety, and self-injury was reported in a patient after taking valerian with fluoxetine (Prozac) for a mood disorder (the person was also drinking alcohol). In theory, valerian may interact with anti-seizure medications, although human data is lacking. Valerian tinctures may contain high alcohol content (15% to 90%) and theoretically may cause vomiting if taken with metronidazole (Flagyl) or disulfiram (Antabuse). Valerian may interact with certain drugs metabolized by the liver or vasopressin.

Interactions with Herbs and Dietary Supplements

- Based on theoretical concerns, valerian may increase the amount of drowsiness caused by some herbs or supplements.
- A brief episode of confusion was reported in one patient during use of valerian with loperamide (Imodium) and St. John's wort (*Hypericum perforatum* L.). Nausea, sweating, muscle cramping, weakness, elevated pulse, and high blood pressure were reported after a single dose of a combination product with St. John's wort, kava, and valerian. Valerian may interact with certain herbs and supplements that are metabolized by the liver.

For a complete list of references, please visit www.naturalstandard.com.

V

Vitamin A
(Retinol)

RELATED TERMS

- 3,7-dimethyl-9-(2,6,6, trimethyl-1-cyclohexen-1-yl)-2,4,6,8-natetraen-1-ol, 3-dehydroretinol, antixerophthalmic vitamin, Aquasol A, axeropthologlum, beta-carotene oleovitamin A, Palmitate-A, retinol, retinaldehyde (RAL), retinyl acetate, retinyl N-formyl aspartamate, retinyl palmitate, Solatene, vitamin A, vitamin A aldehyde, vitamin A1, vitamin A USP, vitaminum A.

BACKGROUND

- Vitamin A is a fat-soluble vitamin that is derived from two sources: preformed retinoids and provitamin carotenoids. Retinoids, such as retinal and retinoic acid, are found in animal sources like liver, kidney, eggs, and dairy products. Carotenoids like beta-carotene (which has the highest vitamin A activity) are found in plants such as dark or yellow vegetables and carrots.

- Natural retinoids are present in all living organisms, either as preformed vitamin A or as carotenoids, and are required for a vast number of biological processes like vision and cellular growth. A major biological function of vitamin A (as the metabolite retinal) is in the visual cycle. Research also suggests that vitamin A may reduce the mortality rate from measles, prevent some types of cancer, aid in growth and development, and improve immune function.

- Recommended daily allowance (RDA) levels for vitamin A oral intake have been established by the U.S. Institute for Medicine of the National Academy of Sciences to prevent deficiencies in vitamin A. At recommended doses, vitamin A is generally considered non-toxic. Excess dosing may lead to acute or chronic toxicity.

- Vitamin A deficiency is rare in industrialized nations but remains a concern in developing countries, particularly in areas where malnutrition is common. Prolonged deficiency can lead to xerophthalmia (dry eye) and ultimately to night blindness or total blindness, as well as to skin disorders, infections (such as measles), diarrhea, and respiratory disorders.

EVIDENCE

Uses Based on Scientific Evidence	Grade
Acne Derivatives of vitamin A, retinoids, are used to treat skin disorders such as acne. Topical and oral prescription medications, such as tretinoin (Avita, Renova, Retina-A, Retin-A Micro) and isotretinoin (Accutane), are available for treatment. Isotretinoin may cause severe side effects and should be used only for severe resistant acne. Isotretinoin must not be used in women who are pregnant, plan to become pregnant, or have a chance of being pregnant because of a risk of severe birth defects. These medications should be prescribed and coordinated by a qualified licensed healthcare professional. Vitamin A supplements should not be used simultaneously because of a risk of increased toxicity.	A
Acute Promyelocytic Leukemia (Treatment, All-Trans-Retinoic Acid) The prescription drug All-*Trans*-Retinoic Acid (ATRA, Vesanoid) is a vitamin A derivative that is an established treatment for acute promyelocytic leukemia and improves median survival in this disease. Treatment should be under strict medical supervision. Vitamin A supplements should not be used simultaneously with ATRA because of a risk of increased toxicity.	A
Eye Disorders (Bitot's Spot) Vitamin A deficiency can lead to Bitot's spot, or the buildup of keratin debris in the conjunctiva. Bitot's spot is a sign of xerophthalmia and may be treated with vitamin A supplementation.	A
Measles (Supportive Agent) Vitamin A should be administered to children diagnosed with measles in areas where vitamin A deficiency may be present. Measles is a viral disease that can lead to serious complications such as diarrhea, pneumonia, and encephalitis. Supplementation with vitamin A in children with measles has been shown to be beneficial, by decreasing the length and impact of the disease. Side effects such as diarrhea, pneumonia, and death have been reduced with the use of vitamin A. Management of measles should be under strict medical supervision.	A
Vitamin A Deficiency Vitamin A deficiency may occur after chronic lack of adequate amounts of vitamin A or beta-carotene. Vitamin A is necessary for vision, and an early sign of vitamin A deficiency is keratomalacia (night blindness). Prolonged deficiency may lead to xerophthalmia (dry eye) and Bitot's spot, or the buildup of keratin debris in the conjunctiva. Eventually, blindness can occur from damage to the retina and cornea. Vitamin A is necessary for healthy growth and development, and recommended daily amounts (RDAs) should be assured, particularly in children.	A
Xerophthalmia (Dry Eye) Oral vitamin A is the treatment of choice for xerophthalmia due to prolonged vitamin A deficiency and should be given immediately once the disorder is established.	A
Malaria (Supportive Agent) Limited research suggests that vitamin A may reduce fever, morbidity, and parasite blood levels in patients with malaria (*Plasmodium falciparum* infection). However, there is a lack of evidence suggesting that vitamin A is equivalent or superior to well-established drug therapies used for the prevention or treatment of malaria. Patients with malaria or those living/	B

Uses Based on Scientific Evidence	Grade
traveling in endemic areas should speak with a physician about appropriate measures.	
Retinitis Pigmentosa Retinitis pigmentosa is a genetic disorder that affects night vision. Early symptoms include night blindness and progressive loss of vision over time. Based on recent findings, vitamin A in the palmitate form has been recommended in patients with retinitis pigmentosa.	B
Antioxidant The benefits to humans of potential antioxidant activity are not clear.	C
Breast Cancer Research results are not clear as to whether vitamin A is beneficial in the treatment or prevention of breast cancer. Patients receiving chemotherapy or radiation therapy for cancer should speak with their doctor(s) before taking antioxidants such as vitamin A during treatment, because of possible interference.	C
Cataract Prevention Vitamin A has been suggested to prevent cataract formation. Carotenoids such as beta-carotene, lutein, and zeaxanthin may decrease the risk of severe cataracts. There is insufficient evidence to form a clear conclusion at this time.	C
Diarrhea Vitamin A may reduce the severity and duration of diarrheal episodes in malnourished children but not in well-nourished children. Since diarrhea is a major cause of morbidity and mortality in developing countries, vitamin A supplementation may be considered in undernourished children with diarrhea.	C
HIV Infection The role of vitamin A in the prevention, transmission, or treatment of HIV is controversial and not well established. A clear conclusion cannot be formed based on the available scientific research.	C
Immune Function Vitamin A deficiency may compromise immunity, but there is no clear evidence that additional vitamin A supplementation is beneficial for immune function in patients who are not vitamin A deficient.	C
Infant Mortality There is a limited amount of research in this area, with mixed results. Some evidence suggests possible decreases in infant mortality with vitamin A supplementation, while other research reports no benefits. A clear conclusion cannot be formed based on the available scientific research.	C
Iron Deficiency Anemia Vitamin A supplementation in combination with iron may have beneficial effects in patients with iron	C

deficiency anemia, including children and pregnant women. It is not clear that there are benefits in people who are not vitamin A deficient. This area remains controversial.

	Grade
Pancreatic Cancer Vitamin A supplementation has not been shown to improve response to gemcitabine in pancreatic cancer. It is unclear whether vitamin A may provide any benefits in patients with pancreatic cancer. More research is needed in this area.	C
Parasite Infection (Acaris Reinfection) After deworming, children supplemented with vitamin A may be less prone to *Ascaris* parasite reinfection. These benefits may be less in children with stunted growth.	C
Photoreactive Keratectomy Photoreactive keratectomy is a type of laser eye surgery used to correct nearsightedness. High-dose vitamin A supplementation in addition to vitamin E has been suggested to help improve ocular healing after surgery and to improve visual acuity, although additional evidence is necessary before a definitive conclusion can be reached.	C
Pneumonia (Children) One study found no effect of a moderate dose of vitamin A supplementation on the duration of uncomplicated pneumonia in underweight or normal-weight children aged younger than five years. However, a beneficial effect was seen in children with high basal serum retinol concentrations.	C
Polyp Prevention Alpha-carotene and vitamin A may protect against recurrence of polyps and adenoma in nonsmokers and nondrinkers or indicate a compliance or another healthy lifestyle factor that reduces risk.	C
Pregnancy-Related Complications Maternal vitamin A deficiency is common in developing countries. Beta-carotene may reduce pregnancy-related complications and mortality in such people. However, excess intake of vitamin A has been reported to increase the risks of some birth defects. Vitamin A supplementation above the RDA is therefore not recommended in pregnancy.	C
Skin Aging (Improving Aging Skin Appearance) Some studies suggest that topical vitamin A may improve the appearance and integrity of aged skin.	C
Skin Cancer Prevention It is not clear if vitamin A or beta-carotene, taken by mouth or used on the skin with sunscreen, is beneficial in the prevention or treatment of skin cancers or wrinkles.	C
Viral Infection (Norovirus [NoV] Infection) Vitamin A supplementation has been suggested to help prevent NoV infection in children and reduce the symptoms associated with NoV infections.	C

V

(Continued)

Uses Based on Scientific Evidence	Grade
Weight Loss Daily vitamin A with calcium has been suggested for weight loss, and in one study an average loss of two pounds was reported after two years of supplementation in young women.	C
Wound Healing In preliminary research, retinol palmitate significantly reduced rectal symptoms of radiation proctopathy, perhaps because of wound-healing effects.	C
Chemotherapy Adverse Effects Vitamin A supplementation does not appear to improve chemotherapy-related side effects including nausea, vomiting, diarrhea, or mouth sores.	D
Lung Cancer Vitamin A has been studied as a possible treatment for lung cancer without evidence of benefits. Available evidence suggests that high-dose Vitamin A and beta-carotene may actually increase the risk of adverse effects, especially among alcohol users and smokers.	D

Uses Based on Tradition or Theory

Aging, allergic rhinitis, asthma, blurred vision, bronchopulmonary dysplasia in premature infants, burns, candidiasis, cellulite (topical retinal), cold sores, conjunctivitis, Crohn's disease, cystic fibrosis, deafness, deficiency (protein), diabetes, eczema, fibrocystic breast disease, glaucoma, headache (persistent), heart disease, hyperthyroidism, increasing sperm count, infections, keratosis follicularis (Darier's disease), kidney stones, leukoplakia, Lichen planus pigmentosus, liver disease, menorrhagia (heavy menstruation), metabolic disorders (Hurler syndrome), neurodegenerative diseases, periodontal disease, pityriasis rubra pilaris, plantar warts, pollutant protection, premenstrual syndrome, psoriasis, rhinitis, sebaceous cysts, sinusitis, skin disorders (ichthyosis), sunburn, tinnitus, ulcers (stress ulcers in severely ill hospitalized patients), urinary tract infections, vaginitis, vision enhancement (nearsightedness).

DOSING
Sources of Vitamin A

- Vitamin A is found in dairy products, fish, and darkly colored fruits and vegetables. Consumption of five servings of fruits and vegetables per day supplies 5 to 6 mg daily of provitamin A carotenoids, which provides about 50% to 65% of the adult RDA for vitamin A.

Adults (18 Years and Older)

- Vitamin A is included in most multivitamins, often in 5,000 IU doses as softgels, capsules, tablets, or liquid. The Recommended Daily Allowance (RDA) for adults established by the U.S. Institute of Medicine of the National Academy of Sciences is: 900 mcg (3,000 IU) daily for men and 700 mcg (2,300 IU) daily for women. For pregnant women 19 years and older, 770 mcg (2,600 IU) daily is recommended. For lactating women 19 years and older, 1,300 mcg (4,300 IU) daily is recommended.

- For vitamin A deficiency not involving xerophthalmia, 100,000 IU orally or intramuscularly administered daily for three days, followed by 50,000 IU daily for two weeks has been used. A maintenance dose of 10,000 to 20,000 IU daily for two months has been recommended.
- Supporting care following chemotherapy may include weekly injections of 100,000 IU vitamin A. Patients receiving vitamin A should be observed carefully for liver toxicity.
- Injections should always be performed by a licensed healthcare provider.

Children (Younger than 18 Years)

- The Recommended Daily Allowance (RDA) established by the U.S. Institute of Medicine of the National Academy of Sciences is: for children 1 to 3 years old, 300 mcg (1,000 IU) daily; for children 4 to 8 years old, 400 mcg (1,300 IU) daily; and for children 9 to 13 years old, 600 mcg/day (2,000 IU) daily. For pregnant women 14 to 18 years old, 750 mcg/day (2,500 IU) is recommended; for lactating women 14 to 18 years old, 1,200 mcg (4,000 IU) daily is recommended.
- The World Health Organization (WHO) has established dosage guidelines for children 6 to 11 months old to receive 100,000 IU of vitamin A. This increases to 200,000 IU every six months from 12 to 59 months of age.

SAFETY
Allergies

- Avoid in people with a known hypersensitivity/allergy to vitamin A.

Side Effects and Warnings

- Vitamin A toxicity, or hypervitaminosis A, is rare in the general population. Vitamin A toxicity can occur with excessive amounts of vitamin A taken over short or long periods of time. Consequently, toxicity can be acute or chronic. An infant with acute toxicity can develop a bulging fontanelle (the soft spot on the head) and symptoms similar to a brain tumor. Adults experience less specific symptoms such as headache, dizziness, fatigue, malaise, blurry vision, bone pain and swelling, nausea, and/or vomiting. Acute vitamin A toxicity may also lead to increased intracranial pressure, pruritus or itching, and bone problems. Severe toxicity can lead to eye damage, high levels of calcium, and liver damage. People with liver disease and high alcohol intake may be at risk for hepatotoxicity from vitamin A supplementation. Smokers who consume alcohol and beta-carotene may be at an increased risk for lung cancer or cardiovascular disease.
- Vitamin A toxicity may lead to intrahepatic cholestasis, a condition in which bile cannot flow from the liver into the intestines. Treatment with ursodeoxycholic acid has been shown to greatly improve the symptoms of cholestasis.

Pregnancy and Breastfeeding

- Vitamin A should be used within the recommended dietary allowance only, because vitamin A excess, as well as deficiency, has been associated with birth defects. Excessive doses of vitamin A have been associated with central nervous system malformations.
- Vitamin A is excreted in human breast milk. Benefits or dangers to nursing infants are not clearly established.

INTERACTIONS
Interactions with Drugs

- Vitamin A supplements should not be taken simultaneously with acitretin (Soriatane), anticoagulants (blood thinners) such as warfarin (Coumadin), bexarotene (Targentin), All-*Trans*-Retinoic Acid (ATRA, Vesanoid), etretinate (Tegison), isotretinoin (Accutane, Amnesteen), or tretinoin (Vesabiod, Avita, Renova, Retin-A, Retin-A Micro, Altinac) because of increased risk of vitamin A toxicity.
- Cholestyramine (Questran) and colestipol (Colestid) may decrease the effectiveness of vitamin A by reducing absorption of this fat-soluble vitamin. Neomycin may interfere with the absorption of vitamin A, although this interaction has not been found to be clinically significant. Oral contraceptives (birth control pills) increase plasma vitamin A levels.
- Vitamin A may reduce seroconversion rates to the measles virus/vaccine, rendering the vaccine less effective. Other vaccines may be enhanced by vitamin A, including the *Haemophilus influenzae* type b vaccine and the diphtheria vaccine. Other vaccines have been demonstrated to be unaffected by vitamin A supplementation. These include the oral polio vaccine (OPV), tetanus toxoid, pertussis, and hepatitis B vaccines. Vitamin A may also alter the immune response to the Bacille Calmette-Guérin (BCG) vaccine, but this interaction is unclear.
- Mineral oil has been reported to reduce absorption of all fat-soluble vitamins. With occasional use, the effect on vitamin A levels does not appear to be significant.
- Orlistat (obesity drug) decreases the absorption of fat-soluble vitamins, although studies suggest that vitamin A is not affected as much by orlistat as other fat-soluble vitamins. Nonetheless, the manufacturer of orlistat recommends that all patients take a multivitamin supplement containing all the fat-soluble vitamins (including vitamins A, D, E, and K unless otherwise contraindicated), separating the dosing time by at least two hours from orlistat.
- Patients who take tetracyclines, specifically minocycline (Minocin), plus vitamin A are at a risk for developing benign intracranial hypertension (pseudotumor cerebri), which can occur with tetracyclines and vitamin A intoxication. Therefore, high doses of vitamin A should be avoided in people taking chromic tetracyclines. Other examples of tetracyclines include demeclocycline (Declomycin) and tetracycline (Achromycin).

Interactions with Herbs and Dietary Supplements

- Carob may increase risk of vitamin A toxicity.
- Vitamin A may improve anemia in people who are deficient in iron and vitamin A. There is likely no benefit in people who are not vitamin A deficient.
- Zinc deficiency may alter vitamin A status, although the mechanism is unclear.

For a complete list of references, please visit www.naturalstandard.com.

V

Vitamin B$_6$

RELATED TERMS

- 2-Methyl-3-hydroxy-4,5-dihydroxymethylpyridine, 5-hydroxy-6-methyl-3,4-pyridinedimethanol [65-23-6], Adermine Hydrochloride, B Complex Vitamin, B$_6$, B (6), Bio Zinc, Beesix, Benadon, Bexivit, Bonadon N, Hexobion 100, Naturetime B6, Pyridoxal, Pyridoxal Phosphate, Pyridoxal-5-Phosphate, Pyridoxamine, Pyridoxine HCl, Pyridoxine Hydrochloride, Pyroxin, Rodex, Vicotrat, Vita-Valu, Vitabee 6, Vitamin B-6.

BACKGROUND

- Vitamin B$_6$ (pyridoxine) is required for the synthesis of the neurotransmitters serotonin and norepinephrine and for myelin formation.
- Pyridoxine deficiency in adults principally affects the peripheral nerves, skin, mucous membranes, and the blood cell system. In children, the central nervous system (CNS) is also affected. Deficiency can occur in people with uremia, alcoholism, cirrhosis, hyperthyroidism, malabsorption syndromes, congestive heart failure (CHF), and in those taking certain medications.
- Mild deficiency of vitamin B$_6$ is common. Major sources of vitamin B$_6$ include cereal grains, legumes, vegetables (carrots, spinach, peas), potatoes, milk, cheese, eggs, fish, liver, meat, and flour.
- Pyridoxine is frequently used in combination with other B vitamins in vitamin B–complex formulations.

EVIDENCE

Uses Based on Scientific Evidence	Grade
Hereditary Sideroblastic Anemia Pyridoxine supplements are effective for treating hereditary sideroblastic anemia under the supervision of a qualified health care provider.	A
Preventing the Adverse Effects of Cycloserine (Seromycin) Cycloserine is a prescription antibiotic that may cause anemia, peripheral neuritis, or seizures by acting as a pyridoxine antagonist or increasing excretion of pyridoxine. Requirements for pyridoxine may be increased in patients receiving cycloserine. Pyridoxine may be recommended by a health care provider to prevent these adverse effects.	A
Pyridoxine Deficiency/Neuritis Pyridoxine supplements are effective for preventing and treating pyridoxine deficiency and neuritis due to inadequate dietary intake, certain disease states, or deficiency induced by drugs such as isoniazid (INH) or penicillamine. Dietary supplements should be taken under the guidance of a qualified health care provider, particularly when an underlying medical condition is present.	A
Pyridoxine-Dependent Seizures in Newborns Pyridoxine-dependent seizures in newborns can result from the use of high-dose pyridoxine in pregnant mothers or from genetic (autosomal recessive) pyridoxine dependency. Refractory seizures in newborns that are caused by pyridoxine dependence may be controlled quickly with intravenous administration of pyridoxine by a qualified health care provider.	A
Akathisia (Movement Disorder) Some neuroleptics, which are used in psychiatric conditions, may cause movement disorders as adverse side effects. Vitamin B$_6$ has been studied for the treatment of acute neuroleptic-induced akathisia (NIA) in schizophrenic and schizoaffective disorder patients. Preliminary results indicate that high doses of vitamin B$_6$ may be useful additions to the available treatments for NIA, perhaps due to its combined effects on various neurotransmitter systems. Further research is needed to confirm these results.	C
Angioplasty There are conflicting findings about the potential benefit or harm of taking folic acid plus vitamin B$_6$ and vitamin B$_{12}$ following angioplasty.	C
Asthma Preliminary research suggests that children with severe asthma might have inadequate pyridoxine status. Theophylline, a prescription drug used to help manage asthma, seems to lower pyridoxine levels. Studies of pyridoxine supplementation in asthma patients taking theophylline yield conflicting results.	C
Attention Deficit Hyperactivity Disorder (ADHD) Some research suggests that pyridoxine supplementation alone or in combination with high doses of other B vitamins might help ADHD. Other studies show no benefit.	C
Birth Outcomes Studies of birth outcomes with vitamin B$_6$ supplementation during pregnancy have yielded mixed results.	C
Cardiovascular Disease/Hyperhomocysteinemia High homocysteine levels in the blood (hyperhomocysteinemia) are a risk factor for cardiovascular disease, blood clotting abnormalities, myocardial infarction (heart attack), and ischemic stroke. Taking	C

Uses Based on Scientific Evidence	Grade
pyridoxine supplements alone or in combination with folic acid has been shown to be effective for lowering homocysteine levels. However, it is not clear if lowering homocysteine levels results in reduced cardiovascular morbidity and mortality. Until definitive data is available, the current recommendation is screening of 40-year-old men and 50-year-old women for hyperhomocysteinemia. Decreased pyridoxine concentrations are also associated with increased plasma levels of C-reactive protein (CRP). CRP is an indicator of inflammation that is associated with increased cardiovascular morbidity in epidemiological studies. Investigation of more renal transplant recipients undergoing longer treatment with Vitamin B6 is needed as study results conflict.	
Carpal Tunnel Syndrome Preliminary data suggests that large doses of vitamin B$_6$ may be helpful for carpal tunnel syndrome. However, this has not been shown conclusively.	C
Depression Preliminary evidence suggests that because pyridoxine increases serotonin and gamma-aminobutyric acid (GABA) levels in the blood, it may benefit people in dysphoric mental states. However, this has not been shown conclusively.	C
Hyperkinetic Cerebral Dysfunction Syndrome There is preliminary evidence that pyridoxine supplementation might benefit hyperkinetic children who have low levels of blood serotonin. Further research is warranted.	C
Immune System Function Vitamin B$_6$ is important for immune system function in older adults. There is some evidence that the amount of vitamin B$_6$ required to reverse immune system impairments in older adults was more than the current recommended dietary allowance (RDA).	C
Kidney Stones (Nephrolithiasis) Pyridoxine alone, or taken with magnesium, may decrease urinary oxalate levels, which can contribute to a certain type of kidney stones. Higher pyridoxine intake has been associated with decreased risk of kidney stone formation in women but not in men with no history of stone formation. Benefit has not been proven in other types of kidney stones such as those associated with high urinary calcium, phosphorus, and creatinine.	C
Lactation Suppression Study results of pyridoxine used to suppress lactation yield mixed results.	C
Lung Cancer Epidemiological research suggests that male smokers with higher serum levels of pyridoxine may have a lower risk of lung cancer. Effectiveness has not been	C

	Grade
clearly demonstrated, and supplementation is not standard therapy at this time.	
Pregnancy-Induced Nausea and Vomiting Studies of the use of pyridoxine alone or in combination with other anti-nausea treatments in pregnant women have yielded conflicting results.	C
Premenstrual Syndrome (PMS) There is some evidence (though not conclusive) that taking pyridoxine orally may improve symptoms of PMS such as breast pain or tenderness (mastalgia) and PMS-related depression or anxiety in some patients.	C
Preventing Vitamin B$_6$ Deficiency Associated with Taking Birth Control Pills The need for vitamin B$_6$ supplementation in women taking birth control pills has not been proven, although some studies show decreased pyridoxine levels in these women. B$_6$ supplementation should be approached cautiously since the long-term effect of such therapy is uncertain.	C
Autism Studies of B$_6$ supplementation alone or in combination with magnesium have not been shown to benefit autism. Autism should be treated by a qualified health care provider.	D
Stroke Reoccurrence Pyridoxine alone or in combination with B$_{12}$ and folic acid orally does not seem to be useful for preventing stroke recurrence.	D
Tardive Dyskinesia Pyridoxine has some antioxidant effects, which theoretically may benefit patients with tardive dyskinesia. There is promising evidence that vitamin B$_6$ may improve symptoms of tardive dyskinesia; however, further research is warranted.	C

V

Uses Based on Tradition or Theory

Acne, alcohol intoxication, allergies, appetite stimulation, arthritis, cancer prevention, chorea, conjunctivitis (pinkeye), cystitis, diabetic neuropathy, diuresis (increased urine production), dizziness, Down's syndrome, high cholesterol, improving dream recall, infertility, menopausal symptoms, migraine headaches, motion sickness, muscle cramps, night leg cramps, poisoning (mushroom), psychosis, radiation sickness, sickle cell anemia, skin conditions.

DOSING
Adults (18 Years and Older)

- Recommended dietary allowances (RDAs) of vitamin B$_6$: Males (19-50 years) 1.3 mg; males (51 years and older) 1.7 mg; females (19-50 years) 1.3 mg; females (51 years and older) 1.5 mg. Some researchers believe that the RDA for women 19-50 years should be increased to

1.5-1.7mg/day. Pregnant women, 1.9 mg; and lactating women, 2 mg.

- Recommended maximum daily intake of vitamin B$_6$: Adults, pregnant, and lactating women (over 18 years) 100 mg. A doctor and pharmacist should be consulted for dosing in other conditions.

Children (Younger than 18 Years)

- Recommended dietary allowances (RDAs) of vitamin B$_6$: Infants (0-6 months) 0.1 mg; infants (7-12 months) 0.3 mg; children (1-3 years) 0.5 mg; children (4-8 years) 0.6 mg; children (9-13 years) 1 mg; males (14-18 years) 1 mg per day; females (14-18 years) 1.2 mg per day.
- Recommended maximum daily intake of vitamin B$_6$: Children (1-3 years) 30 mg; (4-8 years) 40 mg, (9-13 years) 60 mg. Males; females; and pregnant and lactating females (14-18 years) 80 mg.

SAFETY
Allergies

- Patients should avoid vitamin B$_6$ products if they are sensitive or allergic to any of their ingredients.

Side Effects and Warnings

- Some individuals seem to be particularly sensitive to vitamin B$_6$ and may have problems at lower doses. Overall, pyridoxine is generally considered safe in adults and children when used appropriately at recommended doses. Avoid excessive dosing.
- Acne, skin reactions, allergic reactions, and photosensitivity have been reported.
- Nausea, vomiting, abdominal pain, loss of appetite, and increased liver function test results (serum aspartate transaminase [AST, SGOT]) have been reported.
- Headache, paresthesia, somnolence, and sensory neuropathy have been reported.
- Breast soreness or enlargement, decreased serum folic acid levels, seizures after large doses, hypotonia, and respiratory distress in infants have also been reported.

Pregnancy and Breastfeeding

- Vitamin B$_6$ is likely safe when used orally in doses not exceeding the recommended dietary allowance (RDA). Vitamin B$_6$ is possibly safe when used orally and appropriately in amounts exceeding the recommended dietary allowance. A special sustained-release multi-ingredient product has been approved by the U.S. Food and Drug Administration (FDA) for use in pregnancy. However, it should not be used long-term or without medical supervision and close monitoring or in more excessive doses. There is some concern that high-dose maternal pyridoxine can cause neonatal seizures.
- Vitamin B$_6$ is likely safe when used orally in doses not exceeding the recommended dietary allowance (RDA).

There is insufficient reliable information about the safety of pyridoxine when used in higher doses in lactating women. Because most breastfeeding women do not consume the RDA of vitamin B$_6$ in their normal diets and do not provide totally breastfed infants with the RDA of this vitamin, higher doses of vitamin B$_6$ may be recommended although benefits have not been well proven.

INTERACTIONS
Interactions with Drugs

- Preliminary research suggests that pyridoxine may exacerbate amiodarone (Cordarone)-induced photosensitivity. Other research suggests a protective effect. Despite conflicting information, concomitant use is cautioned.
- Destruction of normal gastrointestinal flora by antibiotics can cause decreased production of the B vitamins. Clinical significance is unknown.
- Cycloserine is an antibiotic that may cause anemia or peripheral neuritis by acting as a pyridoxine antagonist or increasing renal excretion of pyridoxine. Requirements for pyridoxine may be increased in patients receiving cycloserine.
- Use of estrogens and estrogen-containing oral contraceptives can interfere with pyridoxine metabolism, reducing serum pyridoxine levels. The need for pyridoxine supplementation has not been adequately studied.
- Hydralazine (Apresoline) can increase pyridoxine requirements. The need for pyridoxine supplementation has not been adequately studied.
- Isoniazid (INH, Rifamate) can increase pyridoxine requirements.
- Pyridoxine enhances the metabolism of levodopa (Sinemet), reducing its anti-parkinsonism effects. Carbidopa and levodopa used together may avoid this interaction.
- Penicillamine (Cuprimine, Depen) can increase pyridoxine requirements.
- Preliminary data suggests that pyridoxine can reduce plasma levels of phenobarbital (Luminal), possibly by increasing metabolism. Patients taking phenobarbital should avoid high doses of pyridoxine.
- Preliminary data suggests that pyridoxine can reduce plasma levels of phenytoin (Dilantin), possibly by increasing metabolism. Patients taking phenytoin should avoid high doses of pyridoxine.
- Theophylline (Theo-Dur), a medication used for asthma, interferes with pyridoxine metabolism. Study results of supplemental pyridoxine in these patients are inconclusive.

Interactions with Herbs and Dietary Supplements

- Theoretically, herbs and supplements with estrogen-like activity may interact with pyridoxine. The need for pyridoxine supplementation has not been adequately studied.

For a complete list of references, please visit www.naturalstandard.com.

Vitamin B$_{12}$
[Alpha-(5,6-dimethylbenzimidazolyl)cobamidcyanide]

RELATED TERMS

- B-12, B Complex, B Complex Vitamin, bedumil, cobalamin, cobalamins, cobamin, cyanocobalamin, cyanocobalaminum, cycobemin, hydroxocobalamin, hydroxocobalaminum, hydroxocobemine, idrossocobalamina, methylcobalamin, vitadurin, vitamin B-12.

BACKGROUND

- Vitamin B$_{12}$ is an essential water-soluble vitamin that is commonly found in a variety of foods such as fish, shellfish, meat, and dairy products. Vitamin B$_{12}$ is frequently used in combination with other B vitamins in a vitamin B complex formulation. It helps maintain healthy nerve cells and red blood cells and is also needed to make DNA, the genetic material in all cells. Vitamin B$_{12}$ is bound to the protein in food. Hydrochloric acid in the stomach releases B$_{12}$ from protein during digestion. Once released, B$_{12}$ combines with a substance called intrinsic factor (IF) before it is absorbed into the bloodstream.

- The human body stores several years' worth of vitamin B$_{12}$, so nutritional deficiency of this vitamin is extremely rare. Older adults are the most at risk. However, deficiency can result from being unable to use vitamin B$_{12}$. Inability to absorb vitamin B$_{12}$ from the intestinal tract can be caused by a disease known as pernicious anemia. Additionally, strict vegetarians or vegans who are not taking in proper amounts of B$_{12}$ are also prone to a deficiency state.

- A day's supply of vitamin B$_{12}$ can be obtained by eating 1 chicken breast plus 1 hard-boiled egg plus 1 cup plain low-fat yogurt, or 1 cup milk plus 1 cup raisin bran.

EVIDENCE

Uses Based on Scientific Evidence	Grade
Megaloblastic Anemia due to Vitamin B$_{12}$ Deficiency Vitamin B$_{12}$ deficiency is a cause of megaloblastic anemia. In this type of anemia, red blood cells are larger than normal and the ratio of nucleus size to cell cytoplasm is increased. There are other potential causes of megaloblastic anemia, including folate deficiency or various inborn metabolic disorders. If the cause is B$_{12}$ deficiency, then treatment with B$_{12}$ is the standard approach. Patients with anemia should be evaluated by a physician in order to diagnose and address the underlying cause.	A
Vitamin B$_{12}$ Deficiency Studies have shown that a deficiency of vitamin B$_{12}$ can lead to abnormal neurologic and psychiatric symptoms. These symptoms may include: ataxia (shaky movements and unsteady gait), muscle weakness, spasticity, incontinence, hypotension (low blood pressure), vision problems, dementia, psychoses, and mood disturbances. Researchers report that these symptoms may occur	A

when vitamin B$_{12}$ levels are just slightly lower than normal and are considerably above the levels normally associated with anemia. People at risk for vitamin B$_{12}$ deficiency include strict vegetarians; older adults; and people with increased vitamin B$_{12}$ requirements associated with pregnancy, thyrotoxicosis, hemolytic anemia, hemorrhage, malignancy, and liver or kidney disease.

Administering vitamin B$_{12}$ orally, intramuscularly, or intranasally is effective for preventing and treating dietary vitamin B$_{12}$ deficiency.

Pernicious Anemia Pernicious anemia (blood abnormality) is a form of anemia that occurs when there is an absence of intrinsic factor, a substance normally present in the stomach. Vitamin B$_{12}$ binds with intrinsic factor before it is absorbed and used by the body. An absence of intrinsic factor prevents normal absorption of B$_{12}$ and may result in pernicious anemia. Pernicious anemia treatment is usually lifelong; supplemental vitamin B$_{12}$ given intramuscularly, intranasally, or by mouth.	A
Alzheimer's Disease Some patients diagnosed with Alzheimer's disease have been found to have abnormally low vitamin B$_{12}$ levels in their blood. However, vitamin B$_{12}$ deficiency itself often causes disorientation and confusion and thus mimics some of the prominent symptoms of Alzheimer's disease. It is unclear whether vitamin B$_{12}$ supplementation may benefit Alzheimer's disease.	C
Angioplasty Some evidence suggests that folic acid plus vitamin B$_{12}$ and pyridoxine daily can decrease the rate of restenosis in patients treated with balloon angioplasty. But this combination does not seem to be as effective for reducing restenosis in patients after coronary stenting. Because of the lack of evidence of benefit and potential for harm, this combination of vitamins should not be recommended for patients receiving coronary stents.	C
Breast Cancer Researchers at Johns Hopkins University report that women with breast cancer tend to have lower vitamin B$_{12}$ levels in their blood serum than do women without breast cancer. In a subsequent review of these findings, it was hypothesized that vitamin B$_{12}$ deficiency may lead to breast cancer because it could result in less folate being available to ensure proper DNA replication and repair. Higher dietary folate intake is associated with a reduced risk of breast cancer. The risk may be further reduced in women who also consume high amounts of	C

V

(Continued)

Uses Based on Scientific Evidence	Grade
dietary vitamin B$_{12}$ in combination with dietary pyridoxine (vitamin B$_6$) and methionine. However, there is no evidence that dietary vitamin B$_{12}$ alone reduces the risk of breast cancer.	
Cardiovascular Disease/Hyperhomocysteinemia Hyperhomocysteinemia (high homocysteine levels in the blood) is a risk factor for coronary, cerebral, and peripheral atherosclerosis, recurrent thromboembolism, deep vein thrombosis, myocardial infarction (heart attack), and ischemic stroke. Elevated homocysteine levels may be a marker instead of a cause of vascular disease. However, it is not clear if lowering homocysteine levels results in reduced cardiovascular morbidity and mortality. Folic acid, pyridoxine (vitamin B$_6$), and vitamin B$_{12}$ supplementation can reduce total homocysteine levels; however, this reduction does not seem to help with secondary prevention of death or cardiovascular events such as stroke or myocardial infarction in people with prior stroke. More evidence is needed to fully explain the association of total homocysteine levels with vascular risk and the potential use of vitamin supplementation.	C
Fatigue There is some evidence that intramuscular injections of vitamin B$_{12}$ given twice per week might improve the general well-being and happiness of patients complaining of tiredness or fatigue. However, fatigue has many potential causes. Well-designed clinical trials are needed before a recommendation can be made.	C
High Cholesterol Some evidence suggests that vitamin B$_{12}$ in combination with fish oil might be superior to fish oil alone when used daily to reduce total serum cholesterol and triglycerides. Well-designed clinical trials of vitamin B$_{12}$ supplementation alone are needed.	C
Imerslund-Grasbeck Disease Administering vitamin B$_{12}$ intramuscularly seems to be effective for treating familial selective vitamin B$_{12}$ malabsorption (Imerslund-Grasbeck disease). Further research is needed.	C
Shaky-Leg Syndrome There is some evidence that cyanocobalamin may help relieve tremor associated with shaky-leg syndrome. Further research is needed.	C
Sickle Cell Disease One study suggests that a practical daily combination may include folic acid, vitamin B$_{12}$, and vitamin B$_6$. This combination may be a simple and relatively inexpensive way to reduce these patients' inherently high risk of endothelial damage. Further research is needed to confirm these results.	C

	Grade
Circadian Rhythm Sleep Disorders Taking vitamin B$_{12}$ orally, in methylcobalamin form, does not seem to be effective for treating delayed sleep phase syndrome. Supplemental methylcobalamin, with or without bright light therapy, does not seem to help people with primary circadian rhythm sleep disorders.	D
Lung Cancer Preliminary evidence suggests that there is no relationship between vitamin B$_{12}$ status and lung cancer.	D
Stroke In people with a history of stroke, neither high-dose vitamin B$_{12}$ combinations containing pyridoxine, vitamin B$_{12}$, and folic acid nor low-dose combinations containing pyridoxine, vitamin B$_{12}$, and folic acid seem to affect risk of recurring stroke.	D
Leber's Disease Vitamin B$_{12}$ is contraindicated in early Leber's disease, which is a hereditary optic nerve atrophy.	F

Uses Based on Tradition or Theory

Aging, AIDS, allergies, amyotrophic lateral sclerosis, asthma, chronic fatigue syndrome, depression, depressive disorder (major), diabetes, diabetic peripheral neuropathy, energy level enhancement, growth disorders (failure to thrive), hemorrhage, immunosuppression, improving concentration, inflammatory bowel disease, kidney disease, liver disease, male infertility, malignant tumors, memory loss, mood (elevate), mouth and throat inflammation (atrophic glossitis), multiple sclerosis, myoclonic disorders (spinal myoclonus), osteoporosis, periodontal disease, protection from tobacco smoke, psychiatric disorders, seborrheic dermatitis, seizure disorders (West syndrome), tendonitis, thyrotoxicosis/thyroid storm (adjunct iodides), tinnitus, tremor, vitiligo.

DOSING

Adults (over 18 years old)

- Recommended Daily Allowances (RDAs) are 2.4 mcg daily for adults and adolescents age 14 years and older, 2.6 mcg daily for adult and adolescent pregnant females, and 2.8 mcg daily for adult and adolescent lactating females. Because 10% to 30% of older adults do not absorb food-bound vitamin B$_{12}$ efficiently, those over 50 years of age should meet the RDA by eating foods fortified with B$_{12}$ or by taking a vitamin B$_{12}$ supplement. Supplementation of 25 to 100 mcg daily has been used to maintain vitamin B$_{12}$ levels in older adults. A doctor and pharmacist should be consulted for use in other indications. Vitamin B$_{12}$ has been taken by mouth and given by intramuscular (IM) injection by healthcare professionals. One clinical trial tested patients' acceptance of intranasal vitamin B$_{12}$ replacement therapy (500 mcg weekly).

Children (Younger than 18 Years)

- Recommended Daily Allowances (RDAs) have not been established for all pediatric age groups; therefore Adequate

Intake (AI) levels have been used. The RDA and AI of vitamin B$_{12}$ are: infants 0 to 6 months, 0.4 mcg (AI); infants 7 to 12 months, 0.5 mcg (AI); children 1 to 3 years, 0.9 mcg; children 4 to 8 years, 1.2 mcg; and children 9 to 13 years, 1.8 mcg.

SAFETY

Allergies

- Vitamin B$_{12}$ supplements should be avoided in people sensitive or allergic to cobalamin, cobalt, or any other product ingredients.

Side Effects and Warnings

- Caution should be used in patients undergoing angioplasty since an intravenous loading dose of folic acid, vitamin B$_6$, and vitamin B$_{12}$ followed by oral administration taken daily after coronary stenting might actually increase restenosis rates. Because of the potential for harm, this combination of vitamins should not be recommended for patients receiving coronary stents.
- Itching, rash, transitory exanthema, and urticaria have been reported. Vitamin B$_{12}$ and pyridoxine have been associated with cases of rosacea fulminans, characterized by intense erythema with nodules, papules, and pustules. Symptoms may persist for up to four months after the supplement is stopped and may require treatment with systemic corticosteroids and topical therapy.
- Diarrhea has been reported.
- Peripheral vascular thrombosis has been reported. Treatment of vitamin B$_{12}$ deficiency can unmask polycythemia vera, which is characterized by an increase in blood volume and the number of red blood cells. The correction of megaloblastic anemia with vitamin B$_{12}$ can result in fatal hypokalemia and gout in susceptible people, and it can obscure folate deficiency in megaloblastic anemia. Caution is warranted.
- Vitamin B$_{12}$ is contraindicated in early Leber's disease, which is hereditary optic nerve atrophy. Vitamin B$_{12}$ can cause severe and swift optic atrophy.

Pregnancy and Breastfeeding

- Vitamin B$_{12}$ is likely safe when used orally in amounts that do not exceed the Recommended Daily Allowance (RDA).
- There is insufficient reliable information available about the safety of larger amounts of vitamin B$_{12}$ during pregnancy.

INTERACTIONS

Interactions with Drugs

- Excessive alcohol intake lasting longer than two weeks can decrease vitamin B$_{12}$ absorption from the gastrointestinal tract.
- Aminosalicylic acid can reduce oral vitamin B$_{12}$ absorption, possibly by as much as 55%, as part of a general malabsorption syndrome. Megaloblastic changes, and occasional cases of symptomatic anemia, have occurred. Vitamin B$_{12}$ levels should be monitored in people taking aminosalicylic acid for more than one month.
- An increased bacterial load can bind significant amounts of vitamin B$_{12}$ in the gut, preventing its absorption. In people with bacterial overgrowth of the small bowel, antibiotics such as metronidazole (Flagyl) can actually improve vitamin B$_{12}$ status. The effects of most antibiotics on gastrointestinal bacteria are unlikely to have clinically significant effects on vitamin B$_{12}$ levels.

- The data regarding the effects of oral contraceptives on vitamin B$_{12}$ serum levels are conflicting. Some studies have found reduced serum levels in birth control pill users, but others have found no effect despite the use of birth control pills for up to six months. When birth control pill use is stopped, normalization of vitamin B$_{12}$ levels usually occurs. Lower vitamin B$_{12}$ serum levels seen with birth control pills probably are not clinically significant.
- Limited case reports suggest that chloramphenicol can delay or interrupt the reticulocyte response to supplemental vitamin B$_{12}$ in some patients. Blood counts should be monitored closely if this combination cannot be avoided.
- Cobalt irradiation of the small bowel can decrease gastrointestinal (GI) absorption of vitamin B$_{12}$.
- Colchicine can disrupt normal intestinal mucosal function, leading to malabsorption of several nutrients, including vitamin B$_{12}$. Lower doses do not seem to have a significant effect on vitamin B$_{12}$ absorption after three years of colchicine therapy. The significance of this interaction is unclear. Vitamin B$_{12}$ levels should be monitored in people taking large doses of colchicine for prolonged periods.
- Colestipol (Colestid) and cholestyramine (Questran) resins can decrease gastrointestinal (GI) absorption of vitamin B$_{12}$. It is unlikely that this interaction will deplete body stores of vitamin B$_{12}$ unless there are other factors contributing to deficiency. In a group of children treated with cholestyramine for up to 2.5 years, there was no change in serum vitamin B$_{12}$ levels. Routine supplements are not necessary.
- H2-blockers include cimetidine (Tagamet), famotidine (Pepcid), nizatidine (Axid), and ranitidine (Zantac). Reduced secretion of gastric acid and pepsin produced by H2 blockers can reduce absorption of protein-bound (dietary) vitamin B$_{12}$, but not of supplemental vitamin B$_{12}$. Gastric acid is needed to release vitamin B$_{12}$ from protein for absorption. Clinically significant vitamin B$_{12}$ deficiency and megaloblastic anemia are unlikely, unless H2-blocker therapy is prolonged (two years or more) or the person's diet is poor. It is also more likely if the person is rendered achlorhydric (lacking hydrochloric stomach acid), which occurs more frequently with proton pump inhibitors than H2 blockers. Vitamin B$_{12}$ levels should be monitored in people taking high doses of H2 blockers for prolonged periods.
- Metformin may reduce serum folic acid and vitamin B$_{12}$ levels. These changes can lead to hyperhomocysteinemia (abnormally large levels of homocysteine in the blood), adding to the risk of cardiovascular disease in people with diabetes. There are also rare reports of megaloblastic anemia in people who have taken metformin for five years or more. Reduced serum levels of vitamin B$_{12}$ occur in up to 30% of people taking metformin chronically. However, clinically significant deficiency is not likely to develop if dietary intake of vitamin B$_{12}$ is adequate. Deficiency can be corrected with vitamin B$_{12}$ supplements even if metformin is continued. The metformin-induced malabsorption of vitamin B$_{12}$ is reversible by oral calcium supplementation. A multivitamin preparation may also be valuable for some patients. Patients should be monitored for signs and symptoms of vitamin B$_{12}$ and folic acid deficiency. People taking metformin chronically should be advised to include adequate amounts of vitamin B$_{12}$ in their diet, and have their serum vitamin B$_{12}$ and homocysteine levels checked annually.

V

- Absorption of vitamin B$_{12}$ can be reduced by neomycin, but prolonged use of large doses is needed to induce pernicious anemia. Supplements are not usually needed with normal doses.
- Nicotine can reduce serum vitamin B$_{12}$ levels. The need for vitamin B$_{12}$ supplementation has not been adequately studied.
- Nitrous oxide inactivates the cobalamin form of vitamin B$_{12}$ by oxidation. Symptoms of vitamin B$_{12}$ deficiency, including sensory neuropathy, myelopathy, and encephalopathy, can occur within days or weeks of exposure to nitrous oxide anesthesia in people with subclinical vitamin B$_{12}$ deficiency. Symptoms are treated with high doses of vitamin B$_{12}$, but recovery can be slow and incomplete. People with normal vitamin B$_{12}$ levels have sufficient vitamin B$_{12}$ stores to make the effects of nitrous oxide insignificant, unless exposure is repeated and prolonged (nitrous oxide abuse). Vitamin B$_{12}$ levels should be checked in people with risk factors for vitamin B$_{12}$ deficiency prior to using nitrous oxide anesthesia.
- Phenytoin (Dilantin), phenobarbital, and primidone (Mysoline) anticonvulsants have been associated with reduced vitamin B$_{12}$ absorption and reduced serum and cerebrospinal fluid levels in some patients. This may contribute to the megaloblastic anemia, primarily caused by folate deficiency, associated with these drugs. It has also been suggested that reduced vitamin B$_{12}$ levels may contribute to the neuropsychiatric side effects of these drugs. Patients should be encouraged to maintain adequate dietary vitamin B$_{12}$ intake. Folate and vitamin B$_{12}$ status should be checked if symptoms of anemia develop.
- Proton pump inhibitors (PPIs) include omeprazole (Prilosec, Losec), lansoprazole (Prevacid), rabeprazole (Aciphex), pantoprazole (Protonix, Pantoloc), and esomeprazole (Nexium). The reduced secretion of gastric acid and pepsin produced by PPIs can reduce absorption of protein-bound (dietary) vitamin B$_{12}$, but not supplemental vitamin B$_{12}$. Gastric acid is needed to release vitamin B$_{12}$ from protein for absorption. Reduced vitamin B$_{12}$ levels may be more common with PPIs than with H2 blockers, because they are more likely to produce achlorhydria (complete absence of gastric acid secretion). However, clinically significant vitamin B$_{12}$ deficiency is unlikely, unless PPI therapy is prolonged (two years or more) or dietary vitamin intake is low. Vitamin B$_{12}$ levels should be monitored in people taking high doses of PPIs for prolonged periods.
- Reduced serum vitamin B$_{12}$ levels may occur when zidovudine (AZT, Combivir, Retrovir) therapy is started. This adds to other factors that cause low vitamin B$_{12}$ levels in people with HIV and might contribute to the hematologic toxicity associated with zidovudine. However, data suggests that vitamin B$_{12}$ supplements are not helpful for people taking zidovudine.

Interactions with Herbs and Dietary Supplements

- Folic acid, particularly in large doses, can mask vitamin B$_{12}$ deficiency. In vitamin B$_{12}$ deficiency, folic acid can produce hematologic improvement in megaloblastic anemia, while allowing potentially irreversible neurologic damage to progress. Vitamin B$_{12}$ status should be determined before folic acid is given as a monotherapy.
- Potassium supplements can reduce absorption of vitamin B$_{12}$ in some people. This effect has been reported with potassium chloride and, to a lesser extent, with potassium citrate. Potassium might contribute to vitamin B$_{12}$ deficiency in some people with other risk factors, but routine supplements are not necessary.
- Preliminary evidence suggests that vitamin C supplements can destroy dietary vitamin B$_{12}$. However, other components of food, such as iron and nitrates, might counteract this effect. Clinical significance is unknown, and it can likely be avoided if vitamin C supplements are taken at least two hours after meals.

For a complete list of references, please visit www.naturalstandard.com.

Vitamin C
(ascorbic acid)

RELATED TERMS

- Antiscorbutic vitamin, ascorbate, ascorbic acid (AA), ascorbyl palmitate, calcium ascorbate, cevitamic acid, iso-ascorbic acid, L-ascorbic acid, sodium ascorbate.

BACKGROUND

- Vitamin C (ascorbic acid) is a water-soluble vitamin that is necessary in the body to form collagen in bones, cartilage, muscle, and blood vessels and aids in the absorption of iron. Dietary sources of vitamin C include fruits and vegetables, particularly citrus fruits such as oranges.
- Severe deficiency of vitamin C causes scurvy. Although rare, scurvy includes potentially severe consequences and can cause sudden death. Patients with scurvy are treated with vitamin C and should be under medical supervision.
- Many uses for vitamin C have been proposed, but few have been found to be beneficial in scientific studies. In particular, research in asthma, cancer, and diabetes remains inconclusive, and no benefits have been found in the prevention of cataracts or heart disease.
- The use of vitamin C in the prevention/treatment of the common cold and respiratory infections remains controversial, with ongoing research. For *cold prevention*, more than 30 clinical trials including over 10,000 participants have examined the effects of taking daily vitamin C. Overall, no significant reduction in the risk of developing colds has been observed. In people who developed colds while taking vitamin C, no difference in severity of symptoms has been seen overall, although a very small significant reduction in the duration of colds has been reported (approximately 10% in adults and 15% in children). Notably, a subset of studies in people living in extreme circumstances, including soldiers in sub-arctic exercises, skiers, and marathon runners, have found a significant reduction in the risk of developing a cold by approximately 50%. This area merits additional study and may be of particular interest to elite athletes or military personnel.
- For *cold treatment*, numerous studies have examined the effects of starting vitamin C after the onset of cold symptoms. So far, no significant benefits have been observed.

EVIDENCE

Uses Based on Scientific Evidence	Grade
Vitamin C Deficiency (Scurvy) Scurvy is caused by a dietary deficiency of vitamin C. Although scurvy is uncommon, it may occur in malnourished people, those with increased vitamin C requirements (such as pregnant or breastfeeding women), or infants whose only source of nourishment is breast milk. Vitamin C administered by mouth or injection is effective for curing scurvy. If vitamin C is not available, orange juice can be used for infantile scurvy. Symptoms should begin to improve within 24 to 48 hours, with resolution within seven days. Treatment should be under strict medical supervision.	A
Common Cold Prevention (Extreme Environments) Scientific studies generally suggest that vitamin C does not prevent the onset of cold symptoms. However, in a subset of studies in people living in extreme climates or under extraordinary conditions, including soldiers in sub-arctic exercises, skiers, and marathon runners, vitamin C significantly reduced the risk of developing colds by approximately 50%. This area merits more study and may be of particular interest to elite athletes or military personnel.	B
Iron Absorption Enhancement Based on scientific research, vitamin C appears to improve oral absorption of iron. Concurrent vitamin C may aid in the absorption of iron dietary supplements.	B
Urinary Tract Infection (During Pregnancy) Vitamin C may decrease the risk of developing urinary tract infections during pregnancy. It is unclear whether vitamin C is effective for treating urinary tract infections.	B
Asthma It has been suggested that low levels of vitamin C (or other antioxidants) may increase the risk of developing asthma. The use of vitamin C for the treatment of asthma has been studied since the 1980s (particularly exercise-induced asthma), although the evidence in this area remains inconclusive. More research is needed before a clear conclusion can be drawn.	C
Bleeding Stomach Ulcers Caused by Aspirin Preliminary evidence suggests that vitamin C may help aspirin-induced gastric damage. More research is needed before a clear conclusion can be drawn.	C
Cancer Prevention Dietary intake of fruits and vegetables high in vitamin C has been associated with a reduced risk of various types of cancer in population studies (particularly cancers of the mouth, esophagus, stomach, colon, or lung). However, it is not clear that a benefit comes specifically from the vitamin C in these foods, and vitamin C supplements have not been found to be associated with this protective effect. Experts have recommended increasing dietary consumption of fruits and vegetables high in vitamin C, such as asparagus, berries, broccoli, cabbage, melon (cantaloupe, honeydew, watermelon), cauliflower, citrus fruits (lemons, oranges), fortified breads/grains/cereal, kale, kiwi, potatoes, spinach, and tomatoes.	C
Cancer Treatment Vitamin C has a long history of adjunctive use in cancer therapy, and although there has not been any definite	C

V

(Continued)

Uses Based on Scientific Evidence	Grade
evidence of a benefit from injected (or oral) vitamin C, there is evidence that it has benefit in some cases. More well-designed studies are needed before a firm recommendation can be made.	
Complex Regional Pain Syndrome Clinical research suggests that vitamin C may prevent complex regional pain syndrome among elderly female patients with wrist fracture. This area merits additional study.	C
***Helicobacter pylori* Infection** Adding vitamin C to triple therapy with omeprazole, amoxicillin, and clarithromycin for *Helicobacter pylori* gastric ulcer treatment may allow the dose of clarithromycin to be lower. Further research is needed to confirm these results.	C
Ischemic Heart Disease Because of its antioxidant properties, vitamin C has been used in patients with ischemic heart disease. Preliminary data suggest that vitamin C may have a benefit on blood flow in the heart, but more research is needed to confirm these findings.	C
Metabolic Abnormalities (Alkaptonuria) Alkaptonuria is a disorder characterized by the absence of the enzyme homogentisic acid oxidase, which causes homogentisic acid to collect in the blood and urine. Limited research reports that daily high-dose vitamin C may provide relief of symptoms and slow progression of complications of this disorder. More study is merited in this area.	C
Plaque/Calculus on Teeth In preliminary studies, reduced amounts of calculus, visible plaque, and bleeding gum sites were observed after the use of vitamin C chewing gum. Further research is needed to confirm these results.	C
Pneumonia (Prevention) Vitamin C may play a role in the prevention of pneumonia. However, further research is needed to confirm these results.	C
Pregnancy There is not enough evidence to conclude if vitamin C supplementation alone or combined with other supplements is beneficial during pregnancy. Preterm birth may increase with vitamin C supplementation. Some study results show that daily supplementation can effectively lessen the incidence of premature rupture of chorioamniotic membranes (PROM). A gynecologist and pharmacist should be consulted before taking any herbs or supplements during pregnancy.	C
Prostate Cancer Vitamin C has been used in prostate cancer, but there is currently a lack of evidence to determine its effect in this disease.	C
Skin Damage Caused by the Sun (UVA-Induced) Vitamin C and vitamin E applied to the skin may not prevent UVA-induced skin damage (suntan). Further research is needed to confirm these findings.	C
Skin Pigmentation Disorders (Perifollicular Pigmentation) Limited evidence suggests a role for vitamin C in perifollicular pigmentation, which is characterized by increased color pigment near the hair follicle.	C
Stroke Prevention There are variable results of studies that have measured the association of vitamin C intake and risk of stroke. Some studies have reported no benefits, while others report that daily low-dose vitamin C may reduce the risk of death from stroke. More research is merited in this area. People at risk of having a stroke should speak with their healthcare provider about the role of vitamin C supplements in stroke prevention.	C
Vaginitis Preliminary human research shows that vitamin C vaginal tablets given once a day may help patients suffering from non-specific vaginitis. Further research is needed to confirm these findings.	C
Cataracts (Prevention/Progression) Although preliminary population research suggested a reduction in cataract formation among people taking vitamin C for at least 10 years, subsequent research found no reduction in the seven-year risk of age-related cataract formation or progression with the use of daily vitamin C.	D
Common Cold Prevention (General) More than 30 clinical trials including more than 10,000 participants have examined the effects of taking daily vitamin C on cold prevention. Overall, no significant reduction in the risk of developing colds has been observed. In people who developed colds while taking vitamin C, no difference in severity of symptoms has been seen overall, although a very small significant reduction in the duration of colds has been reported (approximately 10% in adults and 15% in children). Laboratory experiments in which volunteers were infected with respiratory viruses while taking vitamin C have yielded conflicting results, but overall they reported small or no significant differences in symptom severity following infection. Notably, a subset of studies in people living in extreme circumstances, including soldiers in subarctic exercises, skiers, and marathon runners, have reported a significant reduction in the risk of developing a cold of approximately 50%. This area merits additional study and may be of particular interest to elite athletes or military personnel.	D
Common Cold Treatment Numerous studies have examined the effects of starting vitamin C after the onset of cold symptoms. Overall, no	D

Uses Based on Scientific Evidence	Grade
significant benefits have been observed. Initial evidence from one study reports possible benefits with high doses of vitamin C taken at the onset of symptoms, but without additional evidence this remains indeterminate. At this time, the scientific evidence does not support this use of vitamin C.	
Heart Disease Prevention Vitamin C does not appear to lower cholesterol levels or reduce the risk of heart attacks. Effects on cholesterol plaques in heart arteries (atherosclerosis) remain unclear, and some studies suggest possible beneficial vasodilation (artery opening) properties. Based on the current scientific evidence, vitamin C is generally not recommended for this use. People at risk of heart attacks should speak with their healthcare provider to consider preventive measures such as aspirin.	D
Premature Infants In a randomized controlled trial, no significant benefits or harmful effects were associated with ascorbic acid supplementation throughout the first 28 days of life.	D

Uses Based on Tradition or Theory

Acne, Alzheimer's disease, anemia, anemia in hemodialysis patients, antiviral, antioxidant, atherosclerosis (hardening of the arteries), attention deficit hyperactivity disorder, autism, bronchitis, capillary fragility, cervical dysplasia, Chédiak-Higaski syndrome, constipation, cystic fibrosis, delayed onset muscle soreness, dental cavities, dermatitis, diabetes, eye disorders, fluorosis (discoloration of tooth enamel), furunculosis (recurrent boils), gallbladder disease, gastric ulcer, hay fever, high blood pressure, high cholesterol, histamine detoxification, idiopathic thrombocytopenic purpura, immune stimulation, infertility, jellyfish stings, lead toxicity, male infertility, macular degeneration, melasma, menorrhagia, heavy metal/lead toxicity (mercury elimination), nitroglycerin activity prolongation (nitrate tolerance prevention), osteoporosis, pressure sores, reduction of levodopa side effects, reflex sympathetic dystrophy, skin conditions (wrinkles), stomach ulcers, tuberculosis, urinary acidification, wound healing.

DOSING
Adults (18 Years and Older)

- Recommended daily intake by the U.S. Food and Nutrition Board of the Institute of Medicine for men older than 18 years is 90 mg daily; for women older than 18 years is 75 mg daily; for pregnant women older than 18 years is 85 mg daily; and for breastfeeding women older than 18 years is 120 mg daily. Recently, some experts have questioned whether the recommended daily intake should be raised. Others have recommended higher intake in some people, such as smokers, in whom an additional 35 mg daily has been recommended by some.
- Upper limit of intake (UL) should not exceed 2,000 mg daily in men or women older than 18 years old (including pregnant or breastfeeding women).

- Vitamin C administered by mouth or injection is effective for curing scurvy. In adults, 100 to 250 mg by mouth four times daily for one week is generally sufficient to improve symptoms and replenish body vitamin C stores. Some experts have recommended 1 to 2 g daily for two days followed by 500 mg daily for one week. Symptoms should begin to improve within 24 to 48 hours, with resolution within seven days. Treatment should be under strict medical supervision. For asymptomatic vitamin C deficiency, lower daily doses may be used.

Children (Younger than 18 Years)

- Adequate Intakes (AIs) and U.S. Dietary Reference Intakes (DRIs) for infants ages 0 to 6 months old is 40 mg daily, and for infants 7 to 12 months old is 50 mg daily. The DRI for children 1 to 3 years old is 15 mg daily; 4 to 8 years old is 25 mg daily; 9 to 13 years old is 45 mg daily; 14- to 18-year-old males is 75 mg daily; 14- to 18-year-old females is 65 mg daily; 14- to 18-year-old pregnant females is 80 mg daily; and 14- to 18-year-old breastfeeding females is 115 mg daily. Recently, some experts have questioned whether recommended daily intakes should be raised.
- Tolerable Upper Intake Levels (UL) have not been determined for infants ages 0 to 12 months, and vitamin C in this group should be derived only from food intake to avoid excess doses. The UL for children ages 1 to 3 years old is 400 mg daily; ages 4 to 8 years old is 650 mg daily; ages 9 to 13 years old is 1,200 mg daily; and ages 14 to 18 years old is 1,000 mg daily (including pregnant or breastfeeding females).
- For scurvy/deficiency in children, 100 to 300 mg daily by mouth in divided doses for two weeks has been used. Older or larger children may require doses closer to adult recommendations. If vitamin C is not available, orange juice may be used for infantile scurvy. Symptoms should begin to improve within 24 to 48 hours, with resolution within seven days. Treatment should be under strict medical supervision. For asymptomatic vitamin C deficiency, lower daily doses may be used.

SAFETY
Allergies

- Patients should avoid vitamin C products if they are sensitive or allergic to any of their ingredients.

Side Effects and Warnings

- Vitamin C is Generally Regarded as Safe in amounts obtained from foods. Vitamin C supplements are also Generally Regarded as Safe for most people in recommended amounts, although there are rarely reported side effects including nausea, vomiting, heartburn, abdominal cramps, and headache. Dental erosion may occur from chronically chewing vitamin C tablets.
- High doses of vitamin C have been associated with multiple adverse effects. These include kidney stones, severe diarrhea, nausea, and gastritis. Rarely, flushing, faintness, dizziness, and fatigue have been noted. Large doses may precipitate hemolysis (red blood cell destruction) in patients with glucose 6-phosphate dehydrogenase deficiency. High doses of vitamin C should be avoided in people with conditions aggravated by acid loading, such as cirrhosis, gout, renal tubular acidosis, or paroxysmal nocturnal hemoglobinuria. Parenteral (injected) vitamin C may cause dizziness, faintness, injection site discomfort,

V

and in high doses may lead to renal insufficiency (kidney function problems). In cases of toxicity due to massive ingestions of vitamin C, forced fluids and diuresis may be beneficial.

- Healthy adults who take chronic large doses of vitamin C may experience low blood levels of vitamin C when they stop taking the high doses and resume normal intake. To avoid this potential complication, people who are taking high doses who wish to reduce their intake should do so gradually rather than acutely. There are rare reports of scurvy due to tolerance or resistance following cessation after long-term high-dose use, such as in infants born to mothers taking extra vitamin C throughout their pregnancy.

Pregnancy and Breastfeeding

- Vitamin C intake from food is generally considered safe during pregnancy. However, it is not clear if vitamin C supplementation in amounts exceeding Dietary Reference Intake recommendations is safe or beneficial. There are rare reports of scurvy due to tolerance/resistance in infants born to mothers taking extra vitamin C throughout their pregnancy. The data are too few to say if vitamin C supplementation alone or combined with other supplements is beneficial during pregnancy. Preterm birth may increase with vitamin C supplementation.

- Vitamin C is present in breast milk. Vitamin C intake from food is generally considered safe in breastfeeding mothers. Limited research suggests that vitamin C in breast milk may reduce the risk of developing childhood allergies. It is not clear if vitamin C supplementation in amounts exceeding Dietary Reference Intake recommendations is safe or beneficial.

INTERACTIONS
Interactions with Drugs

- Vitamin C may increase adverse effects associated with acetaminophen or aluminum-containing antacids such as aluminum hydroxide (Maalox, Gaviscon).
- Vitamin C may increase blood levels and adverse effects of aspirin, whereas aspirin may decrease blood levels of vitamin C.
- The effects of vitamin C may be decreased by barbiturates including phenobarbital (Luminal, Donnatal), pentobarbital (Nembutal), or secobarbital (Seconal).

- Vitamin C supplementation may decrease levels of the drug fluphenazine in the body.
- Concomitant administration of high doses of vitamin C can reduce steady-state indinavir plasma concentrations.
- There is limited case report evidence that high-dose vitamin C may reduce side effects of levodopa therapy such as nausea or malcoordination.
- Nicotine products such as cigarettes, cigars, chewing tobacco, or nicotine patches may decrease the effects of vitamin C.
- Oral estrogens may decrease the effects of vitamin C in the body. When taken together, vitamin C may increase blood levels of ethinyl estradiol.
- The effects of vitamin C may be decreased by tetracycline antibiotics such as doxycycline (Vibramycin), minocycline (Minocin), or tetracycline (Sumycin).
- Vitamin C in high doses appears to interfere with the blood-thinning effects of warfarin by lowering prothrombin time (PT), as noted in case reports in the 1970s. Complications have not been reported (such as increased blood clots).
- High doses of vitamin C are not recommended in patients with kidney failure. Caution is advised when taking vitamin C and drugs that may damage the kidneys because of an increased risk of kidney failure.

Interactions with Herbs and Dietary Supplements

- When taken together, vitamin C may increase the absorption of iron in the gastrointestinal tract, although this effect appears to be variable and may not be clinically significant.
- Vitamin C may increase absorption of lutein vitamin supplements.
- Large doses of vitamin C may interfere with the absorption and metabolism of vitamin B_{12}.
- In theory, large doses of vitamin C may also interact with herbs and supplements with hormonal, antibacterial, and blood-thinning (anticoagulant) activity.
- Caution is advised when taking vitamin C and agents that may damage the kidneys because of an increased risk of kidney failure.

For a complete list of references, please visit www.naturalstandard.com.

Vitamin D
(ergocalciferol, cholecalciferol, calcitriol, 1,25=dihydroxycholecalciferol)

RELATED TERMS

- 1 alpha (OH) D_3, 19-nor-1, 1 alpha-hydroxyvitamin D_2, 1,25-DHCC, 1,25-dihydroxy-22-ovavitamin D(3), 1,25-dihydroxycholecalciferol, 1,25-dihydroxyvitamin D_3, 1,25-diOHC, 1,25(OH) 2D3, 1-alpha-hydroxycholecalciferol, 22-oxacalcitriol (OCT), 25-dihydroxyvitamin D_2, 25-dihydroxyvitamin D_2, 19-nor-1, 25-HCC, 25-hydroxycholecalciferol, 25-hydroxyvitamin D_3, 25-OHCC, 25-OHD$_3$, activated 7-dehydrocholesterol, activated ergosterol, alfacalcidol, calcifediol, calcipotriene, calcipotriol, calcitriol, cholecalciferol, colecalciferol, dichysterol, dihydrotachysterol 2, dihydrotachysterol, ecocalcidiol, ED-21 (vitamin D analogue), ED-71 (vitamin D analogue), ergocalciferol, ergocalciferolum, hexafluoro-1,25dihydroxyvitamin D_3, irradiated ergosterol, MC903, paracalcin, paricalcitol, viosterol, vitamin D_2, vitamin D_3.

BACKGROUND

- Vitamin D is found in many dietary sources such as fish, eggs, fortified milk, and cod liver oil. The sun also contributes significantly to the daily production of vitamin D, and as little as 10 minutes of exposure is thought to be enough to prevent deficiencies. The term *vitamin D* refers to several different forms of this vitamin. Two forms are important in humans: ergocalciferol (vitamin D_2) and cholecalciferol (vitamin D_3). Vitamin D_2 is synthesized by plants. Vitamin D_3 is synthesized by humans in the skin when it is exposed to ultraviolet-B (UVB) rays from sunlight. Foods may be fortified with vitamin D_2 or D_3.
- The major biologic function of vitamin D is to maintain normal blood levels of calcium and phosphorus. Vitamin D aids in the absorption of calcium, helping to form and maintain strong bones. Recently, research also suggests vitamin D may provide protection from osteoporosis, hypertension (high blood pressure), cancer, and several autoimmune diseases.
- Rickets and osteomalacia are classic vitamin D deficiency diseases. In children, vitamin D deficiency causes rickets, which results in skeletal deformities. In adults, vitamin D deficiency can lead to osteomalacia, which results in muscular weakness in addition to weak bones. Populations who may be at a high risk for vitamin D deficiencies include older adults, obese people, exclusively breastfed infants, and those who have limited sun exposure. Also, people who have fat malabsorption syndromes (e.g., cystic fibrosis) or inflammatory bowel disease (e.g., Crohn's disease) are at risk.

EVIDENCE

Uses Based on Scientific Evidence	Grade
Familial Hypophosphatemia Familial hypophosphatemia (low blood levels of phosphate in the blood) is a rare inherited disorder that consists of impaired phosphate transport in the blood and diminished vitamin D metabolism in the kidneys. Familial hypophosphatemia is a form of rickets. Taking calcitriol or dihydrotachysterol by mouth along with phosphate supplements is effective for treating bone disorders in people with familial hypophosphatemia. Management should be under medical supervision.	A
Fanconi Syndrome–Related Hypophosphatemia Fanconi syndrome is a defect of the proximal tubules of the kidney and is associated with renal tubular acidosis. Taking ergocalciferol orally is effective for treating hypophosphatemia associated with Fanconi syndrome.	A
Hyperparathyroidism due to Low Vitamin D Levels Some patients may develop secondary hyperparathyroidism due to low levels of vitamin D. The initial treatment for this type of hyperparathyroidism is vitamin D. For patients with primary or refractory hyperparathyroidism, surgical removal of the parathyroid glands is commonly recommended. Studies also suggest that vitamin D supplementation may reduce the incidence of hypoparathyroidism following surgery for primary hyperparathyroidism (partial or total removal of the parathyroid glands).	A
Hypocalcemia due to Hypoparathyroidism Hypoparathyroidism (low blood levels of parathyroid hormone) is rare, and is often due to surgical removal of the parathyroid glands. High oral doses of dihydrotachysterol (DHT), calcitriol, or ergocalciferol can assist in increasing serum calcium concentrations in people with hypoparathyroidism or pseudohypoparathyroidism.	A
Osteomalacia (Adult Rickets) Adults with severe vitamin D deficiency lose bone mineral content (hypomineralization) and experience bone pain, muscle weakness, and osteomalacia (soft bones). Osteomalacia may be found among older adults with vitamin D–deficient diets, people with decreased absorption of vitamin D, people with inadequate sun exposure (such as those living in latitudes with seasonal lack of sunlight), patients with gastric or intestinal surgery, patients with aluminum-induced bone disease, patients with chronic liver disease, or patients with kidney disease with renal osteodystrophy. Treatment for osteomalacia depends on the underlying cause of the disease and often includes pain control and orthopedic surgical intervention, as well as vitamin D and phosphate binding agents.	A
Psoriasis A number of different approaches are used in the treatment of psoriasis skin plaques. Mild approaches include light therapy, stress reduction, moisturizers, or salicylic acid to remove scaly skin areas. For more	A

V

(Continued)

Uses Based on Scientific Evidence	Grade
severe cases, treatments may include UV-A light, psoralen plus UV-A light (PUVA), retinoids such as isotretinoin (Accutane), corticosteroids, or cyclosporine (Neoral, Sandimmune). The synthetic vitamin D_3 analogue calcipotriene (Dovonex) appears to control skin cell growth and is used for moderately severe skin plaques, particularly for skin lesions resistant to other therapies or located on the face. Vitamin D_3 (tacalcitol) ointment has been reported as being safe and well-tolerated. High doses of becocalcidiol (a vitamin D analogue) used on the skin may be beneficial in the treatment of psoriasis.	
Rickets Rickets develops in children with vitamin D deficiency due to a vitamin D–deficient diet, a lack of sunlight, or both. Infants fed only breast milk (without supplemental vitamin D) may also develop rickets. Although now rare, partially due to the availability of vitamin D–fortified milk, there has been a recent increase in rickets among children in latitudes with periodic, seasonal lack of sunlight. Ergocalciferol or cholecalciferol is effective for treating vitamin D deficiency rickets. Calcitriol should be used in patients with renal (kidney) failure. Treatment should be under medical supervision.	A
Muscle Weakness/Pain Vitamin D deficiency has been associated with muscle weakness and pain in both adults and children. Limited research has reported vitamin D deficiency in patients with low-back pain, and supplementation may reduce pain in many patients.	B
Osteoporosis (General) Without sufficient vitamin D, inadequate calcium is absorbed and the resulting elevated parathyroid (PTH) secretion causes increased bone resorption. This may weaken bones and increase the risk of fracture. Vitamin D supplementation has been shown to slow bone loss and reduce fracture, particularly when taken with calcium.	B
Renal Osteodystrophy Renal osteodystrophy is a term that refers to all of the bone problems that occur in patients with chronic kidney failure. Oral calcifediol or ergocalciferol may help manage hypocalcemia and prevent renal osteodystrophy in people with chronic renal failure undergoing dialysis.	B
Anticonvulsant-Induced Osteomalacia Supplementation with vitamin D_2 has been reported to reduce seizure frequency in initial research. Further research is needed to confirm these results.	C
Breast Cancer Prevention High-dose vitamin D supplementation may be associated with a slightly reduced risk of developing breast cancer. Additional research in this area is warranted.	C
Cancer Prevention Limited research suggests that synthetic vitamin D analogues may play a role in the treatment of human cancers. However, it remains unclear if vitamin D deficiency raises cancer risk, or if an increased intake of vitamin D is protective against some cancers. Until additional trials are conducted, it is premature to advise the use of regular vitamin D supplementation to prevent cancer.	C
Colorectal Cancer Data from a meta-analysis suggest that supplemental vitamin D may prevent the development of colorectal cancer. More research is needed in this area.	C
Corticosteroid-Induced Osteoporosis Some evidence implies that steroids may impair vitamin D metabolism, further contributing to the loss of bone and development of osteoporosis associated with steroid medications. There is limited evidence that vitamin D may be beneficial to bone strength in patients taking long-term steroids.	C
Diabetes (Type 1/Type 2) Type 1 diabetes: It has been reported that infants given calcitriol during the first year of life are less likely to develop type 1 diabetes than infants fed lesser amounts of vitamin D. Other related studies have suggested using cod liver oil as a source of vitamin D to reduce the incidence of type 1 diabetes. There is currently insufficient evidence to form a clear conclusion in this area. Type 2 diabetes: In recent studies, adults given vitamin D supplementation were shown to improve insulin sensitivity. Further research is needed to confirm these results.	C
Fall Prevention Multiple trials have found conflicting results for the effects of vitamin D in the prevention of falls. More studies are needed.	C
Hepatic Osteodystrophy Metabolic bone disease is common among patients with chronic liver disease, and osteoporosis accounts for the majority of cases. Varying degrees of calcium malabsorption may occur in patients with chronic liver disease because of malnutrition and vitamin D deficiency. Oral or injected vitamin D may play a role in the management of this condition.	C
High Blood Pressure (Hypertension) Low levels of vitamin D may play a role in the development of high blood pressure. It has been noted that blood pressure is often elevated under the following conditions: during the winter season, at a further distance from the equator, and in people with dark skin pigmentation (all of which are associated with lower production of vitamin D via sunlight). However, evidence is not clear, and a comparison with more proven methods to reduce blood pressure	C

Uses Based on Scientific Evidence	Grade
has not been conducted. Patients with elevated blood pressure should be managed by a licensed healthcare professional.	
Hypertriglyceridemia There is insufficient evidence in this area.	C
Immunomodulation Preliminary human evidence suggests that vitamin D and its analogues, such as alfacalcidol, may act as immunomodulatory agents. More studies are needed to confirm these results.	C
Mortality Reduction Intake of vitamin D may be associated with a reduction in total mortality. Additional evidence is needed to confirm this association.	C
Multiple Sclerosis (MS) Scientists have detected MS rates to be lower in areas with greater sunlight and higher consumption of vitamin D–rich fish. Preliminary research suggests that long-term vitamin D supplementation decreases the risk of MS; however, additional research is necessary before a firm conclusion can be reached.	C
Myelodysplastic Syndrome There is insufficient evidence in this area.	C
Osteogenesis Imperfecta (OI) OI is a genetic disease that consists of unusually fragile bones that break easily (often under loads that normal bones bear daily) because of a malfunction in the body's production of collagen. Proper calcium and vitamin D intake is essential to maintaining strong bones.	C
Osteoporosis (Cystic Fibrosis Patients) Osteoporosis is common in patients with cystic fibrosis (because of fat malabsorption, which leads to a deficiency of fat-soluble vitamins such as vitamin D). Oral calcitriol administration appears to increase the absorption of calcium and decrease parathyroid concentrations.	C
Proximal Myopathy There is insufficient evidence in this area.	C
Rickets (Hypophosphatemic Vitamin D-Resistant) There are insufficient data to support a role of vitamin D in this condition.	C
Seasonal Affective Disorder (SAD) Seasonal affective disorder (SAD) is a form of depression that occurs during the winter months, possibly due to reduced exposure to sunlight. Some research found vitamin D to be better than light therapy in the treatment of SAD. Further studies are necessary to confirm these findings.	C

	Grade
Senile Warts In preliminary research, senile warts have been treated with topical vitamin D_3.	C
Skin Pigmentation Disorders (Pigmented Lesions) Application of vitamin D_3 ointment on the skin, in combination with intense pulsed-radio frequency, may be beneficial in the treatment of pigmented lesions associated with neurofibromatosis 1 (NF1).	C
Tooth Retention Oral bone and tooth loss are correlated with bone loss at non-oral sites. Research suggests that intake levels of calcium and vitamin D aimed at preventing osteoporosis may have a beneficial effect on tooth retention.	C
Vitamin D Deficiency (Infants and Nursing Mothers) High-quality clinical trial evidence suggests that high doses of supplemental vitamin D provided to breast feeding mothers may improve the vitamin D status of both mother and child. More research is needed to confirm these findings.	C
Weight Gain (Postmenopausal) Vitamin D supplementation (in combination with calcium) may have an effect on post-menopausal weight gain. Evidence suggests that this may be particularly true in women consuming inadequate calcium and warrants further research.	C
Muscle Strength Oral cholecalciferol does not appear to increase muscle strength or improve physical performance in healthy older men who are not vitamin D deficient.	D
Prostate Cancer There is preliminary evidence based on laboratory and human studies that high-dose vitamin D may be beneficial in the treatment of prostate cancer. This area is under active investigation, but clear evidence of benefit is not yet available.	D

Uses Based on Tradition or Theory

Actinic keratosis, Alzheimer's disease–associated hip fractures, ankylosing spondylitis, autoimmune disorders, Graves disease, hyperparathyroidism in renal dialysis, hypocalcemia, hypocalcemic tetany, kidney transplant–related bone loss, metabolic disorders (metabolic syndrome), nervous system disorders (hemichorea), osteitis fibrosa in dialysis, rheumatoid arthritis, scleroderma, squamous cell carcinoma, systemic lupus erythematosus, vaginal disorders (atrophy), vitiligo.

DOSING
Adults (18 Years and Older)
- Vitamin D is included in most multivitamins, usually in strengths from 50 IU to 1,000 IU as softgels, capsules, tablets, and liquids. The Adequate Intake (AI) levels have

V

been established by the U.S. Institute of Medicine of the National Academy of Sciences. Recommendations are: 5 mcg (200 IU or International Units) daily for all people (males, females, pregnant/lactating women) under the age of 50 years old. For all people 50 to 70 years old, 10 mcg/day (400 IU) is recommended. For those who are over 70 years old, 15 mcg/day (600 IU) is suggested. Some authors have questioned whether the current recommended adequate levels are sufficient to meet physiologic needs, particularly for people deprived of regular sun exposure. The upper limit (UL) for vitamin D has been recommended as 2,000 IU daily because of toxicities that can occur when taken in higher doses.

- Not all doses have been found effective for conditions that have been studied. However, ergocalciferol has been used in an oral dose of 400 to 800 IU/day (sometimes higher doses are used in conjunction with calcium) for osteoporosis prevention and treatment.
- Calcitriol has been used in an initial oral dose of 0.25 mcg/day; dosing may be increased by 0.25 mcg/day at four- to eight-week intervals in patients with hypocalcemia from chronic dialysis.
- Dihydrotachysterol has been used in an oral initial dose of 750 mcg (0.75 mg) to 2.5 mg/day for several days for the treatment of hypoparathyroidism. A maintenance dose is typically 200 mcg (0.2 mg) to 1 mg/day. Ergocalciferol has also been used in an oral dose of 50,000 to 200,000 IU units daily concomitantly with calcium lactate 4 grams, six times per day.
- Rickets may be treated gradually over several months or in a single day's dose. Gradual dosing may be 125 to 250 mcg (5,000 to 10,000 IU) taken daily for two to three months, until recovery is well established and alkaline phosphatase blood concentration is close to normal limits. Single-day dosing may be 15,000 mcg (600,000 IU) of vitamin D, taken by mouth divided into four to six doses. Intramuscular injection is also an alternative for single-day dosing. For resistant rickets, some authors suggest a higher dose of 12,000 to 500,000 IU/day, although this has not yet been proven effective.

Children (Younger than 18 Years)

- Adequate Intake (AI) levels have been established by the U.S. Institute of Medicine of the National Academy of Sciences. The recommendation from birth until 50 years old is 5 mcg/day (200 IU or International Units per day). Children older than 1 year should not exceed the upper limit (UL) of 50 mcg (2,000 IU) per day; children younger than 1 year should not exceed the UL of 25 mcg (1,000 IU) per day. Vitamin D is possibly unsafe when used orally in excessive amounts, with adverse effects including hypercalcemia (high blood calcium levels). Some authors have questioned whether the current recommended adequate levels are sufficient to meet physiologic needs, particularly for people deprived of regular sun exposure. A 2008 review recommends 400 IU/day for all infants and children, including adolescents, based on evidence from new clinical trials and the historical precedence.
- Not all doses have been found effective for conditions that have been studied. However, for hypoparathyroidism, ergocalciferol has been used orally in an initial dose of 8,000 units/kg/day for one to two weeks. For maintenance, a dose of 2,000 units/kg/day has been used.

- Rickets may be treated gradually over several months or in a single day's dose. Based on one clinical trial, a single dose of 600,000 IU of oral vitamin D$_3$ was comparable to a dose of 20,000 IU per day of oral vitamin D$_3$ for 30 days. Gradual dosing may be 125 to 250 mcg (5000 to 10,000 IU) taken daily for two to three months, until recovery is well established and alkaline phosphatase blood concentration is close to normal limits. Single-day dosing may be 15,000 mcg (600,000 IU) of vitamin D, taken by mouth divided into four to six doses. Intramuscular injection is also an alternative for single-day dosing. For resistant rickets, some authors suggest a higher dose of 12,000 to 500,000 IU/day.

SAFETY
Allergies

- Avoid or use caution with known hypersensitivity to vitamin D or any of its analogues and derivatives.

Side Effects and Warnings

- Vitamin D is generally well tolerated in recommended Adequate Intake (AI) doses. Some research has found a greater likelihood of daytime sleepiness for patients given vitamin D analogues.
- Vitamin D toxicity can result from regular excess intake of this vitamin and may lead to hypercalcemia and excess bone loss. People at particular risk include those with hyperparathyroidism, kidney disease, sarcoidosis, tuberculosis, or histoplasmosis. Chronic hypercalcemia may lead to serious or even life-threatening complications and should be managed by a physician. Early symptoms of hypercalcemia may include nausea, vomiting, and anorexia (appetite/weight loss), followed by polyuria (excess urination), polydipsia (excess thirst), weakness, fatigue, somnolence, headache, dry mouth, metallic taste, vertigo, tinnitus (ear ringing), and ataxia (unsteadiness). Kidney function may become impaired, and metastatic calcifications (calcium deposition in organs throughout the body) may occur, particularly affecting the kidneys. Treatment involves stopping the intake of vitamin D or calcium, and lowering the calcium levels under strict medical supervision, with frequent monitoring of calcium levels. Acidification of urine and corticosteroids may be necessary.

Pregnancy and Breastfeeding

- The recommended Adequate Intake for pregnant women is the same as for non-pregnant adults. Some authors have suggested that requirements during pregnancy may be greater than these amounts, particularly in sun-deprived people, although this has not been clearly established. Because of the risks of vitamin D toxicity, any consideration of higher daily doses of vitamin D should be discussed with a physician.
- Vitamin D is typically low in maternal milk, and to prevent deficiency and rickets in exclusively breastfed infants, supplementation may be necessary, starting within the first two months of life.

INTERACTIONS
Interactions with Drugs

- Hypermagnesemia (high blood magnesium levels) may develop when magnesium-containing antacids are used concurrently with vitamin D, particularly in patients with chronic renal failure.

- Decreased vitamin D effects may occur with the use of certain anti-seizure drugs, as they may induce hepatic microsomal enzymes and accelerate the conversion of vitamin D to inactive metabolites.
- Based on mechanism of action, use of vitamin D and calcium together may alter inflammatory response.
- Intestinal absorption of vitamin D may be impaired with the use of these agents. Patients on cholestyramine or colestipol should be advised to allow as much time as possible between the ingestion of these drugs and vitamin D.
- Use of corticosteroids can cause osteoporosis and calcium depletion with long-term administration. This calcium depletion creates a greater need for both supplemental calcium and vitamin D (which is necessary for calcium absorption).
- Vitamin D should be used with caution in patients taking digoxin, because hypercalcemia (which may result with excess vitamin D use) may precipitate abnormal heart rhythms.
- Intestinal absorption of vitamin D may be impaired with the use of mineral oil.
- Orlistat (an obesity drug) can reduce vitamin D levels. Patients should consider taking a multivitamin with fat-soluble vitamins at least two hours before or after orlistat or at bedtime.
- Rifampin increases vitamin D metabolism and reduces vitamin D blood levels. The need for vitamin D supplementation with rifampin has not been thoroughly studied, although additional supplementation may be necessary.
- Stimulant laxatives can reduce dietary vitamin D absorption. Stimulant laxatives should be limited to short-term use if possible.
- Concurrent administration of thiazide diuretics and vitamin D to hypoparathyroid patients may cause hypercalcemia, which may be transient or may require discontinuation of vitamin D. Examples of thiazide diuretics include chlorothiazide (Diuril), chlorthalidone (Hygroton, Thalitone), hydrochlorothiazide (HCTZ, Esidrix, HydroDIURIL, Ortec, Microzide), indapamide (Lozol), and metolazone (Zaroxolyn).

Interactions with Herbs and Dietary Supplements

- Based on mechanism of action, the use of vitamin D and calcium together may alter inflammatory response.
- Vitamin D should be used with caution in patients taking herbs with similar properties on the heart as digoxin, because hypercalcemia (which may result with excess vitamin D use) may precipitate abnormal heart rhythms.
- Vitamin D is necessary for calcium absorption. Vitamin D is often included in calcium supplement products.

For a complete list of references, please visit www.naturalstandard.com.

V

RELATED TERMS

- All rac-alpha-tocopherol, alpha-tocopherol, alpha tocopherol acetate, alpha tocopheryl acetate, alpha tocotrienol, antisterility vitamin, beta-tocopherol, beta-tocotrienol, d-alpha-tocopherol, d-alpha-tocopheryl, d-alpha-tocopheryl acetate, d-alpha-tocopheryl succinate, d-beta-tocopherol, d-delta-tocopherol, delta-tocopherol, delta-tocotrienol, d-gamma-tocopherol, dl-alpha-tocopherol, dl-alpha-tocopheryl acetate, dl-tocopherol, d-tocopherol, d-tocopheryl acetate, dl-tocopherol, gamma-tocopherol, gamma-tocotrienol, mixed tocopherols, RRR-alpha-tocopherol, Spondyvit, tocopherol, tocotrienol, tocotrienol concentrate, tocopheryl succinate.

BACKGROUND

- Vitamin E is a fat-soluble vitamin with antioxidant properties. Vitamin E exists in eight different forms ("isomers"): alpha, beta, gamma, and delta tocopherol; and alpha, beta, gamma, and delta tocotrienol. Alpha-tocopherol is the most active form in humans. Dosing and daily allowance recommendations for vitamin E are often provided in Alpha-Tocopherol Equivalents (ATE) to account for the different biological activities of the various forms of vitamin E, or in International Units (IU), which food and supplement labels may use. Vitamin E supplements are available in natural or synthetic forms. The natural forms are usually labeled with the letter *d* (for example, d-gamma-tocopherol), whereas synthetic forms are labeled *dl* (for example, dl-alpha-tocopherol).

- Vitamin E has been proposed for the prevention or treatment of numerous health conditions, often based on its antioxidant properties. However, aside from the treatment of vitamin E deficiency (which is rare), there are no clearly proven medicinal uses of vitamin E supplementation beyond the recommended daily allowance. There is ongoing research in numerous diseases, particularly in cancer and heart disease.

- Recent concerns have been raised about the safety of vitamin E supplementation, particularly in high doses. An increased risk of bleeding has been proposed, particularly in patients taking blood-thinning agents such as warfarin, heparin, or aspirin, and in patients with vitamin K deficiency. Recent evidence suggests that regular use of high-dose vitamin E supplements may increase the risk of death (from "all causes") by a small amount, although a different study found no effects on mortality in women who took vitamin E daily. Caution is warranted.

EVIDENCE

Uses Based on Scientific Evidence	Grade
Vitamin E Deficiency Vitamin E deficiency is rare and may occur in people with diminished fat absorption through the gut (due to surgery, Crohn's disease, or cystic fibrosis),	A

malnutrition, very low fat diets, several specific genetic conditions (abetalipoproteinemia, ataxia and vitamin E deficiency [AVED]), very low birth weight premature infants, or infants taking unfortified formulas. Vitamin E supplementation is accepted as an effective therapy for vitamin E deficiency to halt progression of complications. Diagnosis of this condition and management should be under the care of a physician and nutritionist.

Allergic Rhinitis Although thought to aid in reducing the nasal symptoms of allergies, vitamin E intake may not be effective. Current evidence is limited, however, and more studies are needed before a firm conclusion can be drawn.	C
Altitude Sickness Vitamin E may offer some benefits in exposure to high altitude. Antioxidant supplementation (vitamin E with beta carotene, vitamin C, selenium, and zinc) may improve ventilatory threshold at high altitudes; however, antioxidants may not reduce inflammation after exercise at high altitudes. More research is needed before conclusions can be drawn.	C
Anemia Studies of vitamin E supplementation for anemia have yielded mixed results. Further research is needed before a firm recommendation can be made.	C
Angina Vitamin E has been suggested and evaluated in patients with angina, although possible benefits remain unclear. Further evidence is necessary before a clear conclusion can be drawn. Patients with known or suspected angina should be evaluated by a physician.	C
Antioxidant Vitamin E possesses antioxidant activity, but it is not clear if there is any benefit of this property in humans. The American Heart Association has recommended obtaining antioxidants such as vitamin E by eating a well-balanced diet high in fruits, vegetables, and whole grains, rather than from supplements, until further scientific evidence is available.	C
Atherosclerosis Vitamin E has been proposed to have a role in preventing or reversing atherosclerosis by inhibiting oxidation of low-density lipoprotein ("bad cholesterol"). Several population studies have suggested that a high dietary intake of vitamin E and high blood concentrations of alpha-tocopherol are associated with lower rates of heart disease. However, while the	C

Uses Based on Scientific Evidence	Grade
Cambridge Heart Antioxidant Study supported this hypothesis, the more recent prospective Heart Outcomes Prevention Evaluation (HOPE) study did not. This area remains controversial.	
Bladder Cancer There is preliminary evidence of possible benefits of long-term vitamin E supplementation to reduce the risk of mortality in bladder cancer patients.	C
Breast Cancer Vitamin E has been suggested as a possible therapy for the prevention or treatment of breast cancer. Published studies have included measurement of vitamin E levels, laboratory experiments, and population studies. Evidence remains inconclusive.	C
Breast Cancer–Related Hot Flashes A study of oral vitamin E reports a very small reduction in hot flash frequency (approximately one less hot flash per day), but no preference among patients for vitamin E over placebo.	C
Cancer Treatment There is a lack of reliable scientific evidence that vitamin E is effective as a treatment for any specific type of cancer. Caution is merited in people undergoing treatment with chemotherapy or radiation because it has been proposed that the use of high-dose antioxidants may actually reduce the anti-cancer effects of these therapies. This remains an area of controversy, and studies have produced variable results. High doses of vitamin E may also cause harm in cancer patients. Patients interested in using high-dose antioxidants such as vitamin E during chemotherapy or radiation should discuss this decision with their medical oncologist or radiation oncologist.	C
Cardiovascular Disease in Dialysis Patients It has been suggested that hemodialysis patients may be under increased oxidative stress, and therefore may benefit from the chronic use of antioxidants (particularly for the reduction of risk of heart disease). There is some research on the use of high-dose chronic vitamin E in dialysis patients for heart disease prevention, although benefits or risks remain unclear in this population. Recent concern has been raised that regular use of high-dose vitamin E supplements may actually increase the risk of death (from "all causes") by a small amount, although this remains an area of controversy and active investigation.	C
Cataract Prevention There is conflicting evidence regarding the use of vitamin E to prevent cataracts. Although some studies across populations have suggested some protective effects (which may take up to 10 years to yield benefits), other studies in humans report a lack of benefits	C

when used either alone or in combination with other antioxidants. Additional research is necessary before a clear conclusion can be reached.

Chemotherapy Nerve Damage (Neurotoxicity) Like other antioxidants, vitamin E has been suggested as a therapy to prevent complications due to chemotherapy, such as nerve damage (neuropathy). There is some evidence of benefits, for example, when it is used with cisplatin. However, caution is merited because it is not known if the use of high-dose antioxidants during chemotherapy may actually reduce the anti-cancer effects of some chemotherapy agents or radiation therapy. This remains an area of controversy, and patients interested in using antioxidants during chemotherapy should discuss this decision with their oncologist.	C
Colon Cancer Prevention There is insufficient scientific evidence to determine if vitamin E prevents colon cancer. In patients with previous colon cancer, a combination of vitamins A, C, and E has been reported to reduce the risk of developing a new colon cancer. Preventive benefits have also been suggested in those with no prior colon cancer when vitamin E is used in a multivitamin, but not when used alone. Recent results of the Women's Health Study report no overall reduction in cancer risk with daily use of vitamin E, although this study was not large enough to look at colon cancer specifically.	C
Dementia/Alzheimer's Disease Vitamin E has been proposed and evaluated for the prevention or slowing of dementia (including Alzheimer's type), based on antioxidant properties and findings of low vitamin E levels in some people with dementia. There is some evidence that all-rac-alpha-tocopherol (synthetic vitamin E) is similar in efficacy to selegiline (Eldepryl) and superior to placebo for slowing cognitive function decline in patients with moderately severe Alzheimer's disease, but no additive effect was observed when used in combination with selegiline. Retrospective data suggests that long-term combination therapy with donepezil (Aricept) may help slow cognitive decline in patients with Alzheimer's disease. Overall, the evidence remains inconclusive in his area. Other research suggests that vitamin E from dietary sources or supplements does not affect the risk of developing Alzheimer's disease or vascular dementia.	C
Diabetes Mellitus Vitamin E has been proposed for the prevention of types I or II diabetes; for the improvement of abnormal sugar control in diabetes; for prevention of platelet dysfunction and atherosclerosis in diabetes; for the correction of vitamin E deficiency in diabetic patients; and for the prevention of diabetic complications of the eye, kidneys, and nervous system	C

(Continued)

Uses Based on Scientific Evidence	Grade
(neuropathy, retinopathy, nephropathy). It is not clear that vitamin E is beneficial in any of these areas.	
Dysmenorrhea There is preliminary evidence of possible benefits of vitamin E supplementation to reduce chronic menstrual pain.	C
G6PD Deficiency Vitamin E supplementation has been studied for the inherited disorder G6PD deficiency with conflicting evidence.	C
Glomerulosclerosis (Kidney Disease) It has been suggested that proteinuria (protein in the urine) may be reduced with the use of vitamin E in patients with focal segmental glomerulosclerosis, which is refractory to standard medical management.	C
Healing after Photorefractive Keratectomy High-dose vitamin E plus vitamin A (taken by mouth) may improve healing of the cornea and improve visual acuity (sharpness) following laser surgery for vision correction. Animal research suggests that topical vitamin E on the eye may be helpful.	C
Hepatitis (Hepatitis C) In patients with hepatitis C on antiviral therapy, vitamin E has been proposed to prevent inflammation. More studies are needed to examine the effects of vitamin E in chronic hepatitis.	C
High Cholesterol The effects if vitamin E on cholesterol levels and atherosclerosis have been studied in numerous laboratory, population, and clinical trials. It remains unclear if there are clinically meaningful benefits of vitamin E, and it is not known what the effects of vitamin E are compared to (or in combination with) other agents that have been clearly demonstrated as beneficial for lowering lipids.	C
Immune System Function Studies of the effects of vitamin E supplementation on immune system function have yielded mixed results. Further research is needed before a clear conclusion can be drawn.	C
Intermittent Claudication Multiple studies have evaluated the use of vitamin E in patients with peripheral vascular disease, to improve exercise tolerance and intermittent claudication (pain in the legs with walking due to cholesterol buildup in blood vessels). Although some results have been promising, most studies have been small and poorly designed. It remains unclear if vitamin E is beneficial in this condition.	C
Macular Degeneration Like other antioxidants, vitamin E has been suggested to prevent, slow progression of, or improve macular degeneration. The scientific evidence in this area is not conclusive, although there is some suggestion that vitamin E alone may not be beneficial. In combination with beta-carotene and vitamin C, it may similarly not be significantly beneficial.	C
Parkinson's Disease The scientific evidence is inconclusive in this area.	C
Premenstrual Syndrome The scientific evidence is inconclusive in this area.	C
Prostate Cancer Prevention The role of vitamin E supplementation for the prevention of prostate cancer is controversial. There are numerous laboratory studies that support possible anti-cancer properties. However, the results of population research and human research have been mixed, with some studies reporting benefits and others finding no effects.	C
Respiratory Infection Prevention Daily supplementation with oral vitamin E does not appear to affect the incidence, duration, or severity of pneumonia (lower respiratory tract infections) in elderly nursing home residents or alter patterns of antibiotic use, although there may be a protective effect against colds (upper respiratory tract infections).	C
Seizure Disorder Vitamin E has been evaluated as an addition to other drugs used to prevent seizures, particularly in refractory epilepsy. This evidence is not conclusive enough to make a clear recommendation. The management of seizure disorder should be under medical supervision.	C
Steatohepatitis There is some evidence suggesting possible benefits in the management of steatohepatitis in children.	C
Stomach Cancer (Prevention) Vitamin supplementation has been proposed to reduce the rate of stomach (gastric) cancer. However, there is some evidence suggesting that vitamin E does not reduce the rates of gastric cancer or precancerous gastric lesions. More research is needed to examine whether vitamin E has any effects on gastric cancer.	C
Supplementation in Preterm and Very Low Birthweight Infants Premature infants are at risk of vitamin E deficiency, particularly when they are born with very low birth weight. There are numerous studies of vitamin E	C

Uses Based on Scientific Evidence	Grade
given to premature infants to try to prevent potentially serious complications such as intraventricular hemorrhage (bleeding into the brain), retinopathy (eye damage), or death. The quality of published research is variable, and is not clearly conclusive. Premature infants should be under strict medical supervision, and decisions regarding vitamin supplementation should be made with the infant's physician.	
Tardive Dyskinesia Vitamin E has been studied in the management of tardive dyskinesia and has been reported to significantly improve abnormal involuntary movements, although the results of existing studies are not conclusive enough to form a clear recommendation. Vitamin E may be more effective in higher doses and in people who have had tardive dyskinesia for less than five years.	C
Uveitis Four-month oral supplementation with vitamin E had no apparent effect on uveitis-associated macular edema or visual acuity in one small study.	C
Venous Thromboembolism (VTE) Data suggests that supplementation with vitamin E may reduce the risk of VTE in women, and those with a prior history or genetic predisposition may particularly benefit.	C
Asthma There is preliminary evidence that vitamin E does not provide benefits in people with asthma.	D
Cancer Prevention (General) Recent evidence from a well-conducted randomized controlled trial (the Women's Health Study) reports no reduction in the development of cancer with the use of natural-source vitamin E taken daily. Previously, there have been laboratory, population, and other human trials examining whether vitamin E is beneficial in preventing various types of cancer, including prostate, colon, or stomach cancer. Results of these prior studies have been variable. At this time, based on the best available scientific evidence, and recent concerns about the safety of vitamin E supplementation, vitamin E cannot be recommended for this use.	D
Heart Disease Prevention Numerous studies of vitamin E oral supplementation have suggested no benefits in the prevention of cardiovascular disease, and there is recent evidence to suggest that regular use of high-dose vitamin E increases the risk of death (from "all causes") by a small amount. These conclusions have been criticized by some experts. Recently, the Women's Health Study reported a reduction in cardiovascular deaths in women taking	D

	Grade
vitamin E daily (with 10-year follow-up), but no change in total death rate or number of heart attacks or strokes. Based on the balance of available scientific evidence, and in light of recent safety concerns, chronic use of vitamin E cannot be recommended for this purpose, and high-dose vitamin E should be avoided.	
Osteoarthritis Vitamin E does not appear to reduce symptoms or prevent cartilage loss in knee osteoarthritis. There is a lack of evidence supporting the use of vitamin E in the management of osteoarthritis.	D
Peyronie's Disease One study did not show significant improvement in pain, curvature, or plaque size in patients with Peyronie's disease (PD) treated with vitamin E, propionyl-L-carnitine, or vitamin E plus propionyl-L-carnitine compared with those treated with placebo.	D
Retinitis Pigmentosa Oral vitamin E does not appear to slow visual decline in people with retinitis pigmentosa and may be associated with more rapid loss of visual acuity, although the validity of this finding has been questioned. Until further evidence is available, vitamin E may not be advisable in this condition. Therapy decisions should be under medical supervision.	D
Scar Prevention Application of topical vitamin E does not appear to reduce surgical wound scarring. Because of a risk of contact dermatitis, some authors have recommended against the use of this therapy.	D
Stroke Recent evidence from the Women's Health Study suggests that regular vitamin E supplementation daily does not reduce the risk of stroke. Prior evidence was indeterminate for stroke prevention or stroke recovery. At this time, based on the best available scientific evidence and recent safety concerns, vitamin E cannot be recommended for this use.	D

Uses Based on Tradition or Theory

Abortifacient, acne, aging (prevention), aging skin, air pollution protection, allergies, amiodarone pulmonary toxicity prevention, bee stings, benign prostatic hypertrophy, beta-thalassemia, blood disorders (porphyria), breast pain/inflammation (mastitis), bronchopulmonary dysplasia in premature infants, bursitis, cardiomyopathy, chemotherapy extravasation, chorea (chronic progressive hereditary), congestive heart failure, Crohn's disease, cystic fibrosis, dermatitis, diaper rash, digestive enzyme/pancreatic insufficiency, doxorubicin hair loss prevention, Duchenne muscular dystrophy, dyspraxia, energy enhancement, frostbite, gastric ulcer, granuloma annulare (topical vitamin E), hair loss, heart attack, transplant rejection prevention (heart), hereditary spherocytosis,

Uses Based on Tradition or Theory—Cont'd

Huntington's disease, hypertension, impotence, inflammatory skin disorders, leg cramps, liver spots, lung cancer prevention, male fertility, menopausal symptoms, menstrual disorders, miscarriage, mucositis, muscle strength, myotonic dystrophy, neuromuscular disorders, nitrate tolerance, oral leukoplakia, labor pain, peptic ulcers, physical endurance, poor posture, post-operative recovery (post-angioplasty restenosis prevention), pre-eclampsia prevention (high blood pressure in pregnancy), radiation-induced fibrosis, reperfusion injury protection during heart surgery, restless leg syndrome, rheumatoid arthritis, sickle cell disease, skeletal muscle damage, skin disorders, sperm motility, sunburn, thrombophlebitis (vein inflammation).

DOSING

Dietary Sources of Vitamin E

- Foods that contain vitamin E include: eggs, fortified cereals, fruit, green leafy vegetables (such as spinach), meat, nuts/nut oils, poultry, vegetable oils (corn, cottonseed, safflower, soybean, sunflower), argan oil, olive oil, wheat germ oil, and whole grains. Cooking and storage may destroy some of the vitamin E in foods.

Adults (18 Years and Older)

- Most people in the United States are believed to obtain sufficient vitamin E from dietary sources, although those with very-low-fat diets or intestinal malabsorption disorders may require supplementation. Recommended Daily Allowances (RDAs) for vitamin E are provided in Alpha-Tocopherol Equivalents (ATE) to account for the different biological activities of the various forms of vitamin E, as well as in International Units (IU), which food and supplement labels often use. For conversion, 1 mg ATE = 1.5 IU. The RDA for men or women older than 14 years is 15 mg (or 22.5 IU); for pregnant women of any age is 15 mg (or 22.5 IU); and for breastfeeding women of any age is 19 mg (or 28.5 IU).
- For adults older than 18 years, the tolerable upper limit of dosing for supplementary alpha-tocopherol recommended by the U.S. Institute of Medicine is 1,000 mg/day (equivalent to 1,500 IU). This limit recommendation is not altered during pregnancy or breastfeeding.
- Treatment of vitamin E deficiency should be under medical supervision, tailored to the underlying cause of the deficiency, and may include either oral or injected vitamin E. If the cause is due to chronic malnutrition and there is no evidence of malabsorption, an oral dose that is 2 to 5 times greater than the RDA may be considered. If the cause is malabsorption that cannot be corrected, then injections of vitamin E may be necessary. Dosing recommendations vary by the underlying cause.
- No specific dosing of vitamin E has been established for other conditions, and there is recent evidence suggesting possible adverse health effects of long-term supplementation with 400 IU or more per day. Although controversial, the use of long-term vitamin E supplementation should be approached cautiously until further evidence from prospective clinical trials is available. Various doses and durations have been evaluated in clinical trials, although many have not been proven as effective or safe. Patients are recommended to discuss the choice of dosing and duration with a licensed healthcare professional.

Children (Younger than 18 Years)

- Recommended Daily Allowances (RDAs) for vitamin E are provided in Alpha-Tocopherol Equivalents (ATE) to account for the different biological activities of the various forms of vitamin E, as well as in International Units (IU), because food and supplement labels often use this system. For conversion, 1 mg ATE = 1.5 IU. There is no RDA for infants, but there is a recommended Adequate Intake (AI) for healthy breastfeeding infants ages 0 to 6 months old of 4 mg (6 IU) daily and for infants ages 7 to 12 months old of 5 mg (7.5 IU) daily. The RDA for children ages 1 to 3 years old is 6 mg (9 IU) daily; for ages 4 to 8 years old 7 mg (10.5 IU) daily; for ages 9 to 13 years, 11 mg (16.5 IU) daily; for ages older than 14 years, 15 mg (22.5 IU) daily; for pregnant women of any age 15 mg (22.5 IU) daily; and for breastfeeding women of any age, 19 mg (28.5 IU).
- An upper limit for infants up to 12 months of age has not been established. The tolerable daily upper limit of dosing for ages 1 to 3 years old is 200 mg (300 IU); for ages 4 to 8 years old, 300 mg (450 IU); for ages 9 to 13 years old, 600 mg (900 IU); and for ages 14 to 18 years old, 800 mg (1,200 IU).
- Treatment of vitamin E deficiency should be under medical supervision, tailored to the underlying cause of the deficiency, and may include either oral or injected vitamin E. Selected doses in specific conditions are noted above under adult dosing. Vitamin E absorption may improve if given with meals, and in small doses.
- No specific dosing of vitamin E has been well established for other conditions.

SAFETY

Allergies

- Skin reactions such as contact dermatitis and eczema have been reported with topical vitamin E preparations, such as ointments or vitamin E–containing deodorants. People with a known or suspected hypersensitivity to vitamin E should avoid these products.

Side Effects and Warnings

- Recent evidence suggests that regular use of high-dose vitamin E may increase the risk of death (from "all causes") by a small amount. These conclusions have been criticized by some experts because they are based on re-calculations (meta-analyses) of the results of prior smaller studies, which were of mixed quality, with variable results, and often in patients with chronic illnesses. Nonetheless, this is the best available current scientific evidence, and therefore chronic use of vitamin E should be managed cautiously and high-dose vitamin E should be avoided. Acute overdose of vitamin E is very uncommon.
- For short periods of time, vitamin E supplementation is generally considered safe at doses up to the recommended tolerable upper intake level (UL). However, vitamin E is possibly unsafe when used orally at doses exceeding the tolerable upper intake level. The Recommended Daily Allowance (RDA) obtained through food consumption is considered to be safe and beneficial.

- Skin reactions, such as contact dermatitis and eczema, have been reported with topical vitamin E preparations such as ointments or vitamin E–containing deodorants.
- In rare cases, vitamin E supplementation has been associated with abdominal pain, nausea, diarrhea, or flulike symptoms (particularly when taken at high doses). The risk of necrotizing enterocolitis may be increased with large doses of vitamin E.
- In rare cases, vitamin E supplementation has been associated with gonadal dysfunction and diminished kidney function.
- High doses of vitamin E might increase the risk of bleeding, due to inhibition of platelet aggregation and antagonism of vitamin K–dependent clotting factors (particularly in patients with vitamin K deficiency). In studies of vitamin E, a small increase in rate of hemorrhagic (bleeding) stroke and gum bleeding has been observed, particularly when used with aspirin in humans. Increased risk of bleeding when used with warfarin (Coumadin) has been noted in animal studies. However, other studies have not observed a greater incidence of bleeding. Bleeding has been observed in patients given high repeated doses of intravenous all-rac-alpha-tocopherol (synthetic vitamin E). Caution is advised in patients with bleeding disorders or taking drugs that may increase the risk of bleeding. Dosing adjustments may be necessary.
- In rare cases, vitamin E supplementation has been associated with dizziness, fatigue, headache, weakness, or blurred vision (particularly when used in high doses).
- Oral vitamin E should be avoided in patients with retinitis pigmentosa, as is does not appear to slow visual decline, and may be associated with more rapid loss of visual acuity. This remains a topic of controversy.

Pregnancy and Breastfeeding

- Many prenatal vitamins contain small amounts of vitamin E. Natural forms of vitamin E may be preferable to synthetic forms.
- Use beyond the Recommended Daily Allowance (RDA) level in otherwise healthy pregnant women is generally not recommended. There is otherwise insufficient evidence regarding the safety of higher doses of oral, topical, or injected vitamin E during pregnancy and breastfeeding, and therefore it is not recommended.

INTERACTIONS
Interactions with Drugs

- The amount of bleeding risk associated with vitamin E remains an area of controversy, and caution is warranted in patients with a history of bleeding disorders or taking blood-thinning drugs such as aspirin, anticoagulants such as warfarin (Coumadin) or heparin, anti-platelet drugs such as clopidogrel (Plavix), and non-steroidal anti-inflammatory drugs such as ibuprofen (Motrin, Advil) or naproxen (Naprosyn, Aleve).

- Concern has been raised that antioxidants may interfere with some chemotherapy agents (such as alkylating agents, anthracyclines, or platinums), which themselves can depend on oxidative damage to tumor cells for their anti-cancer effects. Studies on the effects of antioxidants on cancer therapies have yielded mixed results, with some reporting interference, others noting benefits, and most suggesting no significant interaction. However, until additional scientific evidence is available, high-dose antioxidants should be avoided during chemotherapy administration, unless otherwise decided in discussion with the treating oncologist.
- Cholestyramine (Questran), colestipol (Colestid), orlistat (Xenical), isoniazid (INH, Lanizid, Nydrazid), olestra (Olean fat substitute), and sucralfate (Carafate) can reduce dietary vitamin E absorption and blood levels of vitamin E. Gemfibrozil (Lopid) may decrease serum levels of both alpha- and gamma-tocopherol, although clinical significance is not clear. Anticonvulsant drugs such as phenobarbital, phenytoin, or carbamazepine may decrease blood levels of vitamin E.
- Vitamin E use with cyclosporine appears to increase the area under the blood concentration time curve of cyclosporine. A water-soluble form of vitamin E, tocopheryl succinate polyethylene glycol, may improve the absorption of cyclosporine (observed after liver transplantation).
- Vitamin E may have additive effects with cholesterol-lowering medications.

Interactions with Herbs and Dietary Supplements

- High doses of oral or injected vitamin E may increase the risk of bleeding including hemorrhagic stroke (bleeding into the brain), and caution is warranted in patients with a history of bleeding disorders or those taking herbs or supplements that may also increase the risk of bleeding. For example, multiple cases of bleeding have been reported with the use of *Ginkgo biloba* and fewer cases with garlic or saw palmetto.
- Vitamin E may have additive effects with cholesterol-lowering herbs and supplements.
- Mineral oil may reduce dietary vitamin E absorption. Blood levels of vitamin E may be decreased with zinc deficiency. Increased intake of omega-6 fatty acids may increase vitamin E requirements, particularly at high doses.
- Vitamin E is involved in the absorption, storage, and utilization of vitamin A in the body and contributes to avoiding toxicity with vitamin A intake. Large doses of vitamin E may deplete vitamin A stores.
- Aloe is reported to slow the rate of vitamin E absorption, allowing sustained release of vitamin E into the bloodstream.
- Vitamin E has been proposed to improve the bioavailability of iron.

For a complete list of references, please visit www.naturalstandard.com.

Vitamin K
(2-Methyl-1,4-naphthoquinone derivatives)

RELATED TERMS

- 2-methyl-1,4-naphthoquinone, AquaMEPHYTON, Konakion, menadiol (not available in United States), menadiol diphosphate (vitamin K_3), menadione, menaquinones, menatetrenone, Mephyton, Phylloquinone, Phytomenadione, phytonadione.

BACKGROUND

- The name "vitamin K" refers to a group of chemically similar fat-soluble compounds called *naphthoquinones*. Vitamin K_1 (phytonadione) is the natural form of vitamin K, which is found in plants and provides the primary source of vitamin K to humans through dietary consumption. Vitamin K_2 compounds (menaquinones) are made by bacteria in the human gut and provide a smaller amount of the human vitamin K requirement. Vitamin K_1 is commercially manufactured for medicinal use under several brand names (Phylloquinone, Phytonadione, AquaMEPHYTON, Mephyton, Konakion). A water-soluble preparation is available for adults only as vitamin K_3 (menadione).
- Vitamin K is necessary for normal clotting of blood in humans. Specifically, vitamin K is required for the liver to make factors that are necessary for blood to properly clot (coagulate), including factor II (prothrombin), factor VII (proconvertin), factor IX (thromboplastin component), and factor X (Stuart factor). Other clotting factors that depend on vitamin K are protein C, protein S, and protein Z. Deficiency of vitamin K or disturbances of liver function (for example, severe liver failure) may lead to deficiencies of clotting factors and excess bleeding.
- Vitamin K deficiency is rare but can lead to defective blood clotting and increased bleeding. People at risk for developing vitamin K deficiency include those with chronic malnutrition (including those with alcohol dependency) or conditions that limit absorption of dietary vitamins such as biliary obstruction, celiac disease or sprue, ulcerative colitis, regional enteritis, cystic fibrosis, short bowel syndrome, or intestinal resection (particularly of the terminal ileum, where fat-soluble vitamins are absorbed). In addition, some drugs may reduce vitamin K levels by altering liver function or by killing intestinal flora (normal intestinal bacteria) that make vitamin K (for example, antibiotics, salicylates, anti-seizure medications, and some sulfa drugs). Vitamin K is routinely given to newborn infants to prevent bleeding problems related to birth trauma or when surgery is planned.
- Warfarin is a blood-thinning drug that functions by inhibiting vitamin K-dependent clotting factors. Warfarin is prescribed by doctors for people with various conditions such as atrial fibrillation, artificial heart valves, history of serious blood clot, clotting disorders (hypercoagulability), or placement of indwelling catheters/ports. Usually, blood tests must be done regularly to evaluate the extent of blood thinning, using a test for prothrombin time (PT) or International Normalized Ratio (INR). Vitamin K can decrease the blood-thinning effects of warfarin and will therefore lower the PT or INR value. This may increase the risk of

clotting. Therefore, people taking warfarin are usually warned to avoid foods with high vitamin K content (such as green leafy vegetables) and to avoid vitamin K supplements. Conversely, vitamin K is used to treat overdoses or excess anticoagulant effects of warfarin and to reverse the effects of warfarin prior to surgery or other procedures.

EVIDENCE

Uses Based on Scientific Evidence	Grade
Hemorrhagic Disease of Newborn (Vitamin K Deficiency Bleeding, VKDB) Vitamin K deficiency in infants can lead to hemorrhagic disease of the newborn, also known as vitamin K deficiency bleeding (VKDB). Although up to half of newborns may have some degree of vitamin K deficiency, serious hemorrhagic disease with bleeding is rare. Because vitamin K given by injection has been shown to prevent VKBD in newborns and young infants, the American Academy of Pediatrics recommends administering a single intramuscular injection of vitamin K_1 to all newborns. Oral dosing is not considered adequate as prevention, particularly in breastfeeding infants. Initial concerns of cancer risk were never proven and are generally not considered clinically relevant. Treatment: In cases of true VKDB, bleeding may occur at injection sites, at the umbilicus, or in the gastrointestinal tract. Life-threatening bleeding into the head (intracranial) or in the area behind the lower abdomen (retroperitoneum) can also occur. Evaluation by a physician is imperative.	A
Vitamin K Deficiency Vitamin K deficiency is rare in adults but can lead to defective blood clotting and increased bleeding, as well as osteoporosis. People at risk for developing vitamin K deficiency include those with chronic malnutrition (including those with alcohol dependency) or conditions that limit absorption of dietary vitamins such as biliary obstruction, celiac disease or sprue, ulcerative colitis, regional enteritis, cystic fibrosis, short bowel syndrome, or intestinal resection (particularly of the terminal ileum, where fat-soluble vitamins are absorbed). In addition, some drugs may reduce vitamin K levels by altering liver function or by killing intestinal flora (normal intestinal bacteria) that make vitamin K (for example, antibiotics, salicylates, anti-seizure medications, and some sulfa-drugs). Evaluation by a physician should be sought.	A
Warfarin Reversal (Elevated INR/Pre-Procedure) Warfarin is a blood-thinning drug that inhibits vitamin K–dependent clotting factors. Warfarin is prescribed by doctors for people with various conditions such as atrial fibrillation, artificial heart valves, history of	A

Uses Based on Scientific Evidence	Grade
serious blood clot, clotting disorders (hypercoagulability), or placement of indwelling catheters/ports. Usually, blood tests are done regularly to evaluate the extent of blood thinning, using a test for prothrombin time (PT) or International Normalized Ratio (INR). The range for the PT/INR depends on the condition being treated. The PT/INR can become elevated for many reasons and sometimes can get dangerously high and increase the risk of serious bleeding. Patients taking warfarin should be aware of these potential causes, which include many drugs that interact with warfarin, liver disorders, or accidental warfarin overdose. Because the effects of warfarin on anticoagulation are usually delayed by several days, the PT/INR may not increase immediately at the time of overdose. If a person's blood becomes too "thin," management should be under strict medical supervision and may include oral or injected vitamin K to help reverse the effects of warfarin.	
Bleeding Disorders (Prevention of Bleeding or Thrombotic Events in Anticoagulant Therapy) Agents that block vitamin K, such as warfarin and phenprocoumon, are often used in anticoagulant therapy. Because dietary intake of vitamin K can affect anticoagulant function, inconsistent levels of vitamin K in the diet may make it difficult to control anticoagulant stability. Some studies suggest that daily, low-dose vitamin K supplementation may help stabilize anticoagulant therapy.	C
Osteoporosis Prevention Vitamin K appears to prevent bone resorption, and adequate dietary intake is likely necessary to prevent excess bone loss. Elderly or institutionalized patients may be at particular risk, and adequate intake of vitamin K–rich foods should be maintained. Unless patients have demonstrated vitamin K deficiency, there is no evidence that additional vitamin K supplementation is helpful. Some studies show that vitamin K supplements may increase bone mineral density and bone strength, while others show that vitamin K has no effect on bone turnover. However, vitamin K may play a role in the prevention and treatment of glucocorticoid-induced bone loss. Furthermore, vitamin D and calcium supplementation may enhance the beneficial effects of vitamin K. Further research is needed to confirm these results.	C
Hepatocellular Carcinoma (Recurrent Hepatocellular Carcinoma Prevention) Infection with the hepatitis C virus (HCV) may lead to hepatocellular carcinoma (HCC), a form of liver cancer. So far, the results from clinical studies are unclear and do not indicate any beneficial effects of vitamin K in preventing HCC recurrence.	D

Uses Based on Tradition or Theory
Cancer, celiac disease, cystic fibrosis, liver function testing, osteoporosis treatment.

DOSING

Dietary Intake

- Foods rich in vitamin K include green leafy vegetables such as spinach, broccoli, asparagus, watercress, cabbage, cauliflower, green peas, beans, olives, canola, soybeans, meat, cereals, and dairy products. Cooking does not remove significant amounts of vitamin K from these foods.

Adults (18 Years and Older)

- Vitamin K deficiency management should be under medical supervision. If the PT is only slightly elevated and poor dietary intake is thought to be the cause, increasing the ingestion of vitamin K–rich foods can be tried. In nonemergency situations, oral vitamin K_1 (Phytonadione, AquaMEPHYTON, Mephyton, Konakion) can be given in a daily dose of 5 to 10 mg (single doses up to 25 mg are given in some cases). If there is a concern of bile salt deficiency or malabsorption in the ileum, a water-soluble oral form of vitamin K can be considered. If necessary, vitamin K_1 can be injected at a dose of 10 mg, repeated after 8 to 12 hours, or administered daily until the deficiency is corrected.
- Elevated PT/INR (warfarin reversal) or acute liver dysfunction management should be under medical supervision.

Children (Younger than 18 Years)

- Vitamin K1 given by injection has been shown in newborns and young infants to prevent "hemorrhagic disease of newborn," also known as *vitamin K deficiency bleeding* (VKDB). The American Academy of Pediatrics therefore recommends administering a single intramuscular injection of 0.5 to 1 mg of vitamin K_1 to all newborns. Oral dosing is generally not regarded as adequate for prevention, particularly in breastfeeding infants.
- Warfarin toxicity/reversal should be under strict medical supervision.
- Menadiol (not available in the United States) should not be given to infants or children because of rare reports of liver damage and blood cell toxicity (hemolytic anemia).

SAFETY

Allergies

- Intravenous or intramuscular vitamin K has been associated rarely with anaphylactoid reactions, including shock, heart attack, respiratory arrest, and death. Therefore, these routes of administration should be avoided if possible. If given intravenously, preparations should be dilute and administration should be slow under strict medical supervision.
- Skin hypersensitivity reactions are rare and may occur in particular with injections of vitamin K_1 (Phytonadione, AquaMEPHYTON). A raised, itchy plaque may arise at the injection site that may take 1 to 2 months to resolve and can cause a scar.

Side Effects and Warnings

- An unusual taste in the mouth has been rarely reported with vitamin K injections. Liver damage has been reported rarely in infants and children with use of the vitamin K preparation Menadiol (not available in the United States). Conditions that interfere with absorption of ingested vitamin K may lead to deficiency, including short gut, cystic fibrosis, malabsorption (various causes), pancreas or gall bladder disease, persistent diarrhea, sprue, or ulcerative colitis.

- Red, painful swelling at vitamin K injection sites has been reported. A raised, itchy plaque can arise at the injection site that may take 1 to 2 months to resolve and can cause a scar. Transient flushing has been reported.
- Dizziness has rarely been reported with vitamin K injections.
- Damage to red blood cells causing anemia (hemolysis) has been reported rarely in infants and children with the use of the vitamin K preparation Menadiol (not available in the United States). This type of vitamin K should be avoided in people with glucose-6-phosphate dehydrogenase (G6PD) deficiency because vitamin K may cause hemolytic episodes. Vitamin K deficiency decreases blood factors needed for clotting and increases the risk of bleeding.
- Although initial concerns were voiced about the possible cancer risk of universally administering vitamin K by injection to newborns, there is no scientific evidence to support this risk. This is generally considered not to be a concern in the medical community.

Pregnancy and Breastfeeding

- The U.S. Food and Drug Administration (FDA) has categorized vitamin K as Pregnancy Category C. There is insufficient scientific evidence in animals or humans to clearly conclude the effects on the fetus. Vitamin K given to mothers soon before birth is generally not recommended. Regular supplementation with vitamin K during pregnancy (beyond normal dietary intake) may increase the risk of jaundice in the newborn.
- The American Academy of Pediatrics recommends administering a single intramuscular injection of vitamin K_1 to all newborns to prevent vitamin K deficiency bleeding (VKDB), a potentially life-threatening condition. Excessive amounts of vitamin K supplementation in newborns may lead to serious complications, including hemolytic anemia, hemoglobinuria, kernicterus, brain damage, or death. Reactions may be particularly severe in premature infants.
- Vitamin K ingested by mothers is generally considered to be safe during breastfeeding. There is very little vitamin K transmitted to infants through breast milk (as opposed to many infant formulas, which do include vitamin K). It is not known if the amount of vitamin K in breast milk is increased if mothers take vitamin K supplements, but the scientific evidence suggests that this likely would make little if any difference. If an infant formula is used that is not fortified with vitamin K, a physician should be consulted to find another way for the infant to receive vitamin K.

INTERACTIONS
Interactions with Drugs

- Warfarin is a blood-thinning drug that functions by inhibiting vitamin K-dependent clotting factors. Warfarin is prescribed by doctors for people with various conditions such as atrial fibrillation, artificial heart valves, history of serious blood clot, clotting disorders (hypercoagulability), or placement of indwelling catheters/ports. Usually, blood tests must be done regularly to evaluate the extent of blood thinning using a test for prothrombin time (PT) or International Normalized Ratio (INR). Vitamin K can decrease the blood-thinning effects of warfarin and will therefore lower the PT or INR value. This may increase the risk of clotting. Therefore, people taking warfarin are usually warned to avoid foods with high vitamin K content (such as green leafy vegetables) and to avoid vitamin K supplements. Conversely, vitamin K is used to treat overdoses or excess anticoagulant effects of warfarin and to reverse the effects of warfarin prior to surgery or other procedures. Over-the-counter vitamin K1-containing multivitamin supplements disrupt warfarin anticoagulation in vitamin K_1–depleted patients. Vitamin K–depleted patients are sensitive to even small changes in vitamin K_1 intake.
- Some antibiotics may decrease the bacteria in the human gut (which synthesize a small amount of the human vitamin K requirement). Broad-spectrum antibiotics, particularly sulfonamides such as Bactrim, may lower vitamin K levels and increase the risk of deficiency in people not ingesting adequate amounts.
- High doses of salicylates (aspirin) may increase vitamin K requirements.
- Sucralfate or high doses of aluminum hydroxide antacids may decrease absorption of fat-soluble vitamins such as vitamin K.
- Cholestyramine (Questran) mineral oil may decrease the absorption of oral vitamin K and increase vitamin K requirements.
- Quinine, or quinidine, may increase vitamin K requirements.
- Dactinomycin, a cancer chemotherapy drug, may decrease the effects of vitamin K and increase vitamin K requirements.
- Menadiol sodium diphosphase is a form of vitamin K that is not used in the United States. Multiple drugs may cause complications when taken with menadiol.

Interactions with Herbs/Supplements

- Vitamin K may decrease the blood-thinning effects of herbs that act like warfarin (Coumadin) in the body by decreasing clotting factors made in the liver. In particular, this may apply to herbs with coumarin constituents, such as alfalfa (*Medicago sativa*), American ginseng (*Panax quinquefolius*), and angelica (*Angelica archangelica*).
- While the effects of vitamin K on bone density are still unclear, beneficial effects may be enhanced with vitamin D and calcium supplementation.

For a complete list of references, please visit www.naturalstandard.com.

Vitamin O
(Oxygen)

RELATED TERMS

- Aerobic oxygen, bis-beta-carboxyethyl germanium sesqui-oxide, Ge-132, germanium, organic germanium, organic germanium-132, oxygen, salt water, stabilized oxygen.
- **Note:** This review does not cover vitamin O that contains germanium. Please see the chapter on germanium for more information.

BACKGROUND

- Oxygen is an integral part of human existence. Some have dubbed this element as "vitamin O," even though it is not a true vitamin. Proponents of vitamin O claim that disease occurs because the body is lacking in oxygen. Therefore, by ingesting oxygen through vitamin O supplements, these ailments can be reversed.
- There appears to be two types of vitamin O products on the market. The first is an expensive health supplement that is composed largely of salt water and "stabilized" or "aerobic" oxygen. Companies, such as RGarden, marketed vitamin O (without germanium) claiming that it could cure or prevent serious diseases such as cancer, heart disease, and lung disease and when taken by mouth, enrich the bloodstream with supplemental oxygen. These claims were never substantiated with scientific evidence; however, numerous testimonials mention the effects of vitamin O on a variety of conditions. The second vitamin O product contains germanium, which when synthetically derived may be nontoxic and safe at high doses.
- There is no scientific evidence currently available regarding the effectiveness of vitamin O or the benefit of ingesting stabilized or aerobic oxygen. Vitamin O (oral or topical oxygen) has not been proven to be an effective treatment for its claimed uses.

EVIDENCE

Uses Based on Scientific Evidence

No available studies qualify for inclusion in the evidence table.

Uses Based on Tradition or Theory

Alzheimer's disease, amyloidosis (rare disease that causes the buildup of amyloid, a protein and starch, in tissues and organs), antibacterial, antifungal, antiviral, atherosclerosis (hardening of the arteries), asthma, cancer, canker sores, cataracts, chronic bronchitis, common cold, cough, diabetes mellitus, diabetic ulcers, ear infections, energy booster, fatigue, flu, glaucoma, headaches, heart disease, hemorrhoids, hypertension (high blood pressure), immunostimulation, improving breathing, lung disease, memory loss, metabolic disorders, obesity, pain, prostate problems, shingles, sleep disorders.

DOSING

Adults (18 Years and Older)

- There is insufficient evidence to recommend a dose for vitamin O in adults.

Children (Younger than 18 Years)

- There is insufficient evidence to recommend a dose for vitamin O in children.

SAFETY

Allergies

- There are no known reports of allergy to vitamin O.

Side Effects and Warnings

- Vitamin O, although not a proven treatment for any condition, is theoretically safe. However, vitamin O may not be safe when purchased from certain sellers as some products marketed as vitamin O have been known to contain inorganic germanium, which can cause kidney damage and toxicity.
- Manufacturers have reported side effects of slight headache or too much energy following too much vitamin O at one time.
- Use cautiously in patients who are likely to replace proven, effective medications with vitamin O.
- Use cautiously in patients with high blood pressure who are watching their sodium intake, as some vitamin O products contain salt.

Pregnancy and Breastfeeding

- Vitamin O is not recommended in pregnant or breast-feeding women because of a lack of available scientific evidence.

INTERACTIONS

Interactions with Drugs

- Vitamin O products may contain sodium chloride (salt); therefore, patients with high blood pressure should be aware. Use cautiously if taking blood pressure–lowering agents because of possible additive effects.

Interactions with Herbs and Dietary Supplements

- Vitamin O products may contain sodium chloride (salt); therefore, patients with high blood pressure should be aware. Use cautiously if taking blood pressure–lowering herbs or supplements because of possible additive effects.

For a complete list of references, please visit www.naturalstandard.com.

V

Wasabi
(Wasabia japonica)

RELATED TERMS

- Allyl isothiocyanate, alpha-tocopherol, Brassicaceae (family), *Cochlearia wasabi*, desulfosinigrin, *Eutrema japonica*, *Eutrema wasabi* Maxim, isothiocyanates, Japanese domestic horseradish, Japanese spice, Japanese wasabi, Korean wasabi, wasabi-derived 6-(methylsulfinyl)hexyl isothiocyanate, *Wasabi japonica*, *Wasabi japonica* Matsum, wasabi leafstalk, wasabi powder, wasabi roots, *Wasabia japonica*.
- **Note**: This monograph does not include horseradish *(Armoracia rusticana)*, which is a common substitute for wasabi.

BACKGROUND

- The wasabi plant grows naturally along stream beds in mountain river valleys in Japan, but it is cultivated in certain regions in Japan and North America. Traditionally, the root is shredded to create a pungent condiment used with fish, especially sushi. In laboratory studies, wasabi has inhibited cancer cell growth and survival. However, one wasabi constituent also promoted cancer cell growth. Wasabi has also shown anti-inflammatory activity, antiplatelet activity, and anabolic bone metabolism activity in laboratory tests. However, there is currently insufficient available evidence in humans to support the use of wasabi for any indication.

EVIDENCE

Uses Based on Scientific Evidence

No available studies qualify for inclusion in the evidence table.

Uses Based on Tradition or Theory

Analgesia, antibacterial, antioxidant, anti-platelet agent (blood thinner), cancer, detoxification, food preservation, food uses, gastric ulcers, leukemia, melanoma prevention, osteoporosis.

DOSING

Adults (18 Years and Older)

- There is insufficient evidence to recommend a dose for wasabi in adults.

Children (Younger than 18 Years)

- There is insufficient evidence to recommend a dose for wasabi in children.

SAFETY

Allergies

- Avoid in people with a known allergy or hypersensitivity to wasabi *(Wasabia japonica)* or its constituents.

Side Effects and Warnings

- Wasabi is likely safe when ingested in food amounts, based on use in Japanese cuisine. However, in the currently available literature, reports of adverse effects due to wasabi are lacking. Wasabi is commonly used for its sharp, spicy flavor, which is due to the stimulation of neurons associated with painful cold sensations. Use cautiously in patients using capsaicin-based analgesics applied to the skin, as topical wasabi may produce pain and activate the same neurons as capsaicin.
- Wasabi may have anti–*H. pylori* activity.
- Use cautiously in patients with cancer or a predisposition to cancer, those taking agents metabolized by the liver, or those with coagulation (blood) disorders.

Pregnancy and Breastfeeding

- Wasabi is not recommended in pregnant or breastfeeding women because of a lack of available scientific evidence.

INTERACTIONS

Interactions with Drugs

- Wasabi applied on the skin may produce pain and activate the same neurons as topical analgesics, especially capsaicin-based analgesics. Caution is advised when using wasabi with other pain-relieving agents applied on the skin.
- All parts of the wasabi plant may have antibiotic activity. Thus, using wasabi with other agents that have antibacterial effects may result in additive effects.
- Although not well studied in humans, wasabi may increase the risk of bleeding. Caution is advised in patients with bleeding disorders or those taking drugs that may increase the risk of bleeding. Dosing adjustments may be necessary.
- Wasabi may inhibit COX-1 enzyme activity. Caution is advised in patients taking wasabi plus other anti-inflammatory agents.
- Several constituents in wasabi have shown anticancer activity. However, the evidence is currently mixed. Nonetheless, caution is advised when taking wasabi and any anticancer agent. Consult with a qualified healthcare professional, including a pharmacist, to check for interactions.
- All parts of the wasabi plant may have anti–*H. pylori* activity.
- Wasabi may interact with drugs metabolized by the liver. Caution is advised when using wasabi with other agents that are metabolized by the liver or are potentially liver damaging.
- Extracts from wasabi leafstalk (*Wasabi japonica* Matsum) may have an anabolic effect on bone metabolism. Caution is advised when taking wasabi with selective estrogen receptor modulators (SERMs), hormonal agents, or bisphosphonates.

Interactions with Herbs and Dietary Supplements

- All parts of the wasabi plant may have antibacterial activity. Thus, using wasabi with other herbs that have antibacterial effects may result in additive effects.
- Although not well studied in humans, wasabi may inhibit platelet aggregation, thus increasing the risk of bleeding. Caution is advised in patients with bleeding disorders or those taking herbs or supplements that may increase the risk of bleeding. Multiple cases of bleeding have been reported

with the use of *Ginkgo biloba* and fewer cases with garlic and saw palmetto.

- Wasabi may inhibit COX-1 enzyme activity. Caution is advised in patients taking wasabi plus other anti-inflammatory herbs.
- Several constituents in wasabi have shown anticancer activity. However, the evidence is currently mixed. Nonetheless, caution is advised when taking wasabi and any anticancer agent. Consult with a qualified healthcare professional, including a pharmacist, to check for interactions.
- Based on laboratory research, all parts of the wasabi plant may have anti–*H. pylori* activity.

- Wasabi applied to the skin may produce pain and activate the same neurons as capsaicin and *Cannabis sativa*.
- Wasabi may interact with herbs metabolized by the liver. Caution is advised when using wasabi with other agents that are metabolized by the liver or are potentially liver damaging.
- Extracts from wasabi leafstalk (*Wasabi japonica* Matsum) may have an anabolic effect on bone metabolism. Caution is advised when taking wasabi with phytoestrogens or hormonal herbs or supplements.

For a complete list of references, please visit www.naturalstandard.com.

W

Watercress
(Nasturtium officinale)

RELATED TERMS

- Agrião, Berro, Berro de Agua, Brassicacae, Brunnendresenkraut, Brunnenkresse, *Cochleria officinalis,* Crescione Di Fonte, Cresson au Poulet, Cresson D'eau, Cresson de Fontaine, Garden cress, Glucosinolates, Isothiocyanates (ITCs), Herba nasturtii Aquatici, Herbe aux Chantes, Indian Cress, Mizu-Garashi, Nasilord, Nasturii herba, *Nasturtium officinale, Nasturtium officinale* R. Br., Oranda-Garashi, Phenethyl isothiocyanate (PEITC) (PEITC-NAC), *Rorripa, Rorripa nasturtium aquaticum,* scurvy grass, scrubby grass, Selada-Air, Spoonwort, Tall Nasturtium, Tropaeolaceae, Tropaeolum majus, Wasserkresse, waterkres.

BACKGROUND

- Watercress originates from the eastern Mediterranean and adjoining areas of Asia. It is cultivated commercially for its small, pungent leaves that may be used as a salad green or garnish. Greek, Persian, and Roman civilizations ate watercress for its health-related properties. The Greeks believed watercress was beneficial to the brain. Applied externally, it has a reputation as an effective hair tonic, helping to promote the growth of thick hair.
- Watercress is a member of the Brassicaceae family, which includes cabbage, broccoli, cauliflower, Brussels sprouts, kale, mustard greens, collard greens, bok choy, and turnips. These plants contain specific indoles (aromatic organic compounds) that activate enzymes in the body; these enzymes then deactivate and dispose of excess estrogen. Heavy cooking destroys indoles and is not recommended for medicinal purposes.
- Watercress also contains phenethyl isothiocyanate (PEITC), which is a dietary compound present in cruciferous vegetables that has cancer-preventive properties.
- Watercress was formerly used as a domestic remedy against scurvy. The species *Cochlearia officianalis* is commonly referred to as scurvy grass; sailors would consume this plant to prevent scurvy from developing. Although this plant is referred to as *watercress,* scurvy grass has flowers with a strong fragrance and taste.

EVIDENCE

Uses Based on Scientific Evidence

No available studies qualify for inclusion in the evidence table.

Uses Based on Tradition or Theory

Abortifacient (inducing abortion), acne, alopecia (hair loss), anthelminthic (expels worms), antibiotic, anti-inflammatory, antimicrobial, antimutagenic (inhibiting mutations), antimycotic (destroys fungi), appetite stimulant, arthritis, bactericide, blood purifier, bronchitis, cancer risks, canker sores, cellular regeneration, chemoprotective, choleretic preparations, chronic marginal parodontopathies, colon cancer, cold, coughs, detoxification, digestive disorders, diuretic, earaches, eczema, esophageal tumorigenesis, flu, forestomach tumorigenesis, gastrointestinal disorders, gingivitis, gland tumors, goiter, gout (foot inflammation), gum disease, improves bone and joint problems, digestion, laxative, lethargy, lung cancer, lung tumorigenesis, polyps, rashes, respiratory tract mucous membrane inflammation, restorative, rheumatoid arthritis, scabies, scurvy, skin infections, soreness, stimulant, swelling, tuberculosis, tumorigenesis (tumor development), urinary tract infection, vascular deficiencies, vitamin deficiencies, warts.

DOSING
Adults (18 Years and Older)

- There is insufficient evidence to recommend a dose for watercress. 4-6 g of dried herb has been used, as has 20-30 g of fresh herb or 60-150 g as a juice or tea.

Children (Younger than 18 Years)

- There is insufficient evidence to recommend a dose for watercress, and use in children is not recommended.

SAFETY
Allergies

- Avoid in people with a known allergy or hypersensitivity to watercress, or members of the Brassicaceae family, which includes cabbage, broccoli, cauliflower, Brussels sprouts, kale, mustard greens, collard greens, bok choy, and turnips. True *Nasturtium officinale* is known to cause contact dermatitis. Watercress may cause breathing problems or tightness in the throat or chest in allergic people.

Side Effects and Warnings

- Watercress is generally well tolerated; however some adverse effects have been reported. Use caution when gathering watercress from the wild because of the risk of plant infestation with liver fluke parasites.
- Watercress may cause hives, rash, itching, or swollen skin. True *Nasturtium officinale* is known to cause contact dermatitis. Watercress may also cause breathing problems or tightness in the throat or chest in allergic people.
- Large amounts of watercress may cause gastrointestinal irritation. Although not well studied, excessive or prolonged use of watercress may cause kidney damage. Use cautiously in patients with gastric or duodenal ulcers or kidney disease.

Pregnancy and Breastfeeding

- Watercress is not recommended in pregnant or breastfeeding women because of a lack of scientific available evidence. Although not well-studied, watercress may be unsafe when used in pregnancy because of its possible abortifacient (abortion-inducing) effects. Watercress may also stimulate menstruation.

INTERACTIONS
Interactions with Drugs

- Consumption of watercress decreases the levels of oxidative metabolites of acetaminophen. Use cautiously in patients taking acetaminophen (Tylenol), and consult with a qualified healthcare professional, including a pharmacist, before combining therapies.
- Watercress contains a high vitamin K content and may increase the risk of bleeding when taken with drugs that increase the risk of bleeding. Some examples include aspirin, anticoagulants (blood thinners) such as warfarin (Coumadin) or heparin, anti-platelet drugs such as clopidogrel (Plavix), and non-steroidal anti-inflammatory drugs (NSAIDS) such as ibuprofen (Motrin, Advil) or naproxen (Naprosyn, Aleve).
- Concomitant use with chlorazoxazone (Parafon Forte, Paraflex) may alter the effects because of reduced metabolism and elimination. Caution is advised.
- Early evidence suggests that watercress may interfere with the way the body processes certain drugs using the liver's cytochrome P450 enzyme system. As a result, levels of these drugs may be increased in the blood and may cause increased effects or potentially serious adverse reactions. Patients using any medications should check the package insert and speak with a qualified healthcare professional, including a pharmacist, about possible interactions.

Interactions with Herbs and Dietary Supplements

- Watercress contains a high vitamin K content and may increase the risk of bleeding when taken with herbs and supplements that are believed to increase the risk of bleeding. Multiple cases of bleeding have been reported with the use of *Ginkgo biloba* and fewer cases with garlic and saw palmetto. Numerous other agents may theoretically increase the risk of bleeding, although this has not been proven in most cases.
- Watercress may interfere with the way the body processes certain herbs or supplements using the liver's cytochrome P450 enzyme system. As a result, levels of other herbs or supplements may become too high in the blood. It may also alter the effects that other herbs or supplements possibly have on the P450 system.

For a complete list of references, please visit www.naturalstandard.com.

W

Wheatgrass
(Triticum aestivum)

RELATED TERMS

- *Agropyron,* bread wheat, bugday, cheng ping, common wheat, *Elytrigia, Eremopyrum,* fou mai, frumint, Gramineae (family), Hsiao mai, hui mai, hui mien, ka shih tso, lai, mai ch'ao, mai fu, mai fu tzu, man tou, mien, mien chin, mien fen, mo mo, pai mien, *Pascopyrum,* Poaeceae (family), *Pseudoroegneria,* tarwe, trigo, *Triticum aestivum, Triticum hybernum, Triticum vulgar, Triticummacha, Triticummuticum, Triticumsphaerococcum,* vegan diet, wheat, wheat berry, wheat grass.

BACKGROUND

- There are several plants that may be referred to as wheatgrass, including the plant genera *Agropyron, Elytrigia, Eremopyrum, Pascopyrum,* and *Pseudoroegneria.* The common wheat plant, *Triticum aestivum,* is most commonly known as wheatgrass. Wheatgrass is often used in vegan diets or other "living food" diets. Wheatgrass has become popularized in the United States and is marketed toward health conscious people. In folk medicine, practitioners used wheatgrass to treat cystitis, gout, rheumatic pain, chronic skin disorders, and constipation.
- Despite its name, wheatgrass is gluten-free and is suitable for patients with gluten intolerance. Fresh leaf buds of this plant can be crushed to create a juice or dried to make a powder. The unprocessed plant contains high levels of cellulose, which cannot be digested. Wheatgrass juice is the juice extracted from the pulp of wheatgrass and has been used as a general-purpose health tonic for several years.
- Wheatgrass is a complete protein with about 30 enzymes, and it is about 70% crude chlorophyll. The chlorophyll molecule is similar in structure to hemoglobin, leading some to believe that wheatgrass helps blood flow, digestion, and general detoxification of the body. However, despite its popularity in the United States, there are no high-quality clinical trials for wheatgrass.

EVIDENCE

Uses Based on Scientific Evidence	Grade
Beta-Thalassemia (Transfusion Dependent) Preliminary evidence suggests that wheatgrass may be beneficial for patients with beta thalassemia, and decrease the number of blood transfusions needed.	C
Ulcerative Colitis There is preliminary evidence that wheatgras may be beneficial in the treatment of ulcerative colitis.	C

Uses Based on Tradition or Theory

AIDS, acne, alcohol dependence, antibilious (removes excess bile), antiperspirant, antipyretic (fever reducer), blood flow disorders, bruises, burns, cancer (peritoneal), chronic skin disorders, circulation, constipation, cough, cystitis, detoxification, diabetes, digestion, eczema, energy enhancement, eye strain, fever, gout (foot inflammation), hypertension (high blood pressure), infection, gingivitis, malaise, pain (abdominal), poison ivy, psoriasis, scar healing, rheumatoid arthritis, sedative, skin ailments, sore throat, sterility, thirst, tooth disease prevention, weight loss aid, wound healing.

DOSING

Adults (18 Years and Older)

- For transfusion-dependent beta thalassemia (blood disorder) or ulcerative colitis, 100 ml of wheatgrass juice daily has been found effective. Traditionally, 8 to 32 ounces of wheatgrass juice has been administered via enemas, rubber bulb syringes, or colonics for colon cleansing.

Children (Younger than 18 Years)

- There is insufficient evidence to recommend a dose for wheatgrass, and use in children is not recommended.

SAFETY

Allergies

- Avoid in people with a known allergy or hypersensitivity to wheatgrass. Most wheat allergies are due to the gluten found in the wheatberry. However, wheatgrass does not have any gluten because it is cut before the plant forms a grain (berry).
- Some individuals have reported nausea, headaches, hives, or swelling in the throat within minutes of drinking its juice. Hives and swollen throat are often signs of a serious allergic reaction and should be handled as an emergency. Anyone having these kinds of symptoms after ingesting wheatgrass may have even more severe reactions to it later.

Side Effects and Warnings

- Wheatgrass is generally considered safe. No serious side effects were found in several studies using wheatgrass juice daily for up to one month. There have been no other reports of adverse effects in the available literature. Because it is grown in soils or water and consumed raw, wheatgrass may be contaminated with bacteria, molds, or other substances.

- Some individuals have reported hives, nausea, or swelling in the throat within minutes of drinking its juice.

Pregnancy and Breastfeeding

- Because it is grown in soils or water and consumed raw, wheatgrass may be contaminated with bacteria, molds, or other substances. Wheatgrass is not recommended in pregnant or breastfeeding women because of a lack of available scientific evidence.

INTERACTIONS

Interactions with Drugs

- There is insufficient available evidence.

Interactions with Herbs and Dietary Supplements

- There is insufficient available evidence.

For a complete list of references, please visit www.naturalstandard.com.

W

White horehound

(Marrubium vulgare)

RELATED TERMS

- Acylated flavonoid, andorn, blanc rubi, bonhomme, bouenriblé, bull's blood, common hoarhound, eye of the star, grand bon-homme, grand-bonhomme, haran haran, herbe aux crocs, herbe vierge, hoarhound, horehound, hound-bane, houndsbane, labdane diterpene marrubiin, Labiatae (family), Lamiaceae (family), lectins, Llwyd y cwn, maltrasté, mapiochin, mariblé marinclin, marrochemin, marroio, marroio-branco, marromba, marrube, marrube blanc, marrube commun, marrube des champs, marrube officinal, marrube vulgaire, marrubenol, marrubii herba, marrubiin, marrubio, marrubium, *Marrubium vulgare*, marruboside, maruil, marvel, mastranzo, mont blanc, phenylethanoid glycosides, phenylpropanoid esters, Ricola, seed of horus, sesquiterpene, soldier's tea, sterol, weisser Andorn.
- **Note**: White horehound should not be confused with black horehound *(Ballota nigra)* or water horehound *(Lycopus americanus*, also known as bugleweed).

BACKGROUND

- Since ancient Egypt, white horehound (*Marrubium vulgare* L.) has been used as an expectorant (to facilitate removal of mucus from the lungs or throat). Ayurvedic, Native American, and Australian Aboriginal medicines have traditionally used white horehound to treat respiratory (lung) conditions. The U.S. Food and Drug Administration (FDA) banned horehound from cough drops in 1989 because of insufficient evidence supporting its efficacy. However, horehound is currently widely used in Europe, and it can be found in European-made herbal cough remedies sold in the United States (for example, Ricola).
- There is a lack of well-defined clinical evidence to support any therapeutic use of white horehound. The expert German panel, the Commission E, has approved white horehound for lack of appetite, dyspepsia (heartburn), and as a choleretic. There is promising early evidence favoring the use of white horehound as a hypoglycemic agent for diabetes mellitus and as a non-opioid pain reliever.
- There is limited evidence on the safety or toxicity in humans. White horehound has been reported to cause hypotension (low blood pressure), hypoglycemia (low blood sugar), and arrhythmias (abnormal heart rhythms) in animal studies.

EVIDENCE

Uses Based on Scientific Evidence	Grade
Cough Since ancient Egypt, white horehound has been used as an expectorant. Ayurvedic, Native American, and Australian Aboriginal medicines have traditionally used white horehound to treat respiratory (lung)	C

conditions. The U.S. Food and Drug Administration (FDA) banned horehound from cough drops in 1989 because of insufficient evidence supporting its effectiveness. However, horehound is currently widely used in Europe, and it can be found in European-made herbal cough remedies sold in the United States (for example, Ricola).

Diabetes Animal studies and preliminary human studies suggest that white horehound may lower blood sugar levels. White horehound has been used for diabetes in some countries, including Mexico. Clinical evidence, however, is sufficient to support this use.	C
Heartburn/Poor Appetite In Germany, white horehound is approved for the treatment of heartburn and lack of appetite, based on historical use. There is not enough information from scientific studies to evaluate the effectiveness of white horehound for these conditions.	C
High Cholesterol Early research shows that white horehound may lower cholesterol and triglyceride blood levels. Further research is needed to confirm these results.	C
Intestinal Disorders/Antispasmodic White horehound has been used traditionally to treat intestinal disorders. However, there are few well-designed studies in this area, and little information is available about the effectiveness of white horehound for this use.	C
Pain White horehound has traditionally been used for pain and spasms from menstruation or intestinal conditions. There is a lack of reliable human studies on safety or effectiveness for this use.	C

Uses Based on Tradition or Theory

Antioxidant, asthma, bile secretion, bloating, blood vessel dilation (relaxation), bronchitis, cancer, cathartic, chronic obstructive pulmonary disease (COPD), colic, congestion, constipation, debility, diarrhea, emetic, fever reduction, flatulence, food flavoring, gallbladder complaints, heart rate abnormalities, high blood pressure, indigestion, intestinal parasites, jaundice (yellowing of the skin), laxative, liver disease, lung congestion, morning sickness, pneumonia, rabies, respiratory (lung) spasms, skin conditions, snake poisoning, sore throat, sweat stimulation, tuberculosis, upper respiratory tract infection, warts, water retention, wheezing, whooping cough, wound healing.

DOSING
Adults (18 Years and Older)

- Safety and effectiveness of doses has not been proven. Doses that have been used for cough/throat ailments include 10 to 40 drops of extract in water up to three times a day or lozenges dissolved in the mouth as needed. Ricola drops are recommended by the manufacturer at a maximum of 2 lozenges every 1 to 2 hours as needed.
- Doses recommended by the expert German panel, the Commission E, for treating heartburn or stimulating appetite include 4.5 g daily of cut herb or 2 to 6 tbsp of fresh plant juice. Other traditional dosing suggestions are 1 to 2 g of dried herb or infusion three times daily.

Children (Younger than 18 Years)

- There is insufficient evidence to recommend the safe use of white horehound in children.

SAFETY
Allergies

- In theory, white horehound may cause an allergic reaction in people with a known allergy or hypersensitivity to members of the Lamiaceae family (mint family) or any white horehound components.

Side Effects and Warnings

- White horehound is generally considered to be safe when used as a flavoring agent in foods. However, there is limited scientific study of safety, and most available information is from animal (not human) research. Reported side effects include rash at areas of direct contact with white horehound plant juice, abnormal heart rhythms, low blood pressure, and decreased blood sugar (seen in animals with high blood sugar). White horehound may cause vomiting and diarrhea. Caution is warranted in people with heart disease or gastrointestinal disorders. Caution may also be advisable in people with diabetes or hypoglycemia and in those taking drugs, herbs, or supplements that affect blood sugar. Serum glucose levels may need to be monitored by a healthcare professional, and medication adjustments may be necessary.
- Theoretically, white horehound may interfere with the body's response to the hormone aldosterone, which affects the ability of the kidneys to control the body's levels of water and electrolytes. These theoretical effects may cause high blood pressure, high blood sodium, low potassium, leg swelling, and muscle weakness. People who have high or unstable blood pressure, high sodium, or low potassium or who are taking medications that reduce the amount of water in the body (diuretics, or "water pills") should use caution. White horehound may contain estrogen-like chemicals that either have stimulatory or inhibitory effects on estrogen-sensitive parts of the body. It is unclear what effects may occur in hormone-sensitive conditions such as some cancers (breast, ovarian, uterine) and endometriosis or in people using hormone replacement therapy/birth control pills.

Pregnancy and Breastfeeding

- White horehound is not recommended during pregnancy or breastfeeding. Animal studies suggest that white horehound may cause miscarriage.

INTERACTIONS
Interactions with Drugs

- Because white horehound is thought to be an expectorant in the treatment of cough or congestion, its use with cold medications that have expectorant ingredients may cause added effects. Theoretically, white horehound may reduce the effects of some medications given for vomiting (serotonin receptor antagonist drugs such as granisetron and ondansetron), migraine headache (ergot alkaloids such as bromocriptine, dihydroergotamine, or ergotamine), and antidepressants that possess serotonin activity (selective serotonin reuptake inhibitors [SSRIs] like Prozac, Paxil, or Zoloft). White horehound may interact with the ability of the body to excrete penicillin. The reported ability of white horehound to cause diarrhea may cause an excessive response when combined with stool softeners or laxatives.
- Large amounts of white horehound may increase the risk of abnormal heart rhythms and should be avoided by people treated with drugs that affect heart rhythm. Animal studies suggest that the use of white horehound with medications that lower blood pressure may cause a larger than expected drop in blood pressure. White horehound contains glycoside compounds that act on the heart, and these theoretically could affect the activity of glycoside medications such as digoxin (Lanoxin). Theoretically, white horehound may increase the action of the hormone aldosterone on the kidneys, and it may interact with some diuretic medications.
- Based on animal studies, white horehound may lower blood sugar levels. Caution is advised when using medications that may also lower blood sugar levels. Patients taking drugs for diabetes by mouth or insulin should be monitored closely by a qualified healthcare professional. Medication adjustments may be necessary. In theory, white horehound may also interact with medications used to treat thyroid disorders such as iodine, liothyronine (T_3, Cytomel), methimazole (Tapazole), propylthiouracil (PTU), thyroxine (T_4, Levoxyl, Synthroid), and Thyrolar (T_4 plus T_3).
- White horehound may contain estrogen-like chemicals that either have stimulatory or inhibitory effects on estrogen-sensitive parts of the body. It is unclear what effects may occur in people using hormonal therapies such as birth control pills or hormone replacement therapy. Based on early animal study, white horehound may lower cholesterol or triglyceride blood levels and therefore may have additive effects with other drugs with similar actions.

Interactions with Herbs and Dietary Supplements

- In theory, white horehound may lower blood pressure and may cause increased urine production. Caution is advised when using herbs or supplements that lower blood pressure or increase urination.
- White horehound may contain glycoside chemicals that affect the heart and therefore should be used with caution by people taking other supplements that have glycoside ingredients. Notably, bufalin/Chan Suis is a Chinese herbal formula that has been reported as toxic or fatal when taken with cardiac glycosides.
- Because white horehound may cause diarrhea, use caution if combining it with other laxative herbs.
- Animal studies suggest that white horehound may lower blood sugar levels. Caution is advised when using herbs or

W

supplements that may also lower blood sugar levels. Blood glucose levels may require monitoring, and doses may need adjustment.

- Because white horehound may contain estrogen-like chemicals, the effects of other agents believed to have estrogen-like properties may be altered. In theory, white horehound may interact with agents that affect the thyroid, such as bladderwrack. Based on early animal study, white horehound may lower cholesterol or triglyceride blood levels and therefore may have additive effects with other herbs and supplements with similar actions.

- White horehound may interact with herbs and supplements taken to treat cough, vomiting, migraine headache, and depression; use cautiously.

For a complete list of references, please visit www.naturalstandard.com.

Wild indigo
(*Baptisia* spp.)

RELATED TERMS

- *Baptisia australis, Baptisia tinctoria* (L.) R. B., *Baptisia tinctoria* (L.) R. Br., *Baptisia tinctoria* radix, blue false indigo, blue wild indigo, Fabaceae (family), horse fly weed, indigo carmine, indigo weed, rattlebush, rattleweed, wild indigo root.

BACKGROUND

- Wild indigo (*Baptisia australis*) has deep blue to violet flowers, similar to sweet pea flowers. When the plant's sap is exposed to air, it turns purple. Although this sap has been used for dyeing, it is not as colorfast as true indigo (*Indigofera tinctoria*). Some Native Americans tribes used a tea of blue indigo root as an emetic (induces vomiting) and purgative.
- Wild indigo is considered toxic and is on the U. S. Food and Drug Administration's (FDA) list of toxic plants. However, two studies in humans found no adverse effects when it was used in a combination of *Baptisia tinctoria* root, *Echinaca pallida/purpurea* root, and *Thuja occidentalis* leaf. Currently, wild indigo seems most promising as an immunomodulator, as both laboratory studies and clinical studies using combination products have noted some benefit. However, more studies are needed using wild indigo as a monotherapy before its safety and efficacy can be determined.

EVIDENCE

Uses Based on Scientific Evidence	Grade
Respiratory Tract Infections Preliminary evidence has shown immunostimulative properties in wild indigo extracts. However, the available clinical studies have been conducted using the combination called Esberitox N (*Echinacea purpurea* and *pallida* root, *Baptisia tinctoria* root, and *Thuja occidentalis* leaf). Additional research is needed using wild indigo alone to determine effectiveness for respiratory tract infections.	C

Uses Based on Tradition or Theory
Antiviral, emetic (induces vomiting), immunomodulation, laxative (purgative).

DOSING

Adults (18 Years and Older)

- There is insufficient evidence to recommend a dose for wild indigo in adults. Wild indigo is considered toxic and is on the U.S. Food and Drug Administration's (FDA's) list of toxic plants.

Children (Younger than 18 Years)

- There is insufficient evidence to recommend a dose for wild indigo in children. Wild indigo is considered toxic and is on the U.S. Food and Drug Administration's (FDA's) list of toxic plants.

SAFETY
Allergies

- Avoid in people with a known allergy or hypersensitivity to wild indigo (*Baptisia australis*) or its constituents.

Side Effects and Warnings

- There is little information available on the adverse effects of wild indigo in the literature. However, when used in a combination of *Echinacea purpura* and *pallida* root, *Baptisia tinctoria* root, and *Thuja occidentalis* leaf, two studies in humans found no adverse effects. Wild indigo is considered toxic and is on the U.S. Food and Drug Administration's (FDA's) list of toxic plants. Use cautiously in patients on immunosuppressive therapy because wild indigo may be an immunostimulator or immunomodulator.

Pregnancy and Breastfeeding

- Wild indigo is not recommended in pregnant or breastfeeding women because of a lack of available scientific evidence.

INTERACTIONS
Interactions with Drugs

- The combination of an herbal preparation composed of Echinacea, wild indigo, and white cedar mat have antiviral characteristics. Caution is advised when taking wild indigo with other antiviral agents.
- Preliminary evidence suggests that wild indigo may have immunostimulative or immunomodulating effects. Use cautiously with other immunosuppressive agents.

Interactions with Herbs and Dietary Supplements

- The combination of an herbal preparation comprised of Echinacea, wild indigo, and white cedar mat have antiviral characteristics. Caution is advised when taking wild indigo with other antiviral herbs or supplants.
- Preliminary evidence suggests that wild indigo may have immunostimulative or immunomodulating effects. Use cautiously with other immunosuppressive herbs or supplements.

For a complete list of references, please visit www.naturalstandard.com.

W

Wild yam
(Dioscorea villosa)

RELATED TERMS

- Atlantic yam, barbasco, batata silvestre, black yam, China root, colic root, devil's bones, *Dioscorea, Dioscorea barbasco, Dioscorea hypoglauca, Dioscorea macrostachya, Dioscorea opposita, Dioscorea villosa,* Dioscoreae (family), diosgenin, Mexican yam, natural DHEA, phytoestrogen, potassium, rheumatism root, shan yao, white yam, wild yam root, yam, yellow yam, yuma.
- **Note**: "Yams" sold in the supermarket are members of the sweet potato family and are not true yams.

BACKGROUND

- It has been widely believed that wild yam (*Dioscorea villosa* and other *Dioscorea* species) possesses dehydroepiandrosterone (DHEA)-like properties and acts as a precursor to human sex hormones such as estrogen and progesterone. Based on this proposed mechanism, extracts of the plant have been used to treat painful menstruation, hot flashes, and headaches associated with menopause. However, these uses are based on a misconception that wild yam contains hormones or hormonal precursors, largely due to the historical fact that progesterone, androgens, and cortisone were chemically manufactured from Mexican wild yam in the 1960s. It is unlikely that this chemical conversion to progesterone occurs in the human body. The hormonal activity of some topical wild yam preparations has been attributed to adulteration with synthetic progesterone by manufacturers, although there is limited supportive evidence.
- The effects of the wild yam constituent diosgenin on lipid metabolism are well documented in animal models and are possibly due to impaired intestinal cholesterol absorption. However, its purported hypocholesterolemic effect in humans, and the feasibility of long-term use warrant further investigation.
- There are few reported contraindications to the use of wild yam in adults. However, there is a lack of reliable safety or toxicity studies during pregnancy, lactation, or childhood.

EVIDENCE

Uses Based on Scientific Evidence	Grade
High Cholesterol Animal studies have shown that wild yam can reduce the absorption of cholesterol from the gut. Early studies in humans have shown changes in the levels of certain sub-types of cholesterol, including decreases in low-density lipoprotein (LDL, or "bad cholesterol") and triglycerides and increases in high-density lipoprotein (HDL, or "good cholesterol"). However, no changes in the total amount of blood cholesterol have been found. More studies are needed in this area.	C
Menopausal Symptoms Most studies have not shown a benefit from wild yam given by mouth or used as a vaginal cream in reducing menopausal symptoms. However, replacing two thirds of staple food with yam for 30 days was shown to improve the status of sex hormones, lipids, and antioxidants in a recent study in postmenopausal women. The authors suggest that these effects might reduce the risk of breast cancer and cardiovascular diseases in postmenopausal women. Further research is needed before a recommendation can be made.	C
Hormonal Properties (to Mimic Estrogen, Progesterone, or DHEA) Despite popular belief, biologically active progestins, estrogens, or other reproductive hormones do not naturally occur in wild yam. Its active ingredient, diosgenin, is not converted to hormones in the human body. Artificial progesterone has been added to some wild yam products. The belief that there are hormones in wild yam may be due to the historical fact that progesterone, androgens, and cortisone were chemically manufactured from Mexican wild yam in the 1960s.	D

Uses Based on Tradition or Theory

Antifungal, anti-inflammatory, antiviral, asthma, bile flow improvement, biliary colic, breast cancer, breast enlargement, cancer prevention, cardiovascular disease, carminative (prevents gas), childbirth, cramps, croup, decreased perspiration, diverticulitis, energy improvement, excessive perspiration, expectorant, intestinal spasm, irritable bowel syndrome, joint pain, libido, liver protection, low blood sugar, menstrual pain or irregularities, morning sickness, nerve pain, osteoporosis, pancreatic enzyme inhibitor, pelvic cramps, postmenopausal vaginal dryness, premenstrual syndrome (PMS), rash, rheumatic pain, spasms, urinary tract disorders, uterus contraction, vomiting.

DOSING
Adults (18 Years and Older)

- There is insufficient evidence to recommend a dose for wild yam.

Children (Younger than 18 Years)

- There is insufficient evidence to recommend use in children.

SAFETY
Allergies

- Rubbing the skin with *Dioscorea batatas* (a yam species related to *Dioscorea villosa*) has been reported to cause allergic rash. Workers exposed to *Dioscorea batatas* in large amounts and for a prolonged time have developed asthma that is made worse by exposure to the yam. A person who is known to have an allergy to *Dioscorea batatas* may also be allergic to other *Dioscorea* types.

Side Effects and Warnings

- Rubbing the skin with *Dioscorea batatas,* a related yam species, has been reported to cause a rash at the site of contact. Wild yam cream did not cause rash in 23 healthy women in one reported study. In another study, wild yam given by mouth was reported to cause stomach upset at high doses.

- Wild yam was believed in the past to have properties similar to the reproductive hormone progesterone, but this has not been supported by scientific studies. It has been suggested that some wild yam creams might be tainted with artificial progesterone. Based on theoretical hormonal properties and possible progesterone contamination, people with hormone-sensitive conditions should use wild yam products with caution. This caution applies to people who have had blood clots or strokes and to women who take hormone replacement therapy or birth control pills. In addition, women with fibroids, endometriosis, or cancer of the breast, uterus, or ovary should be aware that these are hormone-sensitive conditions that may be affected by agents with hormonal properties.

- Caution is advised in patients with diabetes or low blood sugar and in those taking drugs, herbs, or supplements that affect blood sugar. Blood sugar levels may need to be monitored by a healthcare provider, and medication adjustments may be necessary.

Pregnancy and Breastfeeding

- Use of wild yam is not recommended during pregnancy or breastfeeding because of a lack of safety information. Wild yam is believed to cause uterine contractions, and therefore use is discouraged during pregnancy. Wild yam was once thought to have effects similar to those of reproductive hormones, although this has not been proven in scientific studies. Artificial progesterone may be added to some products.

INTERACTIONS

Interactions with Drugs

- It is not clear whether blood sugar is lowered by *Dioscorea villosa* (wild yam). Dioscoretine, a compound found in the related species *Dioscorea dumentorum* (bitter or African yam), has been shown to lower blood sugar levels, but this has not been shown for *Dioscorea villosa*. Effects on blood sugar in humans have not been reported. Nonetheless, caution is advised when using medications that may also lower blood sugar levels. People taking diabetes drugs by mouth or insulin should be monitored closely by a qualified healthcare provider. Medication adjustments may be necessary.

- Early evidence suggests that wild yam lowers blood levels of indomethacin, a non-steroidal anti-inflammatory drug, and reduces irritation of the intestine caused by indomethacin. Human studies have not been reported in this area, and it is not clear if wild yam affects the blood levels of other anti-inflammatory drugs such as ibuprofen (Advil, Motrin).

- Diosgenin, thought to be the active substance in wild yam, has been found in animals to reduce absorption of cholesterol from the intestine and to lower total cholesterol levels in the blood. Studies in humans show no change in the total amount of cholesterol in the blood, although the amounts of specific types of cholesterol in the blood may be changed; low-density lipoprotein (LDL, or "bad cholesterol") and triglycerides may be lowered and high-density lipoprotein (HDL, or "good cholesterol") may be increased. It is thought that wild yam may enhance the effects of other cholesterol-lowering medications, including fibric acid derivatives such as clofibrate (Questran), gemfibrozil (Lopid), and fenofibrate (Tricor). In animals, wild yam has been found to improve the effect of clofibrate in lowering cholesterol levels.

- Tinctures of wild yam may contain high amounts of alcohol and may lead to vomiting if taken with disulfiram (Antabuse) or metronidazole (Flagyl).

- An early study suggests that wild yam may interfere with the body's ability to control levels of the reproductive hormone progesterone. Progesterone is a key ingredient in some hormone replacement and birth control pills. There are reports that some wild yam products may be tainted with artificial progesterone. Women taking birth control pills or hormone replacement therapy should speak with a licensed healthcare provider before taking wild yam.

- Wild yam may also interact with steroids, although clinical evidence is lacking.

Interactions with Herbs and Dietary Supplements

- It is not clear whether *Dioscorea villosa* (wild yam) lowers blood sugar levels. Although dioscoretine, produced by the related species *Dioscorea dumentorum* (bitter or African yam), has been shown to lower blood sugar, this reaction has not been seen with *Dioscorea villosa* and has not been reported in humans. Nonetheless, caution is advised when using herbs or supplements that may also lower blood glucose. Blood glucose levels may require monitoring, and doses may need adjustment.

- Diosgenin, thought to be the active substance in wild yam, has been found in animals to reduce absorption of cholesterol from the intestine and to lower total cholesterol levels in the blood. Studies in humans show no change in the total amount of cholesterol in the blood, although the amounts of specific types of cholesterol in the blood may be changed; low-density lipoprotein (LDL, or "bad cholesterol") and triglycerides may be lowered and high-density lipoprotein (HDL, or "good cholesterol") appears to be increased.

- In an early study, a wild yam preparation was reported to block the body's natural production of progesterone. However, this finding was not supported by later research. There have been several reports that some wild yam products are tainted with synthetic progesterone. Because wild yam may contain progesterone-like chemicals, the effects of other agents believed to have hormone-like properties, in particular those with estrogen-like properties, may be altered.

- Wild yam may also interact with potassium, vitamin C, or steroids, although clinical evidence is lacking.

For a complete list of references, please visit www.naturalstandard.com.

W

Willow bark
(Salix spp.)

RELATED TERMS

- Acetylsalicylic acid, aspirin, Assalix, Assplant, basket willow, bay willow, beta-salicin, black willow, brittle willow, cadmium, caffeic acid, crack willow, daphne willow, ecorce de saule (French), ferulic acid, flavonoids, fragilin, glycosides, isosalicin, isosalipurposide, knackweide, laurel willow, lorbeerweide, osier rouge, picein, populin, purple osier, purple osier willow, purple willow, purpurweide, reifweide, rheumakaps, Salicaceae (family), salice (Italian), salicin, salicis cortex, salicortin, salicoylsalicin, salicyl alcohol, salicylate, salicylic acid, salicyluric acid, salidroside, saligenin, salipurposide, *Salix alba, Salix daphnoides, Salix fragilis* L., *Salix pentandra, Salix purpurea* L., sauce (Spanish), syringin, tannins, tremulacin, triandrin, vanillin, violet willow, Weidenrinde (German), white willow, white willow bark, willow, willow tree, willowbark, willowprin.
- **Note:** This review covers salicin-containing species of *Salix,* which includes *Salix alba, Salix fragilis, Salix purpurea,* and *Salix pentandra.*

BACKGROUND

- Willow (*Salix* spp.) is a source of salicin, which is metabolized to salicylic acid in the body. Salicin and salicylic acid are chemical precursors to aspirin (*N*-acetyl salicylic acid), a popular analgesic and antiinflammatory agent. However, the side effects of salicylic acid (unpleasant taste and gastric upset) precluded its widespread use. Aspirin, the acetylated version of salicylic acid, is better tolerated. In the United States, willow bark is used by herbalists as an antipyretic (fever reducer), a mild analgesic (pain reliever), and an anti-inflammatory. There is currently strong scientific evidence that willow bark is effective for osteoarthritis and lower back pain. Early study suggests that willow bark extracts may not be helpful for rheumatoid arthritis, but further study is warranted to confirm these recommendations. Taking willow bark may increase the risk of bleeding; however, this risk may be less than taking aspirin.
- Several countries in Europe have approved willow bark for pain and inflammatory disorders. The German Commission E has approved willow bark for fever, rheumatic ailments, and headaches. The British Herbal Compendium indicates that willow bark can be used for rheumatic and arthritic conditions, and fever associated with cold and influenza. In France, willow bark has been approved as an analgesic to treat headache and toothache pain, as well as painful articular (joint) conditions, tendonitis, and sprains. The European Scientific Cooperative on Phytotherapy (ESCOP) has approved willow bark extract for the treatment of fever, pain, and mild rheumatic complaints.

EVIDENCE

Uses Based on Scientific Evidence	Grade
Osteoarthritis Willow bark is a traditional analgesic (pain-relieving) therapy for osteoarthritis. Several studies have confirmed this finding; however, the side effects of salicylic acid (unpleasant taste and gastric upset) precluded its widespread use. Aspirin, the acetylated version of salicylic acid, is better tolerated.	A
Lower Back Pain White willow has been compared to placebo and to cyclooxygenase-2 inhibitors, and many of the studies found willow bark to be as effective or superior to other methods. Cost-effectiveness studies have also been performed between white willow bark and conventional treatment, and found that willow bark was more cost-effective. Additional research would help make a strong recommendation.	B
Headache Willow bark has traditionally been used to treat an array of inflammatory conditions, including headache. One study investigated a salicin topical cream for the treatment and/or prevention of migraine and tension-type headache. Although preliminary evidence is promising, the overall evidence is insufficient to support this use.	C
Rheumatoid arthritis There is good evidence that willow bark may be effective in treating chronic pain from osteoarthritis; however, willow bark extract did not show efficacy in treating rheumatoid arthritis. Additional study is needed to make a firm recommendation.	D

Uses Based on Tradition or Theory

Analgesic (pain reliever), ankylosing spondylitis (arthritis of the spine), anti-inflammatory, antioxidant, antiplatelet, antipyretic (fever reducer), antiseptic, antiviral, cancer, colds, colorectal cancer, connective tissue disorders, coronary artery disease prevention, diabetes, fever, gout (foot inflammation), headache, inflammation, joint inflammation, labor pain, leukemia, malaria, menstrual cramps, myocardial infarction (heart attack), sore throat, sprains, tendonitis, toothache, warts.

DOSING

Adults (18 Years and Older)

- The German Commission E monograph (BGA, Commission E) recommends doses of willow bark extract of 60 to 120 mg of total salicin daily. Clinical studies have used 120 to 240 mg willow bark extract (Assalix) for four weeks to treat lower back pain. For osteoarthritis pain, an effective dose of willow bark extract has been reported as 1,360 to 2,160 mg (containing 240 mg of salicin) daily for 2 weeks.

Children (Younger than 18 Years)

- There is insufficient evidence to recommend a dose for willow bark in children. Because of the potential for Reye's syndrome from salicylates, children with influenza, varicella (chickenpox), or any suspected viral infection should avoid willow bark.

SAFETY
Allergies

- Avoid in people with a known allergy or hypersensitivity to aspirin, willow bark (*Salix* species), or any of its constituents, including salicylates. Symptoms of allergy may include swollen eyes, pruritus (itching), eczema, anaphylaxis, cough, hoarseness, and dysphonia (abnormal voice).

Side Effects and Warnings

- Willow bark extract has been reported to cause various gastrointestinal problems, headaches, and allergic reactions. Plants containing salicylates have a very bitter taste, so willow bark tea may be unpalatable (unpleasant) for most patients, particularly for children.
- Side effects of willow bark may include blood pressure instability, edema (swelling), rash, hypertriglyceridemia (an excess of triglycerides in the blood), diarrhea, heartburn, vomiting, and dyspepsia (upset stomach). Willow bark may also lead to hyperuricemia (high levels of uric acid in the blood), which may precipitate an attack of gout in susceptible patients. Willow bark may cause hepatic dysfunction, dizziness, fatigue, swollen eyes, bronchospam, papillary necrosis, or headaches.
- Although not well studied in humans, combination products containing willow may cause acute weakness, hematemesis (blood in the vomit), melena (black stools), abdominal pain, pale mucous membranes, and panhypoproteinemia (low levels of protein in the blood), indicating severe gastrointestinal bleeding.
- The salicylates present in willow bark may also impair platelet function, resulting in an increased bleeding time. However, daily consumption of salicis cortex extract is thought to affect platelet aggregation to a far lesser extent than acetylsalicylate. Caution is advised in patients with bleeding disorders or those taking drugs that may increase the risk of bleeding. Dosing adjustments may be necessary.

Pregnancy and Breastfeeding

- Willow bark is not recommended in pregnant or breastfeeding women because of a lack of available scientific evidence. Salicylates are listed as a pregnancy category D; there is positive evidence of human fetal risk with use. Salicylates in breast milk may cause rash in breastfed babies.

INTERACTIONS
Interactions with Drugs

- Use of acetazolamide and salicylates may cause lethargy, incontinence, and confusion. Caution is advised in patients taking acetazolamide, a carbonic anhydrase inhibitor, which is often used in treating glaucoma or acute mountain sickness. Taking carbonic anhydrase inhibitors with willow bark may increase the therapeutic and toxic effects of both the carbonic anhydrase inhibitor and the salicylate.
- The combination of salicin, which is found in willow bark, and alcohol may increase the risk of gastrointestinal bleeding and gastritis.

- Salicis cortex extract may increase the risk of bleeding when taken with drugs that increase the risk of bleeding. Some examples include aspirin, anticoagulants (blood thinners) such as warfarin (Coumadin) or heparin, anti-platelet drugs such as clopidogrel (Plavix), and non-steroidal anti-inflammatory drugs (NSAIDS) such as ibuprofen (Motrin, Advil) or naproxen (Naprosyn, Aleve). Willow bark may also have anti-inflammatory effects. When willow bark is taken in combination with sulfinpyrazone, it may theoretically result in additive anti-platelet effects, which may increase bleeding time.
- Willow bark extract may induce hypertriglyceridemia (excess of triglycerides in the blood) or cause blood pressure instability. Patients taking blood pressure medications should consult with a qualified healthcare professional, including a pharmacist. Monitoring may be necessary. Theoretically, the concomitant use of willow bark with diuretics reduces diuretic effects and may enhance the risk for salicylic acid toxicity.
- Theoretically, the concomitant use of diuretics with willow bark may reduce the effectiveness of diuretics and may enhance the risk for salicylic acid toxicity. White willow may also decrease the renal (kidney) excretion of methotrexate resulting in toxic levels due to its salicin content.
- Theoretically, the concomitant use of phenytoin (Dilantin) with willow bark's salicylates may increase the Dilantin levels in the blood, resulting in toxicity.
- Theoretically, the concomitant use of probenecid with willow bark may impair the effectiveness of probenecid.
- Because of the plasma protein-binding salicylate component of white willow bark, some other plasma protein-bound drugs may be displaced, possibly resulting in altered drug levels. Consult with a qualified healthcare professional, including a pharmacist, for a full list of these agents.
- Willow bark plus spironolactone may result in antagonistic or additive effects.
- Theoretically, the concomitant use of sulfonylureas with willow bark may increase the effect of sulfonylureas, possibly increasing the side effects and toxicity.
- Theoretically, white willow bark may impair the effectiveness of valproic acid.

Interactions with Herbs and Dietary Supplements

- Willow bark extract may induce hypertriglyceridemia (excess of triglycerides in the blood) or cause blood pressure instability. Patients taking herbs and supplements that affect blood pressure or cholesterol should use willow bark cautiously.
- Willow bark may be contaminated with high levels of cadmium, which may increase concentrations of cadmium in the body. Consumers should select tested brands to avoid using contaminated products.
- Theoretically, the concomitant use of willow bark with diuretic herbs or supplements may reduce diuretic effects and may enhance the risk for salicylic acid toxicity. Consult with a qualified healthcare professional, including a pharmacist, before combining therapies.
- Willow bark may increase the risk of bleeding when taken with herbs and supplements that are believed to increase the risk of bleeding. Multiple cases of bleeding have been reported with the use of *Ginkgo biloba* and fewer cases

W

with garlic and saw palmetto. Numerous other agents may theoretically increase the risk of bleeding, although this has not been proven in most cases.

- Willow bark may have anti-inflammatory effects and may interact positively with guaiacum resin, black cohosh, sarsaparilla, and poplar bark to reduce chronic arthritic pain symptoms.

- The concomitant administration of tannin-containing herbs or supplements may result in the malabsorption of salicylic acid.

For a complete list of references, please visit www.naturalstandard.com.

Witch hazel
(Hamamelis virginiana)

RELATED TERMS

- Aldehydes, aliphatic alcohols, catechins, epicatechin, epigallo-catechin, flavone aglycones, gallate, gallic acid, gallocatechin, galloylhamameloses, Hamamelidaceae (family), *Hamamelis japonica, Hamamelis mollis,* hamamelis ointment, *Hamamelis vernalis, Hamamelis virginiana,* hamamelitannin, hamame-lose, kaempferol, monoterpenoids, phenolic acids, phenylpro-panoids, polymeric proanthocyanidins, polysaccharides, proanthocyanidin fractions, proanthocyanidins, Prrikweg gel, quercetin, safrole, sesquiterpenoids, snapping hazel, snapping tobacco wood, spotted elder, tannin, tincture of witch hazel, volatile fractions, winter bloom, winterbloom, witchazel, witch hazel distillate, witch hazel extract.

BACKGROUND

- Witch hazel *(Hamamelis virginiana)* is a flowering shrub native to Eastern North America. Other related species exist in North America, Asia, and Europe. Witch hazel has tradi-tionally been used as a facial cleanser/toner and for the treatment of skin irritations, bruises, hemorrhoids, and to stop bleeding.
- Preliminary research has shown that the leaves, stems, and bark of witch hazel contain compounds that may have astringent, anti-irritant, antioxidant, and antiinflammatory properties.
- Although witch hazel is widely available and has been used for a variety of medical conditions, there is currently little human evidence supporting the comparative effectiveness of witch hazel in many of these conditions.

EVIDENCE

Uses Based on Scientific evidence	Grade
Eczema Based on clinical research witch hazel was less effective than hydrocortisone cream, and no more effective than a placebo in relieving inflammation associated with atopic eczema.	C
Hemorrhoids Witch hazel is a common ingredient in over-the-counter hemorrhoid preparations for the skin; how-ever, clinical research evaluating the effectiveness for this indication is currently lacking.	C
Insect Bites A homeopathic formulation containing an extract of witch hazel and tinctures of other botanicals was studied for its effects in relieving redness and itching associated with mosquito bites. According to study results, the formulation did not provide effective relief from mosquito bite symptoms. However, because of the lack of information, the effectiveness of this use remains unclear.	C

Perineal Discomfort after Childbirth Witch hazel has a long history of use for treating inflammation and hemorrhage when applied to the skin. Its use to reduce perineal discomfort associated with childbirth requires well-designed human study before recommendations can be made.	C
Skin Irritation (Minor/Pediatric Patients) Although witch hazel has been commonly used to relieve minor skin irritations, there are few human studies evaluating its use for this purpose, especially in children. Witch hazel as an oil-based formulation may be safe and well tolerated when applied to the skin in children with minor skin irritations. High-qual-ity human research is needed for a conclusion to be made.	C
Ultraviolet Light Skin Damage Witch hazel has a long history of use for treating skin irritations. Human study evaluating the effects of witch hazel formulations applied to the skin have demonstrated some antiinflammatory effects. Until better quality studies are conducted, the efficacy of witch hazel for this indication cannot be determined.	C
Varicose Veins Witch hazel has been studied for the treatment of varicose veins and improving venous tone. Additional research is needed in this area.	C

W

Uses Based on Tradition or Theory
Abnormal menstrual bleeding, acne, anti-aging, anti-inflammatory, antibacterial, antioxidant, anxiety, athlete's foot, bruising, burns, cancer prevention, circulatory disorders, colds, colitis, cosmetic uses, dermatitis, diarrhea, edema, eye disorders, fevers, headache, hemorrhage, herpes simplex virus, high blood sugar/glucose intolerance, itching, pain, gum disease, poison ivy, psoriasis, seborrheic dermatitis, skin rash, tuberculosis, vaginal dryness, venereal disease, vomiting, wrinkle prevention.

DOSING

Adults (18 Years and Older)

- Witch hazel has been used on the skin as an astringent, for first aid, facial cleansing, and inflammatory topical condi-tions in the following forms: compress, steam distillate (undiluted or diluted with water), poultice, gargle or mouthwash, salve, tincture, and fluid extract. Witch hazel suppositories, prepared with leaves or bark of witch hazel in combination with cocoa butter, have been used rectally or vaginally. Witch hazel can also be applied to toilet paper to wipe the anal area.

- For the treatment of moderately severe atopic eczema, 5.35 g of hamamelis distillate with 0.64 mg of ketone per 100 g was used for 14 days.
- For skin damage induced by ultraviolet (UV) light, the following single doses were used: 0.64 mg or 2.56 mg of witch hazel with ketone per 100 g; pH5 Eucerin Aftersun Lotion with 10% witch hazel; and 10% witch hazel distillate.

Children (Younger than 18 Years)

- For minor skin injuries/irritation, an oil-based witch hazel preparation was applied to the skin in a thin layer several times daily.

SAFETY
Allergies

- Avoid with a known allergy or sensitivity to witch hazel.

Side Effects and Warnings

- Witch hazel is recommended for use on the skin only. If redness or burning of the skin after use of witch hazel occurs, it is recommended to dilute with water. A healthcare provider should be contacted if symptoms of diarrhea or constipation persist while using witch hazel.
- Use with caution in patients with liver or kidney disorders, as witch hazel may potentially cause damage to these organs when taken by mouth in large doses.
- Witch hazel may lower blood sugar levels. Caution is advised in patients with diabetes or hypoglycemia, and in those taking drugs, herbs, or supplements that affect blood sugar. Blood glucose levels may need to be monitored by a qualified healthcare professional, including a pharmacist, and medication adjustments may be necessary.
- Use with caution in children, because of limited evidence of safety. In a study of children 27 months to 11 years of age with minor skin irritations, treatment with an oil-based witch hazel preparation was well tolerated.

Pregnancy and Breastfeeding

- Avoid in women who are pregnant or breastfeeding, because of a lack of safety evidence.

INTERACTIONS
Interactions with Drugs

- Witch hazel may lower blood sugar levels. Caution is advised when using medications that may also lower blood sugar levels. Patients taking drugs for diabetes by mouth or insulin should be monitored closely by a qualified healthcare professional, including a pharmacist. Medication adjustments may be necessary.
- Witch hazel may add to the effects of antibiotic, antifungal, antiinflammatory, antiviral, and antiulcer drugs.

Interactions with Herbs and Dietary Supplements

- Witch hazel may lower blood sugar levels. Caution is advised when using herbs or supplements that may also lower blood sugar levels. Blood glucose levels may require monitoring, and doses may need adjustment.
- Witch hazel may add to the effects of anti-inflammatory, antibacterial, antifungal, antiviral, antioxidant, antiulcer, or tannin-containing herbs and supplements.

For a complete list of references, please visit www.naturalstandard.com.

Yarrow
(Achillea millefolium)

RELATED TERMS

- *Achillea millefolium*, arrowroot, Asteraceae (family), bad man's plaything, carpenter's weed, Compositae (family), death flower, devil's nettle, eerie, field hops, gearwe, hundred leaved grass, knight's milefoil, knyghten, milefolium, milfoil, millefoil, noble yarrow, nosebleed, nosebleed plant, old man's mustard, old man's pepper, polyacetylenes, sanguinary, sesquiterpene lactones, seven year's love, snake's grass, soldier, soldier's woundwort, stanch weed, thousand seal, woundwort, yarroway, yerw.

BACKGROUND

- Yarrow *(Achillea millefolium)* has a long history as an herbal remedy applied to the skin for wounds, cuts, and abrasions. The genus name *Achillea* is derived from the mythical Greek character, Achilles, who reportedly carried it with his army to treat battle wounds. Dried yarrow stalks are used as a randomizing agent in I Ching divination.
- Currently, there is a lack of research investigating yarrow. Although a laboratory study demonstrated yarrow's antibacterial effects, one poor-quality study using an herbal combination of yarrow, juniper, and nettle did not find any benefit on plaque or gingivitis inhibition.

EVIDENCE

Uses Based on Scientific Evidence	Grade
Plaque/Gingivitis Based on laboratory research, yarrow grass water extract showed antibacterial effects on *Staphylococcus aureus*. However, clinical research using a combination formula (including yarrow, juniper, and nettle) found no effect on gingivitis or plaque inhibition. Additional human study is needed in this area.	C

Uses Based on Tradition or Theory
Abortifacient (induces abortion), antibacterial, anti-inflammatory, bleeding, blood clots, blood purifier, catarrh, colds, chicken pox, contraceptive, cosmetic uses, cystitis, diarrhea, diabetes, digestion, dyspepsia (upset stomach), eczema, emmenagogue (induces menstruation), fever, hypertension (high blood pressure), insect repellant, measles, piles (hemorrhoids), smallpox, stomach sickness, thrombosis (blood clots), toothache, ulcers, urinary tract health (antiseptic), varicose veins, vision.

DOSING
Adults (18 Years and Older)

- There is insufficient evidence to recommend a dose for yarrow in adults. A rinse with 10 ml of mouthwash twice a day for a period of three months as been studied in human volunteers; however, the rinse did not show any beneficial effects on plaque growth and gingival health.

Children (Younger than 18 Years)

- There is insufficient evidence to recommend a dose for yarrow in children.

SAFETY
Allergies

- Avoid in people with a known allergy or hypersensitivity to yarrow *(Achillea millefolium)*, its constituents, or members of the Compositae/Asteraceae family. Cases of allergic contact dermatitis have been described since 1899. There have been reports of occupational asthma and atopic dermatitis from dried yarrow flowers. Yarrow contains sesquiterpene lactones and is often used in patch testing for allergies. Potential side effects of allergy may include skin irritation or light sensitivity.
- Cross-reactions between chrysanthemum and yarrow have been reported, and sesquiterpene lactones are thought to be the cause of the cross-reaction and sensitization.

Side Effects and Warnings

- There is limited high-quality evidence available describing the adverse effects of yarrow. Yarrow may cause atopic dermatitis or urticaria (hives) due to its sesquiterpene lactone content. Yarrow may also cause skin irritation or light sensitivity. Use cautiously in patients with photosensitivity.
- Use cautiously in patients who are pregnant or planning to become pregnant, based on animal research showing reduced fetal weight and increased placental weight. Yarrow has traditionally been used as an abortifacient (induces abortion), emmenagogue (induces menstruation), contraceptive, and for stimulating uterine contractions.

Pregnancy and Breastfeeding

- Yarrow is not recommended in pregnant or breastfeeding women, as it has traditionally been used as an abortifacient (induces abortion), emmenagogue (induces menstruation), contraceptive, and for stimulating uterine contractions.

INTERACTIONS
Interactions with Drugs

- Based on its coumarin content, yarrow may increase the risk of bleeding when taken with drugs that increase the risk of bleeding. Some examples include aspirin, anticoagulants (blood thinners) such as warfarin (Coumadin) or heparin, anti-platelet drugs such as clopidogrel (Plavix), and non-steroidal anti-inflammatory drugs (NSAIDs) such as ibuprofen (Motrin, Advil) or naproxen (Naprosyn, Aleve).
- Yarrow may interfere with blood pressure medications.
- Potential side effects of yarrow allergy may include phytodermatitis, including irritant plant dermatitis, phototoxic and photo-allergic dermatitis, allergic dermatitis, and airborne contact dermatitis. Caution is advised when taking other photosensitizing agents, as side effects may increase.

Y

Interactions with Herbs and Dietary Supplements

- Based on its coumarin content, yarrow may increase the risk of bleeding when taken with herbs and supplement that are believed to increase the risk of bleeding. Multiple cases of bleeding have been reported with the use of *Ginkgo biloba* and fewer cases with garlic and saw palmetto. Numerous other agents may theoretically increase the risk of bleeding, although this has not been proven in most cases.

- Yarrow may interfere with blood pressure agents.
- Potential side effects of yarrow allergy may include phyto-dermatitis, including irritant plant dermatitis, phototoxic and photo-allergic dermatitis, allergic dermatitis, and airborne contact dermatitis. Caution is advised when taking other photosensitizing agents, such as St. John's wort, as side effects may increase.

For a complete list of references, please visit www.naturalstandard.com.

Yellow dock
(Rumex crispus)

RELATED TERMS

- Curled dock, curley dock, curly dock, Polygonaceae (family), *Rumex crispus*, *Rumex obtusifolius*, yellow dock root.

BACKGROUND

- Yellow dock is often used to help "strengthen" the blood; however, very few studies have been conducted to confirm this traditional use.
- Yellow dock is one of the original plants in the Native American anticancer herbal formula now known as Essiac. In some versions of Essiac, yellow dock is substituted for the sheep's sorrel.
- The roots have been taken internally to build healthy blood, protect the liver, or act as an antifungal or laxative. As a seed tea, yellow dock may heal mouth sores and help diarrhea. Externally, yellow dock has been used to dissolve lumps and as an antitumor and antifungal. Yellow dock root (herb and salad green) is an astringent that has been banned in Canada.

EVIDENCE

Uses Based on Scientific Evidence

No available studies qualify for inclusion in the evidence table.

Uses Based on Tradition or Theory

Acne, anemia, antifungal, anorexia, arthritis, choleretic (bile flow stimulant), blood purifier (tonic), cancer, candidal infection (rash), chronic fatigue syndrome, common cold, constipation, cramps, detoxification, diarrhea, energy booster, exhaustion, hepatitis, high cholesterol, inflammatory skin disorders (eczema, psoriasis), laxative, lymphatic disorders, menopause, mouth sores, oral hygiene, premenstrual syndrome (PMS), skin conditions (dark circles under the eyes), tonic (liver).

DOSING

Adults (18 Years and Older)

- There is insufficient evidence to recommend a dose for yellow dock in adults. Herbalists have recommended the roots and seeds daily for up to 12 months. As a tincture of the fresh roots, 10 to 60 drops has been used (20 drops, two or three times a day). A fresh root vinegar preparation (1 to 2 tbsp or 30 mg) has also been used. Based on expert opinion, no more than 1 cup (250 mg) of the dried seed tea should be taken per day.

Children (Younger than 18 Years)

- There is insufficient evidence to recommend a dose for yellow dock in children.

SAFETY

Allergies

- Avoid in people with a known allergy or hypersensitivity to yellow dock or its constituents. People who are allergic to ragweed pollen may also be allergic to yellow dock pollen.

Side Effects and Warnings

- There are very few available reports on the safety of yellow dock. A report exists of a fatal poisoning, with liver and kidney poisoning, after the consumption of large quantities of the leaves (several hundred grams). Use cautiously in patients with compromised renal (kidney) or hepatic (liver) function.
- Yellow dock contains anthraquinones, which act as laxatives. Anthraquinone laxative abuse may be associated with colon cancer.

Pregnancy and Breastfeeding

- Yellow dock is not recommended in pregnant or breastfeeding women because of a lack of available scientific evidence. Based on expert opinion, pregnant women should not ingest harsh laxatives. Yellow dock is thought to fall into this category, perhaps because of the anthraquinone content. However, other herbal experts have recommended yellow dock in pregnancy because of its iron content, although this has not been proven in clinical trials.

INTERACTIONS

Interactions with Drugs

- Yellow dock may have estrogenic activity, although more research is needed to clarify the exact mechanism of action. Caution is advised when taking drugs with estogenic activity because of possible additive effects.
- A fatal poisoning from yellow dock *(Rumex crispus)* occurred after ingestion of a large quantity of the fresh leaves as a salad vegetable. Pathologic findings included liver and kidney damage, which may have been caused by the tannins found in the leaves. Caution is advised in patients with liver or kidney problems, or in patients who are taking drugs that affect the liver or kidneys.
- Yellow dock contains anthraquinones. In theory, yellow dock may have additive effects with other laxative agents.
- Yellow dock contains tannins and may increase the risk of side effects when taken with other agents that contain tannins.

Interactions with Herbs and Dietary Supplements

- A fatal poisoning from yellow dock *(Rumex crispus)* occurred after ingestion of a large quantity of the fresh leaves as a salad vegetable. Pathologic findings included liver and kidney damage, which may have been caused by the tannins found in the leaves. Caution is advised in patients with liver or kidney problems, or in patients who are taking herbs or supplements that affect the liver or kidneys.
- Yellow dock contains anthraquinones. In theory, yellow dock may have additive effects with other laxative agents.
- Yellow dock may have estrogenic activity, although more research is needed to clarify the exact mechanism of action. Caution is advised when taking herbs or supplements with estogenic activity because of possible additive effects.
- Yellow dock contains tannins and may increase the risk of side effects when taken with other herbs or supplements that contain tannins.

For a complete list of references, please visit www.naturalstandard.com.

Y

Yerba santa
(Eriodictyon californicum)

RELATED TERMS

- Consumptive's weed, bear's weed, eriodictyol, *Eriodictyon californicum*, *Eriodictyon glutinosum*, gum bush, holy herb, mountain balm, sacred herb, tarweed, Wigandia californicum.
- Note: Not to be confused with other herbs that share the same common name(s). For example, the common name *mountain balm* is also used for *Ceanothus velutinus*, *Satureja chandleri*, and *Calamintha nepeta*. The common name *consumptive's weed* is associated with three different *Eriodictyon* species. The common name *gum bush* is also associated with several different *Eriodictyon* species. The common name *bear's weed* is also used for *Arctostaphylos uva-ursi*. The common name *tarweed* is associated with many species of *Hemizonia* and *Madia*. The common name *holy herb* is used for marijuana (*Cannabis sativa*), hyssop (*Sorghum vulgare*), basil (*Ocimum basilicum*), verbena (*Verbena officinalis*) and aloe (*Aloe barbadensis*). The common name *sacred herb* is used for marijuana and tobacco (*Nicotiana tabacum*).

BACKGROUND

- Chumash Indians and other California Indians have used yerba santa (*Eriodictyon californicum*) and other related species (*Eriodictyon crassifolium*, *Eriodictyon trichocalyx*) for many centuries in the treatment of pulmonary (lung) conditions, saliva production, and to stop bleeding of minor cuts and scrapes.
- In the United States and Britain, *Eriodictyon californicum* was formerly used for conditions including influenza, bacterial pneumonia, asthma, bronchitis, and tuberculosis starting in the late 1800s until the 1960s (when drug regulations became more stringent around proof of efficacy). Subsequently, the extracts remained GRAS (Generally Regarded as Safe) as a flavor for foods, beers, and pharmaceuticals (such as to hide the bitterness of quinine). *Eriodictyon* plant extracts have also been used in cosmetics.
- *Eriodictyon* species contain flavones with free radical scavenging (antioxidant) properties, and have therefore been proposed as being beneficial for a number of health conditions. However, there is little scientific study of yerba santa in humans, and effectiveness has not been demonstrated for any specific condition.

EVIDENCE

Uses Based on Scientific Evidence	Grade
Pulmonary Conditions (Lung Conditions) There is an extensive clinical history of use of *Eriodictyon* extracts in pulmonary conditions such as influenza, bacterial pneumonia, asthma, bronchitis, and tuberculosis. However, there is a lack of clinical research to support this use.	C

Uses Based on Tradition or Theory

Allergies, antibacterial, antifungal, anti-inflammatory, anti-parasitic, antioxidant, antiviral, arthritis, asthma, blood coagulation disorders, cancer, cosmetics, dry mouth, excipient (inactive ingredient) for drug delivery, food flavoring, hypercholesterolemia (high cholesterol), hypertension (high blood pressure), malaria, saliva production, skin scrapes, smooth muscle relaxant, tuberculosis, urinary tract infections.

DOSING

Adults (18 Years and Older)

- There is insufficient evidence to recommend a dose for yerba santa in adults. Traditionally, 1 to 2 ml of fluid extract has been taken by mouth with a spoon every 3 to 4 hours for no more than ten days.
- Poultices have been made by crushing 0.2 kg of the leaves in 1,000 ml of water. The leaves have been used traditionally as a treatment for pulmonary (lung) congestion by placing the slightly wet leaves on the chest. The poultice is usually used once or twice every day for up to two weeks.

Children (Younger than 18 Years)

- There is insufficient evidence to recommend a dose for yerba santa in children. Traditionally, 1 ml of the alcohol extract has been used in children. Caution is warranted in children because of the presence of ethanol. Poultices have also been applied on the skin.

SAFETY

Allergies

- Avoid in people with a known allergy or hypersensitivity to *Eriodictyon* species.

Side Effects and Warnings

- There are no published reports of toxicity clearly attributable to yerba santa (*Eriodictyon californicum*), although this herb has been used for centuries by California Indians with a belief in its safety. However, there are no available scientific evaluations of toxicity or safety.

Pregnancy and Breastfeeding

- Yerba santa is not recommended in pregnant or breastfeeding women because of a lack of available scientific evidence.

INTERACTIONS

Interactions with Drugs

- The flavonoids homoeriodictyol and eriodictyol found in yerba santa may interfere with the way the body processes certain drugs using the liver's cytochrome P450 enzyme system. As a result, the levels of these drugs may be increased in the blood and may cause increased effects or potentially serious adverse reactions. Patients using any medications should check the package insert and speak with a qualified healthcare professional, including a pharmacist, about possible interactions.

Interactions with Herbs and Dietary Supplements

- The flavonoids homoeriodictyol and eriodictyol found in yerba santa may interfere with the way the body processes certain herbs or supplements using the liver's cytochrome P450 enzyme system. As a result, the levels of other herbs or supplements may become too high in the blood. It may also alter the effects that other herbs or supplements possibly have on the P450 system.

For a complete list of references, please visit www.naturalstandard.com.

Y

Yew

(Taxus spp.)

RELATED TERMS

- Chinwood, common yew, Coniferae (family), docetaxel, Eibe (German), euar (Manx), European yew, hagina (Basque), idegran (Swedish), if (French), Himalayan yew, Irish yew, iubhar (Scottish Gaelic), iúr (Irish), ivenenn (Breton), marjakuusi (Finnish), Japanese yew, Pacific yew, paclitaxel, phloroglucindimethylether (3,5-dimethoxyphenol), porsukagaci (Turkish), snottle berries, snotty grogs, *T. bourcieri* Carrière, taks (Danish), tasso (Italian), Taxaceae (family), taxine, taxis (Dutch), Taxol, *Taxomyces andreanae*, Taxotere, *Taxus baccata* L., *Taxus brevifolia*, *Taxus canadensis*, *Taxus cuspidata*, *Taxus wallichiana*, Taxuspine C., tejo (Spanish), tisa (Romanian), tis (Czech), western yew, ywen (Welsh), ywenn (Cornish).

BACKGROUND

- There are several species of yew, including the English or European yew *(Taxus baccata)*, Pacific yew *(Taxus brevifolia)*, and Japanese yew *(Taxus cuspidata)*. All species are considered poisonous; however, there is some debate about the medicinal value of the fruits (arils). The name *taxus* may be related to the Greek *toxon* (bow) and *toxicon* (the poison with which the arrowheads were dressed).
- Traditionally, the fruit of yew has been used as an antitussive (preventing or relieving cough), menstrual stimulant, abortifacient (induces abortion), diuretic, and laxative. It is reported that the Native Americans used yew extracts to treat rheumatism, fever, and arthritis.
- Paclitaxel (Taxol) was isolated from the bark of the Pacific yew tree *(Taxus brevifolia)* as early as 1971 and is now approved by the U.S. Food and Drug Administration (FDA). Since 1971, Taxol has been used as an antitumor drug in clinical trials run by the U.S. National Cancer Institute and has been hailed as one of the most significant advances in cancer chemotherapy in recent history. Since 1990, clinical trials using Taxol have succeeded in treating advanced ovarian and breast cancers.

EVIDENCE

Uses Based on Scientific Evidence

No available studies qualify for inclusion in the evidence table.

Uses Based on Tradition or Theory

Abortifacient (induces abortion), antispasmodic (bark), antitussive (cough suppressing), arthritis, astringent, blood clot treatment, bowel diseases, breast cancer, cancer, cardiovascular health, childbirth (expelling afterbirth), colds, diaphoretic (promotes sweating), diphtheria, diuretic, emmenagogue (menstrual stimulant), epilepsy, eruptions, fevers, gout (foot inflammation), headache, laxative, leukemia, liver conditions, lung cancer, lung conditions, malignant melanoma, nerve damage, neuralgia (nerve pain), ovarian cancer, pain, rabies, rheumatism, scurvy, snakebites, tonsillitis, urinary tract infection, vision enhancement, worms, wound healing.

DOSING

Adults (18 Years and Older)

- There is insufficient evidence to recommend a dose for yew, and use in adults is not recommended.

Children (Younger than 18 Years)

- There is insufficient evidence to recommend a dose for yew, and use in children is not recommended. One chewed berry may be lethal.

SAFETY

Allergies

- Avoid in people with a known allergy or hypersensitivity to yew. There has been at least one report of anaphylaxis following yew *(Taxus)* needle ingestion.

Side Effects and Warnings

- There is little documentation of adverse effects. However, of those reported, the most common adverse effects include dermal rash, tachycardia (increased heart rate), bradycardia (decreased heart rate), arrhythmia (altered heart rhythm), upset stomach, and neurologic effects. Death secondary to cardiac arrest has also been reported. There is mixed evidence regarding the prevalence of such effects, and caution is advised. Use berries (fruits, arils) with caution.
- Pale and cyanotic skin and other skin effects have been reported. Queasiness, dry mouth, vomiting, severe abdominal pain, dyspepsia, and reddening of the lips have also been associated with yew. *Taxus baccata* L. may also cause gastric lavage.
- Although not well studied, yew may cause hypotension (low blood pressure), nasal allergy, mydriasis (dilation of the pupil), or adverse effects on the liver or kidneys. Vertigo, weakness, nervousness, unconsciousness, trembling, discoordination, artificial respiration, and coma may also occur.

Pregnancy and Breastfeeding

- Yew is not recommended in pregnant or breastfeeding women because of a lack of available evidence. Caution is advised as yew has traditionally been used to induce abortion.

INTERACTIONS

Interactions with Drugs

- Japanese yew, *Taxus cuspidata*, has been shown to increase the cellular accumulation of vincristine in multidrug-resistant tumor cells. Patients taking anti-cancer drugs should use yew or its derivative product, Taxol, with caution.
- Yew may interact with calcium channel blockers. Caution is advised.

- Although not well studied, yew may lower blood pressure. Patients taking blood pressure–lowering medications should consult with a qualified healthcare professional, including a pharmacist.

Interactions with Herbs and Dietary Supplements

- Japanese yew, *Taxus cuspidata*, has been shown to increase the cellular accumulation of vincristine in multidrug-resistant tumor cells. Patients taking herbs or supplements for cancer should use yew or its derivative product, Taxol, with caution.
- Although not well studied, yew may lower blood pressure. Patients taking blood pressure–lowering herbs and supplements should consult with a qualified healthcare professional, including a pharmacist.

For a complete list of references, please visit www.naturalstandard.com.

Yohimbe bark extract
(*Pausinystalia yohimbe*)

RELATED TERMS

- Aphrodien, Corynanthe johimbi, *Corynanthe yohimbi*, corynine, johimbi, Pausinystalia johimbe, *Pausinystalia yohimbe*, quebrachine, Rubiaceae (family), yohimbehe, yohimbehe cortex, yohimbeherinde, yohimbene, yohimbime, yohimbine.

BACKGROUND

- The terms *yohimbine, yohimbine hydrochloride,* and *yohimbe bark extract* are related but not interchangeable. Yohimbine is an active chemical (indole alkaloid) found in the bark of the *Pausinystalia yohimbe* tree. Yohimbine hydrochloride is a standardized form of yohimbine that is available as a prescription drug in the United States and has been shown in clinical studies to be effective in the treatment of male impotence. Yohimbine hydrochloride has also been used for the treatment of sexual side effects caused by some antidepressants (SSRIs), female hyposexual disorder, as a blood pressure–boosting agent in autonomic failure, for xerostomia, and as a probe for noradrenergic activity.

EVIDENCE

Uses Based on Scientific Evidence	Grade
Dry Mouth (Xerostomia) Studies report that yohimbine can increase saliva in animals and humans. Based on these few studies, yohimbine has been used for the treatment of dry mouth caused by medications such as antidepressants. However, yohimbe bark extract may not contain significant amounts of yohimbine and therefore may not have these effects.	C
Erectile Dysfunction (Male Impotence) Yohimbine hydrochloride is a prescription drug that has been shown in multiple clinical trials to effectively treat male impotence. Although yohimbine is present in yohimbe bark extract, levels are variable and often very low. Therefore, although yohimbe bark has been used traditionally to reduce male erectile dysfunction, there is not enough scientific evidence to support this use.	C
Inhibition of Platelet Aggregation Preclinical studies report that yohimbine alkaloid, isolated from yohimbe bark, may inhibit platelet aggregation. Clinical research is not sufficient to support this use.	C
Libido (Women) Yohimbine has been proposed to increase female libido (sexual interest). There is only limited research to support this use.	C

Nervous System Dysfunction (Autonomic Failure) It is theorized that yohimbine may improve orthostatic hypotension (lowering of blood pressure with standing) or other symptoms of autonomic nervous system dysfunction. However, yohimbe bark extract may not contain significant amounts of yohimbine and therefore may not have these proposed effects.	C
Sexual Side Effects of Selective Serotonin Reuptake Inhibitor (SSRI) Antidepressants Yohimbine hydrochloride, a standardized form of yohimbine that is available as a prescription drug in the United States, has been suggested to treat sexual dysfunction due to SSRI antidepressants. However, research in this area is limited, and more research is needed before a recommendation can be made. In addition, yohimbe bark extract may not contain significant amounts of yohimbine and therefore may not have these proposed effects.	C

Uses Based on Tradition or Theory

Alzheimer's disease, anesthetic, angina, aphrodisiac, atherosclerosis, clonidine overdose, cognition, coronary artery disease, cough, depression, diabetic complications, diabetic neuropathy, exhaustion, feebleness, fevers, hallucinogenic, high cholesterol, insomnia, leprosy, low blood pressure, narcolepsy, obesity, panic disorder, Parkinson's disease, postural hypotension, pupil dilator, schizophrenia, syncope.

DOSING

Adults (18 Years and Older)

- The following doses are based on clinical trials of pharmaceutical standardized yohimbine hydrochloride (available by prescription in the United States). No reliable clinical studies are available for administration of yohimbe bark extract. For erectile dysfunction (male impotence), 15 to 42 mg of yohimbine hydrochloride daily in three divided doses (for example, 5.4 to 10 mg three times daily) has been studied. For libido in women, 5.4 mg three times daily of yohimbine hydrochloride has been studied. For sexual side effects caused by antidepressant drugs, 2.7 to 16.2 mg of yohimbine hydrochloride has been studied. For autonomic dysfunction/orthostatic hypotension, 5.4 to 12 mg of daily yohimbine has been studied. For dry mouth (xerostomia), 6 mg three times daily of yohimbine hydrochloride has been studied.

Children (Younger than 18 Years)

- Yohimbe and yohimbine hydrochloride are not recommended for use in children.

SAFETY
Allergies

- In theory, allergy/hypersensitivity to yohimbe, any of its constituents, or yohimbine-containing products may occur.

Side Effects and Warnings

- Yohimbe bark extract is traditionally said to cause occasional skin flushing, piloerection (body hair standing up), painful urination, genital pain, reduced appetite, agitation, dizziness, headache, irritability, nervousness, tremors, or insomnia.
- Multiple adverse effects have been associated with the use of the drug yohimbine hydrochloride, although in recommended doses it is usually tolerated. If adverse effects occur, discontinuing the drug will likely stop the effects. In theory, these same side effects may also occur with the use of yohimbe bark extract, which contains variable (usually low) amounts of yohimbine.
- There are reports of rash, flushing, breathing difficulty, cough, runny nose, nausea, vomiting, increased salivation, diarrhea, increased urinary frequency, kidney failure, muscle aches, and a lupus-like syndrome with the use of yohimbine hydrochloride. Yohimbine has also been associated with tremulousness, insomnia, anxiety, irritability, and excitability. Yohimbine may precipitate panic attacks, anxiety, manic episodes, or psychosis in patients with a history of mental illness.
- In animal research, yohimbine has been associated with increased motor activity and seizures at higher doses. In humans, yohimbine may change the seizure threshold (the likelihood that a seizure will happen in some people) and may cause blood pressure/heart rate increases, fluid retention, chest discomfort, and heart rhythm abnormalities. Higher doses may lower blood pressure. Yohimbine can enter the brain through the bloodstream. Yohimbine may increase the risk of bleeding by altering platelet function, and may dangerously reduce the number of white blood cells (agranulocytosis).
- Symptoms of toxicity from yohimbine can include paralysis, dangerously low blood pressure, heart rhythm abnormalities, heart failure, and death. These same risks theoretically may also exist with yohimbe bark extract, depending on the concentration of yohimbine present and the amount ingested. Beta-blocker drugs such as metoprolol (Lopressor, Toprol) may be protective against yohimbine toxicity.

Pregnancy and Breastfeeding

- Yohimbe should be avoided during pregnancy because it may relax the uterus and may be toxic to the fetus. Yohimbe should be avoided during breastfeeding, because of reports of deaths in children.

INTERACTIONS
Interactions with Drugs

- Multiple drug interactions may occur with the use of yohimbine hydrochloride. In theory, these effects may also apply to yohimbe bark extract, which contains variable (usually low) amounts of yohimbine.
- Based on clinical research, yohimbine has been reported to block the effects of alpha-adrenergic drugs. Yohimbine may increase the effects of drugs that are anti-adrenergic, such as clonidine or guanabenz. Use of yohimbine with central nervous system stimulants may have additive effects. In theory, because of inhibition of monoamine oxidase (MAOI activity), use of yohimbine with drugs like isocarboxazid (Marplan), phenelzine (Nardil), tranylcypromine (Parnate), or linezolid (Zyvox) may produce additive side effects, such as an increased risk of extremely high blood pressure.
- Based on clinical research, use of ethanol (alcohol) with yohimbine may produce an additive effect of increasing intoxication. Based on clinical research, yohimbine may increase pain relief from morphine and may increase or decrease withdrawal symptoms caused by the medication naloxone. According to historical use and animal research, yohimbine may increase the effects of diabetic medications, including insulin, although there is no reliable scientific evidence in this area. Caution is advised when using medications that may lower blood sugar. Patients taking drugs for diabetes by mouth or insulin should be monitored closely by a qualified healthcare provider. Medication adjustments may be necessary.
- Based on clinical research, use of yohimbine with physostigmine in patients with Alzheimer's disease may be associated with anxiety, agitation, restlessness, and chest pain. Use of yohimbine with antihistamines is cautioned, although there is no reliable scientific evidence in this area. The combination of yohimbine with anti-muscarinic agents may result in increased risk of toxicity. In theory, yohimbine may add to the effects of drugs that lower blood pressure.
- In theory, yohimbine may interfere with the way the body processes certain drugs using the liver's cytochrome P450 enzyme system. As a result, levels of these drugs (and yohimbine) in the blood may be altered and may cause increased or decreased effects or potentially serious adverse reactions. Patients using any medications should check the package insert and speak with a qualified healthcare professional or pharmacist about possible interactions.
- Yohimbine may also interact with benzodiazepines (tranquilizers), antibiotics such as linezolid, phenothiazines, and tricyclic antidepressants (TCAs). Patients using any medications should check the package insert and speak with a qualified healthcare professional or pharmacist about possible interactions.

Interactions with Herbs and Dietary Supplements

- Multiple interactions may occur between the drug yohimbine hydrochloride and herbs/supplements. In theory, these effects may also apply to yohimbe bark extract, which contains variable (usually low) amounts of yohimbine.
- In theory, other over-the-counter products containing stimulants, including caffeine, phenylephrine, and phenylpropanolamine (removed from the U.S. market), may lead to additive effects when used in combination with yohimbine. Yohimbine theoretically may interfere with blood pressure control and should be used cautiously with other herbs or supplements that affect blood pressure.
- Because of inhibition of monoamine oxidase, use of yohimbine with herbs/supplements with possible similar properties may produce additive effects, such as an increased risk of dangerously high blood pressure (hypertensive crisis). In theory, caffeine-containing agents such as coffee, tea, cola, guarana, and mate may also increase the risk of hypertensive crisis when taken with yohimbine.
- Yohimbine theoretically may add to the effects of herbs or supplements that may lower blood sugar. Blood glucose levels may require monitoring, and doses may need adjustment.

- In theory, yohimbine may interfere with the way the body processes herbs or supplements using the liver's cytochrome P450 enzyme system. As a result, levels of herbs or supplements (and yohimbine) in the blood may be altered and may cause increased or decreased effects or potentially serious adverse reactions. It may also alter the effects that other herbs or supplements possibly have on the P450 system.
- In theory, yohimbine may also interact with goldenseal or berberine-containing herbs.

For a complete list of references, please visit www.naturalstandard.com.

Yucca
(*Yucca* spp.)

RELATED TERMS

- Adam's needle, Agavaceae (family), alexin, resveratrol, *Yucca aloifolia*, *Yucca gloriosa* L., *Yucca recurvifolia* Salisb., *Yucca schidigera*, yuccaols.

BACKGROUND

- Yucca is the common name for the more than 40 species of perennials in the *Yucca* genus. The plants are well known for their tough, swordlike leaves and a large spike of whitish flowers. They are native to the hot and dry parts of North America, Central America, and the West Indies, although they are popular landscaping plants and can be found worldwide.
- There is insufficient clinical evidence to support the use of yucca for any indication. One clinical study indicates that a blend of *Yucca schidigera* and *Quillaja saponaria* extracts may reduce cholesterol levels in hypercholesterolemic patients. Preliminary studies also indicate that yucca may have antioxidant, antifungal, and anti-inflammatory properties.
- **Note:** Yucca should not be confused with cassava (*Manihot esculenta*), which is commonly known as yucca.

EVIDENCE

Uses Based on Scientific Evidence	Grade
Hypercholesterolemia A blend of partially purified *Yucca schidigera* and *Quillaja saponaria* extracts may reduce cholesterol levels in hypercholesterolemic patients. However, additional research is needed with yucca studied alone.	C

Uses Based on Tradition or Theory
Antifungal, anti-inflammatory, antioxidant, antiviral, cancer.

DOSING

Adults (18 years and older):

- There is insufficient evidence to recommend a dose for yucca.

Children (younger than 18 years):

- There is insufficient evidence to recommend a dose for yucca in children.

SAFETY

Allergies

- Avoid in people with a known allergy or hypersensitivity to yucca (*Yucca schidigera*) or its constituents.

Side Effects and Warnings

- There are very few reports of yucca and its adverse effects. Of the available literature, there is some information on contact urticaria (hives) and allergic rhinitis (hay fever) caused by yucca. Use cautiously in patients taking antihyperlipidemia (cholesterol-lowering) agents.

Pregnancy and Breastfeeding

- Yucca is not recommended in pregnant or breastfeeding women because of a lack of available scientific evidence.

INTERACTIONS

Interactions with Drugs

- Alexin extracted from *Yucca gloriosa* flowers may have a broad spectrum of antifungal activity. Use cautiously when taking yucca with other antifungal agents.
- Yuccaols and resveratrol from yucca may reduce inflammation. Use cautiously when taking yucca with other anti-inflammatory agents.
- Ingestion of a blend of *Yucca schidigera* and *Quillaja saponaria* extract filtrates may decrease total and LDL cholesterol levels in hypercholesterolemic patients. Caution is advised when taking yucca with other cholesterol-lowering agents.
- Although not well studied in humans, yuccaols and resveratrol from yucca may reduce cell proliferation. Caution is advised in patients with cancer and those taking anticancer agents.
- Yucca may have antioxidant activity. Caution is advised when taking yucca with other antioxidant agents.
- Although not well studied in humans, yucca leaf protein isolated from the leaves of *Yucca recurvifolia* Salisb. inhibited herpes simplex virus type 1, herpes simplex virus type 2, and human cytomegalovirus. Use cautiously in patients taking antiviral agents.

Interactions with Herbs and Dietary Supplements

- Alexin extracted from *Yucca gloriosa* flowers may have a broad spectrum of antifungal activity. Use cautiously when taking yucca with other antifungal agents.
- Yuccaols and resveratrol from yucca may reduce inflammation. Use cautiously when taking yucca with other anti-inflammatory herbs or supplements.
- Although not well studied in humans, yuccaols and resveratrol from yucca may reduce cell proliferation. Caution is advised in patients with cancer and in those taking anticancer herbs or supplements.
- Yucca may have antioxidant activity. Caution is advised when taking yucca with other antioxidant herbs or supplements.
- Although not well studied in humans, yucca leaf protein isolated from the leaves of *Yucca recurvifolia* Salisb. inhibited herpes simplex virus type 1, herpes simplex virus type 2, and human cytomegalovirus. Use cautiously in patients taking antiviral herbs or supplements.
- Based on a clinical trial, ingestion of a blend *Yucca schidigera* and *Quillaja saponaria* extract filtrates may decrease total and LDL cholesterol levels of hypercholesterolemic patients. Caution is advised in patients with hypercholesterolemia or hyperlipidemia, and those taking herbs or supplements such as red yeast rice for these conditions.

For a complete list of references, please visit www.naturalstandard.com.

Y

Zinc (Zn)

RELATED TERMS

- Atomic number 30, Indian tin, pewter, polaprezinc, zinc acetate, zinc acexamate, zinc aspartate, zinc carbonate, zinc citrate, zinc chloride, zinc gluconate, zinc methionate, zinc methionine, zinc monomethioine, zinc oxide, zinc picolinate, zinc sulfate ($ZnSO_4$), Zink, ZN, Zn.
- **Brands used in clinical trials**: A-84, Articulin-F, Astra, Curiosin (zinc and hyaluronic acid), Herpigon, Nels Cream, Orazinc, Solvezink, Virudermin Gel, Zeta N, Zicam Nasal Gel, Zincolak, Zincomed, Zineryt, Zinvit-C250.

BACKGROUND

- Zinc has been used since ancient Egyptian times to enhance wound healing, although the usefulness of this approach is only partially confirmed by current clinical evidence.
- Zinc is necessary for the functioning of more than 300 different enzymes and plays a vital role in an enormous number of biological processes. Zinc is a cofactor for the antioxidant enzyme superoxide dismutase (SOD) and is in a number of enzymatic reactions involved in carbohydrate and protein metabolism.
- Its immune-enhancing activities include regulation of T lymphocytes, CD4, natural killer cells, and interleukin II. In addition, zinc has been claimed to possess antiviral activity. It has been shown to play a role in wound healing, especially following burns or surgical incisions. Zinc is necessary for the maturation of sperm and normal fetal development. It is involved in sensory perception (taste, smell, and vision) and controls the release of stored vitamin A from the liver. Within the endocrine system, zinc has been shown to regulate insulin activity and promote the conversion of the thyroid hormone thyroxine to triiodothyronine.
- Based on available scientific evidence, zinc may be effective in the treatment of (childhood) malnutrition, acne vulgaris, peptic ulcers, leg ulcers, infertility, Wilson's disease, herpes, and taste or smell disorders. Zinc has also gained popularity for its use in the prevention of the common cold.
- The role for zinc is controversial in some cases, as the results of published studies provide either contradictory information or the methodological quality of the studies does not allow for a confident conclusion regarding the role of zinc in those diseases.

EVIDENCE

Uses Based on Scientific Evidence	Grade
Diarrhea (Children) Multiple studies in developing countries found that zinc supplementation in malnourished children with acute diarrhea may reduce the severity and duration of diarrhea, especially in children with low zinc levels.	A
Gastric Ulcers The healing process of gastric ulcers may be enhanced through treatment with zinc, although further studies will be needed to determine to what extent zinc may be beneficial for patients with this condition. Most studies report no or few adverse effects associated with its use.	A
Sickle Cell Anemia (Management) There is strong scientific evidence to suggest that zinc may help manage or reduce symptoms of sickle cell anemia. Most of these studies reported increased height, weight, immune system function, and testosterone levels and decreased numbers of crises and sickled cells following zinc treatment.	A
Zinc Deficiency Causes: Zinc deficiency is caused by inadequate intake or absorption, increased zinc excretion, or increased bodily need for zinc. Symptoms: Zinc deficiency symptoms include growth retardation, hair loss, diarrhea, delayed sexual maturation, impotence, eye and skin conditions, and loss of appetite. Additional symptoms may include weight loss, delayed wound healing, taste changes, and mental lethargy. Diagnosis: Zinc can be measured in plasma, red blood cells, white blood cells, and hair.	A
Acne Vulgaris Based on high-quality studies, topical or oral use of zinc seems to be a safe and effective treatment for acne vulgaris; however, some studies report no or negative effects of zinc. Additionally, many studies used combination treatments. Several studies have identified a positive correlation between serum zinc levels and severity of acne, while others did not, and it remains to be determined to what degree internal zinc levels may correlate with the severity of acne.	B
Attention Deficit Hyperactivity Disorder (ADHD) Preliminary studies have shown a correlation between low serum free fatty acids and zinc serum levels in children with attention deficit hyperactivity disorder. Additional studies found that zinc supplements reduced hyperactive, impulsive, and impaired socialization symptoms, but did not reduce attention deficiency symptoms. Zinc supplementation may be a more effective treatment for older children with higher body mass index (BMI) scores.	B
Down's Syndrome In several studies, zinc supplements seemed to counteract hypothyroidism and slightly reduce the number of infections in children with Down syndrome. However, zinc did not seem to improve depressed immune systems. Additional human research is needed before a firm conclusion can be made.	B

Uses Based on Scientific Evidence	Grade
Fungal Infections (Scalp) Evidence from human trials suggests that zinc pyrithione shampoo may be an effective treatment for tinea versicolor fungal infections of the scalp. No side effects were noted.	B
Herpes Simplex Virus Low-quality studies have been conducted to assess the effects of zinc (topical or taken by mouth) on herpes type I or II. Several of these studies used combination treatments or permitted the continued use of other medications, so the exact role of zinc in those studies is unclear. However, the positive results obtained in most trials suggest that zinc may represent a safe and effective alternative treatment for herpes type I and II and should encourage further research into the topic using well-designed studies.	B
High Cholesterol Zinc may improve blood cholesterol levels in hemodialysis patients. There is some evidence that zinc may improve cholesterol ratio of HDL "good cholesterol" versus LDL "bad cholesterol," which would be considered a positive effect.	B
Immune Function Zinc appears to be an essential trace element for the immune system, but research on the effect of zinc supplementation on immune function is scant and mostly focuses on patients with specific diseases. Zinc gluconate appears to have beneficial effects on immune cells. There are relatively few studies that examine zinc levels and the effects of zinc supplementation on the health of the elderly population.	B
Plaque/Gingivitis A few studies have reported significant reduction in plaque accumulation following treatment with zinc rinses and dentifrices. Preliminary research suggests that zinc citrate dentifrice may reduce the severity and occurrence of supragingival calculus formation. However, more well-designed studies are needed to confirm such benefits. More research might help to determine zinc's potential efficacy in other dental applications.	B
Wilson's Disease Wilson's disease is an inherited disorder of copper metabolism characterized by a failure of the liver to excrete copper, which leads to its accumulation in the liver, brain, cornea, and kidney, with resulting chronic degenerative changes. Preliminary research suggests that zinc treatment may be effective in the management of Wilson's disease. Relatively few cases of adverse effects have been reported, including one case report presenting a fatality; however, it is unclear whether or not the death was caused by zinc. Several studies have been conducted by the same authors, resulting in possible bias. More well-	B

designed trials are needed to confirm these preliminary results.

	Grade
Alopecia (Hair Loss) A few studies that examined the efficacy of zinc in treating alopecia report conflicting results.	C
Anorexia Nervosa Reports of zinc's effectiveness in treating symptoms of anorexia nervosa observed in young adults are based on small, low-quality studies, but all agree on the beneficial effects of zinc. Well-designed trials with a larger number of participants are needed to confirm these results.	C
Bad Breath Chewing gum containing zinc or rinsing out the mouth with a solution containing zinc seemed to reduce bad breath (halitosis) in preliminary studies.	C
Beta-Thalassemia (Hereditary Disorder) One small study noted that children with beta-thalassemia who took oral zinc supplements for 1 to 7 years increased in height more than those who did not take zinc. More studies are needed to confirm these findings.	C
Blood Disorders (Aceruloplasminemia) Data from case reports suggest a potential role for zinc supplementation in aceruloplasminemia, a neurodegenerative disease caused by a gene mutation.	C
Boils In one study, patients with recurrent boils (furunculosis) treated with zinc found their furuncles did not reappear. Well-designed clinical trials are needed to confirm this potential benefit.	C
Burns Study results of zinc sulfate supplements given to burn victims to increase healing rate yield mixed results.	C
Chronic Prostatitis (CP) Preliminary studies suggest that zinc supplements taken with antibiotics may be more effective than antibiotics alone in reducing pain, urinary symptoms, quality of life, and maximum urethra closure pressure for patients with chronic prostatitis. Further research is needed to confirm these results.	C
Closed Head Injuries Preliminary poorly designed studies indicate that zinc supplementation may enhance neurological recovery in patients with closed head injuries. Further research is needed to confirm these results.	C
Cognitive Deficits (Children) Preliminary studies indicate that daily supplementation with zinc may be of limited usefulness for improving cognition in lead-exposed schoolchildren. Further research may be warranted in this area.	C

(Continued)

Uses Based on Scientific Evidence	Grade
Common Cold There are conflicting results regarding the effect of zinc formulations in treating duration and severity of common cold symptoms. Although zinc might be beneficial in the treatment of cold symptoms, more studies are needed to clarify which zinc formulations may be most effective, which rhinoviruses are affected by zinc, and if nasal sprays provide a useful alternative application route for zinc treatment. A recent study found no significant differences between zinc nasal spray and placebo. Negative results may be caused by using doses of zinc that are too low or they may be affected by the presence of compounds like citric or tartaric acid, which may reduce efficacy because of chelating of the zinc ion.	C
Crohn's Disease Preliminary studies of zinc supplements in patients with Crohn's disease have found positive results. Well-designed clinical trials are needed to confirm these results.	C
Dandruff Shampoo containing 1% of zinc pyrithione has been shown to reduce dandruff in some people.	C
Diabetes (Type 1 and Type 2) Diabetic patients typically have significantly lower serum zinc levels compared with healthy controls. In preliminary high-quality studies, zinc supplementation for type 2 diabetics may have beneficial effects in elevating serum zinc level and in improving glycemic control that is shown by decreasing HbA1c concentration.	C
Diabetic Neuropathy (Nerve Damage) Oral zinc supplementation may improve glycemic control and severity of peripheral neuropathy. However, clinical evidence is not sufficient to support this use.	C
Diaper Rash Zinc may reduce the incidence of diaper rash and have a preventative effect.	C
Eczema There are conflicting data regarding the correlation of zinc serum levels and eczema. One study noted that zinc might have caused an increase in itching after several weeks of supplementation. Additional information is needed to help clarify these results.	C
Exercise Performance Zinc may improve exercise performance in athletes with low serum zinc or zinc deficiencies. Additional evidence is needed before a recommendation can be made.	C
Gilbert's Syndrome Gilbert's syndrome is a common, often inherited disorder that affects processing by the liver of the greenish-brown pigments in bile (called *bilirubin*). The resulting abnormal increase of bilirubin in the bloodstream can lead to yellowing of the skin (jaundice), but the liver itself remains normal. It is more common in men than women and is named after a French gastroenterologist. Zinc sulfate supplementation seemed to decrease serum unconjugated bilirubin levels in a small study. Well-designed clinical trials are needed to confirm these results.	C
Growth (Stunted Infants) Evidence suggests that supplementation with zinc plus iron (but not with zinc alone) may improve linear growth (length) of stunted infants with low hemoglobin.	C
Hepatic Encephalopathy Hepatic encephalopathy is abnormal brain function caused by passage of toxic substances from the liver to the blood. Preliminary high-quality trials of zinc for this indication have yielded conflicting results.	C
Hepatitis C Viral Infection (Chronic) Preliminary studies have shown that zinc in combination with interferon or interferon and ribavirin for hepatitis C viral infection patients did not show significant benefits, except for lower incidence of gastrointestinal side effects in one study. Further study may be warranted in this area. Recent high-quality evidence suggests that supplementation with polaprezinc in patients undergoing treatment with pegylated interferon alpha-2b and ribavirin may decrease damage to the liver cells.	C
HIV/AIDS Patients with HIV/AIDS, especially those with low zinc levels, may benefit from zinc supplementation. Some low-quality studies cite reduction in infections, enhanced weight gain, and immune system function, including increased CD4 and CD8 cells. However, conflicting results have been reported.	C
Hypothyroidism Case report data suggest zinc supplementation may improve thyroid hormone levels (particularly T_3) among women with hypothyroidism.	C
Incision Wounds Although zinc is frequently thought to have beneficial effects on incision wound healing, few studies have investigated this use.	C
Infertility Many studies report beneficial results of zinc supplements on infertility, as expressed in improved sperm quality and number, although this effect may depend on the cause of infertility. A minor increase in abnormal spermatozoa in subfertile males taking zinc was noted in one study.	C

Uses Based on Scientific Evidence	Grade
Kidney Function Preliminary studies show potential improvement in uremic patients taking zinc supplements. Further research is needed to confirm these results. Zinc supplementation may be recommended only in the patients with proven zinc deficiency, but for all chronic renal failure patients it is questionable.	C
Kwashiorkor (Malnutrition From Inadequate Protein Intake) Short-term zinc supplementation may increase weight gain and decrease infections, swelling, diarrhea, anorexia, and skin ulcers in children with extreme malnourishment.	C
Leg Ulcers There are conflicting findings regarding the potential benefit of zinc for healing leg ulcers. All studies, however, reported no or few adverse effects.	C
Leprosy A few studies have examined the efficacy of zinc treatment in leprosy. Studies of zinc taken by mouth report positive results, while one study of topical zinc reports negative results.	C
Liver Cirrhosis People with alcoholic liver cirrhosis may be deficient in zinc. Preliminary studies suggest that zinc may benefit these patients. Further evidence is needed to confirm these findings.	C
Lower Respiratory Infections in Children Results from large clinical trials suggest that supplementation with zinc may reduce the incidence and severity of lower respiratory infections. Some studies suggest these effects to be apparent only in boys and not girls. A trend toward increased respiratory infections in children has been noted in one study. A recent study does not support the use of zinc supplementation in the management of acute lower respiratory infections requiring hospitalization in indigenous children living in remote areas. Study results are conflicting.	C
Macular Degeneration Most studies examining the relationship between dietary zinc intake over many years and macular degeneration have not reported positive correlations. However, one large high-quality study, which examined the efficacy of zinc supplements in preventing loss of visual acuity, found that zinc supplements helped prevent the occurrence of age-related macular degeneration. Study results are conflicting.	C
Malaria Results are contradictory for the effect of zinc on malaria symptoms. Some high-quality studies suggest no effect of zinc supplementation on the severity of malaria. Other studies suggest that zinc supplementation may reduce the number of stays in hospital	C

and death rate due to *P. falciparum* infection. Further well-designed trials are required to address these discrepancies.

Menstrual Cramps Case report data suggest a possible role for zinc supplementation in menstrual cramps. Additional research is needed to confirm these findings.	C
Muscle Cramps (Cirrhosis) The results of one case series suggest that zinc supplementation may improve muscle cramps in patients with cirrhosis. Further research is needed to confirm these results.	C
Mortality Evidence from high-quality studies found no association between zinc supplementation and mortality among children. Additional research is needed in this area.	C
Parasites In a few studies of varying quality, patients with cutaneous leishmaniasis were injected with zinc sulfate intralesionally. One study found that zinc sulfate was better than meglumine antimoniate for the first four weeks, but no statistical differences were observed after six weeks. Zinc may decrease the severity of infection and re-infection of *S. mansoni* but does not seem to prevent initial infection. More research should be done in this area to examine how zinc affects the *S. mansoni* life cycle and whether this data can be extrapolated to other species of *Schistosoma*. The effects of zinc on the rate of parasitic re-infestation have been examined in children. No significant effect of zinc treatment was found. Recent high-quality study data suggest that supplementation with zinc and vitamin A may favorably alter infection rate and duration among children. Study results are conflicting.	C
Poisoning (Arsenic) Results from one study show that a combination of spirulina extract plus zinc may be useful for the treatment of chronic arsenic poisoning with melanosis and keratosis. More research is needed to confirm the effects of zinc alone.	C
Pregnancy According to multiple reviews, there is no evidence to suggest that zinc supplementation offers benefits during pregnancy, although there is a possible reduction in labor complications and preterm deliveries. However, results from individual studies suggest a possible benefit of zinc supplementation on blood pressure during pregnancy.	C
Psoriasis There are only a few studies that examine the efficacy of zinc treatment on symptoms of psoriasis, including psoriasis-induced arthritis-like symptoms. One trial	C

Z

(Continued)

Uses Based on Scientific Evidence	Grade
noted a reduction in pain and joint swelling. Other studies do not support a role for zinc in alleviating the symptoms of psoriasis.	
Radiation-Induced Mucositis Radiation has the potential side effect of mucositis, which is inflammation of mucous membranes inside of the mouth, nose, and throat. Two trials suggest that zinc may lower the degree of mucositis in patients on radiation.	C
Respiratory Disease (Juvenile-Onset Recurrent Respiratory Papillomatosis) Evidence from case reports suggests a possible role for zinc supplementation as adjuvant therapy in juvenile-onset recurrent respiratory papillomatosis (JORRP).	C
Rheumatoid Arthritis Most trials do not show significant improvements in arthritis symptoms following zinc treatment. Interpretation of some data is difficult because patients in the studies were permitted to continue their previous arthritis medication and most studies used a small number of participants.	C
Skin Damage Caused by Incontinence Preliminary evidence suggests that topical zinc oxide oil may help manage perianal and buttock skin damage in incontinent patients.	C
Stomatitis Zinc sulfate has been studied for the treatment of recurrent aphthous stomatitis (RAS, mouth ulcer). Study results conflict.	C
Taste Perception (Hemodialysis, Cancer) Results from studies investigating the potential role of zinc in treating taste and smell disorders are contradictory. Recently, a large high-quality trial showed no evidence of a benefit of zinc supplementation on taste alterations among patients undergoing radiation therapy for head and neck cancer.	C
Tinnitus Studies on the efficacy of zinc in treating tinnitus yield contradictory results based on subjective findings.	C
Trichomoniasis Little research is available on the efficacy of zinc for the treatment of trichomoniasis, a sexually transmitted disease (STD). One very small study suggests that a zinc sulfate douche and the prescription antibiotic metronidazole may effectively treat patients with recalcitrant trichomoniasis.	C
Viral Warts Studies have found conflicting results of the effect of zinc on viral warts. Well-conducted studies are needed to clarify these early results.	C

	Grade
Celiac Disease In a very small study, oral zinc supplements did not seem to improve the clinical condition of patients with unresponsive celiac syndrome.	D
Chronic Inflammatory Rheumatic Disease Preliminary studies found that zinc supplementation did not seem to benefit patients with chronic inflammatory rheumatic disease.	D
Continuous Ambulatory Peritoneal Dialysis (CAPD) Zinc supplementation did not improve the nutritional status in patients on CAPD based on one well-designed trial.	D
Cystic Fibrosis Zinc supplementation does not seem to affect clinical status, growth velocity, or lung function in children with cystic fibrosis.	D
Inflammatory Bowel Disease Preliminary studies have found that zinc supplementation does not seem to improve inflammatory bowel disease.	D
Pneumonia (Children) Studies have found that zinc supplementation does not seem to lessen the duration of abnormally fast breathing, hypoxia (inadequate oxygen), chest indrawing, inability to feed, lethargy, severe illness, or hospitalization in children.	D

Uses Based on Tradition or Theory

Acrodermatitis enteropathica, alcoholism, Alzheimer's disease, benign prostate hyperplasia, bladder cancer, bulimia, cancer, diabetic retinopathy, diarrhea (AIDS), encephalopathy, eye disorders (night blindness, retinol pigmentation abnormalities), hypoxia, human papilloma virus, hypogonadism, hyperprolactinemia, liver enlargement and disorders, menopause, nutritional deficiencies (consumption of dirt), pancreatitis, psychosis, Parkinson's disease, poisoning (nickel), schizophrenia, seizures, skin disorders (parakeratosis), smell disorders, spleen disorders (enlargement), tuberculosis, wound healing.

DOSING
Adults (18 Years and Older)
Oral

- **Acetazolamide side effects**: 0.2 g zinc sulfate three times daily has been studied in those with grave acetazolamide-induced side effects.
- **Acne vulgaris**: Doses ranging from 45 to 220 mg of zinc sulfate (Orazinc or effervescent), three times daily, up to 12 weeks have been studied. Doses of 45 to 135 mg of zinc in divided doses have been studied for up to 12 weeks, and 30 to 200 mg zinc gluconate has been used for three months.

- **Acrodermatitis enteropathica**: Various doses have been studied: 100 mg zinc, three times daily; 45 mg, two times daily; 30 to 65 mg daily; 200 mg daily (Solvezink, Tika AB); 135 mg zinc sulfate daily; 220 mg, three times daily, or 50 mg, twice daily; 45 mg zinc, three times daily (Solvezink, Tika AB); and 45 mg zinc, three times daily for two months.
- **Acute lymphoblastic leukemia**: 0.02 mg/kg body weight of zinc has been studied as an adjunct therapy for leukemia.
- **Alopecia areata**: Zincomed, 220 mg zinc sulfate twice daily has been studied for three months.
- **Anorexia**: 45 to 100 mg daily of zinc, zinc sulfate, or zinc acetate have been studied. 15 mg zinc (as sulfate), three times daily for two weeks, followed by 50 mg, three times daily, has also been used.
- **Burns**: A dose of 660 mg of zinc sulfate ($ZnSO_4$) has been used.
- **Cancer**: 90 mg daily zinc sulfate for five days, with a maintenance dose of 180 mg daily, has been used to treat pustules in a woman with squamous cell carcinoma and a zinc deficiency.
- **Chronic inflammatory rheumatic disease**: 45 mg zinc as gluconate has been used daily for two months.
- **Cirrhosis/alcoholism**: 200 mg as sulfate has been used three times daily. A daily oral intake of 200 mg of zinc sulfate for two months has been studied for its immune-enhancing effects in these patients.
- **Common cold/lower respiratory infection**: Doses ranged from 4.5 to 23.7 mg zinc/lozenge and were taken every half hour during waking hours. Lozenges containing 5 mg or 11.5 mg zinc acetate or 13.3 mg zinc gluconate (Quigley Corporation, PA) were taken every 2 to 3 waking hours (total of six lozenges daily). Zinc lozenges (Heiko Chemicals, PA) containing zinc acetate, 42.96 mg, 12.8 mg zinc) have been studied. Zinc lozenges with 10 mg zinc (Quigley Corporation) have been used three times daily. 23 mg zinc (as gluconate) lozenges have been taken daily for seven days. Lozenges (Quigley Corporation, PA) containing zinc (13.3 mg zinc gluconate trihydrate with molar concentrations of glycine) have been used every two hours of waking time. Effervescent lozenges (containing 10 mg zinc acetate) taken for three days, and at least four lozenges a day, have also been studied. 23 mg zinc lozenges containing 2% citric acid were taken every half hour while awake. 23 mg zinc lozenges (Truett Laboratories, TX) were used in one study where patients were instructed to let them dissolve in their mouth. Initial dose consisted of two lozenges, then one every two hours.
- **Continuous ambulatory peritoneal dialysis (CAPD)**: 100 mg daily of elemental zinc for three months has been studied.
- **Crohn's disease**: 60 mg daily $ZnSO_4$; 200 mg daily $ZnSO_4$ for three months has been studied for thyroid function in Crohn's disease patients. 200 mg of zinc sulfate daily for six weeks has also been studied.
- **Cutaneous leishamaniasis**: 2.5 to 10 mg of zinc sulfate has been used (Analar [BDH]).
- **Dental application**: One or two pieces of a zinc chewing gum for at least 10 minutes, three times daily for one week has been studied to treat halitosis. 0.5% zinc citrate dentifrice has also been studied for three months.
- **Diabetes**: 30 mg daily as amino acid chelate for three weeks. 30 mg of zinc (as glycine), for three weeks, has been given to alleviate oxidate stress in diabetics; 30 mg of zinc (as gluconate) has been studied; 50 mg zinc has been used daily for 28 days.
- **Diabetic neuropathy**: Zinc sulfate (660 mg) for six weeks has been studied.
- **Dialysis**: 50 mg daily as acetate has been used in dialysis patients for effects on lymphocyte and granulocyte function.
- **Diaper rash**: 10 mg zinc gluconate supplements have been used as an adjunct to anti-fungal cream for diaper rash.
- **Down syndrome/hypothyroidism**: Zinc supplements (1 mg/kg of body weight) for two months, followed by a 10-month break, and then again for two months of zinc treatment. 135 mg zinc (as sulfate) daily for two months.
- **Dysgeusia**: Zinc gluconate 140 mg daily has been used.
- **Eczema**: 220 mg of daily oral zinc treatment as sulfate has been studied.
- **Exercise performance**: Zinc at 3 mg/kg body weight has been studied for four weeks.
- **Furunculosis**: 45 mg has been used three times daily (Solvezink, Tika) for four weeks.
- **Gastroduodenal ulcers**: Doses of zinc acexamate 300 to 1,800 mg, three times daily have been studied for five weeks with maintenance doses of 600 mg for up to six months. 220 mg zinc sulfate taken three times daily for three weeks has also been used.
- **Gastrointestinal disease**: 300 mg zinc acexamate has been taken daily.
- **Gastric/gastroduodenal ulcers**: A-84, 300 mg, three times daily for three weeks. Doses of zinc acexamate 300 to 600 mg daily. 220 mg as sulfate, three times daily for four weeks.
- **Gilbert's syndrome**: 40 mg of $ZnSO_4$ in a single dose has been used for acute conditions, and 100 mg $ZnSO_4$ in a single dose has been given for seven days for chronic conditions.
- **Hepatic encephalopathy**: Zinc sulfate or zinc acetate, 600 mg, has been used for seven to ten days.
- **Hypercholesterolemia**: 7.7 micromoles zinc sulfate (50 mg elemental zinc) for 90 days has been studied.
- **Hyperlipidemia**: 150 mg zinc daily for 12 weeks has been studied.
- **Hyperprolactinemia**: 37.5 mcg oral zinc as sulfate and 15.9 mg as sulfate has been used three times daily for 60 days.
- **HIV/AIDS**: 200 mg of zinc sulfate has been used daily for four weeks as an aid in immune response. 125 mg of zinc gluconate has been used twice daily for three weeks.
- **Immune function**: 30 mg zinc daily for 14 weeks has been investigated. 200 mg of zinc sulfate has been used for two months.
- **Immune function in the elderly**: 25 mg of zinc phosphate has been investigated. 220 mg zinc sulfate, twice daily for one month. 50, 100, and 150 mg elemental zinc has been used daily. 12 mg of Zn+ has been used daily for one month in infected elderly subjects.
- **Infertility**: 50 mg zinc daily. 66 mg zinc sulfate daily for 26 weeks has been used to improve sperm count in fertile and subfertile males. 250 mg of zinc sulfate has been used twice daily for three months. 220 mg of zinc sulfate has been used once daily, for four months (Cap, ZINCOLAK, Shalaks Chemicals). 440 mg zinc sulfate for 12 months. 220 mg zinc sulfate for impotence and hypogonadism in hepatic cirrhosis patients. 500 mg zinc has been used daily as a supplement with hydrochlorothiazide and sexual side effects.

Z

- **Inflammatory bowel disease**: 300 mg zinc aspartate (equal to 60 mg elemental zinc) has been used daily for four weeks.
- **Intestinal malabsorption**: 100 mg, three times daily and 19 mg daily have been used.
- **Leg ulcers**: 220 mg zinc sulfate, 1 to 3 times daily for up to 10 months, has been studied. 200 mg zinc sulfate, three times daily (Solvezink, Astra), for up to one year.
- **Leprosy**: 220 mg zinc sulfate daily has been studied as an adjunct to leprosy medication for up to 18 months.
- **Macular degeneration**: 100 mg, two times daily for up to two years.
- **Muscle cramps (cirrhosis)**: 220 mg twice daily oral zinc sulfate three times weekly for 12 weeks has been used.
- **Nickel-positive patients**: Zinc sulfate 100 mg, three times daily, for 30 days has been studied.
- **Pancreatitis/home parenteral nutrition**: 30 mg zinc sulfate for the first three days of total parenteral nutrition has been used.
- **Pregnancy**: 30 mg elemental zinc has been studied during the last two trimesters of pregnancy, but did not improve birth outcome in Bangladeshi urban poor. 14 mg iron and 250 micrograms folate with 15 mg zinc has been studied in pregnancy.
- **Psoriasis**: 220 mg, three times daily for the first for six weeks, then six months. 220 mg zinc sulfate three times daily for two months. 50 mg of zinc, three times daily (Mericon Industries, IL).
- **Rheumatoid arthritis**: 220 mg of zinc sulfate (Mericon Industries, IL) three times daily has been used up to 12 weeks. 220 mg has been used three times daily for six months (356). 200 mg has been used three times daily. 220 mg zinc sulfate, three times daily for at least two months (Solvezink, Astra). 600 mg has been used every 24 hours (divided up into three doses) for eight months, but showed little success.
- **Sickle cell anemia**: 220 mg zinc, three times daily has been used. 75 mg of zinc supplements have been used daily for up to three years. A solution of 1% of zinc sulfate in distilled water has been used. 15 mg zinc as acetate has been used twice daily. 25 mg every four hours has been studied to enhance healing of leg ulcers and control sickling of erythrocytes in people with sickle cell anemia. 15 mg zinc as acetate has been used three times daily for 12 months to treat serum testosterone deficiency in adults with sickle cell anemia.
- **Skin lesions**: 400 mg zinc sulfate has been used daily.
- **Stomatitis**: A dose of 200 mg zinc sulfate once daily for up to 12 weeks has been studied.
- **Supplementation**: 15 mg or 100 mg daily for three months has been studied in healthy elderly people.
- **Supragingival calculus formation**: Denifrices containing 0.5% zinc citrate have been used.
- **Taste disorders**: 45 mg zinc sulfate, three times daily, has been used as an adjunct to external radiotherapy. 100 mg zinc ion has been used daily for three months. 220 mg of zinc sulfate has been used daily for six weeks. 29 mg of zinc picolinate capsules have been used three times daily for three months. 100 mg zinc sulfate has been used daily for six months. 50 mg of zinc acetate has been used daily.
- **Tinnitus**: 22 mg of zinklet tablets (slow-release tablets) have been taken three times daily for over eight weeks. 50 mg of zinc has been taken daily. Zinc (34 to 68 mg daily, for 2 weeks) has been taken.

- **Trichomoniasis**: 220 mg Zincaps has been used twice daily for three weeks to treat trichomoniasis infection that was unresponsive to metronidazole.
- **Viral warts**: Oral zinc sulfate has been given at doses ranging from 10 to 600 mg/kg, 1 daily for up to six months.
- **Wilson's disease**: Various maintenance doses have been studied. For example, 25 to 150 mg zinc acetate in divided doses has been taken for up to one year. Doses of 25 to 50 mg three times daily have been investigated for maintaining copper balance in those with Wilson's disease. For zinc sulfate, doses used have ranged from 100 to 400 mg, three times daily.
- **Wound healing**: 220 mg zinc sulfate, three times daily has been used following surgery to promote wound healing.

Topical

- **Acne vulgaris**: Erythromycin (4%) plus 1.2% zinc for 12 weeks is a commonly studied dose. This dose has been studied for up one year in clinical studies.
- **Dandruff**: Shampoo containing 1% zinc pythione (ZPT) has been shown to reduce the number of PAS-positive microorganisms (but not Gram-positive microorganisms).
- **Dental application**: 0.5% zinc citrate has been used.
- **Herpes**: Two applications daily of 0.3% zinc oxide/glycine cream has been studied. Virunderim Gel, containing 10 mg zinc sulfate, has also been used up to 12 days. 0.01% to 0.05% zinc sulfate solution has been applied often during a breakout and once a week during remission. Immersion treatment with liquid soap containing 1% zinc sulfate has been used for three months followed by weekly application. A 4% zinc sulfate solution in water has also been used.
- **Immune enhancement**: 10 mg zinc gluconate has been studied, and during diarrhea, 20 mg of zinc gluconate has been reported.
- **Leg ulcers**: Topical 250 to 510 mcg/cm^2 topical zinc oxide in polyvinyl pyrrolidone has been studied for eight weeks. Zinc oxide dressings (Mezinc) have been investigated for eight weeks. Gauze compress medicated with zinc oxide (ZnO) 400 mcg/cm^2 has been studied for eight weeks.
- **Psoriasis**: Cow udder ointment (containing zinc) has been studied for psoriasis.
- **Sebum levels**: Erythromycin lotions (4%) with (1.2%, Zineryt lotion) have been studied for three months for effects on sebum levels.
- **Sickle cell anemia**: 10 mg daily of zinc in a 5-mL cherry soup has been taken for one year.
- **Trichomoniasis**: Zinc sulfate douche (1%) and metronidazole has been used.

Intravenous, Intramuscular

- **Anorexia**: 40 micromoles of zinc daily, intravenously for seven days, followed by 15 mg daily for 60 days has been reported.
- **Cutaneous leishmaniasis**: Intralesional injections of 2% zinc sulfate (ZnSO$_4$) have been studied.

Nasal

- **Common cold**: 0.12% zinc sulfate nasal spray administered four times daily into each nostril has been reported. Gels containing zinc gluconate (Zicam) have been used at the recommended dose of one spray (120 microliters) into each nostril, every four hours.

Children (under 18 years old)

- **Childhood malnutrition**: 10 mg daily or 1 mg/kg body weight daily by mouth has been studied.
- **Common cold**: 10 mg daily taken by mouth or 23 mg zinc lozenges (Truett Laboratories, TX) have been studied with initial dose consisting of one lozenge (half of the adult dose) every two hours, not to exceed six daily.
- **Diarrhea**: Children aged six months to two years received zinc (20 mg as acetate, in syrup) for treatment of dehydration and diarrhea; 14.2 mg zinc acetate or 40 mg zinc acetate has also been studied in six-month-old to two-year-old children, respectively. In 3- to 24-month-old infants, 20 mg zinc acetate daily for two weeks has been used. Zinc syrup containing 15 mg zinc was used on 6- to 11-month-old children and 30 mg with 12- to 35-month-old children. 15 mg (in children younger than or equal to 12 months old) or 30 mg (in children older than 12 months old) elemental zinc daily in three divided doses has been studied for 14 days. Another study reported using 10 mg zinc daily for five days of the week or 50 mg zinc once weekly for 16 weeks. Other doses used in children include 20 mg zinc daily for up to two weeks; 20 mg of zinc as sulfate, two times daily; 10 to 20 mg zinc in a multivitamin formula for six months; multivitamin juice with 15 mg zinc acetate per kg body weight; 10 mg zinc sulfate in 4 ml liquid daily, for seven months; and zinc gluconate (elemental zinc 10 mg) to infants and 20 mg to older children.
- **Down syndrome**: 20 mg/kg zinc daily for two months showed an increase in DNA synthesis. 50 mg (for up to six months) and 1 mg/kg/daily (for up to four months) zinc have shown a reduction in the number of infections.
- **Eczema**: 22.5 mg zinc, three times per day (in sustained-release capsules), for eight weeks, has been reported.
- **HIV/AIDS**: 1.8 to 2.2 mg/kg body weight daily, for three to four weeks, has been studied as an immune response aid in children.
- **Infection**: 20 mg zinc for one year has been studied for stunted growth and episodes of infectious disease.
- **Infection with *Schistosoma mansoni***: 30 to 50 mg, as zinc sulfate five times a week for 12 months, has been studied for *S. mansoni* infection in children.
- **Kwashiorkor**: Doses of 2 to 5 mg/kg zinc supplements have been studied for one week in children.
- **Lower respiratory tract infections**: Studied doses include 10 mg zinc gluconate six times a week; 10 mg zinc sulfate in 4 ml liquid daily, for seven months; 10 mg to infants and 20 mg to older children or placebo for four months; and 10 mg zinc as acetate (twice daily for five days).
- **Malaria**: Studied doses include 12.5 mg zinc sulfate for six days per week for six months; 10 mg zinc gluconate per day, six days per week; 10 mg elemental zinc, six days per week for 46 weeks; and zinc 20 mg daily for infants or 40 mg daily for older children for four days.
- **Parasites**: Zinc supplements 10 mg as amino acid chelate have been used.
- **Sickle cell anemia**: Zinc 10 mg daily in 5 ml cherry soup has been used in children.
- **Taste perception**: Zinc chelate 1 mg/kg daily for three months has been used in children.
- **Wilson's disease**: Pediatric patients of 1 to 5 years of age were given 25 mg of zinc twice daily; patients of 6 to 15 years of age, if under 125 pounds body weight, were given 25 mg of zinc three times daily; and patients 16 years of age or older were given 50 mg of zinc three times daily.

SAFETY

Allergies

- Case study evidence reports a patient with zinc oxide allergy.

Side Effects and Warnings

- Zinc is regarded as relatively safe and generally well tolerated when taken at recommended doses, and few studies report side effects. Occasionally, adverse effects such as nausea, vomiting, or diarrhea have been observed.
- Sideroblastic anemia, leukopenia, microcytic anemia, and neutropenia have been reported in individual case reports following the ingestion of large amounts of zinc.
- Reduced levels of high-density lipoprotein (HDL; "good" cholesterol) have been observed following daily supplementation with zinc.
- Unpleasant taste, taste distortion, and abdominal cramping have been occasionally reported, especially in studies examining the efficacy of zinc containing lozenges in treating symptoms of common cold or treatment of diarrhea in children. Bleeding gastric erosion, hepatitis (liver inflammation), liver failure, and intestinal bleeding have been reported in individual case reports following the ingestion of higher zinc doses.
- Acute tubular necrosis and interstitial nephritis have been reported following the ingestion of large amounts of zinc (doses not specified). Patients with severe kidney disease should reduce or omit taking zinc because it is primarily eliminated in urine.
- There is one case report of a fatal outcome from cystic degeneration in putamen and necrosis in the hypothalamus. It was reported as a consequence of zinc treatment for Wilson's disease; however, the patient had received penicillamine, followed by a relatively high dose of zinc per day for several weeks, followed by penicillamine again for an unspecified time, so it remains unclear if zinc was responsible for the death.
- Slight tingling or burning sensation in the nostril has been reported from zinc nasal gel. A trend toward increased respiratory infections in children has been noted. One case of hypersensitivity pneumonitis has been reported.
- Reports of skin conditions have been noted. In one study, worsening of an acne condition was observed following topical application of zinc, although many studies show positive effects of zinc on acne. A case report suggested the presence of dermatitis due to zinc deficiency.
- High-quality studies have found evidence of an association between high-dose zinc supplement use and hospitalization for urinary complications, including benign prostatic hyperplasia/urinary retention, urinary tract infection, and urinary lithiasis. This was especially evident among males.
- There is one report of death following the ingestion of 400 coins (mostly pennies). Pennies are composed mostly of zinc. Reduced immune responses have also been observed in a small study.

Pregnancy and Breastfeeding

- **Pregnancy, Category A**: Zinc is categorized as Pregnancy Category A. If this drug is used during pregnancy, the possibility of fetal harm appears remote. Because studies cannot

Z

rule out the possibility of harm, however, zinc acetate should be used during pregnancy only if clearly needed. Zinc appears to be safe in amounts that do not exceed the established tolerable upper intake level.

- **Pregnancy, Category C**: Animal reproduction studies have not been conducted with zinc chloride. It is also not known whether zinc chloride can cause fetal harm when administered to a pregnant woman or can affect reproduction capacity. Zinc chloride should be given to a pregnant woman only if clearly needed under medical supervision.

INTERACTIONS

Interactions with Drugs

- Hormone replacement therapy and cholestyramine may reduce zinc excretion in the urine. Amiloride (Midamor) reduces urinary zinc excretion and increases zinc blood levels. Theoretically, concurrent use of amiloride with zinc supplementation could cause zinc toxicity. Chlorthalidone (Hygroton) may increase serum zinc levels.
- Caffeine and alcohol may decrease zinc concentrations. Birth control pills and diuretics (loop or thiazide) may decrease zinc absorption.
- Deferoxamine (Desferal) increases urinary zinc elimination. Captopril (Capoten) and enalapril (Vasotec) might increase urinary zinc excretion in patients with high blood pressure. Data on other ACE-inhibitor (ACEIs) drugs is lacking. The clinical consequence of urinary zinc loss in patients with high blood pressure is unknown.
- Zinc sulfate may interact with carbenoxolone analog (BX24).
- Supplementation with zinc has the potential to improve the efficacy of oral cholera vaccine in children.
- Zinc may interact with LDL, HDL lipoproteins, and triglycerides, reducing HDL "good" cholesterol levels. Use cautiously with cholesterol medications, because of possible additive effects.
- Zinc may increase the cytotoxicity of cisplatin (Platinol-AQ) when in the presence of the chelate ethylenediaminetetraacetic acid (EDTA), as compared to cisplatin treatment alone.
- Zinc may decrease the absorption of erythromycin. However, in a study comparing erythromycin with and without added zinc, the results showed a significant reduction in severity and number of acne vulgaris lesions (including inflamed lesions) in the zinc treated group compared to those taking erythromycin alone.
- Zinc may decrease the effectiveness of fluoroquinolone antibiotics (e.g., Cipro). Zinc decreases the absorption and serum levels of demeclocycline, minocycline, and tetracycline because of zinc binding. Doxycycline does not seem to interact with zinc. Penicillamine (Cuprimine) chelates zinc and can reduce the effects of supplemental zinc. Dosing time should be separated by at least two hours.
- Zinc may improve both insulin secretion and insulin sensitivity and may exert insulin-like effects. Use cautiously with diabetes medications.
- High amounts of zinc may result in the prevention of interferon release, and interact with Interferon Alfa-2B (Intron A).
- Pancreatic enzyme replacements may improve absorption of zinc compared to pancreatic insufficiency.
- Zinc supplementation has been shown to alter thyroid hormone metabolism in disabled patients with zinc deficiency.

Interactions with Herbs and Dietary Supplements

- Zinc may interact with LDL, HDL lipoproteins, and triglycerides, reducing HDL "good" cholesterol levels. Use cautiously with herbs and supplements taken for cholesterol, because of possible additive effects.
- Zinc may interfere with copper metabolism. However, one study indicates no detrimental effects of zinc on plasma copper levels in healthy volunteers over a period of six weeks.
- Non-heme iron may decrease zinc absorption. Non-heme iron and zinc compete for a common absorption pathway in the gut. However, when iron and zinc are taken with food, this interaction is not likely to occur. When taken with food, zinc absorption is facilitated by proteins in food through an alternate pathway that does not compete with iron. Protein-bound heme iron (found in red meats) does not seem to affect zinc absorption.
- Zinc supplementation has been shown to alter thyroid hormone metabolism in disabled patients with zinc deficiency.
- Zinc may interact with herbs and supplements that contain caffeine or have blood pressure–altering, antibiotic, hormonal, diabetic, hypoglycemic, or diuretic effects.

For a complete list of references, please visit www.naturalstandard.com.

POTENTIAL HYPOGLYCEMIC OR HYPERGLYCEMIC EFFECTS

Note: This is not an all-inclusive list of herbs and supplements with hypoglycemic or hyperglycemic properties. A pharmacist should be consulted with specific questions or concerns regarding potential effects or interactions.

Possible Hypoglycemic Effects

- Abuta, acacia, acerola, aconite, African wild potato, agave, agrimony, alfalfa, algin, aloe *(Aloe vera)*, alpha-linolenic acid, alpha-lipoic acid, alpinia, amaranth, American pennyroyal, andiroba, andrographis *(Andrographis paniculata)*, annatto, antineoplastons, arnica, ashwagandha, asparagus, astaxanthin, astragalus, bael fruit, bamboo, banaba, barberry, barley, bay leaf, beet, beta carotene, beta-glucan, beta-sitosterol, sitosterol, betel nut, betony, bilberry, bitter melon, bitter orange, black seed, black walnut, bladderwrack, buchu, bupleurum, burdock, cajeput, calamus, calendula, caper, carob, carqueja, carrageenan, carrot, cat's claw, celery, chamomile, chaparral, chia, chicory, chlorella, chlorophyll, chromium, chrysanthemum, clove, codonopsis, coleus, cordyceps, corn silk, couch grass, cowhage, cranberry, creatine, damiana, dandelion, danshen, devil's claw, devil's club, dogwood, dong quai, elder, elecampane, Essiac herbal combination tea, eucalyptus, euphorbia, evening primrose, eyebright, false pennyroyal, fenugreek, fig, fish oil, flax, fo-ti, galega, gamma oryzanol, garcinia, garlic, germanium, ginger, ginkgo, ginseng, glucomannan, glucosamine, goji, goldenrod, goldenseal, gotu kola, grape seed, grapefruit, greater celandine, guggul, gymnema, hawthorn, heartsease, holy basil, hop, horse chestnut, horsetail, hydrangea, hyssop, ispaghula, jackfruit, java tea, jequirity, jiaogulan, juniper, katuka, kudzu, lady's mantle, lavender, lemongrass, licorice, lycopene, maitake mushroom, mangosteen, marshmallow, meadowsweet, milk thistle, morus nigra, mugwort, myrcia, myrrh, neem, niacin (vitamin B$_3$), noni, nopal, onion, oregano, peony, peppermint, perilla, policosanol, pomegranate, psyllium, pycnogenol, quercetin, red clover, red yeast rice, rehmannia, reishi mushroom, rhodiola, rose hip, rosemary, safflower, sage, sarsparilla, saw palmetto, schisandra, seaweed, senega, shark cartilage, shiitake, Siberian ginseng, soy, spirulina, stevia, stinging nettle, sweet marjoram, tamarind, tansy, turmeric, uva ursi, wheatgrass, white horehound, white oak, wild yam, witch hazel, yarrow, yohimbine

Possible Hyperglycemic Effects

- Agave, arginine (L-arginine), carnitine, cocoa, DHEA, elecampane, ephedra, ginseng, holy basil, hydrocotyle, licorice, melatonin, myrcia, rosemary, scarlet gourd, water pennywort

POTENTIAL INCREASED RISK OF BLEEDING OR CLOTTING

Note: This is not an all-inclusive list of herbs and supplements that affect bleeding or clotting. A pharmacist should be consulted with specific questions or concerns regarding potential effects or interactions.

Reported to Cause Clinically Significant Bleeding in Case Report(s)

- Garlic, ginger, ginko *(Ginkgo biloba)*, saw palmetto *(Serenoa repens)*

Herbs, Constituents, and Supplements that May Increase the Risk of Bleeding When Taken Alone or Concomitantly with Other Agents, Based on Known Mechanism of Action, Basic Science Studies, Human Case Reports/Trials, and/or Expert Opinion

- Acacia, acerola, aconite, agrimony, alfalfa,* aloe, alpha-linolenic acid, alpinia, American ginseng, American pawpaw, andrographis, angelica,* anise,* annatto, arabinogalactan, arginine (L-arginine), aristolochia, arnica, asafoetida,* ashwagandha, aspen,[†] astragalus, avocado, babassu, barley, bear's garlic, beta-sitosterol, sitosterol, bilberry, birch,[†] black cohosh,[†] black currant, bladderwrack, blessed thistle, bogbean, boldo, borage, breviscapine, bromelain, bupleurum, burdock, calamus, calendula, red pepper, cat's claw, celery,* chamomile,* chaparral, chia, chlorella, chondroitin sulfate, cinnamon, clove, clove, codonopsis, coleus, coltsfoot, cordyceps, cowhage, cranberry, daisy, dandelion,* danshen, desert parsley, devil's claw, dong quai, elder, EPA, evening primrose,[‡] fennel, fenugreek,* feverfew,[‡] fig, fish oil, flax (seed, not oil), forskolin, gamma oryzanol, garlic,[‡] German chamomile, ginger,[‡] ginkgo,[‡] ginseng,[‡] globe artichoke, goldenseal, grape seed, grapefruit, green tea, guarana, guggul, gymnema, hawthorn, horny goat weed, horse chestnut,* horseradish, jequirity, jiaogulan, juniper, kava, kinetin, kudzu, lady's mantle, lavender, lemongrass, leopard's bane, licorice,[‡] ling zhi, lovage root, male fern, marjoram, meadowsweet,[†] mistletoe, modified citrus pectin, niacin (vitamin B$_3$), nopal, nordihydroguairetic acid (NDGA), northern prickly ash, octacosanol, omega-3 fatty acids, onion, oregano, papain, papaw, papaya, parsley, passion flower, PC-SPES, peony, policosanol, polypodium, poplar,[†] prickly ash,* Pycnogenol, quassia,* quercetin, quinine, red clover,* red yeast rice, rehmannia, reishi, resveratrol, rhubarb, Roman chamomile, rose hip, rosemary, rue, rutin, safflower, sage, sassafras, savory, saw palmetto, schisandra, Scotch broom, sea buckthorn, seaweed, shea, shiitake mushroom, Siberian ginseng, sorrel, Southern prickly as, soy,[‡]; Spanish bayonet, spirulina, stinging nettle, strawberry, sweet birch,[†] sweet clover,* sweet marjoram, tamanu, tarragon, tea, thyme, tonka bean, turmeric, usnea, vitamin A, vitamin C,[‡] vitamin E,[‡] wasabi, watercress, wheatgrass, wild carrot, wild lettuce, willow,[†] wintergreen,[†] yarrow, yew, yohimbe

Possible Pro-Coagulant Agents

- Abuta, acerola, aconite, African wild potato, agrimony, alfalfa, annatto, apricot, arnica, astragalus, bael, bilberry, black haw, blessed thistle, cat's claw, chlorella, coenzyme Q10, cordyceps, dehydroepiandrosterone (DHEA), dong quai, ginseng, goldenrod, goldenseal, guggul, horsetail, jequirity, jiaogulan, lime, melatonin, milk thistle, mistletoe, myrcia, nopal, psyllium, raspberry, rhubarb, sage, Scotch broom, shepherd's purse, skunk cabbage, stinging nettle, tamanu, tea, white oak, white water lily, yarrow

Because passion flower *(Passiflora incarnata)*, hydroalcoholic extracts, juniper *(Juniperus communis)*, and verbena *(Verbena officinalis)* supply variable quantities of vitamin K, they may lessen the effect of oral anticoagulant therapy. Vitamin K–rich foods/herbs such as green leafy vegetables (e.g., collards, kale, and spinach) may decrease the anticoagulant effects of warfarin (Coumadin).

*Agents with coumarin constituents.

†Agents with salicylate constituents.

‡Agents that inhibit platelets.

POTENTIAL HEPATOTOXIC EFFECTS

Note: This is not an all-inclusive list of herbs and supplements with hepatotoxic properties. A pharmacist should be consulted with specific questions or concerns regarding potential effects or interactions. Potential hepatotoxic agents should be used cautiously with other possibly hepatotoxic agents, and monitoring of transaminase levels should be considered.

- Ackee, American pennyroyal, antineoplastons, bee pollen, birch oil, blessed thistle,† borage, bush tea,* butterbur, celandine, chaparral, coltsfoot, comfrey, creatine, dehydroepiandrosterone (DHEA), echinacea, English plantain,† false pennyroyal, germander, greater celandine, groundsel,* heliotropes, horse chestnut, jin-bu-huan, kava, lobelia, L-tetrahydropalmatine (THP), mate,* mistletoe, niacin (vitamin B₃), niacinamide, Paraguay tea, periwinkle, pride of Madeira,* ragwort,* rosy periwinkle, rue, sassafras, skullcap, sorrel, tansy ragwort,* tea,† turmeric, tu-san-chi,* uva ursi, valerian, viper's bugloss,* white chameleon

*Contains pyrrolizidine alkaloids, which may account for hepatotoxicity.

†Contains tannins and may be hepatotoxic in large quantities.

POTENTIAL HYPOTENSIVE OR HYPERTENSIVE EFFECTS

Note: This is not an all-inclusive list of herbs and supplements with hypotensive or hypertensive properties. A pharmacist should be consulted with specific questions or concerns regarding potential effects or interactions.

Possible Hypotensive Effects

- Abuta, aconite/monkshood, agrimony, algina, alpha-linolenic acid, andrographis, alpha-lipoic acid, alpinia, amaranth, andrographis, annatto, apple, arabinoxylan, arnica, asafoetida, asarum, ashwagandha, astaxanthin, astragalus, avens, bamboo, baneberry, barberry, barley, beet, berberine, beta-glucan, betel nut, betony, bilberry, birthwort, black cohosh, black currant, black seed, black walnut, bladderwrack, blood root, boldo, bromelain, bryony, buchu, cajeput, calamus, calendula, California poppy, caper, carrageenan, cat's claw, celery, chia, chlorella, chrysanthemum, cinnamon, cove, codonopsis, coenzyme Q10, coleus, coltsfoot, comfrey, common polypody, cordyceps, corn silk, couch grass, cowslip, cramp bark, curcumin, dandelion, danshen, deer velvet, devil's claw, dong quai, elecampane, eucalyptus, evening primrose, false hellebore, fenugreek, fish oil, flax, forskolin, fo-ti, bladderwrack, fumitory, gamma linolenic acid, garlic, germanium, ginger, ginkgo, ginseng, goji, goldenrod, goldenseal, gotu kola, green

hellebore, green tea, gymnema, hawthorn, hibiscus, horny goat weed, horse chestnut, horseradish, hyssop, Indian snakeroot, Indian tobacco, jaborandi, jasmine, java tea, juniper, kudzu, ladies mantle, lavender, lemon balm, lemongrass, lotus, lutein, lycopene, maitake mushroom, melatonin, mistletoe, morus nigra, mugwort, myrcia, neem, niacin (vitamin B₃), night blooming cereus, noni, nopal, northern prickly ash, octacosanol, oleander, olive leaf, omega-3 fatty acids, onion, parsley, pasque flower, passion flower, peony, perilla, periwinkle, plantain, pleurisy root, pokeroot, polypodium, pokeroot, Pycnogenol, pomegranate, psyllium, red yeast rice, rehmannia, reishi mushroom, rhodiola, rhubarb, rooibos, rosemary, rutin, safflower, sage, saw palmetto, schisandra, Scotch broom, sea buckthorn, shepherd's purse, shiitake, southern prickly ash, soy, spirulina, squill, St. John's wort, stevia, stinging nettle, sweet marjoram, Texas milkweed, thyme, tribulus, turmeric, uva ursi, valerian, verbena, wheatgrass, white horehound, wild carrot, wild cherry, yarrow, yerba santa

Possible Hypertensive Effects

- Andrographis, arnica, bayberry, betel nut, bloodroot, blue cohosh, broom, cayenne, cola, coltsfoot, cramp bark, ephedra, gentian, ginger, ginseng, grape seed, green tea, hawthorn, kola nut, lavender, licorice, mate, mistletoe, red pepper, rehmannia, schisandra, Scotch broom, shepherd's purse, Siberian ginseng, tea, verbena, yerba mate, yohimbe

POTENTIAL HORMONAL EFFECTS

Note: This is not an all-inclusive list of herbs and supplements with hormonal properties. A pharmacist should be consulted with specific questions or concerns regarding potential effects or interactions.

Possible Androgenic Effects

- Abuta, aizarin, angel's trumpet, anise, annatto, apricot, arnica, asarum, ashwagandha, asparagus, avocado, bacopa, bael fruit, bee pollen, beet, betel nut, black cohosh, burdock, calamus, cardamom, carqueja, chasteberry, cinnamon, clove, coleus, comfrey, cordyceps, creatine, damiana, deer velvet, ephedra, fennel, fenugreek, fo-ti, garlic, ginger, ginkgo, ginseng, goji, gotu kola, guarana, gymnema, hop, horny goat weed, jasmine, jequirity, jimson weed, kava, khat, lavender, lotus, lovage, maca, marshmallow, muira puama, nux vomica, parsnip, passion flower, pomegranate, Pycnogenol, pygeum, rhodiola, rose hip, saw palmetto, schisandra, shiitake, star anise, stinging nettle, sundew, sweet almond, tribulus, wild yam, yohimbe

Possible Antiandrogenic Effects

- Ephedra, PC-SPES, saw palmetto, yohimbine

Possible Estrogenic or Progestogenic Effects

- Aconite, agrimony, alfalfa, alizarin, allspice, alpha-linolenic acid, amaranth, American pennyroyal, anise, apple cider vinegar, arabinogalactan, arginine (L-arginine), arnica, asarum, ashwagandha, astragalus, avocado, bay leaf, bee pollen, belladonna, beta-sitosterol, sitosterol, betel nut, betony, bilberry, black cohosh,‡ black currant, black haw, black hellebore, black horehound, black seed, bladderwrack, blessed thistle, bloodroot, blue cohosh, blue flag, boldo, boneset, borage, boron, boswellia, bromelain, bugleweed, bupleurum, burdock, butterbur, calabar bean, calendula, camphor, canada balsam, cannabis, carrot, cat's claw, chamomile, chasteberry, cherry, chia, chicory, cinnamon, cleavers, comfrey, cordyceps, cornflower, daisy, damiana, dandelion, danshen, deer velvet, devil's claw, dill, dogwood, dong quai, echinacea, Essiac herbal combination tea, eucalyptus, evening primrose, fennel, fenugreek, feverfew, flax, fo-ti, gamma linolenic acid, gamma oryzanol, garcinia, garlic, ginger, ginkgo, ginseng, goji, goldenseal, gotu kola, green tea, ground ivy, guggul, hawthorn, hops,* horny goat weed, horse chestnut, horsetail, hyssop, ignatia, jointed flatsedge, kava, kelp, kudzu,† lady's mantle, lady's slipper, lavender, lemongrass, licorice,* lotus, lovage, maca, meadowsweet, melatonin, milk thistle, mistletoe, moxibustion, mugwort, muira puama, mullein, neem, niacin (vitamin B₃), noni, nux vomica, oreganoovaraden, ovariin, passion flower, peony, peppermint, physostigma, pleander, pleurisy, pokeweed, pomegranate,* Pycnogenol, pygeum, quassia, quercetin, quercetin, raspberry, red clover,† rehmannia, resveratrol, rhodiola, rhubarb, rose hip, rosemary, safflower, sage, sarsaparilla, saw palmetto, schisandra, Scotch broom, sea buckthorn, seaweed, shepherd's purse, Siberian ginseng, skullcap, slippery elm, soy,† St. John's wort, star anise, stinging nettle, sweet almond, sweet marjoram, sweet woodruff, tansy, tea, thyme, tribulus, turmeric, vervain, white horehound, wild yam, yucca

---

*Estriol, estrone, estradiol, or estrogen constituents.

†Isoflavone constituents.

‡Estrogen and isoflavone constituents.

POTENTIAL DIURETIC EFFECTS

Note: This is not an all-inclusive list of herbs and supplements with diuretic properties. A pharmacist should be consulted with specific questions or concerns regarding potential effects or interactions.

- Abuta, aconite, agave, agrimony, alfalfa, alizarin, aloe, alpinia, amaranth, American pennyroyal, anise, annatto, antineoplastons, arginine (L-arginine), arnica, artichoke, asarum, ashwagandha, asparagus, astragalus, bacopa, Baikal skullcap, barberry, bay leaf, bee pollen, belladonna, betel nut, betony, birch, black currant, black horehound, bladderwrack, blessed thistle, bloodroot, blue cohosh, blue flag, boldo, boneset, boswellia, bromelain, broom, buchu, bugleweed, bupleurum, burdock, butterbur, calcium, calendula, Canada balsam, caper, celery, chamomile, chaparral, chicory, cinnamon, cleaver, club moss, coleus, copper, corn silk, couch grass, cranberry, creatine, daisy, damiana, dandelion, dandelion, danshen, devil's claw, dong quai, Eastern hemlock, elder flower, ephedra, foxglove, garcinia, garlic, ginger, ginkgo, ginseng, globe artichoke, glucomannan, glucosamine, goldenrod, goldenseal, gotu kola, grape seed, green tea, ground ivy, guaiacum, guarana, gumweed, gymnema, hawthorn, heartsease, horse chestnut, horseradish, horsetail, hydrangea, hyssop, java tea, jequirity, jewelweed, juniper, kava, khella, labrador tea, ladies mantle, lavender, lemongrass, licorice, lignum-vitae, lime, lovage, marshmallow, mastic, meadowsweet, mistletoe, morus nigra, mullein, nopal, oleander, passion flower, pokeroot, polypodium, raspberry, red clover, rehmannia, rhubarb, rose hip, rosemary, rutin, saw palmetto, Scotch broom, seaweed, shepherd's purse, Siberian ginseng, skunk cabbage, slippery elm, sorrel, squill, St. John's wort, star anise, stevia, stinging nettle, sweet marjoram, sweet woodruff, tansy, tea, thiamin, thyme, tribulus, uva ursi, uva ursi, valerian, watercress, white horehound, yarrow, yew

POTENTIAL SEDATING EFFECTS

Note: This is not an all-inclusive list of herbs and supplements with sedating properties. A pharmacist should be consulted with specific questions or concerns regarding potential effects or interactions.

- 5-HTP (5-hydroxytryptophan), aconite, agrimony, American pennyroyal, angel's trumpet, anise, annatto, ashwagandha, asparagus, astragalus, bacopa, Baikal skullcap, bay leaf, belladonna, berberine, betony, bitter almond, bitter orange, black cohosh, black haw, black horehound, black mulberry, blood root, blue cohosh, boldo, borage, boswellia, boxwood, bugleweed, bulbous buttercup, bupleurum, butterbur, calamus, calamus, calendula, California poppy, cardamom, catnip, celery, centaury, chamomile, chasteberry, chicory, codonopsis, coleus, cordyceps, corn poppy, corydalis, couch grass, cowslip, daisy, danshen, deer velvet, devil's claw, dogwood, dong quai, Eastern hemlock, elder, elecampane, eucalyptus, euphorbia, false pennyroyal, fennel, feverfew, garlic, German chamomile, germanium, ginkgo, ginseng, goldenrod, goldenseal, gotu kola, ground ivy, guarana, hawthorn, holy basil, hops, horsetail, hydrocotyle, hyssop, ignatia, Jamaica dogwood, jasmine, jequirity, jimson weed, jointed flatsedge, kava (believed to be hypnotic/anxiolytic without significant sedation), labrador tea, lady's mantle, lady's slipper, lavender, lemon balm, lemongrass, lousewort, lovage, maca, meadowsweet, melatonin, mistletoe, mugwort, muira puama, mullein, neem, nux vomica, passion flower, passion flower, pennywort, perilla, polypodium, quassia, raspberry, red pepper, rehmannia, reishi, rhodiola, sage, sassafras (*Sassafras* spp.), saw palmetto, schisandra, Scotch broom, sea buckthorn, senega, shepherd's purse, Siberian ginseng, skullcap, skunk cabbage, spirulina, St. John's wort, stinging nettle, sweet almond, sweet woodruff, tamanu, tansy, tea, valerian, wheatgrass, white water lily, wild carrot, wild lettuce, yerba mansa, yohimbe

POTENTIAL CARDIOACTIVE EFFECTS

Note: This is not an all-inclusive list of herbs and supplements with cardioactive properties. A pharmacist should be consulted with specific questions or concerns regarding potential effects or interactions.

- Abuta, aconite, adonis, agrimony, aloe vera, alpha-linolenic acid, American hellebore, annatto, apple, apple cider vinegar, arnica, ashwagandha, astragalus, bacopa, bael, balloon cotton, barberry, berberine, betel nut, bilberry, bitter orange, black cohosh, black hellebore, black Indian hemp, bloodroot, broom, bufalin/chan su, bugleweed, bushman's poison, cactus, calamus, cat's claw, cereus, chamomile, chia, chicory, cinnamon, codonopsis, cola, coleus, coltsfoot, convallaria, cordyceps, corydalis, danshen, devil's claw, dong quai, elecampane, ephedra, Essiac herbal combination tea, evening primrose, eyebright, false hellebore, fenugreek, feverfew, figwort, flax, fo-ti, foxglove/digitalis, frangipani, fumitory, garlic, ginger, ginkgo, ginseng, goldenseal, green hellebore, guarana, hawthorn, hedge mustard, hellebore, hemp/Canadian hemp, horehound, horny goat weed, horsetail, jasmine, katuka, kava, khella, king's crown, kola nut, kudzu, lavender, lemon balm, licorice, lily-of-the-valley, lime, lotus, mangosteen, mate, milk thistle, mistletoe, motherwort, muira puama, myrcia, neem, nopal, northern prickly ash, oleander, omega-3 fatty acids, oregano, parsley, pheasant's eye, plantain, pleurisy, policosanol, polypodium, pomegranate, psyllium, pycnogenol, quassia, quercetin, red clover, redheaded cotton-bush, resveratrol, rhodiola, rhubarb, rosemary, rubber vine, rutin, safflower, schisandra, Scotch broom, sea buckthorn, sea mango, seaweed, senna, shepherd's purse, shiitake, skullcap, southern prickly ash, squill, St. John's wort, strophanthus, sweet woodruff, tea, uzara, valerian, vitamin D, wallflower, white horehound, wild carrot, willow, wintersweet, yellow dock, yellow oleander

POTENTIAL CYTOCHROME P450 ENZYME ACTIVITY

Note: This is not an all-inclusive list of herbs and supplements with cytochrome P450 enzyme activity. A pharmacist should be consulted with specific questions or concerns regarding potential effects or interactions.

General Agents

- Alpha-lipoic acid, antineoplastons, cat's claw, chaparral, eyebright, ginseng, grapefruit, kava, red yeast rice, yerba santa

May Induce CYP1A2

- Beta-glucan, broccoli, Brussels sprouts, cabbage, cauliflower, Essiac herbal combination tea, tobacco

May Inhibit CYP1A2

- Chaparral, dandelion, Essiac herbal combination tea, ginger, nordihydroguairetic acid (NDGA), shiitake mushroom, turmeric

Possible CYP2A6 Substrates

- European pennyroyal, false pennyroyal, watercress

May Induce CYP2B

- Hop

May Inhibit CYP2C19

- Chaparral, red yeast rice

May Inhibit CYP2C9

- Cat's claw, chamomile, chaparral, clove, ginger, gotu kola, kava, milk thistle, oregano, sage, Siberian ginseng, St. John's wort, tea, thyme, turmeric

May Inhibit CYP2D6

- Cat's claw, chamomile, chaparral, clove, carlic, ginger, gotu kola, kava, oregano, sage, St. John's wort, tea, thyme, turmeric

May Inhibit CYP2E1

- Dandelion, chaparral

Possible CYP3A (4,5,7) Substrates

- Eucalyptus, tea tree, yohimbe

May Induce CYP3A (4,5,7)

- Bloodroot, chasteberry, damiana, garlic, hop, oregano, phytoprogestins, St. John's wort, yucca

May Inhibit CYP3A (4,5,7)

- Cannabinoids, chaparral, Essiac herbal combination tea, ginseng, goldenseal, grapefruit, milk thistle, peppermint, Siberian ginseng, St. John's wort

May Inhibit CYP4A

- Cat's claw, chamomile, clove, echinacea, ginger, goldenseal, gotu kola, kava, licorice, oregano, red clover, sage, saw palmetto, tea, thyme, turmeric, wild cherry

POTENTIAL SELECTIVE SEROTONIN REUPTAKE INHIBITOR (SSRI) EFFECTS

Note: This is not an all-inclusive list of herbs and supplements with selective serotonin reuptake inhibitor properties. A pharmacist should be consulted with specific questions or concerns regarding potential effects or interactions.

- 5-Hydroxytryptophan (5-HTP), adrenal extract, chromium, dehydroepiandrosterone (DHEA), DL phenylalanine (DLPA), ephedra, evening primrose, fenugreek, ginkgo, hop, hydrazine sulfate, kali bromatum, lemon balm, passion flower, S-adenosylmethionine (SAMe), St. John's wort, tyrosine, valerian, vitamin B$_6$, white horehound, yohimbe

POTENTIAL MONOAMINE OXIDASE INHIBITOR (MAOI) EFFECTS

Note: This is not an all-inclusive list of herbs and supplements with monamine oxidase inhibitor properties. A pharmacist should be consulted with specific questions or concerns regarding potential effects or interactions.

- 5-Hydroxytryptophan (5-HTP), adrenal extract, avocado, betel nut, California poppy, chaparral, chromium, dehydroepiandrosterone (DHEA), DL phenylalanine (DLPA), ephedra, evening primrose, fenugreek, ginkgo, ginseng, hop, hydrazine sulfate, kali bromatum, kava, L-phenylalanine, mace, passion flower, red pepper, S-adenosylmethionine (SAMe), St. John's wort, valerian, vitamin B$_6$, yohimbe

Note: Tyramine/tryptophan–containing foods may induce hypertensive crisis when taken concomitantly with MAOIs and should be avoided by people taking MAOIs. These include protein foods that have been aged/preserved. Specific examples of foods include anchovies, avocados, bananas, bean curd, beer (alcohol-free/reduced), caffeine (large amounts), caviar, champagne, cheeses (particularly aged, processed, or strong varieties [e.g., camembert, cheddar, stilton]), chocolate, dry sausage/salami/bologna, fava beans, figs, herring (pickled), liver (particularly chicken), meat tenderizers, papaya, protein extracts/powder, raisins, shrimp paste, sour cream, soy sauce, wine (particularly Chianti), yeast extracts, and yogurt.

POTENTIAL LAXATIVE/STIMULANT-LAXATIVE EFFECTS

Note: This is not an all-inclusive list of herbs and supplements with laxative properties. A pharmacist should be consulted with specific questions or concerns regarding potential effects or interactions.

- Alder buckthorn, aloe, apple cider vinegar, black root, blue flag rhizome, butternut bark, calcium, cascara, castor oil, chasteberry, colocynth, dandelion, dong quai, elder, Essiac herbal combination tea, eyebright, fenugreek, flax, gamboges, horsetail, jalap, manna, oleander, plantain, podophyllum, psyllium, rhubarb, senna, squill, wild cucumber, yellow dock

POTENTIAL IMMUNOMODULATING ACTIVITY

Note: This is not an all-inclusive list of herbs and supplements with immunomodulating properties. A pharmacist should be consulted with specific questions or concerns regarding potential effects or interactions.

Possible Immunostimulants

- Acerola, aconite, African wild potato, aloe, alpha-lipoic acid, alpinia, amaranth, andrographis, apple, arabinogalactan, arabinoxylan, arnica, ash, ashwagandha, asparagus, astaxanthin, astragalus, babassu, bacopa, barley, bee pollen, berberine, beta-carotene, beta-glucan, beta-sitosterol, sitosterol, birthwort, bitter melon, black currant, black seed, black tea, blessed thistle, bloodroot, boneset, borage, boswellia, boxwood, bromelain, bupleurum, calamus, calendula, caper, cardamom, carrageenan, carrot, cascara sagrada, cat's claw, catnip, chamomile, chaparral, chlorella, chromium, chrysanthemum, cinnamon, cleaver, codonopsis, coenzyme Q10, coleus, cordyceps, dandelion, danshen, deer velvet, dong quai, echinacea, elder, elecampane, Essiac herbal combination tea, euphorbia, fenugreek, focusing, foti, gamma linolenic acid, gamma oryzanol, garlic, germanium, ginger, ginkgo, ginseng, goji, goldenseal, gotu kola, grape seed, grapefruit, greater celandine, green tea, ground ivy, holy basil, horny goat weed, jackfruit, katuka, lemon balm, lemongrass, licorice, lime, lutein, lycopene, maca, maitake mushroom, mangosteen, marshmallow, milk thistle, mistletoe, modified citrus pectin, MSM, neem, noni, nopal, pagoda tree, papain, peony, peppermint, perilla, peyote, polypodium, polypodium (*Polypodium leucotomos*), propolis, propolis, PSK, Pycnogenol, quercetin, red yeast rice, rehmannia, reishi mushroom, rhodiola, rhubarb, rose hip, rosemary, rutin, safflower, sage, sarsaparilla, saw palmetto, schisandra, sea buckthorn, seaweed, shiitake, Siberian ginseng, skullcap, slippery elm, sorrel, soy, spirulina, St. John's wort, stevia, stinging nettle, sweet Annie, tea, tea tree, tribulus, turmeric, wild indigo

Possible Immunosuppressants

- Beta-glucan, bupleurum, cat's claw

HERBS AND SUPPLEMENTS WITH POTENTIAL HYPOLIPEMIC OR HYPERLIPEMIC EFFECTS

Note: This is not an all-inclusive list of herbs and supplements with hypolipemic or hyperlipemic properties. A pharmacist should be consulted with specific questions or concerns regarding potential effects or interactions.

Possible Hypolipemics

- Alfalfa, artichoke, beta-carotene, beta-glucan, beta-sitosterol, bilberry, biotin, bitter melon, black cohosh, black currant, black hellebore, black horehound, black seed, black tea, black walnut, bladderwrack, bloodroot, blue flag, borage, boswellia, bromelain, bupleurum, butterbur, calamus, calendula, Canada balsam, caper, capsicum, cardamom, carob, carrageenan, cat's claw, chamomile, cherry, chia, chicory, chlorella, chlorophyll, cinnamon, clove, codonopsis, coleus, comfrey, cordyceps, corydalis, cowslip, cranberry, dandelion, danshen, devil's claw, devil's club, dogwood, dong quai, elder, elecampane, euphorbia, evening primrose, false hellebore, fenugreek, feverfew, fish oil, flax, fo-ti, gamma oryzanol, garlic, germanium, ginger, ginkgo, ginseng, globe artichoke, goji, goldenseal, grape seed, grapefruit, guggul, gymnema, hawthorn, hibiscus, holy basil, honey, hop, horny goat weed, hyssop, ispaghula, jiaogulan, jimson weed, katuka, kelp, khella, kiwi, kudzu, lavender, lemongrass, licorice, lotus, lutein, lycopene, maitake mushroom, mangosteen, meadowsweet, milk thistle, mistletoe, modified citrus pectin, muira puama, myrcia, myrrh, neem, noni, nopal, nux vomica, octacosanol, oleander, omega-3 fatty acids, onion, peony, perilla, plantain, policosanol, pomegranate, PSK, psyllium, Pycnogenol, quercetin, quinoa, raspberry, red clover, red pepper, red yeast rice, rehmannia, reishi mushroom, resveratrol, rhodiola, rhubarb, riboflavin, rose hip, rosemary, rutin, safflower, salvia, schisandra, Scotch broom, sea buckthorn, senega, shea, shiitake mushroom, Siberian ginseng, sitosterol, skullcap, soy, spirulina, squill, stinging nettle, sweet almond, sweet basil, sweet marjoram, tamarind, tangerine, tansy, tea, tribulus, trumpet tree, turmeric, valerian, white horehound, wild yam, willow, yellow dock, yerba santa, yew, yohimbe, yucca

Possible Hyperlipemics

- Pennywort

POTENTIAL ANTISPASMODIC EFFECTS

Note: This is not an all-inclusive list of herbs and supplements with antispasmodic properties. A pharmacist should be consulted with specific questions or concerns regarding potential effects or interactions.

- Angelica (*Angelica archangelica*), aniseed (*Pimpinella anisum*), asafoetida (*Ferula asafetida*), blue cohosh (*Caulophyllum thalictroides*), calendula (*Calendula officinalis*), red pepper (*Capsicum*), cassia (*Cinnamomum* spp.), celery (*Apium graveolens*), cinnamon, clove (*Eugenia aromatica*), cowslip (*Primula veris*), echinacea (*Echinacea* spp.), elecampane (*Inula helenium*), euphorbia (*Euphorbia* spp.), German chamomile (*Matricaria recutita*), Jamaica *dogwood* (*Piscidia erythrina, Piscidia piscipula*), lime flower (*Tilia europea*), raspberry (*Rubus idaeus*), Roman chamomile (*Anthemis nobilis*), rosemary (*Rosmarinus officinalis*), sage (*Salvia officinalis*), skullcap (*Scutellaria lateriflora*), tansy (*Tanacetum vulgare*), thyme (*Thymus vulgaris*), valerian (*Valeriana officinalis*)

POTENTIAL ANTI-INFLAMMATORY EFFECTS

Note: This is not an all-inclusive list of herbs and supplements with anti-inflammatory properties. A pharmacist should be consulted with specific questions or concerns regarding potential effects or interactions.

- Abuta, acacia, acai, ackee, aconite, African wild potato, alfalfa, alkanna, allspice, aloe, alpha-lipoic acid, alpinia, amaranth oil, American pawpaw, American pennyroyal, andiroba, andrographis, angel's trumpet, angelica, anise, annatto, arabinogalactan, arnica, arrowroot, asafoetida, asarum, ash, asparagus, astaxanthin, astragalus, avocado, babassu, Bach flower remedies, bacopa, bael fruit, Baikal skullcap, bamboo, barberry, bay leaf, belladonna, berberine, betony, bilberry, birch, birthwort, bitter almond, bitter melon, bitter orange, black bryony, black cohosh, black currant, black hellebore, black pepper, black seed, black walnut, blessed thistle, bloodroot, blue cohosh, blue flag, boldo, boneset, borage, boswellia, bromelain, buchu, bulbous buttercup, bupleurum, burdock, butterbur, cajeput oil, calamus, calendula, calendula, camphor, Canada balsam, cardamom, carqueja, carrageenan, cascara sagrada, cassia, cat's claw, centaury, chamomile, chaparral, chasteberry, cherry, chia, chicory, chlorella, chrysanthemum, cinnamon, cleaver, clove, coleus, coltsfoot, comfrey, cordyceps, cornflower, corydalis, couch grass, cowslip, cramp bark, cranberry, daisy, damiana, dandelion, danshen, deer velvet, devil's claw, devil's club, dong quai, Eastern hemlock, echinacea, elder, elecampane, English ivy, ephedra, eucalyptus, euphorbia, evening primrose, eyebright, false hellebore, fenugreek, feverfew, figwort, flax, gamma oryzanol, garcinia, garlic, gentian, German chamomile, germanium, ginger, ginseng, goji, goldenrod, goldenseal, gotu kola, grape seed, greater celandine, ground ivy, guarana, guggul, gumweed, heartsease, hibiscus, holy basil, hop, horny goat weed, horse chestnut, horseradish, hydrangea, hydrocotyle, hyssop, ignatia, jequirity, jiaogulan, jimson weed, jointed flatsedge, jojoba, juniper, kava, khella, kudzu, Labrador tea, lady's mantle, lady's slipper, lavender, lemon balm, lemongrass, lesser celandine, licorice, lime, lingonberry, lotus, mangosteen, marshmallow, mastic, meadowsweet, milk thistle, mistletoe, morus nigra, muira puama, mullein, myrrh, neem, nettle, noni, nopal, northern prickly ash, nux vomica, oleander, oregano, pagoda tree, passion flower, PC-SPES, pennywort, peony, peppermint, perilla, plantain, pokeroot, pokeweed, polypodium, pomegranate, populus, Pycnogenol, pygeum, quassia, quercetin, raspberry, red yeast rice, rehmannia, reiki, reishi mushroom, resveratrol, rhodiola, riboflavin, Roman chamomile, rose hip, rosemary, rutin, safflower, sage, salvia, sarsaparilla, saw palmetto, schisandra, Scotch broom, sea buckthorn, shea, shepherd's purse, shiitake, skunk cabbage, slippery elm, sorrel, southern prickly ash, soy, spirulina, St. John's wort, star anise, stevia, stinging nettle, strawberry, sweet basil, sweet marjoram, sweet woodruff, tamanu, tangerine, tansy, tea, tea tree oil, thyme, tree tobacco, tribulus, turmeric, tylophora, usnea, uva-ursi, valerian, verbena, warrow, wasabi, water hemlock, watercress, wheatgrass, white horehound, white oak, white water lily, wild yam, willow, witch hazel, yarrow, yerba santa, yew, yohimbe, yucca

NATURAL STANDARD DOES NOT RECOMMEND SPECIFIC THERAPIES OR PRACTITIONERS.

GRADE: A (Strong Scientific Evidence)

Therapy	Specific Therapeutic Use(s)
Alpha-lipoic acid	Diabetes, neuropathy (nerve pain or damage)
Andrographis, Kan Jang, SHA-10	Upper respiratory tract infection (treatment)
Arginine	Growth hormone reserve test/pituitary disorder diagnosis, inborn errors of urea synthesis
Beta-carotene	Erythropoietic protoporphyria
Beta-glucan	Hyperlipidemia
Biotin	Biotin deficiency, biotin-responsive inborn errors of metabolism
Calcium	Antacid (calcium carbonate), bone loss (prevention), cardiopulmonary resuscitation (CPR), deficiency (calcium), High blood phosphorous level, osteoporosis, toxicity (magnesium)
Chondroitin sulfate	Osteoarthritis
Coenzyme Q10	Coenzyme Q10 deficiency
Copper	Copper deficiency
Creatine	Enhanced muscle mass/strength
Ephedra	Weight loss
Feverfew	Migraine headache prevention
Folate	Folate deficiency, megaloblastic anemia due to folate deficiency, pregnancy complications (prevention)
Ginkgo	Dementia (multi-infarct and Alzheimer's type)
Glucosamine	Knee osteoarthritis (mild to moderate)
Grape seed	Edema
Hawthorn	Congestive heart failure
Horse chestnut	Chronic venous insufficiency
Iodine	Goiter prevention, iodine deficiency, radiation emergency (potassium iodide thyroid protection), skin disinfectant/sterilization, water purification
Iron	Anemia of chronic disease, iron deficiency anemia
Kava	Anxiety
L-Carnitine	Nutritional deficiencies (primary and secondary carnitine deficiency in adults)
Liver extract	Pernicious anemia
Niacin	Pellagra

(Continued)

NATURAL STANDARD DOES NOT RECOMMEND SPECIFIC THERAPIES OR PRACTITIONERS.—CONT'D

GRADE: A (Strong Scientific Evidence)

Therapy	Specific Therapeutic Use(s)
Omega-3 fatty acids, fish oil, alpha-linolenic acid	Hypertension, secondary cardiovascular disease prevention (fish oil/EPA plus DHA)
Pantothenic acid	Pantothenic acid deficiency
Phosphates, phosphorus	Constipation, hypercalcemia (high blood calcium levels), hypophosphatemia (low blood phosphorus level), kidney stones (calcium oxalate stones), laxative/bowel preparation for procedures
Policosanol	Platelet aggregation inhibition
Probiotics	Antibiotic-related adverse effects, atopic dermatitis (eczema), *Helicobacter pylori* infection
Psyllium	High cholesterol
Pygeum	Benign prostatic hyperplasia/BPH symptoms
Red yeast rice	High cholesterol
Riboflavin	Neonatal jaundice, riboflavin deficiency (ariboflavinosis)
Saccharomyces boulardii	Diarrhea (antibiotic associated)
Sage	Mood enhancement
Saw palmetto	Enlarged prostate (benign prostatic hyperplasia/BPH)
Soy	Dietary source of protein, high cholesterol
St. John's wort	Depressive disorder (mild-to-moderate)
Thiamin	Metabolic disorders (subacute necrotizing encephalopathy, maple syrup urine disease, pyruvate carboxylase deficiency, hyperalaninemia), thiamin deficiency (beriberi, Wernicke's encephalopathy, Korsakoff's psychosis, Wernicke-Korsakoff syndrome)
Vitamin A	Acne, acute promyelocytic leukemia (treatment, all-trans retinoic acid), eye disorders (Bitot's spot), measles (supportive agent), vitamin A deficiency, xerophthalmia (dry eye)
Vitamin B_{12}	Megaloblastic anemia due to vitamin B_{12} deficiency, pernicious anemia, vitamin B_{12} deficiency
Vitamin B_6	Hereditary sideroblastic anemia, cycloserine (Seromycin)–related adverse effects (prevention), pyridoxine deficiency/neuritis, pyridoxine-dependent seizures in newborns
Vitamin C	Vitamin C deficiency (scurvy)
Vitamin D	Familial hypophosphatemia, Fanconi syndrome–related hypophosphatemia, hyperparathyroidism due to low vitamin D levels, hypocalcemia due to hypoparathyroidism, osteomalacia (adult rickets), psoriasis, rickets
Vitamin E	Vitamin E deficiency
Vitamin K	Hemorrhagic disease of newborns (vitamin K deficiency bleeding/VKDB), vitamin K deficiency, warfarin reversal (elevated INR/pre-procedure)
Willow bark	Osteoarthritis
Zinc	Diarrhea (children), gastric ulcers, sickle cell anemia (management), zinc deficiency

NATURAL STANDARD DOES NOT RECOMMEND SPECIFIC THERAPIES OR PRACTITIONERS.—CONT'D

GRADE: B (Good Scientific Evidence)

Therapy	Specific Therapeutic Use(s)
5-HTP	Depression, fibromyalgia, headache, obesity
Aloe	Genital herpes, psoriasis vulgaris, seborrheic dermatitis
Aortic acid	Intermittent claudication
Arginine	Coronary artery disease/angina, critical illness, heart failure, migraine headache, peripheral vascular disease/claudication
Avocado	Osteoarthritis (knee and hip)
Bacopa	Cognition
Barley	Coronary heart disease (CHD)
Berberine	Heart failure
Beta-glucan	Diabetes
Betaine anhydrous	Hyperhomocysteinemia, hyperhomocysteinemia (in chronic renal failure patients), steatohepatitis (non-alcoholic)
Beta-sitosterol, Sitosterol	Benign prostatic hyperplasia (BPH)
Bloodroot	Plaque/gingivitis
Borage seed oil	Periodontitis/gingivitis, rheumatoid arthritis
Boswellia	Brain tumors
Bromelain	Sinusitis
Butterbur	Migraine prophylaxis
Calcium	Black widow spider bite, hyperkalemia (high blood potassium level), hypertension, premenstrual syndrome (PMS)
Calendula	Radiation skin protection
Carob	Hypercholesterolemia (high cholesterol)
Chasteberry	Hyperprolactinemia (excessive prolactin in the blood)
Cherry	Muscle strains/pain (exercise-induced muscle damage prevention)
Chia	Cardiovascular disease prevention/atherosclerosis
Chitosan	Obesity/weight loss
Choline	Asthma, fatty liver (hepatic steatosis), nutritional supplement (infant formula), total parenteral nutrition (associated liver dysfunction)
Chondroitin sulfate	Urinary incontinence/detrusor instability
Chromium	Polycystic ovary syndrome (glucose intolerance)
Clove	Dental pain
Coenzyme Q10	Hypertension
Coleus	Cardiomyopathy, glaucoma
Comfrey	Pain

(Continued)

NATURAL STANDARD DOES NOT RECOMMEND SPECIFIC THERAPIES OR PRACTITIONERS.—CONT'D

GRADE: B (Good Scientific Evidence)

Therapy	Specific Therapeutic Use(s)
Cordyceps	Liver disease (cirrhosis/chronic hepatitis B)
Cranberry	Urinary tract infection prophylaxis
Creatine	Congestive heart failure (chronic)
Devil's claw	Low back pain
DHEA	Depression, obesity, systemic lupus erythematosus
DMSO	Interstitial cystitis (chronic bladder infection)
Echinacea	Upper respiratory tract infections: treatment (adults)
Elderberry and elder flower	Influenza
Ephedra	Asthmatic bronchoconstriction
Evening primrose oil	Atopic dermatitis (eczema)
Fennel	Infantile colic
Folate	Methotrexate toxicity
Gamma linolenic acid	Diabetic neuropathy
Gamma oryzanol	Hyperlipidemia (high cholesterol)
Garlic	High cholesterol
Ginger	Nausea and vomiting of pregnancy (hyperemesis gravidarum)
Ginkgo	Cerebral insufficiency
Ginseng	Hyperglycemia (healthy people), immune system enhancement, type 2 diabetes
Globe artichoke	Lipid lowering
Glucosamine	Osteoarthritis (general)
Gotu kola	Chronic venous insufficiency/varicose veins
Grape seed	Diabetic retinopathy, vascular fragility
Green tea	Genital warts
Gymnema	Type 2 diabetes mellitus
Hibiscus	Hypertension (high blood pressure)
Horsetail	Diuresis (increased urine)
Iodine	Bacterial conjunctivitis, Graves' disease (adjunct iodine/iodides), hearing loss (iodine deficiency), ocular surgery infection prevention/cataract surgery antisepsis, ophthalmia neonatorum (prevention), oral mucositis, thyrotoxicosis/thyroid storm (adjunct)
Iron	ACE inhibitor–associated cough, menstruation-induced iron deficiency (prevention), iron-deficiency anemia in pregnancy (prevention)
Lactobacillus acidophilus	Bacterial vaginosis

NATURAL STANDARD DOES NOT RECOMMEND SPECIFIC THERAPIES OR PRACTITIONERS.—CONT'D

GRADE: B (Good Scientific Evidence)

Therapy	Specific Therapeutic Use(s)
L-Carnitine	Angina (chronic stable), peripheral vascular disease
Lemon balm	Herpes simplex virus infections
Melatonin	Delayed sleep phase syndrome (DSPS), insomnia in the elderly, sleep disturbances in children with neuro-psychiatric disorders, sleep enhancement in healthy people
Milk thistle	Cirrhosis
Niacin	Atherosclerosis (as an adjunct therapy; niacin), cardiovascular disease (niacin)
Omega-3 fatty acids, fish oil, alpha-linolenic acid	Primary cardiovascular disease prevention (fish intake), protection from cyclosporine toxicity in organ transplant patients, rheumatoid arthritis (fish oil)
Pantethine	Hyperlipidemia (high cholesterol)
Para-aminobenzoic acid	Melasma (prevention), recurrent herpes labialis infection (prevention)
Peony	Heart disease (pulmonary)
Peppermint	Cough, dyspepsia, irritable bowel syndrome (IBS), tension headache treatment (topical)
Phenylalanine	Vitiligo
Phosphates, phosphorus	Refeeding syndrome prevention
Podophyllum	Warts (genital warts, plantar warts)
Policosanol	Coronary heart disease (CHD), intermittent claudication (IC)
Probiotics	Cirrhosis, colon cancer, dental caries, diarrhea in children (nosocomial), diarrhea (prevention), diarrhea treatment (children), growth, immune enhancement, infections (gastrointestinal/respiratory), infectious diarrhea, irritable bowel syndrome (IBS), pancreatitis (acute), radiation-induced colitis/diarrhea, sinusitis (hypertrophic), ulcerative colitis
Psyllium	Constipation, diarrhea
Pycnogenol	Asthma, chronic venous insufficiency
Rhubarb	Gingivitis, renal failure (chronic)
Rose hip	Dysmenorrhea, osteoarthritis
Rutin	Edema
Saccharomyces boulardii	Diarrhea in children
Safflower	Deficiency (fatty acid)
Sage	Acute pharyngitis, Alzheimer's disease, herpes, menopausal symptoms
SAMe	Osteoarthritis
Selenium	Antioxidant, Keshan disease, prostate cancer (prevention)

(Continued)

NATURAL STANDARD DOES NOT RECOMMEND SPECIFIC THERAPIES OR PRACTITIONERS.—CONT'D

GRADE: B (Good Scientific Evidence)

Therapy	Specific Therapeutic Use(s)
Soy	Diarrhea (acute) in infants and young children, menopausal symptoms
St. John's wort	Somatoform disorders
Stevia	Hypertension
Strawberry	Antioxidant
Sweet almond	High cholesterol (whole almonds)
Taurine	Nutritional supplement (infant formula)
Thiamin	Acute alcohol withdrawal, total parenteral nutrition (TPN)
Vitamin A	Malaria (supportive agent), retinitis pigmentosa
Vitamin C	Common cold prevention (extreme environments), iron absorption enhancement, urinary tract infection (during pregnancy)
Vitamin D	Muscle weakness/pain, osteoporosis (general), renal osteodystrophy
Willow bark	Lower back pain
Zinc	Acne vulgaris, attention deficit hyperactivity disorder (ADHD), Down's syndrome, fungal infections (scalp), herpes simplex virus, hypercholesterolemia, immune function, plaque/gingivitis, Wilson's disease

GRADE: C (Unclear or Conflicting Scientific Evidence)

Therapy	Specific Therapeutic Use(s)
5-HTP	Alcoholism (withdrawal symptoms), anxiety, Down's syndrome, neurologic disorders (Lesch-Nyhan syndrome), psychiatric disorders, sleep disorders
Acacia	Plaque
Aconite	Heart failure, post-operative pain (in infants)
African wild potato	Benign prostate hyperplasia
Agrimony	Gastrointestinal disorders
Alfalfa	Diabetes, hyperlipidemia
Alizarin	Viral infections
Aloe	Aphthous stomatitis, cancer (prevention), diabetes (type 2), dry skin, HIV infection, lichen planus, skin burns, skin ulcers, ulcerative colitis (including inflammatory bowel disease), wound healing
Alpha-lipoic acid	Alcoholic liver disease, cognitive function (HIV), glaucoma, kidney disease, pain (burning mouth syndrome), pancreatic cancer, postoperative tissue injury prevention (ischemia; reperfusion injury after liver surgery), radiation injuries, skin aging, wound healing (in patients undergoing hyperbaric oxygen therapy)
Amaranth oil	Coronary heart disease, immunomodulation, night vision
American hellebore	Hypertension, pre-eclampsia/pregnancy-induced hypertension

NATURAL STANDARD DOES NOT RECOMMEND SPECIFIC THERAPIES OR PRACTITIONERS.—CONT'D

GRADE: C (Unclear or Conflicting Scientific Evidence)

Therapy	Specific Therapeutic Use(s)
American pawpaw	Lice
American pennyroyal	Emmenagogue (menstrual flow stimulant)
Amylase inhibitors	Obesity/weight loss
Andrographis paniculata Nees, Kan Jang, SHA-10	Familial mediterranean fever, influenza (flu), upper respiratory tract infection (prevention), familial Mediterranean fever, influenza, upper respiratory tract infection (prevention)
Anhydrous crystalline maltose	Dry mouth (Sjögren's syndrome)
Antineoplastons	HIV, sickle cell anemia/thalassemia
Aortic acid	Atherosclerosis, cerebral ischemia, thrombosis (deep vein thrombosis), venous disorders
Arabinogalactan	Immune stimulation, kidney disease (chronic renal failure), lipid lowering (cholesterol and triglycerides)
Arabinoxylan	Diabetes (type 2)
Arginine	Adrenoleukodystrophy (ALD), anal fissures, autonomic failure, breast cancer, burns, chemotherapy adjuvant, chest pain (non-cardiac), circulation problems (critical limb ischemia), dental pain (ibuprofen arginate), diabetes (type 1/type 2), diabetic complications, erectile dysfunction, gastrointestinal cancer surgery, heart protection during coronary artery bypass grafting (CABG), hypertension, hypercholesterolemia, immunomodulator, intrauterine growth retardation, kidney disease or failure, MELAS syndrome, myocardial infarction (heart attack), pre-eclampsia (pregnancy-induced hypertension), pressure ulcers, prevention of restenosis after coronary angioplasty (PTCA), Raynaud's phenomenon, recovery after surgery, respiratory infections, senile dementia, transplants, wound healing
Arnica	Coagulation, diabetic retinopathy, diarrhea in children (acute), Ileus (post-operative), osteoarthritis, pain (post-operative), stroke, trauma
Arrowroot	Diarrhea
Ashwagandha	Diuretic, hypercholesterolemia, longevity/anti-aging, osteoarthritis, Parkinson's disease
Asparagus	Galactagogue
Aspartic acid	Chronic fatigue syndrome
Astaxanthin	Hyperlipidemia (LDL oxidation), male infertility, muscle strength, musculoskeletal injuries, rheumatoid arthritis
Astragalus	Athletic performance, burns, chemotherapy adjuvant, coronary artery disease, diabetes, heart failure, hepatitis, herpes, HIV, immunostimulant, liver protection, mental performance, renal failure, smoking cessation, tuberculosis, upper respiratory tract infection, viral myocarditis
Avocado	Psoriasis
Bach flower remedies	Attention deficit hyperactivity disorder, major depressive disorder, pain

(Continued)

NATURAL STANDARD DOES NOT RECOMMEND SPECIFIC THERAPIES OR PRACTITIONERS.—CONT'D

GRADE: C (Unclear or Conflicting Scientific Evidence)

Therapy	Specific Therapeutic Use(s)
Bacopa	Anxiety (clinical), epilepsy, irritable bowel syndrome, memory
Baikal skullcap	Cancer
Banaba	Diabetes
Barley	Constipation, hyperglycemia, ulcerative colitis, weight loss
Bee pollen	Cancer treatment side effects
Beet	Peritonitis, type 2 diabetes (gastric hormone secretion)
Belladonna	Autonomic nervous system disturbances, headache, irritable bowel syndrome, menopausal symptoms, otitis media, premenstrual syndrome, radiodermatitis, sweating (excessive)
Bellis perennis	Bleeding (postpartum, mild)
Berberine	Chloroquine-resistant malaria, diabetes (type 2), Glaucoma, *H. pylori* infection, hypercholesterolemia, infectious diarrhea, parasitic infection (leishmania), thrombocytopenia, trachoma
Beta-carotene	Carotenoid deficiency, cataract (prevention), chemotherapy toxicity, chronic obstructive pulmonary disease (COPD), cognitive performance, cystic fibrosis, exercise-induced asthma (prevention), immune system enhancement, oral leukoplakia, osteoarthritis, polymorphous light eruption (PLE), pregnancy-related complications, UV-induced erythema (prevention)/sunburn
Beta-glucan	Antioxidant, burns, cancer, cardiovascular disease, diagnostic procedure, heart protection during coronary artery bypass grafting (CABG), hypertension, immune stimulation (breast cancer), infection, weight loss
Betaine anhydrous	Cholesterol levels, weight loss
Beta-sitosterol, Sitosterol	Androgenetic alopecia (treatment), HIV, immune suppression, rheumatoid arthritis, Tuberculosis (adjunct treatment)
Betel nut	CNS stimulant, dental caries, salivary stimulant, schizophrenia, stroke recovery, ulcerative colitis
Bilberry	Cataracts, chronic venous insufficiency, diabetes mellitus, diarrhea, dysmenorrhea, fibrocystic breast disease, glaucoma, peptic ulcer disease (PUD), retinopathy (diabetic, vascular)
Biotin	Brittle fingernails, cardiovascular disease risk (in diabetics), diabetes mellitus (type 2), hepatitis (in alcoholics), pregnancy supplementation, total parenteral nutrition (TPN)
Birch	Actinic keratosis
Bishop's weed	Tinea versicolor, vitiligo (leukoderma)
Bitter melon	Diabetes, human immunodeficiency virus (HIV)
Bitter orange	Fungal infections, weight loss
Black cohosh	Breast cancer, menopausal symptoms, migraine (menstrual)
Black currant	Chronic venous insufficiency, hypertension, immunomodulation, musculoskeletal conditions (stiffness), night vision, nutrition supplementation (phenylketonuria), rheumatoid arthritis, stress

NATURAL STANDARD DOES NOT RECOMMEND SPECIFIC THERAPIES OR PRACTITIONERS.—CONT'D

GRADE: C (Unclear or Conflicting Scientific Evidence)

Therapy	Specific Therapeutic Use(s)
Black pepper	Stroke recovery (difficulty swallowing)
Black tea	Asthma, cancer (prevention), colorectal cancer, dental cavity (prevention), diabetes, heart attack (prevention)/cardiovascular risk, memory enhancement, mental performance/alertness, metabolic enhancement, methicillin-resistant *Staphylococcus aureus* (MRSA) infection, oral leukoplakia/carcinoma, osteoporosis (prevention), stress, weight loss
Blackberry	Antioxidant
Blessed thistle	Dyspepsia/indigestion/flatulence, viral infections
Bloodroot	Periodontal disease
Boneset	Colds/flu
Borage seed oil	Alcohol-induced hangover, asthma, atopic dermatitis, cystic fibrosis, hyperlipidemia, infant development/neonatal care (in preterm infants), malnutrition (inflammation complex syndrome), seborrheic dermatitis (infantile), stress, supplementation in preterm and very low birthweight infants (fatty acids)
Boron	Improving cognitive function, osteoarthritis, osteoporosis, vaginitis (topical)
Boswellia	Crohn's disease, osteoarthritis, rheumatoid arthritis (RA), ulcerative colitis
Bovine cartilage	Skin care (laser resurfacing adjunct)
Bovine colostrum	Diarrhea, exercise performance enhancement, *Helicobacter pylori* infection, immune function, immune system deficiencies (cryptosporidiosis), infections (rotavirus), multiple sclerosis, oral hygiene, recovery from surgery, sore throat, upper respiratory tract infection
Boxwood	HIV/AIDS
Bromelain	Burn debridement, cancer, chronic obstructive pulmonary disease (COPD), digestive enzyme/pancreatic insufficiency, knee pain, muscle soreness, nutritional supplement, osteoarthritis (OA) of the knee, rash (unknown cause), rheumatoid arthritis (RA), steatorrhea (fatty stools due to poor digestion), urinary tract infection
Bupleurum	Fever, hepatitis, hepatocellular carcinoma (prevention), thrombocytopenic purpura
Burdock	Quality of life (breast cancer)
Butterbur	Allergic skin disease, asthma
Calcium	Bone stress injury (prevention), colorectal cancer, growth (mineral metabolism in very low birth weight infants), hypertension, (pregnancy-induced), hyperparathyroidism (secondary), lead toxicity (acute symptom management), osteomalacia/rickets, osteoporosis prevention (steroid-induced), prostate cancer (increased risk), weight loss
Calendula	Otitis media, skin inflammation, venous leg ulcers, wound healing
Caper	Cirrhosis

(Continued)

NATURAL STANDARD DOES NOT RECOMMEND SPECIFIC THERAPIES OR PRACTITIONERS.—CONT'D

GRADE: C (Unclear or Conflicting Scientific Evidence)

Therapy	Specific Therapeutic Use(s)
Caprylic acid	Epilepsy (children)
Carob	Diarrhea in children, gastroesophageal reflux disease (in infants)
Carrageenan	Hyperlipidemia
Carrot	Antioxidant, vitamin A deficiency
Cascara sagrada	Constipation
Cat's claw	Anti-inflammatory, arthritis (osteoarthritis, rheumatoid arthritis), cancer, immunostimulation
Cedar	Alopecia areata (hair loss)
Celery	Mosquito repellent
Chamomile	Common cold, diarrhea in children, eczema, gastrointestinal conditions, hemorrhagic cystitis (bladder irritation with bleeding), hemorrhoids, Infantile colic, mucositis from cancer treatment (mouth ulcers/irritation), quality of life in cancer patients, skin inflammation, Sleep aid/sedation, vaginitis, wound healing
Chaparral	Cancer
Chasteberry	Corpus luteum deficiency/luteal phase deficiency, cyclic mastalgia, irregular menstrual cycles, premenstrual dysphoric Disorder (PMDD), premenstrual syndrome (PMS)
Chicory	Chronic hepatitis
Chitosan	Dental plaque, renal failure, wound healing
Chlorella	Adjunct in surgery, hypertension, skin cancer, ulcerative colitis, vaccine adjunct
Chlorophyll	Fibrocystic breast disease, herpes (simplex and zoster), pancreatitis (chronic), pneumonia (active destructive), poisoning (reduce Yusho symptoms), protection from aflatoxins, reduction of odor from incontinence/bladder catheterization, rheumatoid arthritis, tuberculosis
Choline	Acute viral hepatitis, allergic rhinitis, brain injuries (craniocerebral), coma, ischemic stroke, muscle mass/body mass, Parkinson's disease, post-surgical recovery
Chondroitin sulfate	Coronary artery disease, interstitial cystitis, iron absorption enhancement, ophthalmologic uses, psoriasis
Chromium	Bipolar disorder, bone loss (postmenopausal women), cardiovascular disease, cognitive function, depression, diabetes mellitus (glucose intolerance), hyperlipidemia, immunosuppression, Parkinson's disease, schizophrenia (body composition and mental states)
Chrysanthemum	Diabetes
Cinnamon	Diabetes (type 2), *Helicobacter pylori* infection
Clay	Functional gastrointestinal disorders, mercuric chloride poisoning, protection from aflatoxins
Clove	Fever reduction, mosquito repellent, premature ejaculation

NATURAL STANDARD DOES NOT RECOMMEND SPECIFIC THERAPIES OR PRACTITIONERS.—CONT'D

GRADE: C (Unclear or Conflicting Scientific Evidence)

Therapy	Specific Therapeutic Use(s)
Coenzyme Q10	Age-related macular degeneration, alzheimer's disease, angina, asthma, breast cancer, cancer, cardiomyopathy (dilated, hypertrophic), chemotherapy toxicity (anthracycline), chronic fatigue syndrome, cocaine dependence, coronary heart disease, exercise performance, Friedreich's ataxia, gum disease (periodontitis), heart attack (acute myocardial infarction), heart failure (CHF), heart protection during surgery, HIV/AIDS, hypertriglyceridemia, idiopathic asthenozoospermia, lipid lowering (adjunct to statin therapy), migraine, mitochondrial diseases and Kearns-Sayre syndrome, mitral valve prolapse (children), muscular dystrophies, myelodysplastic syndrome, Parkinson's disease, post-surgical recovery (adjuvant), prostate cancer, renal failure, tinnitus
Coleus	Anti-inflammatory action after cardiopulmonary bypass, breast milk stimulant, breathing aid for intubation, depression and schizophrenia, erectile dysfunction
Comfrey	Myalgia
Copper	Arthritis, dental plaque, malnutrition (marasmus), Menkes' kinky-hair disease, metabolic disorders (trimethylaminuria), systemic lupus erythematosus (SLE)
Coral	Bone healing (reconstructive surgery and grafting)
Cordyceps	Anti-aging, asthma, exercise performance enhancement, immunosuppression, liver disease (hepatic cirrhosis), nephrotoxicity (drug-induced), reduction of adverse effects of chemotherapy and radiation, renal failure (chronic), respiratory disorders, sexual dysfunction
Cornflower	Urolithiasis (urinary tract stones)
Corydalis	Antiparasitic, arrhythmia, *Helicobacter pylori* infection (with chronic atrophic gastritis), pain (cold-induced)
Cowhage	Parkinson's disease
Cranberry	Achlorhydria and B_{12} absorption, antibacterial (pediatric), antioxidant, antiviral and antifungal, cancer (prevention), dental (oral) plaque, memory enhancement, radiation-induced urinary symptoms, reduction of odor associated with incontinence/bladder catheterization, urinary tract infection treatment, urine acidification, urolithiasis, urostomy care
Creatine	Adjunct in surgery (coronary heart disease), apnea (of prematurity), athletic performance enhancement (aging), athletic performance enhancement (cyclists), athletic performance enhancement (females), athletic performance enhancement (high-intensity endurance), athletic performance enhancement (rowers), athletic performance enhancement (runners), athletic performance enhancement (specific sports), athletic performance enhancement (sprinters; general), athletic performance enhancement (swimmers), bone density, chronic obstructive pulmonary disease, depression, dialysis (hemodialysis), GAMT deficiency, Huntington's chorea/disease, hyperlipidemia, hyperornithinemia, ischemic heart disease, mcArdle's disease, memory, multiple sclerosis, muscular dystrophies, myocardial infarction, neuromuscular disorders (general; mitochondrial disorders), spinal cord injury
Damiana	Weight loss (obese patients)

(Continued)

NATURAL STANDARD DOES NOT RECOMMEND SPECIFIC THERAPIES OR PRACTITIONERS.—CONT'D

GRADE: C (Unclear or Conflicting Scientific Evidence)

Therapy	Specific Therapeutic Use(s)
Dandelion	Antioxidant, cancer, colitis, diabetes, diuretic, hepatitis B
Danshen	Burn healing, Cardiovascular disease/angina, diabetic complications (diabetic foot), dialysis (peritoneal), glaucoma, hyperlipidemia, ischemic stroke, kidney disease, liver diseases (cirrhosis, fibrosis, hepatitis B), pancreatitis (acute), prostatitis, syncope (vasovagal), tinnitus, weight loss
Date palm	Skin aging (wrinkles)
Devil's claw	Appetite stimulant, Cancer (bone metastases), Digestive tonic
Devil's club	Diabetes
DHEA	AIDS, cardiovascular disease, cervical cancer, chronic fatigue syndrome, cocaine withdrawal, Crohn's disease, dementia, erectile dysfunction, fibromyalgia, induction of labor, infertility, libido (premenopausal women), perimenopausal symptoms, psoriasis, rheumatoid arthritis, schizophrenia, Sjögren's syndrome
DMSO	Amyloidosis, anesthesia (for kidney and gallbladder stone removal), diabetic ulcers, extravasation, gastritis, herpes zoster, inflammatory bladder disease, intracranial pressure, pressure ulcers (prevention), reflex sympathetic dystrophy, rheumatoid arthritis, surgical skin flap ischemia, tendopathies
Dogwood	Postmenopausal symptoms
Dong quai	Amenorrhea (lack of menstrual period), angina pectoris/coronary artery disease, arthritis, dysmenorrhea (painful menstruation), glomerulonephritis, idiopathic thrombocytopenic purpura (ITP), menstrual migraine headache, nerve pain, pulmonary hypertension
Echinacea	Cancer, immune system stimulation, radiation-associated leucopenia, uveitis, vaginal yeast infections
Elderberry and elder flower	Bacterial sinusitis, bronchitis, hyperlipidemia
Emu oil	Cosmetic uses
English ivy	Chronic obstructive pulmonary disease
Ephedra	Allergic rhinitis, hypotension, sexual arousal
Essiac	Cancer
Eucalyptus oil	Asthma, decongestant-expectorant/upper respiratory tract infection (oral/inhalation), dental plaque/gingivitis (mouthwash), headache (topical), skin ulcers, smoking cessation, tick repellant (topical)
Euphorbia	Eczema, epilepsy, inflammation (oral)
Evening primrose oil	Acute bronchitis, breast cancer, breast cysts, breast pain (mastalgia), diabetes, diabetic peripheral neuropathy, ichthyosis vulgaris, multiple sclerosis, obesity/weight loss, osteoporosis, postviral/chronic fatigue syndrome, pre-eclampsia/pregnancy-induced hypertension, Raynaud's phenomenon, rheumatoid arthritis
Eyebright	Conjunctivitis, anti-inflammatory, hepatoprotection
Fennel	Cough (ACE inhibitor–induced), dysmenorrhea, ultraviolet light skin damage protection

NATURAL STANDARD DOES NOT RECOMMEND SPECIFIC THERAPIES OR PRACTITIONERS.—CONT'D

GRADE: C (Unclear or Conflicting Scientific Evidence)

Therapy	Specific Therapeutic Use(s)
Fenugreek	Diabetes mellitus type 2, galactagogue (breast milk stimulant), hyperlipidemia
Feverfew	Rheumatoid arthritis
Fig	Diabetes (Type 1)
Flax	Attention deficit hyperactivity disorder (flaxseed oil), breast cancer (flaxseed), constipation/laxative (flaxseed), cyclic mastalgia (breast pain) (flaxseed), HIV/AIDS, hyperglycemia/diabetes (flaxseed), hyperlipidemia (flaxseed and oil), hypertension (flaxseed), keratoconjunctivitis sicca (dry eye), lupus nephritis (flaxseed), menopausal symptoms, obesity, pregnancy (spontaneous delivery), prostate cancer (flaxseed)
Folate	Alzheimer's disease, arsenic poisoning (arsenic-induced illnesses), cancer, chronic fatigue syndrome, depression, folate deficiency in alcoholics, hearing loss (age-associated), nitrate tolerance, phenytoin-induced gingival hyperplasia, pregnancy-related gingivitis, stroke, vascular disease/hyperhomocysteinemia, vitiligo
Gamma linolenic acid	Acute respiratory distress syndrome, atopic dermatitis, attention deficit hyperactivity disorder, blood pressure control, cancer treatment (adjunct), immune enhancement, mastalgia, menopausal hot flashes, migraine, osteoporosis, pre-eclampsia, premenstrual syndrome, pruritis, rheumatoid arthritis, Sjögren's syndrome, ulcerative colitis
Gamma oryzanol	Gastritis, hypothyroidism, menopausal symptoms, prevention of restenosis after coronary angioplasty (PTCA), skin conditions
Garcinia	Weight loss
Garlic	Anti-fungal (topical), anti-platelet effects, atherosclerosis, cancer (prevention), cardiac secondary (prevention), cryptococcal meningitis, familial hyperlipidemia, hypertension, peripheral vascular disease, tick repellant, upper respiratory tract infection
Germanium	Multiple myeloma
Ginger	Anti-platelet agent, migraine, motion sickness/sea sickness, nausea and vomiting (chemotherapy-induced), nausea and vomiting (postoperative), osteoarthritis, rheumatoid arthritis, shortening labor, urinary disorders (post-stroke), weight loss
Ginkgo	Acute hemorrhoidal attacks, acute ischemic stroke, age-associated memory impairment (AAMI), altitude (mountain) sickness, asthma, cardiovascular disease, chemotherapy adjunct (reduce adverse vascular effects), chronic cochleovestibular disorders, chronic venous insufficiency, cocaine dependence, decreased libido and erectile dysfunction (drug related), depression and seasonal affective disorder (SAD), diabetic neuropathy, dyslexia, gastric cancer, glaucoma, Graves' disease (adjunct iodine/iodide), macular degeneration, memory enhancement (in healthy patients), mood and cognition in post-menopausal women, multiple sclerosis (MS), premenstrual syndrome (PMS), pulmonary interstitial fibrosis, quality of life, Raynaud's disease, retinopathy, schizophrenia, tinnitus, vertigo, vitiligo

(Continued)

NATURAL STANDARD DOES NOT RECOMMEND SPECIFIC THERAPIES OR PRACTITIONERS.—CONT'D

GRADE: C (Unclear or Conflicting Scientific Evidence)

Therapy	Specific Therapeutic Use(s)
Ginseng	Aplastic anemia, attention deficit hyperactivity disorder (ADHD), birth outcomes (anoxemic encephalopathy), cancer (chemotherapy adjunct), cancer (prevention), chronic hepatitis B, congestive heart failure, coronary artery disease, dementia, diabetic nephropathy, exercise performance, fatigue, fistula, hepatoprotection, hyperlipidemia, hypertension, Idiopathic thrombocytopenic purpurea (ITP), intracranial pressure, kidney dysfunction (hemorrhagic fever with renal syndrome), menopausal symptoms, mental performance, methicillin-resistant *Staphylococcus aureus* (MRSA), neurologic disorders, postoperative recovery (breast cancer), pregnancy (intrauterine growth retardation), premature ejaculation, pulmonary conditions, quality of life, radiation therapy side effects, sexual arousal (in women), sexual function/libido/ erectile dysfunction, viral myocarditis, well-being
Globe artichoke	Alcohol-induced hangover, antioxidant, dyspepsia, irritable bowel syndrome
Glucosamine	Chronic venous insufficiency, diabetes (and related conditions), inflammatory bowel disease (Crohn's disease, ulcerative colitis), pain (leg pain), rehabilitation (after knee injury), rheumatoid arthritis, temporomandibular joint (TMJ) disorders
Glyconutrients	Failure to thrive
Goji	Cancer, vision
Goldenseal	Heart failure, hypercholesterolemia, immunostimulant, infectious diarrhea, narcotic concealment (urine analysis), trachoma (*Chlamydia trachomatosis* eye infection), upper respiratory tract infection
Gotu kola	Anxiety, cognitive function, diabetic microangiopathy, liver cirrhosis, wound healing
Grape seed	Agitation in dementia, antioxidant, cancer, hypercholesterolemia, inhibition of platelet aggregation, melasma (chloasma), pancreatitis, premenstrual syndrome, radiation skin protection (UV), skin aging (postmenopausal women), vision problems
Grapefruit	Endocrine disorders (metabolic syndrome), heart disease, kidney stones
Greater celandine	Biliary colic, esophageal cancer, lung cancer, pancreatic cancer, tonsillitis
Green tea	Anxiety, arthritis, asthma, cancer (general), cardiovascular conditions, common cold (prevention), dental caries (prevention), diabetes, fertility, human T-cell lymphocytic virus (carriers), hypercholesterolemia, hypertension, hypertriglyceridemia, menopausal symptoms, mental performance/alertness, photoprotection, weight loss
Green-lipped mussel	Osteoarthritis
Guarana	Mood enhancement, weight loss
Guggul	Acne, obesity, osteoarthritis, rheumatoid arthritis
Gymnema	Hyperlipidemia, weight loss
Hawthorn	Anxiety, coronary artery disease (angina), functional cardiovascular disorders, hypertension (in patients with type 2 diabetes), orthostatic hypotension

NATURAL STANDARD DOES NOT RECOMMEND SPECIFIC THERAPIES OR PRACTITIONERS.—CONT'D

GRADE: C (Unclear or Conflicting Scientific Evidence)

Therapy	Specific Therapeutic Use(s)
Hibiscus	Lice
Holy basil	Diabetes mellitus
Honey	Dermatitis (dandruff), diabetes mellitus type 2, Fournier's gangrene, gastroenteritis (infantile), herpes, hypercholesterolemia, hypertension, leg ulcers, Plaque/gingivitis, radiation mucositis, rhinoconjunctivitis, skin graft healing (split thickness), wound healing
Hops	Menopausal symptoms, rheumatic diseases, sedation
Horny goat weed	Sexual dysfunction (in renal failure patients)
Horseradish	Sinusitis, urinary tract infection
Horsetail	Osteoporosis
Hoxsey formula	Cancer
Hydrazine sulfate	Cancer treatment
Ignatia	Emotional disorders (emergency use)
Iodine	Bladder irrigation, bleeding, bowel irrigation, cancer, cognitive function, corpus vitreous degeneration, goiter treatment, Lymphedema (filarial), molluscum contagiosum, oral intubation, pelvic infection, periodontitis/gingivitis, pneumonia, postcesarean endometritis, renal pelvic instillation sclerotherapy (RPIS), septicemia (serious bacterial infections in the blood), wound healing
Iron	Attention deficit hyperactivity disorder (ADHD), fatigue in women with low ferritin levels, improving cognitive performance related to iron deficiency, lead toxicity, preventing anemia associated with preterm/low birth weight infants, preventing iron deficiency in exercising women, iron deficiency after blood donation (prevention), iron deficiency anemia due to gastrointestinal bleeding (prevention), treatment of predialysis anemia
Jackfruit	High blood sugar/glucose intolerance
Jasmine	Lactation suppression, memory improvement, stroke
Jewelweed	Contact dermatitis (Poison ivy/oak skin rash)
Jiaogulan	Fatty liver (nonalcoholic)
Jojoba	Mosquito repellent
Kava	Insomnia, Parkinson's disease, stress
Khat	Cognitive function
Khella	Vitiligo
Kinetin	Meniere's disease, ocular disorders (blood pressure)
Kiwi	Respiratory problems (prevention)
Kudzu	Cardiovascular disease/angina, deafness, diabetes (insulin resistance), diabetic retinopathy, glaucoma, menopausal symptoms

(Continued)

NATURAL STANDARD DOES NOT RECOMMEND SPECIFIC THERAPIES OR PRACTITIONERS.—CONT'D

GRADE: C (Unclear or Conflicting Scientific Evidence)

Therapy	Specific Therapeutic Use(s)
Lactobacillus acidophilus	Allergy treatment (Japanese cedar pollen), asthma, diarrhea (prevention), diarrhea treatment (children), hepatic encephalopathy (confused thinking due to liver disorders), hypercholesterolemia, irritable bowel syndrome, lactose intolerance, necrotizing enterocolitis (prevention in infants), vaginal candidiasis (yeast infection)
Lavender	Alopecia/hair loss (topical), antibiotic (topical), anxiety (aromatherapy), cancer (perillyl alcohol), cognitive performance, dementia, depression (mild to moderate), ear pain, eczema, hypnotic/sleep aid (aromatherapy), overall well being (lavender used in a bath), pain (vascular injury, cancer, back and neck pain), perineal discomfort following childbirth (bathing), quality of life (postpartum), rheumatoid arthritis pain, spasmolytic (oral)
L-Carnitine	ADHD, AIDS, alcoholism, Alzheimer's disease, arrhythmia, cerebral ischemia, congestive heart failure, dementia (elderly), depression, diabetes mellitus, diabetic neuropathy, dialysis (CAPD), dialysis (hemodialysis), diphtheria, erectile dysfunction, exercise performance, fatigue, fragile X syndrome, hepatic encephalopathy, huntington's chorea/disease, hyperlipoproteinemia, hyperthyroidism, infertility (asthenospermia), lactic acidosis, liver disease (cirrhosis), memory, myocardial infarction, nutritional deficiencies (adults), nutritional deficiencies (full-term infants), nutritional deficiencies (premature infants), obesity, peripheral neuropathy, Peyronie's disease, pregnancy (miscarriage), respiratory distress (adults), respiratory distress (infants), rett's syndrome, sickle cell disease, surgical uses (bypass), tuberculosis
Lemon balm	Agitation in dementia, anxiety, cognitive performance, colitis, dyspepsia, sleep quality
Lemongrass	Sedation
Licorice	Aplastic anemia, apthous ulcers/canker sores, atopic dermatitis, bleeding stomach ulcers caused by aspirin, dental hygiene, dyspepsia (functional), familial mediterranean fever (FMF), herpes simplex virus, high potassium levels resulting from abnormally low aldosterone levels, HIV, Hyperprolactinemia (neuroleptic-induced), idiopathic thrombocytopenic purpura, inflammation, polycystic ovarian syndrome, reducing body fat mass, upper respiratory tract infections, viral hepatitis (SNMC)
Lime	Iron deficiency
Lingonberry	Urinary tract infection (UTI) prevention
Liver extract	Chronic fatigue syndrome, chronic hepatitis (hepatitis C), hepatic disorders, surgical uses (urological operation adjunct)
Lutein	Atherosclerosis, cancer, cataracts, diabetes mellitus, eye disorders (lens opacities), eye disorders (macular degeneration), eye disorders (retinal degeneration), lung function, muscle soreness, obesity, pre-eclampsia, UV-induced erythema (prevention)/sunburn
Lycopene	Asthma (exercise-induced), atherosclerosis (coronary artery disease), benign prostatic hypertrophy (BPH), breast cancer (prevention), cancer prevention (general), cervical cancer (prevention), Eye disorders (age-related macular degeneration and cataract), gingivitis, hypertension, infertility, kidney disease (renal cell cancer), lung cancer (prevention), oral mucositis (oral submucous fibrosis), ovarian cancer (prevention), pre-eclampsia/pregnancy-induced hypertension, prostate cancer (treatment and prevention), sun protection, upper gastrointestinal tract and colorectal cancer (prevention)

NATURAL STANDARD DOES NOT RECOMMEND SPECIFIC THERAPIES OR PRACTITIONERS.—CONT'D

GRADE: C (Unclear or Conflicting Scientific Evidence)

Therapy	Specific Therapeutic Use(s)
Maca	Hormone regulation (male), spermatogenesis
Maitake mushroom	Diabetes, immune stimulation
Marshmallow	Inflammatory skin conditions (eczema, psoriasis)
Mastic	Duodenal ulcer, gastric ulcer
Melatonin	Alzheimer's disease (sleep disorders), antioxidant (free radical scavenging), attention deficit hyperactivity disorder (ADHD), benzodiazepine tapering, bipolar disorder (sleep disturbances), cancer treatment, chemotherapy side effects, circadian rhythm entraining (in blind persons), depression (sleep disturbances), glaucoma, headache (prevention), hypertension, HIV/AIDS, insomnia (of unknown origin in the non-elderly), Parkinson's disease, periodic limb movement disorder, preoperative sedation/anxiolysis, REM sleep behavior disorder, Rett's syndrome, schizophrenia (sleep disorders), seasonal affective disorder (SAD), seizure disorder (children), sleep disturbances due to pineal region brain damage, smoking cessation, stroke, tardive dyskinesia, thrombocytopenia (low platelets), ultraviolet light skin damage protection, work-shift sleep disorder
Milk thistle	Acute viral hepatitis, *Amanita phalloides* mushroom toxicity, cancer, diabetes mellitus (associated with cirrhosis), drug/toxin–induced hepatotoxicity, dyspepsia, hyperlipidemia, menopausal symptoms
Mistletoe	Cancer, hepatitis, HIV, immunomodulation, respiratory disease (recurrent)
Modified citrus pectin	Prostate cancer
MSM	Osteoarthritis
Muira puama	Sexual dysfunction (females)
Mullein	Earache (associated with acute otitis media)
Myrcia	Diabetes (type 2)
Neem	Mosquito repellent, psoriasis vulgaris, ulcers (gastroduodenal)
Niacin	Age-related macular degeneration, Alzheimer's disease/cognitive decline, headaches, hyperphosphatemia, osteoarthritis (niacinamide), skin conditions (topical), type 1 diabetes mellitus: preservation of beta-islet cell function (niacinamide), type 2 diabetes
Noni	Hearing loss
Nopal	Diabetes, hyperlipidemia
Oleander	Congestive heart failure
Omega-3 fatty acids, fish oil, alpha-linolenic acid	Angina pectoris, asthma, atherosclerosis, bipolar disorder, cancer (prevention), cardiac arrhythmias (abnormal heart rhythms), colon cancer, Crohn's disease, cystic fibrosis, depression, dysmenorrhea, eczema, IgA nephropathy, infant eye/brain development, lupus erythematosus, nephrotic syndrome, preeclampsia, prevention of graft failure after heart bypass surgery, prevention of restenosis after coronary angioplasty (PTCA), primary cardiovascular disease prevention (alpha-linolenic acid [ALA]), psoriasis, schizophrenia, secondary cardiovascular disease prevention (alpha-linolenic acid [ALA]), stroke (prevention), ulcerative colitis

(Continued)

NATURAL STANDARD DOES NOT RECOMMEND SPECIFIC THERAPIES OR PRACTITIONERS.—CONT'D

GRADE: C (Unclear or Conflicting Scientific Evidence)

Therapy	Specific Therapeutic Use(s)
Onion	Alopecia areata, diabetes, hypertension, scar prevention
Oregano	Parasites
Pantethine	Ischemic heart disease
Pantothenic acid	Athletic performance, attention deficit hyperactivity disorder (ADHD), burns, hypercholesterolemia, osteoarthritis, rheumatoid arthritis, wound healing
Papain	Gastrointestinal disorders (phytobezoar), jellyfish stings, pulmonary conditions (lung abscess), radiation therapy side effects, recovery from surgery (prevention of postoperative adhesion formation), rheumatic disorders, skin conditions (xerotic skin), sore throat, wound healing
Para-aminobenzoic acid	Asthma, autoimmune disorders (pemphigus vulgaris adjuvant), cancer pain, hair loss, inflammatory skin disorders (lichen sclerosus), Peyronie's disease, photoprotection, scleroderma
Passion flower	Congestive heart failure (exercise capacity)
PC-SPES	Prostate cancer
Peony	Allergic dermatitis, antioxidant, chronic hepatitis (liver cirrhosis), coronary heart disease (prevention), coronary heart disease (treatment), gastric disorders (*Campylobacter pyloridis*), hemolytic disease of the newborn, hormone regulation, hypertension (gestational), lipid-lowering effects, lung cancer, Menstrual irregularities, nephritis (crescentic), rheumatoid arthritis, uterine fibroids (myomas), wrinkle prevention
Peppermint	Abdominal distention, asthma, bad breath, breast tenderness (preventing cracked nipples), functional bowel disorders, nasal congestion, post-herpetic neuralgia, post-operative nausea (inhalation), stroke recovery (hemiplegic shoulder pain), tuberculosis, urinary tract infection, vigilance improvement in brain injury
Perilla	Aphthous stomatitis, asthma
Perillyl alcohol	Cancer
Phenylalanine	Attention deficit hyperactivity disorder (adults), dental anesthesia
Phosphates, phosphorus	Bone density (bone metabolism), burns, diabetic ketoacidosis, hypercalciuria (high urine calcium levels), hyperparathyroidism, total parenteral nutrition (TPN), vitamin D–resistant rickets
Podophyllum	Leukoplakia (HIV-related), rheumatoid arthritis, uterine cancer
Policosanol	Hypercholesterolemia, reactivity/brain activity
Polypodium leucotomos extract and anapsos	Atopic dermatitis (eczema), dementia (memory loss, disorientation), Alzheimer's disease, psoriasis, skin damage (UV-induced), vitiligo (loss of pigment in the skin), dementia, psoriasis, skin damage caused by the sun
Pomegranate	Antioxidant, atherosclerosis, chronic obstructive pulmonary disease (COPD), dental conditions (plaque, periodontitis), erectile dysfunction, hypercholesterolemia, hypertension, menopausal symptoms, prostate cancer, sunburn

NATURAL STANDARD DOES NOT RECOMMEND SPECIFIC THERAPIES OR PRACTITIONERS.—CONT'D

GRADE: C (Unclear or Conflicting Scientific Evidence)

Therapy	Specific Therapeutic Use(s)
Probiotics	Allergy, amoebiasis, asthma, bacterial infection, bacterial vaginosis, cardiovascular disease, cardiovascular risk reduction (smokers/atherosclerosis), colitis (collagenous), constipation, diarrhea (acute), diarrhea (antibiotic-associated), diarrhea (chronic bacterial overgrowth-related), diarrhea (*Clostridium difficile*), ear infections, hepatic encephalopathy (confused thinking due to liver disorders), hypercholesterolemia, infections (complications), infections (rotavirus nosocomial), inflammatory bowel disease (IBD), lactose intolerance, necrotizing enterocolitis (NEC) (prevention), nutrition, peptic ulcers, pneumonia, pouchitis, premature labor (prevention), rheumatoid arthritis (RA), supplementation in preterm and very low birthweight infants, thrush, urinary tract infection, vaccine adjunct, vaginal candidiasis (yeast infection)
Propolis	Burns, dental analgesia (and wound healing), dental plaque and gingivitis (mouthwash), genital herpes simplex virus (HSV) infection, *Helicobacter pylori* infection, infections (bacterial, parasitic, fungal), Legg-Calve-Perthes disease/avascular hip necrosis, post-herpetic corneal complications, recurrent aphthous stomatitis, rheumatic diseases, rhinopharyngitis prevention (children), upper respiratory tract infection (children), vaginitis
PSK	Colorectal cancer (adjuvant), esophageal cancer (adjuvant), gastric cancer (adjuvant), leukemia (adjuvant), liver cancer (adjuvant), lung cancer (adjuvant), nasopharyngeal carcinoma (adjuvant), non–small cell lung cancer (NSCLC) (adjuvant)
Psyllium	Anal fissures, colon cancer, colonoscopy preparation, fat excretion in stool, gas (flatulence), hemorrhoids, hyperglycemia, induction of labor/abortion (cervical dilator), inflammatory bowel disease (Crohn's disease, ulcerative colitis), irritable bowel syndrome, obesity
Pycnogenol	Attention deficit hyperactivity disorder (ADHD), chronic venous insufficiency, diabetes (type 2), diabetic microangiopathy, erectile dysfunction, gingival bleeding/plaque, hypertension, platelet aggregation (smokers), prevention of blood clots during long airplane flights, retinopathy, systemic lupus erythematosus (SLE), venous leg ulcers
Quassia	Head lice
Quercetin	Immune function (after intense exercise), pancreatic cancer prevention, Prostatitis
Raspberry	Childbirth
Red clover	Cardiovascular blood flow, diabetes, high cholesterol, hormone replacement therapy (HRT), menopausal symptoms, osteoporosis, prostate cancer, prostate enlargement (benign prostatic hypertrophy), benign prostatic hypertrophy (BPH), hormone replacement therapy (HRT), hypercholesterolemia, osteoporosis, prostate cancer
Red yeast rice	Coronary heart disease, diabetes
Rehmannia	Hypopituitarism (Sheehan's syndrome)
Reishi mushroom	Cancer, chronic hepatitis B, coronary heart disease, diabetes mellitus type 2, hypertension, poisoning (Russula subnigricans), postherpetic neuralgia, Proteinuria

(Continued)

NATURAL STANDARD DOES NOT RECOMMEND SPECIFIC THERAPIES OR PRACTITIONERS.—CONT'D

GRADE: C (Unclear or Conflicting Scientific Evidence)

Therapy	Specific Therapeutic Use(s)
Resveratrol	Cardiovascular disease, longevity/anti-aging
Rhodiola	Exercise performance enhancement, hypoxia, lung disease (acute injury), mental performance
Rhubarb	Age-associated memory impairment (AAMI)
Rhubarb	Aplastic anemia, constipation (chronic), fatty liver (non-alcoholic), gastrointestinal cancer surgery, gastrointestinal tract disorders, hemorrhage (nephritic syndrome), hepatitis, herpes, hypercholesterolemia, nasopharyngeal carcinoma, nephritis (mid-advanced crescentic), obesity (simple), pre-eclampsia, sepsis (systemic inflammation reaction syndrome; SIRS)
Riboflavin	Anemia, anorexia/bulimia, cataracts, cognitive function, depression, esophageal cancer (prevention and treatment), ethylmalonic encephalopathy, malaria, migraine headache (prevention), pre-eclampsia
Rose hip	Dermatoses, immune function, ophthalmologic disorders, wound healing
Rosemary	Anxiety/stress
Rutin	Hemorrhoids, Ménière's syndrome, microangiopathy, retinal vein occlusion, retinopathy, schizophrenia, skin conditions, thrombosis, varicose leg ulcers, varicose veins, venous hypertension
Saccharomyces boulardii	Antibacterial (amebiasis), Crohn's disease, diarrhea (*Clostridium difficile*), diarrhea (HIV-associated), diarrhea (prevention during tube feeding), diarrhea (traveler's), irritable bowel syndrome (IBS), nutritional support (premature infants)
Safflower	Angina pectoris/coronary artery disease, atherosclerosis (lipid peroxidation), cardiovascular disorders (chronic cor pulmonale), chronic hepatitis (hepatitis C), cystic fibrosis, diabetes mellitus type 2, familial hyperlipidemia, Friedreich's ataxia, hypercholesterolemia, hypertension, kidney disorders (type II nephritic syndrome), malnutrition (protein-energy), nutritional supplement (infant formula), skin conditions (phrynoderma), total parenteral nutrition, toxicity (lithium)
Sage	Lung cancer (prevention)
SAMe	Attention deficit hyperactivity disorder, cholestasis (non-pregnant), cholestasis (pregnancy), depression, fibromyalgia, liver disease (general)
Sandalwood	Anxiety
Sanicle	Atopic eczema, otitis media (recurrent)
Saw palmetto	Androgenetic alopecia (topical), hypotonic neurogenic bladder, prostate cancer, prostatitis/chronic pelvic pain syndrome (CP/CPPS)
Schisandra	Eczema, familial Mediterranean fever (FMF), liver disease, vision
Scotch broom	Diuretic (increased urine flow), labor induction (oxytocic)
Sea buckthorn	Atopic dermatitis, burns, cardiovascular disease, cirrhosis, common cold, gastric ulcers, hypertension, pneumonia

NATURAL STANDARD DOES NOT RECOMMEND SPECIFIC THERAPIES OR PRACTITIONERS.—CONT'D

GRADE: C (Unclear or Conflicting Scientific Evidence)

Therapy	Specific Therapeutic Use(s)
Seaweed, kelp, bladderwrack	Antibacterial/antifungal, anticoagulant, antioxidant, cancer, goiter (thyroid disease), hyperglycemia (diabetes)
	Asthma, blood disorders, bronchitis, cancer (prevention), cancer treatment, cardiomyopathy, cardiovascular disease (prevention), central nervous system disorders, chemotherapy side effects, critical illness, cystic fibrosis, dandruff, dialysis, eye disorders, fatigue, hypertension, HIV/AIDS, infection (prevention), infertility, intracranial pressure symptoms, liver disease, longevity/anti-aging, low birth weight, malabsorption, pancreatitis, physical endurance, post-operative recovery, pre-eclampsia, quality of life, radiation side effects, rheumatoid arthritis, seizures, sepsis (severe bacterial infection in the blood), skin disorders, sunburn (prevention), thyroid conditions, trauma, yeast infections
Shark cartilage	Arthritis, cancer (solid tumors), macular degeneration, psoriasis
Shea butter	Decongestant (nasal), lipid-lowering effects (cholesterol and triglycerides)
Shiitake	Genital warts (*Condyloma acuminatum*), HIV (adjunct therapy), immunomodulator
Slippery elm	Diarrhea, gastrointestinal disorders, sore throat
Sorrel	Antibacterial, antiviral, bronchitis, cancer, quality of life (cancer), sinusitis
Soy	Breast cancer (prevention), cancer treatment, cardiac ischemia, cardiovascular disease, cognitive function, colon cancer (prevention), Crohn's disease, cyclical breast pain, diarrhea in adults, endocrine disorders (metabolic syndrome), endometrial cancer (prevention), exercise capacity improvement (spinal cord injury patients), gallstones (cholelithiasis), hypertension, kidney disease (chronic renal failure, nephrotic syndrome, proteinuria), menstrual migraine, obesity/weight reduction, osteoporosis, post-menopausal bone loss, prostate cancer (prevention), skin aging, skin damage caused by the sun, stomach cancer, thyroid disorders, tuberculosis, type 2 diabetes
Spirulina	Arsenic poisoning, diabetes mellitus (type 2), eye disorders (blepharospasm), hypercholesterolemia, malnutrition, oral leukoplakia/cancer, weight loss
Squill	Coronary artery disease
St. John's wort	Anxiety disorder, atopic dermatitis, depression (children), obsessive-compulsive disorder (OCD), perimenopausal symptoms, premenstrual syndrome (PMS), seasonal affective disorder (SAD), social phobia
Stinging nettle	Arthritis, benign prostatic hyperplasia (BPH), insect bites, joint pain, plaque/gingivitis
Strawberry	Colorectal cancer prevention
Sweet almond	Anxiety (in palliative care patients)
Sweet annie	Malaria
Tamarind	Bone diseases (skeletal fluorosis prevention)

(Continued)

NATURAL STANDARD DOES NOT RECOMMEND SPECIFIC THERAPIES OR PRACTITIONERS.—CONT'D

GRADE: C (Unclear or Conflicting Scientific Evidence)

Therapy	Specific Therapeutic Use(s)
Taurine	Congestive heart failure (CHF), cystic fibrosis, diabetes mellitus (type 2), energy, epilepsy (seizure), hypercholesterolemia, hypertension, iron-deficiency anemia, liver disease, myotonic dystrophy, nutritional support (TPN), obesity, Surgery (coronary bypass), vaccine adjunct, vision problems (fatigue)
Tea tree oil	Allergic skin reactions, bad breath, dandruff, dental plaque/gingivitis, eye infections (ocular demodex), lice, methicillin-resistant *Staphylococcus aureus* (MRSA) colonization, onychomycosis, recurrent herpes labialis infection, thrush (oral *Candida albicans*), tinea pedis (athlete's foot), vaginal infections (yeast and bacterial)
Thiamin	Alzheimer's disease, atherosclerosis (prevention in patients with acute hyperglycemia, impaired glucose tolerance [IGT], and diabetes mellitus), athletic performance, cancer, cataract (prevention), coma/hypothermia of unknown origin, Crohn's disease, Didmoad (Wolfram) syndrome, heart failure (cardiomyopathy), leg cramps (during pregnancy), pyruvate dehydrogenase deficiency (PDH), subclinical thiamin deficiency in the elderly
Thyme	Bronchitis/cough, dental plaque, inflammatory skin disorders, paronychia/onycholysis/antifungal
Thymus extract	Alopecia, anxiety/stress, arthritis, asthma, burns, cancer, cancer (chemotherapy adjunct), cancer (radiotherapy side effects), cardiomyopathy, chronic obstructive pulmonary disease, dermatomyositis, diabetes, eczema, encephalitis, gastritis, glaucoma, HIV/AIDS, human papilloma virus, immunostimulation, keratitis, liver disease, myelodysplastic syndrome, psoriasis, respiratory tract infections, skin conditions, systemic lupus erythematosus, tuberculosis, urinary tract infection, warts
Tribulus	Exercise performance enhancement, infertility (female), infertility (male)
Turmeric	Cancer, cholelithiasis prevention/cholagogue, cognitive function, dyspepsia, hepatoprotection, HIV/AIDS, hyperlipidemia, inflammation, irritable bowel syndrome, oral leukoplakia (oral submucous fibrosis), osteoarthritis, peptic ulcer disease, rheumatoid arthritis, scabies, uveitis, viral infection
Tylophora	Asthma
Usnea	Oral hygiene
Uva ursi	Urinary tract infection (UTI)
Valerian	Depression, insomnia, menopausal symptoms, sedation
Vitamin A	Antioxidant, breast cancer, cataract (prevention), diarrhea, HIV infection, immune function, infant mortality, iron-deficiency anemia, pancreatic cancer, parasite infection (*Acaris* reinfection), photoreactive keratectomy, pneumonia (children), polyp (prevention), pregnancy-related complications, skin aging (improving aging skin appearance), skin cancer (prevention), Viral infection (Norovirus [NoV] infection), weight loss, wound healing
Vitamin B_{12}	Alzheimer's disease, angioplasty, breast cancer, cardiovascular disease/hyperhomocysteinemia, fatigue, hypercholesterolemia, Imerslund-Grasbeck disease, shaky-leg syndrome, sickle cell disease

NATURAL STANDARD DOES NOT RECOMMEND SPECIFIC THERAPIES OR PRACTITIONERS.—CONT'D

GRADE: C (Unclear or Conflicting Scientific Evidence)

Therapy	Specific Therapeutic Use(s)
Vitamin B_6	Akathisia (movement disorder), angioplasty, asthma, attention deficit hyperactivity disorder (ADHD), birth outcomes, cardiovascular disease/hyperhomocysteinemia, carpal tunnel syndrome, depression, hyperkinetic cerebral dysfunction syndrome, immune system function, kidney stones (nephrolithiasis), lactation suppression, lung cancer, pregnancy-induced nausea and vomiting, premenstrual syndrome (PMS), preventing vitamin B_6 deficiency associated with taking birth control pills, tardive dyskinesia
Vitamin C	Asthma, bleeding stomach ulcers caused by aspirin, cancer (prevention), cancer treatment, complex regional pain syndrome, *Helicobacter pylori* infection, ischemic heart disease, metabolic abnormalities (alkaptonuria), plaque/calculus on teeth, pneumonia (prevention), pregnancy, prostate cancer, skin damage caused by the sun (UVA-induced), skin pigmentation disorders (perifollicular pigmentation), stroke (prevention), vaginitis
Vitamin D	Anticonvulsant-induced osteomalacia, breast cancer (prevention), cancer (prevention), colorectal cancer, corticosteroid-induced osteoporosis, diabetes (type 1/type 2), fall (prevention), hepatic osteodystrophy, hypertension, hypertriglyceridemia, immunomodulation, mortality reduction, multiple sclerosis (MS), myelodysplastic syndrome, osteogenesis imperfecta (OI), osteoporosis (cystic fibrosis patients), proximal myopathy, rickets (hypophosphatemic vitamin D–resistant), seasonal affective disorder (SAD), senile warts, skin pigmentation disorders (pigmented lesions), tooth retention, vitamin D deficiency (infants and nursing mothers), weight gain (postmenopausal)
Vitamin E	Allergic rhinitis, altitude sickness, anemia, angina, antioxidant, atherosclerosis, bladder cancer, breast cancer, breast cancer–related hot flashes, cancer treatment, cardiovascular disease in dialysis patients, cataract (prevention), chemotherapy nerve damage (neurotoxicity), colon cancer (prevention), dementia/Alzheimer's disease, diabetes mellitus, dysmenorrhea, G6PD deficiency, glomerulosclerosis (kidney disease), healing after photorefractive keratectomy, hepatitis (hepatitis C), hypercholesterolemia, immune system function, intermittent claudication, macular degeneration, parkinson's disease, premenstrual syndrome, prostate cancer (prevention), respiratory infection (prevention), seizure disorder, steatohepatitis, stomach cancer (prevention), supplementation in preterm and very low birthweight infants, tardive dyskinesia, uveitis, venous thromboembolism (VTE)
Vitamin K	Bleeding disorders (prevention of bleeding or thrombotic events in anticoagulant therapy), osteoporosis prevention
Wheatgrass	Ulcerative colitis
White horehound	Cardiovascular disease prevention/atherosclerosis, choleretic (dyspepsia, appetite stimulation), cough, diabetes, pain
Wild indigo	Respiratory tract infections
Wild yam	Menopausal symptoms
Willow bark	Headache
Witch hazel	Hemorrhoids, insect bites, perineal discomfort after childbirth, skin irritation (minor/pediatric patients), ultraviolet light skin damage protection, varicose veins
Yarrow	Plaque/gingivitis

(Continued)

NATURAL STANDARD DOES NOT RECOMMEND SPECIFIC THERAPIES OR PRACTITIONERS.—CONT'D

GRADE: C (Unclear or Conflicting Scientific Evidence)

Therapy	Specific Therapeutic Use(s)
Yerba santa	Pulmonary conditions (lung conditions)
Yohimbe bark extract	Autonomic failure, inhibition of platelet aggregation, libido (women), sexual side effects of SSRIs, xerostomia (psychotropic drug-induced)
Yucca	Hypercholesterolemia
Zinc	Alopecia (hair loss), anorexia nervosa, bad breath, beta-thalassemia (hereditary disorder), blood disorders (aceruloplasminemia), boils, burns, chronic prostatitis (CP), closed head injuries, cognitive deficits (children), common cold, crohn's disease, dandruff, diabetes (type 1 and type 2), diabetic neuropathy (nerve damage), diaper rash, eczema, exercise performance, Gilbert's syndrome, growth (stunted infants), hepatic encephalopathy, hepatitis C viral infection (chronic), HIV/AIDS, hypothyroidism, incision wounds, infertility, kidney function, kwashiorkor (malnutrition from inadequate protein intake), leg ulcers, leprosy, liver cirrhosis, lower respiratory infections in children, macular degeneration, malaria, menstrual cramps, mortality, muscle cramps (cirrhosis), parasites, poisoning (arsenic), pregnancy, psoriasis, radiation-induced mucositis, respiratory disease (respiratory papillomatosis), rheumatoid arthritis, skin damage caused by incontinence, stomatitis, taste perception (hemodialysis, cancer), tinnitus, trichomoniasis, viral warts

GRADE: D (Fair Negative Scientific Evidence)

Therapy	Specific Therapeutic Use(s)
5-HTP	Seizures/epilepsy (myoclonic disorders)
Acacia	Hypercholesterolemia
Aloe	Mucositis, pressure ulcers, radiation dermatitis
Arginine	Altitude sickness, cyclosporine toxicity, exercise performance, infertility, interstitial cystitis, kidney protection during angiography
Arnica	Muscle soreness
Beta-carotene	Abdominal aortic aneurysm (AAA) (prevention), Alzheimer's disease, angioplasty, birthmark/mole (dysplastic nevi) (prevention), cancer, cardiovascular disease, *Helicobacter pylori* bacteria eradication, macular degeneration, mortality reduction, postoperative tissue injury (prevention), stroke
Bilberry	Night vision
Bitter almond	Cancer (Laetrile)
Bitter orange	Dementia (behavior challenges)
Boron	Bodybuilding aid (increasing testosterone), menopausal symptoms, prevention of blood clotting (coagulation effects), psoriasis (topical)
Calcium	Vaginal disorders (atrophy, wasting or thinning of the vaginal tissue)
Chamomile	Post-operative sore throat/hoarseness due to intubation
Choline	Alzheimer's disease/cognitive decline, cerebellar ataxia, improving sports performance (endurance sports), schizophrenia
Chondroitin sulfate	Muscle soreness (delayed onset)

NATURAL STANDARD DOES NOT RECOMMEND SPECIFIC THERAPIES OR PRACTITIONERS.—CONT'D

GRADE: D (Fair Negative Scientific Evidence)

Therapy	Specific Therapeutic Use(s)
Coenzyme Q10	Diabetes, Huntington's disease
Copper	Neural tube defect prevention
Cranberry	Chronic urinary tract infection prophylaxis (children with bladder dysfunctions)
Creatine	Amyotrophic lateral sclerosis (ALS), athletic performance enhancement (endurance; general), surgical recovery (soft tissue)
Deer velvet	Sexual function/libido/erectile dysfunction
DHEA	Memory, muscle strength
DMSO	Scleroderma
Dong quai	Menopausal symptoms
Echinacea	Genital herpes, upper respiratory tract infections: treatment (children)
Evening primrose oil	Asthma, attention deficit hyperactivity disorder (ADHD), cardiovascular health, menopause (flushing/bone metabolism), premenstrual syndrome (PMS), psoriasis, schizophrenia
Folate	Down's syndrome, lometrexol toxicity
Gamma oryzanol	Bodybuilding
Garlic	*Helicobacter pylori* infection, type 2 diabetes
Ginkgo	Mental performance (post-prandial dip)
Glucosamine	Hypercholesterolemia (diabetes)
Grape seed	Allergic rhinitis, radioprotection
Green-lipped mussel	Rheumatoid arthritis
Iodine	Kidney problems (kidney cysts), visual outcomes in corneal ulceration
Iron	Therapy for anemia after orthopedic surgery
Licorice	Peptic ulcer disease
Lycopene	Immune stimulation (cell-mediated), lung function after exercise
Niacin	type 1 diabetes mellitus prevention (niacinamide)
Octacosanol	Amyotrophic lateral sclerosis (ALS)
Omega-3 fatty acids, fish oil, alpha-linolenic acid	Appetite/weight loss in cancer patients, diabetes, hypercholesterolemia, transplant rejection prevention (kidney and heart)
Pantethine	Athletic performance, cystinosis
Pantothenic acid	Radiation skin irritation
Papain	Insect bites (fire ants)
Phenylalanine	Attention deficit hyperactivity disorder (children), chronic pain, low back pain

(Continued)

NATURAL STANDARD DOES NOT RECOMMEND SPECIFIC THERAPIES OR PRACTITIONERS.—CONT'D

GRADE: D (Fair Negative Scientific Evidence)

Therapy	Specific Therapeutic Use(s)
Phosphates, phosphorus	Exercise performance
Probiotics	Bacterial infection (translocation), diarrhea (HIV patients on antiretroviral therapy), fertility
PSK	Breast cancer (adjuvant)
Selenium	Arthritis (osteoarthritis, rheumatoid arthritis), diabetes (prevention), Kashin-Beck osteoarthropathy, muscle and joint disorders, skin cancer (nonmelanoma) prevention
Spirulina	Chronic fatigue syndrome, chronic viral hepatitis
St. John's wort	Human immunodeficiency virus (HIV)
Sweet almond	Radiation therapy skin reaction (topical)
Thiamin	Fractures (hip)
Vitamin A	Chemotherapy adverse effects, lung cancer
Vitamin B_6	Autism, stroke reoccurrence
Vitamin B_{12}	Circadian rhythm sleep disorders, lung cancer, stroke
Vitamin C	Cataracts (prevention/progression), common cold prevention (general), common cold treatment, heart disease (prevention), premature infants
Vitamin D	Muscle strength, prostate cancer
Vitamin E	Asthma, cancer prevention (general), heart disease prevention, osteoarthritis, Peyronie's disease, retinitis pigmentosa, scar (prevention), stroke
Vitamin K	Hepatocellular carcinoma (recurrent hepatocellular carcinoma prevention)
Wild yam	Hormonal properties (estrogenic, progestinic, DHEA-like)
Willow bark	Rheumatoid arthritis
Zinc	Celiac disease, chronic inflammatory rheumatic disease, continuous ambulatory peritoneal dialysis (CAPD), cystic fibrosis, inflammatory bowel disease, pneumonia (children)

GRADE: F (Strong Negative Scientific Evidence)

Therapy	Specific Therapeutic Use(s)
Arginine	Asthma
Bael fruit	Dysentery (shigellosis)
Chromium	Obesity/weight loss (body composition)
Folate	Fragile X syndrome
Phenylalanine	Multiple sclerosis
Vitamin B_{12}	Leber's disease

Index

Contents